Life Care Planning and Case Management Handbook

Fourth Edition

Life care planning is an advanced collaborative case management specialty practice focused on assessing, evaluating, coordinating, consulting, planning for, and monitoring necessary services for individuals with complex medical care needs over their lifetime. This handbook provides a comprehensive resource for all people involved with catastrophic impairments and chronic medical care case management.

The *Life Care Planning and Case Management Handbook*, Fourth Edition, begins by defining the roles played by each of the key team members working with the life care planner. It provides planners with insights critical to successful interactions with medical and health-related professionals as well as the team members they are most likely to encounter as they work to build an accurate and reliable life care plan. Next, the text offers up-to-date information on the disabilities most frequently encountered by the life care planner. The contributors, who are recognized experts in their disciplines, also address issues in forensic settings, ethics, standards, research, and credentials.

The fourth edition includes numerous chapters on general issues, as well as updated standards of practice from the International Academy of Life Care Planners (IALCP), Life Care Planning Consensus Statements, and Valuable step-by-step charts and checklists. Completely updated and expanded, this revised handbook now includes new chapters on multicultural considerations in life care planning, admissibility of life care plans in U.S. Courts, and Canadian life care planning practice. Additionally, infused in other chapters is new information on medical coding and costing for life care planners, life care planning in non-litigated contexts, as well as research and education within life care planning.

Life Care Planning and Case Management Handbook

Fourth Edition

Edited by
Roger O. Weed
Debra E. Berens

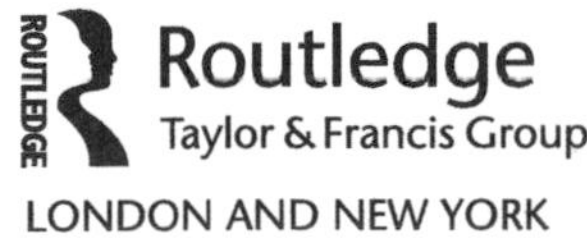

LONDON AND NEW YORK

Fourth edition published 2018
by Routledge
4 Park Square, Milton Park, Abingdon, Oxon OX14 4RN
605 Third Avenue, New York, NY 10017

First issued in paperback 2023

Routledge is an imprint of the Taylor & Francis Group, an informa business

Publisher's Note
The publisher has gone to great lengths to ensure the quality of this reprint but points out that some imperfections in the original copies may be apparent.

Third edition published by CRC Press 2009

Library of Congress Cataloging-in-Publication Data
A catalog record has been requested for this book

ISBN 13: 978-1-03-265229-0 (pbk)
ISBN 13: 978-1-4987-3110-2 (hbk)
ISBN 13: 978-1-315-15728-3 (ebk)

DOI: 10.4324/9781315157283

Typeset in Adobe Garamond Pro
by Nova Techset Private Limited, Bengaluru & Chennai, India

Contents

Foreword ... ix
Acknowledgments and Tributes ... xi
Editors ... xv
Contributors ... xvii

SECTION I THE ROLES OF LIFE CARE PLAN TEAM MEMBERS

1 **Life Care Planning: Past, Present, and Future** ... 3
Roger O. Weed

2 **The Role of the Physiatrist in Life Care Planning** ... 21
Richard Paul Bonfiglio

3 **The Role of the Rehabilitation Nurse in Life Care Planning** ... 29
Amy M. Sutton

4 **The Role of the Vocational Rehabilitation Counselor in Life Care Planning** ... 41
Debra E. Berens and Roger O. Weed

5 **The Role of the Psychologist in Life Care Planning** ... 61
Harvey E. Jacobs

6 **The Role of the Neuropsychologist in Life Care Planning** ... 79
Carol Walker

7 **The Role of the Occupational Therapist in Life Care Planning** ... 105
Nancy L. Mitchell and Courtney V. Mitchell

8 **The Role of the Physical Therapist in Life Care Planning** ... 135
Kathie Allison and Kirsten Potter

9 **The Role of the SLP and Assistive Technology in Life Care Planning** ... 149
Carolyn Wiles Higdon

10 **The Role of the Audiologist in Life Care Planning** ... 255
William D. Mustain and Carolyn Wiles Higdon

11 **The Role of the Economist in Life Care Planning** ... 317
Everett G. Dillman

SECTION II SELECTED DISABILITIES: TOPICS AND ISSUES

12 **Life Care Planning for the Amputee** 335
Robert H. Meier, III

13 **Life Care Planning for Acquired Brain Injury** 367
David L. Ripley and Roger O. Weed

14 **Life Care Planning for the Burn Patient** 401
Ruth B. Rimmer and Kevin N. Foster

15 **Life Care Planning for Depressive Disorders, Obsessive-Compulsive Disorder, and Schizophrenia** 443
Nicole M. Wolf

16 **Life Care Planning for People with Chronic Pain** 469
Denise D. Lester

17 **Life Care Planning for Spinal Cord Injury** 497
David J. Altman and Dan M. Bagwell

18 **Life Care Planning for Organ Transplantation** 533
Dan M. Bagwell and Lisa Norris

19 **Life Care Planning for the Visually Impaired** 571
Roger O. Weed and Rasheeda Wilkins

20 **Elder Care Management Life Care Planning Principles** 591
Dorothy J. Zydowicz-Vierling

SECTION III FORENSIC CONSIDERATIONS

21 **Forensic Issues for Life Care Planners** 609
Roger O. Weed

22 **A Personal Perspective of Life Care Planning** 631
Raymond L. Arrona, and Mamie Walters, as told to Anna N. Herrington

23 **A Plaintiff's Attorney's Perspective on Life Care Planning** 641
Katherine A. Brown-Henry

24 **A Defense Attorney's Perspective on Life Care Planning** 655
Tracy Raffles Gunn

25 **Life Care Planning and the Elder Law Attorney** 669
Terry C. Cox and F. Auston Wortman, III

26 **Day-in-the-Life Video Production in Life Care Planning** 681
J. Mat Hunt, Jr.

27 **Ethical Issues for the Life Care Planner** 691
Debra E. Berens and Roger O. Weed

SECTION IV GENERAL ISSUES

28 Reliability of Life Care Plans: A Comparison of Original and Updated Plans........703
Amy M. Sutton, Paul M. Deutsch, Roger O. Weed, and Debra E. Berens

29 Americans with Disabilities Act (ADA): From Case Law to Case Management and Life Care Planning Practice 711
Lewis E. Vierling

30 Life Care Planning Resources 729
Ann Maniha and Leslie L. Watson

31 Medical Equipment Choices and the Role of the Rehab Equipment Specialist in Life Care Planning...759
Paul Amsterdam

32 Home Assessment in Life Care Planning 787
Jim Karl and Roger O. Weed

33 Vehicle Modifications: Useful Considerations for Life Care Planners 799
C. Dan Allison, Jr.

34 Credentialing and Other Issues in Life Care Planning.......................................813
Debra E. Berens and Roger O. Weed

35 Admissibility Considerations in Life Care Planning 819
Timothy F. Field

36 Cultural Considerations for Life Care Planning...833
Mary Barros-Bailey

37 Life Care Planning in Canada... 843
Dana M. Weldon

Appendix I: Standards of Practice for Life Care Planners, 3rd Edition...........................865

Appendix II: Consensus and Majority Statements Derived from Life Care Planning Summits Held in 2000, 2002, 2004, 2006, 2008, 2010, 2012, and 2015...875

Appendix III: *Journal of Life Care Planning* Title Index...879

Author Index...897

Subject Index... 909

Foreword

This 2018 edition of the *Life Care Planning and Case Management Handbook* represents the fourth edition of one of the pillars of reference texts in the practice of life care planning. In the Foreword for the 2010 edition, I indicated that a number of important and valuable contributors within the practice of life care planning had been brought together to advance this practice specialty. Co-editors Dr. Weed and Dr. Berens have accomplished no less a feat for this current edition in bringing together specialists in their practice areas to present readers with the most important updates to aid in plan development and case management. Perhaps the most important change for the fourth edition is the addition of several relevant and contemporary chapters that make this text a timely and necessary contribution to the ongoing practice of life care planning.

From an historical perspective, Dr. Weed and I first met in 1984. This was approximately 8 years after I had begun working on the development of the basic tenets, methodologies, and principles of life care planning and 3 years after the publication of *Damages in Tort Actions.* No one to that point in time had come to life care planning with greater enthusiasm or interest. Since that time, no one has proven to share my vision for life care planning with greater dedication and effort. Dr. Weed has been a dedicated colleague, researcher, writer, lecturer, teacher, and a tremendous overall contributor to the advanced practice of life care planning. In recognition of his work, he was invited to participate in *A Guide to Rehabilitation* (Deutsch & Sawyer, 1985–2007, AHAB Press, White Plains, New York). That text was retired in 2007 and the *Life Care Planning and Case Management Handbook,* along with Susan Riddick Grisham's *Pediatric Life Care Planning and Case Management* text (2010), represent the two most comprehensive texts on the topics of Life Care Planning and Case Management currently on the market. Dr. Weed has, without question, been a major moving force in the advancement of life care planning for the past two and one half decades. He has done this by always remaining a team player who stays focused on what is good for life care planning and the practitioners as a whole. We have always shared a philosophy of openly contributing in our lectures and our texts all of the latest information and research we have available. Dr. Weed never holds anything back, and, even in his retirement today, this latest text continues to hold to that philosophy.

The 2018 edition of the *Life Care Planning and Case Management Handbook* will continue to be a necessary desktop reference for every advanced practitioner of life care planning. New chapters included in the fourth edition are on topics such as Admissibility Considerations Life Care Planning, Cultural Considerations for Life Care Planning, and Life Care Planning in Canada, and these will prove to be exceptionally important and relevant to today's practitioner. The reader will also find that chapters upon which they have depended in the past have been carefully reviewed and updated to reflect present day or contemporary issues in life care planning. In some cases, past contributors have aptly fulfilled this role, but in other instances new contributors with proven, specialized skills and insights have been tapped to provide their insights to completely rewrite or update some of the chapters.

What is most important for readers such as myself is we can still find what we have so come to rely on in past editions. For example:

In the opening 10 chapters, the text continues to define the roles played by each of the key team members working with the life care planner, with a completely revised chapter on the nursing role. It provides life care planners with the insights critical to successful interaction with medical, health-related professionals, and economic team members they are most likely to encounter as they work to build a successful and accurate life care plan.

In the next nine chapters, the book provides up-to-date information on the disabilities most frequently encountered by the life care planner. Most importantly, we are not just lecturing on current information, but we are providing critical resources for being able to bring ourselves up to date on a day-to-day and case-by-case basis. This is what makes this book a critical desktop reference.

The *Handbook* then moves on to address issues typically left out of similar texts—issues made critical by *Daubert v. Merrell Dow* in the forensic setting and issues that should be critical even in the nonforensic setting. I refer to ethics, standards, research, credentials, and a review of litigation-related case law, all of which are thoroughly and professionally addressed within these pages. In addition, the text includes a chapter on updated and present day resources used most commonly by life care planning practitioners in conducting their work, followed by separate chapters that address medical equipment, home assessments, and vehicle modifications.

It is easy to see that this text continues to illustrate the progression of a career, in which Drs. Weed and Berens have both written and edited many other books, chapters, and articles. With a combined career of 70 years in the field of rehabilitation, this text has been instrumental in not only helping to develop and advance the specialized practice of life care planning but also helping to develop the market for the work product we produce. Once again, I extend my congratulations to co-editors Dr. Weed and Dr. Berens, and all of the contributors on an excellent work. I also continue to congratulate those with the insight to be working with a copy of this text on their desktops.

Paul M. Deutsch, PhD, CRC, CCM, CLCP, FIALCP
Past Chair: Foundation for Life Care Planning Research
(Editor's note: Dr. Deutsch is founder of the Life Care Planning movement)

Acknowledgments and Tributes

There are a number of people who have contributed to helping this fourth edition become a reality. First to be recognized is Dr. Paul Deutsch, acknowledged as the father of life care planning, who, although now retired, has for many years maintained strong support for our work in this field. We are truly honored to have him write the Foreword to this edition. His lifelong dedication of promoting and enhancing the specialty practice is unmatched. He has been a prolific author, generous sharer of practice details through numerous presentations, the founder of the Foundation for Life Care Planning Research, and all-around powerhouse for developing established protocol and methodology of life care planning practice. Furthermore, there are numerous contributors to this text who represent a major powerhouse of knowledgeable movers and shakers in the life care planning specialty practice from a wide range of specialties.

In addition, there are some former contributors who sadly are no longer with us. As we go to print with the fourth edition of the *Life Care Planning and Case Management Handbook*, we want to make a special tribute to these authors. Since publishing the first edition of the *Life Care Planning and Case Management Handbook* in 1999, several superb contributors have passed on, but their legacies and contributions not only to the *Handbook* but to the life care planning community continue. The following is intended to thank these extraordinary professionals, once again, for their contributions to the promotion of life care planning. All are greatly missed!

Paul Amsterdam was a Nationally Certified Assistive Technology Professional (ATP) who specialized in wheelchair mobility and adaptation. With more than 35 years of experience in the medical equipment industry, Paul specialized in complex rehabilitation diagnoses and served as an expert in wheelchair mobility and adaptive seating as well as consulted with life care planners to ensure the equipment and technology recommendations in their plan were appropriate and well-supported. In addition to his full-time medical equipment work, Paul helped to create more than 100 wheelchair clinics and volunteered his time to raise funds and awareness of people with disabilities, including awareness for wheelchair sports. However, he is perhaps most known within the life care planning community for his knowledge about purchase, modification, maintenance, repair, and life expectancy of rehabilitation-related equipment. He contributed to all editions of this text, authored several articles and chapters, and freely agreed to speak at many life care planning and rehabilitation organization conferences. Most recently, Paul contributed a standing column to the *Journal of Life Care Planning* titled "The Medical Equipment Corner."

Tyron C. Elliott, JD, was primarily a practicing plaintiff's trial lawyer where he focused on the area of neurolaw, which emphasized brain and spinal cord injuries. He was an adjunct professor at Emory University School of Medicine in Atlanta, where he lectured on legal-medical issues. He was also a popular speaker on litigation-related topics and presented at numerous life care planning conferences. Tyron was the executive editor of the *Neurolaw Letter* and contributed several articles on brain injury and related litigation. Tyron filled a unique niche in the life care planning community as attorney and a true "counselor" of the law. He contributed the former chapter on A Plaintiff's Attorney's Perspective on Life Care Planning. (*From Roger*: I enjoyed consulting with Tyron for many years but finally decided that I valued him as my own personal attorney, thus we agreed that I would no longer provide expert witness services for his clientele.)

Randall W. Evans, PhD, ABPP, was president and CEO of Learning Services Corporation, a national provider of neurorehabilitation and supported living services. A practicing neuropsychologist, Dr. Evans published extensively in the areas of neuropsychology, neuropharmacology, and neurorehabilitation. Randy was a surveyor for the Commission on Accreditation of Rehabilitation Facilities and also served as a clinical associate professor of psychiatry at the University of North Carolina School of Medicine at Chapel Hill. He was one of the first rehabilitation professionals in the United States to receive Diplomate status from the American Board of Rehabilitation Psychology. Randy contributed the initial chapter on The Role of the Neuropsychologist in Life Care Planning.

Patricia McCollom, RN, MS, CRRN, CDMS, CCM, CLCP, was president and nurse consultant for LifeCare Economics, LTD, Management Consulting & Rehabilitation Services, Inc., and was the founding CEO of the American Academy of Nurse Life Care Planners and the International Academy of Life Care Planners. She was past national president of the Association of Rehabilitation Nurses, former chair of the National Task Force on Case Management, and past chair of the Commission for Case Manager Certification. At the national level, she taught case management practice and life care planning. She was vice president of the Board of Directors of the Foundation for Life Care Planning Research. The author of many articles on rehabilitation, case management, and life care planning, she was one of three principle developers of the certificate course in Life Care Planning, to be initiated by Kaplan College. In recognition of her visionary talents she was the first editor of the *Journal of Life Care Planning*. She also was a life care planning lifetime achievement award winner and, in honor of her dedication to research and education, the Patti McCollom Research Award (which included cash) was created and continues to be awarded by the Foundation for Life Care Planning Research. Patti contributed the original chapter on Elder Care Management.

Terry Winkler, MD, CLCP, was a Board Certified Physiatrist (PM&R) physician and, due to his popularity as a speaker and charming personality, he was one of the first physician repeat educators for the National Life Care Planning training program. He was past medical director of Cox Hospital Rehabilitation Programs and medical director of Springfield Park Care Sub-Acute Rehabilitation Program and Curative Rehabilitation Center. Terry contributed numerous life care planning publications. As an active practicing physician he specialized in traumatic/acquired brain injury, spinal cord injury, amputations, and life care planning consulting. Terry was also Clinical Associate Faculty at the University of Florida, Gainesville and LSU Medical Center, Department of Rehabilitation, New Orleans. Past honors included a Lifetime Achievement Award for life care planning, the America Award, Alumnus of the Year at Louisiana Tech University, and the Jean Claude Belot Award for Academic Achievement from Harvard University. Terry contributed the chapters on Spinal Cord Injury and Visual Impairment in life care planning.

Sheri Jasper was not a direct contributor to this publication but contributed to the specialty practice of life care planning in many other ways. Those of us who have participated in or even just explored life care planning training programs probably encountered her at some point in the process. Her professional background was centered around sales, customer service, and operational management, and she was hired as the contact point person at the beginning of the nationwide life care planning training in the early 1990s. Sheri initially worked for the Rehabilitation Training Institute, Intelicus, and later Medipro Seminars, all providers of the first nationwide life care planning training program that led to certification in Life Care Planning. An absolute joy to work with, Sheri was always exuberant and helpful and could be found coordinating and implementing the initial on-site training programs and conferences. She was the first contact for professionals seeking training and the heartbeat of life care planning training behind the scenes. When she lost her battle with cancer, the Sheri Jasper Award was created to honor others who embodied her spirit of positive, supportive, friendly, and encouraging attitude toward colleagues and exemplified a willingness to go the extra mile with good humor and perseverance.

As life care planning practitioners, we are eternally grateful for the contributions of the above-mentioned authors (and Sheri) who laid the foundation for what was to come.

We also think it is valuable to recognize others who have been instrumental in our careers.

From Roger: My parents have primary credit for urging me to break the mold of local tradition by continuing my education. I was raised in a very small town where high school graduates commonly went to work in the timber industry. In fact, one of my peers could not understand why I would go to college when I could make almost as much money as a college graduate right out of high school. At the time, I did not have a good answer for him. However, the last time I saw him, now years ago, he was chronically "between jobs" due to the massive turndown in the local economy, which is based almost entirely on wood products and logging.

Dr. Timothy Field, who in 1984 was a professor at the University of Georgia, agreed to be my PhD major advisor after a few years of mentoring and advising me in my professional life. I can truly convey that Dr. Field has been a major positive factor in my professional life. He has opened many doors, been supportive beyond the call of duty, and shown me new horizons. As mentioned above, Dr. Paul Deutsch has also been very supportive in my professional career by including me in his life care planning training, writing, and volunteer-related activities as well as being available for consultation. Julie Kitchen, who retired from life care planning within the past year, has also been available for an enormous number of contacts for information and was always a pleasure to work with. I also acknowledge my co-editor, Debbie Berens, who at the time of this edition has, for close to 30 years, been a major cheerleader, editor, organizer, co-author, and overall superb and talented colleague.

Last, but certainly not least, my wife, Paula, has always encouraged me to pursue professionally whatever I wanted. This support resulted in many moves and job changes for her, and she has never wavered. Now that I am enjoying retirement, looking back over an amazing career of teaching and consulting reminds me that what unfolded surpassed all expectations. All in all, I believe that many people have observed more capability in me than I saw in myself. Through good fortune, outstanding resources, and a lot of assistance, this fourth edition text has come to fruition.

From Debbie: It is thrilling to realize that for almost 30 years I have had the incredible experience of mentorship from co-editor, Roger Weed, even as he has retired from his academic career and active life care planning and consulting practice and is enjoying his "second career" as an avid traveler and forever champion of the rehabilitation profession. Roger continues to be the epitome of a mentor, colleague, professional confidante, sounding board, motivator, and friend. And although he is now retired, I hope for many continued years of professional association.

Another major driving force in my life for over 30 years has been Mark, my husband, who gets the most credit for endurance and perseverance throughout my professional career. His unfaltering belief in me and unwavering support of all my activities has allowed me to take risks and to grow in professional ways that I would have never imagined. And for our two sons, Matt and Jacob, whose strength and constant love and support, even as they enjoy their college years, is the backbone of who I am. Every step on the journey to bring this text together has been made with each of them by my side and in my heart.

For my extended family, Mom and Dad, who have been there at all the right times throughout my life as only parents know how to do, and to my sisters and their families who shower me with support from across the miles, my world is so much better with each of you in it.

With appreciation, we recognize that this book is the culmination of many contributors within the specialty practice of life care planning who have given of their valuable time, energy, and expertise to write a chapter. In our daily practices, we are continuously reminded of the good that goes on in life care panning and the collective energy of life care planning professionals who produce quality work and are committed to advancing the practice. It is hoped that this book will play a small part in continuing the life care planning and case management momentum.

Roger O. Weed

Debra E. Berens

Editors

Roger O. Weed, PhD, CRC/R, LPC/Ret, CCM/R, CDMS/R, CLCP/R, FNRCA, FIALCP/R, Professor Emeritus, is retired as professor and graduate rehabilitation counseling coordinator at Georgia State University. He also held doctoral student graduate faculty status in Counseling Psychology as well as Counselor Education and Practice doctoral programs. He has authored or co-authored about 150 books, reviews, articles, and book chapters, approximately 80 of which were specific to life care planning.

During his more than 42 years in the profession, Dr. Weed was honored several times for his work including the 2006 Distinguished Professor Award from Georgia State University's Alumni Association (sole recipient), the 2011 Lifetime Appreciation Award from the International Commission on Health Care Certification, the 2009 Larry Huggins Lifetime Achievement Award from the Private Rehabilitation Specialists of Georgia, the 2005 Lifetime Achievement Award from the sponsors of the International Life Care Planning Conference, the 2004 Lifetime Achievement Award from the International Association of Rehabilitation Professionals (as well as recognition in 1997 and 1991 as the Outstanding Educator), the 1993 National Professional Services Award from the American Rehabilitation Counseling Association, and the 2003 Research Excellence Award from the College of Education at Georgia State University.

Dr. Weed is one of the five founders of the original, nationwide training program leading to Life Care Planning certification. He is also past chair of the Georgia State Licensing Board for professional counselors, marriage and family therapists, and social workers, as well as past president of the International Association of Rehabilitation Professionals.

Debra E. Berens, PhD, CRC, CCM, CLCP, maintains a nationwide consulting practice specializing in life care planning for children and adults with catastrophic injuries, disabilities, or chronic medical conditions since 1989. She has authored/co-authored more than 40 articles/chapters and given more than 50 presentations on topics of life care planning, rehabilitation consulting, and case management, and served for 16 years as moderator of the International Symposium for Life Care Planning. Dr. Berens also is a clinical assistant professor in the Clinical Rehabilitation Counseling graduate program at Georgia State University and is recipient of industry awards including the 2010 Faculty Excellence Award by Georgia State University College of Education, the 2010 Outstanding Life Care Planning Educator, and the 2013 Lifetime Achievement Award in Life Care Planning.

Editors

Contributors

Kathie Allison, PT, MS, CLCP, obtained her BS in physical therapy from the University of Kansas in 1972 and her MS in education from the University of Kansas in perceptual motor development in 1979. She was certified as a Life Care Planner in 2000. She worked as a physical therapy clinician for 35 years. She was on faculty at the University of Kansas from 1979–1986 where she taught in the Physical Therapy Education program. Her emphasis was on clinical techniques and cardiopulmonary physical therapy. From 1986–1993, she was in health care management. She started her independent practice of life care planning in 1993. She has presented at both the IALCP and AALNCP conferences and has written chapters for the *AALNC Journal*. Her area of specialty is transplantation.

C. Dan Allison, Jr., MS, OTR/L, ATP, CDRS, is an occupational therapist with a certification in Driving Rehabilitation, as well as assistive technology. He is currently employed in Atlanta, Georgia, at the Shepherd Center, a rehabilitation hospital specializing in medical treatment, research, and rehabilitation for people with spinal cord injury and brain injury, where he works full time in the driving program. Prior to that, he was a research associate at the T.K. Martin Center for Technology and Disability of Mississippi State University. Allison received his BS degree in supervision from Purdue University, and a MSc degree in occupational therapy from Western Michigan University, with an emphasis on disabled driver rehabilitation. He is currently president of the Association for Driver Rehabilitation Specialists (ADED), with memberships in the American Occupational Therapy Association (AOTA), the GA Occupational Therapy Association, the Rehabilitation Engineering and Assistive Technology Society of North America (RESNA), and the National Mobility Equipment Dealers Association (NMEDA).

David J. Altman, MD, CLCP, is a physician specializing in neurology with an active clinical practice in San Antonio, Texas. Dr. Altman completed his undergraduate training at Brandeis University in 1992, after which he attended medical school at the University of Connecticut, receiving his medical degree in 1996. After completing his internship at Hartford Hospital in 1997, Dr. Altman completed his neurology residency at the University of Texas Health Science Center in San Antonio in 2000. He also completed a fellowship in clinical neurophysiology at Brown University in 2001 before returning to San Antonio to begin his clinical practice in neurology. Dr. Altman provides inpatient clinical services as a neuro-hospitalist for the Methodist Healthcare System. In this capacity, he provides neurology consultation services for diagnosis, emergency management, and follow-up inpatient care of patients who have suffered stroke, brain injury, spinal cord injury, peripheral nerve injury, and other neurologic injuries or diseases in all departments at this Level I Trauma Center and Joint Commission Certified Stroke Center, as well as other hospitals within this system of care throughout South Texas. He has taken an active role in developing and building the stroke program for the Methodist Healthcare System. Dr. Altman serves as the regional neurology advisor for the Warm Springs Healthcare System in San Antonio. He has also served as the medical director for Global Rehabilitation Hospital in San Antonio and partnered with the Neurology Center of San Antonio, as well as the neurology director of Access Quality Therapy Services. In addition to his clinical neurology practice, Dr. Altman is a Certified Life Care Planner and provides life care planning services as a consultant with Rehabilitation Professional Consultants, Inc. in San Antonio.

Paul Amsterdam, ATS, was a specialist in the field of rehabilitation medical equipment. He comes from a family of three generations in this industry, starting in 1929 with the founding of Amsterdam Bros., one of the country's first orthotic and surgical supply stores. Amsterdam was a Nationally Certified Assistive Technology Specialist. He helped to create and participated in more than 100 wheelchair clinics in rehabilitation hospitals, developmental centers, and schools for people with disabilities throughout the New York–New Jersey metropolitan area. He was been a featured columnist for *Case Manager* magazine and other publications for more than 5 years. Amsterdam was considered an expert in wheelchair mobility and adaptive seating. He made full assessments of functional needs, designed custom positioning seating systems, and offered alternatives in decubitus prevention as well as manual and power mobility options. As a nationwide consultant he provided complete evaluations for both adults and pediatrics with a wide range of physical disabilities.

Raymond L. Arrona began his career in 1967 as an independent contractor with Wear-Ever Aluminum, Inc., Alcoa Aluminum's first subsidiary, which marketed Wear-Ever Cookware and Cutco Cutlery. He quickly achieved one of the company's coveted positions as division manager and relocated from Arizona to Georgia in 1976 where he was president and CEO until 1997 of RASAR Management Services, Inc./dba Vector Marketing, which represents the Cutco Cutlery product. He also operated as Vector's southern zone division manager for the states of Georgia and South Carolina. In late 1997, he joined a start-up company, QuestCom, which develops websites for businesses. Since the publication of the first edition of this book, he has relocated with his daughter, Anita (now deceased), to Mesa, Arizona, where he owns Pride of the Valley, an upscale shared direct mail card deck, an affiliate of Pride of the City. Arrona experienced every father's nightmare when his daughter, Anita, was tragically injured in an accident caused by a drunk driver. "The impact of Anita's accident has been far reaching in all areas of my family's life, including the personal, financial, spiritual, educational, judicial, professional, and friendship levels. No emotion has been immune from the effects of that tragic day. It is my wish that by telling Anita's story, it will in some way help others through similar situations, or assist in allowing life care planners to gain insight into our family as we continue to deal with this life-changing event."

Dan M. Bagwell, BSN, RN, CLCP, CCM, CDMS, is chief executive officer of Rehabilitation Professional Consultants, Inc. and president of Dan Bagwell & Associates, both of which are located in San Antonio, Texas. Bagwell is a registered nurse, licensed to practice in the State of Texas. He received a bachelor of science in nursing in 1978 from the University of Mississippi School of Nursing. He is a Certified Life Care Planner, Certified Case Manager, and Certified Disability Management Specialist. Bagwell provides adult and pediatric catastrophic case management and life care planning services for individuals in Texas and many other states throughout the country. His clinical nursing experience spans nearly four decades, with the majority of his professional services dedicated to medical case management, professional consultation in health care, and life care planning services involving litigated and non-litigated matters. His clinical experience has included critical care nursing and service as an officer in the United States Air Force Nurse Corps and medical crew director in Tactical Aeromedical Evacuation with the USAF Reserves. Bagwell previously served as president and co-founder of Life Care Personal Living Centers and co-founder and vice president of MediSys Rehabilitation, Inc. He has given numerous presentations, lectures, and symposiums concerning life care planning at regional, national, and international conferences, and he has authored peer-reviewed journal articles and textbook chapters on life care planning.

Mary Barros-Bailey, PhD, CRC, CLCP, is a Spanish- and Portuguese-speaking life care planner and vocational expert. Her caseload often includes multicultural and international cases. She has presented on a variety of professional topics throughout the country and on three continents. Beyond her forensic and clinical practice and professional publishing, presenting, and research, Dr. Barros-Bailey is adjunct teaching and clinical faculty with the University of Idaho's rehabilitation counseling program and teaches a global child advocacy class at Winona State University. She holds dual citizenship in the United States and the European Union and has traveled to every continent, including Antarctica.

Debra E. Berens, PhD, CRC, CCM, CLCP, maintains a nationwide consulting practice specializing in life care planning for children and adults with catastrophic injuries, disabilities, or chronic medical conditions since 1989. She has authored/co-authored more than 40 articles/chapters and given more than 50 presentations on topics of life care planning, rehabilitation consulting, and case management, and served for 16 years as Moderator of the International Symposium for Life Care Planning. Dr. Berens also is a Clinical Assistant Professor in the Clinical Rehabilitation Counseling graduate program at Georgia State University and is recipient of industry awards including the 2010 Faculty Excellence Award by Georgia State University College of Education, 2010 Outstanding Life Care Planning Educator, and 2013 Lifetime Achievement Award in Life Care Planning.

Richard Paul Bonfiglio, MD, is board certified by the American Board of Physical Medicine and Rehabilitation. Dr. Bonfiglio has previously served as the medical director of several nationally recognized rehabilitation facilities, including the Lake Erie Institute of Rehabilitation and the Bryn Mawr Rehabilitation Hospital. He has also maintained close academic ties, including having served as residency program director at the Schwab Rehabilitation Center. He is an adjunct faculty member at Lake Erie College of Osteopathic Medicine. Dr. Bonfiglio's clinical practice within the field of physical medicine and rehabilitation has included providing care to children and adults with traumatic brain injuries, spinal cord injuries, amputations, and acute and chronic pain problems. He is an internationally recognized speaker on rehabilitation topics. Dr. Bonfiglio has been involved for years in the review and critical analysis of life care plans. His interests include the development of a strong medical foundation to enhance the accuracy and reliability of these plans. He is also an expert in life expectancy determinations for individuals following catastrophic illnesses and injuries. He has been on the faculty of the Rehabilitation Training Institute and MediPro Seminars for life care planning. Dr. Bonfiglio has sustained a strong clinical practice within the field of physical medicine and rehabilitation, providing care to children with a variety of physical and cognitive impairments, and children and adults with traumatic brain injuries, spinal cord injuries, amputations, and acute and chronic pain problems.

Katherine (Kate) A. Brown-Henry, Esq., is an associate with Cline Farrell Christie & Lee located in Indianapolis, Indiana. Brown-Henry's practice focuses in the areas of personal injury, wrongful death, premises liability, automobile and trucking incidents, product liability, and medical malpractice. She is a 2002 graduate of DePauw University with a BA in political science and a minor in German. She is a 2006 graduate of the Valparaiso University School of Law and was admitted to the Indiana bar the same year. Brown-Henry was named a Super Lawyers Rising Star (2014–2017), was listed as a National Trial Lawyer's Association Top 40 under 40 (2013), a Top 100 Trial Lawyer (2014–2017) for Indiana, and an Up and Coming Lawyer (2013) by *The Indiana Lawyer*. She contributes time as a mentor with the Walker Foundation, and as a "We the People" Judge for high school, middle school, and elementary school district competitions. Brown-Henry is a member of the American Association for Justice where she serves on the Board of Governors, the Indiana State Bar Association, Indiana Trial Lawyers Association where she serves on the Board of Directors, and the Indianapolis Bar Association.

Terry C. Cox, JD, is an elder law attorney in private practice in Collierville, Tennessee. He has represented individual and business clients in a broad range of civil and criminal cases in various courts, and is committed to providing advice and counsel to elders and their families on issues of aging to help clients protect their interests, plan for their future legal needs, and plan for their future health care needs.

Paul M. Deutsch, PhD, LMHC, CRC, CLCP, retired, is a licensed mental health counselor with a PhD in rehabilitation counseling and counseling psychology. He specialized in working with catastrophic disabilities resulting from either birth or a trauma. Dr. Deutsch is best known for having developed the basic tenets, methodologies, and processes of life care planning. He first published on life care planning as a fundamental tool of case management in his 1981 text (*Damages in Tort Actions,* Deutsch and Raffa). Dr. Deutsch has authored or co-authored 12 volumes and more than 50 peer-reviewed journal articles and chapters. Dr. Deutsch has taught as an adjunct professor at several universities and lectured widely through the United States and Europe. In the 1980s and early 1990s, he worked extensively in the former Soviet Union with colleagues of Alexander Romanovich Luria. He has worked extensively in brain injury and spinal cord injury rehabilitation, among other areas. His experience includes co-ownership and directorship of a brain injury rehabilitation center in the 1980s and later ownership and management of a long-term residential and supported work program for severe brain injury patients. He remained active in research efforts until retirement and helped to spearhead the formation of the Foundation for Life Care Planning Research along with Dr. Roger Weed, Dr. Christine Reid, Patricia McCollom, MS, RN, and Susan Riddick, RN. The primary work of this foundation is research on the reliability and validity of the life care planning process. Related areas of research may include life expectancy as it is influenced by effective life care planning, as well as case management and all appropriate related life care planning research. The foundation has forged multiple university relationships and developed successful fundraising efforts. Funding has allowed the foundation to support several doctoral dissertation projects, other research efforts, and offer recognition awards to professionals who contribute to the advancement of life care planning. Dr. Deutsch also was a prime author of the core materials for the profession's amicus curiae brief that was filed in the Texas Seventh District Court of Appeals which became a major foundation for the specialty practice of life care planning. He also was instrumental in establishing ongoing education (Kaplan online, University of Florida, and others), training, and certification (certificate #1) for Life Care Planners.

Everett G. Dillman, PhD, is an educator and business consultant, and president of International Business Planners, Inc. Dr. Dillman has been active in governmental, business, and financial circles in the Southwest for more than 50 years. During this period he has served on the advisory board of the Lubbock Division of the Small Business Administration, as well as on the board of directors of several profit and civic organizations. Dr. Dillman has served on the Board of Directors of the National Association of Forensic Economists and on the Steering Committee for Forensic Rehabilitation of the National Association of Rehabilitation Professionals in the private sector. He has published extensively in both the vocational and economic areas.

Timothy F. Field, PhD, a former educator in rehabilitation counseling at the University of Georgia, is founder and president of Elliott & Fitzpatrick, Inc., a consulting and publishing company in Athens, Georgia. E & F produces resources (books, journals, and related materials) for the practicing forensic rehabilitation consultant and life care planners. Dr. Field also is a frequent conference speaker on forensic topics including transferable skills, estimating lost earnings, expert testimony and the law, and more recently, the Affordable Care Act, collateral sources and implications for the life care planners. He has been recognized several times for his contributions to the profession including the Lifetime Achievement Award from the International Association of Rehabilitation Professionals. Dr. Field continues to author manuscripts and pamphlets related to the above topics.

Kevin N. Foster, MD, MBA, FACS, is the director of the Arizona Burn Center and program director, director of Surgical Research and former director of General Surgery Residency, as well as Maricopa Medical Center. Dr. Foster is a graduate of the Medical College of Ohio and completed a general surgery residency at the University of Wisconsin, followed by burn surgery and trauma research fellowships at the University of Washington. He also completed an MBA at Indiana University School of Business.

Tracy Raffles Gunn, JD, is the founder of Gunn Appellate Practice, PA, in Tampa, Florida. Dr. Gunn is board certified by the Florida Bar as a specialist in appellate practice and is AV rated by Martindale Hubbell. She is chair of the Florida Supreme Court Committee on Standard Jury Instructions in Civil Cases, is an elected member of the American Law Institute, and serves on the Executive Council of the Appellate Practice Section of the Florida Bar. She has been recognized as one of the "Best Lawyers in America" in the specialty of appellate practice, and was named one of the Top 50 Female Attorneys in Florida by Florida Superlawyers.

Anna N. Herrington, PhD, is a graduate of the rehabilitation counselor training and counseling psychology programs at Georgia State University and is a counseling psychologist in Atlanta, Georgia.

Carolyn Wiles Higdon, PhD, CCC-SLP, owns and operates a national/international private practice in assistive technology and speech-language pathology services, based in Georgia, licensed in multiple states. Her practice includes assistive technology for all ages, as well as educational consulting, forensics, and life care planning, catastrophic health care of acquired brain injury and trach- and ventilator-dependent patients, tele-practice/tele-supervision and mediation and legal consulting. Dr. Higdon testifies as an expert witness in all areas of communication sciences and disorders (hearing, speech, language, swallowing, technology) for all ages, is a past chair of the Georgia Board of Examiners for Speech Pathology and Audiology, and is a past chair of Division

12 of the American Speech-Language-Hearing Association (ASHA), the AAC Division. Dr. Higdon is a fellow of the ASHA, is active in multiple professional organizations, and has taught and consulted in Russia, Eastern Europe, Hong Kong, China, Costa Rica, and Thailand. Dr. Higdon is an ASHA consultant to the American Medical Association in the areas of augmentative and alternative communication and current procedural terminology (CPT) codes. Dr. Higdon is the past chair of the Department of Communicative Disorders and the past director of the Center for Speech and Hearing Research in the School of Applied Sciences at the University of Mississippi (Oxford, Mississippi), and is an adjunct clinical associate professor at the University of Mississippi Medical Center in Jackson, Mississippi. Dr. Higdon has been vice president of finances on the American Speech-Language-Hearing Association's board of directors (2011–2014), and has received the Mississippi Speech and Hearing (MSHA) Honors of the Association with recognition as the MSHA Clinician of the Year in 2017. Dr. Higdon is active in developing universal licensure for speech-language pathology and audiology, and is current chair of the Council of Academic Programs Committee on InterProfessional Practice and InterProfessional Education.

J. Mat Hunt, Jr., CLVS, after years of electronic media experience as a television news and weather reporter, anchor, and documentary producer/writer/editor, founded in 1982 what is now Huntridge LVS (www.huntridge.com), a legal video service firm in Elberton, Georgia and Greenville, South Carolina. In addition to the usual video depositions and day-in-the-life presentations, his settlement documentaries are credited with helping to turn the corner in settlement negotiation and mediation. Permitted works have received multiple Telly Awards and Silver Reels—a rarity in court-related media. An invited guest lecturer with authentic "Show & Tell" in conferences and continuing legal education seminars, Hunt's more than three-decade profession has been the humanizing of litigation.

Harvey E. Jacobs, PhD, CLCP, is a Licensed Clinical Psychologist and Certified Life Care Planner. He graduated from Florida State University, was a post-doctoral fellow at the Johns Hopkins University School of Medicine, and a Mary Switzer Research Fellow at the National Institute of Handicapped Research. Dr. Jacobs has served on multiple medical school faculties, hospitals, programs and facilities, and as a principal investigator on federal, state, and private grants. He lectures and publishes widely on rehabilitation for neurological, psychiatric, medical, and intellectual impairments; life care planning; behavior analysis; and complex treatment issues across the life span. Dr. Jacobs currently serves on the national boards of the North American Brain Injury Society, the United States Brain Injury Alliance, and the editorial boards of the *Journal of Head Trauma Rehabilitation*, the *Rehabilitation Professional*, and the *Journal of Life Care Planning*. He is one of 50 professionals helping the Brain Injury Association of America draft national guidelines for the treatment of adults with traumatic brain injury.

Jim Karl, BS, GC, CEAC, CAPS, has a degree in industrial arts education with a K–12 certificate and additional hours toward a master in course curriculum development. Karl has more than 20 years of hands-on experience in construction and accessible renovations and is an owner of All In One Accessibility based in Marietta, Georgia (www.allinoneaccess.com). He is a Certified Aging-in-Place Specialist with the National Home Builders Association, a Certified Environmental Access Contractor through U.S. Rehab, and a general contractor. He has volunteered his time to several organizations including service on the Board of Directors of Professional Resources in Management Education, Inc., the previous certifying organization for CEAC now operated by U.S. Rehab. He has consulted nationally on Life Care Plan Home Assessment and has an extensive speaking resume.

Denise D. Lester, MD, received her medical degree from the New Jersey Medical School, then completed her residency in anesthesiology as well as pain management training at the Thomas Jefferson University Hospital. Dr. Lester is an assistant professor of anesthesiology and an assistant professor of physical medicine and rehabilitation at the Medical College of Virginia, Virginia Commonwealth University and practicing physician of pain management at the Hunter Holmes McGuire Veterans Affairs Medical Center in Richmond, Virginia. A Diplomat of the American Board of Anesthesiology and the American Board of Pain Medicine, Dr. Lester holds specialty certifications in Spinal Cord Stimulation, SPRINT Peripheral Nerve Stimulation, Intraspinal Pump Management, Radiofrequency Ablation, Percutaneous Discectomy (Dekrompressor), Vertebroplasty, Kyphoplasty, and Minimally Invasive Decompression (MILD procedure). She has been honored with numerous awards, is a teacher and speaker, as well as a volunteer to various committee and professional organizations. When not working, she is a fitness instructor.

Sylvia "Ann" Maniha, RN, CLCP, CMC, obtained her CLCP in 1998 and CMC in 2004. Her background includes experience in life care planning, medical case management, research and specialty nursing care including orthopedics, post-anesthesia care unit, outpatient surgery, medical-surgical, substance abuse, and psychiatry. She developed "Life Care Planning for the PC," a life care planning software for Microsoft Word and Corel WordPerfect. She has published two articles pertaining to medical coding and pricing associated with life care planning, is a member of the International Academy of Life Care Planning (IALCP), a section of the International Association of Rehabilitation Professionals (IARP), and the proud recipient of the Cheryl L. Jasper Memorial Recognition Award in September 2015.

Robert H. Meier, III, MD, is a physiatrist who has practiced in the specialty of physical medicine and rehabilitation for 44 years. He completed his medical school and residency training in physical medicine and rehabilitation at the Temple University School of Medicine in Philadelphia, Pennsylvania. Dr. Meier began his professional career at The Institute for Rehabilitation and Research (TIRR) and at the Baylor College of Medicine in 1973 where he provided comprehensive rehabilitation services for persons with spinal cord injury, amputation, burn injury, and brachial plexus injuries. He moved to Denver and the University of Colorado Health Sciences Center in 1986. He was chairman of the Department of Rehabilitation Medicine until 1996. He has served as the president of both the American Congress of Rehabilitation Medicine and the Association of Academic Physiatrists. In 1996, he entered private practice to concentrate on developing a comprehensive center of excellence for persons with amputations now called the Amputee Services of America. In 2005, he moved his practice to the Presbyterian/St. Luke's Medical Center in Denver to focus on the rehabilitation needs of complex limb dysfunction including amputation nerve injury, burns, and tumors. He is the physiatric consultant for the Institute for Limb Preservation that deals with complex extremity injuries, vascular problems, and tumors that threaten the function of an extremity. In this setting, he has every level and type of rehabilitation, acute medical and surgical service that a person would need to regain function of a threatened or damaged extremity. During his extensive career, Dr. Meier has provided comprehensive rehabilitation services for more than 4000 adults and children with amputations and limb deficiencies. Dr. Meier is also involved with life care planning for persons with amputation, burns, and neurologic injury. He actively participates in the teaching of life care planners and in their summit meetings for education and development of the field of life care planning. In the past, Dr. Meier has been a surveyor for the Commission on the Accreditation of Rehabilitation Facilities and in 2011, he became a Paradigm Medical Director for Amputee Care. In March 2012, Dr. Meier became the president of the Active Medical Staff for the Spalding Rehabilitation Hospital, a CARF-accredited facility in Denver, Colorado. He now continues an outpatient practice and medico-legal practice dealing with complex limb injuries and amputations.

Nancy L. Mitchell, MA, OTR/L, CLCP, FIALCP, is an occupational therapist with more than 40 years of experience in various rehabilitation settings. She became a Certified Life Care Planner in 1998. Mitchell co-owns a private practice, Mitchell Disability Assessments and Life Care Planning. The practice specializes in the assessment, research, and development of life care plans for children and adults with a broad scope of disabilities, as well as performing disability and home nursing assessments. Mitchell holds a master's degree in gerontology with an emphasis on aging with a disability. She was named a Fellow International Academy of Life Care Planners in 2005. Mitchell presents locally and nationally. She has published articles in the *Journal of Life Care Planning* and *Journal of Legal Nurse Consultants* as well as a previous chapter for the *Life Care Planning and Case Management Handbook.* Mitchell writes the quarterly "Ethics Interface" article for the *Journal of Life Care Planning* and chairs the Ethics Committee for the column. She is currently director at large for the International Academy of Life Care Planners to the International Academy of Rehabilitation Professionals organization.

Courtney V. Mitchell, MS, OTR/L, CLCP, is an occupational therapist with experience treating various diagnoses in a variety of treatment settings. She is currently working at Hennepin County Medical Center in occupational therapy as well as her co-ownership of Mitchell Disability Assessments and Life Care Planning. She became a Certified Life Care Planner in 2016. She has presented on evaluation and treatment of visual deficits secondary to brain injuries, neurorehabilitation techniques for the upper extremities, and multidisciplinary approaches to traumatic brain injury.

William D. Mustain, PhD, CCC-A, CNIM, BCS-IOM, is currently professor, Department of Otolaryngology and Communicative Sciences and professor, Department of Neurology, at the University of Mississippi Medical Center in Jackson. He is also an adjunct professor in the Department of Communicative Sciences and Disorders at the University of Mississippi (Oxford Campus). Dr. Mustain received a BA in psychology from the College of William and Mary, and a MEd in deaf education and PhD in audiology from the University of Virginia. He has been involved in the evaluation and management of hearing- and balance-impaired patients of all ages for more than 30 years.

Lisa Norris, MS, MBA, has more than 20 years of experience in health care management and more than 16 years of experience in the field of transplantation administration. She is currently the managing director and principal of Transplant Leadership Institute LLC, the leading recruitment and search firm serving the fields of transplantation and organ procurement. She has served as a transplant administrator at a number of prestigious institutions: CHRISTUS Transplant Institute in San Antonio, Texas; UNC Center for Transplant Care at the University of North Carolina Health Care System in Chapel Hill, North Carolina; the University of Maryland Medical System in Baltimore; and the University of Colorado Hospital in Denver. She has been a Region 8 administrator on the UNOS Transplant Administrator's Committee and has held various board positions with other transplant-related organizations. Norris is a graduate of the University of Colorado, Boulder and earned an MS degree from Northeastern University and an MBA from the Leeds School of Business at the University of Colorado. She is also the editor of the first book on the business of transplantation entitled *Transplant Administration* published by Wiley Blackwell.

Kirsten Potter, PT, DPT, MS, obtained her BS in physical therapy from the University of Buffalo in 1985, a masters in physical therapy from the University of Health Sciences/Chicago Medical School (now the Rosalind Franklin University of Medicine & Science), and a Doctor of Physical Therapy from MGH Institute of Health Professions. Dr. Potter's clinical experience and specialization is in adult neurologic rehabilitation. She has provided care to clients in acute care and rehabilitation hospitals, outpatient clinics, and home settings. She has been an educator in PT programs since 1993 and is currently an associate professor in the Department of Physical Therapy at Rockhurst University in Kansas City where she teaches students in the DPT program, conducts research on outcome measurements, and provides service to local organizations supporting people with multiple sclerosis and Parkinson's disease.

Ruth B. Rimmer, PhD, CLCP, is the owner of Care Plans for Life, LLC. She served as the director of Psychological/Social Research and Family Service at the Arizona Burn Center for 15 years. Dr. Rimmer received her PhD in Life-Span Developmental Psychology and Certification in Gerontology from Arizona State University and a Certificate in Life Care Planning from MediPro and the University of Florida. She has been working in the field of burns for 24 years and continues to research issues associated with the psycho/social and rehabilitation needs of burn survivors. Dr. Rimmer is an active member of the American Burn Association and has served on the Ethics and Rehabilitation committees and as the chair of the Psycho/Social Special Interest Group. She is a published children's author, an accomplished ventriloquist, and fluent in Spanish.

David L. Ripley, MD, MS, CRC, FAAPM&R, is section chief of Brain Injury Medicine and Rehabilitation at the Shirley Ryan Ability Lab and associate professor of Physical Medicine and Rehabilitation in the Feinberg School of Medicine of Northwestern University. He is the program director for the O'Boyle Fellowship in Brain Injury Medicine and Rehabilitation. He is board certified in Physical Medicine and Rehabilitation (PM&R) and Brain Injury Medicine. He is a Fellow of the American Academy of Physical Medicine and Rehabilitation. Prior to entering medical school, Dr. Ripley worked as a vocational rehabilitation counselor and retains his certification (Certified Rehabilitation Counselor). His clinical practice at the Shirley Ryan Ability Lab involves providing medical and rehabilitation care to individuals with brain injury.

Amy M. Sutton, PhD, RN, BSN, MA, CLCP, is a Certified Life Care Planner in private practice. She obtained her doctorate in counseling psychology from Georgia State University with a focus on rehabilitation, health and neuropsychology. She received two Bachelor's degrees in Psychology and Nursing from Purdue University and Indiana University and a master's degree in Psychology from Ludwig Maximillian's University in Munich, Germany. Dr. Sutton lived and worked as a home health nurse in Germany for four years. During her graduate studies in Germany, Dr. Sutton conducted an internship/research project in South Africa on AIDS education in the public school system. During and after her graduate studies in Georgia, Dr. Sutton published several articles and textbook chapters in life care planning as well as publishing the first life care plan validation study. She was awarded the Rosalynn Carter Caregiver Fellowship in 2004 and 2005 and earned the

Outstanding Doctoral Dissertation Award in 2009. As a registered nurse, Dr. Sutton has worked in critical care, home health, and inpatient rehabilitation. Dr. Sutton is currently working as a life care planner in southern California.

Lewis E. Vierling, MS, NCC, NCCC, CRC, CCM, is president and is, with a masters degree in counseling from Drake University, a vocational rehabilitation counselor and consultant for Vierling & Associates Inc. in Johnston, Iowa. With relevance to the contributed chapter, he has authored multiple articles, chapters, and a book on the American with Disabilities Act (ADA). He has also been an invited speaker and educator to numerous local, regional, and national conferences. Further, in 1982, Vierling was appointed by the Governor of Iowa to the Commission on Persons with Disabilities, where he served for 10 years, including as elected chairperson. He was also personally invited by the White House to attend the signing into law of the Americans with Disabilities Act, by President George H.W. Bush, on July 26, 1990. For 6 years, Vierling was a board member of the National Commission for Case Manager Certification serving as ethics chair and as a member of the Research and Examination Committee. In recognition of his prominence, the National Institute on Disability and Rehabilitation Research, Department of Education, in July 2011, selected Vierling to be a reviewer for a national grant proposal project related to the ADA. He was also a founding member of the original Board of Directors for the Foundation for Life Care Planning Research and served from 2007 to 2013.

Carol Walker, PhD, ABPP-CN, CLCP, completed her PhD in clinical/medical psychology at the University of Alabama at Birmingham mentored by Thomas J. Boll, PhD, ABPP, who is a nationally recognized leader in the field of neuropsychology. Her primary interests in her graduate training were neuropsychology, chronic pain, and cardiovascular disease. Dr. Walker completed an internship at the Medical College of Georgia in Augusta, where she received specialized training in post-traumatic stress disorder. Her postdoctoral training was completed in an acute rehabilitation hospital setting under the supervision of Dr. Boll. Dr. Walker is board certified in Clinical Neuropsychology by the American Board of Professional Psychology (ABPP). She received specialized training in Life Care Planning from the University of Florida/Intelicus, which is known as the most extensive and comprehensive training program for life care planning in the nation. She is a Certified Life Care Planner (CLCP) and past board member of the Foundation for Life Care Planning Research. She has 27 years of combined experience as a clinician treating patients with traumatic brain injury, spinal cord injury, and other catastrophic injuries in an acute rehab setting and is currently in full-time private practice. She also provides treatment to patients suffering from cardiovascular accidents, Alzheimer's disease, and other neurological conditions. Dr. Walker has an active Chronic Pain Program and furnishes Independent Medical Examinations for patients, insurance companies, and attorneys. She has given numerous invited lectures to a variety of audiences in professional communities locally and nationally. She is also a lecturer for the University of Florida's Online Life Care Planning curriculum, offering specialized expertise to life care planners in the University of Florida's online training program, proceeds of which Dr. Walker donates to the Foundation for Life Care Planning Research.

Mamie Walters, CNHP, pursued a career in music theory and composition until 1981 when she became co-owner and successfully operated a cutlery distributorship for 6 years. During this period, she met Ray Arrona, who was with Vector Marketing Corporation. Her business acumen led to a national promotion as senior assistant to the executive vice president of sales and marketing for the southern zone with Vector. In March 1994, this position ended and Walters pursued her education full time. In January 1995, she began working as a private hire for Ray Arrona, natural and legal guardian of Anita Arrona for several years. Walters is a Certified Natural Health Professional and is currently enrolled and active in the Doctor of Naturopathy Program. She is also a member of the American Naturopathic Practitioners Association and EarthSave International.

Leslie L. Watson, MA, CRC, CDME, received her master's in rehabilitation counseling in 1984 and has been a Certified Rehabilitation Counselor (CRC) since 1985. She obtained her Durable Medical Equipment Specialist (CDME) certification in 2017. She has more than 26 years of experience providing medical cost research services in the life care planning field. She worked with Paul M. Deutsch & Associates for 10 years and for the past 16 years has provided medical cost research services as a private consultant for life care planners across the United States. She is experienced in researching medical costs for physician services, therapies, medical equipment and supplies, surgical procedures, home health care, diagnostic testing, short-term and long-term care, and other needs associated with the life care plan. Additional work experience includes case manager, neuropsychological testing administrator, and group facilitator with an outpatient traumatic brain injury day program. She has co-authored several articles and poster presentations. She has been a presenter for life care planning training and conferences, including the Institute for Rehabilitation Education and Training (IRET).

Roger O. Weed, PhD, CRC/R, LPC/Ret, CCM/R, CDMS/R, CLCP/R, FNRCA, FIALCP/R, Professor Emeritus, is retired as professor and graduate rehabilitation counseling coordinator at Georgia State University. He also held doctoral student graduate faculty status in Counseling Psychology as well as Counselor Education and Practice doctoral programs. He has authored or co-authored approximately 150 books, reviews, articles, and book chapters, approximately 80 of which were specific to life care planning. During his more than 42 years in the profession, Dr. Weed was honored several times for his work including the 2006 Distinguished Professor Award from Georgia State University's Alumni Association (sole recipient), the 2011 Lifetime Appreciation Award from the International Commission on Health Care Certification, the 2009 Larry Huggins Lifetime Achievement Award from the Private Rehabilitation Specialists of Georgia, the 2005 Lifetime Achievement Award from the sponsors of the International Life Care Planning Conference, the 2004 Lifetime Achievement Award from the International Association of Rehabilitation Professionals (as well as recognition in 1997 and 1991 as the Outstanding Educator), the 1993 National Professional Services Award from the American Rehabilitation Counseling Association, and the 2003 Research Excellence Award from the College of Education at Georgia State University. Dr. Weed is one of the five founders of the original, nation-wide training program leading to Life Care Planning certification. He is also past chair of the Georgia State Licensing Board for professional counselors, marriage and family therapists, and social workers, as well as past president of the International Association of Rehabilitation Professionals.

Dana M. Weldon, MS, CRC, CLCP, CCLCP, currently maintains a private practice as a rehabilitation consultant and life care planner. Weldon's formal education includes a master of science in vocational rehabilitation with a concentration in vocational rehabilitation counseling obtained through the University of Wisconsin–Stout; bachelor of environmental studies; bachelor of education; Ontario Teacher's Certificate; and Life Care Planning Post Graduate Certificate. She was a member of the IARP Board of Directors from 1997 to 2001 and a member of the IARP Ethics Committee from 2001 to 2007. Weldon also held an appointment to the editorial board of the peer-reviewed *Journal of Life Care Planning* from 2015 to 2017. Weldon is currently a member of the faculty at the Institute of Rehabilitation Education and Training (IRET) as the Canadian instructor for the on-site training module. She also sits on the board as a Commissioner of Life Care Planning with the International Commission on Health Care Certification (ICHCC).

Rasheeda Wilkins, MS, CRC, is the program director for the Adult Facility Based Services (New View) program at the Center for the Visually Impaired in Atlanta, Georgia. The Center for the Visually Impaired (CVI) is a fully accredited organization providing rehabilitation services. CVI serves individuals of all ages who are blind or visually impaired. She graduated from Southern University and A&M College, where she received a bachelor of science degree in psychology. She received her masters of science degree in rehabilitation counseling at Georgia State University. After graduation, Wilkins earned the designation of CRC (Certified Rehabilitation Counselor) by the Commission on Rehabilitation Counselor Certification. Wilkins began working with the Georgia Department of Labor as a Certified Rehabilitation Counselor serving individuals with sensory impairments. After a year of helping clients return to the competitive labor market, she took a position as a vocational evaluator in the Career Services Department at CVI. Since that time, Wilkins has grown with the agency over the past 11 years. As the program director for Adult Facility Based Services, Wilkins is responsible for planning, directing, and supervising the delivery of rehabilitation services for all working-age clients.

Nicole M. Wolf, MS, CRC, LPC, CPRP, has a masters degree in rehabilitation counseling and is a certified rehabilitation counselor, licensed professional counselor, and certified psychiatric rehabilitation practitioner. She is employed as a quality improvement specialist at United Behavioral Health where she focuses on improving quality and effectiveness for members in the areas of mental health and substance. Previously she worked as a clinician and research assistant at the Promedica Research Center in Tucker, GA. Her research interests include pharamacologic and nonpharmacologic interventions in mental illness and vocational strategies in severe and persistent mental illness.

F. Auston Wortman, III, JD, MPT, has a master's degree in physical therapy and was an elder law attorney in Tennessee.

Dorothy J. Zydowicz-Vierling, RN, BSN, CCM, CDMS, is a Certified Case Manager and Certified Disability Management Specialist. Professionally she is a nurse consultant as well as the vice president and director of operations for Vierling and Associates Inc., in Johnston, Iowa. A Summa Cum Laude graduate of Elmhurst College in nursing and psychology, Vierling has more than 27 years of experience in the health care and managed care industries. She has worked in many specialty areas in life care planning and case management such as case manager and supervisor, secondary, tertiary, and catastrophic group health case management, utilization management, transplantation services, medical consultation, retrospective reviews, independent medical reviews, disease management, as well as nationwide consultation and training. Vierling is a past board member of the National Commission for Case Manager Certification. She has also been recognized for her contributions in several ways including the 2010/2011 National Association of Professional Women's "Women of the Year" award. Further, Vierling has contributed to the professional literature with many journal articles and chapters.

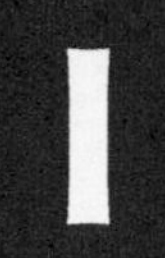

THE ROLES OF LIFE CARE PLAN TEAM MEMBERS

Chapter 1

Life Care Planning: Past, Present, and Future

Roger O. Weed

Contents

Introduction 3
The Past 4
The Present 6
Step-by-Step Procedures 9
The Future 13
Conclusion 15
Appendix: Life Care Planner: Secretary, Know-It-All, or General Contractor? One Person's Perspective 15
Two Apparent Self-Serving Views 16
A Critical Review of Educational Requirements 16
A Third View—By Analogy 18
Conclusion 19
References 19

Introduction

In the previous editions of this text, I wrote that life care planning has become a major buzzword in the field of professional rehabilitation. Many people who have little knowledge about published concepts in life care planning continue to use the term *life care plans* to generate business. Several years ago, I recall reading a deposition from a PhD-level "life care planner" who, when asked by the opposing attorney about resources in life care planning, revealed that it was his opinion there were no written resources or training programs in life care planning. This discourse occurred in 1996, after there already existed a national certification in life care planning. It was repeated in 2003 by two "experts," one of whom claimed there were no training programs but also claimed to be one of the founders of the life care planning practice. Since the second edition, there have been fewer similar occasions, suggesting, in this author's opinion, that life care planning has become mainstream underscored by references in the legal literature (Field & Weed, 2015). Although more professionals are aware of the life care planning concepts, many life care planners have faced deposition and courtroom challenges in personal injury litigation, which have further refined the requirements for successful presentation of information (for more information see Weed & Johnson, 2006, as well as the forensics chapter in this text).

Clearly, life care planning continues to be the standard by which other plans are to be measured with regard to the management of catastrophic impairments, complex health care needs, or opinions for various litigation venues. The published methods, concepts, and procedures are an effective means to determine the road map of care as well as to identify reasonable needs and costs associated with an impairment (as an example, see Deutsch et al. 1989a). However, not everyone is demonstrating quality practice; many do not know of existing standards of practice (IALCP, 2015), and many professionals are resisting standardization of the concept. As with previous editions, it is helpful to review the specialty practice of life care planning as a foundation for this book.

The Past

The original issuance of life care plans appeared in a legal publication, *Damages in Tort Actions* (Deutsch & Raffa, 1981), which established the guidelines for determining damages in civil litigation cases. By 1985, the life care plan was introduced to the health care industry in the *Guide to Rehabilitation* (Deutsch & Sawyer, 1985). One of the first nationwide rehabilitation professional training programs was organized by Dr. Paul Deutsch and offered on September 16–17, 1986, in Hilton Head, South Carolina, where more than 100 rehabilitation professionals from throughout the United States assembled to begin the process of learning about life care plans. Initially the training comprised approximately 2 days to introduce rehabilitation professionals to the overall concepts and the format that was published in the *Guide to Rehabilitation*. It also became evident that many people were practicing life care planning in a variety of ways, some of which appeared to be contrary to the intended goals and purposes of ethical rehabilitation practices (Weed, 1995b). In addition, as previously mentioned, many people were using the term *life care planning* as it became more popular, but had little or no awareness of the appropriate uses or practices associated with this emerging industry.

In the fall of 1992, five rehabilitation professionals, Richard Bonfiglio, MD; Paul Deutsch, PhD; Julie Kitchen, CDMS; Susan Riddick, BS, RN; and Roger Weed, PhD, met to discuss the apparent problems associated with the life care planning practices. Concerned that fragmentation and poor standardization would result in the overall decline of the specialty practice, they decided to develop a concentrated training program consisting of eight 2-day modules representing the various aspects of life care planning.

Module I was a basic overview of life care planning process methods, standards, and formats. Module II was designed to include the vocational aspects of clients whose life care plans appropriately included work-related opinions. Module III addressed effective case management strategies within the complex medical environment. Module IV outlined the various forensic rehabilitation issues to which many rehabilitation professionals, willingly or unwillingly, are subjected. Module V focused specifically on spinal cord injury issues, and Module VI identified brain injury issues. Module VII was an overview of the long-term care issues for other physical and emotional disabilities as well as some disease processes. Module VIII focused more explicitly on business and ethical practices, including the use of technology in life care planning.

Following this process, a management company (Rehabilitation Training Institute) was contracted to set up training programs throughout the United States. Before the first flyers were fully distributed, the first of the organized modules (scheduled for November 1993) was filled. Two introductory courses were developed: one on the West Coast and the other on the East Coast. It became obvious that there were a number of rehabilitation professionals who were interested in pursuing continuing education related to life care planning, and several participants requested official recognition for their educational efforts. Dr. Horace Sawyer of the University of Florida was approached, and he agreed to pursue an official certificate of completion through the University of Florida's Continuing Education Department. A private-public partnership between the Rehabilitation Training Institute and the University of Florida was formed and named Intelicus. The five founders donated the program content to Intelicus, which was purchased by Medipro Seminars in 2003. However, Medipro has since ceased operations. Most of the founders continue to donate time and services in support of online training through the University of Florida and the annual life care planning symposium (visit the website for the International Academy of Life Care Planners—https://connect.rehabpro.org/lcp/home—for the current schedule).

Although an initial description of life care planning was offered by Drs. Deutsch and Raffa in *Damages in Tort Action*, collaboration with leaders and organizations resulted in an agreed upon definition:

> A *Life Care Plan* is a dynamic document based upon published standards of practice, comprehensive assessment, data analysis, and research, which provides an organized concise plan for current and future needs with associated costs, for individuals who have experienced catastrophic injury or have chronic health care needs. [Combined definition of the University of Florida and Intelicus Annual Life Care Planning Conference and the American Academy of Nurse Life Care Planners (now known as the International Academy of Life Care Planners) presented at the Forensic Section meeting, NARPPS annual conference, Colorado Springs, Colorado, and agreed upon April 3, 1998.]

Although the certificate of completion from such programs as the University of Florida and Kaplan University underscored the value of obtaining education specific to this specialized profession, it did not provide the assurance of ethical practice or the professional identity that was desired by people who had invested thousands of dollars and much of their time in the training process. Several certification boards were contacted, with three indicating an interest in leading the way to certification. Eventually the Commission on Disability Examiner Certification (now known as the International Commission on Health Care Certification, or ICHCC) based in Midlothian, Virginia, and owned by V. Robert May, RhD, assumed the responsibility, and the first certifications were offered in the spring of 1996. Although the ICHCC also certifies nurses, for nurses who wish to affiliate with an organization that only certifies nurses, the American Association of Nurse Life Care Planners was formed.

Occasionally, there are questions about who did what first. The chronology below is intended to "lay out" the development of the specialty practice of life care planning as it is known today. As noted previously, Paul Deutsch, in the mid-1980s, was the first rehabilitation professional to formally teach "life care planning" concepts, methodology, and such. He is considered the "founder" of the life care planning process and was the first one to publish on the topic in the rehabilitation literature (with Fred Raffa) in 1981 (*Damages in Tort Action*).

Susan Riddick-Grisham was the first nurse to formally teach other nurses an organized series of life care planning classes when she was hired by Crawford & Company in the early 1990s to educate their consultants nationwide. It may be obvious, but she underwent specific life care planning training prior to teaching the methodology to others. She was also the only nurse to help develop the original nationwide training program curriculum launched by the Rehabilitation

Training Institute (which later became Intelicus and, through the years, has been reformatted to be today's life care planning certificate training program offered by the University of Florida).

Patti McCollom was the first nurse to start an organization specifically for nurses and life care planning in the mid-1990s when she founded the American Academy of Nurse Life Care Planners. Under Patti's direction and at the urging of others, the organization was expanded to include life care planners from disciplines including and outside of nursing (i.e., multidisciplinary) and is now known as the International Academy of Life Care Planners (IALCP), a section of the International Association of Rehabilitation Professionals (IARP). Later, there was another "nurse only" group founded by Kelly Lance, known as the American Association of Nurse Life Care Planners (AANLCP).

Finally, life care plans have historically been subject to intense scrutiny in a variety of rehabilitation fields, including managed care, workers' compensation claims, civil litigation, mediation, reserve setting for insurance companies, and federal vaccine injury fund cases.

The Present

At present, the life care planning specialty practice continues to grow, change, and modify the scope of practice associated with catastrophic case management. The International Academy of Life Care Planners is well established and has published the third edition of basic standards of practice (IALCP, 2015). The *Journal of Life Care Planning* was launched in 2002. Kaplan University, Capital Law School's paralegal program, and the University of Florida's Distance Education program offered online training programs leading to certification. At the time of this publication, Kaplan University has discontinued training and the University of Florida's Distance Education program transferred ownership of their Life Care Planning Pre-Certification Program to the Institute of Rehabilitation Education and Training (IRET) which continues to offer on-line life care planning training programs. Also new since the third edition is the American Academy of Physician Life Care Planners (AAPLCP), founded in 2013, which held their inaugural conference in San Antonio in April 2016 chaired by Joe Gonzales, MD (aaplcp.org, 2016). Reportedly, this physician focused group is a professional organization of board certified physicians *and* other qualified clinical and forensic professionals dedicated to the practice and advancement of life care planning. According to the website, only life care planning certified physicians (CPLCP™) will be members with the "Fellow" designation. Qualified physicians and nonphysicians may join as a "member," "associate member," or "resident member" (see website for criteria). Although there may be other purported credentials for life care planning, "exams," if any, may not be based on reliable/valid data, backed by legitimate role and functions studies, and an exam *administered* by a well-known organization does not constitute due diligence for a valid credential. An additional training program is FIG Services, independently owned and established in 2005 to provide education in Nurse Life Care Planning, Life Care Planning, and Medicare Set-Asides (FIG Services, 2017).

In addition to training programs, the Foundation for Life Care Planning Research (FLCPR), established in 2002, is a nonprofit research group that supports graduate students and other qualified research efforts in life care planning, including reliability and validity studies. The Foundation has held national Life Care Planning Summits on a biennial basis since 2002 with representation and endorsements from multiple life care planning and related organizations. Outcomes from the Summits have led to transdisciplinary and transorganizational consensus and majority views on more than 100 statements relevant to important topics and issues within life care planning (Johnson, 2015). At the time of this edition, the primary task of organizing the Summits has been assumed by the IALCP.

Although life care planning principles can be used in almost any aspect of care management, they are particularly useful in complex medical cases because the principles and methods that have been developed:

- Provide for needed quality care
- Reduce errors and omissions
- Allow fewer clients to drop through the cracks
- Reduce the failure to consider various aspects that can influence the ultimate outcome of the client's medical care (Weed & Riddick, 1992; Weed, 1995a)

Complex case management has become a specialty area, and, indeed, the *Certified Case Manager* (CCM) designation became established in 1993. Good case managers—professionals who are able to work consistently in a complex and often adversarial system—are very valuable professionals.

Since the third edition of this textbook, certification continues to attract a variety of health care professionals, and there are now certified life care planners in Canada and most of the United States. Sometimes arguments continue to be raised that life care planners should be people with nursing backgrounds only (Weed, 1989 as cited in Weed & Berens, 2010). In addition, one article proposed that only professionals with at least a doctorate should be considered qualified to develop life care plans (Weed, 1997). However, in the view of many practicing life care planners as well as the organizers of the initial national life care planning training program, it is the expectation that various professionals are qualified to practice in areas of their knowledge, skills, and abilities. For example, a rehabilitation nurse who has recently graduated from nursing school is ill prepared to effectively manage catastrophic cases. On the other hand, a master's-level vocational counselor who has spent several years working specifically in spinal cord injury rehabilitation may be extremely qualified to develop life care plans for that population. In addition, it is expected that life care planning members are part of a team, and it is further expected that team members will practice within their knowledge area. Historically, it has been common for vocational counselors and rehabilitation nurses to work together to develop vocational and medical rehabilitation plans (Riddick & Weed, 1996). Occasionally, nurses who author life care plans have been at a disadvantage since they are not educated or trained in vocational planning aspects. For helpful hints, see the chapter regarding the Role of the Rehabilitation Nurse in Life Care Planning where a checklist is available on questions the life care planner should ask the vocational expert.

In current practice, many organizations and hospitals have adopted life care planning procedures for discharge planning (Weed & Riddick, 1992; Riddick & Weed, 1996; Weed & Field, 2012). There are also health care professionals (such as physiatrists/physicians, occupational therapists, physical therapists, speech/language pathologists, nurses, dietitians, counselors, psychologists, audiologists, etc.) who develop projected care based on the published formats used in life care planning. Although it is important that the various participants in the training have a rehabilitation education and relevant certification in their area of specialty before engaging in the life care planning process, this by itself is certainly not enough; additional education and experience specific to life care planning are necessary (Weed, 1989, 1997). To identify some of the basic methodologies used in the profession and to underscore the relevance of the chapters included in this book, a review of the peer-reviewed current standards, developed in 2001, revised in 2006 and 2015, is appropriate (IALCP, 2015). Additionally, life care planning includes various topics that assure the effectiveness of the overall plan. Items included are listed in Table 1.1.

Table 1.1 Life Care Plan Checklist

Projected Evaluations: Have you planned for different types of nonphysician evaluations (e.g., physical therapy, speech therapy, recreational therapy, occupational therapy, music therapy, dietary assessment, audiology, vision screening, swallow studies, etc.)?
Projected Therapeutic Modalities: What therapies will be needed (based on the previous evaluations)? Will a case manager help control costs and reduce complications? Is a behavior management or rehab psychologist, pastoral counseling, or family education appropriate?
Diagnostic Testing/Educational Assessment: What testing is necessary and at what ages? Vocational evaluation? Neuropsychological? Educational levels? Educational consultant to maximize PL 94–142 and/or Individuals with Disabilities Education Act (IDEA)?
Wheelchair Needs: What types and configuration of wheelchairs will the client require? Power? Shower? Manual? Specialty? Ventilator? Reclining? Quad pegs? Recreational?
Wheelchair Accessories and Maintenance: Has each chair been listed separately for maintenance and accessories (bags, cushions, trays, etc.)? Have you considered the client's activity level?
Aids for Independent Functioning: What can this individual use to help himself or herself? Environmental controls? Adaptive aids? Omni-reachers?
Orthotics/Prosthetics: Will the client need braces? Have you planned for replacement and maintenance?
Home Furnishings and Accessories: Will the client need a specialty bed? Portable ramps? Hoyer or other lift?
Drug/Supply Needs: Have prescription and nonprescription drugs been listed, including size, quantity, and rate at which to be consumed? All supplies such as bladder and bowel program, skin care, etc.?
Home Care/Facility Care: Is it reasonable for the client to live at home? How about specialty programs such as yearly camps? What level of care will he or she require?
Future Medical Care—Routine: Is there a need for an annual evaluation? Which medical specialties? Orthopedics? Urology? Internist? Vision? Dental? Lab?
Transportation: Are hand controls sufficient or is a specialty van needed? Can local transportation companies be used?
Health and Strength Maintenance: What specialty recreation is needed? Blow darts? Adapted games? Row cycle? Annual dues for specialty magazines? (Specialty wheelchairs should be placed on wheelchair page.)
Architectural Renovations: Have you considered ramps, hallways, kitchen, fire protection, alternative heating/cooling, floor coverings, bath, attendant room, equipment storage, etc.?
Potential Complications: Have you included a list of potential complications likely to occur such as skin breakdown, infections, psychological trauma, contractures, etc.?
Future Medical Care/Surgical Intervention or Aggressive Treatment: Are there plans for aggressive treatment? Or additional surgeries such as plastic surgery?
Orthopedic Equipment Needs: Are walkers, standing tables, tilt tables, and/or body support equipment needed?
Vocational/Educational Plan: What are the costs of vocational counseling, job coaching, tuition, fees, books, supplies, technology, etc.?

After it is determined that a life care plan is appropriate, locating a qualified life care planner is necessary. Certainly, individuals who have completed the programs through the American Association of Nurse Life Care Planners, IRET, IARP, and others who have achieved the national board certified life care planner designation should be qualified, and visiting the certification boards' websites (www.ichcc.org/clcp.html and www.aanlcp.org) will provide a list of certified individuals. The person seeking a qualified life care planning professional should inquire as to the source of the credential, the published peer reviewed research foundation for establishing the criteria, and whether the organization is recognized by credible overseers such as the National Commission for Certifying Agencies (see www.credentialingexcellence.org/ncca, 2016). Alternatively, there are other people who have been practicing in their respective fields for decades and have extensive experience that may supplant the need for a designated or certified life care planner (such as a fellow of the International Academy of Life Care Planners or those with extensive experience). Questions regarding the planner's qualifications, which include education, work experience, life care planning experience, research knowledge and experience, certifications in legitimate rehabilitation areas, and, in the area of civil litigation, forensic experience, would be relevant (Table 1.2). It may also be important to determine the consultant's awareness of life care planning with regard to his or her expertise or knowledge about the methodology of life care planning, courses completed on life care planning, references and publications relevant to life care planning, and knowledge of professionals who have been movers and shakers in the life care planning field.

It is also relevant to determine the consultant's commitment to the profession by inquiring into which organizations he or she participates in. Many professionals pay monetary dues to associations but do not participate in professional development, committee work, or other profession-enhancing activities. It is pertinent to determine if the professional has contributed time and effort by either volunteering to work with clients, speaking on relevant issues, holding office within professional organizations, or writing for relevant publications. Receiving awards, honors, or peer recognition is also pertinent.

Other questions to ask may include the consultant's jurisdictional experience. If the practitioner is expected to work in personal injury litigation, then experience in this arena seems appropriate. Other specialty practices exist and the rules differ, such that it is often extremely important to ensure that the practitioner's experience covers these specialized fields (Weed, 1994, 1996; Weed & Field, 2012).

Reviewing a sample life care plan may be appropriate to determine if the prospective professional establishes a generally accepted foundation for his or her opinions and uses checklists and forms for other health professionals in their specific area of expertise. In *general*, it is expected that a physician be involved in the plan's medical opinions, although there are many ways to establish a medical foundation for diagnosis and treatment if a qualified physician is not available. Other types of miscellaneous information may help determine if the consultant has a current vita that outlines his or her experiences, as well as any history of ethics or malpractice complaints.

Step-by-Step Procedures

Assuming that the rehabilitation professional is qualified to assess and project a lifetime care plan for a client and is knowledgeable in the topics to be covered, the next step is to begin the process of the life care plan (Table 1.3). First, of course, the referral must be made to the life care planner and basic information, including time frames, billing agreements, retainer information, and information release topics, must be discussed (Weed & Field, 2012). Second, it is important to obtain as complete a copy of the medical records as possible, including nurses' notes, physicians'

Table 1.2 Checklist for Selecting a Life Care Planner

Professional's Qualifications

• **Education**, including degrees and continuing education? If doctorate, was the university accredited? (Some have mail-order graduate degrees or diplomas from universities that are less than stellar.) • **Work** experience? • **Life care planning** experience? • **Research** knowledge and experience? • **Certifications or licenses**? Generally accepted rehabilitation certifications include **CLCP** (certified life care planner), **CRC** (certified rehabilitation counselor), **CDMS** (certified disability management specialist), **CVE** (certified vocational evaluator), **CRRN** (certified rehabilitation registered nurse), **CCM** (certified case manager), diplomate, or fellow **ABVE** (American Board of Vocational Experts). • **Forensic experience** (if appropriate)? Familiar with the rules pertaining to experts? Have they testified? Do they have a list of cases in which they testified at deposition or trial for the previous 4 years? Plaintiff/defense ratio?
Prospective consultant's awareness of life care planning
• Are they a board **certified** or qualified life care planner? • Have they achieved the **certificate** in life care planning offered through one of the recognized training programs? • Have they completed **courses** offered by a noted program on life care planning? (e.g., Kaplan University, Intelicus if previous to the 3rd edition of this text, University of Florida, International Association of Rehabilitation Professionals, AANLCP, et al.) • Can they cite life care planning **references**? • Do they subscribe to the *Journal of Life Care Planning*? • Do they know some of the **professionals** associated with life care planning publications and training (e.g., Dr. Debbie Berens, Dr. Terry Blackwell, Dr. Richard Bonfiglio, Dr. Paul Deutsch, Julie Kitchen, Dr. Robert Meier, Dr. Ann Neulicht, Karen Preston, Dr. Fred Raffa, Susan Riddick-Grisham, Dr. Horace Sawyer, Dr. Randall Thomas, Dr. Roger Weed, Dr. Terry Winkler)?
Commitment to the profession
• Are they a member of the International Academy of Life Care Planners? What professional and disability-specific **organization**(s) do they belong to? (Are these legitimate or fringe organizations such as a for-profit owned by an individual or group with little recognition or substance?) • Do they **participate** in professional development? • Have they **contributed** their time and effort by volunteering services to clients in need, speaking, holding office with professional organizations, writing articles, chapters, or books? • Have they received **awards, honors, and/or peer recognition**?
Specialty practice experience?
• Workers' compensation or federal Office of Workers' Compensation Programs? • Personal injury? • Social Security? • State rehabilitation? • Longshore workers? • Jones Act? • Federal Employees Liability Act (FELA)? • Long-term and short-term disability? • Specialize in a particular disability?

(*Continued*)

Table 1.2 (Continued) Checklist for Selecting a Life Care Planner Professional's Qualifications

Medical foundation for opinions established
• Use established published **checklists** and **forms**? • Routinely consult with a **physician** as part of the team and/or use clinical practice guidelines, medical records, medical depositions, or other recognized sources? • Include other **health professionals** as appropriate (e.g., OT, PT, SLT, RT, audiology, neuropsych, etc.)?
Other
• What and how do they **bill** for their services? Do they charge different rates for interview, records review, deposition, or trial? • Do they have a current curriculum **vita**? • History of **ethics** complaints or **arrests**?

orders, ambulance reports, emergency records, consultants' reports, admission and discharge reports, and laboratory and radiographic reports.

It is also useful to obtain additional information from the client or family in the form of depositions, interrogatories, or other records. Employment records, tax records, and school records are usually helpful if there are vocational issues to be included in the report. If the client is a young child with no educational or medical history, then it would be of value to survey in extensive detail the family history, including mother and father, aunts and uncles, and grandparents (Weed, 1996, 2000). In some situations, siblings may have school and other history that may be useful. Occasionally, videotapes of the client prior to the injury or day-in-the-life videos may be compiled by the attorney and can be useful, particularly in civil litigation defense cases or insurance consulting where the client is not readily accessible to the consultant.

An initial interview should occur at the client's residence if possible (whether facility or home), and appropriate people should be invited to the interview, which may include parents, spouse, siblings, or caregivers. In general, initial interviews will last from 3 to 5 hours. When the professional attends the interview, it is important to use interview forms or checklists that will help structure the interview and ensure that topics appropriate to be discussed are encompassed. There may be supplemental forms for pediatric cases, brain injury, assistive technology, Activities of Daily Living, and others. It is useful to obtain a copy of the life care plan checklist (see Table 1.1) to educate the client and family members as to the purpose of the life care plan and the general components that make up the care plan. It is also recommended that a camera or video recorder be used to record the living situation, medications, supplies, and equipment used for the client. For example, a home may need to be modified and photographs are beneficial for documentation.

In general, it is valuable to consult with the therapeutic team members, if possible. As noted previously, there may be personal injury litigation defense cases or insurance consulting where this is not possible. It is also reasonable to retain the services of a physician or other individuals as appropriate when treatment team members are not available to discuss the case or the caregivers are not specialized. Also, some treating physicians are not experts in the particular disability or are reluctant to provide recommendations, in which case it may be appropriate to arrange for specialty evaluations by other qualified medical professionals.

There is a special note that should be made with regard to medical foundation for cases that have some or many medically based needs. There are people who are not physicians who claim that they need not have any more medical foundation than their own experience. There are others who

Table 1.3 Step-by-Step Procedure for Life Care Planning

1. **Case Intake:** When you talked with the referral source, did you record the basic referral information? Time frames discussed? Financial/billing agreement? Retainer received (if appropriate)? Arrange for information release?
2. **Medical Records:** Did you request a **complete** copy of the medical records? Nurses' notes? Doctors' orders? Ambulance report? Emergency room records? Consultants' reports? Admission and discharge reports? Lab/X-ray/etc.?
3. **Supporting Documentation:** Are there depositions of the client, family, or treatment team that may be useful? Day-in-the-life videotapes? And if vocational issues are to be included in report, school records (including test scores), vocational and employment records, tax returns?
4. **Initial Interview Arrangements:** Is the interview to be held at the client's residence? Have you arranged for all appropriate people to attend the initial interview (spouse, parents, siblings)? Did you allow 3 to 5 hours for the initial interview? (Some consultants or defense experts may not be permitted direct access to the client or treating health care professionals.)
5. **Initial Interview Materials:** Do you have the initial interview form for each topic to be covered? Supplemental form for pediatric cases, CP, traumatic brain injury (TBI), spinal cord injury (SCI) as needed? Do you have a copy of the life care plan checklist? Example plan to show the client? Camera or camcorder to record living situation, medications, supplies, equipment, and other documentation useful for developing a plan?
6. **Consulting with Therapeutic Team Members:** Have you consulted with and solicited treatment recommendations from appropriate therapeutic team members (if appropriate or able to do so)?
7. **Preparing Preliminary Life Care Plan Opinions:** Do you have information that can be used to project future care costs? Frequency of service or treatment? Duration? Base cost? Source of information? Vendors?
8. **Filling in the Holes:** Do you need additional medical or other evaluations to complete the plan? Have you obtained the approval to retain services of additional sources from the referral source? Have you composed a letter outlining the right questions to assure you are soliciting the needed information, as appropriate?
9. **Researching Costs and Sources:** Have you contacted local sources for costs of treatment, medications, supplies, equipment? Or do you have catalogs or flyers? For children, are there services that might be covered, in part, through the school system?
10. **Finalizing the Life Care Plan:** Did you confirm your projections with the client and family (if appropriate)? Treatment team members (if appropriate)? Can the economist project the costs based on the plan if one is used? Do you need to coordinate with a vocational expert?
11. **Last But Not Least:** Have you distributed the plan to all appropriate parties (client, if appropriate, referral source, attorney, economist, if there is one)?

Source: Roger O. Weed and Susan Grisham. Handout at various professional training sessions.

assert they merely are administratively writing down the notes dictated to them by physicians and are not making independent judgments about the efficacy of recommendations. In this author's opinion, a qualified life care planner must be a collaborator, participant, and author of the life care plan. For a detailed review of this issue, see the Appendix at the end of this chapter entitled "The Life Care Planner: Secretary, Know-It-All, or General Contractor? One Person's Perspective" (Weed, 2002a), as well as additional comments made in the forensic chapter later in this book.

After preliminary life care plan needs are assessed, information should include frequency of the service or treatment, duration of the treatment, cost, source of information, and perhaps vendors for the services or products listed.

It is not uncommon for basic evaluations to reveal various holes that may require additional medical or other evaluations to be appropriate. For example, a neuropsychologist may be required in brain injury cases. It is important that the consultant compose a list of questions that will assist the evaluator in addressing questions that are specific to the life care plan (Blackwell et al., 1994a, 1994b; Weed & Field, 2012). For example, neuropsychologists may perform an outstanding job in writing reports and listing the results of tests but may be less than adequate in identifying functional limitations that result from the disability, as well as revealing specific treatment options with costs so that a projection of its estimated value can be determined.

After a life care plan has been completed, it is common for the planner to research the costs of treatment, medications, supplies, and equipment. There are occasions when catalogs will provide the necessary resource, particularly for products that are commonly available through mail order or for remote locations where the services or products are limited. In some states, depending on the jurisdiction (e.g., civil litigation, workers' compensation, long-term disability, etc.), there may be a need to identify collateral sources. A common collateral source is a "free and appropriate education" often offered through the public school system for eligible students with a qualified disability under the federal Individuals with Disabilities Education Act (IDEA). There may also be special rules regarding the costs associated with products. One state, California, for example, proposes linking products and services for workers' compensation insurance cases to Medicare/Medicaid reimbursement schedules.

As the life care plan is approaching finalization, it *may* be appropriate to consult with the client and family to determine that historical information is accurate and that the topics included in the life care plan are suitable and reasonable in accordance with the rules of the jurisdiction. Once the life care plan is complete, it is the responsibility of the life care planner to distribute the life care plan to appropriate resources. The life care planner should be mindful of the rules within the jurisdiction to avoid distribution of a plan to inappropriate sources. In the case of civil litigation, the attorney who retains the consultant's service typically determines the appropriate recipient(s).

One more contemporary task in which some life care planners who are retained by plaintiff's attorneys in civil litigation participate is to help develop day-in-the-life videos in support of settlement or trial exhibits. In recognition of this growing opportunity, a chapter on this topic has been added to this edition.

The Future

Life care planning continues to realize new horizons. Since the life care plan first emerged in the rehabilitation literature in the 1980s, the concept has grown immensely to represent the most effective case management method within the specialty practice, particularly with regard to complex medically challenging cases (Deutsch et al., 1989b; Kitchen et al., 1989; Weed & Sluis, 1990, Blackwell et al., 1997; Weed, 2007). As this book goes to press, many of the topics that were considered the future of life care planning just a few years ago have already become the present (Deutsch, 1994). Life care planning in the areas of reserve setting for insurance companies, managed care organizations, workers' compensation, personal injury, facility discharge planning, and government-funded vaccine injury programs have strongly endorsed the concept. In civil injury litigation, the *Daubert* (1993) and *Kumho* rulings (see the new Chapter 36 on Admissibility as well as Weed & Johnson, 2006) will continue to affect how some professionals develop life care plans by encouraging the practice of using consistent, researched, and critiqued methods of developing opinions (see chapters on forensics and perspectives by defense and plaintiff attorneys for more information).

It was predicted that areas of mental health (especially serious lifelong psychiatric illness such as schizophrenia), geriatrics, mediation, facility-based life care planning, special needs trusts for children, divorce cases, and assisting families with financial and estate planning will increase. However, there is more room for growth in all of these areas. An example was a divorce case where the settlement was based somewhat on the cost of a persistent vegetative-state client living at home; the soon-to-be ex-wife was aware that the child's father planned to place the client in a facility because it was less expensive and therefore would reduce his obligation for child support. The care planner was initially asked to identify a reasonable care plan. Another example is that attorneys who identify themselves as elder care lawyers are now practicing a recognized specialty (see Chapter 25, Life Care Planning and the Elder Law Attorney, as well as the new chapter on Elder Care Management Life Care Planning Principles in this book).

In addition, based on participants in recent training programs, experts from a variety of health care–related occupations (physicians, neuropsychologists, occupational therapists, physical therapists, and speech and language pathologists) will participate individually as life care planners and as members of a team. Furthermore, life care planners are participating in training programs and certification specific to the development of Medicare set-aside plans used primarily in the workers' compensation arena (ICHCC, 2016). Gaining knowledge and expertise in medical coding procedures for determining medical charges for various services included in a life care plan also appears to be an emerging area. Health maintenance organizations will use this methodology to assist with the projection of costs for their catastrophically impaired patient population. Managed care is a current phenomenon that has special application to life care planning. If the goal is to manage care, then using life care planning procedures is a viable option. The design is an excellent method to avoid errors and omissions. Unfortunately, the term *managed care* often really means *managed costs*. If health maintenance organizations truly wish to enhance care outcomes for their patients, then we will observe many case management professionals involved in training programs focused on life care planning. At least one nationwide case management firm (General RE Corporation) has adopted the basic life care planning procedure to work with insurance companies for catastrophic injuries in an attempt to assist them with overall rehabilitation planning and projection of costs. Structured settlement companies use the life care plan to develop proposals for settlements and estate planning. Facility and hospital discharge planners will use the method for more effective patient and family education as well as for assurance of comprehensive care. Another area that appears on the horizon but is slow to catch on is provision for the care of children who have complex health care needs and who are in the foster care system or are adopted (Buckles et al., 2008).

Another exceptionally relevant specialty area has to do with the care of wounded warriors. One source estimates more than 35,000 injured military personnel, with substantial numbers requiring long-term medical care (Leskin et al., 2007). However, it appears that veterans' specific life care planning has been slow to "catch on." Several life care planners have also become a person's case manager and end-of-life and hospice choices training and education may be another emerging need.

With the Affordable Care Act, many life care planners in litigation venues have been challenged to consider the collateral source and financially offset appropriate categories (Field & Weed, 2015). With the changing and undetermined future of health care insurance in the United States, life care planning professionals should be prepared to answer challenging questions regarding cost of future care needs.

Additionally, life care planning research already completed (Sutton et al., 2002, and reprinted in this text), has and will continue to increase in number and sophistication with an eye toward underscoring reliability and validity criteria, as well as enhancing the standards of practice. At the time this book went to press, the most comprehensive role and function study of life care planning was being updated and was in the data collection stage with results expected to be published in the *Journal of Life Care Planning*. For a current list of research projects completed or underway, visit the FLCPR website at http://www.flcpr.org/research.html.

Conclusion

Life care planning has emerged as an effective method for identifying and outlining future care needs and costs. The specialty practice continues to grow and develop new horizons. It is of specific importance that a coordinated effort with standardized approaches be promoted so that the practice as a whole progresses and becomes more useful in an ever-increasing number of venues. As more professionals, including allied health professionals, become involved in this process, the specialty practice will mature and develop more effective outcome measurements. Some universities are developing doctoral programs to endorse or encompass life care planning procedures and methods. A 2003 unpublished study of accredited graduate rehabilitation counselor training programs revealed that two-thirds offer training in life care planning (Isom et al., 2003). Indeed, beginning with its exam administration in October 2017, the Commission on Rehabilitation Counselor Certification has included life care planning as one of its knowledge domain areas under the category of Community Resources and Partnerships for which applicants will be tested (Commission on Rehabilitation Counselor Certification, 2017; see Section 11: The Certification Examination, https://www.crccertification.com/filebin/pdf/CRCCertificationGuide102017.pdf). In civil litigation, both plaintiff and defense attorneys have increasingly turned to rehabilitation professionals to consult on life care planning issues. It is incumbent upon the life care planning professional to assure that services offered are consistent with the standards of the profession and the methodologies that have been endorsed by practitioners. Building on the work of others, rather than reinventing the wheel, will assist in achieving this goal.

Appendix: Life Care Planner: Secretary, Know-It-All, or General Contractor? One Person's Perspective

Some professionals have criticized life care planners for the way in which they conduct the process of accumulating the data required for projecting future care of clients. For consistency in this appendix, the life care plan definition is as follows: A Life Care Plan is a dynamic document based upon published standards of practice, comprehensive assessment, data analysis, and research, which provides an organized concise plan for current and future needs, with associated costs, for individuals who have experienced catastrophic injury or have chronic health care needs. Source: Combined definition of the University of Florida and Intelicus annual life care planning conference and the American Academy of Nurse Life Care Planners (now known as the International Academy of Life Care Planners) presented at the Forensic Section meeting, NARPPS annual conference, Colorado Springs and agreed upon April 3, 1998 and cited in Weed, 1999; available at www.internationalacademyoflifecareplanners.com. Consistent with the definition of life care planning, standards of practice, ethics, and procedures have been developed over the years to assure effective elucidation of client needs and published in peer-reviewed journals (McCollom & Weed, 2002; Weed 2002b). How one accomplishes this task has been refined to the extent that certified life care planners (CLCP) have been trained to review medical records, depositions, and all other available information, conduct interviews where possible, contact treating professionals when accessible, or otherwise obtain a foundation for the entries in the plan (such as hiring consultants to provide recommendations within their scope of practice and expertise or relying upon research). It is recognized that many life care planners are consultants in litigation, assist insurance companies to set reserves in workers' compensation or health insurance cases, or work in other settings where they may not have access (either direct or indirect) to the treating professionals involved in the client's care, and alternative approaches have been developed to assure accurate assessment of client needs. For purposes of this appendix, the focus will be on litigation-related plans.

Two Apparent Self-Serving Views

Varying criticism has been launched by some with regard to procedures used by life care planners for obtaining recommendations. This appendix is intended to address two well-known criticisms. The first is the rehabilitation consultant who stated in testimony that the life care planner's role is essentially one of a "secretary." The professional meets with the doctor or others and simply writes down their opinions, researches costs, and then publishes a report with the entries. The person presenting this assertion portrays the life care planner as merely a conduit for information. (It should be noted that the individual making this assertion is not a CLCP but was criticizing a life care plan—not this author's, by the way. Reportedly, at least one CLCP has also presented this opinion.)

The second argument is by the professional who has "been there, done that" and based on his/her experience expresses that they do not need to consult anyone about projected needs. These individuals contend that a review of the records and perhaps an interview is all that is necessary to develop a comprehensive and accurate care plan for an individual with a catastrophic injury. Within this argument, several depositions reviewed reveal that these individuals believe their nursing degree uniquely qualifies him/her, or the CRC credential or PhD degree is adequate for him/her to complete a life care plan. Conferring with physicians or treating professionals (if available) is deemed unnecessary because, at least implicitly, "they *know it all*" or, alternatively, *ipse dixit* (loosely interpreted as "I said it so it must be true"). Also, the representation that one group of health care professionals is superior or more "uniquely qualified" to develop life care plans (assuming they have the credentials to seek certification) smacks of prejudice which sets up a foundation for conflict and strife (not unlike diversity bias). In fact, rehabilitation practice is built upon the foundation of teamwork to maximize outcomes.

A Critical Review of Educational Requirements

After reviewing various cases in litigation, workers' compensation, and other disability related treatment venues, there seems to be a rather clear picture of what is acceptable with regard to developing an expert opinion that is "valid." The "secretary" view can be easily dismissed since it is incumbent upon the qualified life care planner to:

- Know and understand medical terminology, basic anatomy, physiology, and the functional meaning of a diagnosis.
- Know what questions need to be asked of providers in order to get appropriate information regarding future needs.

- Know how to work within the medical system and access the needed information.
- Know which specialties and specialists should be included in care plans.
- Know how to conduct relevant research about medical conditions and costs.
- Be able to critically analyze and synthesize information from a variety of sources.
- Know when information received is not credible or the professionals providing the information are not adequate.
- Know when consultation by a specialist or specialists is indicated.
- Know how to identify qualified specialists and coordinate the consultation.
- Offer opinions within his/her professional expertise as a part of the overall plan.
- Other… (Updated resources: For more information on role and function studies for life care planners, see https://www.ichcc.org/certified-life-care-planner-clcp.html and https://connect.rehabpro.org/lcp/home).

Like a secretary, life care planners use the telephone and often the computer to author letters and reports. However, "secretarial" work is a minor part of the process. Indeed, master's degree students in rehabilitation counseling at Georgia State University must develop a comprehensive rehabilitation plan with a "real" client as part of their program. Even with specialized instruction, it is rare that a student can offer a professional quality product until they have gained real-world experience. In fact, students have available to them example projects as well as a textbook with step-by-step procedures yet most need "hand-holding" throughout the semester in order to complete the project. The point to the above is to underscore that the job of accumulating future care data for a person with a catastrophic injury or complex health problems cannot be delegated to someone who does not have specialized knowledge and training.

With regard to the "know-it-all" professional, in this author's experience the individual commonly is not a CLCP. Two recent depositions reviewed were by nurses who admitted in deposition to never having any training in life care planning but, nonetheless, offered opinions for the plaintiff without the benefit of physician or therapist participation or endorsement of recommendations. The nurses claimed that their nursing education and experience was sufficient as the foundation for opinions. Three others, two of whom held doctorates and one master's level CRC, opined that his/her experience was adequate to express opinions, with one stating that his/her rehabilitation counselor training was essentially equivalent to the CLCP. In an attempt to survey these assertions more closely, the accreditation agencies for nursing (National League for Nursing Accreditation Commission, www.nlnac.org) and rehabilitation counselor training (Council on Rehabilitation Education, www.core-rehab.org) were contacted. First, according to a survey of accredited rehabilitation counselor master's degree programs, 54 percent offer some training specifically in life care planning and all are required to offer training in case management skills (Countiss & Deutsch, 2002). Other required curricula include medical aspects of disability (including anatomy and physiology), psychosocial aspects of disability, functional capabilities of people with disabilities, assistive technology, counseling and helping skills, vocational and career development, assessment, job development, research, and foundations of rehabilitation counseling. Nursing programs require education in anatomy and physiology, theoretical and clinical applications, nursing theory, nursing process, critical thinking, health assessment, technical skills, health promotion/disease prevention, concepts of illness and disease management, nursing research, nursing role, leadership/management, health systems and policy, and trends and issues in community based, acute care, and long-term care settings. A baccalaureate nursing curriculum typically includes courses on medical surgical nursing, obstetrics/women's health, pediatrics, gerontology, psychiatry, and community health. There are other liberal arts courses with an emphasis in the sciences included, which is similar to the baccalaureate programs the rehabilitation counselors must accomplish before embarking on a graduate degree. The bottom line: Although both education curricula include a foundation for working within the medical system, both have strengths and weaknesses. Nurses generally have more in-depth medical education than most rehabilitation counselors and may have some case management training but certainly are not trained as physicians or therapists. Rehabilitation counselors generally have more education and a broader perspective with medical case management, rehabilitation planning, and vocational planning training but likewise are not trained as physicians or therapists either. In addition, rehabilitation counselors with doctorates have more than twice the higher education than nurses and have additional specific rehabilitation training with a heavy emphasis on research. In this author's view, all life care planners must have an adequate foundation for expressing medical or other expert opinions and just knowing what degree they possess is not enough. Indeed, many physicians will defer to other physicians when opinions are outside of his/her specialty area, so the nonphysician offering recommendations that are, in effect, prescriptions seems well outside his/her scope of practice. It should be recognized that this appendix does not address the training of the many other health care–related professionals who author life care plans, but many of the points are relevant to them as well.

In summary, the life care planner who portrays him- or herself as able to identify the details of lifetime needs of clients who require a physiatrist, neurologist, orthopedist, gastroenterologist, ophthalmologist, internist, neuropsychologist, occupational therapist, physical therapist, speech/language therapist, as well as nursing care, diagnostic studies, vocational needs, case management, and so on, is not credible. Even if the life care planner is a physician, he or she is not qualified to address many of the areas listed above (for example, case management and vocational needs) (Deutsch, 2002). The punch line of this discussion is that in order for the life care planner, retained as an expert witness, to offer a well-founded plan, he/she must rely upon many sources (medical records, literature, as well as solicited medical recommendations) for his/her opinions.

A Third View—By Analogy

An alternative comparison might be encapsulated in the analogy of the general contractor. In this author's experience, general contractors come from a wide variety of educational and experiential backgrounds. The range of training includes engineering and architecture, as well as the person with a GED who worked up through the ranks by building homes. However, it is a rare person who knows every specialty. Think about some of the tasks that go into building a quality home: Architectural design, drafting, site preparation, foundation planning and forming, framing, electrical, plumbing, sheet rock, roofing, security systems, cabinetry, tile, bricklaying, wallpapering, flooring, painting, heating/air conditioning, landscaping, irrigation planning and installation, deck building, budgeting, and facilitating the permit process. The experienced general contractor probably has a "good idea" of what is involved in building a home but rarely knows all of the details especially when it involves troubleshooting, anticipating problem areas, or knowing the latest in building techniques and materials in all subspecialty areas. Likely, the general contractor will rely upon the opinions of experts within the various specialties to attend to those details which he/she is not qualified to do. In commercial construction where a bid is required, the general contractor will usually solicit bids from subcontractors and then compile the estimates into a proposal. The competent contractor knows who to hire or how to locate an expert in order to end up with a product that can be sold. However, we all know stories of failures in this industry where housing is not according to code or is substandard—not unlike some life care plans.

Conclusion

The qualified life care planner is neither a secretary nor all-knowing. He or she is more akin to a general contractor who has much to offer the health care industry in many settings. Like a general contractor, most states allow life care planners to hang out their shingle without anything other than a business license. However, most competent general contractors who build homes will join a local chapter of the Home Builders Association and agree to a set of ethics which adds a measure of comfort for the customer. Likewise, the foundation of a qualified life care planner is embedded in the individual professional's education, related experience, and personal history. Receiving training specific to life care planning, joining an organization specific to life care planning, and achieving CLCP certification where standards and ethics are specific to the profession further supports that foundation and is the beginning to enhancing a valued profession. Since qualified life care planners are more alike than different and must rely on other professionals within his/her respective areas of expertise in developing a solid plan, it is incumbent upon all life care planning professionals to work together in this coordinated effort and to build consensus for uniformly accepted standards, ethics, and purposes.

Note: Thanks to Debbie Berens, for her editorial and consulting assistance. Thanks to Patricia McCollom, Linda Shaw, Amy Sutton, Tim Field, and Paul Deutsch for comments on the draft.

References

AAPLCP 2016. About. *Available at* http://aaplcp.org/Default.aspx

Blackwell, T., Kitchen, J., & Thomas, R. 1997. *Life Care Planning for the Spinal Cord Injured.* Athens, GA: E & F Vocational Services.

Blackwell, T., Sluis Powers, A., & Weed, R. 1994a. *Case Management for the Brain Injured (foreword by James S. Brady).* Athens, GA: E & F Vocational Services.

Blackwell, T., Weed, R., & Sluis Powers, A. 1994b. *Case Management for the Spinal Cord Injured.* Athens, GA: E & F Vocational Services.

Buckles, V., Pomeranz, J., & Young, M. E. 2008. The applicability of the life care plan for adopted children with disabilities: What will Medicaid pay? *Journal of Life Care Planning, 75*(3), 107–122.

Commission on Rehabilitation Counselor Certification. 2017. *CRC® Certification Guide.* Schaumburg, IL: Author.

Countiss, R., & Deutsch, P. 2002. The life care planner, the judge and Mr. Daubert. *Journal of Life Care Planning, 1*(1), 35–43.

Daubert v. Merrill Dow Pharmaceuticals. US Sp Ct. 92–102 (1993).

Deutsch, P. 1994. Life care planning: Into the future. *Journal of Private Sector Rehabilitation, 9,* 79–84.

Deutsch, P. 2002. Historical perspective of life care planning. *Topics in Spinal Cord Injury Rehabilitation, 7*(4), 1–4.

Deutsch, P., & Raffa, F. 1981. *Damages in Tort Action* (Vols. *8 & 9*). New York: Matthew Bender.

Deutsch, P., & Sawyer, H. 1985. *Guide to Rehabilitation.* New York: Ahab Press.

Deutsch, P., Weed, R., Kitchen, J., & Sluis, A. 1989a. *Life Care Plans for the Head Injured: A Step by Step Guide.* Athens, GA: Elliott & Fitzpatrick.

Deutsch, P., Weed, R., Kitchen, J., & Sluis, A. 1989b. *Life Care Plans for the Spinal Cord Injured: A Step by Step Guide.* Athens, GA: Elliott & Fitzpatrick.

Field, T., & Weed R. 2015. Will the Affordable Care Act and tort reform render the collateral source doctrine obsolete in resolving the issue of damages in cases involving personal injury and life care planning? *RehabPro, 23*(3), 133–148.

FIG Services 2017. Available at https://www.figeducation.com/

International Academy of Life Care Planners. 2015. *Standards of practice for life care planners*, 3rd ed. Available at http://www.rehabpro.org/sections/ialcp/life-care-planning/standards.
ICHCC 2016. *Certification programs*. Available at http://ichcc.org/index.htm.
Isom, R., Marini, I., & Reid, C. 2003. Life care planning: Rehabilitation education curricula and faculty needs. *Journal of Life Care Planning, 2*, 171–174.
Johnson, C. 2015. Life care planning consensus statements. *Journal of Life Care Planning, 13*(4), 34–38.
Kitchen, J., Cody, L., & Deutsch, P. 1989. *Life Care Plans for the Brain Damaged Baby: A Step by Step Guide*. Orlando, FL: Paul M. Deutsch Press.
Leskin, G., Lew, H., Queen, H., Reeves, D., & Bleiberg, J. 2007. Adaptation of life care planning to patients with polytrauma in a VA inpatient setting: Implications for seamless care coordination. *Journal of Rehabilitation Research & Development, 44*, xxiii–xxvi.
McCollom, P., & Weed, R. 2002. Life care planning: Yesterday, and today. *Journal of Life Care Planning, 1*(1), 3–7.
Riddick, S., & Weed, R. 1996. The life care planning process for managing catastrophically impaired patients. In *Case Studies in Nursing Case Management* (pp. 61–91). Gaithersburg, MD: Aspen.
Sutton, A., Deutsch, P., Weed, R., & Berens, D. 2002. Reliability of life care plans: A comparison of original and updated plans. *Journal of Life Care Planning, 1*, 187–194.
Weed, R. 1989. Life care planning questions and answers. *Life Care Facts, 1*, 5–6.
Weed, R. 1994. Life care plans: Expanding the horizons. *Journal of Private Sector Rehabilitation, 9*, 47–50.
Weed, R. 1995a. Life care plans as a managed care tool. *Medical Interface, 8*, 111–118.
Weed, R. 1995b. Objectivity in life care planning. *Inside Life Care Planning, 1*, 1–5.
Weed, R. 1996. Life care planning and earnings capacity analysis for brain injured clients involved in personal injury litigation utilizing the RAPEL method. *Journal of NeuroRehabilitation, 7*, 119–135.
Weed, R. 1997. Comments regarding life care planning for young children with brain injuries. *The Neurolaw Letter, 6*, 112.
Weed, R. 1999. Life care planning: Past present and future. In R. Weed (ed.). *Life Care Planning and Case Management Handbook*. Winter Park FL: CRC Press, pp. 1–13.
Weed, R. 2000. The worth of a child: Earnings capacity and rehabilitation planning for pediatric personal injury litigation cases. *The Rehabilitation Professional, 8*, 29–43.
Weed, R. 2002a. The life care planner: Secretary, know-it-all, or general contractor? One person's perspective. *Journal of Life Care Planning, 1*, 173–177.
Weed, R. 2002b. Life care plan development. *Topics in Spinal Cord Injury, 7*(4), 5–20.
Weed, R. 2007. *Life Care Planning: A Step-by-Step Guide*. Athens, GA: E & F Vocational Services.
Weed, R., & Berens, D. (Eds.) 2010. *Life Care Planning and Case Management Handbook* (3rd ed.) Boca Raton, FL: St. Lucie/CRC Press.
Weed, R., & Field, T. 2012. *The Rehabilitation Consultant's Handbook* (4th ed.). Athens, GA: E & F Vocational Services.
Weed, R., & Johnson, C. 2006. *Life Care Planning in Light of Daubert and Kumho*. Athens, GA: E & F Vocational Services.
Weed, R., & Riddick, S. 1992. Life care plans as a case management tool. *The Individual Case Manager Journal, 3*, 26–35.
Weed, R., & Sluis, A. 1990. *Life Care Plans for the Amputee: A Step by Step Guide*. Boca Raton, FL: CRC Press.

Chapter 2

The Role of the Physiatrist in Life Care Planning

Richard Paul Bonfiglio

Contents

Introduction 21
Life Care Planning Implications 22
Choosing the Right Physiatrist 23
Role of the Physiatrist 24
Common Medical Scenarios for Which Life Care Plans Are Developed 24
Spinal Cord Injury 24
Brain Injury 25
Chronic Pain 25
Amputation 26
Prognosis 26
Example Case 26
Summary and Conclusions 27
References 27

Introduction

Physicians specializing in the field of physical medicine and rehabilitation (also known as physiatrists and rehabilitation physicians) through their education and training are uniquely qualified to evaluate and treat persons who have suffered catastrophic illness or injuries for whom life care plans are most often developed. According to the American Board of Physical Medicine and Rehabilitation, physicians in the field focus on restoring "functions in persons whose abilities have been limited by disease, trauma, congenital disorders, or pain to achieve their maximum functional abilities" (Braddom, 1996). The goals of rehabilitation and life care planning include enhancing functional capabilities, reducing suffering, preventing secondary complications, increasing independence with Activities of Daily Living, improving cognitive and linguistic capabilities, and enhancing psychological adjustment to impairments (Weed & Owens, 2018). Physiatrists understand the unique physiologies of persons with spinal cord and brain injuries that can cause severe impairments and potential secondary medical conditions and complications (Fletcher et al., 1992; DeLisa et al., 1993; Sinaki et al., 1993; Downey et al., 1994). The team approach that is essential to life care planning development and implementation is also key to rehabilitation physicians' approaches to patient care.

Life Care Planning Implications

Nonphysician life care planners generally depend on physician input to develop medically appropriate plans. All of the elements of a life care plan must be medically necessary and appropriate (Bonfiglio, 2010). Treating physicians including primary care physicians, orthopedic or neurosurgeons, neurologists, and other medical specialists can provide this medical foundation. However, treating physicians may not understand or value the life care planning process and may not have the time or inclination to provide needed medical recommendations. Therefore, when a life care plan is being developed for a medicolegal case, the referring attorney may hire an expert medical witness to provide the medical foundation. For reasons already delineated, a physician in the field of physical medicine and rehabilitation may be best suited to provide this medical foundation.

The individual preferences, unique needs, desires, and aspirations of the person for whom a life care plan is developed should be taken into account during the planning process. An appropriate life care plan must also consider the long-term consequences of medical conditions and impairments and the impact of the aging process. Physiatrists routinely direct rehabilitation teams that address the acute and chronic rehabilitation needs of individuals with a variety of disabling conditions including brain injuries, spinal cord injuries, amputations, strokes, organ system failures, and chronic pain issues. Individuals with functional limitations often require additional assistance with daily activities later in life. The need for supportive services can vary from a few hours per day of attendant care to 24 hours per day of nursing care.

The plan recommendations should also reflect technological advancements. Ambulation and even stair climbing for persons with paraplegia is now possible with the provision of computerized and powered bionic external support systems like ReWalk. Marked improvements with prostheses include computerized control of key components like the knee joint for above the knee amputees; these sophisticated joints allow amputees to ambulate with a variable cadence and enhanced stability and safety. Lower limb orthoses utilizing functional electrical stimulation allow persons with hemiplegia following strokes to ambulate with more normal gait patterns with reduced energy demands. There have also been significant improvements in wheelchairs, environmental control systems, and augmentative communication devices. Thus, ongoing development of assistive and medical technology should be reflected in life care plans. Forward-looking life care plans that provide the most up-to-date equipment can greatly improve function and quality of life.

Life care plan components should also reflect current clinical practice including changes in health care delivery that are not always to the benefit of patients. Shorter hospital stays and increased use of outpatient settings for surgery and comprehensive rehabilitation should be reflected in life care plans. For example, standard care for persons' status post spinal cord injury often included annual hospitalizations for neurogenic bladder evaluation and management and review of rehabilitation efforts. Such routine admissions no longer occur. The quicker discharge of persons with complex care needs often greatly increases their daily care needs at home or in extended care facilities.

Thus, physicians specializing in physical medicine and rehabilitation can facilitate the development of life care plans with solid medical foundations that address the person's individual medical condition, premorbid medical issues, patient and family preferences, and desired functional outcomes. A physiatrist can help project future care needs based on the impact of the aging process, likely secondary medical complications, future care needs, and prognoses.

There are physiatrists who independently develop life care plans. The insight of a rehabilitation physician developed through training and experience may improve the quality of the plan. However, in this author's experience, nonphysician life care planners often develop more detailed plans with greater specificity and more accurate associated cost figures.

Choosing the Right Physiatrist

Although rehabilitation physicians are uniquely qualified to provide accurate and sound medical foundations for life care plans, the experience and expertise of individual physiatrists can vary widely. Matching the right physician with a particular case can significantly affect the process. Review of a physiatrists' *curriculum vitae* and available online information can serve as an initial assessment.

The following list can help with the selection of a physiatrist for a specific case, especially for an individual's status of post-catastrophic illness or injury:

1. Completion of medical school and residency from recognized leading programs
2. Board certification in physical medicine and rehabilitation and subspecialty in applicable area
3. Training and experience in applicable area of subspecialization like traumatic brain injury or spinal cord injury
4. Previous publications and national or international presentations, especially on related topics
5. Academic appointment
6. Research experience
7. Recognized expertise by rehabilitation peers
8. Testimony experience
9. Comfort with litigation process
10. Reputation for objective and comprehensive assessments, compassionate and effective treatment, and ethical practices

In this author's opinion, physicians who maintain a clinical practice in addition to medicolegal work are usually more credible than those who exclusively provide medicolegal opinions.

Initial contact with the physiatrist can be done by the life care planner or referring attorney. Determining the physician's accessibility, availability, and ability to articulate the key issues in establishing the extent of future care needs and prognosis is essential. Requesting a sample report is appropriate for judging the physiatrist's documentation thoroughness and suitability. Reviewing the physician's past testimony, especially regarding comparable cases, may also be helpful in identifying the physician's opinions regarding key areas.

Role of the Physiatrist

A thorough review of medical records, deposition testimony, opposing expert reports, and other documents and a comprehensive patient evaluation are essential components of a physiatric case analysis that can provide the basis for the determination of lifelong daily, medical, and rehabilitative care needs to be delineated in a life care plan and the individual's prognosis. The expert physiatrist should understand that a financial settlement can allow the affected individual to receive the ongoing care that is needed over a lifetime by someone with a catastrophic injury or illness.

For cases that go to trial, the expert physiatrist must provide testimony to educate the jury about the full extent of the individual's lifetime daily, medical, and rehabilitative care needs (Cooper & Vernon, 1996; Council on Ethical and Judicial Affairs, 1997; Culver, 1990; Romano, 1996). The physiatrist must also explain all of the physiologic changes, medical conditions, and impairments caused by the index injury or illness including its physical, cognitive, and psychological implications. The additional energy requirements and time for performing tasks with a disability often take a toll, and there may also be an impact on family dynamics. Both the physical and psychological stress of caring for a family member with significant needs can negatively impact family members.

Common Medical Scenarios for Which Life Care Plans Are Developed

Spinal Cord Injury

Paraplegia and tetraplegia are delineated based on the lowest intact neurological level and the completeness of the spinal cord injury. For those persons with complete or nearly complete injuries, especially cervical-level injuries, virtually every organ system is affected. Loss of autonomic nervous system control below the level of injury can cause marked hypotension during the initial period of spinal shock. Postural hypotension can be especially problematic during the acute hospitalization and rehabilitation process, but may become a chronic issue. Over time, some persons following spinal cord injury, especially with injuries above the T6 level, develop autonomic dysreflexia or hyperreflexia. Sensory stimulation below the level of injury as commonly triggered by bladder overdistention, excessive and prolonged skin pressure, and constipation can trigger dysreflexia causing dramatic hypertension, facial flushing, sweating, and headache. Untreated, this condition can cause life-threatening hypertension and cardiac arrhythmias.

Designing a life care plan for a person who has suffered a spinal cord injury also necessitates neurogenic bladder management. Needed diagnostic testing includes laboratory testing including blood urea nitrogen (BUN), creatinine, creatinine clearance, electrolytes, urinalysis, and urine culture. Bladder and renal ultrasound and cystoscopy are also frequently needed (Blackwell et al., 2001).

Additional alterations in physiology after a spinal cord injury may cause spasticity, constipation, and impaired sweating and thermal regulation. Additional possible secondary complications include contractures, osteoporosis, heterotopic ossification, pressure ulcers, urinary tract stones, cancer, reduced respiratory reserve, coronary artery disease, hyperlipidemia, gallstones, and a perforated abdominal viscus. Designing a life care plan that addresses the altered physiology, functional limitations, and potential secondary complications necessitates the medical input of a physician with experience taking care of persons with similar issues.

Brain Injury

The extent of a brain injury can range from a transient concussion to a persistent vegetative state. Determining the nature and extent of the brain injury guides the development of an appropriate life care plan (Ripley & Weed, 2010; Rosenthal et al., 1990). The recommendations must be specific to the individual's needs and can be influenced by many factors including the family support system, available community resources, and architectural considerations.

Distinguishing between a person being in a persistent vegetative state and a minimally conscious state can be difficult, but may be very important from a medicolegal context. A person in a persistent vegetative state is completely detached from the environment and unable to appreciate pleasure, pain, and suffering. In contrast, an individual in a minimally conscious state has some awareness of the environment and limited ability to make thoughts, desires, and preferences known. The level of alertness on a given day for such a person can be impacted by acute medical conditions, the effects of medications, and fatigue. The life care plan for a person in a status of post-catastrophic brain injury generally requires lifelong ongoing daily, medical, and rehabilitative care.

Brain injuries with children, especially birth-related hypoxic ischemic injuries, can necessitate extensive, lifelong daily, medical, and rehabilitative care. The life care planning process is further complicated for these children by the impact of the brain injury on developmental and growth processes, new learning, and socialization. Designing a lifelong plan to meet the needs of these children is bolstered by a physiatrist who has experience taking care of children and adults with childhood onset impairments and functional limitations.

A person with a mild to moderate traumatic brain injury may experience significant disruption of daily activities and may be unable to normally function at home, school, or work. Neuropsychological testing may be helpful in determining the nature and extent of ongoing impairments and strengths. Ongoing assistance with daily activities, medications, therapies, physician visits, and psychological counseling may be needed. A physiatrist can help to translate functional limitations to life care planning components.

Chronic Pain

Determining the etiology and pathophysiology of chronic pain for an individual can be difficult (see also the chapter on pain elsewhere in this text). Defining the extent of pain and its functional implications can be problematic. Pain cannot be measured, compared, or even validated. The impact of pain physically, cognitively, and psychologically is quite variable. Pain for all of us becomes a common occurrence with the aging process. However, some individuals are profoundly affected due to the nature and extent of the pain, previous pain experiences, and the presence of contributing medical conditions like depression, an anxiety disorder, post-traumatic stress disorder, sleep disorder, peripheral neuropathy, and traumatic brain injury. Thus, the input of a physiatrist can be helpful in designing a life care plan for a person with a chronic pain problem due to the training and experience of a physiatrist in looking at the functional implications of disease and disability.

Amputation

A physiatrist can determine the most appropriate prosthesis for a person with an amputation. Recognizing the extent of impairments and medical conditions caused by the amputation is within the experience of many physiatrists. The impact of an amputation goes beyond the loss of the affected limb since amputations also cause increased energy demands with mobility and daily activities, chronic phantom and stump pain, psychological issues due to loss of body image, and increased mechanical stress on adjacent joints.

Prognosis

Rehabilitation physicians can provide testimony regarding the prognosis for individuals' status of post-catastrophic injuries and illnesses. In addition to projecting future care needs, physiatrists can also opine about the impact of the care on quality of life issues, functional improvements, vocational potential, work life expectancy, and life expectancy.

Rehabilitation goals typically include improving an individual's quality of life when possible. The impact of a life care plan on improving a person's functional capabilities is another common rehabilitation goal and often includes improving mobility, increasing independence with Activities of Daily Living, and enhancing communication.

For those persons with vocational potential, rehabilitation physicians can opine about the individual's medical capabilities and limitations to do work with or without restrictions (Weed & Owens, 2018). Determining if reasonable accommodations can facilitate return to work can also be evaluated. The aging process and injury-induced impairments may reduce the person's work life expectancy.

To accurately project lifetime daily, medical, and rehabilitative care in a life care plan, an accurate prediction of life expectancy is needed. However, there is no medical literature for individuals with catastrophic injuries or illnesses that projects life expectancy *based on the level of care* that is typically outlined in a life care plan. Additional medical literature limitations include the use of statistical projections without medical foundation and lack of current health care provision or technological advances. Additionally, population studies do not address the unique medical and personal situations of individual persons. Therefore, in this author's opinion, an opinion provided by an experienced physiatrist can better predict life expectancy. However, such determinations require a thorough review of available medical records to recognize underlying medical conditions, catastrophic injury or illness impact, and potential complications. A comprehensive evaluation including a physical examination provides further basis for life expectancy projections. Thus, a physiatrist can utilize a comprehensive medical assessment to provide a life expectancy determination for individuals' status of post-catastrophic injuries or illnesses.

Example Case

Each entry in the life care plan requires certain data. Each recommendation must include the medical specialty, start date, stop date, frequency of service, and duration. A base or procedure cost is added that will allow an economist to estimate the total value of the services or procedures. Table 2.1 provides an example of a few entries associated with the care of a 73-year-old woman with C5–C6 tetraplegia, which is within the domain of the physiatrist.

Table 2.1 Example Physiatrist Recommendation for a Life Care Plan

Recommendation[a]	*Dates*	*Frequency*	*Expected Cost*
Outpatient spinal cord injury reevaluation to include MD, RN, OT, PT, RT, dietary	2017 to life expectancy	1 time per year	$850–1,200 each
IVP or renal ultrasound, CBC, UA, and others as needed	2017 to life expectancy	1 time per year	Included in yearly evaluation
Physiatrist	2017 to life expectancy	4 times per year	$156 per visit
Urologist	2017 to life expectancy	2 times per year	$120–150 per visit
KUB	2017 to life expectancy	1 time per year	$65.77 each
Orthopedist	2017 to life expectancy	1 time per year	$100–125 per visit

[a] Partial plan only. Illustration of physician-related minimum data needed.

Summary and Conclusions

An expert physiatrist can provide the framework for establishing the extent of damages in medicolegal cases. Expert opinions can be provided regarding:

1. Nature and extent of a person's impairment and residual functional capabilities
2. Future natural history of a person's disease and disabilities including impact of aging process
3. Potential future medical complications
4. Medical basis of vocational potential and functional limitations
5. Delineation of a person's functional limitations including physical, cognitive, emotional, and fatigue components
6. Medical basis for need for medications, medical and adaptive equipment, supplies, home modifications, transportation needs, therapies, daily care, and other care services
7. Life expectancy

These opinions provide the medical basis for the life care plan and associated prognostic information.

References

Blackwell, T., Krause, J., Winkler, T., & Stiens, S. 2001. *Spinal Cord Injury Desk Reference: Guidelines for Life Care Planning and Case Management.* New York, NY: Demos.

Bonfiglio, R. P. 2010. The role of the physiatrist. In R. Weed (Ed.), *Life Care Planning and Case Management Handbook* 3rd ed. Boca Raton, FL: CRC Press, pp. 17–25.

Braddom, R. L. 1996. *Physical Medicine & Rehabilitation.* Philadelphia, PA: W.B. Saunders.

Cooper, J., & Vernon, S. 1996. *Disability and the Law.* London: Jessica Kingsley Publishers.

Council on Ethical and Judicial Affairs. 1997. *American Medical Association: Code of Medical Ethics.* Chicago, IL: American Medical Association.

Culver, C. M. 1990. *Ethics at the Bedside.* Hanover, NH: University Press of New England.

DeLisa, J. A. et al. 1993. *Rehabilitation Medicine Principles and Practice,* 2nd ed. Philadelphia, PA: J.B. Lippincott.

Downey, J. A. et al. 1994. *The Physiologic Basis of Rehabilitation Medicine*, 2nd ed. Stoneham, MA: Butterworth-Heinemann.

Fletcher, C. F. et al. 1992. *Rehabilitation Medicine: Contemporary Clinical Perspectives*, Philadelphia, PA: Lea & Febiger.

Ripley, D., & Weed, R. 2010. Life care planning for acquired brain injury. In R. Weed (Ed.), *Life Care Planning and Case Management Handbook* (3rd ed.). Boca Raton, FL: CRC Press, pp. 349–381.

Romano, J. L. 1996. *Legal Rights of the Catastrophically Ill and Injured*, Norristown, PA: Rosenstein & Romano.

Rosenthal, M. et al. 1990. *Rehabilitation of the Adult and Child with Traumatic Brain Injury*, 2nd ed. Philadelphia, PA: F.A. Davis.

Sinaki, M. et al. 1993. *Basic Clinical Rehabilitation Medicine*, 2nd ed. St. Louis, MO: Mosby.

Weed, R., & Owens, T. 2018. *Life Care Planning: A Step-by-Step Guide*, Athens, GA: E & F Vocational Services.

Chapter 3

The Role of the Rehabilitation Nurse in Life Care Planning

Amy M. Sutton

Contents

Introduction 29
The Nursing Process and Care Plan Development 30
The Contributions of the Rehabilitation Nurse in Life Care Planning 32
Research Issues for the Rehabilitation Nurse in Life Care Planning 34
Other Roles of the Rehabilitation Nurse in Life Care Planning 35
Related Certifications and Organizations 37
Conclusion 38
References 39

Introduction

Qualified life care planners present with a variety of backgrounds and experiences, as well as various medical, psychological, and nursing licensures and certifications. These professionals include, but are not limited to, nurses, physiatrists, psychologists, rehabilitation counselors, and physical, occupational, and speech therapists. The life care planning training programs and certification processes were designed to train specialists to practice in the field of life care planning utilizing standards of practice to guide the life care planning process and set expectations with regard to methodology and an ethical approach (Weed, 2010). This chapter will outline the advantages and expected roles of involving the rehabilitation nurse in consultation and/or the development of a life care plan. Many areas covered in this chapter will be discussed in further detail in subsequent chapters of this text as some of these issues apply to life care planners from all rehabilitation backgrounds.

The Nursing Process and Care Plan Development

Nurses from every field of health care delivery share the basic tenets of the nursing process (Wilkerson, 2012). They are the foundation for patient-focused care, and they include:

Assessment: This step involves physical assessment of the patient, as well as psychological, sociological, economic, life-style, past and current health history, and past and present stressors and coping strategies assessment.

Nursing Diagnoses: While nurses do not make medical diagnoses, they are expected to diagnose the patient's response to a current or potential diagnosis. These diagnoses are broken down into physical and psychological components including diagnoses such as "at risk for falls," "impaired skin integrity," "adjustment difficulties," "nutritional deficits," "ineffective airway clearance," "anxiety," etc.

Outcomes/Planning: Following assessment and after the resulting nursing diagnoses are determined, the nurse sets goals, both short- and long-term, to address and ultimately resolve/treat the identified diagnoses. The result of this process is called the nursing care plan which is typically documented so that other nurses and health care professionals can participate in the process and provide continuity of care. The nursing care plan and the process of its development are quite similar to the development and implementation of a life care plan.

Implementation: Once the care plan is developed, the plan is implemented to facilitate progress toward the identified goals.

Evaluation: The care plan is continually evaluated, updated, and modified as it is a living document, just as a life care plan is a dynamic document which is adjusted based on the needs of the patient.

The nursing care plan, resulting from Outcomes/Planning, is an organized list of nursing diagnoses and goals for each patient based on their unique medical and psychosocial diagnoses and the patient's own expectations and family expectations, and considers both the potential of the patient and their limitations. These documents are a means of communication between nurses and other health care professionals and are educational tools for patients, families, and caregivers. Nursing care plans are often utilized as a guide for duration of hospitalization, home health services, and reimbursement by third-party payers. The nursing care plans are updated based on changes in the patient's condition on an as-needed basis. Similarly, the life care plan identifies the needs and goals of a patient, incorporates the services and equipment to achieve these goals, and is updated and reevaluated based on the changing needs of the patient over time (Weed, 2010).

There are many areas of nursing specialties including pediatrics, obstetrics, surgery, home health, critical care, and so on. One such specialty is rehabilitation nursing. The rehabilitation nurse is a nurse who has procured special expertise in maximizing and maintaining function and quality of life in patients with various disabilities or chronic illnesses that have limited their ability to function in their daily lives (Association of Rehabilitation Nurses, 2014a). A rehabilitation nurse may decide to obtain special certification by the Association of Rehabilitation Nurses (ARN) which results in the credentials CRRN (Certified Rehabilitation Registered Nurse). Certainly not all competent rehabilitation nurses are CRRNs. It is an optional credential available and is becoming more popular as rehabilitation facilities encourage their nursing staff to obtain this certification. Information about that certification is included at the end of this chapter. Rehabilitation nurses are employed in inpatient and outpatient rehabilitation hospitals, as well as in the home health industry. They are frequently utilized by insurance companies or practice as case managers to manage long-term care and associated costs for patients with lifelong disabilities or illnesses. The roles of the rehabilitation nurse include:

1. *Educator*: The rehabilitation nurse educates the patient, family, and caregivers about the particular disability or disease. They train the self-care skills necessary to achieve independence, if possible, such as managing bowel and bladder function, monitoring skin condition, safety with mobility, etc. When a family member or caregiver is involved, they will train those individuals to provide the necessary care, assistance, and reminders. The rehabilitation nurse will also educate the family regarding expectations for the future with regard to possible future equipment needs, potential complications, and changing needs over time due to the aging process. For example, a spinal cord injured child may require the caregiver to catheterize him or her while they are too young but with maturity, the child may learn to catheterize him- or herself, thereby achieving increased independence. In contrast, an individual with a disability who has been independent most of their lives may require more assistance than the average person in the later years of their life.
2. *Caregiver*: The rehabilitation nurse, depending on their type of employment, may provide ongoing assessment of the patient, develop and implement a nursing care plan, and evaluate and adjust the care plan as needed (see earlier description of the nursing process).
3. *Collaborator*: The rehabilitation nurse, as with all nurses, works with other specialists to develop goals and facilitate communication between all health care professionals involved with the patient's care. Often, the rehabilitation nurse is working with a large interdisciplinary team given the nature of long-term disability and chronic illness. For example, individuals with spinal cord injury or traumatic brain injury may have multiple therapists (physical, occupational, speech, psychological, vocational, etc.), as well as multiple physicians (physiatrist, neurologist, orthopedist, neurosurgeon, psychiatrist, etc.). The collaboration process in these complex cases often requires team conferences or frequent interdisciplinary communication. The rehabilitation nurse or nurse case manager may be the point of convergence where all of these disciplines are informed about the current plan of care.
4. *Client Advocate*: Depending on the role, the rehabilitation nurse advocates for services and equipment that will promote quality of life for the patient and assist the patient to achieve their maximum potential. When appropriate, they may refer the patient to resources in the community who can provide additional services at low to no cost to the patient or family. They may assist patients and families in the process of finding and obtaining appropriate and affordable equipment, supplies, and services, and negotiating with insurance case managers to fund items and/or services (Association of Rehabilitation Nurses, 2014b).
5. *Consultant*: In addition to the roles outlined by the Association of Rehabilitation Nurses, a new role is emerging. The nurse may be retained by insurance companies, lawyers, families,

trusts, and others to provide expertise and suggestions for management of long-term care needs, referrals to appropriate medical specialists for further evaluation, and other similar functions. In some situations, these consultants are not disclosed but rather work behind the scenes to achieve a variety of goals.

The Contributions of the Rehabilitation Nurse in Life Care Planning

As previously noted, the nursing care plan is a tool very similar to the life care plan. Rehabilitation nurses are trained to develop and implement the nursing care plan early in their nursing career. There are significant advantages to involving a rehabilitation nurse with life care planning training in the development or evaluation of life care plans.

As part of nursing education, student nurses are educated in almost all areas of nursing specialties. There are classes in pediatrics, obstetrics, gerontology, intensive care, cardiology, psychiatry, home health, rehabilitation, and much more. Students are required to participate in practicum experiences in these various areas to learn hands-on care for patients with a variety of conditions. Following graduation, nurses often work in a variety of settings before landing in a specialty area. Clinical nurses in a hospital are frequently required to work in many different areas of the hospital depending on staffing needs and therefore must be proficient in most specialties. This background is especially beneficial in the field of life care planning due to the range of illnesses and disabilities presented to the life care planner during his or her career.

Rehabilitation nurse life care planners who have worked as clinical nurses have hands-on experience with procedures, supplies, equipment, post-operative needs, and so on. For example, a rehabilitation nurse who has catheterized or taught a patient to self-catheterize has firsthand knowledge about the types of supplies necessary, the difference between catheter types, and the amount of training time required to learn this skill. They have utilized a hydraulic lift, a pulse oximeter, a ventilator, and so on. They have dressed, bathed, and transferred a completely dependent patient, and they understand the burden on caregivers and the equipment that can ease that burden. This practical knowledge is an advantage when developing a life care plan and when educating an attorney or a jury about why something should or should not be included in a future care plan.

The life care planning process is collaborative and interdisciplinary, requiring the input from multiple specialists via direct contact or through medical records (International Academy of Life Care Planners, 2015). Nurses in every field have extensive experience collaborating with a variety of specialists. Rehabilitation nurses have regular contact with speech, physical, and occupational therapists, neuropsychologists, physicians, respiratory therapists, and so on, and have at least some training in most of these areas. The development of a life care plan is an extension of this collaborative process. However, the broad experiences and training of the rehabilitation nurse does not allow for him or her to make recommendations in every category of the life care plan. The nurse life care planner must stay within his or her scope of practice. It is essential for the nurse to establish a foundation for recommendations outside of his or her scope. For example, medications, frequency and type of physician visits, surgeries/hospitalizations, and diagnostic testing require input from a medical doctor. If the nurse life care planner has additional expertise in other areas, such as being a physical therapist or psychologist, they may

Table 3.1 Desirable Traits for Rehabilitation Nurse Life Care Planners

1. Know inpatient medical-surgical or acute rehabilitation services
2. Have emergency medical experience
3. Possess verbal and analytical reasoning skills
4. Have the ability to communicate with a variety of cultural, educational, and experiential backgrounds
5. Possess problem-solving, negotiation, and conflict resolution skills
6. Are computer literate for research and communication
7. Have knowledge of professional resources and access to resources
8. Have the ability to critically analyze literature
9. Understand the scope and limitations of medical and allied health fields
10. Have pharmacology knowledge
11. Know normal laboratory values
12. Know drug actions/interactions
13. Know pathophysiology of different disabilities
14. Have basic abnormal psychology knowledge
15. Know the effects of trauma on coping and psychological functioning
16. Deal effectively with stress
17. Pay attention to details
18. Are well organized
19. Document the work in the file
20. Maintain meticulous files
21. See the big picture
22. Have self-confidence
23. Are objective and professional
24. Stay within area of expertise

Source: Riddick-Grisham, S. 2010, reprinted from the 3rd edition of the *Life Care Planning and Case Management Handbook*, p. 34.

include independent recommendations in those areas as well (International Academy of Life Care Planners, 2015).

In many life care plans, the most important and most expensive category of the plan is home/facility care (Sutton et al., 2002). This area of the life care plan is within the scope of a rehabilitation nurse as long as they rely upon the medical experts' or treating physicians' assessment of the patients' abilities and limitations. When needed, the recommendations may include a companion, a nursing assistant (or home health aide), a nurse, a case manager, a nursing home, a group home, an assisted living facility, or some combination of any of these services. Following hospital discharge, the amount and level of care needed is typically determined by a home health or rehabilitation nurse during an initial evaluation based on the medical skills necessary and the level of independence demonstrated by the patient. During the development of a life care plan, the rehabilitation nurse life care planner discusses these issues with the physicians, therapists, and neuropsychologist (depending on the specialists involved) to determine the patients' abilities and limitations. They can then utilize their background and training to determine the appropriate amount and level of care indicated.

Overall, the rehabilitation nurse in the role of a life care planner is expected to have the background, education, and experience to fulfill the aforementioned expectations. The care planner is often in situations that are complex, stressful, and require critical thinking skills and a great deal of patience. See Table 3.1 for additional desirable traits for the rehabilitation nurse life care planner.

Research Issues for the Rehabilitation Nurse in Life Care Planning

The issue of research in the field of life care planning is applicable to all life care planners, not just the nurse life care planner. Some nurse life care planners are conducting or participating in current life care planning research. Others may not be actively involved in research but all life care planners should be familiar with the past and present research in the field and have an understanding of the research process. This is especially relevant in light of *Daubert* challenges, which highlight the importance of scientific and quantifiable life care planning research that can demonstrate the reliability and validity of the life care planning process in the area of forensics (Countiss & Deutsch, 2002). With the availability of the Internet, information has become accessible to everyone, including attorneys who would like to discredit a particular life care planner. The research process assists the nurse life care planner in staying current with standards of practice, expected outcomes of various disabilities and treatment modalities, conducting a market survey of costs, determining replacement frequency of equipment, researching applicable case law depending on where the case is tried, and finding organizations which provide services for various disabilities, cultures, and belief systems.

Although nurse life care planners commonly rely on the input from physicians regarding expected outcomes for medical diagnoses and specific medical interventions, there is a large body of research available to help guide the life care planner with future care recommendations specific to each type of disability. For example, the Consortium for Spinal Cord Medicine (sponsored by the Paralyzed Veterans of America) has published guidelines and expected outcomes for spinal cord injured patients based on the level of injury (Paralyzed Veterans, 2002). Medical journals have published outcome studies for various pain management procedures like spinal cord stimulators and baclofen/morphine pumps. These types of publications can be helpful in guiding discussions with experts or treating physicians regarding the needs of a patient following an intervention or specific injury and facilitate an educated discussion with experts, defending a plan during deposition, or testifying at trial.

The nurse life care planner should be familiar with the services offered by the state in which the patient resides. Some services are federally funded such as IDEA (Individuals with Disabilities Education Act 1990, as amended), which funds a variety of services for school-aged children with disabilities. Some services are privately funded such as Easter Seals, assisting adults and children with disabilities. Each state has programs in place such as Early Intervention for children under age three. Life care planners often practice in multiple states and should research the resources available, as well as the bases for those resources. For example, in California, the Regional Center and California Children's Services are available to assist with therapy needs, parenting needs, medical and equipment needs, respite care, and case management for children (State of California Department of Developmental Services, 2007). The Regional Center also provides group home services for adults with a qualifying diagnosis and who were disabled prior to age 18. The funding for the Regional Center is protected by the Lanternman Act that was passed in 1977 (Department of Developmental Services, 2018). Researching these types of details specific to each source and each state goes a long way in providing the foundation for including these sources in a life care plan.

Researching the costs for the life care plan is a fundamental step in the process of creating a useful tool for future planning, as well as determining the overall cost of funding the life care plan. The Standards of Practice provide the basic tenets of cost research and the life care planner chooses their preferred method of determining the reasonable market rate (International Academy of Life Care Planners, 2015). The Consensus and Majority Statements Derived from Life Care Planning Summits (Johnson, 2015) also provides guidance for the cost research process. Some life care planners prefer using databases, while others conduct a market survey by calling local providers for current prices. Service providers often have different rates depending on the payer source. They may have a specific rate negotiated with each insurance company, which is likely different than the rate they bill the insurance company, and a private pay or cash rate for patients who are uninsured or choose to pay out-of-pocket. Determining which rate to use will likely depend on the payer source that is expected to fund the life care plan. If the life care plan is for litigation and third-party payers are excluded from being named as a collateral source, the cash rate may be appropriate. However, it is not appropriate for the life care planner to negotiate a discounted rate that would not be readily available to the general public (International Academy of Life Care Planners, 2015). Each state has case laws that may help guide the life care planner in selecting the applicable rates. Most states have case law specific to past medical care cost recovery and some have case law that either states or implies future care costs and recovery rates (Field et al., 2015). Each state also has case laws that set forth whether collateral sources may be utilized and may depend upon whether the case is medical malpractice or personal injury. The life care planner should research and be familiar with the applicable case law.

Some nurse life care planners require assistance in collecting data in all of these areas and employ a research assistant. These individuals are not expected to provide expert testimony but, instead, may assist the life care planner with researching costs of services and equipment, identifying resources available in the community, conducting a literature search for applicable publications on a particular topic, and researching availability of specialty services and checking ratings of specialty facilities. The research assistant should be familiar with the nursing/medical field and be educated by the life care planner regarding market survey or cost research methodology. Research assistants must be directed and supervised by the life care plan author to assure they follow the process and methodology of the author and to assure that the patient's confidentiality is protected. When researching the cost of community or medical services, the focus should be on conducting a market survey rather than determining a list of specific locations where the patient must receive future care. The survey is utilized to establish the typical prices in a particular area, not a list of precise referrals. For pricing home/facility care options, private *and* agency hire options should be considered (Johnson, 2015). If a facility or group home is included, the appropriateness for each specific patient should be considered especially with regard to diagnosis, average age of the residents, and the level of care provided.

Other Roles of the Rehabilitation Nurse in Life Care Planning

Rehabilitation nurse life care planners provide a variety of services during the life care planning process, as well as consulting on cases without actually developing a life care plan. See Table 3.2 for a description of some of these services and responsibilities. See Table 3.3 for questions for the attorney. See Table 3.4 for questions the nurse life care planner should ask the vocational expert (if one is involved).

Table 3.2 Additional Roles and Expectations of the Rehabilitation Nurse Life Care Planner

1. Educate attorneys in selecting a life care planner and how to evaluate the background and credentials of the opposing life care planner (see Table 3.3).
2. Assist attorneys in selecting other specialties that could or should be retained or consulted (i.e., vocational expert, physiatrist, urologist, plastic surgeon, neuropsychologist, etc.) depending on the specifics of the case.
3. Assist attorneys in preparing deposition questions for patients, family members, experts, and treating physicians.
4. Review pre- and post-incident medical records to determine services that are unrelated or preexisting, then confirm with appropriate medical experts.
5. Rely upon nursing diagnoses and life care planning standards of practice to assist other retained experts or treating physicians in identifying future care needs:
   a. Collaborate with experts and/or treating providers on expected outcomes of treatment that may affect long-term prognoses (i.e., eventual increase or reduction in medications, increase or decrease in attendant care needs, increase or reduction in palliative care needs, etc.).
   b. Cover all categories of the life care plan with each expert and/or treating provider to promote a thorough future care plan (i.e., an orthopedic expert may recommend follow-up visits and a future surgery only but if asked about future diagnostic testing, post-operative home health, or post-operative physical therapy, he or she may realize that the recommendations exceed just surgery and follow-up visits).
   c. Educate experts and/or treating providers in the legal standards for including services in the life care plan (greater than 50% probability).
   d. Communicate recommendations of all experts and/or treating providers with other involved experts/treating providers to avoid overlap or contradictions in recommendations.
   e. Develop one's own or utilize published lists of questions to guide discussions with other retained experts to maintain consistency in methodology. The types of questions will depend on the area of expertise: vocational expert, psychological or neuropsychological expert, physicians (specific to specialty), therapists (specific to specialty), and the economist (source-example of questions for the vocational expert).
6. Evaluate one's own or the opposing life care plan as a whole, not in parts, to determine whether the plan is reasonable and feasible (i.e., number of hours per day in therapy, caregiver services overlapping with school or day treatment programs, including intensive interventions without reasonable expectation of benefitting from those services).
7. Educate attorneys and other experts regarding the standards of practice in life care planning. The standards of practice can protect one life care planner while highlighting the methodological flaws in another one (Fick & Preston, 2015).

Source: Reprinted in accordance with copyright requirements for members from the *Journal of Life Care Planning*, Vol 13, #3, p. 19. The Life Care Planning Section of the International Association of Rehabilitation Professionals. Publisher: International Association of Rehabilitation Professionals, 1000 Westgate Drive, #252, St. Paul, MN 55114, 888-IARP (888-427-7722), webpage: http://www.rehabpro.org.

Table 3.3 Questions for the Attorney: Life Care Planner Qualifications and Expertise

1. Does the life care planner have specific training in this specialized profession and the type of disability involved?
2. Is the person board certified? (CLCP, CNLCP, or CPLCP)
3. Does the life care planner belong to the International Academy of Life Care Planners (IALCP), the International Association of Rehabilitation Professionals (IARP), the American Association of Nurse Life Care Planners (AANLCP), or the American Association of Physician Life Care Planners (AAPLCP)?
4. Does the life care planner subscribe to the *Journal of Life Care Planning* and/or other relevant journals (i.e., *Rehabilitation Nursing*)?
5. Do they have publications related to life care planning in their library (i.e., *Guide to Rehabilitation* by Deutsch & Sawyer [out of print], *Life Care Planning and Case Management Handbook* (edited by Weed & Berens), *Pediatric Life Care Planning and Case Management* (edited by Grisham & Deming), other relevant publications?
6. Does the life care planner offer vocational and life care planning expertise? If so, do they have the background, training, and credentials to provide both services?
7. Does the life care planner have the medical foundation for necessary recommendations or do they collaborate with medical professionals who *can* provide the foundation?
8. Does the life care planner project *future* needs in addition to current needs (i.e., needs that may increase or decrease over time)?
9. Is the life care planner familiar with and do they subscribe to the published Standards of Practice for life care planning, including methodology, omission, or removal of costs for preexisting conditions, ethical guidelines, etc.?

Source: Adapted from Sutton, A. M. & Weed, R. W. 2004. *Life Care Planning Issues for the Attorney.* The ATLA Docket, Winter, 10–22.

Related Certifications and Organizations

There are a number of organizations that offer credentials for life care planning, rehabilitation nursing, legal nurse consulting, case management, and related certifications. This is a list of many of the credentials that are related to nursing and life care planning:

- CRRN: Certified Rehabilitation Registered Nurse, offered by the Association of Rehabilitation Nurses (ARN); www.rehabnurse.org
- CLCP: Certified Life Care Planner, offered by the International Commission on Health Care Certification (ICHCC); www.ichcc.org
- CNLCP: Certified Nurse Life Care Planner, offered by the American Association of Nurse Life Care Planners (AANLCP); www.aanlcp.org
- CPLCP: Certified Physician Life Care Planner; www.aaplcp.org
- LNC: Legal Nurse Consultant, offered by the American Association of Legal Nurse Consultants (AALNC); www.aalnc.org
- CCM: Certified Case Manager, offered by the Commission for Case Manager Certification (CCMC); www.ccmcertification.org
- CMCN: Certified Managed Care Nurse, offered by the American Board of Managed Care Nursing (ABMCN); www.abmcn.org
- CMC: Care Manager, Certified, offered by the National Academy of Certified Care Managers (NACCM); www.naccm.net
- COHN: Certified Occupational Health Nurse, offered by the American Board for Occupational Health Nurses (ABOHN); www.abohn.org

Table 3.4 Questions the Nurse Life Care Planner Should Ask the Vocational Expert

First determine if vocational aspects have been considered or are already underway (e.g., already initiated by insurance company or attorney).

- What vocational interview information has been obtained from the client (e.g., work skills, leisure activities, education, work, functional abilities based on O*Net, Department of Labor and/or physician)?
- Have you obtained copies of relevant medical records?
- Have you obtained work related information (such as tax returns, job evaluations, school and test records, training history, and treating or consulting MD comments)?
- Does the client need testing before determining vocational potential (e.g., vocational evaluation, psychological, neuropsychological or physical capacities testing)? Also, is the evaluation a "quality" and "valid" appraisal which can stand the scrutiny of talented reviewers/opposing experts?
- If there is work potential, is there a need for justifying a plan by performing a Labor Market Survey, aka Labor Market Research? If LMS, what method is used (e.g., direct contact with employers vs. statistics, computer program and/or publications)?
- What is the client's expected income including benefits? (If personal injury litigation, then pre- vs. post-injury capacity.)
- If there is an apparent market for the client's labor, is there a need for a job analysis? (And if an analysis was completed, was it compliant with the Americans with Disabilities Act guidelines?)
- What are the estimated costs of the vocational plan? For example:
  1. Counseling, career guidance? When does it start/stop, frequency, and cost, (e.g., 30 hrs. over 6 months at $65/hr)?
  2. Job placement, job coaching, or supported employment costs?
  3. Tuition or training, books, supplies? Include dates for expected costs (e.g., technical training 2 years, @ $400/yr. for 1997–1999.)
  4. Rehabilitation or assistive technology, accommodations, or aids, costs for work, education and/or training (e.g., computer, printer, work station, tools, tape recorder, attendant care, transportation—include costs and replacement schedules)?
- What effect, if any, does the injury have on work life expectancy (e.g., delayed entry into workforce, less than full-time, earlier retirement, expected increased turnover, or time off for medical follow-up or treatment)?

Source: © Roger O. Weed, PhD (1997, rev, 2002, 2016), with permission.

Conclusion

The rehabilitation nurse can offer a variety of services in the ongoing treatment, future care planning, and long-term maintenance of patients with catastrophic injuries and chronic health concerns. The combined rehabilitation and nursing expertise with the life care planning training allows nurse life care planners to apply their broad nursing training and experience to future care plan development. The nurse life care planner has extensive clinical experience in collaborating across multiple disciplines to achieve patients' goals and maximum potential. The nursing care plan process is both similar and complementary to the process of developing life care plans and designed to predict needs and prevent complications. When the rehabilitation nurse incorporates the nursing process with standards of practice in life care planning and has the attributes, skill set, and qualifications described in Tables 3.1–3.3, he or she can be an excellent choice for providing life care planning services in forensics or the private sector.

References

Association of Rehabilitation Nurses 2014a. *Standards and Scope of Rehabilitation Nursing Practice*, 6th Edition. Rehabilitation Nursing Foundation of the Association of Rehabilitation Nurses, Chicago, IL.

Association of Rehabilitation Nurses 2014b. *ARN Position Statement—Role of the Nurse in the Rehabilitation Team*. Chicago, IL, http://www.rehabnurse.org/uploads/files/PS-Role.pdf.

Countiss, R. N., & Deutsch, P. M. 2002, The life care planner, the judge, and Mr. Daubert. *Journal of Life Care Planning, 1*, 35–43.

Department of Developmental Services 2018. *Lanternman Developmental Disabilities Services Act and Related Laws*. Sacramento CA, 1–346. https://www.dds.ca.gov/statutes/docs/LantermanAct_2018.pdf.

Fick, N., & Preston, K. 2015. An attorney perspective on standards of practice: a weapon or a shield? *Journal of Life Care Planning, 13*(3), 17–20.

Field, T. F., Choppa, A. J., & Johnson, C. B. 2015. *The Affordable Care Act, Collateral Sources, and Tort Reform: Implications for the Life Care Planner*. Athens, GA: Elliot & Fitzpatrick.

Individuals with Disabilities Education Act. 1990. (Public Law No. 94-142).

International Academy of Life Care Planners 2015. *Standards of Practice for Life Care Planners*, 3rd Edition. Glenview, IL: IARP.

Johnson, C. B. 2015. Consensus and majority statements derived from life care planning summits held in 2000, 2002, 2004, 2006, 2008, 2010, 2012, & 2015. *Journal of Life Care Planning, 13*(4), 35–38.

Paralyzed Veterans of America 2002. *Expected Outcomes: What you should know—A guide for people with spinal cord injury. Consortium for Spinal Cord Injury Medicine*- Clinical Practice Guidelines.

Riddick-Grisham, S. 2010. The Role of the Nurse Case Manager in Life Care Planning, in *Life Care Planning and Case Management Handbook*, Weed, R. O., & Berens, D. E. Eds. Boca Raton, FL: CRC Press.

State of California Department of Developmental Services; last updated 2007. http://www.dds.ca.gov.

Sutton, A. M., Deutsch, P. M., Weed, R. O., & Berens, D. E. 2002. Reliability of life care plans: A comparison of original and updated plans. *Journal of Life Care Planning, 1*(3), 187–194.

Sutton, A. M., & Weed, R. W. 2004. *Life Care Planning Issues for the Attorney*. The ATLA Docket, Winter, Little Rock, Arkansas, 10–22.

Weed, R. 2010, Life Care Planning: Past, Present, and Future, in *Life Care Planning and Case Management Handbook*, 3rd Edition. Weed, R. O., & Berens, D. E. Eds. , Boca Raton, FL: CRC Press.

Wilkerson, J. M. 2012. *Nursing Process and Critical Thinking*, 5th Edition, Prentice Hall, Upper Saddle River, NJ.

References

Association of Rehabilitation Nurses. [illegible] *Professional and Advanced Rehabilitation Nursing Practice*, 6th Edition. Rehabilitation Nursing Foundation of the Association of Rehabilitation Nurses, [illegible], IL.

Association of Rehabilitation Nurses. [illegible] *Role of the Nurse in the Rehabilitation* [illegible] Role.pdf

Centers for [illegible] 2009 [illegible] life care planning [illegible]

[illegible]

Chapter 4

The Role of the Vocational Rehabilitation Counselor in Life Care Planning

Debra E. Berens and Roger O. Weed

Contents

Introduction....41
Vocational Rehabilitation Counselor as Team Member....42
Vocational Assessment/Evaluation....44
Neuropsychological Evaluations in Return-to-Work Assessment....49
Pediatric: Neuropsychological Evaluations....51
Adult: Neuropsychological Evaluations....52
Wage Loss and Earnings Capacity Analysis....53
Labor Market Survey and Job Analysis....55
Collaborating with the Rehabilitation Nurse....57
Vocational Resources....58
Conclusion....59
References....59

Introduction

The *Dictionary of Occupational Titles* (*DOT*), 4th edition (U.S. DOL, 1991a, p. 52), defines a vocational rehabilitation counselor as one who "counsels handicapped individuals to provide vocational rehabilitation services." Such services generally include interviewing and evaluating clients, conferring with medical and professional personnel and analyzing records to determine type and degree of disability, developing and assisting clients throughout the rehabilitation plan (or program), and aiding clients in outlining and obtaining appropriate medical and social services. The *DOT* further states that vocational rehabilitation counselors may specialize in a type of disability (e.g., spinal cord injury, traumatic brain injury, amputation, burn, visual impairment, hearing impairment, chronic pain, etc.). The role of the vocational rehabilitation counselor in life care planning expands this definition and is specific to persons who are catastrophically impaired or have complex medical needs and limited access to the labor market. This role has become more defined since the early 1980s, when life care planning was first introduced into the literature (Deutsch & Raffa, 1981). In today's climate, vocational rehabilitation counselors serve as instrumental members of the rehabilitation team to coordinate assessments in an effort to measure a person's aptitude, achievement levels, and transferable work skills. These assessments help determine one's potential for future work activity, such as full- or part-time employment, sheltered or supported employment, or, in cases where work activity is not a realistic goal, achieving their highest level of productivity or independent living. The essential premise underlying vocational rehabilitation is that involvement in work or some productive, meaningful activity is the goal of one's rehabilitation program (Marme & Skord, 1993; Weed & Field, 2012). And if return to work or productive activity is appropriate, then the needs and steps to achieve that goal must be included in the life care plan (Weed, 2007).

Vocational rehabilitation counselors who work within the life care planning arena generally are rehabilitation professionals who have a minimum of a master's degree in rehabilitation counseling, hold one or more national certifications in the field of rehabilitation, and have extensive training and experience in the areas of evaluation and assessment, catastrophic case management, transferable work skills, earnings capacity analysis, and job placement (Weed & Field, 2012). Vocational rehabilitation counselors can be credentialed in a number of areas, most notably CRC (Certified Rehabilitation Counselor), CDMS (Certified Disability Management Specialist), CCM (Certified Case Manager), CVE (Certified Vocational Evaluator), and ABVE (American Board of Vocational Experts). Credentials can also be obtained from other organizations that, on the surface, appear to be based more on profit-making than on advancing the role and function of the rehabilitation professional. While some of these credentials may be valuable, the authors strongly encourage those professionals interested in pursuing further credentials to thoroughly research the history of the organization, assure the credential is founded upon published role and function research, and scrutinize the validity of the offer.

Vocational Rehabilitation Counselor as Team Member

Vocational rehabilitation counselors with advanced degrees and appropriate credentials are properly trained, qualified, and fully prepared to complete life care plans. They can be found working in a variety of fields, including workers' compensation, personal injury, health or disability insurance/managed care, federal Office of Workers' Compensation programs, and state vocational rehabilitation agencies. Additionally, many facilities (e.g., specialty centers of excellence such as the Shepherd Center in Atlanta, Georgia) employ rehabilitation counselors to assist in the evaluation and, when appropriate, transition of a client into other services for return-to-work assistance or to achieve productivity.

Vocational rehabilitation counselors must be knowledgeable and stay within the accepted standards and guidelines of the particular jurisdiction for which they are preparing the life care plan. For instance, in the workers' compensation arena, the vocational counselor must work within the established definitions of disability and return-to-work hierarchy (see Weed & Field, 2012). This also includes the "odd lot" doctrine that has been defined by case law as "any work that the client may be able to perform which would be of limited quantity, dependability or quality, and for which there is no reasonably stable market for their labor activities" (*Gil Crease v. J.A.*

Jones Construction Company, 1982; *Clark v. Aqua Air Industries*, 1983). In comparison, vocational rehabilitation counselors within the disability insurance arena, such as long-term disability/short-term disability (LTD/STD), will be expected to provide information on the status of the client's "any/own occupation," as well as the client's vocational potential and the cost of future vocational/educational needs. Similarly, vocational rehabilitation counselors within the personal injury arena will need to determine if the client has vocational potential and to what degree. They will also need to provide information on the cost of the client's expected future vocational/educational needs in an effort to identify vocational damages associated with the injury or disability.

Regardless of the specific jurisdiction, vocational rehabilitation counselors in life care planning must be able to determine first if a client can work and, if so, what work the client can perform. This determination would include providing information on not only the types of vocational activity a client can be expected to perform, but also the cost, frequency, and duration or replacement of any training or assistance (such as job coach, vocational counseling, rehabilitation technology, modified or custom-designed workstation, supported employment, tuition/books, or other specialized education programs) that may be required to reach the goal (Weed & Riddick, 1992). Depending on the type of disability, the vocational rehabilitation counselor will work with a variety of medical and allied health professionals in determining the client's vocational potential and providing information for the life care plan.

Professionals such as physicians and medical specialists, physical therapists, occupational therapists, speech/language pathologists, recreation therapists, nurses, psychologists, neuropsychologists, audiologists, counselors or other mental health professionals, and, in the case of school-age clients, school personnel, all work with the vocational rehabilitation counselor to provide information for the life care plan. Generally, team members whose primary responsibilities are for cognitive and psychosocial remediation interact more with vocational counselors than do other team members, and interactions are more effective when focused on adaptive work behaviors, such as the ability to relate with coworkers and supervisors (Sbordone & Long, 1996). In some cases, the rehabilitation nurse for a client with a catastrophic injury will be the primary author of the life care plan, and the vocational rehabilitation counselor must work in conjunction with the nurse to gather and disseminate vocationally relevant information. It is common for the vocational rehabilitation counselor to rely on the client's primary physician (if available to the expert based on legal protocol), typically a physiatrist, also known as a specialist in physical medicine and rehabilitation (PM&R), in determining a client's functional level and potential to perform vocational activity. In appropriate cases, the vocational counselor may request a functional capacity evaluation (FCE), which may also be known as a physical capacity evaluation or functional capacity assessment, to objectively delineate a client's physical functioning. Although there are arguments about the validity of FCEs, in the authors' opinion, an appropriately trained examiner can provide objective data regarding the client's ability to perform various physical demands (lifting, standing, walking, sitting, pushing/pulling, etc.), which are usually performed in a facility that specializes in occupational health information. The FCE provides a snapshot of a client's functional abilities on one particular day (although evaluation may be conducted over 2 days), and given the outcome of the testing, the client's work capacity from a physical standpoint is determined. Additional factors that the vocational rehabilitation counselor must take into consideration in assessing a client's physical capacities are the client's ability to perform work activity over time (endurance), the client's subjective complaints, test validity/reliability (often associated with the examiner as well as the tests), and secondary gain issues (Matheson et al., 2002). In summary, the FCE is just one of many pieces of information used by the vocational rehabilitation counselor in assessing a client's vocational potential.

It is the responsibility of the vocational rehabilitation counselor to maintain a vocational focus on issues related to the life care plan. Most importantly, the counselor needs to collaborate with the team to establish a medical or psychological foundation to support a client's work potential opinion. A case in which the authors consulted illustrates the need to establish a medical foundation. The case involved a 50-year-old iron-metal construction worker who fell 70 to 90 feet from scaffolding and received multiple orthopedic injuries. The nurse assigned to the case referred the client for a vocational evaluation to determine his work potential. Results from the vocational evaluation coupled with the client's reported high motivation to return to work seemed to suggest that he had the capacity to return to work in some area related to his previous work experience. The vocational rehabilitation counselor (not one of the authors of this chapter) then proceeded to conduct a labor market survey to identify actual jobs in his area. Although on the surface it appeared that the case was progressing appropriately (at least from the case manager's perspective), it was learned through contacts with the client's treating physician that it was his opinion the client was permanently and totally disabled from work. Indeed, the client applied for and was approved for Social Security Disability Insurance (SSDI) benefits, which supported the doctor's opinion that the client was disabled from work activity. Furthermore, the physician indicated that his recommendations with regard to the client's vocational potential had not been solicited by the vocational counselor. In fact, the physician was unaware that a vocational rehabilitation plan had been developed to return the client to work, and he obviously did not support the plan. This is a clear example of the importance of interacting with a client's medical care providers (when able) to establish a foundation to support the vocational plan.

Vocational Assessment/Evaluation

The terms *vocational assessment* and *vocational evaluation* have been used over the years in rehabilitation literature to generally describe the process of gathering data and determining a person's potential for work activity. Botterbusch (1987) defines vocational assessment as "more limited in scope" than vocational evaluation and cites the Vocational Evaluation and Work Adjustment Association (1983) definition of vocational evaluation, which "incorporates medical, psychological, social, vocational, educational, cultural, and economic data" (p. 191). In Siefker (1992), it is noted that the two phrases "do not describe a significantly different process and can be considered synonymous" (p. 1). For purposes of this chapter, the phrases will be used interchangeably to describe the comprehensive evaluation of a client's biographical and social history, education and work history, medical and other pertinent records (employment/personnel records, school records, parents' school records in pediatric cases, etc.), psychological/neuropsychological records, and actual vocational test results in determining vocational potential.

In compiling data for the life care plan, it is within the role of the vocational counselor to recommend and obtain a formal vocational assessment/evaluation, particularly in the case of a client who:

- Is of working age (generally age 16 to 67)
- Has no or an unclear vocational goal
- Has no work history or a series of short, sporadic jobs
- Has not been determined permanently and totally disabled (i.e., is thought to have some vocational potential)

It may be interesting to note that there has been an increase in the Social Security Administration's (SSA) determination of full or normal retirement age. The age at which SSA full retirement benefits may begin is now considered to be 67 years old for people born in or after 1960. For individuals born in 1937 or earlier, the full retirement age is 65 and increases incrementally to age 67 for individuals born between 1937 and 1960. Individuals may still begin taking retirement at age 62; however, their SSA retirement benefits will be reduced by an amount greater than that for individuals retiring at age 62 today (see www.ssa.gov). Obviously, rules apply to normal SSA retirement benefits, which are different from Social Security Disability Insurance (SSDI) benefits and Supplemental Security Income (SSI) benefits that may be received by some clients with a disability.

For clients who are catastrophically injured, it is important for the vocational evaluation to be as specific as possible and to take into account the client's personality traits, interests, aptitudes, and physical capabilities so as to adequately identify appropriate vocational options (Weed & Field, 1994, 2001). In their book *Counseling the Able Disabled*, Deneen and Hessellund (1986) describe some of the most common reasons for vocational testing. Below is a modified version of the list that is felt to be most relevant to life care planning:

1. Provide information about a person's interests, mental and physical abilities, and temperament with respect to work.
2. Support, clarify, and document impressions gained during interviews.
3. Discover job interests and potential vocational objectives.
4. Objectively and accurately describe the client's likes, dislikes, needs, and abilities rather than rely solely on verbal interview information.
5. Observe and evaluate the client's physical stamina, endurance, agility, and ability as related to work performance.
6. Evaluate the degree to which a particular impairment is a physical disability or handicap.

Vocational assessments can vary depending on the particular jurisdiction in which the case is involved. For example, vocational evaluations performed for workers' compensation cases typically do not include personality testing in determining suitable* employment (Weed & Field, 2012). These evaluations generally focus on aptitudes and physical capacities (and sometimes interests) as well as the client's demonstrated work history. It is the authors' opinion that vocational evaluations

* Suitable employment is defined as "Employment or self-employment which is reasonably attainable in light of the individual's age, education, previous occupation, and injury and which offers an opportunity to restore the individual as soon as practical and nearly as possible to [his] average weekly earnings at the time of injury." Some clients have successfully challenged the assumption that because they are able to perform the physical functions and they possess the aptitude to perform an occupation that it constitutes suitable employment. One case demonstrates the issue. A licensed practical nurse was injured on the job. The employer offered her a clerical position which she turned down. Although the clerical job was within her physical limitations, it was not considered suitable employment because "Woods is a nurse, and she never expressed any interest in doing clerical work" (*Workers Compensation Law Bulletin*, 1992, 15 [10A], p. 7).

Maryland similarly defines suitable, gainful employment as: "… employment, excluding self-employment, that restores the disabled covered employee, to the extent possible, to the level of support at the time that the disability occurred" (Workers Comp Law, LE, 9-670, p 212). The law further states that in determining whether employment is suitable, gainful employment, the following shall be considered: (1) the qualifications, interests, incentives, pre-disability earnings, and future earnings capacity of the covered employee; (2) the nature and extent of the disability of the covered employee; and (3) the current and future condition of the labor market. Other states including Oregon, California, and Minnesota, have also adopted guidelines which include personality and interest factors which often are over looked by vocational evaluations (Oregon's code OAR 436-120-005 [6]; California Workers' Compensation Code L.C. 4635 [f]; Minnesota MS 176.102 [13]).

that do not address personality factors or testing should be closely scrutinized as to why such assessment tools are not included. Is it an oversight on the part of the evaluator? Is the evaluator not qualified to administer personality tests? Is the evaluator relying upon government data associated with the job history as published in the *DOT* and the *Transitional Classification of Jobs* (Field & Field, 2004)? Or is there a deliberate attempt not to define personality traits, which may have a positive or negative effect on the client's vocational potential? Even in workers' compensation cases, at least one court ruled on appeal that a client's vocational interests were relevant and necessary (Weed & Field, 2012).

When referring for a vocational evaluation, the vocational rehabilitation counselor must review the evaluator's credentials and specify which areas to assess. (See also the section on referring for neuropsychological testing later in this chapter.) The vocational rehabilitation counselor should be concerned not only with the expertise and experience of the evaluator, but also with the technical or scientific aspects of a particular assessment tool and the way in which the test results will be used (Kapes & Mastie, 1988; Siefker, 1992). In developing a life care plan, the vocational rehabilitation counselor must be able to translate results from the vocational evaluation into requirements for the life care plan (Weed & Field, 1994, 2001; Weed, 2007). Such requirements may include cost for training, transportation, tuition, specialized or adaptive equipment, and maintenance and replacement schedules of needed equipment (Siefker, 1992; Weed, 2007). For example, the authors were involved in identifying the costs associated with completing a master's degree and pursuing a PhD for a triple amputee who was a teacher at the time of his electrical injury. Not only were costs included in the life care plan for education requirements, but also costs of transportation, prosthetic devices, maintenance and replacement, clothing allowance (due to increased wear and tear on garments as a result of prosthetic use), and computer and other assistive technology needed to assist the client in attaining his vocational goal of education administrator. This case example also demonstrates that a client's ability to achieve a vocational goal is closely related to other life care plan issues such as ability to perform Activities of Daily Living (ADLs), accessible housing and transportation, psychological adjustment to disability, home/attendant care, wheelchair or mobility needs, and others. This case also provides an example of the inclusive approach the vocational rehabilitation counselor must use in conducting a comprehensive assessment of the client and interrelating realistic occupational goals with all other aspects of the client's care.

In addition to having a comprehensive evaluation performed, the vocational rehabilitation counselor must be sensitive to how the specific tests are administered. For example, group vs. individual; timed, speeded, or untimed; paper and pencil vs. computer administered vs. work sample; short vs. long form; normed vs. nonnormed; and objective vs. subjective, to name a few (see Table 4.1). In general, group tests are not as specific as individual tests (Anastasi, 1982; Siefker, 1992), and speeded or timed tests are usually biased against catastrophically impaired persons. In clients who are motorically or cognitively impaired, tests that are timed may reveal a lower score than is intellectually indicated given that the score is based on speed more than ability. Additionally, situational or job specific tests that evaluate a person's ability for work activity in an actual work environment typically are more favorable and yield more accurate results than a work sample assessment in which job tasks are simulated. Some authors suggest that a client's vocational potential can be most effectively determined when the workplace is used as the primary site of all rehabilitation activity. They further indicate that no other location can be compared to the workplace for face validity and actual job activities (Sbordone & Long, 1996).

Table 4.1 Selected Issues Related to Vocational Assessment

Speeded, timed, and untimed tests	Speed and timed tests may be biased against physically impaired clients. Untimed tests may not reveal how competitive a client may be.
Individual vs. group tests	Usually, the group test is offered for economic reasons and is more general. Individually administered tests allow for examiner comment regarding effort and behavioral observation.
Short "screening" vs. in-depth testing	Vocational evaluators often use short tests for achievement, intelligence, aptitude, and interest screening. Tests such as the Wide Range Achievement Test and current revision (WRAT), Self-Directed Search, General Aptitude Test Battery (GATB), Slosson Intelligence Test, and others are not as precise as more detailed tests (e.g., Wechsler). Many evaluators are not qualified to administer more precise tests.
Tests vs. on-the-job evaluation	In order of general priority for best assessment: • On the job with an employer • On the job based on general standard by professional evaluator • Work sample • Individually administered test • Group test
Leaving out personality factors	It is common in workers' compensation to leave out interest and personality factors when developing an opinion. Basic information with regard to interests, work values, and personality as it relates to work is recommended.

Much has been written on the various vocational assessment tools given to persons with a disability (see *Vocational Assessment & Evaluation Systems: A Comparison*, 1987; *A Counselor's Guide to Career Assessment Instruments*, 1988; *Vocational Evaluation in the Private Sector*, 1992; and *A Guide to Vocational Assessment*, 2006). The following list is provided to give an overview of some of the more common or well-known tools used in the vocational assessment/evaluation of persons who are catastrophically impaired. The reader is referred to the publications referenced previously for a description of each test and information regarding its usefulness for specific populations of persons with a disability.

Intelligence:

- Wechsler Intelligence Scales (preschool, child, and adult versions; the standard of the industry)
- Stanford–Binet Scales (child and adult)
- Slosson Intelligence Test (brief and very general)
- Raven Progressive Matrices (emphasis on reasoning ability)

Personality:

- Minnesota Multiphasic Personality Inventory (MMPI) (also in Spanish)
- 16 Personality Factors (16 PF)
- Myers–Briggs Type Indicator (MBTI)
- Personality Assessment Inventory (PAI)
- Rorschach Inkblot Test

Interest:

- Strong–Campbell Interest Inventory (SCII)
- Career Assessment Inventory (CAI)
- Self-Directed Search (SDS)
- Kuder Occupational Interest Inventory

Aptitude:

- General Aptitude Test Battery (GATB) (out of print but some still use)
- Apticom (rarely used)
- Armed Services Vocational Aptitude Battery (ASVAB)
- Differential Aptitude Tests (DAT)
- McCarron Dial System
- Crawford Small Parts Dexterity
- Hester Evaluation System
- Purdue Pegboard

Achievement:

- Wide Range Achievement Test (WRAT as revised)
- Woodcock–Johnson Psychoeducational Battery (as revised)
- Peabody Individual Achievement Test
- Basic Occupational Literacy Test (BOLT)

Work Sample:

- VALPAR
- Jewish Employment and Vocational Service (JEVS)

Assessment of Physical Functioning:

- Vineland Social Maturity Scale
- PULSES (*p*hysical condition, *u*pper limb, *l*ower limb, *s*ensory, *e*xcretory, *s*upport factors)
- Barthel Inventory of Self-Care Skills

In conjunction with objective test results, the vocational rehabilitation counselor should consider the client's behavior during the interview and test session. Behavioral observation is an integral part of the vocational assessment process and should always be interpreted with the actual test results and client's history, assuming the test is one that lends itself to such observation (Siefker, 1992). The qualified vocational evaluator is attuned to behavioral issues that may affect test results (e.g., pain behaviors, visual/hearing difficulties, need for medication or rest breaks, fatigue, cultural issues and language barriers, and environmental issues, such as: Is the room too hot or cold? Is it early or late in the day?). Likewise, the client's behavior may reveal areas of concern or discrepancy that may warrant further investigation (e.g., Was the client late for the testing session? What are the nonverbal behaviors? Are the client's appearance and grooming appropriate?). Behavior is a valid indication of how one will respond in certain situations, whether it is in a work environment or social/community setting.

In addition to behavioral observations, information about a client's abilities and skills obtained through educational and work experience may be more valid than test results (Siefker, 1992; Weed & Field, 2012). For this reason, a transferable skills analysis may be an essential component of the vocational evaluation and for determining a client's vocational potential. Simply described, a transferable skills analysis is based upon a profile of the worker traits required of a specific occupation. It is used primarily for clients with a documented work history and takes into consideration one's work experience and residual functional capacities to determine appropriate vocational options. The *DOT* and *Transitional Classification of Jobs* (*COJ*) are necessary to compile a transferable skills analysis, and some experts utilize various computer programs to assist with managing large amounts of data (Truthan, 1997; McCroskey, 2001; Weed & Field, 2001; Gibson, 2003). Also, the Occupational Information Network (O*Net) has been designed to eventually replace the *DOT*; however, the O*Net does not yet offer a way to conduct a transferability analysis that can reliably be used in formulating opinions for Social Security disability determinations and personal injury cases, and the *DOT* continues to be the vocational resource of choice at the present time. See the vocational resources section later in this chapter for a description of these and other relevant vocational publications.

Neuropsychological Evaluations in Return-to-Work Assessment

Neuropsychological evaluations are performed on clients following a brain injury or neurological disease and are essential in identifying the relationships that exist between one's brain and behavior or, more specifically, between one's actions and abilities and higher-level cognitive processes (Gabel et al., 1986; Evans, 2004). It is within the role of the vocational rehabilitation counselor to refer a client for a neuropsychological evaluation in cases where there is documented or suspected brain injury/impairment. According to Gabel et al. (1986), referral to a neuropsychologist is appropriate to assess problems of a more long-standing nature and includes areas such as visual, auditory, or tactile processing difficulties; constructional apraxia (copying designs or free drawing); abstract reasoning or concept formation; receptive or expressive language deficits; attention/concentration deficits; and short- or long-term memory problems. Neuropsychological testing is valuable not only to assess a client's current behavioral and learning problems (i.e., to establish a functional baseline), but also to establish prognoses, monitor and document changes over time, and assist in the planning of the rehabilitation program (Evans, 1999).

Historically, the focus of neuropsychological testing has been on the determination of brain damage and its location. Over the past decade, there is a growing interest within neuropsychology to focus on the client's capacity to function in everyday life. The prediction of work behavior is the second most frequent reason for referral to neuropsychological evaluations. However, such evaluations are somewhat limited by a lack of norms based on specific job types and specific client population, and more work is needed in this area (Sbordone & Long, 1996).

Neuropsychologists and vocational rehabilitation counselors generally share the goal of facilitating the client's transition to an active and productive life. Vocationally speaking, neuropsychological evaluations should assist the vocational counselor in identifying the client's vocational capabilities and behaviors and in planning for a successful entrance into an appropriate work environment or, at minimum, to achieve the highest level of functioning/productivity (Sbordone & Long, 1996). For this reason, neuropsychological evaluations are helpful for both adult and pediatric clients and, as with vocational evaluations, must be as specific as possible.

For purposes of life care planning, results from neuropsychological evaluations must relate specifically to the client's function and ability and must also provide recommendations for future care needs. Problems in thinking and reasoning, information processing speed, attention/concentration, and long- or short-term memory are vocational barriers that need to be accurately assessed (Sbordone & Long, 1996). Additionally, psychosocial and interpersonal relationship skills need to be assessed such that there is an obvious need for strong communication and collaboration between vocational rehabilitation counselors and neuropsychologists in the interest of maximizing return to work and identifying life care planning recommendations.

Neuropsychological testing helps determine how much assistance is needed in the home, on the job, at school, and within the community. When referring for a neuropsychological evaluation, it is prudent for the vocational rehabilitation counselor to know to whom a referral is being made and the credentials of the neuropsychologist. Experience has shown that the most qualified neuropsychologist not only has a PhD in clinical psychology and is board certified as a neuropsychologist, but also has experience in evaluating persons across all levels of severity of brain injury and has demonstrated a commonsense approach to evaluation and test interpretation.

Once a referral is made to a neuropsychologist, it is recommended that the vocational counselor provide specific questions to the neuropsychologist, which, when answered, would provide information needed specifically for the life care plan. The effects of brain trauma can be found in any or all aspects of one's life, including interpersonal, vocational, educational, recreational, and Activities of Daily Living. It is the role of the neuropsychologist to evaluate the long-term or lifelong effects of brain injury on the client's ability to function (Weed, 1994; Evans, 2004). Suggested questions specifically pertinent for the life care planning process are listed in Table 4.2. Rehabilitation counselors should ask neuropsychologists to answer the questions as part of their evaluation for life care planning.

As stated previously, neuropsychological evaluations are useful in both adult and pediatric cases. The interested reader is referred to *Neuropsychological Assessment* (Lezak, 1995) for detailed information on neuropsychological evaluations. According to Lezak (1976), the basic neuropsychological battery contains both individually administered tests and paper-and-pencil tests that are self-administered. The individually administered tests can take up to 3 hours, and the paper-and-pencil tests can take from 3 to 6 hours, depending on the extent of the client's impairment(s). The paper-and-pencil tests typically are not timed; however, the individually administered tests are usually timed. Especially in the case of pediatric clients, neuropsychological evaluations are often given over two sittings in order to avoid fatigue factors. Again, the vocational rehabilitation counselor is cautioned to be sure the neuropsychologist provides a comprehensive evaluation that is sensitive to the client's particular needs and provides information that is relevant for life care planning. Similar to vocational evaluations, neuropsychological evaluations are not done with a single test but instead are a compilation of data based on test results and interpretation and behavioral observations. It is recommended, and good practice, for the vocational counselor to establish a mechanism to meet or speak directly with the neuropsychologist to discuss test results and solicit input for life care planning.

Table 4.2 Neuropsychologist Questions

In addition to the standard evaluation report, add the following as appropriate:

1. Please describe, in layman's terms, the damage to the brain.
2. Please describe the effects of the accident on the client's ability to function.
3. Please provide an opinion on the following topics:
   a. Intelligence level (include pre- vs. post-incident if able)
   b. Personality style with regard to the workplace and home
   c. Stamina level
   d. Functional limitations and assets
   e. Ability for education/training
   f. Vocational implications on style of learning
   g. Level of insight into present functioning
   h. Ability to compensate for deficits
   i. Ability to initiate action
   j. Memory impairments (short-term, long-term, auditory, visual, etc.)
   k. Ability to identify and correct errors
   l. Recommendations for compensation strategies
   m. Need for companion or attendant care
4. What is the proposed treatment plan?
   a. Counseling (individual and family)?
   b. Cognitive therapy?
   c. Reevaluations?
   d. Referral to others (e.g., physicians)?
   e. Other?
5. How much and how long? (Include the cost per session or hour and reevaluations.)

Source: Roger O. Weed, partially adapted by R. Frazier.

For purposes of this chapter, a brief overview of some of the more common evaluation tools for each age group is given. For additional information, refer to Chapter 6, The Role of the Neuropsychologist in Life Care Planning.

Pediatric: Neuropsychological Evaluations

Pediatric cases present many unique challenges for the life care planner (Weed, 2000). One challenge is that there is little, if any, history on which to rely, and practitioners are often hesitant to offer future care recommendations. For this reason, neuropsychological evaluations are particularly helpful with children to qualify and quantify the impact of a child's brain injury on functioning and behavior (Weed, 1996). Although there are many assessment tools to evaluate pediatric clients, the Halstead–Reitan and Luria–Nebraska batteries are the most frequently used in the neuropsychological assessment of children (Gabel et al., 1986).

According to Gabel et al. (1986), perhaps the greatest usefulness of the Halstead–Reitan batteries is the establishment of objective baseline data that can clarify a child's strengths and weaknesses and be helpful in outlining educational strategies and programs to enhance capabilities. In comparison, the Luria–Nebraska Children's Neuropsychological Test Battery can be administered to children ages 8 to 12 years and focuses on functional systems involved in brain–behavior relationships. A third common assessment battery for children is the Kaufman Assessment Battery for Children (K-ABC)

(1983 and revisions), which is individually administered to children ages 2 to 12 years and measures intelligence and achievement. Also, for academic assessment, it is common for the Woodcock–Johnson Tests of Achievement or Cognitive Abilities test to be administered. Last, a useful tool to assess infants who have experienced brain trauma from age 2 months to 30 months is the Bayley Scales of Infant Development (1969 and revisions). The scales are considered to be the best measure of infant development and provide valuable data regarding early mental and motor development and developmental delay. Other scales of infant developmental attainment are the Cattelle Scales of Infant Development and the Vineland Adaptive Behavior Scales (1984 and revisions).

Adult: Neuropsychological Evaluations

Whereas there are numerous neuropsychological assessment tools from which to choose when evaluating children for life care planning, there are significantly more tests for adult assessments. Below is a brief list of some of the more common neuropsychological tools for adults and areas they evaluate. For more information and descriptions regarding the listed tests, refer to Lees-Haley's *Last Minute Guide to Psychological and Neuropsychological Testing* (1993).

- Wechsler Adult Intelligence Scale, 3rd edition (WAIS-III) (intelligence)
- Wisconsin Card Sorting Test (executive or higher-order functions)
- Boston Naming Test (language)
- Rey Auditory Verbal Learning (memory)
- Wechsler Memory Scale–Revised (WMS-III) (memory)
- Stroop Color Test (mental control)
- Serial 7s or Serial 3s (attention)
- Benton Visual Retention Test (visual memory)
- Gates–MacGinitie Reading Tests (reading academic skills)
- Hooper Visual Organization Test (visual perception)
- Woodcock–Johnson (academic and cognitive assessment)
- Haptic Intelligence Test (intelligence); used for clients with visual impairment
- Leiter Intelligence Test (intelligence); used for clients with hearing impairment
- Hisky–Nebraska Aptitude Test (aptitude); used for clients with hearing impairment

In summary, neuropsychological evaluations for clients with brain impairment are usually essential in the field of life care planning to assess both the near- and long-term effects of brain damage on one's functioning and developmental levels. Information obtained through neuropsychological testing can be crucial in developing the appropriate future care planning of a client with a traumatic brain injury. Inasmuch as neuropsychological evaluations are vital to life care planning, test results for young children are very variable. Generally, IQ test results are not considered of substantial value until the child reaches school age. Additionally, it is generally more preferable to rely on schoolchildren's standardized achievement test scores than on actual grades as a true measure of their achievement. In referring a client for neuropsychological testing, the vocational counselor should ensure that the evaluator reviews all available medical and academic records and that the evaluation includes developmental assessments in addition to the standardized test batteries. It is common to include in the life care plan provisions for neuropsychological reevaluations at specific life stages in the client's development or at specific time intervals throughout one's life expectancy in order to assess and monitor the client's functioning abilities. This also applies to the assessment of aging on brain injury or neurological impairment (Weed, 1998).

Wage Loss and Earnings Capacity Analysis

In addition to contributing information relevant to a client's vocational and educational outlook with regard to life care planning, the vocational counselor also may be asked to assess the client's loss of earnings capacity. According to one source, future medical care and loss of earnings capacity are directly related to the education and experience of most vocational counselors. The vocational counselor can offer valuable input in three critical areas: lost capacity to earn an income, loss of opportunity to be employed (loss of access to the labor market), and cost of future medical care (Weed & Field, 1994, 2001; Weed, 2000; Weed, 2002). The first and second areas will be described in this chapter. The third area, establishing the cost of future medical care, is referenced throughout this book and will not be covered specifically in this section. Refer to Table 4.3 for a summary of the relevant factors to consider in establishing a foundation for earnings capacity for both pediatric and adult clients.

With regard to lost earnings capacity, it is first necessary to establish the client's wages at the time of injury. This can be fairly simple for a client who was working at the time of injury in a job that is considered representative of his or her earnings potential. In pediatric cases or for young clients who may have been working but had not yet established a clear vocational identity, the process can be more challenging. The issue of identifying earnings capacity can be divided into four client populations (Weed, 1996; Weed & Field, 2001):

1. Clients injured at birth or in the neonatal period
2. Clients injured before they reach school age (and have no academic grades or standardized test scores)
3. Clients injured before establishing a career identity
4. Clients injured after having an established work history representative of their vocational potential

Clearly, there are differences in the way the vocational rehabilitation counselor considers information based on the age of the client at the time of injury.

Table 4.3 Establishing a Foundation for Earnings Capacity

Client Age	*Factors to Consider*
0–1 year of age	Review of family history (i.e., parents, older siblings, aunts/uncles, and grandparents) to include education and work records as a way to establish family patterns.
2–5 years of age	Same as previous, plus daycare records/observations, church/school observations, preschool records, pediatrician records, family videotapes, baby books if well maintained by parents, developmental records, neuropsychological evaluations, or other relevant records.
6–18 years of age	Review of family history, school records (including standardized test scores, academic grades, honors, disciplinary records, and extracurricular activities), pediatrician records, neuropsychological testing, vocational testing, or other relevant records.
18+ years of age	Review of employment/personnel records, school records, tax records, military records, community/civic involvement, neuropsychological testing, vocational testing, or other relevant information.

The listed factors can be a good predictor or give a reasonable approximation of what the client could have done prior to the injury (preinjury earnings or capacity). Obviously, the more history and documentation there is, the better and more accurate a foundation can be established with regard to earnings capacity.

The vocational rehabilitation counselor must determine the level of the client's functioning both before the injury (preinjury) and after the injury (post-injury) as it relates to the types of jobs the client could hold now or in the future. In general, wage loss refers to the amount of money (wages) lost by the client as a result of the injury and is based on his or her actual past work history. Earnings capacity, on the other hand, refers to the loss of future earnings related to what would be considered a reasonable estimation of the client's work potential (capacity) (Weed & Field, 1994, 2001; Weed, 2000).

In some cases, it may be possible to determine that a client is permanently and totally disabled from the workforce based on work history and type of injury. Such an example includes the case of a 58-year-old career truck driver who was involved in a motor vehicle accident and has tetraplegia resulting from a spinal cord injury at the C4 level. Although it may be arguable that the client could possibly be employed as a dispatcher or in some other related job in the trucking industry, it is not likely given his advanced age and the fact that he would require extensive job modification and rehabilitation technology, as well as an employer willing to make the modifications and employ the client. In such cases, the actual earnings of the client would be the basis on which to project wage loss (Blackwell et al., 1992).

In other cases, it may be more appropriate to identify a client's pre- vs. post-injury earnings capacity in categories of jobs rather than specific job titles (Weed, 2000). For example, in cases where the client is a child or young adult with no clearly established work history, the vocational expert can identify categories of jobs that are representative of types of workers (such as skilled or unskilled) and can then identify certain jobs that fall under those categories (such as lawyer or laborer) to determine the client's earnings capacity. Another alternative is to estimate the client's pre- vs. post-injury educational capacity. For example, if the client is expected to have the educational capacity of a high school graduate, average earnings representative of a high school graduate can be used. Similarly, average earnings of individuals with a 4-year degree, master's degree, and doctorate or professional-level degree can be determined based on education level.

To determine wage loss or loss of earnings capacity, the vocational expert essentially evaluates the client's pre- and post-injury employability (defined in Weed & Field, 1994, 2001, as possessing the skills, abilities, and traits necessary to perform a job) and compares the two. Once the counselor has evaluated the difference in pre- and post-injury earnings capacity, the economist then calculates the total amount of lost earnings capacity over the client's work life expectancy (Siefker, 1992). See the chapter on the role of the economist in life care planning for further information.

There are many factors and approaches to consider when determining future wage loss and earnings capacity analysis. Of the many approaches, the RAPEL method considers most of the factors (Weed & Field, 1994, 2001). The RAPEL method, developed by Weed (1994), offers a comprehensive approach to determining earnings capacity analysis, particularly in forensic cases. (See the chapter on forensic issues for additional information.) The approach incorporates a *rehabilitation* plan (or life care plan for the client who is more catastrophically impaired), information with regard to the client's *access* to the labor market (employability), information with regard to the client's *placeability* (defined as the likelihood that the client could successfully be placed in a job), *earnings* capacity, and *labor* force participation or work life expectancy. Generally, if there is a reduction in the client's life expectancy as a result of his or her injury, there also will be a reduction in the work life expectancy. The experienced vocational counselor would express this reduction in a percentage of loss or number of years lost in the labor market. For more information on the topic of wage loss/earnings capacity analysis, refer to Dillman (1987) and the chapter on the role of the economist in this text. The reader is also referred to Neulicht and Berens (2005) for a description of PEEDS-RAPEL, a method for determining wage loss/earnings capacity for pediatric clients.

Labor Market Survey and Job Analysis

The labor market survey is designed to reveal current information about a specific job market (Weed & Field, 1994, 2001). Questions include:

1. Do jobs of a particular nature exist in the economy?
2. If these jobs exist, are they available locally?
3. If available locally, are these jobs open to my client?
4. What do these jobs pay (including benefits)?

Part of the opinion regarding an adult client's earnings capacity may be related to the current labor market. Obviously, a pediatric case would not include a specific employer-by-employer analysis; however, data that are collected by the government with regard to the future outlook of an occupation may be included. See Table 4.4 for common topics included in the labor market survey (summarized from Weed & Field, 1994, 2001).

It should be noted that the way in which the consultant asks questions could skew the results toward a desired direction. In an example case, a plaintiff's expert revealed that a client who had chronic pain was unemployable and used as partial justification the results of a labor market survey. She reported that the survey revealed that the client would not be an acceptable candidate for sedentary jobs that were directly in line with her work history. Following the deposition, the defense expert contacted the same employers and distinctly different information was provided. It was hypothesized that the consultant asked questions in a way that solicited support for her conclusions. Ethics, on the part of some consultants, can also be suspect. In another case, contact with the employers listed in another consultant's notes revealed that no employer on the list recalled being contacted with regard to a labor market survey, therefore raising the question of whether a survey had actually been performed.

Once a prospective job is located, it may be appropriate to conduct a job analysis (Weed et al., 1991; Blackwell et al., 1992; Weed & Field, 1994, 2001). The analysis is designed to determine if job traits match the worker's traits and therefore represent a reasonable probability of employment. There are specific guidelines that consultants must follow in order to make sure that they are conducting the analysis according to published standards. Indeed, one successful malpractice lawsuit resulted when a nurse completed a "job analysis" that consisted of less than one page (*Drury v. Corvel*, as cited by Oakes, 1994). The topics covered in the analysis did not follow published standards. In fact, it appeared as if the nurse was unaware that the government and others have published on this topic.

It is important that the life care planner, who may not be a vocational expert, be aware that when working with the vocational aspects of the plan, the vocational expert must provide a proper foundation for an opinion. For more information, the reader is encouraged to review these topics in the *Rehabilitation Consultant's Handbook* (Weed & Field, 1994, 2001), the *Revised Handbook for Analyzing Jobs* (U.S. DOL, 1991c), and *Methods and Protocols: Meeting the Criteria of General Acceptance and Peer Review under Daubert and Kumho* (Field, Johnson, Schmidt, & Van de Bittner, 2006).

Table 4.4 Labor Market Survey Checklist

Introduction (include the following identifying information for report) Name Age Date of injury Type of injury & medical limitations Work experience Education Other historical information Vocational test results
Method(s) used (What methods were used to obtain the information? Suggest starting with residual employability profile by Vocational Diagnosis and Assessment of Residual Employability Process [VDARE] for worker traits.)
Personal contacts (as appropriate) with: Personal network Yellow Pages City Directory or Haynes Directory Chamber of Commerce Professional and trade associations Job service
Vocational rehabilitation Other
Publications Wage rates for selected occupations (state) Occupational supply and demand (state Department of Industry and Trade or Labor) State career information systems (or similar) Manufacturing directory (Standard Industrial Classification [SIC] codes) Bureau of Labor Statistics; e.g., Area Wage Survey (federal) Census Bureau (federal) Job Service/posted jobs (state) Classified ads or job flyers Identified discrete jobs related to client's experience Labor Market Access Analysis Other
Results Employer/s contacted—approximately 10 Job(s) available Wages and benefits (holidays, vacation, sick, medical, dental, personal leave, etc.) Training/education needed Willingness to work with disabled Accessibility/architectural barriers Other
Conclusions (the professional's opinion) Placeability Expected income Other related comments

Collaborating with the Rehabilitation Nurse

Unless specifically trained in life care planning, vocational counselors often are teamed with a medical expert, typically a rehabilitation nurse. Many rehabilitation counselors either are not qualified or not comfortable as the primary author of a life care plan unless they have received specific training. Some attorneys also are concerned that juries may be hesitant to accept opinions from one who claims multiple credentials and therefore retain different experts for vocational and medical needs identification. The following checklist may be helpful for medical expert/vocational rehabilitation teams (Table 4.5).

Table 4.5 Life Care Planning Questions Regarding Vocational Needs

First determine if vocational aspects have been considered or are already underway (e.g., already initiated by insurance company or attorney).
What interview information have you obtained from the client (e.g., work skills, leisure activities, education, work, functional ability)?
Have you obtained copies of relevant medical records?
Have you obtained work-related information (such as tax returns, job evaluations, school and test records, training history, and treating MD comments)?
Does the client need testing before determining vocational potential (e.g., vocational evaluation, psychological, neuropsychological or physical capacities testing)? Also, is the evaluation a quality and valid appraisal?
If there is work potential, is there a need for justifying a plan by performing a labor market survey? (If LMS, what method is used, e.g., direct contact with employers vs. statistics or publications?)
What is the client's expected income, including benefits? (If personal injury litigation, then pre- vs. post-injury capacity.)
If there is an apparent market for the client's labor, is there a need for a job analysis? (And if an analysis was completed, was it done according to the Americans with Disabilities Act guidelines?)
What are the estimated costs of the vocational plan?
Counseling, career guidance? (When does it start/stop, and what are the frequency and cost, e.g., 30 hrs. over 6 months at $65/hr.?)
Job placement, job coaching, or supported employment costs?
Tuition or training, books, supplies? (Include dates for expected costs, e.g., technical training 2 years @ $400/yr. for 1997–1999.)
Rehabilitation or assistive technology, accommodations or aides, costs for work, education, and/or training (e.g., computer, printer, workstation, tools, digital recorder, attendant care, transportation—include costs and replacement schedules)?
What effect, if any, does the injury have on work life expectancy (e.g., delayed entry into workforce, less than full-time, earlier retirement, expected increased turnover, or time off for medical follow-up or treatment)?

Source: © Roger O. Weed, PhD (1997, rev, 2002, 2016).

Vocational Resources

The vocational rehabilitation counselor has many resources available to assist in assessing a client's vocational potential and making appropriate recommendations for the life care plan. The following lists a few of the more valuable reference materials used by the vocational rehabilitation counselor:

- *Dictionary of Occupational Titles* (*DOT*), 4th Edition (1991). Contains definitions of 12,741 job titles and descriptions of jobs found in the national economy. Data compiled by the U.S. Department of Labor. Although dated, the data are available through the SkillTRAN website since the O*Net is not usable for true transferability of skills analysis required by Social Security disability determination and forensic consultation.
- *Transitional Classification of Jobs (COJ)* (2004). Contains worker trait profiles of the 72 U.S. Department of Labor worker traits for each of the 12,741 *DOT* job titles. The worker traits are assigned a code and rated. Also includes information on the O*Net database.
- *Occupational Outlook Handbook* (*OOH)* (2003). Clusters jobs by occupation and gives information with regard to employment potential, labor market trends, salary, requirements, and training needed to enter the occupation. Updated versions available at www.bls.gov/oco/.
- *The Enhanced Guide for Occupational Exploration (GOE)* (1991b). Provides descriptions of all jobs organized within related job clusters and includes information pertaining to academic and physical requirements, work environment, salary and outlook, typical duties, skills and abilities required, and where to obtain additional information.
- *The Revised Handbook for Analyzing Jobs* (*RHAJ*) (1991c). Gives descriptions on how to examine individual jobs to determine suitability for a client. The process continues to be relevant for analyzing jobs in forensic consultation.
- *Job Analysis and the ADA: A Step-by-Step Guide* (1992). This is another option for a comprehensive guide for determining the suitability of a job for clients with disabilities.
- O*NET, the Occupational Information Network. A comprehensive database of worker attributes and job characteristics. Contains hundreds of occupational units (OUs) and is intended as the replacement for the *Dictionary of Occupational Titles.* O*NET is the nation's primary source of occupational information. However, it is not usable in its present form for transferability of skill analysis (manual or computerized). Available at http://online.onetcenter.org.

The previously listed resources use data compiled by the federal government, with many published by the government. In addition to the ones listed, there are other state, regional, and local publications specific to occupations found in certain geographic areas. For various approaches to transferable skills analysis, see Weed (2002) and the associated special issue journal on this subject.

For additional print and computer resources available to the vocational rehabilitation counselor, the following may be useful:

- SkillTRAN (Truthan, 1997). An online and telephonic system of ordering job search and transferable skills information, as well as other resources for purchase; (800) 827–2182 or www.skilltran.com.
- Vertek, Inc. (Gibson, 2003). Developed the OASYS computerized job-matching program; (800) 220–4409 or www.Vertekinc.com.
- McCroskey Vocational Quotient System (MVQS) (McCroskey, 2001, updated 2005). Job–person matching, transferable skills analysis, values, needs, vocational interest and personality

reinforcer (VIPR) type indicator, and earning capacity estimation system; (612) 569–0680 or www.vocationology.com.

- Job Accommodation Network (JAN), Office of Disability Employment Policy, U.S. Department of Labor (1984). Offers free consulting service that provides information about job accommodations, the Americans with Disabilities Act (ADA), and the employability of people with disabilities; (800) 526–7234 or www.jan.wvu.edu.

For other websites, see Weed and Field (2012).

Conclusion

This chapter outlines some of the vocational factors that a life care planner may encounter if a client is expected to have the capability for work activity. If the life care planner does not have the expertise to develop opinions in this specialized area, it may be reasonable to obtain services of a vocational expert and ensure that the vocational expert includes the relevant areas, as described in this chapter, and has sufficient expertise to develop reasonable opinions. Some of the topics included in this chapter are designed to assist the nonvocational expert with an overview so that appropriate questions can be asked in order to enhance the life care plan, reduce overlap or duplication in services, and facilitate the client's return to employment and achievement of a highest level of functioning. Table 4.5 summarizes some issues, topics, and questions that a life care planner who is not a vocational expert can ask the professional on whom the life care planner is relying for a vocational opinion and recommendations.

References

Anastasi, A. 1982. *Psychological Testing* (5th ed.). New York, NY: Macmillan.

Blackwell, T., Conrad, D., & Weed, R. 1992. *Job Analysis and the ADA: A Step-by-Step Guide*. Athens, GA: E & F Vocational Services.

Botterbusch, K. F. 1987. *Vocational Assessment and Evaluation Systems: A Comparison*. Menomonie, WI: University of Wisconsin Materials Development Center.

Clark v. Aqua Air Industries. 1983. 435 So. 2d 492.

Crease, G. v. J. A. 1982. Jones Construction Company, 425 So. 2d 274 (LA App. 1982).

Deneen, L., & Hessellund, T. 1986. *Counseling the Able Disabled*. San Francisco, CA: Rehab Publications.

Deutsch, P., & Raffa, F. 1981. *Damages in Tort Actions* (*Vol. 8*). New York, NY: Matthew Bender.

Dillman, E. 1987. The necessary economic and vocational interface in personal injury cases. *Journal of Private Sector Rehabilitation*, *2*, 121–142.

Evans, R. 1999. The role of the neuropsychologist in life care planning. In R. Weed (Ed.), *Life Care Planning and Case Management Handbook* (pp. 65–76). Boca Raton, FL: CRC Press.

Evans, R. 2004. The role of the neuropsychologist in life care planning. In R. Weed (Ed.), *Life Care Planning and Case Management Handbook* (pp. 77–87). Boca Raton, FL: CRC Press.

Field, J. E., & Field, T. F. 2004. *Transitional Classification of Jobs*. Athens, GA: Elliott & Fitzpatrick.

Field, T., Johnson, C., Schmidt, R., & Van de Bittner, E. 2006. *Methods and Protocols: Meeting the Criteria of General Acceptance and Peer Review under Daubert and Kumho*. Athens, GA: Elliott & Fitzpatrick.

Gabel, S., Oster, G., & Butnik, S. 1986. *Understanding Psychological Testing in Children*. New York, NY: Plenum Publishing.

Gibson, G. 2003. *Oasys*. Bellevue, WA: Vertek, Inc. (computer program).

Kapes, J., & Mastie, M. (Eds.). 1988. *A Counselor's Guide to Career Assessment Instruments* (2nd ed.). Alexandria, VA: National Career Development Association.

Lees-Haley, P. 1993. *The Last Minute Guide to Psychological and Neuropsychological Testing: A Quick Reference for Attorneys and Claims Professionals.* Athens, GA: Elliott & Fitzpatrick.

Lezak, M. D. 1976. *Neuropsychological Assessment.* New York, NY: Oxford University Press.

Lezak, M. D. 1995. *Neuropsychological Assessment* (3rd ed.). New York, NY: Oxford University Press.

Marme, M., & Skord, K. 1993. Counseling strategies to enhance the vocational rehabilitation of persons after traumatic brain injury. *Journal of Applied Rehabilitation Counseling, 24*, 19–25.

Matheson, L., Rogers, L., Kaskutas, V., & Dakos, M. 2002. Reliability and reactivity of three new functional assessment measures. *Work, 18*, 41–50.

McCroskey, B. (2001, updated 2005). *The McCroskey Vocational Quotient System 2005, version 2005.03.* Brooklyn Park, MN: Vocationology, Inc. (computer program).

Neulicht, A. T., & Berens, D. E. 2005. PEEDS-RAPEL: A case conceptualization model for evaluating pediatric cases. *Journal of Life Care Planning, 4*(1), 27–36.

Oakes, M. 1994. *Drury v. Corvel.* Retrieved June 20, 2003, from www.oakes.org/webdoc14.htm.

Sbordone, R. J., & Long, C. J. (Eds.). 1996. *Ecological Validity of Neuropsychological Testing.* Delray Beach, FL: St. Lucie Press.

Siefker, J. M. (Ed.). 1992. *Vocational Evaluation in Private Sector Rehabilitation.* Menomonie, WI: University of Wisconsin Materials Development Center.

Truthan, J. 1997. *SkillTRAN, LLC.* Spokane, WA: SkillTRAN, LLC (computer program).

U.S. Department of Labor (U.S. DOL). 1984. *Job Accommodation Network.* Washington, DC. Retrieved 4/30/18, https://www.dol.gov/general/topic/disability/jobaccommodations

U.S. Department of Labor (U.S. DOL). 1991a. *Dictionary of Occupational Titles.* Lanham, MD: Bernan Press.

U.S. Department of Labor (U.S. DOL). 1991b. *Enhanced Guide for Occupational Exploration.* St. Paul, MN: Jist Works.

U.S. Department of Labor (U.S. DOL). 1991c. *Revised Handbook for Analyzing Jobs.* Washington, DC: United States Government Printing Office.

U.S. Department of Labor (U.S. DOL). 2002–2003. *Occupational Outlook Handbook.* Washington, DC: United States Government Printing Office.

Weed, R. 1994. Evaluating the earnings capacity of people with acquired brain injury. In C. Simkins (Ed.), *Analysis, Understanding and Presentation of Cases Involving Traumatic Brain Injury*, (pp. 213–228). Washington, DC: National Head Injury Foundation.

Weed, R. 1996. Life care planning and earnings capacity analysis for brain injured clients involved in personal injury litigation utilizing the RAPEL method. *Journal of Neurorehabilitation, 7*, 119–135.

Weed, R. 1998. Aging with a brain injury: The effects on life care plans and vocational opinions. *The Rehabilitation Professional, 6*, 30–34.

Weed, R. 2000. The worth of a child: Earnings capacity and rehabilitation planning for pediatric personal injury litigation cases. *The Rehabilitation Professional, 8*, 29–43.

Weed, R. 2002. The assessment of transferable work skills in forensic settings. *Journal of Forensic Vocational Analysis, 5*, 1–4 (special issue editorial).

Weed, R. 2007. *Life Care Planning: A Step-by-Step Guide.* Athens, GA: E & F Vocational Services.

Weed, R., & Field, T. 1994. *Rehabilitation Consultant's Handbook* (2nd ed.). Athens, GA: Elliott & Fitzpatrick.

Weed, R., & Field, T. 2001. *Rehabilitation Consultant's Handbook* (3rd ed.). Athens, GA: Elliott & Fitzpatrick.

Weed, R., & Field, T. 2012. *Rehabilitation Consultant's Handbook* (4th ed.). Athens, GA: Elliott & Fitzpatrick.

Weed, R., & Riddick, S. 1992. Life care plans as a case management tool. *The Individual Case Manager Journal, 3*, 26–35.

Weed, R., Taylor, C., & Blackwell, T. 1991. Job analysis for the private sector. *NARPPS Journal and News, 6*, 153–158.

Workers' Compensation Law Bulletin. 1992. 15 [10A], p. 7.

Chapter 5

The Role of the Psychologist in Life Care Planning

Harvey E. Jacobs*

Contents

Introduction 62
Psychologist Credentialing and Orientations 62
Psychological Issues Common to Rehabilitation 63
The Client 63
Traumatic Brain Injury 64
Spinal Cord Injury 64
Burn Injuries 65
Other Forms of Impairment 66
The Family/Social Support Network 66
Adjustment to Disability 67
The Psychologist's Role in Assessment and Diagnosis 68
Therapeutic Strategies 69
Types of Psychological Treatment 69
Methods of Treatment Delivery 70
Selected Therapeutic Techniques 71
The Interface between Life Care Planner and Psychologist 72
Case Example 73
List of Items and Services 74
Conclusion 75
References 75

* This chapter is adapted from previous editions of this topic authored by Dr. Randall L. Thomas and Dr. Anne Sluis Powers.

Introduction

With customary experience in interdisciplinary processes, psychologists can serve numerous life care planning related roles. This chapter focuses on ways psychologists work with individuals with disabilities, their support systems, and the rehabilitation team. Several different topics will be considered: (1) choosing a psychologist, (2) psychological issues common to rehabilitation, (3) the psychologist's role in assessment and diagnosis, (4) psychological testing, (5) types of psychological treatment, and (6) the interface between the psychologist and life care planner.

Psychologist Credentialing and Orientations

It is important to understand a psychologist's academic training, licensing credentials, theoretical orientation and experience, especially when making a referral.

Regulations vary across states, but a licensed psychologist has typically earned a doctoral degree (PhD, PsyD) from an accredited university program or professional psychology school that has been approved by the American Psychological Association (or deemed equivalent, in some cases). Psychologists are typically required to complete a 1500–2000 hour pre-doctoral internship, followed by a minimum of 1 year of approved post-doctoral supervision (typically 2000 hours) by a qualified licensed psychologist. This may be completed through a post-doctoral fellowship or cumulative hours of supervision on the job.

After completing the previous requirements, the candidate petitions his or her state board of psychological examiners for the right to take the national written examination (Evaluation of Professional Practice in Psychology), which must be passed within his or her state-legislated parameters. The candidate then takes a separate written or oral examination based on legal and ethical issues in that state. Successfully passing examinations and a background check typically allows licensure within that state. It is only upon formal licensure that the person may use the title *psychologist* and be compensated for his or her services. All states require psychologists to subsequently participate in continuing education activities and maintain adherence to state professional and ethics regulations to sustain licensure. Most states maintain an online log of all licensed psychologists and their standing, including past violations.

Use of the title without proper licensure constitutes violation of legal statutes and ethical principles. Please note there are some exceptions that allow the use of the term *psychologist* by nonlicensed employees of universities or state agencies. Some states also have specialization of psychology licensure for such areas as neuropsychology, medical/prescribing psychology, school psychology, industrial psychology, etc.

Psychologists practice within the scope of their training and experience, which may vary widely, hence the need to understand the psychologist's academic and professional experience. Oftentimes a psychologist (or psychologists) may have already been involved in the case when the life care planner is retained. Sometimes, the life care planner may be asked to help find a psychologist who has specialized in health, medical, or rehabilitation psychology and experience working on clinical issues similar to the presenting case. In such situations, it is also desirable to identify psychologists who endorse collaborative team approaches and understand the roles of other rehabilitation professionals. It also important to understand that in some cases more than one psychologist may be concurrently involved or required relative to issues of assessment, treatment, or even treatment of specific clinical concerns.

The American Psychological Association presently recognizes 56 different areas of psychology, and clearly not all of these are relevant to rehabilitation. The following are brief descriptions of some of the different areas of psychology that a life care planner may encounter (Altmaier, 1991).

1. *Rehabilitation psychologists* provide services on behalf of individuals with disabilities and society through such activities as research, assessment, treatment, program development, teaching, public education, development of social policy, and advocacy.
2. *Neuropsychologists* have special expertise understanding relationships between brain and behavior, particularly as these relationships can be applied to the diagnosis of brain disorder, assessment of cognitive and behavioral functioning, and the design of effective treatment.
3. *Behavioral psychologists* analyze environmental factors and functional relations that can be empirically identified and altered to help the individual optimize his or her capabilities and moderate dysfunctional or problematic behaviors. Over the past decade many states have also begun licensing behavior analysts who may focus more specifically on functional analyses of behavior, training, and environmental management. These professionals may have different training than psychologists.
4. *Cognitive-behavioral psychologists* incorporate behavioral principles and involve the roles of thoughts and feelings in acquiring and maintaining successful behaviors.
5. *Prescribing psychologists* have specialized training in medicine and pharmacology and can prescribe selected medications for specific clinical issues. This relatively new specialty is currently only licensed in New Mexico, Louisiana, Illinois, and Ohio. Additionally, trained psychologists may now be credentialed to prescribe in the U.S. Defense Department, the U.S. Public Health Service, and the Indian Health Service.
6. *Health psychologists* incorporate biosocial models and emphasize systems approaches; no part of a system operates exclusively of others. Health psychologists often develop and implement rehabilitation interventions related to specific health related issues in concert with other professionals.
7. *Developmental psychologists* examine cognitive, social, and psychomotor development of individuals relative to their age-related peers. Developmental psychologists often evaluate children, and their findings may be useful following catastrophic events occurring before adulthood. However, they are sometimes used in adult cases to understand the client's current psychological presentation relative to earlier developmental issues or to characterize a client's current psychological presentation relative to developmental templates.
8. *Psychodynamic/Psychoanalytic psychologists* incorporate the theories of Sigmund Freud, Alfred Adler, Harry Stack Sullivan, Karen Horney, Erik Erikson, and others. They also focus on dynamic aspects of relationships presumed to originate in infancy and childhood.

Psychological Issues Common to Rehabilitation

The Client

Rehabilitation clients often face dynamic and diverse physical, cognitive, emotional, behavioral, financial, and social challenges. These vary according to the nature and intensity of the person's impairment/disability, entry into treatment, recovery trajectory, supports, premorbid presentation, and other factors. It is important to recognize the full person and their social support systems in any assessment and treatment formulation rather than objectify the individual on the basis of their impairment. Each person and the nature of their presentation is unique. However, different types of primary injuries are often associated with selected signature challenges.

Traumatic Brain Injury

Following traumatic brain injury (TBI), the client may experience significant changes as a result of altered brain functioning (Ripley & Weed, 2010). Systemically this might include cognitive, motoric, behavioral, emotional/psychiatric, medical, metabolic, sensory, and perceptual challenges. These factors may individually or conjointly affect diverse functional abilities ranging from primary physiological/medical stability to basic self-care, primary and advanced Activities of Daily Living, sleep, productive daily activity patterns such as work and education, social and intimate relationships, communication, community access/integration, resource management, competency, and most aspects of daily life (Jacobs, 2010). Behavioral and cognitive factors are often cited among the most common sequelae following traumatic brain injury (McAllister, 2008). They may be revealed through subtle or obvious problems regarding attention, concentration, memory, problem solving, insight, concrete thinking, awareness, impulse control, judgment, anxiety, depression, emotional lability, irritation, irritability, and anger. There are many other considerations including social isolation, exaggerated or degraded self-image, drug/alcohol abuse, altered sexual functioning/behavior, and post-traumatic stress disorder, to name a few. It is important to consider that individuals with other types of primary injuries may have also experienced a concurrent brain injury if significant physical forces or oxygen restriction were associated with the primary injury. Similarly, the client with TBI may have sustained other injuries at the time of the index event that could contribute to noted dysfunction. These may include skeletal/muscular injury, pain syndromes, damage to internal organs, other neurological impairments, and so on.

Psychological services following TBI can vary considerably due to the diversity and variability of challenges associated with this class of impairments. Psychological assessment may involve areas of intellectual, cognitive, perceptual, sensory, clinical, emotional, personality, psychopathological, and behavioral functioning. Special considerations may require assessment of pain and health issues, suicidality, substance use/abuse, competency/capacity, and differentiation of the contribution of premorbid versus index-related factors of specific challenges. Neuropsychological assessment is most often associated with TBI, but other forms of evaluation including clinical and personality assessments, status screenings, and both functional and ecological analyses of behavior are also valuable. Psychiatric evaluation may also be beneficial in selected cases.

Psychological treatment will vary widely according to the client's functional presentation. Individuals who retain awareness and insight may benefit from more traditional forms of individual psychotherapy/counseling, cognitive behavioral therapy, and group therapies with adjunctive supports for problems involving memory, executive functioning, comprehension, language, processing speed, and other challenges. Individuals with limited awareness and insight and greater impairment in the above noted areas may require more concrete approaches including social and environmental management, the use of mentors or life skills coaches in their daily situations, and involvement by key members of their social support network.

Spinal Cord Injury

Motor impairments involving paralysis, paraplegia, or tetraplegia are only one of the prominent challenges that individuals with spinal cord injury experience. Sensory alterations, both numbness/ insensitivity and pain syndromes involving radicular, muscular/skeletal, and neuropathic origins are equally frequent. Issues regarding organ system functioning, especially as it relates to bowel and bladder control, respiration, skin integrity, circulation, sexual functioning, and sexuality are also of concern (Fichtenbaum & Kirshblum, 2011). Early psychological reactions often involve dealing with sudden and oftentimes permanent changes in physical capacities. Return to premorbid roles and function at home, work, and community may require changes in routines, including the acceptance and incorporation of adaptive equipment, living with decreased spontaneity/freedom and increased dependency, managing social stigma, reconceptualization of intimacy, changes in body image and self-esteem, and rebuilding a personal sense of control. The roles and relationships of other key people in the person's life may also change, creating additional stressors. Key aspects of psychological support focus on adaptation, personal integrity, and life quality. Age of onset will affect course and outcome.

Psychological issues can include adjustment reaction, complicated grieving, depression, suicidality, anxiety disorders, post-traumatic stress disorder, pain syndromes, noncompliance, social phobia, body image distortion, fear or actual loss of intimacy, addictive disorders, self-neglect, and personal degradation (Richards et al., 2010). Cognitive factors may also be of concern when there is concurrent TBI. Early psychological assessment and treatment typically involves assessing and managing the client's reaction to being newly and oftentimes profoundly impaired, their relative participation in treatment modalities, and adapting to possibly invasive care procedures for often-considered private personal functions. This is also a time for establishing early foundations of adaptation such as beginning the steps of transition from a sick to an injured or impaired role (Larson et al. 1998).

Longer term psychological services may require formal assessment of personality factors that may encourage or impede adaptation; assessment of mood, pain, anxiety, and other associated disorders; as well as screening for substance abuse and other self-defeating behaviors. Psychological interventions are ultimately most effective when they are proactive and facilitate adaptation and positive role definition. They may include counseling and psychoeducational treatment to help reduce distorted perceptions (Chung et al., 2006); cognitive behavioral therapy to improve adjustment and problem-solving skills; training in coping skills; peer counseling (Tate et al., 1992); use of meaning-based strategies (Pollard & Kennedy, 2007); referral for psychopharmacological treatment for refractory issues, especially depression and anxiety; biofeedback; couples' counseling; intervention for addictive and self-defeating behaviors; and helping the client redefine and reestablish a sense of meaning and life quality. At times the psychologist's role may also involve advocating for the client when the client's goals are reasonably at odds with *common medical/psychological practices and wisdom.*

Burn Injuries

Burn injury is often a devastating event with long-term physical and psychosocial effects (Van Loey & Van Son, 2003). Wiechman & Patterson (2007) note three phases of physiological recovery—resuscitative or critical, acute, and long-term rehabilitation with differing psychological needs at each stage. During the resuscitative or critical stage medical treatment is focused on basic survival. The procedures, medications, and intensive care environments can add to confusion, delirium, and brief psychotic reactions. Psychological intervention may be limited to helping patients utilize basic defense mechanisms, use of nonmedical pain control such as hypnosis and relaxation, and helping to facilitate sleep. During the acute phase, patients continue to endure painful treatments but are generally more alert, start to realize the nature of their injuries, and face uncertainty about their future. Problems of acute stress disorders, post-traumatic stress disorder, and depression may evolve. Psychological treatment may focus on psychological counseling, cognitive behavioral therapy, hypnotherapy, and relaxation techniques for both pain control and to help patients consolidate information and experiences. Long-term rehabilitation typically begins after hospital discharge. Psychological treatment may focus on helping clients sustain continuing medical and physical treatments, adapt to functional capacities and limitations in daily life, and develop proactive strategies to optimize opportunity and life quality.

Psychological distress is among the most frequent and debilitating complications post-burn injury (Dalal et al., 2010) with common sequelae of depression, generalized stress disorders, post-traumatic stress disorder, anxiety, pain, negative body image, anger, alienation, a sense of loss of control, and suicidal ideation (Williams et al., 2003; Fauerbach et al., 2007; Askay & Patterson, 2008). Problems related to social interaction and sexual life may also require treatment (Thombs et al., 2007). Neuropsychological consequences such as memory and attention deficits, sensory and motor deficits, speech and language difficulties, problems with executive functioning, and intellectual impairments may also occur, especially in electrical injuries (Duff & McCaffrey, 2001; Pliskin et al., 1994), though smoke inhalation may also contribute to such presentations.

The type and frequency of psychological treatment for long-term issues may vary in frequency and approach. Cognitive behavioral therapy (CBT) and/or pharmacological treatment may help to reduce depression, as well as manage anxiety and pain. Patients suffering from post-traumatic stress disorder may also respond to CBT in addition to desensitization techniques and eye movement desensitization reprocessing (EMDR) treatment. Positive psychological approaches along with social skills training, support groups, and community interventions may assist with treating self-image and body image, alienation, avoidance, and adverse social interactions. Counseling and sexual health education may help promote sexuality. More frequent psychological intervention may be required at times of crisis or when the client is facing recurring medical procedures, such as surgical scar revision or affiliated complications such as neuropathies, amputation, thermoregulation, and so on. It is important for the psychologist to adequately account for these recurring issues over the client's life span.

Other Forms of Impairment

There are clearly many other forms of impairment and disability that life care plans address; the previous three examples highlight that psychological concerns and services can vary greatly. In each case it is incumbent upon psychologists to holistically understand the client's presentation as a "full person" rather than objectify the individual according to sequelae of an index event. It is also important to provide recommendations for long-term, as well as acute psychological services, as applicable to the case.

The Family/Social Support Network

Families and social support networks are dynamic and naturally change over one's lifespan as the person transitions from infant, to child, to adolescent/teen, to young adult, to middle age, to elderly, and so on. These key relationships evolve as capacities, roles, resources, and goals reciprocally change. Illness, injury, and disability naturally change roles, resources, and relationships for all parties. Hence, people within a client's primary social support network are directly affected by the client's injury/illness onset, treatment, and long-term course as his or her needs and capacities change, thereby effecting changes in their own lives. Social support network members can also affect a client's outcome by their reactions, support, or abdication.

Understanding who constitutes a person's support network is critical, and customary assumptions are not always valid. Biological/marital families are frequently identified as the primary support network, but it may actually consist of others such as close friends, significant others, stepfamily members, and so on. In some cases there may be little social support, or professional caregivers may fill such roles. Some close relationships may be defined within legal documents such as durable powers of attorney, living wills, or service contracts. External forces such as legal statutes may also influence the support network constellation, relative to rights of access, decision making, and property. In some cases, a person may have multiple primary support clusters, and if so, these clusters may be cooperative or antagonistic with associated effects.

Each member of a client's social support network is unique and possesses their own strengths and challenges. Divergence or synchrony across members can affect communication, resources, support, and outcomes. Each network member has his or her own responsibilities and needs relative to his or her own life, which can alter his or her relationships and support to the client. Premorbidly, there is often a reciprocal balance of giving and receiving between the client and key members of his or her support network. However, illness/injury and associated disability/handicap skews this balance, which can dramatically affect long-term network membership and structure. Individual members may remain or leave for many different reasons as they seek their own homeostasis. Some people may cyclically appear, or primary caretakers may similarly change over time due to stress, burnout, changes in their own lives, needs of other individuals in their own social support networks, per client preferences, and so on. (Ergh et al., 2002). It is important to clarify the pragmatic and psychological ramifications of these dynamics.

Adjustment to Disability

Most descriptions of adjustment to disability are based on adaptations of Kubler-Ross's 1969 seminal book *On Death and Dying*. Dr. Kubler-Ross proposed a five-stage model of grieving, incorporating phases of (1) *denial* of the reality of the situation, (2) *anger* or other intense emotional expression when the reality of the situation becomes evident, (3) *bargaining* as a means to find an alternative to the likely course or situation, (4) *depression* as a reaction to the practical implications of loss, and (5) *acceptance* of the loss and the ability to move on. Though powerful, this model has limits of applicability in rehabilitation. First, onset of disability generally reflects a change in life trajectory, rather than death. Second, there is greater understanding that the first stage of reaction is as likely based on having to rapidly process overwhelming and divergent information, lack of knowledge, or incomplete communication as much as denial. Each of these is a dynamically different situation that requires different intervention approaches. Third, rehabilitation psychology often promotes accommodation versus acceptance (5th stage), recognizing that people may successfully adapt to current circumstances while still seeking future opportunities. Fourth, not all people progress through all five stages, in the same order, or at the same time.

Muir & Haffey (1984), promoted the concept of *mobile mourning* in which individuals move back and forth between stages on a lifetime basis as new opportunities or challenges arise. Hence, an individual successfully living with long-standing burn injuries who now faces infection may find themselves again facing anger and depression; the primary partner of an individual with TBI may revisit denial when the person has been arrested for an unintended but significant social boundary violation; and the person with spinal cord injury may face new challenges regarding adaptation after being diagnosed with overuse syndrome and having to face moving from a manual to an electric wheel chair. Cohn (1961) also modified the five stages. The first stage is *shock*, where denial or minimization is common. In the second stage, *expectancy for recovery*, the client may admit to current deficits but continue to expect a quick and complete recovery. As the extent of the disability becomes apparent, *mourning* occurs. Depression, suicidal ideation, suicidal attempts, and disengagement from or active resistance to the therapy process are common during this stage and should be identified. During the fourth stage, *defense*, the adjustment process begins. The person reaches a critical point where either denial or movement toward independence tends to occur. The final stage, *adjustment*, occurs when the client has a realistic appraisal of his or her strengths and/or weaknesses and begins to focus on moving forward with life.

It is important to recognize that both the client and individual members of his or her social support network are likely to experience these processes, though not all at the same time, with the same intensity, or via the same dynamics—each person responds to challenges and stress differently. Sometimes, social support network members may begin progressing through selected stages earlier than the client, especially if the client initially experiences periods of prolonged unconsciousness, amnesia, or sedation. Problems involving lack of awareness or anosognosia may minimize a client's own reactions as the extent of the changes and challenges are muted. At the same time, the client may face later stages with greater intensity than others, as he or she has to deal with the challenges on a long-term, daily basis. People closest to the client may similarly experience stronger effects than more-remote network members. Selected social support network members may, at times, require their own psychological and educational services to help them respond to these issues, for the benefit of the client.

The Psychologist's Role in Assessment and Diagnosis

Multiple forms of psychological assessment may be required over a client's lifespan. As a result, the life care planner may have to consider a variety of data from different sources in formulating psychological treatment recommendations. Early assessments may involve basic screenings for individuals who have been acutely hospitalized. Depending on the nature of the injury or illness, more comprehensive assessments may occur in a rehabilitation facility or on an outpatient basis, especially if the client's illness or injury did not require hospitalization. These assessments often incorporate multifactorial and multidimensional approaches to evaluate cognitive functions, emotional state, behavior, personality, support systems dynamics, and the environment to which the client will return. Serial evaluations may also be used to assess changes in performance over time, including initial recovery and screening for subsequent possible deterioration.

In each situation, some of the key goals of psychological assessments include: (1) providing information about the client's current cognitive, neurobehavioral, and psychological functioning, (2) identifying cognitive and behavioral strengths and weaknesses that can be respectively engaged and remediated to promote a positive treatment response, and (3) noting indications of potential future functioning to assist in long-term planning (Reid-Arndt et al., 2011).

Most assessments begin with a comprehensive review of the client's history and present status. This may be accomplished via records reviews or interviews with the client or other informants. Topical issues may include: medical diagnosis, psychological/psychiatric diagnosis, preexisting conditions (medical conditions, mental health issues, legal issues), past psychological and psychiatric treatment history, premorbid health beliefs and behaviors, educational background, employment history, medications (including side effects and interactions), substance use/abuse history, abuse history (physical, emotional, and/or sexual), legal history, premorbid personality characteristics, extent of social support network, marital status/stability of primary relationship, role within family prior to injury or illness, financial resources, community resources, religious/

spiritual beliefs, cultural and ethnic considerations, daily activity patterns, functional capacities/limitations (daily living skills, intellectual functioning, and cognitive skills), notable behavioral patterns, affective status, suicidal/homicidal potential, and other key issues (Thomas & Powers, 2010). Behavioral observations are also noted during the course of the interview and assessment.

Testing protocols are dependent on the referral questions. They may include, individually or combined, structured interviews, functional and ecological analyses of behavior, projective testing, self-report measures completed by the client and/or collaterals, standardized assessment, biofeedback, and other protocols. While there are many commonly used tests, there is no singular battery of assessments or process for all cases, even within a similar impairment or disability. Statistical validation of a test does not assure that it is a reliable and valid instrument for the presenting referral question(s). Issues related to underlying constructs and hypotheses used in test design, the sample used to standardize the instrument versus client presentation, retrospective versus predictive accuracy, validity profile, the context and process by which the test is administered, methods of data analysis, relationship to other tests used in assessment, time since last administration, and other factors can all affect interpretation (Pope et al., 2006). It is incumbent upon the psychologist to provide a valid and coherent rationale for selected assessment procedures to answer Gordon Paul's (1967) question: "What treatment, by whom, is most effective for this individual with that specific problem, and under which set of circumstances?"

Therapeutic Strategies

From whatever point of introduction or need that psychological intervention may originate, rehabilitation psychology ultimately seeks to promote the possible over the pathological. Early services, especially in catastrophic cases, may focus on short-term risk management, moderation of fear and anxiety, emotional debridement, managing behavioral outbursts, providing as-needed information, affirmation, and supportive problem-solving to both the client and social support network members. Over time, intervention ultimately transitions to capitalizing on strengths and helping the client reestablish life quality, meaning, and self-determination within personal and social support network capacities. With strong foundations in bio-social models of behavior, anticipated rehabilitation psychology services recognize the dynamic experiences, both positive and negative, that the client may face over a lifetime, but sustains an emphasis on competencies, masteries, and strengths. Hence, while psychological setbacks may sometimes require more intensive treatment, especially in the presence of severe behavioral/emotional decompensation, suicidal, or violent behavior, treatment remains focused on promoting dignity and social capital. The biosocial model also recognizes the importance of social and physical environments in promoting well-being and promotes proactive productive activities and incorporation of social and community supports as required to optimize outcomes.

Types of Psychological Treatment

Psychotherapeutic treatment needs to reflect the client's ethnic and cultural beliefs, social support network, community, capacities, challenges, and goals. Often a mixture of therapeutic approaches is required that will likely change over time according to treatment efficacy, life experiences, aging, and other factors. It is also important to clarify what each form of treatment addresses, noting that in some cases there may be concurrent or complementary services. The type of therapist may also vary depending on the nature of the treatment and available resources in the client's community. This may include psychologists, licensed clinical therapists, social workers, or other accredited professional counselors with the requisite training, credentialing, and experience. The rationale for such selection should be provided in the life care plan.

Methods of Treatment Delivery

Individual therapy sessions involving a variety of different treatment modalities may initially be the most frequent mode of treatment. They provide the greatest focus and privacy and are amenable to a wide range of techniques and clinical concerns.

Conjoint treatment, a modification of individual sessions, involves an additional party of the client's choosing. This is helpful when the client may benefit from individual therapy sessions, but needs help reporting events to the therapist, following through on treatment-prescribed tasks or homework assignments, or applying techniques in their daily environments.

Group therapy can be used for many different purposes, including skills training, psychoeducational treatment, and peer counseling. Effective therapy group structures reinforce treatment goals and remain focused. Without such organization, groups can fall fallow and promulgate despair rather than aspiration and achievement.

Milieu therapy uses therapeutic environments to facilitate the functional capacities of its participants. Neurobehavioral treatment programs (Eames & Wood, 1989) serving individuals with significant behavioral sequelae following brain injury use specially trained staff and modified environments to help moderate triggers to behavioral dysfunction while facilitating other capacities. Substance abuse programs may use milieu approaches involving explicit guidelines, modeling by staff or more senior patients, and supports for adaptation to more effective coping strategies. Short-term milieu programs can also help people to test out new skills, perceptions, or coping skills within realistic but supportive environments.

Experiential or *in vivo therapy* involves directly working with the client in his or her natural environment where the therapist is able to more accurately observe situational nuances and develop more contextually relevant skills through coaching or modeling. This approach is sometimes used when treating fears and phobias but can also be used for skills development such as in social skills training, community integration, educational, or vocational settings. It is also effective for individuals who have problems with memory, impulsivity, initiation, transitions, or carryover skills. Here, the therapist can serve as a "prosthesis," filling in the missing links to help the client perform more successfully. Mentors or life skills coaches are also sometimes used when this approach is needed on a regular basis.

Telehealth services connect the provider with the client via phone, Internet, or other technological means. This offers opportunities for more frequent outreach to individuals who live in remote areas, are housebound, or have time and transportation limitations. Positive factors include convenience, scheduling flexibility, and possible cost savings, and a number of studies have reported good efficacy (Novotney, 2011; Jenkins-Guarnieri et al., 2015). However, not all clients respond favorably, and the lack of in situ involvement may obliterate important cues, contextual opportunities, communication, and trust (Rozenthal et.al., 2015). Licensure laws may also limit provision of services across states (APA, 2013).

Inpatient or other intensive treatment may be required in cases of severe psychological decompensation, with a goal of helping the client return to a less restrictive and more community inclusive environment upon stabilization.

Selected Therapeutic Techniques

The range of psychological techniques is as broad as the diversity of psychological orientations and clinical challenges. Several more-common approaches include, but are not limited to, the following:

Cognitive behavioral therapy (CBT) is a goal-oriented treatment that takes a hands-on and practical approach to problem-solving and personal optimization. Its goal is to change patterns of thinking or behavior that contribute to a person's difficulties and thereby change the way the person feels (Martin, 2015). Developed from the work of Aaron T. Beck (1967), CBT techniques have continued to evolve in process and clinical issues addressed (Follette et al., 2009). Therapeutic techniques that share some components of CBT include rational emotive therapy, acceptance and commitment therapy, behavioral activation, self-monitoring, response prevention, interoceptive exposure, functional communication training, cognitive restructuring, motivational interviewing, assertiveness skills training, habit reversal training, distress tolerance, communication/problem-solving skills training, cognitive delusion, progressive relaxation, etc. Key aspects of CBT include a proactive skills focus, direct reappraisal of cognitions, experiential exposure, and empirical evaluation (O'Donohue & Fisher, 2009).

Desensitization/exposure therapies (Wolpe, 1958) help individuals gain mastery over stimuli and events that cause fear or panic. The basic process is based on gradually and systematically exposing the client to aspects of the feared situation while also aiding the development of effective coping strategies. Stimuli presented in treatment can be presented in a variety of modalities. Systematic desensitization involves the individual visualizing or discussing the phobic stimuli in a safe therapeutic environment. *In vivo* desensitization involves direct exposure to the feared stimulus in a graduated manner. Virtual reality desensitization uses computer graphics to create the phobic situation with progressive presentation as the client gains mastery.

Biofeedback techniques help the client learn about his or her responses to stressors and how to moderate their adverse effects, often without using medications or other medical interventions (Basmajian, 1989). The technique may be considered for psychophysiological problems such as hypertension, muscle tension, pain, and stress disorders. Physical and occupational therapists have also found biofeedback to be a helpful adjunct in neuromuscular reeducation programs.

Family (social support network) therapy can cover a wide range of areas and it is important to prioritize those areas that are directly related to the client's functioning. This may include educating key support members regarding the nature and course of the client's needs so that they can optimize function and life quality, how to address major life transitions, boundary/personal rights issues, legal matters, and effective communication strategies. Counseling may also be required when the client is involved in an enduring relationship, including marriage. Some key social network members may also require their own psychotherapeutic intervention, and it will be important to determine if this is directly related to the client's benefit, in which case it might be included in the life care plan. Or it might be a secondary issue that could become that person's own and financial responsibility.

Pain management strategies often focus on helping the client reduce his or her reliance on potentially addictive pain medications and increasing functional independence. Treatment approaches include relaxation techniques, mindfulness, cognitive defusion, reactivation steps, and other processes collectively referred to as psychological flexibility (McCracken & Turk, 2002; Vowles & McCracken, 2010).

Contingency management and behavioral contracting techniques involve increasing or decreasing the frequency of selected behaviors through management of antecedents and consequences related to the target behavior. These procedures have wide applicability across situations and behaviors (Cooper et al., 2007).

Mentoring/life skills coaching (Powers et al., 1995; Wheeler et al., 2007) involves the engagement of peer mentors or trained staff (life skills coaches) who work collaboratively with a client in his or her daily environment. Peer-mentoring approaches typically focus on socialization and positive self-imaging. Life skills coaches also support sustained productive activity patterns via modeling, counseling, and guidance during the course of daily activities. Life skills coaches have the ability to communicate with requisite professionals and laypeople in the client's life and, working collaboratively with the client, the capacity to comprehend, conceptualize, and integrate disparate information in coherent and operational positive support systems.

The Interface between Life Care Planner and Psychologist

Psychologists may become involved in a case for a variety of reasons and it is important for the life care planner to understand their roles and responsibilities. Treating psychologists are clinically involved with the client, providing assessment and/or treatment. They usually become involved upon referral by another provider or through client self-referral. They may become involved in litigation as a matter of course regarding their treatment and clinical opinions. Expert psychologists are typically retained by one of the attorneys associated with the case to provide testimony or are sometimes engaged via a direct request of the court. Psychologists may also be retained by a trust or insurance company in non-litigated cases to help identify psychological needs and requisite reserves for a specific case. Not all psychologists may be familiar with life care plans, and an explanation of the process can be helpful.

Psychologists are generally oriented toward patient care, and the type of information life care planners solicit is familiar to the psychologist. Five key questions that outline the overall discussion and will help direct more specific recommendations include:

- What is/are the client's diagnosis/diagnoses?
- What are the client's key clinical issues and how do they affect daily functioning and life quality?
- What is the client's current treatment program?
- What is the client's projected course of treatment?
- What is the client's projected prognosis?

Establishing specific assessment and treatment recommendations requires greater focus; that is, general recommendations, such as "the client will need counseling," need to be qualified and quantified regarding frequency and duration. Since psychological treatment is a dynamic process, the need or frequency of therapy may vary over the client's lifespan. For example, he or she may need more intervention during early years of rehabilitation or at times of major disruption during their lifespans. Some psychologists will address this by titrating services across years. For example:

> Mr. Cauthen will require one hour of individual psychotherapy per week for the first year to address severe depression, anger management, and post-traumatic stress disorder; one hour of individual psychotherapy every two weeks in the second and third years; one hour of individual psychotherapy every month in years four through eight; and an average of six hours of psychotherapy per year on a lifetime basis.

Other psychologists may make similar recommendations during the initial years of treatment, for example, similar recommendations as above for the first 3 years, then recommend a "bolus" of treatment hours over the client's remaining life span. The reason for this approach is that the psychologist may not be able to predict precise annual treatment needs over the client's lifespan but can predict the likelihood that dynamic events will occur requiring periods of increased treatment or that needs may change with aging. For example:

> An additional 250 hours of individual psychotherapy to be utilized as needed over the client's remaining life span.

Using an outline can facilitate the discussion with the psychologist. Key topics include:

1. Type, frequency/ages of evaluations (e.g., clinical, neuropsychological, functional assessment, etc.)
2. Type, frequency, and duration of psychological treatment, such as, but not limited to, the types and modalities discussed in this chapter
3. Psychoeducational training and counseling for key members of the client's social support network to both increase members' capabilities to work with the client and as needed for personal adaptation/adjustment
4. Personal care attendant services for issues related to cognitive, behavioral, and mental capacity/incapacity
5. Use of life skills coaches and mentors to facilitate social, community, and productive day activity pattern competencies
6. Recommendations related to restrictive/least restrictive environment
7. Adaptive technology related to cognition, socialization, and independence
8. Case management related to psychological care
9. Psychiatric hospitalization—inpatient or partial hospitalization
10. Substance abuse treatment (as appropriate to the case)
11. Opinions and recommendations relating to vocational outlook (personality, trauma, intelligence, etc.)
12. Opinions regarding the person's pre- versus post-injury functioning
13. Opinions regarding competency/incompetency of person and/or assets
14. Referral to other professionals such as psychiatrist for medication

Once the psychologist has provided his or her list of recommendations, it is advisable for the life care planner to type them up and return them to the psychologist for review and signature. This provides the psychologist the opportunity to review for any areas of miscommunication or omission. The written document also provides documentation of the participation of the professionals involved in the planning process and reduces the potential for a challenge that the life care planner's testimony is based on hearsay in forensic cases.

Case Example

The patient is a 28-year-old unmarried female who is 30 months post-injury from a motor vehicle crash. She sustained significant physical injuries, including a severe onset brain injury, soft tissue injuries, and chronic fatigue. Neuropsychological testing reveals significant impairments in the ability to sustain attention and concentration, judgment, problem solving, auditory and visual memory (both short-term and long-term), expressive language, impulse control, and emotional lability. She has deepening depression, is easily agitated, reports chronic headaches and lower back pain, and requires a cane or walker for ambulation.

In a phone conference with the life care planner, Dr. Mary Smith, the patient's psychologist, provided the following recommendations, which she subsequently sent in a formal letter.

List of Items and Services

1. Diagnoses
   - Major neurocognitive disorder due to traumatic brain injury, with behavioral disturbance (impulse control and agitation).
   - Depressive disorder due to another medical condition—traumatic brain injury, with major depressive-like episode.
   - Anomic aphasia (word finding).
   - Impaired mobility requiring a cane or walker.
   - Chronic pain.
2. Psychological Evaluations
   - Assessment of competency of person or assets: One time.
   - Comprehensive neuropsychological examination: One time every 2 years for the next 4 years, then one time every 10 years on a lifetime basis unless annual clinical screenings indicate anomalies or there are notable changes in functional abilities.
   - Annual psychological screenings of clinical and neuropsychological functioning on a lifetime basis in the years that a comprehensive neuropsychological examination is not scheduled.
3. Client-Focused Services
   - Individual psychotherapy sessions (conjoint sessions per client's approval) involving cognitive behavioral therapy to address mood, problem solving, interpersonal relationships, self-concept, emotional debridement, pain management (biofeedback to also be used for pain management and services will be coordinated with associated medical services), and coordinating services with allied staff. One time per week for 6 months, then one time every 2 weeks for 2 years, then an average of one time per month on a lifetime basis.
   - Life skills coaching to facilitate carryover of therapeutic techniques into the client's daily environment, train personal care attendant staff, and engage the client in community-based productive activity patterns when not involved in milieu treatment. Average of 5 hours a week on a lifetime basis.
   - Participation in a supportive milieu such as the "All Together Brain Injury Clubhouse," or similar program of client's preference to support social skills, relationship building, community integration, and avocational skills development. Average of three times per week for 37 years.
   - Home-based personal care attendant services for an average of 8 hours per day due to cognitive deficits, safety issues, and poor judgment; assuming her regular participation in milieu therapy, otherwise 12 hours a day; on a lifetime basis.
   - Home monitoring system for emergencies (falls, fire, medical emergencies, etc.) on a lifetime basis.
   - Referral to psychiatry for evaluation and possible medication management of behavioral and emotional sequelae.
4. Primary Social Support Network Services
   - Psychoeducational services involving educational counseling, educational materials, and attendance at pertinent meetings and conferences to help key support network members

better understand the client's dynamic challenges as a result of her injuries and how to best facilitate her cognitive, functional, and emotional capacities over time. 100 hours to be used over a lifetime basis.

5. Case Management Services
   - An average of 4 hours per month on a lifetime basis to coordinate services.
6. Other Treatment Considerations
   - The client may require short-term inpatient psychiatric treatment if she demonstrates significant behavioral or emotional decompensation. Average length of stay per admission would be 7–14 days, with one to five such episodes occurring over her lifetime.
   - The client may require full-time tenure in a residentially based brain injury treatment and assistive living program on a lifetime basis if the above-noted services are not successful in sustaining her abilities.
   - The client may require placement in a residential memory center or dementia program if she demonstrates significant cognitive decline as she ages.

Conclusion

This chapter has reviewed roles and responsibilities in the psychological assessment and treatment of individuals who experience disability. A key focus of such efforts involves emphasizing capacities over challenges, facilitating function, and promoting holistic life quality. As a result, treatment and service modalities often expand beyond the individual client, into his or her daily environments and social support networks. It is also important to note that not all psychological intervention may involve a psychologist! Most psychologists will be able to readily collaborate with a life care planner as long as clear and organized questions are provided.

References

Altmaier, E. M. 1991. Research and practice roles for counseling psychologists in health care settings. *The Counseling Psychologist, 19*(3), 342–364.

American Psychological Association 2013. *Guidelines for the practice of telepsychology.* Washington, DC: Author.

Askay, S. W., & Patterson, D. R. 2008. What are the psychiatric sequelae of burn pain? *Current Pain and Headache Reports, 12*(2), 94–97.

Basmajian, J. V. (Ed.). 1989. *Biofeedback: Principles and Practice for Clinicians.* Baltimore, MD: Williams & Wilkins.

Beck, A. T. 1967. *Depression: Clinical, experimental, and theoretical aspects.* Philadelphia, PA: University of Pennsylvania Press.

Chung, M. C., Preveza, E., Papandreou, K., & Prevezas, N. 2006. The relationship between posttraumatic stress disorder following spinal cord injury and locus of control. *Journal of Affective Disorders, 93*(1), 229–232.

Cohn, N. 1961. Understanding the process of adjustment to disability. *Journal of Rehabilitation, 27*(6), 16–22.

Cooper, J. O., Heron, T. E., & Heward, W. L. 2007. *Applied Behavior Analysis.* Columbus, OH: Pearson.

Dalal, P. K., Saha, R., & Agarwal, M. 2010. Psychiatric aspects of burn. *Indian Journal of Plastic Surgery, 43*(3), 136–142.

Duff, K., & McCaffrey, R. J. 2001. Electrical injury and lightning injury: a review of their mechanisms and neuropsychological, psychiatric, and neurological sequelae. *Neuropsychology Review, 11*(2), 101–116.

Eames P., & Wood R. L. 1989. The structure and content of a head injury rehabilitation service. In R. L. Wood & P. Eames (Eds.) *Models of Brain Injury Rehabilitation*. 31–47. London: Chapman & Hall.

Ergh, T. C., Papport, L. J., Coleman, R. D., & Hanks, R. A. 2002. Predictors of caregiver and family functioning following traumatic brain Injury: Social support moderates caregiver distress. *Journal of Head Trauma Rehabilitation, 17*(2), 155–174.

Fauerbach, J. A., McKibben, J., Bienvenu, O. J., Magyar-Russell, G., Smith, M. T., Holavanahalli, R., Patterson, D., Wiechman, S.A., Blakeney, P., & Lezotte, D. 2007. Psychological distress after major burn injury. *Psychosomatic Medicine, 69*(5), 473–482.

Fichtenbaum, J., & Kirshblum, S. 2011. Psychological impact of spinal cord injury. In S. Kirshblum, D.I. Campagnolo, P.H. Gorman, R.F. Heary & M.S. Nash (Eds.) *Spinal Cord Medicine*, 2nd Edition. 382–397. Philadelphia, PA: Lippincott Williams & Wolters.

Follette, W. C., Darrow, S. M., & Bonow, J. T. 2009. Cognitive behavior therapy: A current appraisal. In W.T. O'Donohue & J.E. Fisher (Eds.) *General Principles and Empirically Supported Techniques of Cognitive Behavior Therapy*. 42–62. Hoboken, NJ: John Wiley & Sons.

Jacobs, H. E. 2010. *Understanding Everybody's Behavior after Brain Injury: Don't "Don't!"®*. Author. Originally published: Wake Forest, NC: Lash and Associates Publishing/Training, Inc.

Jenkins-Guarnieri, M. A., Pruitt, L. D., Luxton, D. D., & Johnson, K. 2015. Patient perceptions of telemental health: Systematic review of direct comparisons to in-person psychotherapeutic treatments. *Telemedicine and e-Health, 21*(8), 652–660.

Kubler, R. E. 1969. *On Death and Dying*. New York, NY: Macmillan.

Larson, P. D., Lewis, P. R., & Lubkin, I. M. 1998. Illness and behavior roles. In I. M. Lubkin (Ed.) *Chronic Illness Impact and Interventions*, 4th Edition 23–44. Sudbury, MA: Jones and Bartlett.

Martin, B. 2015. In-Depth: Cognitive Behavioral Therapy. Psych Central. http://psychcentral.com/lib/in-depth-cognitive-behavioral-therapy/.

McAllister, T. W. 2008. Neurobehavioral sequelae of traumatic brain Injury: Evaluation and management. *World Psychiatry, 7*(1), 3–10.

McCracken, L. M., & Turk, D. C. 2002. Behavioral and cognitive–behavioral treatment for chronic pain: outcome, predictors of outcome, and treatment process. *Spine, 27*(22), 2564–2573.

Muir, C. A., & Haffey, W. J. 1984. Psychological and neuropsychological interventions in the mobile mourning process. In B.A. Edelstein & E.T. Coture (Eds.) *Behavioral Assessment and Rehabilitation of the Traumatically Brain-Damaged*. 247–271. New York, NY: Springer.

Novotney, A. 2011. A new emphasis on telehealth. *Monitor on Psychology, 42*(6), 40. Washington, DC: American Psychological Association.

O'Donohue, W. T., & Fisher, J. E. 2009. Introduction. In W.T. O'Donohue & J.E. Fisher (Eds.) *General Principles and Empirically Supported Techniques of Cognitive Behavior Therapy*. 1–3. Hoboken, NJ: John Wiley & Sons, Inc.

Paul, G. L. 1967. Strategy of outcome research in psychotherapy. *Journal of Consulting Psychology, 31*(2), 109–118.

Pliskin, N. H., Meyer, G. J., Dolske, M. C., Heilbronner, R. L., Kelley, K. M., & Lee, R. C. 1994. Neuropsychiatric aspects of electrical injury. *Annals of the New York Academy of Sciences, 720*(1), 219–223.

Pollard, C., & Kennedy, P. 2007. A longitudinal analysis of emotional impact, coping strategies and post-traumatic psychological growth following spinal cord injury: A 10-year review. *British Journal of Health Psychology, 12*(3), 347–362.

Pope, K. S., Butcher, J. N., & Seelen, J. 2006. *The MMPI, MMPI-2, & MMPI-A in court: A practical guide for expert witnesses and attorneys*, 3rd edition. Washington, DC: American Psychological Association.

Powers, L. E., Sowers, J. A., & Stevens, T. 1995. An exploratory, randomized study of the impact of mentoring on the self-efficacy and community-based knowledge of adolescents with severe physical challenges. *Journal of Rehabilitation, 61*(1), 33.

Reid-Arndt, S. A., Caplan, B., Rusin, M. J., Slomine, B. S., Umoto, J. M., & Frank, R. A. 2011. Psychological assessment and intervention in rehabilitation. In R. Braddom (Ed.) *Physical medicine & Rehabilitation*. 65–98. Philadelphia, PA: Elsevier Saunders.

Richards, J. S., Kewman, D. G., Richardson, E., & Kennedy, P. 2010. Spinal cord injury. In R.G. Frank, M. Rosenthal & B. Caplan (Eds.) *Handbook of rehabilitation psychology*, 2nd Edition. 9–28. Washington, DC: American Psychological Association.

Ripley, D., & Weed, R. 2010. Life care planning for acquired brain injury. In R. Weed (Ed.) *Life Care Planning and Case Management Handbook*. 349–381. Boca Raton, FL: CRC Press.

Tate, D. G., Rasmussen, L., & Maynard, F. 1992. Hospital to community: A collaborative medical rehabilitation and independent living program. *Journal of Applied Rehabilitation Counseling, 23*(1), 18–21.

Thomas, R. L., & Powers, A. S. 2010. The role of the psychologist. In R.O. Weed & D.E. Berens (Eds.) *Life Care Planning and Case Management Handbook* 63–82. Boca Raton, FL: CRC Press.

Thombs, B. D., Haines, J. M., Bresnick, M. G., Magyar-Russell, G., Fauerbach, J. A., & Spence, R. J. 2007. Depression in burn reconstruction patients: symptom prevalence and association with body image dissatisfaction and physical function. *General Hospital Psychiatry, 29*(1), 14–20.

Van Loey, N. E., & Van Son, M. J. 2003. Psychopathology and psychological problems in patients with burn scars. *American Journal of Clinical Dermatology, 4*(4), 245–272.

Vowles, K. E., & McCracken, L. M. 2010. Comparing the role of psychological flexibility and traditional pain management coping strategies in chronic pain treatment outcomes. *Behaviour Research and Therapy, 48*(2), 141–146.

Wheeler, S. D., Lane, S. J., & McMahon, B. T. 2007. Community participation and life satisfaction following intensive, community-based rehabilitation using a life skills training approach. *OTJR: Occupation, Participation and Health, 27*(1), 13–22.

Wiechman, S. A., & Patterson, D. R. 2007. Psychosocial aspects of burn injuries. *BMJ*. 329: 391–393.

Williams, N. R., Davey, M., & Klock-Powell, K. 2003. Rising from the ashes: stories of recovery, adaptation and resiliency in burn survivors. *Social Work in Health Care, 36*(4), 53–77.

Wolpe, J. 1958. *Psychotherapy by Reciprocal Inhibition*. Stanford, CA: Stanford University Press.

Chapter 6

The Role of the Neuropsychologist in Life Care Planning

Carol Walker

Contents

Introduction 79
Selecting a Neuropsychologist 83
The Neuropsychological Examination 85
Case Study 91
References 102

Introduction

This chapter will provide a history of the field of neuropsychology beginning with the ancient view, progressing to the present and potential future of the field as the role of technology continues to change, and discussing advancements. It will also address the various roles for a neuropsychologist, focusing on utilization of the evaluation process to assist in treatment planning. The chapter will address how a life care planner might select a neuropsychologist with whom to consult, the elements of the neuropsychological evaluation, and the methods used by neuropsychologists for interpreting data obtained in a neuropsychological examination. Implications for life care planning will be discussed in terms of recommendations that may be made for treatment planning and methods to help to insure the evaluation is useful to the life care planner in developing the plan.

"Clinical neuropsychology is a specialty in professional psychology that applies principles of assessment and intervention based upon the scientific study of human behavior as it relates to normal and abnormal functioning of the central nervous system The specialty is dedicated to enhancing the understanding of brain–behavior relationships and the application of such knowledge to human problems" (CRSPPP, 2010). There is reliance upon the observation of changes in thoughts and behaviors that relates to the structural integrity of the brain, or more simply, a way of studying the brain indirectly by evaluating behaviors. While the field emerged in the 1930s in the United States, the concept of relationships between the brain and behavior predates this by many centuries. The Edwin Smith Papyrus, from 2500 to 3000 BC, represents the oldest written record of medical treatment (Fitzhugh-Bell, 1997). Among the cases described, Fitzhugh-Bell notes there are references to head and brain injuries. The descriptions suggest that brain functions are localized in specific areas of the brain. In the fifth century BC, Hippocrates of Kos (who is considered the father of modern medicine) postulated that diseases are physiological rather than punishment from the gods (Heilman & Valenstein, 1993). There was also recognition that the brain was the controlling center of the body and emotions. He was the first to recognize that paralysis occurred on the side of the body contralateral to the side of a head injury. Galen, a Greek physician, surgeon and philosopher in the Roman Empire, related mental functions to the ventricles of the brain, giving rise to the concept of the "humors" which persisted for 1000 years. Galen assigned mental functions, which were described by Aristotle (memory, attention, fantasy, reason), as well as common sense to locations in the ventricles (Freemon, 1994). Gall (1758–1828), neuroanatomist and physiologist, introduced the concept that the brain was comprised of discrete organs, each localized and responsible for a specific psychological trait. His concept, phrenology, correlated mental abilities to specific brain areas. Followers of Gall characterized individuals on the basis of skull shape and size and, by inference, brain size. Gall postulated that measurements of the skull might allow the deduction of moral and intellectual characteristics since the shape of the skull is modified by the underlying brain (Heilman & Valenstein, 1993). One example was Gall's observation that his student with good verbal memory had prominent eyes. Based on this observation, he suggested that memory for words was localized in the frontal lobes. As was the case with Galen's theory about humors, phrenology was not supported by studies. Despite the erroneous conclusions reached, Gall's phrenology represents the beginning of the modern-day localizationist doctrine.

In the late 1800s, Broca, a French physician, anatomist, and anthropologist, described the well-known case of "Tan," who was Broca's patient and suffered the effects of a left hemispheric stroke. While only able to utter the word "tan," he was able to accurately comprehend language. Broca used this case, in conjunction with others, to demonstrate that the expression of language is subserved by the left frontal lobe. This area subsequently became known as "Broca's area" and individuals with damage to Broca's area are referred to as having "Broca's aphasia."

Several years after Broca presented his findings regarding aphasia in frontal lobe lesions, Wernicke, a German physician, anatomist, psychiatrist, and neuropathologist, presented cases of patients with lesions in the superior posterior portion of the left hemisphere leading to language comprehension deficits. This finding led to the idea that the component processes of language were localized, and on this basis, the modern doctrine of component process localization and disconnection syndromes was begun. The doctrine states that complex mental functions, such as language, represent the combined processing of a number of subcomponent processes that are represented in widely diverse areas of the brain.

The advent of methods to visualize structures of the brain allowed for the opportunity to understand the structural and physiological concomitants of neurocognitive processes and neurological diseases (c.f. Bigler, 1996; Damasio & Damasio, 1989). Neuroimaging has gained widespread use in neuropsychological research and practice. Neuroimaging is not expected to replace neuropsychological testing. The well-established knowledge base of clinical and actuarial inferences derived from neuropsychological approaches is likely to remain salient given that implementations of advances in rehabilitation, forensics, and treatment planning remain basic functions of neuropsychologists (Benitez et al., 2014). Benitez and associates (2014) also caution against the tendency to overlook the inherent limitations of these relatively new neuroimaging technologies and to emphasize the neuroimaging findings over decades of data derived from neuropsychological research.

Ward Halstead (1908–1969) was a primary contributor in the development of the field of neuropsychology. He worked in collaboration with neurological surgeons to perform research that helped form the scientific basis for neuropsychological testing. He set up the first neuropsychology laboratory in the United States in 1935. He used neuropsychological testing to study the effects of different types of brain damage on various cognitive domains, as well as sensory and perceptual functioning. In the beginning, neuropsychological test results were used primarily for lesion localization. Prior to utilizing the testing, Halstead observed individuals with brain damage in a variety of real-world settings in order to determine the types of problems they experienced. He then assembled a battery of 10 tests, which were administered to these patients (Sbordone et al., 2007). In collaboration with his student, the late Ralph Reitan, Halstead created the Halstead–Reitan Battery. In one early study, the Halstead–Reitan Neuropsychological Battery (HNRB) compared computerized tomography, electroencephalograms, and the HNRB and found that the HNRB interpretation had the highest degree of accuracy in identifying brain damage (Yantz et al., 2006). According to a survey of assessment practices and test usage patterns among clinical neuropsychologists completed in 2005, this battery remains the sixth most commonly used assessment instrument (Rabin et al., 2005). The Boston Approach, which was developed at the Boston VA by Harold Goodglass, Edith Kaplan, and Nelson Butters, focuses on a qualitative strategy. This approach relies heavily on behavioral observations during the performance of a task. Another prominent figure in the field of neuropsychology is Alexander Luria. He developed a theory of brain–behavior relationships that postulated complex behavior may be reduced to the individual components and studied to determine what functional system had been damaged (Luria, 1973). In collaboration with Anne-Lise Christensen, a Danish psychologist, his testing method was introduced in the United States, in 1981 by Charles Golden. There is not a commercial source for this battery at present.

Neuropsychology is based in two primary fields of study, neurology and psychometrics (Russell, 1986). Neuropsychology was first recognized as a discipline separate from psychology or neurology in the 1960s when Klove used the term "neuropsychology" in the English biomedical literature and with the inception of the International Neuropsychological Society in 1967 (Bilder, 2011). There has been considerable research in the area of neuropsychology, especially since the 1970s. There are no other areas in psychology where there is a greater empirical research base (Russell, 1986). While diagnosis has remained one focus of neuropsychological testing, it has been supplanted as a primary diagnostic tool to a large degree by the advent of advanced neuroimaging techniques such as CT and MRI (see Bigler, 1996). However, since neuropsychological testing and evaluation remain the most sensitive measure of brain function, there is continuing utilization of evaluations for measuring function since even the most sensitive imaging will not provide the nature and quantification of behavioral strengths and deficits in a particular case.

Additionally, as documented in Lezak et al. (2004), neuropsychological testing can be helpful in discriminating psychiatric versus neurological symptoms, identifying possible neurological disorders, distinguishing between neurological disorders, and providing input regarding localization of lesion sites, at least to a hemispheric level. While the role of neuropsychological evaluation in lesion localization has largely been supplanted by advanced neuroimaging, a neuropsychological evaluation of cognitive abilities and skills that is well-done can provide the foundation for not only accurate diagnosis but also useful recommendations for treatment, which can be applied clinically. Recommendations may include individual psychotherapy, family psychotherapy, psychiatric interventions, behavioral interventions, training and coaching, special education services, and specialized needs such as services provided by other professionals (e.g., occupational therapy, neuro-ophthalmology, speech therapy, neurological consultations, dietary consultations).

Many patients are referred for neuropsychological evaluation to assess their cognitive strengths and weaknesses, and to obtain information about behavioral alterations and personality characteristics. Assisting with adjustment to an individual's disability for the patient, their family, and/or their caregiver is also within the purview of the neuropsychologist. Primarily, this role consists of educating the family, caregiver, and patient regarding the effects of the neurological condition on the individual's behavior. This education and a full description of the patient's abilities, deficits, prognosis, and need for rehabilitation are crucial for the best adjustment of the entire family. Without this information, it is difficult for families and others to make plans for future care, need for and degree of supervision, and other management issues for a patient with acquired brain injury or other neurological dysfunction. The neuropsychologist may answer questions regarding an individual's capacity to care for himself or herself, ability to follow a therapeutic regimen independently, cognitive capacity to operate a motor vehicle, and ability to manage personal financial matters. A neuropsychologist is also frequently called on to assess an individual regarding their cognitive capacity for competence in probate hearings. The American Psychological Association (APA) and the American Bar Association (ABA) have collaborated to develop a document to provide a framework for these evaluations in older adults (ABA/APA, 2008). There are separate documents for psychologists, attorneys, and judges. The overall methodology is often used by neuropsychologists performing capacity evaluations on younger individuals as well. It requires not only that one address cognitive capabilities but link those capabilities to functional tasks as well.

Provision of information to patients regarding their deficits is imperative but must be done in a respectful manner. In those individuals with appreciation of their deficits, there is often depression and mistrust (Lezak et al., 2004). In those individuals who exhibit anosognosia, which is a lack of awareness of deficits (or simply, "I don't know what I don't know"), informing their caregivers and others with whom they routinely interact of deficits may facilitate improved interpersonal relationships. Those individuals with brain injury and lack of self-awareness are at greatest risk for acting-out and self-injurious behaviors. This lack of self-awareness is not analogous to psychological denial. It is more often a function of frontal lobe/executive dysfunction or other brain lesion. These individuals may be at risk of engaging in illegal activities, either due to impulsivity and poor judgment or vulnerability to the influence of others. Because of deficits in executive functioning they may not recognize when others are taking advantage of them. Many of them have lost relationships with people they interacted with prior to the injury and due to loneliness are vulnerable in multiple environmental contexts.

Follow-up neuropsychological testing allows for a determination of changes in the neuropsychological status of an individual. It may also be used to determine the effects of treatment and cognitive remediation strategies. In those individuals whose symptoms are being treated with medications, repeat testing might also help determine the effects of the medication on cognitive functioning. For example, their cognitive abilities may improve due to behavioral stability, better sleep patterns, or reduced depression or anxiety or, conversely, cognitive abilities may decline due to adverse side effects of medications. Neuropsychological testing can also be used to assist in educational placement, curriculum planning, and recommendations to maximize learning. The neuropsychologist may be able to serve as a liaison between the school and the family to provide for a smoother transition for the student, cognitively and behaviorally. It is also the case that the neuropsychologist, particularly one who has been involved with the individual during rehabilitation, is likely to be helpful in developing a behavior management program should one be required.

Neuropsychological assessment can also provide information regarding an individual's ability to participate and, more importantly, benefit from rehabilitation treatment. The questions of whether an individual obtains benefits and of whether that benefit has psychological and social value and is maintained long enough to warrant the cost can be answered by repeat neuropsychological testing (Solberg & Mateer, 1989).

While some neuropsychologists provide assessment only, others provide treatment to individuals with acquired brain injury, other neurological disorders, chronic pain, and post-traumatic stress disorder. In these cases, a primary goal is often to address the behaviors of the patient with a brain injury. Common postmorbid behaviors include irritability, egocentrism, impulsivity, and other behaviors that lead to high levels of stress on the family. Family members are often included in sessions with the patient, or seen independently, to help them better understand changes in their injured family member and to more effectively cope with the effects not only on the injured patient but also on the entire family. Neuropsychologists who practice in rehabilitation settings, whether acute or postacute, are often involved in education with family members throughout the patient's admission, to help pave the way for a smoother transition at discharge. They are also part of the rehabilitation team and provide input regarding behavioral and cognitive issues. They are often called upon during acute and postacute rehabilitation to develop behavior management programs when behaviors interfere with the patient's progress.

Cognitive remediation is an area where some neuropsychologists are involved in either helping to develop treatment strategies or as a provider of service. This is an area where additional research is needed to determine the strategies, duration of treatment, and other factors that influence outcome. A committee from the National Academy of Science found limited evidence regarding the effectiveness of cognitive remediation training (Koehler et al., 2011). However, the committee members opined that this does not indicate the effectiveness of limited and supported ongoing clinical applications of the interventions for individuals with cognitive and behavioral deficits. They also recommended emphasis on functional patient centered outcomes. Ben-Yishay and Diller (2011) describe their holistic neuropsychological rehabilitation program. This program has been providing a therapeutic community type of day program for three decades. The interventions of the program are directed toward helping the person to compensate for basic deficits such as impulse control issues, initiation, persistence, focusing and maintaining attention-concentration, information processing, and problems with emotional adaptation to injury and interpersonal difficulties. They also seek to organize the environment to minimize failure in coping. There are other programs that use the model developed by Dr. Ben-Yishay and Dr. Diller. This approach was described in the book *Over My Head: A Doctor's Own Story of Head Injury from the Inside Looking Out.*

Selecting a Neuropsychologist

How should one go about selecting a neuropsychologist for a specific case? Division 40 of the American Psychological Association (APA) published a definition of a neuropsychologist in *The Clinical Neuropsychologist* (March 22, 1989). This definition was adopted by the Division 40 Executive Committee and reviewed and accepted again in re-approved 2003. The necessary education attributes are listed and a definition of a neuropsychologist is given therein. This definition stressed that attainment of the diplomate in clinical neuropsychology from the American Board of Clinical Neuropsychology "is the clearest evidence of competence as a clinical neuropsychologist assuring that all of these criteria have been met." A listing of clinical neuropsychologists who have obtained this board certification may be found at www.abpp.org under the Directory. The American Board of Professional Neuropsychology, which is another certifying body for neuropsychologists, has a listing of their diplomates at http://abn-board.com. Both of these certifying bodies require appropriate education and training for a neuropsychologist to become certified. This is not to suggest that there are not many excellent, well-trained, and experienced neuropsychologists who are not board certified. However, if seeking a neuropsychologist in a particular area, their peers have evaluated those who are board certified by either of the previously described boards, and their work has been found to meet the established criteria for expertise. This being the case, when there are no personal recommendations available, this allows greater assurance of the training and expertise of the neuropsychologist. It is important to ensure that the neuropsychologist being chosen for referral has not received board certification through a so-called vanity board. These boards provide certifications without regard for competence or training in neuropsychology. Because there are no criteria for determining competency by these vanity boards, any psychologist who holds such credentials should have their qualifications thoroughly assessed before a referral is made to them for an evaluation.

Additional information regarding the necessary education and training in clinical neuropsychology, as well as the description of the scope of practice is available at the following resources:

- Policy Statement, Houston Conference on Specialty Education and Training in Clinical Neuropsychology (1998), www.div40org/pub/Houston_conference.pdf
- National Academy of Neuropsychology, "Definition of a Neuropsychologist," http://nanonline.org/downloads/paio/Position/NAN PositionDefNeuro.pdf

While there are a number of educational requirements for neuropsychologists, the experience each brings to a particular disorder differs. This being the case, it is incumbent when making a referral for a neuropsychological examination to determine the experience of the neuropsychologist in the particular area of interest. In the case of children, it is important that the neuropsychologist have experience in working with children of the same age as the child to be evaluated. In children, not only the disorder but the developmental stage of the child must be considered. The application of adult brain behavior relationship is not consistently appropriate. Family and socio-environmental issues are often more complex with evaluating children or adolescents. While it is helpful to utilize a pediatric neuropsychologist, there is not always an available specialist in every area of the country. The American Board of Clinical Neuropsychology has a subspecialty board certification for Pediatric Neuropsychologists that can be located on the website noted earlier. The American Academy of Pediatric Neuropsychology (AAPdN) also has a listing of their board certified specialists found at www.theaapn.org. If no pediatric specialist is available, it may be useful to determine the number of evaluations provided for children and adolescents in a year performed by the neuropsychologist to whom a referral is to be made.

Sbordone et al. (2007) note that the theoretical orientation of the neuropsychologist influences the outcome of the evaluation. These authors cite information from a 1986 article (Sbordone & Rudd, 1986) which reportedly found that psychologists with certain theoretical treatment orientations were less likely to recognize underlying neurological disorders. Sbordone et al. (2007) also report the 1986 study found that the training environment of the neuropsychologists influenced how they viewed cases. These authors further note that many neuropsychologists have little or no experience in the rehabilitation of individuals with acquired brain injury. Because of the lack of experience, opinions regarding the relative permanence of cognitive problems and ability to return to competitive employment, school, or household responsibilities are opined to be often inaccurate or inappropriate. Sbordone and his colleagues further noted that most psychologists are unfamiliar with cognitive rehabilitation techniques and have minimal to no experience training people to use compensatory strategies and techniques to maximize behavioral and cognitive functioning following brain injury. When these neuropsychologists perform evaluations or make recommendations, Sbordone et al. (2007) state the opinions are often overly pessimistic. These authors note that rehabilitation neuropsychologists, on the other hand, may be overly optimistic about the potential for improvement.

Another issue to address in looking at the opinions of a neuropsychologist is that person's role in the case. This may be particularly important in obtaining information as a life care planner. If the neuropsychologist is the treating neuropsychologist, he or she may have had limited background records, especially pre-injury records, and may not have performed as detailed an evaluation as would be the situation if the injured person was referred for a forensic evaluation and the neuropsychologist was acting as an expert. There are a number of differences between the roles of a treating psychologist and expert psychologist. It is beyond the scope of this chapter to address all of these differences. However, for interested readers, they are delineated in a paper by Greenberg and Shuman (1997).

Overall, when selecting a neuropsychologist, it is important to ensure that the provider is appropriately trained and has the skills necessary to evaluate the individual for whom referral is sought. Client factors to be considered include ethnicity, age, and presenting diagnosis. Important provider factors to consider include the training environment of the neuropsychologist, the experience in clinical neuropsychology, as well as knowledge and experience in the disorder and referral questions, the theoretical orientation of the neuropsychologist, and his or her forensic experience. Board certification, by either ABCN, ABN, or AAPdN, provides external validation that the individual has undergone examination by his or her peers in terms of neuropsychological competence. This is not to suggest they are the only competent neuropsychologists, but it gives one greater confidence when referring to a neuropsychologist about whom one knows very little. In many cases it is important that the neuropsychologist understand the medicolegal issues involved in the case. It is important that the neuropsychologist understand the legal constructs and the case law governing the evaluation. For example, some states allow third-party observers during examinations conducted by the defense. Some states do not allow neuropsychologists to testify regarding the cause of a neurological condition such as brain injury but are limited to opining whether the findings are "consistent with" the diagnosis. The neuropsychologist should be made aware if a case is involved in litigation to ensure a willingness to become involved.

The Neuropsychological Examination

While most neuropsychologists rely largely on standardized test data, these data alone do not provide all of the information needed to fully assess an individual. There is a need to consider information from subjective sources, objective sources, and collateral sources. Subjective information includes information provided by the patient, family members, and caregivers, which cannot be verified with other data. It often includes complaints of physical, emotional, and/or cognitive difficulties. Family members and caregivers often relate the patient's complaints of their feelings or physical distress but may also provide, or be able to provide, with appropriate questioning, objective data. Beyond relating what they have been told about how the patient feels, they may have extensive knowledge of patterns of behavior, sleeping habits, eating habits, personality changes, and interpersonal relationship changes. Objective information includes information from school records, medical records, vocational records, neuropsychological and psychological test data, and any other data from either before the injury, where possible, or post-injury. The individual's social history, including educational and work experiences, provides information about premorbid cognitive potential. Marital history also provides relevant information and may tell a great deal about emotional stability, social judgment, and relationship stability over time. Assessment of the individual's current life circumstances also provides information about how the individual is currently functioning and how they are adapting to changes.

Comparison of an individual's functioning pre- and post-injury helps to delineate the changes since the injury and helps in treatment planning. Medical history and current medical status provide information about the individual's premorbid history. Medications that have been prescribed, or dosage modifications required, may also provide some understanding of how functioning has changed over time. Another important source of information is the observation of the examinee during the testing process. While testing may be performed by either a technician or the neuropsychologist, there is often a large amount of information gathered during the examination process, which lasts from several hours to days in some instances. For instance, how an individual approaches a task may give a significant amount of information beyond that provided by the test score alone. For example, the degree of disrupted behaviors in a quiet, one-to-one setting is likely to be magnified in a work, school, social, or even home environment. How an individual responds to success or failure on testing provides information regarding the potential for perseverance in the face of frustrating tasks. Behaviors that occur during the testing, again in a setting designed to obtain the person's best performance, are highly important in understanding his or her ability to function outside the testing environment. While some neuropsychologists break up the testing sessions over several days to minimize the effects of fatigue, how the person functions early in the day versus when they are tired may be more useful in predicting overall ability to return to school or work. Using all available data allows the neuropsychologist to develop a picture of how the person functioned before and after an injury or illness. Failure to consider this information may lead to spurious conclusions by the neuropsychologist. For example, this author tested an individual who reported having completed 12 years of education. The individual further stated he was a high school graduate and an average student. On testing, his intellect was measured to fall in the low end of the borderline range and academic assessment revealed reading in the extremely low range (no school records were available prior to the examination). When school records were provided, it was determined he had not obtained a diploma but a certificate of attendance. He had also been in special education beginning in elementary school. If only the results of testing had been considered, his deficits would have been overstated. The converse may also occur if the neuropsychologist is not aware of past history; an individual with a high level of functioning may not be identified as having changes in cognitive abilities if there is no attempt to determine premorbid level of function.

The assessment dynamics should be predicated on the referral questions. It is often the case that the referral questions are related to an individual's ability to work or return to school. Questions regarding the need for competency to manage financial affairs or make other cognitive decisions are also often asked of neuropsychologists. Lezak et al. (2004) note that examination questions fall into two categories: diagnostic questions and descriptive questions. Diagnostic questions are generally asked when the etiology of cognitive or behavioral problems is unknown. These are usually questions of differential diagnosis. Descriptive questions are those asking about specific abilities and often arise in vocational and educational planning. These authors note these questions are especially important if the planning involves withdrawal or return of normal adult rights and privileges, such as driving or legal competence. In these cases, the neuropsychological examination will focus on the relevant skills and functions. Other areas of assessment include awareness of one's condition and capacity to incorporate new information and skills.

Tests are typically selected that meet criteria for reliability and validity and have norms appropriate for the individual being assessed. There are some neuropsychologists who use a fixed battery approach; this approach is exemplified by the Halstead–Reitan Battery. Most neuropsychologists use a flexible battery approach to address the referral question(s). In a flexible battery a selection of tests to measure the various domains of cognitive functioning are combined. Rabin et al. (2005) have a list of the tests most commonly used by neuropsychologists. Typically, multiple measures in each cognitive domain are employed. The cognitive domains that are often assessed include intellectual abilities, attention/concentration, speed of cognitive information processing, memory and learning, speech and language, academic functioning, motor functioning, visual spatial functioning, response bias and effort, executive function, mood, personality, and adaptive functioning.

Another element of the examination is determining the pre-injury baseline of the individual. It is relatively unusual to have someone who has had a previous full neuropsychological examination unless they have suffered a previous injury or neurological illness. Neuropsychologists must try to ascertain how the person might have functioned in the past to develop a benchmark to which current test scores are compared. While most of the population functions in the average range, the individuals whose scores premorbidly fall at the ends of the distribution pose a challenge. If an individual functioned at the upper end of the distribution, even milder changes may affect their ability to function, at least in a vocational sense. For example, a neurosurgeon with mild injuries is likely to have greater difficulty vocationally than an individual who does not deal with complex life or death issues on a daily basis. If an individual was functioning marginally pre-injury, then she may have greater difficulty coping than would be the case for someone who functions at a higher level. These individuals have fewer cognitive reserves and thus do not have the cognitive resources to adapt as well. There are several regression equations that have been developed to estimate premorbid intellect (e.g., the Barona equation). Another method frequently used is reading ability (Johnstone et al., 1996). There is an obvious difficulty in using this method in cases of premorbid reading difficulties or where the person has sustained damage to reading centers of the left hemisphere. However, given that reading is learned relatively early in development, and is then overlearned as part of the education process, it provides one measure of premorbid abilities in many cases.

Consideration must also be given to factors other than brain damage, which may affect test results. These include motivation, fatigue, pain, depression, anxiety, and litigation. These factors, either singly or in combination, may affect results of testing to varying degrees. Neuropsychologists are encouraged to use measures of performance validity to assess, to the degree possible, the person's motivation during a neuropsychological examination performed in a forensic context (c.f. National Academy of Neuropsychology [NAN] position paper).

The situation where there is a need for an interpreter is another issue that may impact test results. There are some tests that are available in other languages, for example Spanish, with appropriate norms for populations of individuals who speak that language. However, the use of an interpreter to administer test questions translated from English into another language should be applied judiciously. There is a high likelihood that the test will not render fully valid or reliable results. The problem is multifactorial; first, the accuracy of the interpretation cannot be determined. Second, the tests often have cultural biases inherent in testing. Third, the norms for the test may not be appropriate for the individual being tested. The greater the difference between the individual being tested and the normative sample, the less reliance one may place on the outcome. However, there are situations where it is not possible to find a neuropsychologist who fluently speaks the language of the patient. In these cases, the choice becomes one of either making no attempt to assess the individual or using an interpreter. Some authors have argued there are ethical considerations in testing someone whose language we do not speak (Artiola et al., 1998); this should be given due consideration before doing so. It is the practice of this author to refer to a neuropsychologist who speaks the language of the patient. If this is not possible, a clinical interview is completed using an interpreter. Tests that have been shown to have limited cultural bias are then administered

(Lezak et al., 2004). Even with this caution, the results cannot be considered fully reliable or valid but may provide some useful information regarding function. Knowledge of the individual's culture becomes highly important in these situations as behaviors may be misinterpreted.

There are multiple neurobehavioral variables and diagnostic issues to be considered in the neuropsychological evaluation (Lezak et al., 2004). These variables include lesion characteristics, subject variables, and psychosocial variables. For example, there are changes in cognitive abilities related to the aging process. The relationship between moderate to severe TBI and later development of dementia has been well-documented in the research literature. However, there are epidemiological studies that do not reach this conclusion (Smith et al., 2013). Additional research is needed to elucidate the issue. An individual's premorbid personality and social adjustment also play a role in outcome. Research has shown that premorbid personality is not so often changed as much as it is exaggerated by brain injury. It is easy to see how the impulsivity, difficulty with anger management, and disinhibition associated with frontal lobe damage are complicated in an individual whose premorbid self-regulation of behavior was poor. Emotional difficulties, such as depression, may also complicate the clinical presentation of an individual with brain injury. It is important that the neuropsychologist identify depression, both premorbid and postmorbid, as it may complicate recovery; in addition, the patient may lack the initiative or cognitive ability to seek help on his/her own. The partial or complete loss of independence experienced by an individual with brain injury may also complicate testing, for example, due to uncooperative behavior, passive-aggressive behavior, fear of failure, or fear of additional loss of independence.

It is helpful to have a series of questions for the neuropsychologist to addres. (*Editors' note:* See also the checklist of questions to ask the neuropsychologist in Chapter 4, The Role of the Vocational Rehabilitation Counselor). Ensuring that they are questions that can be appropriately answered is paramount to increase the utility of the examination. Receiving a report that documents the potential location of the lesion is not likely to be as helpful in determining life care planning needs as would be a report detailing the functional abilities of the individual with brain injury. One way to obtain the needed information is to ask the neuropsychologist a series of specific questions. For example, Uomoto (2000) states it is easier for a neuropsychologist to answer whether a person can perform a specific task of a specific job than to answer whether they can return to work. One of the most salient issues in answering questions posed has to do with the ecological validity of testing. Sbordone (1997) defines ecological validity as the "functional and predictive relationship between the patient's performance on a set of neuropsychological tests and behavior in a variety of real-world settings." Providing the neuropsychologists with information regarding the demands of the environment allows for a better assessment of how the demands interact with the individual's cognitive strengths and weaknesses, premorbid abilities and skills, and future goals. Without this information, the predictions made based on test data alone have a significant likelihood of being inaccurate. In his article on ecological validity, Sbordone notes the importance of obtaining a detailed history and interviewing collateral sources, the importance of behavioral observations, using appropriate norms, and the relevance of test scores to real-world settings. Sbordone cites the review of Acker in 1990, which examined the question of how neuropsychological tests related to real-world behavior. Acker reportedly found moderate correlations between test results and various functional assessments. She also noted the findings varied according to when during the recovery period the tests were administered. When attempts are made to correlate neuropsychological test results with Activities of Daily Living, the complex tests appear to be better predictors. It seems that the most effective method to increase predictive ability is to ascertain the degree to which test data are consistent with data from other sources (medical records, family observations, academic records, vocational records, and observation of the patient's behavior in a variety of settings). The degree of agreement between these sources then provides an "operational estimate of our test data" (Sbordone, 1997). If the test data do not fit with the other data, then the ecological validity would be considered low. Neuropsychological test data with a higher level of concordance would be considered to have higher ecological validity.

With these considerations, it is possible to obtain ecologically valid predictions from neuropsychological testing. There have been a number of instances where questions were raised about the value of a neuropsychological examination. In many of those cases, it is likely the neuropsychologist performed a general examination and not one designed to answer specific questions. When a patient is referred by a physician for a clinical evaluation (particularly an outpatient evaluation), the examination may not include review of the objective information and supplemental records listed earlier in this chapter (e.g., educational records, medical records). The neuropsychologist is in the role of treating neuropsychologist and will often complete the examination without collateral information other than that provided by a family member who accompanies the patient (if the patient allows their participation). It is often the case, particularly early in the recovery process, that the family is overwhelmed by changes that have occurred in their lifestyle. This may lead to faulty information being provided. For example, the family may not be able to accurately assess deficits due to their own emotional overload. If the patient lacks insight, his or her view of self has a high probability of being inaccurate. This being the case, records should be provided to the neuropsychologist prior to the testing and reviewed by the neuropsychologist prior to answering the referral questions. Making the questions specific helps the neuropsychologist to answer more helpfully. For example, the individual may be able to sustain attention in an environment with minimal distractions but have difficulty if he is asked to perform in a work cubicle environment where multiple telephone conversations are taking place simultaneously. Describing the environment to the neuropsychologist is likely to increase his or her ability to make accurate predictions. When asked about the need for supervision, it is often helpful to ask rehabilitation neuropsychologists this question in terms of Functional Independence Measure Scores (FIMS) developed by Smith, Hamilton, and Granger in 1990. For neuropsychologists who are unfamiliar with FIMS, using the descriptors from the scale (e.g., unable to perform an activity or independence in performing an activity) may be useful. It may also be useful to ask about specific tasks that may require supervision such as the self-administration of medications, ability to be left alone with a young child, ability to manage finances, ability to make financial decisions, or ability to make safety decisions. Another avenue would be to ask questions that would be necessary to answer if the person were being evaluated with regard to civil competence.

In summary, when choosing a neuropsychologist for referral, determine the best person for the referral based on education and expertise in the area of interest. Ask specific questions. Rather than "Can he/she return to work?"—ask questions about specific tasks and demands in the environment. Provision of a job description may be helpful but often is too general to be useful. Also, ask about potential barriers, such as those imposed by fatigue or behavioral issues. When asking about the ability to live independently, focusing on specific areas requiring independence rather than a global question of independence is likely to yield more precise information.

To avoid receiving a report that does not answer your questions, provide the referral questions before the neuropsychological examination. If not, you may receive a report that describes the person's strengths and deficits and behavioral deficits, which may not be useful for the life care plan recommendations. In many cases, the neuropsychologist may be able to answer your questions after the fact; however, having the questions beforehand may help guide test selection and interview questions. For example, there are specific tests and techniques employed in evaluations of civil competency; knowing that questions regarding independent living skills will be raised may lead test selection in a somewhat different direction. It also ensures that the neuropsychologist does not, after the fact, say they cannot provide specific answers to the questions.

When should neuropsychological testing be administered for use in a life care plan? Most of the natural recovery following acquired brain injury occurs in the first 6 months after an injury. The degree of recovery is affected by a number of factors including premorbid abilities, age, and family support. It is generally the case that an adult with brain injury is reevaluated every 6 months until the end of 2 years or until the treating neuropsychologist determines the patient's deficits are unlikely to significantly change. Research tends to support permanence of deficits at the end of 2 years (Lezak et al., 2004). However, there are studies documenting significant cognitive improvement for up to 3 years post-injury when cognitive remediation is provided (Berrol, 1990).

The course of recovery is more complex in children. Children with moderate to severe brain injury have been shown to have cognitive and behavioral deficits that can persist over a span of several years. As the child matures, and additional cognitive skills and behaviors are expected to develop, a secondary impact of the brain injury may become apparent. In these cases, in addition to follow-up for 2 years post-injury, having evaluations completed at academic transition periods is recommended. Specifically, evaluations at the end of third grade, fifth grade, eighth grade, and tenth grade are likely to be helpful in guiding academics. For those individuals for whom postsecondary education is expected, additional neuropsychological examination is recommended after completion of high school. In the situation where a child is in special education, the results of neuropsychological evaluation may help in developing and/or implementing the individualized education program (IEP). The results of testing can also help to determine services needed, beyond those mandated by the Individuals with Disabilities Education Act (IDEA) and provided by the school system, to maximize the child's ability to benefit from education. (For more information on this technical topic, visit www2.ed.gov/parents/needs/speced/iepguide/index.html.)

Once the patient's deficits have reached a level where additional change is not anticipated, an additional neuropsychological examination is included as the patient ages. There are declines in cognition that occur as a function of normal aging. In addition to these normal changes, those individuals who have experienced a more severe brain injury are found to be at higher risk for developing dementia in some studies (e.g., Fleminger et al., 2003).

Psychotherapy, either with a neuropsychologist or other mental health professional with training and experience in acquired brain injury, is likely to be required. In adults, this is likely to be needed periodically throughout their life expectancy, especially during periods of stress or when they are confronted with situations that are changed by the impact of their injury and subsequent deficits. An example would be a parent who loses custody of a child because of a brain injury or the stress of having to move in with family after living independently.

The disruptive effect of acquired brain injury has been well-documented in the literature (Kreutzer et al., 1992). Family members and other caregivers, particularly in the cases where there are negative behavioral changes, will require education, support, and therapy to cope. Rosenthal and Geckler (1997) note that the primary focus, until more recently, was on the physical aspects of the injury. The issues of psychosocial and family adjustment have since been recognized with regard to the effect on progress in rehabilitation and overall recovery. Family support and pre-injury family environment have been shown to have significant effects on outcome in children following traumatic brain injury (Yeates et al., 1997; Max et al., 1999). Anecdotally, it is the experience of this author that families may have a prolonged period of grief related to the changes that accrue following a brain injury. This may result in their attributing deficits in executive function exhibited by the individual who has residual symptoms of brain damage to volitional behavior. Conversely, feelings of guilt, empathy, or fear may lead them to reinforce negative behaviors to avoid confrontation. There are myriad other family and social difficulties where psychological intervention may help improve the quality of life for the patient and family or caregivers.

In the case where the person with the injury is a child, parents benefit from therapy to help with parenting skills, as well as help in adjusting to changes in the child's current behavior and future goals and aspirations. Additional psychotherapy sessions may be needed during puberty and through the teenage years when sexual issues need to be addressed and if no injury or illness had occurred, the child would have been expected to have become increasingly independent.

Case Study

The following tables are excerpted from a Life Care Plan for a woman who sustained a severe traumatic brain injury in a motor vehicle collision. Since the accident, she has had multiple cognitive symptoms, consistent with diffuse brain injury and specific injury to the right frontal lobe. She also has significant physical limitations that impair her abilities in performance of activities other than basic Activities of Daily Living (ADLs). The recommendations were obtained through consultations with her treating physiatrist and neuropsychologist. Consultation was also held with a medical case manager to determine appropriate recommendations for Ms. Smith's ongoing needs in this domain. The life care planning tables are displayed in SaddlePoint Software, LLC format (format reprinted by permission, William Walker, 256-651-5445).

Life Care Plan Tables
for
Belinda L. Smith

Old Desert Drive
Yuma, AZ

Date of Birth: 04/28/1979

Event Date: 09/30/2015

Primary Disability: Multiple Trauma

Preparation Date: December 12, 2017

NeuroLife, LLC
Carol P. Walker, PhD, ABPP-CN, CLCP
PO Box 4647
Huntsville, AL 35815

256-535-2322

Prepared By: Carol P. Walker, PhD, ABPP-CN, CLCP

Projected Evaluations

Item or Service	Purpose	Replacement Schedule	Start / End	Costs
Case Manager 1 Options 1, 2	The case manager will assist in appointment scheduling and other activities associated with medical care. The case manager will also assist in hiring and monitoring attendant care.	1 Time Only	# Start Age/Year 38 2017 # End Age/Year 38 2017	Cost/Unit $85.00 to $99.00 Cost/Year $340.00 to $396.00

Cost/Year = 4/1 x $85.00 = $340.00
Cost/Year = 4/1 x $99.00 = $396.00
Cost/Year Average = ($340.00 + $396.00) ÷ 2 = $368.00

Item or Service	Purpose	Replacement Schedule	Start / End	Costs
Family/Guardian Counseling and Education 2 Options 1, 2	Assist immediate family with coping skills.	1 Time/ Year	# Start Age/Year 38 2017 # End Age/Year 38 2017	Cost/Unit $198.00 to $248.00 Cost/Year $198.00 to $248.00

CPT 90791

Cost/Year Average = ($198.00 + $248.00) ÷ 2 = $223.00

Growth Trends to be determined by an Economist.
*LE = Life Expectancy **U = Unknown N/A = Not Applicable
All Ages and Dates are Inclusive, e.g. 2000-2006 = 7 Years

Prepared By: Carol P. Walker, PhD, ABPP-CN, CLCP

Projected Evaluations

Item or Service	Purpose	Replacement Schedule	Start End	Costs
Home Assessment 3 Option 1	Professional assessment of home for safety issues.	1 Time Only	# Start Age/Year 38 2017 # End Age/Year 38 2017	Cost/Unit $51.00 to $60.00 Cost/Year $816.00 to $960.00

This is for four hours of either a PT or an OT to assess her home for safety issues that may be addressed in addition to home modifications. Additional assessment may be needed if she moves to another home.
Cost/Year = 16/1 x $51.00 = $816.00
Cost/Year = 16/1 x $60.00 = $960.00
Cost/Year Average = ($816.00 + $960.00) ÷ 2 = $888.00

Item or Service	Purpose	Replacement Schedule	Start End	Costs
Psychologist 4 Options 1, 2	Evaluation in anticipation of therapy and to develop a plan of care.	1 Time Only	# Start Age/Year 38 2017 # End Age/Year 38 2017	Cost/Unit $198.00 to $248.00 Cost/Year $198.00 to $248.00

Cost/Year Average = ($198.00 + $248.00) ÷ 2 = $223.00

Item or Service	Purpose	Replacement Schedule	Start End	Costs
Occupational Therapy Evaluation 5 Option 1	Assess ongoing equipment needs and ADLs.	1 Time/ Year	# Start Age/Year 38 2017 # End Age/Year 70 2049	Cost/Unit $117.00 to $143.00 Cost/Year $117.00 to $143.00

Cost/Year Average = ($117.00 + $143.00) ÷ 2 = $130.00

Life Care PlanTables for Belinda L. Smith

Growth Trends to be determined by an Economist.
*LE = Life Expectancy **U = Unknown N/A = Not Applicable
All Ages and Dates are Inclusive, e.g. 2000-2006 = 7 Years

Prepared By: Carol P. Walker, PhD, ABPP-CN, CLCP

Projected Evaluations

Item or Service	Purpose	Replacement Schedule	Start End	Costs
Physical Therapy Evaluation 6 Option 1	Assess status and make recommendations regarding physical therapy needs.	1 Time/ Year	# Start Age/Year 38 2017	Cost/Unit $121.00 to $148.00
			# End Age/Year 70 2049	Cost/Year $121.00 to $148.00

Cost/Year Average = ($121.00 + $148.00) ÷ 2 = $134.50

Life Care PlanTables for Belinda L. Smith

Growth Trends to be determined by an Economist.

*LE = Life Expectancy **U = Unknown N/A = Not Applicable

All Ages and Dates are Inclusive, e.g. 2000-2006 = 7 Years

Prepared By: Carol P. Walker, PhD, ABPP-CN, CLCP

Projected Therapeutic Modalities

Item or Service	Purpose	Replacement Schedule	Start / End	Costs
Case Management - Home Care Setup 1 Option 1	The case manager will assist in appointment scheduling and other activities associated with medical care. The case manager will also assist in hiring and monitoring attendant care.	1 Time Only	# Start Age/Year 38 2017 # End Age/Year 38 2017	Cost/Unit $85.00 to $99.00 Cost/Year $850.00 to $990.00

This recommendation was obtained from J. Bragg, a Certified Case Manager.

Cost/Year = 10/1 x $85.00 = $850.00
Cost/Year = 10/1 x $99.00 = $990.00
Cost/Year Average = ($850.00 + $990.00) ÷ 2 = $920.00

Item or Service	Purpose	Replacement Schedule	Start / End	Costs
Case Management 2 Option 1	The case manager will assist in appointment scheduling and other activities associated with medical care. The case manager will also assist in hiring and monitoring attendant care.	2 - 4 Hours/ Month	# Start Age/Year 38 2017 # End Age/Year 70 2049	Cost/Unit $85.00 to $99.00 Cost/Year $2,040.00 to $4,752.00

Cost/Year = $85.00 x 2 x 12 = $2,040.00
Cost/Year = $99.00 x 2 x 12 = $2,376.00
Cost/Year = $85.00 x 4 x 12 = $4,080.00
Cost/Year = $99.00 x 4 x 12 = $4,752.00
Cost/Year Average = ($2,040.00 + $4,752.00) ÷ 2 = $3,396.00

Growth Trends to be determined by an Economist.
*LE = Life Expectancy **U = Unknown N/A = Not Applicable
All Ages and Dates are Inclusive, e.g. 2000-2006 = 7 Years

Prepared By: Carol P. Walker, PhD, ABPP-CN, CLCP

Projected Therapeutic Modalities

Item or Service	Purpose	Replacement Schedule	Start / End	Costs
Case Manager Facility Setup	The case manager will assist in arranging aspects of facility care.	1 Time Only	# Start Age/Year 38 2017	Cost/Unit $85.00 to $99.00
3 Option 2			# End Age/Year 38 2017	Cost/Year $510.00 to $594.00

This recommendation was obtained from J. Bragg, a Certified Case Manager.

Cost/Year = 6/1 x $85.00 = $510.00
Cost/Year = 6/1 x $99.00 = $594.00
Cost/Year Average = ($510.00 + $594.00) ÷ 2 = $552.00

Item or Service	Purpose	Replacement Schedule	Start / End	Costs
Case Manager	The case manager will assist in appointment scheduling and other activities associated with medical care. The case manager will also assist in hiring and monitoring attendant care.	6 Hours/ Year	# Start Age/Year 38 2017	Cost/Unit $85.00 to $99.00
4 Option 2			# End Age/Year 70 2049	Cost/Year $510.00 to $594.00

Cost/Year = $85.00 x 6 = $510.00
Cost/Year = $99.00 x 6 = $594.00
Cost/Year Average = ($510.00 + $594.00) ÷ 2 = $552.00

Growth Trends to be determined by an Economist.
*LE = Life Expectancy **U = Unknown N/A = Not Applicable
All Ages and Dates are Inclusive, e.g. 2000-2006 = 7 Years

Prepared By: Carol P. Walker, PhD, ABPP-CN, CLCP

Projected Therapeutic Modalities

Item or Service	Purpose	Replacement Schedule	Start / End	Costs
Family/Guardian Counseling and Education 5 Options 1, 2	Assist family with coping skills.	17 - 23 Times/ Year	# Start Age/Year 38 2017 # End Age/Year 38 2017	Cost/Unit $134.00 to $187.00 Cost/Year $15,946.00 to $30,107.00

This recommendation is based on consultation with Ms. Smith's treating neuropsychologist.

Cost/Year = 7/1 x $134.00 x 17 = $15,946.00
Cost/Year = 7/1 x $187.00 x 17 = $22,253.00
Cost/Year = 7/1 x $134.00 x 23 = $21,574.00
Cost/Year = 7/1 x $187.00 x 23 = $30,107.00
Cost/Year Average = ($15,946.00 + $30,107.00) ÷ 2 = $23,026.50

Item or Service	Purpose	Replacement Schedule	Start / End	Costs
Psychotherapy (Individual) 6 Options 1, 2	This therapy is specifically to address adjustment to changes in her life secondary to her injuries and to address behavioral issues related to her brain injury.	12 - 24 Times/ Year	# Start Age/Year 38 2017 # End Age/Year 38 2017	Cost/Unit $129.00 to $166.00 Cost/Year $1,548.00 to $3,984.00

This recommendation is based on consultation with Ms. Smith's treating neuropsychologist. Ms. Smith was being treated for anxiety and depression prior to the injury.

Cost/Year = $129.00 x 12 = $1,548.00
Cost/Year = $166.00 x 12 = $1,992.00
Cost/Year = $129.00 x 24 = $3,096.00
Cost/Year = $166.00 x 24 = $3,984.00
Cost/Year Average = ($1,548.00 + $3,984.00) ÷ 2 = $2,766.00

Growth Trends to be determined by an Economist.
*LE = Life Expectancy **U = Unknown N/A = Not Applicable
All Ages and Dates are Inclusive, e.g. 2000-2006 = 7 Years

Prepared By: Carol P. Walker, PhD, ABPP-CN, CLCP

Projected Therapeutic Modalities

Item or Service	Purpose	Replacement Schedule	Start End	Costs
Psychotherapy (Individual) 7 Options 1, 2	This therapy is specifically to address adjustment to changes in her life secondary to her injuries and to address behavioral issues related to her brain injury.	1 Time/ Year	# Start Age/Year 39 2018 # End Age/Year 70 2049	Cost/Unit $129.00 to $166.00 Cost/Year $129.00 to $166.00

This recommendation is based on consultation with Ms. Smith's treating neuropsychologist. Ms. Smith was being treated for anxiety and depression prior to the injury.

Cost/Year Average = ($129.00 + $166.00) ÷ 2 = $147.50

Item or Service	Purpose	Replacement Schedule	Start End	Costs
Physical Therapy 8 Options 1, 2	Maintain physical capacity and address balance issues.	12 - 16 Visits/ Year	# Start Age/Year 38 2017 # End Age/Year 70 2049	Cost/Unit $45.00 to $65.00 Cost/Year $2,160.00 to $4,160.00

Recommended by Ms. Smith's treating physiatrist.

Cost/Year = 4/1 x $45.00 x 12 = $2,160.00
Cost/Year = 4/1 x $65.00 x 12 = $3,120.00
Cost/Year = 4/1 x $45.00 x 16 = $2,880.00
Cost/Year = 4/1 x $65.00 x 16 = $4,160.00
Cost/Year Average = ($2,160.00 + $4,160.00) ÷ 2 = $3,160.00

Growth Trends to be determined by an Economist.
*LE = Life Expectancy **U = Unknown N/A = Not Applicable
All Ages and Dates are Inclusive, e.g. 2000-2006 = 7 Years

Item or Service	Purpose	Replacement Schedule	Start / End	Costs
Occupational Therapy 9 Options 1, 2	Maintain ADLs.	12 - 16 Times/ Year	# Start Age/Year 38 2017	Cost/Unit $54.00 to $68.00
			# End Age/Year 70 2049	Cost/Year $2,592.00 to $4,352.00

Recommended by Ms. Smith's treating physiatrist.

Cost/Year = 4/1 x $54.00 x 12 = $2,592.00
Cost/Year = 4/1 x $68.00 x 12 = $3,264.00
Cost/Year = 4/1 x $54.00 x 16 = $3,456.00
Cost/Year = 4/1 x $68.00 x 16 = $4,352.00
Cost/Year Average = ($2,592.00 + $4,352.00) ÷ 2 = $3,472.00

Item or Service	Purpose	Replacement Schedule	Start / End	Costs
Bookkeeper/Financial Manager 10 Options 1, 2	Manage household expenses.	1 Time/ Week	# Start Age/Year 38 2017	Cost/Unit $18.57 to $18.57
			# End Age/Year 70 2049	Cost/Year $1,371.21 to $1,371.21

This service is based on consultations with and recommendations by Ms. Smith's treating physician and neuropsychologist as well as this consultant. The time and hourly costs are from the Dollar Value of a Day, Home Management which includes these services as well as others related to financial management.
Cost/Year = 1.42/1 x $18.57 x 52 = $1,371.21

Growth Trends to be determined by an Economist.
*LE = Life Expectancy **U = Unknown N/A = Not Applicable
All Ages and Dates are Inclusive, e.g. 2000-2006 = 7 Years

Prepared By: Carol P. Walker, PhD, ABPP-CN, CLCP

Diagnostic/Educational Testing

Item or Service	Purpose	Replacement Schedule	Start / End	Costs
Neuropsychological Evaluation 1 Options 1, 2	Monitor cognitive, emotional, and behavioral status.	2 Times/ Year	# Start Age/Year 39 2018 # End Age/Year 40 2019	Cost/Unit $218.00 to $282.00 Cost/Year $3,488.00 to $4,512.00

This item is based on consultation with her treating neuropsychologist.

Cost/Year = 8/1 x $218.00 x 2 = $3,488.00
Cost/Year = 8/1 x $282.00 x 2 = $4,512.00
Cost/Year Average = ($3,488.00 + $4,512.00) ÷ 2 = $4,000.00

Item or Service	Purpose	Replacement Schedule	Start / End	Costs
Neuropsychological Evaluation 2 Options 1, 2	Monitor cognitive, emotional, and behavioral status.	1 Time Only	# Start Age/Year 42 2021 # End Age/Year 42 2021	Cost/Unit $218.00 to $282.00 Cost/Year $1,744.00 to $2,256.00

This item is based on consultation with her treating neuropsychologist.

Cost/Year = 8/1 x $218.00 = $1,744.00
Cost/Year = 8/1 x $282.00 = $2,256.00
Cost/Year Average = ($1,744.00 + $2,256.00) ÷ 2 = $2,000.00

Life Care PlanTables for Belinda L. Smith

Growth Trends to be determined by an Economist.

*LE = Life Expectancy **U = Unknown N/A = Not Applicable

All Ages and Dates are Inclusive, e.g. 2000-2006 = 7 Years

Prepared By: Carol P. Walker, PhD, ABPP-CN, CLCP

Diagnostic/Educational Testing

Item or Service	Purpose	Replacement Schedule	Start / End	Costs
Neuropsychological Evaluation 3 Options 1, 2	Monitor cognitive, emotional, and behavioral status.	1 Time/ 3 Years	# Start Age/Year 45 2024	Cost/Unit $218.00 to $282.00
			# End Age/Year 70 2049	Cost/Year $290.67 to $376.00

This item is based on recommendation by her treating neuropsychologist for ongoing cognitive and behavioral screening. Four hours are included for these evaluations.

Cost/Year = 4/1 x $218.00 x 1÷ 3 = $290.67
Cost/Year = 4/1 x $282.00 x 1÷ 3 = $376.00
Cost/Year Average = ($290.67 + $376.00) ÷ 2 = $333.33

Item or Service	Purpose	Replacement Schedule	Start / End	Costs
Head Injury Foundation 4 Options 1, 2	Provide support to Ms. Smith and her family.		# Start Age/Year	Cost/Unit
			# End Age/Year	Cost/Year

Life Care PlanTables for Belinda L. Smith

Growth Trends to be determined by an Economist.
*LE = Life Expectancy **U = Unknown N/A = Not Applicable
All Ages and Dates are Inclusive, e.g. 2000-2006 = 7 Years

References

American Bar Association/American Psychological Association Assessment of Capacity in Older Adults Project Working Group 2008. *Assessment of Older Adults with Diminished Capacity: A Handbook for Psychologists*. Washington, DC: American Bar Association and American Psychological Association.

Artiola i Fortuny, L., & Mullaney, H. A. 1998. Assessing patients whose language you do not know: Can the absurd be ethical? *The Clinical Neuropsychologist, 12*, 113–126.

Benitez, A., Hassenstab, J., & Bangen, K. J. 2014. Neuroimaging training among neuropsychologists: A survey of the state of current training and recommendations for trainees. *The Clinical Neuropsychologist, 28* (4), 600–613.

Ben-Yishay, Y. & Diller, L. 2011 *Handbook of Holistic Neuropsychological Rehabilitation*. New York, NY: Oxford Press.

Berrol, S. 1990. Issues in cognitive rehabilitation. *Archives of Neurology, 47*, 219–220.

Bigler, E. D. (Ed.). 1996. *Neuroimaging. I Basic Science; I Clinical Applications*. New York, NY: Plenum Press.

Bilder, R. M. 2011. Neuropsychology 3.0: Evidence based science and practice. *Journal International Neuropsycholcial Society, 17* (1), 7–13.

Commission for the Recognition of Specialties and Proficiencies in Professional Psychology. (n.d.) Retrieved 11/13/2016 from http://www.apa.org/ed/graduate/specialize/neuro.aspx.

Damasio, H. & Damasio, A. R. 1989. *Lesion Analysis in Neuropsychology*. New York, NY: Oxford Press.

Fitzhugh-Bell, K. B. 1997. Historical antecedents of clinical neuropsychology. In A. M. Horton, D. Wedding, S. J. Webster (Eds.). *The Neuropsychological Handbook: Volume 1. Foundations and Assessment* (2nd Edition, pp. 67–90). New York, NY: Macmillian.

Fleminger, S., Oliver, D., Lovestone, S., Rabe-Hesketh, S., & Giora, A. 2003. Head injury as a risk factor for Alzheimer's disease: The evidence 10 years on; a partial replication. *Journal Neurology, Neurosurgery & Psychiatry, 74*, 857–862.

Freemon, F. R. 1994. Galen's ideas on neurological function. *Journal of the History of the Neurosciences*, 4, 263–271. Available http://dx.doi.org/10.1080/09647049409526l9/.

Greenberg, S. A., & Shuman, D. W. 1997. Irreconcilable conflict between therapeutic and forensic roles. *Professional Psychology: Research and Practice, 28*, 50–57.

Heilman, K. M. & Valenstein, E. 1993. Introduction. In Heilman, K.M. & Valenstein, E. (Eds.). *Clinical Neuropsychology* (3rd Edition, pp. 1–16). New York, NY: Oxford Press.

Houston Conference on Specialty Education and Training in Clinical Neuropsychology. 1998. *Policy Statement*. Retrieved November 11, 2016, from https://theaacn.org/wp-content/uploads/2015/10/houston_conference.pdf.

Johnstone, B., Callahan, C. D., Kapila, C. J., & Bowman, D. E. 1996. The comparability of the WRAT-R Reading Test and NAART as estimates of premorbid intelligence in neurologically impaired patients. *Archives of Clinical Neuropsychology, 11*, 513–519.

Koehler, R., Wilhelm, E., & Shoulson, I. (Eds.). 2011. *Cognitive Rehabilitation Therapy for Traumatic Brain Injury: Evaluating the Evidence*. Committee on Cognitive Rehabilitation Therapy for Traumatic Brain Injury: Institute of Medicine. Available: http://nap.edu/13220.

Kreutzer, J., Marwitz, J., & Kepler, K. 1992. Traumatic brain injury: Family response and outcome. *Archives of Physical Medicine and Rehabilitation, 73*, 771–778.

Lezak, M. D., Howieson, D. B., & Loring, D. W. 2004. *Neuropsychological Assessment* (4th Edition). New York, NY: Oxford Press.

Luria, A. R. 1973. *The Working Brain: An Introduction to Neuropsychology*. London: Penguin Books.

Max, J. E., Roberts, M. A., Koele, S. L., Lindgren, S. D., Robin, D. A., Arndt, S., Smith, W. L., Jr., & Sato, Y. 1999. Cognitive outcome in children and adolescents following severe traumatic brain injury: Influence of psychosocial, psychiatric, and injury-related variables. *Journal of the International Neuropsychological Society, 5*, 58–68.

National Academy of Neuropsychology. (n.d.). *Definition of a Neuropsychologist*. Retrieved November 2016 from https://nanonline.org/nan/Professional_Resources/Position_Papers/NAN/_ProfessionalResources/Position_Papers.

Rabin, L. A., Barr, W. B., Burton, L. A. 2005. Assessment practices of clinical neuropsychologists in the United States and Canada: A survey of INS, NAN, and APA division 40 members. *Archives of Clinical Neuropsychology, 20*, 33–65.

Rosenthal M., & Geckler C. 1997. Family intervention in neuropsychology. *Brain Injury, 11*, 891–906.

Russell, E. W. 1986. The psychometric foundation of clinical neuropsychology. In S. B. Filskov and T. J. Boll (Eds.), *Handbook of Clinical Neuropsychology* (Vol. 2, pp. 45–81). New York, NY: John Wiley & Sons.

Sbordone, R. J. 1997. The ecological validity of neuropsychological testing. In A. M. Horton, Jr., Danny Wedding, and Jeffrey Wedding (Eds.), *The Neuropsychology Handbook* (Vol. 1, pp. 365–393). New York, NY: Springer Publishing.

Sbordone, R. J., & Rudd, M. 1986. Can psychologists recognize neurological disorders? *Journal of Experimental and Clinical Neuropsychology*, 8(3), 285–291.

Sbordone, R. J., Saul, R. E., & Purisch, A. D. 2007. *Neuropsychology for Psychologists, Health Care Professionals, and Attorneys*. Boca Raton, FL: CRC Press.

Smith, D. H., Johnson, V. E., & Stewart, W. 2013. Chronic neuropathologies of single and repetitive TBI: substrates of dementia? *Nature Reviews Neurology*, 9. Doi:10.1038/nrneurol.2013.29.

Solberg, M. M., & Mateer C. A. 1989. *Introduction to Cognitive Remediation*. New York, NY: Guilford Press.

Uomoto, J. M. 2000. Application of the neuropsychological evaluation in vocational planning after brain injury. In R. T. Fraser and D. C. Clemmons (Eds.), *Traumatic Brain Injury Rehabilitation: Practical Vocational, Neuropsychological, and Psychotherapy Interventions* (pp. 1–94). Boca Raton, FL: CRC Press.

Yantz, C. L., Gavett, B. E., Lynch, J. K., & McCaffrey, R. J. 2006. Potential for interpretation disparities of Halstead–Reitan neuropsychological battery performances in a litigating sample. *Archives of Clinical Neuropsychology, 21*(8), 809–817.

Yeates, K. O., Taylor, H. G., Drotar, D., Wade, S. L., Klein, S., Stancin, T., et al. 1997. Preinjury family environment as a determinant of recovery from traumatic brain injury in school-age children. *Journal of the International Neuropsychological Society, 3*, 617–630.

Chapter 7

The Role of the Occupational Therapist in Life Care Planning

Nancy L. Mitchell and Courtney V. Mitchell

Contents

Introduction....106
Activities of Daily Living....108
Instrumental Activities of Daily Living....114
OT Educational Requirements and Specialization....119
Contents of the Life Care Plan and the Role of the OT....120
Projected Evaluations....120
Projected Therapeutic Modalities....121
Aides for Independent Function/ADL....121
Wheelchair and Wheelchair Maintenance....121
Wheelchair Accessories....121
Durable Medical Equipment....121
Orthotics and Prosthetics....122
Orthopedic Equipment....122
Architectural Modifications....122
Supplies....122
Home and Facility Care....122
Computer....122
Health and Strength Maintenance....122
Transportation....122
Complications....123
Vocational/Worksite Modifications....123
The OT as a Consultant to the Life Care Planner....123
Ethical Standards and Considerations for Occupational Therapists....123
Aging with a Disability....124

Abbreviations Commonly Used in OT 126
Case Study 127
Conclusion 133
References 133

Introduction

Occupational therapists can provide a unique and critical role in the formation of the life care plan. Many of the pages of a life care plan fall under the domain of occupational therapy (OT). The ability to perform daily tasks of self-care, play, school, work, or social participation is the very core of the practice of OT, as well as the basis for some of the contents of a life care plan.

The objective of OT is the essence of the purpose of a life care plan. "In its simplest terms, occupational therapists and occupational therapy assistants help people of all ages participate in the things they want and need to do through the therapeutic use of everyday activities (occupations). Unlike other professions, occupational therapy helps people function in all of their environments (e.g., home, work, school, community) and addresses the physical, psychological, and cognitive aspects of their well-being through engagement in occupation.

> Common occupational therapy interventions include helping children with disabilities to participate fully in school and develop social skills, helping people recovering from injury to regain function through retraining and/or adaptations, and providing support for older adults experiencing physical and cognitive changes. Occupational therapy services typically include:
>
> - An individualized evaluation, during which the client, family, and occupational therapist determine the person's goals,
> - Customized intervention to improve the person's ability to perform daily activities and reach the goals, and
> - An outcomes evaluation to ensure that the goals are being met and/or to modify the intervention plan based on the patient's needs and skills.
>
> "Occupational therapy services may include comprehensive evaluations of the client's home and other environments, recommendations for adaptive equipment and training in its use, training in how to modify a task or activity to facilitate participation, and guidance and education for family members and caregivers" (American Occupational Therapy Association [AOTA], 2015a,b).

Several philosophical assumptions are presented to guide OTs in their profession. The assumptions that parallel those of the life care planner are (Atchinson & Dirette, 2012, p. 2):

- "Each individual has a right to a meaningful existence: the right to live in surroundings that are safe, supportive, comfortable, and over which he or she has some control; to make decisions for himself or herself; to be productive; to experience pleasure and joy; to love and be loved."
- "Each individual has the right to reach his or her potential through purposeful interaction with the human and nonhuman environment."
- "The extent to which intervention is focused on the context, the areas of occupational performance or on the client depends on the needs of the particular individual at any given time."

The World Federation of Occupational Therapists (2012) says, "In occupational therapy, occupations refer to the everyday activities that people do as individuals, in families, and with communities to occupy time and provide meaning and purpose to life. Occupations include things people need to, want to, and are expected to do."

The *Occupational Therapy Practice Framework* (2014) reports, "Occupations are central to a client's (person's, group's or population's) identity and sense of competence and have particular meaning and value to that client" (p. S5). The *Framework* goes on to identify the OT assessment process: "The initial step in the evaluation process provides an understanding of the client's occupational history and experiences, patterns of daily living, interests, values, and needs. The client's reason for seeking services, strengths, and concerns in relation to performing occupations and daily life activities, areas of potential occupational disruption, supports and barriers, and priorities are also identified" (p. S10). This is in harmony with the approach of the life care planner in determining numerous contents of a life care plan.

Occupational Therapy Assessment Tools: An Annotated Index (2014) reviews almost 600 instruments used for evaluation by OTs. Evaluation tools reflect the broad scope of OT. The contents of the *Index* lists assessment tools in the following areas: occupational performance; quality of life assessments; disability status and adaptive behaviors assessments; Activities of Daily Living and Instrumental Activities of Daily Living, including driving, rest and sleep; education; work; play; leisure; social participation; quality of life; developmental skills; motor and praxis; perception; sensory; emotional and psychological regulation; social interaction; cognitive; values, beliefs and spirituality; habits, routines, roles and rituals; assessments of context: social and virtual; and assessments of home and work environments (pp. v–xi). Clearly, it is beyond the scope of this chapter to review all of these assessment tools. Use of a particular instrument is likely to vary by region of the country and OT subspecialty, and it is unlikely any OT will have expertise in administration and knowledge of interpretation of all of these measures. Some of the more frequently used evaluation tools are provided here:

- Canadian Occupational Performance Measure (COPM), 4th Edition (2005; originally published 1991)

Purpose: This individualized clinical outcome measure was designed to detect change in a client's self-perception of occupational performance over time. The COPM fosters collaboration between the client and the OT to design intervention (*Occupational Therapy Assessment Tools: An Annotated Index*, 2014, p. 31).

- FIM System and WeeFIM System II (includes 0-to-3 module) (revised from the Functional Independence Measure and Functional Independence Measure for Children) (FIM 1997; originally published 1987; WeeFIM II 2004; originally published 1998)

Purpose: Designed as individual or group outcome measures of severity of disability. These instruments assess the ability to perform specified self-care, communication, and cognitive tasks. They have been used during initial, periodic, discharge, and follow-up evaluation periods to monitor patient progress and analyze outcomes of rehabilitation in terms of burdens of care. (*Occupational Therapy Assessment Tools: An Annotated Index*, 2014, p. 124).

- WorkWell Systems FCE, version 2 (2006)

Purpose: FCE is designed to identify a person's maximum safe work abilities, identify limitations that prevent safe return to work, and provide recommendations to assist safe return to work (*Occupational Therapy Assessment Tools: An Annotated Index*, 2014, p. 317).

- Bayley Scales of Infant and Toddler Development, 3rd Edition (Bayley III; including the Bayley-III Motor Scale and Bayley-III Screening Test) (2005; originally published 1969, 1984, 1983)

Purpose: This measure of fine and gross motor skills is designed to identify children with developmental delays of motor functioning and provide information to aid intervention planning (*Occupational Therapy Assessment Tools: An Annotated Index*, 2014, p. 446).

- Test of Visual-Motor Skills (TVMS-3) (2010) (originally published 1992, 1995)

Purpose: The TVMS-3 assesses visual-motor skills by visually guided fine motor movements required to copy a design, to determine whether distortions or gross inaccuracies in copied design could result from deficits in visual perception, motor planning, and/or execution. The test can be used for evaluation and diagnostic purposes (*Occupational Therapy Assessment Tools: An Annotated Index*, 2014, p. 424).

- Sensory Profile 2 (SP2) (2014; originally published 1999): Adolescent/Adult SP (2002)

Purpose: The SP2 is designed to measure sensory processing patterns in everyday life that support or interfere with function. This assessment allows caregivers' observations to be used in conjunction with other evaluations, reports, and observations from critical members of the team to plan effective interventions (*Occupational Therapy Assessment Tools: An Annotated Index*, 2014, p. 417).

- Allen Cognitive Level Screen (ACLS-5) (LACLS-5) (2007) (originally published 1995, 1990, 1996, 2000)

Purpose: The ACLS-5 and the larger, easier-to-see version, LACLS-5, are brief screening tests to estimate a client's cognitive functioning and capacity to learn to guide treatment goal setting (*Occupational Therapy Assessment Tools: An Annotated Index*, 2014, p. 557).

- Pediatric Evaluation of Disability Inventory (PEDI) (1992); Pediatric Evaluation of Disability Inventory-Computer Adaptive Test (PEDI-CAT, 2012)

Purpose: The PEDI and PEDI-CAT offer comprehensive clinical assessment of functional capabilities and typical performance in children and adolescents with disabilities. Both versions are used to identify functional delay, monitor improvement after intervention, evaluate outcome of a therapeutic program, and monitor and evaluate group progress for program evaluation and research (*Occupational Therapy Assessment Tools: An Annotated Index*, 2014, p. 137).

Activities of Daily Living

The performance of Activities of Daily Living (ADL) has long been the cornerstone and domain of the OT. While typical self-care skills of dressing, eating, and bathing are often associated with the profession, the scope of ADL is significantly greater. The *Occupational Therapy Practice Framework: Domain and Process* (2014) provides the details (p. S19):

- *Bathing, Showering:* Obtaining and using supplies; soaping, rinsing, and drying body parts; maintaining bathing position; and transferring to and from bathing positions.

- *Toileting and Toilet Hygiene*: Obtaining and using toileting supplies; managing clothing; transferring to and from toileting position; cleaning body; and caring for menstrual and continence needs (including catheters, colostomies, and suppository management), as well as completing intentional control of bowel movements and urination and, if necessary using equipment or agents for bladder control (Uniform Data System for Medical Rehabilitation 1996, pp. III-20, III-24).
- *Dressing*: Selecting clothing and accessories appropriate to time of day, weather, and occasion; obtaining clothing from storage area; dressing and undressing in a sequential fashion; fastening and adjusting clothing and shoes; and applying and removing personal devices, prostheses, or orthoses.
- *Swallowing/Eating*: Keeping and manipulating food or fluid in the mouth and swallowing it; *swallowing* is moving food from the mouth to the stomach.
- *Feeding*: Setting up, arranging, and bringing food (or fluid) from the plate or cup to the mouth; sometimes called *self-feeding*.
- *Functional Mobility:* Moving from one position or place to another (during performance of everyday activities), such as in-bed mobility, wheelchair mobility, and transfers (e.g., wheelchair, bed, car, shower, tub, toilet, chair, or floor). Includes functional ambulation and transportation of objects.
- *Personal Device Care*: Using, cleaning, and maintaining personal care items, such as hearing aids, contact lenses, glasses, orthotics, prosthetics, adaptive equipment, and contraceptive and sexual devices.
- *Personal Hygiene and Grooming*: Obtaining and using supplies; removing body hair (e.g., using razors, tweezers, lotions); applying and removing cosmetics; washing, drying, combing, styling, brushing, and trimming hair; caring for nails (hands and feet); caring for skin, ears, eyes, and nose; applying deodorant; cleaning mouth; brushing and flossing teeth; and removing, cleaning, and reinserting dental orthotics and prosthetics.
- *Sexual Activity*: Engagement in activities that result in sexual satisfaction and/or meet relational or reproductive needs.

Following is one example of a checklist for Activities of Daily Living used by life care planners that can be completed during the life care plan evaluation and addresses many of the ADLs listed previously.

ACTIVITIES OF DAILY LIVING		
*NAME:*__________ *DISABILITY:*__________ *DATE:* __________ CODES: 1 = Can do without difficulty. 2 = Can do with some difficulty. 3 = Can do with great difficulty and/or needs assistance from attendant. 4 = Dependent on someone else to do.		
FEEDING	Code	Comments or amount of time required
Fix meal		
Open cans/jars/tubes/boxes		
Open containers/packages/empty contents		

(*Continued*)

Use manual or electric can opener (note if there is a difference)		
Use microwave		
Use stove/oven (turn on/use)		
Can access refrigerator/cupboard		
Open refrigerator		
Open drawers		
Transport items short distance		
Use fork/spoon/knife (note if adapted utensils are used)		
Cut with knife		
Butter bread		
Eat soup with spoon		
Make sandwich/light meal		
Reach meal area		
Eat meal		
Get drink		
Drink from cup/glass with/without adaption		
Other		
HYGIENE		
Reach sink area		
Reach/turn faucets		
Brush teeth		
Wash and dry self (note if there is a difference with hands/face/entire body)		
Use shower (note if roll-in is required)		
Use tub		
Bed bath		
Apply deodorant		
Comb/brush hair		
Shave		
Apply/remove makeup		

(*Continued*)

Shampoo and dry hair		
Cut/clean nails		
Other		
BOWEL/BLADDER		
Sit balanced without assistance		
Use catheter		
Irrigate catheter/prepare equipment		
Change catheter/prepare equipment		
Handle urinal		
Empty leg bag		
Put leg bag on/off or Don/doff leg bag		
Connect/disconnect tubing		
Perform bowel cares (note if digital stimulation, suppository)		
Cleanse self after toileting		
Flush toilet/empty commode		
Manage clothing before/after toileting		
Transfer to/from toilet/commode		
BED ACTIVITIES		
Transfer to/from bed		
Sit up		
Check skin		
Operate bed controls		
Sit at side of bed		
Roll side to side		
Turn over		
DRESSING		
Select appropriate clothes and match colors		
Button garment with/without adaptive aid		
Fasten closures (slippers, snaps, belt)		
Don/doff shirt		
Don/doff slacks/underpants/skirt		

(*Continued*)

Don/doff corset or binder		
Don/doff socks		
Don/doff shoes		
Tie shoelaces		
Don/doff coat/sweater		
Don/doff elastic or TED hose		
Take clothes in/out of drawers/closet		
COMMUNICATION		
Write		
Speak with normal voice		
Summon emergency assistance		
Use telephone, mobile phone/push-button/cordless		
Use word processor/typewriter		
Use augmentative communications		
ENVIRONMENT		
Use ECU (note brand/options)		
Control temperature		
Open/close door		
Use keys		
Turn light on/off		
Use TV/radio/stereo		
Set and/or read clock/watch		
Manipulate newspaper/book		
Use scissors		
Plug in cord		
Pick up things off floor		
Use adaptive aids		
Open/read mail		
MOBILITY		
Maneuver power/manual wheelchair (note if Quad pegs/one hand/joystick/sip & puff, etc.)		
Transfer from chair to vehicle		

(*Continued*)

Manipulate wheelchair		
Utilize and adjust armrests		
Manage leg rests		
Put brakes on/off		
Put safety belt on/off		
Remove items from wheelchair		
Use lap board/bag/caddy/ashtray		
Utilize cushion		
Do chair maintenance		
Adjust body in chair		
Shift weight		
Get from floor to chair		
Hook arm/reach forward		
Reposition in chair with/without assistance		
Cross/uncross legs		
Negotiate ramps/curbs		
Negotiate rough/smooth terrain		
Get chair in/out of car/van		
Drive		
If drive, any adaptations		
Use public transportation		
ORTHOTICS/PROSTHESIS		
Don/doff upper extremity orthotic/brace		
Don/doff upper extremity prosthesis		
Don/doff lower extremity prosthesis		
Don/doff lower extremity orthotic/brace		
Don/doff/adjust AFO or KAFO		
Don/doff splint/sling		
PERSONNEL/ATTENDANT CARE NEEDS	*X if required*	*Comments*
Independent (no need)		
Needs companion for judgment (due to TBI)		

(*Continued*)

Needs guardian (incl. money management)		
Occasional (e.g., morning/eve/weekends)		
Live-in attendant (10–12 hours per day and night safety)		
24-hour attendant awake		
24-hour skilled/high-tech awake		
Housecleaning/meals/laundry		
House maintenance interior/exterior		
Errands/doctor appointment		
Other		

Instrumental Activities of Daily Living

Hinojosa and Blount (2004) describe Instrumental Activities of Daily Living (IADL) as "complex multi-step activities requiring the integration of higher level cognitive skills (e.g., meal preparation, money management, community travel)" (p. 447). The authors report that these skills are needed to "participate in complex social relationships and societal organizations" (p. 447). The *Occupational Therapy Practice Framework: Domain and Process* (2014) provides the details of what is included in IADL (pp. S19–S21):

- *Care of others (including selecting and supervising caregivers)*: Arranging, supervising, or providing the care for others.
- *Care of pets*: Arranging, supervising, or providing the care for pets and service animals.
- *Child-rearing*: Providing the care and supervision to support the developmental needs of a child.
- *Communication management*: Sending, receiving, and interpreting information using a variety of systems and equipment, including writing tools, telephones (cell phones or smart phones), keyboards, audiovisual recorders, computers or tablets, communication boards, call lights, emergency systems, Braille writers, telecommunication devices for deaf people, augmentative communication systems, and personal digital assistants.
- *Driving and community mobility*: Planning and moving around in the community and using public or private transportation, such as driving and riding in buses, or accessing buses, ride-sharing services like taxi cabs, or other public transportation systems.
- *Financial management*: Using fiscal resources, including alternate methods of financial transaction and planning and using finances with long-term and short-term goals.
- *Health management and maintenance*: Developing, managing, and maintaining routines for health and wellness promotion, such as physical fitness, nutrition, decreasing health risk behaviors, and medication routines.
- *Home establishment and management*: Obtaining and maintaining personal and household possessions and environment (e.g., home, yard, garden, appliances, vehicles), including maintaining and repairing personal possessions (e.g., clothing, household items) and knowing how to seek help or whom to contact.

- *Meal preparation and cleanup*: Planning, preparing, and serving well-balanced, nutricious meals, and cleaning up food and utensils after meals.
- *Religious and spiritual activities and expression*: Participating in religion, "an organized system of beliefs designed to facilitate closeness in the sacred or transcendent", and engaging in activities that allow a sense of connectedness to something larger than oneself or especially meaningful, such as taking time out to play with a child, engaging in activities in nature, and helping others in need.
- *Safety procedures and emergency responses*: Knowing and performing preventive procedures to maintain a safe environment; recognizing sudden, unexpected hazardous situations; and initiating emergency action to reduce the threat to health and safety. Examples include ensuring safety when entering and exiting the home, identifying emergency contact numbers, and replacing items such as batteries in smoke alarms and light bulbs.
- *Shopping*: Preparing shopping lists (grocery and other); selecting, purchasing, and transporting items; selecting method of payment, and completing money transactions; included are Internet shopping and related use of electronic devices such as computers, cell phones, and tablets.

The life care planner must be knowledgeable about the performance of IADL of the life care plan recipient. This information is typically not fully included in the medical records and can change over time. The authors use the following checklist of IADL in the process of evaluation for a life care plan.

IADL ASSESSMENT			
Name: ______________________		**Date:**____________	
Indicate percent of time task was performed by person being assessed pre-/post-disability/illness.			
LAWN			
Task	**Pre**	**Post**	**Comments**
Mowing			
Watering			
Fertilizing			
Aerating			
Seeding			
Trimming			
Edging			
Bush/tree trimming			
Weeding			
Composting			
Raking leaves			

(Continued)

GARDEN			
Task	**Pre**	**Post**	**Comments**
Planting			
Hoeing			
Weeding			
Watering			
Fencing			
Harvesting			

SNOW REMOVAL			
Task	**Pre**	**Post**	**Comments**
Shoveling			
Plowing			
Applying sand/salt			
Maintaining plow			

OUTSIDE CHORES			
Task	**Pre**	**Post**	**Comments**
Put on/take off storms/screens			
Clean gutters			
Wash exterior windows			
Stain deck			
Paint exterior			
Seal driveway			
Maintain A/C			
Get mail			
Clean deck furniture			
Clean garage			
Put in dock			
Feed birds			
Maintain pool			
Maintain boats/ snowmobiles			

(Continued)

Landscape			
Decorate exterior for holidays			
Take out trash			
HOME REPAIRS/MAINTENANCE			
Task	**Pre**	**Post**	**Comments**
Paint/prep			
Wallpaper/Prep			
Plaster/Dry wall repairs			
Repair plumbing			
Repair electrical			
Carpentry			

(Continued)

Replace ceiling light bulbs			
Maintain water softener			
Replace furnace filter			
Test smoke alarms/ change batteries			
AUTO MAINTENANCE			
Task	**Pre**	**Post**	**Comments**
Change oil			
Rotate tires			
Fill fluids			
Pump gas			
Other car repairs			
Change flat tire			
Wash car interior			
Wash car exterior			
DRIVING/TRANSPORTATION			
Task	**Pre**	**Post**	**Comments**
Short distance			
Long distance			

(Continued)

Manual transmission			
Public transportation			
WOOD			
Task	**Pre**	**Post**	**Comments**
Chop			
Split			
Stack			
Haul			
HOUSEHOLD CHORES			
Task	**Pre**	**Post**	**Comments**
Vacuum			
Clean carpet			
Clean interior windows			
Clean floors			
Clean toilet/tub/sink			
Clean oven			
Clean refrigerator			
Dust			
Do dishes			
Do laundry			
Fold laundry			
Put away laundry			
Make bed			
Change sheets			
Flip mattress			
Cook			
Plan meals			
Bake			
Sew			
Repair clothing			
Make appointments			

(*Continued*)

Prepare taxes			
Pay bills			
Balance checkbook			
Buy gifts			
Wrap gifts			
Decorate indoors for holidays			
Send cards/ Correspondence			
Feed pets			
Bathe pets			
Walk pets			
Clean up after pet			
Grocery shopping			
Put groceries away			
Run errands			
Make phone calls			
Use computer			

OT Educational Requirements and Specialization

The educational requirements for the OT have expanded over time. Previously, a registered occupational therapist (OTR) needed a bachelor's degree to enter practice, and working therapists with that level of education continue to practice. However, the current requirement of a beginning OT is a master's degree. A doctor of occupational therapy (DOT) will be needed for entry level practice as of 2027. This is a clinical doctorate with an emphasis on enhanced clinical practice. Some experienced therapists are expanding their credentials with this additional education. Some OTs choose to obtain a PhD in occupational therapy toward a path of research or education. Certified occupational therapy assistants (COTAs) typically have an associate's degree. OT practitioners are licensed by their individual states.

The OT that treats the person for whom the life care plan is being written is certainly the best first contact for obtaining OT recommendations for the plan. If that therapist is unwilling or unable to make the needed projections, additional OT evaluations may be needed. For example, an individual with a spinal cord injury may have had excellent OT interventions during his or her acute rehabilitation but the treating therapist may not have the expertise to provide input into the life care plan about needed driving adaptations. An additional evaluation from an OT specializing in this area may be needed.

Like many other medical professions, OTs tend to specialize in areas of practice. These include pediatrics, geriatrics, hand therapy, cardiac rehabilitation, physical disabilities, mental health, ergonomics, and health and wellness programming. While more OTs are becoming life care planners, the forensic arena is fairly new for the field. In general, OTs are not trained in litigation and may be reluctant to provide opinions that will be used in a legal setting. An inquiry to the state OT association may be a helpful first step.

In addition, while OTs pride themselves on addressing the needs of the whole person, their consideration of therapy and equipment needs tends to address the short-term rather than the lifelong projections that are needed for a life care plan. As a part of therapist training, long-term goals that are a part of the typical therapy plan address needs in a given episode of care, which may mean areas of focus in the weeks or months ahead rather than over a client's entire lifetime. A pediatric therapist treating a child with cerebral palsy, for example, could be encouraged to project therapy and equipment needs throughout childhood and adolescence, but lack the experience or expertise to know what this child will need in his or her adult years. That being said, there are numerous components of the life care plan within the direct expertise of the OT.

Contents of the Life Care Plan and the Role of the OT

OTs are unique in the roles they offer as the health care professional on the team with the knowledge and treatment of allowing people as much independence as possible in their daily lives. Their opinions can include that a person will need the assistance of a caregiver to complete daily activities or for safety and supervision in the home/school/work setting, or the use of equipment for safety or energy conservation. The next section describes many of the areas of a life care plan that could be enhanced with the input of an OT.

In general, costs of an OT evaluation can vary greatly. *Medical Fees in the United States* (PMIC, 2016) reports that the charge for an OT evaluation is $153 (50th percent) to $269 (90th percent), without geographic modifiers. However, in our experience it is not unusual for an OT evaluation at a facility-based practice to be in excess of $500. In many states, OTs have direct access to evaluate a person without a doctor's prescription. However, health care facilities require a doctor's order for an OT evaluation as this is needed for payment by insurance providers.

Projected Evaluations

The OT should be comfortable providing recommendations for ongoing OT evaluations. However, the therapist may be unwilling or unable to project lifelong needs as this is outside of the typical frame of reference for a given therapy episode of care. In this case, the life care planner can defer to the opinions the physiatrist who will likely be more comfortable providing projections for lifelong needs. It is typical for the author to include an annual OT evaluation for people with lifelong disabilities such as spinal cord injury, cerebral palsy, or upper extremity amputation.

Of special note for pediatric clients is the Individuals with Disabilities Education Act (IDEA), reenacted in 2004. The IDEA is a federal law ensuring services to children with disabilities who attend public schools throughout the nation. The IDEA governs how states and public agencies provide early intervention, special education, and related services to students with disabilities (retrieved from http://www.help4adhd.org/education/rights/idea).

As part of the law, the IDEA is mandated to provide OT and other therapeutic services that are educationally related to children ages 3 to 21 who attend a public school. The implication for the life care planner developing a life care plan for a child covered under the IDEA is that, for example, a child with a brain injury may have OT evaluation and treatment services written into the individualized education program (IEP) as it relates to his/her education needs and as provided for by the school system; however, it is important for the life care planner to consider the child's needs outside the school setting as well. In the authors's opinion, it would be unusual for a child who qualifies for school OT not to need additional OT services external to the school setting.

Projected Therapeutic Modalities

The OT should be comfortable providing recommendations for ongoing OT treatment. However, similar to the previous discussion, the therapist may be unwilling or unable to project lifelong needs as this is outside the typical frame of reference for a given therapy episode of care. Again, input from the treating physician is likely to be invaluable.

Aides for Independent Function/ADL

Occupational therapists are experts in daily living activities and should be very helpful in providing specific suggestions of equipment needed to enhance the client's independence and/or to facilitate the caregiver's task of providing care for the client. This will allow a life care planner to include specific items in the life care plan that will be of benefit to the client. In our opinion, rather than providing a general allowance for these items, a method often seen in life care plans that probably have not utilized the services of an OT, specific pieces of equipment and replacement schedules, in most instances, can be recommended. This enhances the credibility of the life care plan. However, it is recognized that itemizing numerous low-cost items, such as each adapted eating utensil, plate, and cup, can be unnecessarily detailed. The OT could also be helpful in projecting equipment needs that, while perhaps not needed currently, will address aging-related factors and enhance abilities as a person ages.

Wheelchair and Wheelchair Maintenance

Many OTs perform wheelchair and seating evaluations as a part of their practice. The OT's input into current and future needs for wheelchairs is likely to be very helpful to the life care planner. The OT who performs these evaluations will be able to make projections about the changing need for wheelchairs over time, such as a child's ability to benefit from powered mobility or a person's future need to move to a power-assisted wheelchair.

Wheelchair Accessories

OTs are often involved in choosing appropriate cushions, wheelchair backs, carrying bags, cup holders, and other accessories. Their input into this portion of the life care plan could be invaluable.

Durable Medical Equipment

OTs are experts on bath, toileting, and transferring equipment. They may also have significant knowledge of bed, transportation, and ambulation aides.

Orthotics and Prosthetics

OTs commonly make splints for the arms, wrists, and hands. They have knowledge about the type of splint that is needed and the frequency of replacement. In some settings, the fabrication of splints is delegated to orthotists. Many OTs also work with upper extremity amputees in their clinical practice. Prosthetists, however, are likely to have a greater depth of knowledge about prosthetic options, costs, and replacement frequencies.

Orthopedic Equipment

OTs will vary in their expertise in this area. Most should have a working knowledge of crutches, canes, walkers, standers, gait trainers, and positioning equipment. Physical therapists are more likely the experts with regard to this equipment.

Architectural Modifications

OTs have a basic education in accessibility needs for people with disabilities. Some have additional training and may be experts on ergonomics and home modifications. It may be very helpful to obtain an evaluation of a home access specialist to provide the details needed to get more exact costs and recommendations. This would need to be discussed with the retaining attorney as there will be a cost for this evaluation. Few OTs have this credential (see Chapter 32 on Home Assessment).

Supplies

Supplies in the life care plan that relate to adaptive clothing and adaptive feeding generally fall under the expertise of the OT. See also the previous discussion on ADLs.

Home and Facility Care

An OT evaluation may be a critical determination of the amount of care and supervision that is needed for a given individual. OTs are trained to evaluate safety and the ability to perform ADLs and IADLs. An OT can also determine when it is important to provide assistance because of limitations due to pain or impaired endurance as well as age-related factors.

Computer

Many OTs are experts in computer use and adaptations that are needed to access the computer.

Health and Strength Maintenance

OTs often evaluate and suggest home exercise programs and equipment needed to maintain strength and endurance. They can also be a resource to identify camps or special recreation programs or activities for individuals with specific disabilities.

Transportation

Some OTs have a Driver Rehabilitation Specialist certification and perform driving evaluations and adapted drivers' training as part of their clinical practice (see www.driver-ed.org). They can provide invaluable input into the need for driving evaluations and adaptations, costs, and replacement schedules for this equipment.

Complications

OTs may be helpful in determining how a given complication may affect functional abilities and the need for equipment in the future. OTs also have knowledge of the risk of overuse injuries for people with disabilities.

Vocational/Worksite Modifications

Some OTs specialize in ergonomics and worksite accommodations. They can provide valuable input about injury and overuse prevention and offer suggestions for equipment to enhance success in the workplace.

The OT as a Consultant to the Life Care Planner

As seen in the preceding section, many of the core components of a life care plan fall under the professional domain of the OT. An evaluation from an OT may be key in making life care plan recommendations. That being said, it will likely be important to communicate to the therapist what information is needed prior to the evaluation. Additionally, an evaluation in the home and, separately, the community, may be particularly helpful. The case study at the end of this chapter will illustrate the value of the OT assessment in the formulation of a life care plan.

Ethical Standards and Considerations for Occupational Therapists

Occupational therapists are expected to uphold and abide by the ethical standards developed for their profession by its national professional organization, the American Occupational Therapy Association (AOTA). "The Ethics Commission (EC) is one of the bodies of the Representative Assembly of the American Occupational Therapy Association (AOTA). The EC is responsible for developing the Ethics Standards for the profession, which apply to occupational therapy personnel at all levels and in all professional and societal roles".

To ensure ethical, safe, and effective care, these standards provide the foundation to guide occupational therapists in their clinical practice and decision making. If occupational therapists fail to abide by these standards, AOTA processes are in place to apply sanctions when a complaint is filed and a member is found to be in violation of these standards (Enforcement Procedures for the Occupational Therapy Code of Ethics, 2015a).

The EC has established the professional Core Values of altruism, equality, freedom, justice, dignity, truth, and prudence (Occupational Therapy Code of Ethics, 2015b). These values "provide a foundation to guide occupational therapy personnel in their interactions with others. Although the Core Values are not themselves enforceable standards, they should be considered when determining the most ethical course of action" (Occupational Therapy Code of Ethics, 2015b). These principles are expected to be present during any occupational therapist interaction, whether with a consumer, a member of the treatment team, or a life care planner seeking assistance and input from a treating therapist.

AOTA has also established six principles and standards of conduct to help clinicians with ethical decision-making, that is, beneficence, nonmaleficence, autonomy, justice, veracity, and fidelity (Occupational Therapy Code of Ethics, 2015b). Of these, autonomy, justice, veracity, and fidelity may impact the life care planner contacting an occupational therapist for input into the life care plan.

Autonomy: "Occupational therapy personnel shall respect the rights of the individual to self-determination, privacy, confidentiality, and consent" (Occupational Therapy Code of Ethics, 2015b). The therapist should follow a client's desire to refuse treatment, temporarily or permanently, despite the likelihood that this will result in poor outcomes (Occupational Therapy Code of Ethics, 2015b). Therefore, even if frequent occupational therapy visits are included in a life care plan, it is not ethical for a therapist to conduct this treatment if the individual does not want to participate. It will be important for the life care planner to determine, with the client and the treatment team, the client's desire and motivation to complete future therapies. The client's current compliance with treatment, therapy recommendations, and home programs can provide insight into the likelihood of future participation in therapy. Case management services may be a critical piece of facilitating future therapy participation. To comply with this standard and federal laws (HIPAA), treating therapists will require a release of information form indicating the individual has signed a consent to allow the occupational therapist to discuss specific treatment and future needs.

Justice: "Occupational therapy personnel shall promote fairness and objectivity in the provision of occupational therapy services" (Occupational Therapy Code of Ethics, 2015b), that is, therapists are expected to discharge a client who is no longer progressing; therapy services cannot be delivered solely by the ability to pay; clients are to be treated equally; and fees for services are to be "fair, reasonable, and commensurate with services delivered" (Occupational Therapy Code of Ethics, 2015b). Justice is also a consideration for the life care planner; a life care plan with funds for excessive therapy will be overreaching and inaccurate.

Veracity: "Occupational therapy personnel shall provide comprehensive, accurate and objective information when representing the profession" (Occupational Therapy Code of Ethics, 2015b). The therapist is expected to provide reliable communication with the life care planner.

Fidelity: "Occupational therapy personnel shall treat clients, colleagues, and other professionals with respect, fairness, discretion, and integrity," and "promote collaborative actions and communication as members of inter-professional teams to facilitate quality care and safety for clients" (Occupational Therapy Code of Ethics, 2015b). The occupational therapist may be unfamiliar with life care planners and the therapist's role to provide client information and make future care projections. Therapists may also have concerns about giving such information to members outside of the direct team. Life care planners should therefore describe their role, its impact on the client, the plan's educational role to guide future care, and how the therapist can provide the most accurate and helpful information.

Occupational therapists like other health care professionals have ethical standards that guide their practice. OTs are accustomed to collaboration with the client, family, and treatment team about the current episode of care but may lack experience or knowledge in providing long-term projections. They may have ethical concerns about being stretched outside of their comfort zones. In that circumstance, future occupational therapy needs may best be provided by a physical medicine and rehabilitation physician.

Aging with a Disability

While much has been written on aging with a disability, Mitchell (2004) reported that aging-related complications such as pain, fatigue, decreased strength and endurance, and subsequent loss of functional abilities occurs 20 to 30 years sooner for people with early-onset disabilities than for their able-bodied peers. The information remains valid and this can have significant impact in the life care plan both for care and equipment. In general, the need for care will increase as functional abilities decline. Changes in equipment and assistive technology are likely to be needed as a person is less able to function in his or her daily routine, and it is important for the life care planner to anticipate and plan for these changes.

Needs related to aging can vary by disability type. Mitchell (2004) provided the following recommendations to consider when developing a life care plan for individuals who have cerebral palsy, spinal cord injury, or amputation.

Summary of implications for the life care plan for a person with cerebral palsy (Mitchell, 2004, pp. 96–97):

- Case management is an important consideration for the person with cerebral palsy. It may be difficult to find or access specialized care. The necessary time and equipment needed for regular preventative care may not be readily available and case management assistance may be critical even for those people with normal cognition.
- Specialized dentistry may be needed lifelong. Special equipment for oral care may be needed.
- Consultation with a dietician at regular intervals will be helpful in problems associated with weight management (over- and underweight), which are common in this disability group.
- Alternative means of mobility should be an early consideration for those with any ambulation impairment. Powered mobility is an important consideration for distance mobility.
- A lifelong fitness routine is critical in maintaining strength, flexibility, endurance, and independence. A physical trainer may not have the needed expertise to meet the specialized needs of this population. Physical therapy or OT evaluations every 2 to 3 years over a lifetime may be a more appropriate choice.
- Consider increased care needs as the person ages.
- Assistive technology needs can change over time (e.g., a normal bed may work well in youth but a bed cane or hospital bed may be needed in later decades).
- An ergonomically correct environment in both the home and work setting is critical in preventing injury. Ergonomic assessments at life phase changes may be appropriate.
- Pain management, while not needed in childhood, may well become important as a person ages.
- Periodic psychology assessments may be helpful in monitoring psychological status.
- Potential aging-related complications such as overuse syndrome and potential for falls should be addressed.

A summary of the implications for the life care plan for a person with spinal cord injury are as follows (Mitchell, 2004, p. 99):

- Periodic assessments with a dietician may be important for weight control.
- Powered mobility should be considered for those needing to travel long distances or on uneven ground (e.g., college campus or rural environment) even with manual wheeling proficiency. Manual assist wheelchairs should typically be introduced 10 to 15 years after injury and powered wheelchairs for spinal cord injured clients using manual wheelchairs 20 years after injury.
- Other assistive technology needs are likely to change over time. Occupational and physical therapy evaluations to assess assistive technology are recommended.

- An ergonomically correct environment in the home and worksite will minimize injury risk. Periodic ergonomic assessments at life phase changes may be indicated.
- A lifelong fitness routine is critical in maintaining strength, flexibility, endurance, and independence. A physical trainer may not have the needed expertise to meet the specialized needs of this population. Physical or OT evaluations every 2 to 3 years over a lifetime may well be a more appropriate choice.
- The life care plan should address the potential need for increased care as the person ages and consider the possible psychological impact of increased dependency.

A summary of the implications for the life care plan for a person with amputation is as follows (Mitchell, 2004, p. 100):

- An ergonomically correct environment in the home and worksite will minimize injury risk. Ergonomic assessments at life phase changes may be helpful.
- Weight control is important for prosthetic fit and to help avoid overstressing joints. Periodic assessments with a dietician for those with a potential for weight control difficulties is recommended.
- A fitness program is essential to minimize injuries related to overuse. Input from therapists or a personal trainer may be a benefit to this disability group.
- Alternative mobility may be needed for those with lower-extremity amputations. Age and mobility environment will need to be considered.
- Pain management may not be a concern early in the disability for the person with amputation. However, it can become a problem as the person ages.

Abbreviations Commonly Used in OT

In review of therapy records, a life care planner may have difficulty deciphering abbreviations used by OTs. While there is a national effort to standardize abbreviations, some may be unique to therapists and some may even be specific to a given organization. Following is a list of abbreviations that may be found in OT medical records:

AAC	Augmentative and alternative communication
AAROM	Active assistive range of motion (person needs assistance to complete the full range of motion)
AD	Alzheimer's disease
ADD	Attention deficit disorder (now replaced by AD/HD)
AD/HD	Attention deficit hyperactivity disorder
ADLs	Activities of Daily Living
A/E	Above elbow
AFO	Ankle foot orthosis
A/K	Above knee
APD	Auditory processing disorder
AROM	Active range of motion (person is able to move through the range of motion but may not be able to do so with resistance)
AS	Asperger's syndrome
ASD	Autism spectrum disorder

AT	Assistive technology
B/E	Below elbow
B/K	Below knee
BMP	Behavior management plan
CD	Conduct disorder
CGA	Contact guard assist (direct contact with the person for safety but no physical assistance)
COTA	Certified occupational therapy assistant (typically an associate degree education)
DCD	Development coordination disorder (DSM-IV 315.4)
DD	Developmentally delayed
ECU	Environmental control unit
FES	Functional electrical stimulation
FNMES	Functional Neuromuscular Electrical Stimulation (see also FES & TENS)
IADL	Instrumental Activities of Daily Living (Activities of Daily Living beyond self-care, such as money management, meal preparation, child or pet care, telephone or computer use, use of public transportation, driving, and home cleaning and maintenance tasks)
KAFO	Knee ankle foot orthosis
LTG	Long-term goal
OT	Occupational therapist or occupational therapy
OTR/L	Occupational therapist licensed (occupational therapists are registered nationally but licensed by the individual states)
PCA	Personal care attendant
PECS	Picture exchange communication system
PT	Physical therapist or physical therapy
SBA	Standby assistance (no direct contact with the person)
SI	Sensory integration
SID	Sensory integrative (or integration) disorder/dysfunction
SLP	Speech language pathologist
STG	Short-term goal
TENS	Transcutaneous electrical nerve stimulation
TX	Treatment
VC	Verbal cue
WFL	Within functional limits (able to move within the limits needed to perform daily activities but may not have full range of motion or normal strength)

Case Study

A life care planner was asked to evaluate Jane, a 46-year-old woman who was diagnosed with a T7 spinal cord injury resulting in complete paraplegia. The life care planner visited Jane in her rural home. She had completed her in-patient rehabilitation over 2 years ago. The life care planner was concerned because Jane was significantly overweight and complained of severe shoulder pain. Jane was resistant to going into the city for physiatry follow-up and had purchased much of her durable medical equipment over the Internet. Jane was struggling to perform her Activities of Daily Living and relying more and more on her family for assistance. It was clear that some of Jane's equipment was no longer appropriate for her needs. Jane did agree to have an OT assessment in her home and the life care planner found a qualified OT to conduct the evaluation.

Childcare/Parenting/Grandparenting ______________________________
Fitness ______________________________
Hobbies ______________________________
Relationship ______________________________
Sexuality ______________________________
Holidays ______________________________
Entertaining ______________________________
Friendships ______________________________
Sleep ______________________________
Worship ______________________________

Source: Distributed by Nancy Mitchell, Mitchell Disability Assessments and Life Care Planning, Apple Valley, MN. Reprinted with permission.

An OT with spinal cord injury and home accessibility expertise evaluated Jane. Numerous issues that would have relevance to the life care plan were discovered by the OT and needed items were added to the preliminary life care plan:

- Not only had transfers become difficult for Jane; they were in fact unsafe. The OT recommended physical therapy intervention after a physiatry or orthopedic consultation to determine if Jane's shoulder pain and consequent strength deficits could be improved. If possible, transfer training would need to be retaught. There was an immediate need for a lift. Physical therapy and later PT or personal care attendant hours needed to be increased to eliminate Jane's need to continue unsafe transfers. See the sample life care plan entries in the following table. (Note: In an actual life care plan, items would be distributed into the appropriate categories. For purposes of this chapter, recommendations have been grouped together and numerous other items not specifically relevant to this chapter have been excluded.)

Item/Service	**Replacement/Service Frequency**	**Purpose**	**Cost**
PM&R or orthopedic visit	1–2x (additional visits are possible)	Evaluate shoulder/strength and provide recommendations.	$121–270/visit

Physical therapy	2–10 sessions	Reassess transfer status, train caregivers in lift use if needed, initiate home exercise program for shoulder. See later in plan for PT or personal trainer long-term follow-up.	$136–$272 per session
Invacare Reliant battery-powered lift	10 years	Caregiver use when independent or assisted transfers were unable to be performed.	$3,024.32
Lift slings	2–3 years	Slings are needed for use with lift.	$308.05
Personal care attendant	4–10 hours/day	These hours are needed to assist with personal cares, homemaking tasks, and eliminate independent transfers while shoulder pain is present. It is possible hours will be reduced if shoulder pain is eliminated.	$21–$30/hour

- A power wheelchair with an elevating seat was recommended. Jane could access her kitchen cupboards, microwave, and refrigerator with an elevating seat. Without it, the OT noted she used poor ergonomics and put further stress on her shoulders. Powered mobility was recommended sooner than what is typical in Jane's case because of her pain and mobility in her home. Typically, a power assist wheelchair is introduced 10–15 years after a spinal cord injury and a power chair 20 years after injury for the manual chair user (Mitchell, 2004). See the following example of a life care plan entry:

Item/Service	Replacement Frequency	Purpose	Cost
Invacare TDX SPCG base with Motion Concepts power seating	5 years	A power chair with elevating seat to fully access kitchen and enhance independence. This chair will need tilt-in-space feature because of inability to perform weight shifts secondary to shoulder pain.	$19,072

Source: Lisa Michaels COTA/L, ATP/SMS, CRTS/Rehab Consultant, Handi Medical, St. Paul, MN.

- A power wheelchair would necessitate a van with a lift. Jane had been going into the community less and less because of her transferring inabilities.

Item/Service	Replacement Frequency	Purpose	Cost
2016 Chrysler Town & Country Touring Van with adaptations	7 years	This van will allow independence in community mobility.	$53,300 (less than the cost of an average vehicle in the United States in 2016)

Source: Cummings Mobility, Albertville, MN.

- A van with a lift necessitates an oversized garage stall to provide needed maneuvering space for the van, the drop-down lift, and needed clear floor space to roll off the lift and maneuver toward the entrance door. This requires an additional 7 to 9 feet of clear width in one vehicle parking area. Jane has an attached single car garage. It is important to maintain an attached garage for the van so Jane does not have to maneuver through extreme weather elements to reach her van (e.g., snow, rain, ice, etc.) and to acknowledge Jane's inability to scrape frost off of windows or to remove snow off the vehicle.

Item/Service	Replacement Frequency	Purpose	Cost
Garage modification	1x or may be needed again with additional moves	To allow parking in garage and allow adequate floor space for exit/entry with van lift.	$13,759

- The OT offered Jane and her family suggestions about rearranging the kitchen, bedroom, and bathroom to improve access and ergonomics. Some OTs have this expertise, but the advice of a home access specialist can also be critical in a life care plan. Although there are several areas in the house to consider, such as vertical access, garage overhead door, access into house, doorways, bathroom, kitchen, hallways, floor surfaces, controls, and so on, for the purpose of this chapter, the kitchen will be addressed to suggest the level of detail and costs appreciated.
- The kitchen did not provide any features to assist Jane in independent or safe meal preparation. The original kitchen layout had not been modified to accommodate needed clear floor space for Jane's wheelchair or to accommodate the need to approach work areas in a forward approach to get close to the task area. Jane has been relying on her family for most meal preparation and cleanup. See the following example life care plan entry for details:

Item/Service	Replacement Frequency	Purpose	Cost
Kitchen modifications	1x (more often may be needed with moves)	• Rearrange cabinet configuration to provide turning space for the wheelchair and approach to each work area. • Replace cabinets with new cabinets. Ergonomically, this will be much easier for Jane to use from a seated position. • Provide clear knee space at the sink, cooktop, and one mix/work area and incorporate dual pull-out cutting boards.	$34,600

		• Replace the kitchen sink with a shallower sink to maximize knee clearance height; drains are to be located at the back of the sink to maximize knee clearance depth. • Conceal or wrap drainpipes to avoid hot water burns to Jane's knees. • Install single-lever faucet hardware at the sink. • Extend the wall cabinet over the dishwasher down to the countertop so dish storage is located within reach range. • Replace the gas range with an electric cooktop that offers front controls. • Rewire the range fan and light switch located within accessible reach range. • Provide a wall-mounted oven with a side-swinging door. • Provide a pull-out board below or adjacent to the oven to rest cool items removed from the oven. • Incorporate pull-out shelves in base cabinets. • Incorporate a pantry, with pull-out shelves. • Replace the existing refrigerator with a side-by-side refrigerator that has water and ice in the door, allowing storage for both compartments in reach range. • Relocate outlets and switches to the front face of countertops. Provide task lighting at each work area. • Replace the kitchen flooring to accommodate newly configured cabinetry and to extend the flooring into each knee space. Ensure the transition to adjacent floor materials is neutral.	

- A tub lift was recommended. While Jane had a shower chair, her spasticity and relaxation were improved with warm water. Jane could not get in the tub without a lift. See the following example of a life care plan entry:

Item/Service	Replacement Frequency	Purpose	Cost
Aqua Tec RSB with reclining lateral support and rotary seat	5 years	Allow for safety and enhanced independence with tub baths.	$3,144.00

Source: Lisa Michaels COTA/L, ATP/SMS, CRTS/Rehab Consultant, Handi Medical, St. Paul, MN.

- Jane's current wheelchair cushion needed replacement. See the following example of a life care plan entry:

Item/Service	Replacement Frequency	Purpose	Cost
Motion Concepts Libra cushion	3 years	Provide pressure relief, comfort, and positioning.	$485.00

Source: Lisa Michaels COTA/L, ATP/SMS, CRTS/Rehab Consultant, Handi Medical, St. Paul, MN.

- Jane was educated about shoulder overuse in people with spinal cord injury. Fitness equipment that could be used without harm was suggested. See the following example of a life care plan entry:

Item/Service	Replacement/Service Frequency	Purpose	Cost
Bowflex Versatrainer[a]	10–12 years	Upper body strengthening from wheelchair.	$1,599
Dura-Band Exercise System[a]	2 years	Exercise bands to be used as an alternative to Bowflex or for out of home use.	$35.95
Personal trainer	4–6 sessions/year	Regular assessment from a personal trainer will be needed to advise regarding exercise/strengthening program as medical status changes and with aging. It is possible to get this same advice from a PT but cost is likely to be greater unless accomplished during annual PT evaluation.	$50–$100/ session

[a] It is possible that a physical trainer/PT may recommend alternative equipment.

- Jane was only 46 years old, 2 years after her injury, and already experiencing shoulder pain. The OT recommended an item, while not currently needed, to be added to the life care plan as Jane aged:

Item/Service	Replacement Frequency	Purpose	Cost
Bed cane	5 years	This device will assist with bed mobility/ transfers. While not currently needed, it should be added to the plan beginning at age 55.	$145

Conclusion

Recommendations from the OT may be vital in the development of a life care plan as many components fall under the expertise of the OT. However, the life care planner should remain aware that OTs typically think about a current episode of care and may be unaccustomed to projecting lifelong needs. Additionally, few have forensic experience and may be reluctant to offer an opinion that may be used in a legal setting if they are not experienced or familiar with litigation issues. They may need education about how the information will be used and what it will mean for them to offer an opinion for the life care plan. Therapists also tend to specialize in specific areas of practice and consultation, and more than one OT may be needed for a specific life care plan. Consultation with OTs who specialize in other professional practice areas can bring added depth and detail to the life care plan.

References

American Occupational Therapy Association. (2015a). Enforcement Procedures for the Occupational Therapy Code of Ethics. *American Journal of Occupational Therapy, 69*(Suppl. 3), 6913410012. http://dx.doi.org/10.5014/ajot.2014.696S19.

American Occupational Therapy Association. (2015b). Occupational Therapy Code of Ethics (2015). *American Journal of Occupational Therapy, 69*(Suppl. 3), 6913410030. http://dx.doi.org/10.5014/ajot.2015.696S03.

Asher, I. E. (2014). *Occupational Therapy Assessment Tools: An Annotated Index* (4th ed.). Bethesda, MD: American Occupational Therapy Association.

Atchinson, B. J., & Dirette, D. K. (2012). *Conditions in Occupational Therapy: Effect on Occupational Performance* (4th ed.). Baltimore, MD: Lippincott Williams & Wilkins.

Hinojosa, J., & Blount, M. (2004). *The Texture of Life: Occupations and Related Activities* (2nd ed.). Bethesda, MD: AOTA Press.

Mitchell, N. (2004). Aging with cerebral palsy, spinal cord injury, and amputation: Implications for life care planners. *Journal of Life Care Planning, 3*, 163–175.

Chapter 8

The Role of the Physical Therapist in Life Care Planning

Kathie Allison and Kirsten Potter

Contents

Introduction 136
Physical Therapists Scope of Practice 136
The PT's Role in Primary Care 138
The PT's Role in Secondary Care, Tertiary Care, Health, and Wellness 138
The Role of Standardized Outcome Measures in PT Practice and Impact on the Life Care Plan 139
Physical Therapy Contributions to the Life Care Plan: The Who, Where, When, and How 142
Case Study: Traumatic Brain Injury (TBI), Spinal Cord Injury (SCI) Client 144
    Life Care Planning from the PT Perspective 144
    Patient History 144
    Hospital Course 144
    Present Status 144
What Is the PT's Contribution in This Life Care Plan? 145
    Future Medical Care 145
    Therapeutic Interventions 145
    Home/Facility Care Recommendations 145
    Durable Medical Equipment 146
    Orthotic and Prosthetic Needs 146
    Physical Therapy Charges 146
Conclusion 146
Acknowledgments 147
References 147

Introduction

Physical Therapists (PTs) play an important and integral role in the delivery of health care in a variety of settings. "Physical therapists help individuals maintain, restore, and improve movement, activity, and functioning, thereby enabling optimal performance and enhancing health, well-being, and quality of life. Their services prevent, minimize, and eliminate impairment of body function and structures, activity limitations, and participation restrictions" (*American Physical Therapy Association*, 2001).

The life care planning process, through its concise methodology, also strives to determine the client's future medical and support care needs that are based on the functional deficits of individuals who have experienced a catastrophic injury or disability. The goals of both services are mutually similar. However, the life care planner also serves to identify the costs of those needs. The PT clinician can serve to provide valuable information to the life care planner in formulating a comprehensive life care plan—based on their standard of practice and their skill. This chapter will identify the role that the physical therapist can play in the formulation of the life care plan.

Physical Therapists Scope of Practice

Physical therapists treat pain, disease, and injury by physical therapeutic means (Stedman, 2000). The professional organization for physical therapist practice is the American Physical Therapy Association (APTA). The association is responsible for establishing standards of practice, code of ethics, and guidelines for the delivery of PT services. Currently, physical therapy education programs award a Doctorate in Physical Therapy. Individuals who previously received degrees at the baccalaureate and master's level have equal standing for the care and treatment of clients. Licensure for physical therapists is regulated by states. Physical therapists take a national examination and can use those test scores for reciprocity among those states for which it is allowed. Physical therapists can choose to become board certified clinical specialists through the American Board of Physical Therapist Specialties.

The *Guide to Physical Therapist Practice* (2001) describes a patient/client management model used for all clients seen by a physical therapist. The model delineates a process as follows: Examination (History, Systems Review, and Tests/Measures)—Evaluation—Diagnosis—Prognosis—Intervention. The PT examination begins with conducting a history (i.e., interview) of the client to gather information related to general demographics, current and past health conditions, living environment, and social history, among others. The systems review is a brief examination of the musculoskeletal, neuromuscular, cardiovascular/pulmonary, and integumentary systems that aims to identify areas needing further testing by PT or a referral to a different health care provider. The final step in the PT examination involves conducting tests and measures that provide specific objective data to:

- Confirm or refute hypotheses about the client's activity limitations or participation restrictions
- Client's activity limitations or participation restrictions
- Determine baseline status
- Inform the PT regarding the evaluation, diagnosis, and prognosis

Following the examination, the PT conducts an evaluation by interpreting the examination data. This leads to the formation of the PT diagnosis, a label that identifies the impact of the client's condition on a system or the whole person. In the PT profession, increasing emphasis is placed on the role of the PT in identifying a diagnosis related to the movement system. The PT prognosis aims to identify the expected goals and outcomes (i.e., short- and long-term goals) that expect to be attained through the client's participation in PT and the time needed to achieve each goal/outcome.

The *Guide to Physical Therapist Practice* has defined the practice of physical therapy to include:

1. Examining (history, system review, tests, and measures) individuals with impairment, functional limitation, and disability or other health-related conditions in order to determine a diagnosis, prognosis, and intervention; tests and measures may include the following:
   - Aerobic capacity/endurance
   - Anthropometric characteristics
   - Assistive technology
   - Balance
   - Circulation (arterial, venous, lymphatic)
   - Community, social, and civic life
   - Cranial and peripheral nerve integrity
   - Education life
   - Environmental factors
   - Gait
   - Integumentary integrity
   - Joint integrity and mobility
   - Mental functions
   - Mobility (including locomotion)
   - Motor function
   - Muscle performance (including strength, power, and endurance)
   - Neuromotor development and sensory processing
   - Pain
   - Posture
   - Range of motion
   - Reflex integrity
   - Self-care and domestic life
   - Sensory integrity
   - Skeletal integrity
   - Ventilation and respiration
   - Work life
2. Alleviating impairment and functional limitation by designing, implementing, and modifying therapeutic interventions that include, but are not limited to:
   - Patient/client instruction
   - Airway clearance techniques

   - Assistive technology
   - Biophysical agents
   - Functional training in self-care and domestic, work, community, social, and civic life
   - Integumentary repair and protective techniques
   - Manual therapy techniques
   - Motor function training
   - Therapeutic exercise

3. Preventing injury, impairment, functional limitation, and disability, including the promotion and maintenance of health, wellness, fitness, and quality of life in all age populations.
4. Engaging in consultation, education, and research.

Relation to Vision 2020: Evidence-Based Practice (State Government Affairs, ext. 8533) [Document updated: 03/06/2014].

The PT's Role in Primary Care

Within the health care spectrum, the physical therapist may represent an entry point to the health care system. The goal of primary care is to direct client care through the health care system and return the individual to their prior level of function in the most efficient and cost-effective way. The physical therapist works as a member of the health care team in this endeavor. Knowledge of the roles that other health care providers play in health care delivery assures that the PT facilitates access to needed care that is appropriately identified and timely. The physical therapist is particularly well qualified to coordinate care related to loss of physical function as a result of musculoskeletal system disorders, but may also play a role in primary care for clients with conditions related to the neuromuscular, cardiopulmonary, or integumentary systems. PTs utilize their skill and knowledge to assess multiple body systems of their clients in order to provide clients with comprehensive PT services and, importantly, make appropriate and timely referrals to other health care providers. In addition, the PT can provide education to the community. In industrial workplace settings the PT also practices at the primary care level by identifying the demands of the work environment placed on the individual and matching therapeutic interventions needed to return the employee to the job. When needed, the physical therapist can work with the employer to identify if possible job modifications will allow the employee to return to the work environment.

The PT's Role in Secondary Care, Tertiary Care, Health, and Wellness

Physical therapists also play major roles in secondary and tertiary care. In these cases, other health care professionals typically refer the client to physical therapy. The PT may play an active and ongoing role throughout the care of a client but may also function as a consultant or educator operating as part of a multispecialty team. Physical therapists are also involved in the promotion of health and wellness; prevention and screening; and providing health education regarding lifestyle factors, home modifications, assessing the development of infants and children, and identifying risk factors (e.g., fall risk) for elderly clients. Physical therapists can provide interventions to slow the progression of functional decline and disability. They can reduce the degree of disability by restoring skills and independence for those with chronic conditions. Physical therapists working with other members of the health care team can be instrumental in helping families to identify the appropriate level of care that is based on the client's function and prognosis.

The Role of Standardized Outcome Measures in PT Practice and Impact on the Life Care Plan

In the rehabilitation arena, various outcome measures have been developed to provide an objective method to document the baseline function of an individual entering rehabilitation and to measure the increments of progress. Outcome measures generate scores that are intended to quantify a client's performance or health status based on standardized evaluation protocols or closed-ended questions (Jette et al., 2009). One of the most commonly used outcome measures in rehabilitation is the Functional Improvement Measure (FIM) (Uniform Data System for Medical Rehabilitation, 2017). The FIM is a standardized interdisciplinary tool used to assess the burden of care needed for the client to perform 18 functional tasks. Each health care professional involved in the client's care contributes to the scoring. The FIM score has been utilized for years to chart a client's progress from rehabilitation admission to discharge. Other resources exist that provide physical therapists with summarized data on outcome measures that can be used in client care. The Rehabilitation Measures Database, an online product of the Rehabilitation Institute of Chicago's Center for Rehabilitation Outcome Measurement (Shirley Ryan AbilityLab, 2017) provides summaries of over 350 measures used in rehabilitation. Task forces of the American Physical Therapy Association Academy of Neurologic Physical Therapy (Academy of Neuro PT, 2015) have developed recommendations on the use of outcome measures for specific client populations: stroke, multiple sclerosis, Parkinson's disease, brain injury, spinal cord injury, and vestibular dysfunction.

Understanding of the purpose and use of these tools helps the life care planner set the foundation for all elements of need in the life care plan. Functional outcome measures can be used to establish the client's prior level of function or independence; it documents progress or regress from that point and it identifies where the client is functioning at the time of the preparation of the life care plan. When the client shows an increase in score or improvement, the life care plan design needs to identify resources that maximize functional independence. When clients demonstrate a decrease in their total score, the life care plan will need to identify the barriers that are prohibiting the client from achieving independence and what the costs are to purchase services that bridge that gap. Perhaps most importantly, the FIM measurement establishes the burden of care required by the client. Many of the costs identified in the life care plan can have their foundation based on the client's change in pre-injury and post-injury functional profiles. Most functional profiles include both self-care activities and Instrumental Activities of Daily Living. It is useful for each activity to have a predicted time-to-accomplish estimate that would be considered within a reasonable time. By using a functional profile tool, the life care planner demonstrates an organized concise method that serves to determine the extent of support care required by the client, what level of skill will be needed in home health support care, and justification for the costs associated with the identified level of care. The functional assessment can document the needed residential care instead of home support care and/or will substantiate the need for transition to a residential care setting. The following is an example of a modified functional profile.

Functional Profile for Home Use Sample			
Client Name ______________	**Date**______________		
Daily Log for Activities			
Activities	*Avg. Time*	*Prior Level of Function*	*Current Level of Function/Modifications*
Bathing			
Shower	15–30 min.		
Tub			
Sponge	15–30 min.		
Hair Care	30 min.		
Skin Care			
Clean Nails			
Apply Lotion			
Support Skin			
Shaving	10 min.		
Oral Care	5 min.		
Brush Teeth			
Denture Care			
Dressing	15–30 min.		
Upper Body			
Lower Body			
Shoes & Socks			
Prosthesis	10–15 min.		
Toileting	15–30 min.		
Bowel & Bladder			
Toilet/Commode			
Catheter Care			
Ostomy Bag			
Transfers	10–20 min.		
Bed			

(*Continued*)

Chair	10–20 min.		
Furniture			
Car/Vehicle			
Ambulation (Walking)			
Independent			
Device-Aided			
Mobility—Wheelchair/ Scooter			
Eating			
Setup/Assist	5 min.		
Food-specialty			
Meal Preparation	30 min.		
All Meals			
Future Meals	30 min.		
Cleanup	15–30 min.		
Safety			
Preparation	15–30 min.		
Shopping			
Groceries	1–3 hr.		
Personal Items	30 min.		
Medication	30 min.		
Clothing	30 min.		
Medication			
Knows All	5 min.		
Takes on Time			
Setup Help	5–10 min.		
Assistance to Take	5–10 min.		
Laundry	2 hrs.		
Housekeeping	2 hrs.		
General	30 min.		

(*Continued*)

Toilet/Bath	30 min.		
Kitchen	30 min.		
Make Bed	5–10 min.		
Change Bed	30 min.		
Trash Removal	5 min.		
Heavy Cleaning			
Telephone Skill	5 min.		
Checkbook Use	1 hr.		
Life Goals/Parenting			
Home Maintenance	1–3 hrs.		
Lawn			
Snow Removal			
Ladders			
Inside Upkeep			
Outside Upkeep			
Ladders			

Persons assisting in this report ____

Prior hobbies ____

Current hobbies ____

Note: This chart can be modified to allow for a daily diary of care to trend needs over time for substantiating home care.

Physical Therapy Contributions to the Life Care Plan: The Who, Where, When, and How

The PT evaluation process can provide the life care planner with information on the client's status in many areas. The PT evaluation also serves to help the life care planner establish reasonable objectives for therapeutic intervention in the future. Physical therapists base their treatment goals on evidence-based practice objectives. Future therapy recommended in the life care plan should be accompanied with specific objectives and/or outcomes that are consistent with the PT diagnosis and reasonable plan of care.

- General strength and range of motion of the extremities and trunk

  Is the client's strength functional to allow independent functioning? Will therapeutic interventions be needed now or in the future to maintain or maximize function?

- Gait and balance

    Does the client demonstrate that he/she can walk for functional distances? Will an assistive device improve gait distance or overall balance? Over time, will the client's mobility status change, requiring added assistance?
- Sensation

    Does the client have adequate sensation? Is there a possibility that skin breakdown will be a recurring future complication? Is there a need for positioning tools now or in the future to compensate for sensory deficits?
- Cognition/psychological abilities

    Does the client exhibit good judgment? Is he/she oriented to their environment? Can he/she follow directions? Is safety a concern? How can the life care plan help to bridge that gap?
- Communication

    Is the client able to adequately express their needs? Are there communication tools that will foster the client's independence? Will there be a need for periodic assessment of communication skills? Does he/she have the strength/range of motion (ROM) in their upper extremities to use assisted communication devices?
- Pain

    Does the client have pain that limits his/her ability to function on a daily basis? Are there therapeutic interventions that can improve the client's ability to function now or in the future? Is there an expectation that the pain will resolve or become chronic in nature? What are appropriate recommendations regarding the use of therapy to alleviate pain? How much therapy is too much or not enough? Are there health maintenance suggestions to foster improvement in pain control? Does the client meet criteria for a pain pump or dorsal column stimulator?
- Cardiopulmonary integrity

    Does the client exhibit an adequate cardiopulmonary functioning to live independently? Are there home modifications needed to decrease the work of living independently? Are there appropriate support care services that will assist in keeping the client independent?
- Neurological integrity

    Does the client exhibit normal muscle tone? Does the client have good coordination of movement? Does the client have adequate neurocognitive function to be independent? What level of assistance will the client require? What therapeutic interventions are needed now or in the future?
- Environment

    Is the client's living situation safe and appropriate? Are there modifications that can be made to the client's home to assure a safe environment? What is the level of supported care needed for the client to stay in their home?
- Community access

    Is the client able to move about in the community without assistance? Are there mobility devices that will improve the client's ability to be out in the community? Are there resources in the community that are available to help the client travel within the community? Will the client benefit from a wheelchair van or other modified vehicle to access the community?
- Work considerations

    Will the client benefit from a vocational evaluation? Are there workplace modifications that will facilitate return to work? Can workplace education provide a safer environment for the client and others?

- Clinical specialty in PT
  Each specialty area of physical therapy practice offers a unique perspective for identifying future client care. Example: Pediatric PTs are uniquely qualified to assist in projecting care needs and equipment needs occurring over the child's developmental spectrum. In addition, their knowledge of public programs and access to those programs is invaluable for the pediatric life care plan.

Case Study: Traumatic Brain Injury (TBI), Spinal Cord Injury (SCI) Client

Life Care Planning from the PT Perspective

The following case study history was initially presented at the International Academy of Life Care Planners (IALCP) summit held 2006. The case history was also used for an example in 2012 for the preconference program Dimensions of Practice: Nursing, OT, and PT Domains in Establishing the LCP. It is presented here to outline the role of the PT clinician in providing recommendations for the life care plan.

Patient History

- 19-year-old male, motor vehicle accident (MVA), ejected from car
- Glasgow Coma Scale (GCS) 14, dropped to 4 during resuscitation
- Hemodynamically unstable at the scene: required 5 L fluid, 6 units packed red blood cells (PRBC)
- Pneumothorax—chest tube in place
- CT brain: compressed right ventricle
- Vertebral body fractures: T9 body, L1 Burst
- Spinal Fusion, thoracic lumbar sacral orthotic (TLSO) brace post-operative (P/O)
- TBI: adjustment disorder, information processing deficit, psychological distress
- Post-op decubitus ulcer, related to weight loss and immobility
- Central pain syndrome
- Neurogenic bowel
- Adjustment disorder

Hospital Course

- Acute hospital stay: 21 days
- Acute inpatient rehabilitation: 46 days
- Outpatient: PT, occupational therapy (OT), counseling, neuropsychological testing
- Returned home to parents and older sibling
- Home modifications included room addition for accessibility

Present Status

- Adjustment issues: anger, despair, withdrawal
- Incontinence; mom provides bulk of care; frequent UTIs
- Sexuality and reproductive issues
- Ongoing weight loss

- High risk of skin breakdown
- Dependent; driving, community access

What Is the PT's Contribution in This Life Care Plan?

Future Medical Care

- Rationale for annual therapy evaluation for lifetime—needed to monitor client status and the status of the plan of care that was established prior to discharge home.
- Use of clinical practice guidelines to identify additional services, tests, etc., for the client over lifetime.
- Future needs not identified by the care team can be recommended by the PT life care planner if that need would have been recommended in a routine discharge planning meeting.
- PT can recommend other appropriate ancillary care. PT can establish frequency of treatments based on clinical standards, their training, education, and experience.
- PT can establish criteria for referral back to physician for assessment.

Therapeutic Interventions

- PTs are the experts in identifying overuse injuries occurring in the SCI population. They can establish the guidelines for recognition of overuse injuries, treatment options, and any equipment modifications needed to decrease occurrence.
- PTs have the training and experience to establish an average number of PT visits for any occurrence of therapy: usually 8–12 visits. PT reevaluation serves to document progress and to justify extension of care. PT's can educate regarding the transition of treatment objectives that change over the course of a client's lifetime: from initial goals of strengthening and independence—to modified goals of health maintenance and supportive care—to palliative goals of minimizing contracture and planning for added care.
- PTs identify the appropriate therapeutic interventions to decrease further skin breakdown; recommend seating modifications; establish criteria for timely transition to a power chair.
- PTs provide education and training for community mobility, and they identify the appropriate mode of transportation for the client.
- PTs create and monitor home programs.

Home/Facility Care Recommendations

- PT assessment of client's function during the preparation of the life care plan will serve to identify the client's capabilities and what level of intervention is needed.
- The functional profile identifies the specific nature of the task and the standard time required for hiring support care.
- The PT can help determine whether home modifications will result in improved independence or ease of caregiver handling, or if alternate living is more appropriate.
- The PT can assist in identifying the appropriate skill level of residential care that the client needs now and what changes may be needed in living situation over the client's lifetime.

Durable Medical Equipment

- PTs, in collaboration with OT, provide invaluable input in identifying adaptive equipment for individuals with SCI.
- The PT evaluation of strength, ROM, and balance is essential for proper wheelchair selection.
- The PT is able to recommend all durable medical equipment (DME) related to bowel and bladder management, bathing, transfers, gait aides, and transportation.

Orthotic and Prosthetic Needs

- PTs evaluate the client to determine appropriate lower extremity orthotics, trunk orthotics, and lower extremity prosthetic prescriptions.
- PTs provide training for prosthetic wearing and orthotic use.
- PTs can provide a blueprint for the future progression of DME needs over the client's lifetime.

Physical Therapy Charges

Physical therapy charges vary widely throughout the country. Basic charges are for evaluation/reevaluation time, treatment intervention time, and modality use. Charges are often dependent on where the service is delivered. Services performed in hospitals are generally charged at a higher rate than services performed at a private practice outpatient facility. The following is only a guideline. The life care planner should contact local facilities to determine regional costs.

- General evaluation charges are billed in 15–30-minute increments. Charges for evaluation range from $200.00–$300.00.
- Therapeutic exercise is generally billed in 15-minute increments in the range of $45.00–$65.00/per unit for free-standing outpatient (OP) clinic charges. Hospital-based charges are billed at $110.00–$145.00/unit. Most PT treatment sessions are for 30–60 minutes.
- Specialized exercise such as cardiac or pulmonary rehabilitation is usually billed at a separate rate.
- Home health PT is billed on a per-visit basis.
- Work hardening/pain management programs are usually billed on a per diem day or half-day fee.

Conclusion

"The strength of the team is each individual member. The strength of each member is the team" (Jackson, no date). It is possible that a life care plan can be accomplished by one individual working alone, making all the decisions. However, a life care planner who works in collaboration with the client's care team and independent experts when indicated has the ability to create a truly comprehensive report. The physical therapist is an important contributor to the life care planning process. The perspective offered by individuals who work daily on function, functional possibilities, and overcoming functional barriers, will add depth to the report. In addition, therapists are often the first clinicians to ask questions and to work with teams members to come up with the answers.

Acknowledgments

At the start of this review, I met with two individuals to discuss where to start this review, Dr. Kirsten Potter and Dr. Amy Foley, both faculty members for the DPT program at Rockhurst University in Kansas City. We quickly came to the conclusion that over the past few years the practice of physical therapy has undergone quantum changes both in scope of practice and accountability of practice. Their insight provided the spring board for the chapter rewrite. Kirsten served as my editor and was the contributor for the section on the Guide to PT Practice. Many thanks to both for their help.

References

Academy of Neuro PT. 2015. Neurology Section Outcome Measure Recommendations. Available at: http://www.neuropt.org/professional-resources/neurology-section-outcome-measures-recommendations.

American Physical Therapy Association. 2001. Guide to Physical Therapist Practice. 3rd ed. Available at: http://guidetoptpractice.apta.org.

American Physical Therapy Association (APTA) vision statement for physical therapy 2020.

Jackson P. (no date). Available at http://www.azquotes.com/quote/475782.

Jette D., Halbert J., Iverson C., Miceli E., & Shah P. 2009. Use of standardized outcome measures in physical therapist practice: Perceptions and applications. *Phys Ther. 89*, 125–135.

Shirley Ryan AbilityLab. 2017 Rehabilitation Measures Database, 2017. Available at: http://www.rehabmeasures.org/default.aspx.

Stedman, T. L. 2000. Stedman's Medical Dictionary. Baltimore, MD, Lippincott Williams & Wilkins.

Uniform Data System for Medical Rehabilitation (no date). About the FIM System. Retrieved 12/8/2017 from: http://www.udsmr.org/WebModules/FIM/Fim_About.aspx.

Acknowledgements

[illegible]

References

[illegible]

Chapter 9

The Role of the SLP and Assistive Technology in Life Care Planning

Carolyn Wiles Higdon

Contents

Introduction....................150
The Role of the SLP in Life Care Planning....................152
Qualifications and Credentials of an SLP for Life Care Planning Purposes....................153
    SLP Training and Preparation....................155
        Interprofessional Education and Interprofessional Practice (IPE and IPP)....................156
        Interpersonal Communication, Human Learning, Counseling Theories and Practices, and Family Systems and Systems Theory....................157
Research in Communication Sciences and Disorders....................161
    Laryngeal Imaging....................161
        Implications for Life Care Plans....................163
    Biofeedback for Acquired Apraxia of Speech....................163
        Implications for Life Care Plans....................165
Terminology in the Field of Communication Sciences and Disorders....................165
    The SLP Review of Records and Intake....................166
Assessment Process....................167
Pediatric and Adolescent Assessments....................167
Federal Mandates and Policies....................168
    Gleason Act....................170
Examples of ATs....................171
Speech-to-Speech Relay System....................175
    Background....................175
    Who Uses STS?....................176
    Using STS....................176
    Alternatives....................176

Mandatory Minimum Standards for STS 176
Filing a Complaint with the FCC 176
Manufacturers' Roles 177
Funding and Economic Issues 177
Medical Coding 178
Neurolitigation 178
Hot Topics in Speech-Language Pathology Update 189
Case Study 190
Conclusion 190
Appendices 191
References 253

Introduction

Individuals with communication disorders present complex, confusing, and often frustrating challenges to the life care planner. Communication is defined as the transmission or exchange of thoughts and information from one individual to another, whatever the means (e.g., speech, manual signs, gestures, or other graphic symbols). Communication may be linguistic or nonlinguistic. Communication itself is an abstract concept, with disorders in communication, defined by brain-monitoring technology, sophisticated differential diagnoses, and an ability to understand normal and abnormal human speech and language. The best-qualified person to evaluate and make recommendations in this specific area is the speech-language pathologist (SLP). The area of study is accurately referred to as communication sciences and disorders, which includes speech-language pathology and audiology. Speech-language pathology includes cognitive communication, speech, language, and swallowing.

As we begin the second century of neuroscience, we have embarrassingly little information about how speech and language develop in the normal human brain, and our understanding of how these processes can be disrupted is also extremely primitive. To a large extent, this predicament results from severe technological limitations in the study of human anatomy and physiology that have prevailed until recently. Either techniques have been too invasive for use with human subjects or, for those less invasive techniques (conventional electroencephalography), the information generated is difficult to interpret, particularly with regard to normal function.

Brain imaging refers to a group of radiological techniques that differentiate abnormal from normal brain structures. Newer imaging techniques permit examining live brain tissue integrity without cranial penetration, now allowing SLPs to gather very sophisticated information about the brain and communication. Brain imaging is divided into static and dynamic techniques. Static techniques identify the anatomical structures of the brain and include computed tomography (CT) and magnetic resonance imaging (MRI). Dynamic techniques examine brain functional anatomy or physiology and include regional cerebral blood flow, single-photon emission computed tomography (SPECT), and positron emission tomography (PET).

In addition to imaging techniques, several other diagnostic techniques may be chosen to gather cognitive and language function information from the brain. The electroencephalogram (EEG) is a graphic representation of the potential differences between two separated points on the scalp surface that represent brain-transmitted electrical potentials or the electrical activity generated by brain cells. Electrical potentials are called brain waves. Brain electrical activity mapping represents a topographic mapping of the temporally recorded EEG activity of the electrical potentials from the brain. Brain electrical activity mapping provides greater clinical insight into brain physiology than an EEG (Bhatnagar, 2012).

Electromyography (EMG) is the visual record of muscular electrical activity during spontaneous and voluntary movements. Electromyography is used to determine the nerve or muscle pathology when clinical evidence is either absent, equivocal, or needs confirmation. An examination of the quality, speed, and magnitude of electrical impulses in muscles can help detect nerve or muscle damage. It can also differentiate among muscle disease (myopathy), atrophy of spinal motor neurons (neuropathy), interruption of nerve supply (denervation), and neuromuscular (myoneural) problems.

Evoked potentials refer to normal electrical activities of the central nervous system that occur in response to specific and controlled sensory stimulation. Whether the sensory stimulus is *visual*, *somatosensory*, or *auditory*, evoked brain responses are recorded using electrodes referred to the spinal cord, brain stem, and scalp. Visual evoked potentials are used to evaluate electrical conduction along the optic nerve, optic tract, lateral geniculate, optic radiations, and visual cortex. Somatosensory evoked responses are elicited by simulation of contralateral peripheral nerves. Clinical conditions in which somatosensory evoked potentials are of diagnostic value include multiple sclerosis, brain injuries, brain death, posterior column spinal cord lesions, and lesions of the peripheral nerves. Evoked response audiometry is the electrophysiological assessment of auditory functions. It measures changes in neural activity that occur in the auditory acoustic stimuli. Evoked response audiometry is used for assessing the functioning of the auditory neural pathway to predict hearing thresholds in patient populations that are difficult to test. In evoked response audiometry, the most commonly measured responses are the *auditory brain stem responses (brain stem auditory evoked response).*

Dichotic listening is a noninvasive neuropsychological tool that involves auditory stimuli and is commonly used for assessing cerebral dominance. It involves presenting simultaneous but partially different auditory stimuli to both ears. The attention factors are minimized by requiring subjects to simultaneously attend to both ears and report the stimuli they perceive. When the linguistic material presented in both ears is largely similar and spoken in the same voice, attending to the stimuli from both ears poses processing difficulties. The neurolinguistic implications of these findings are that right ear performance can serve as an index for determining degrees of language lateralization. Strong support for the stronger contralateral auditory projections in dichotic listening came when the dichotic testing results were supported by the observation of the left language lateralization by hemispheric infusion of sodium amobarbital.

The lumbar puncture (spinal tap) is used for diagnosing various infections and hemorrhages of the central nervous system that are not observable from the CT scan. Chemical analysis of the obtained cerebrospinal fluid helps in the differential diagnosis of multiple sclerosis, neurosyphilis, Guillain–Barre syndrome, carcinomatous meningitis, and neuropathies. Lumbar puncture is contraindicated in cases of increased intracranial pressure because of the possibility of a brain stem herniation (Bhatnagar, 2012). These are a few commonly used radiological diagnostic techniques that directly apply to the management of neurological patients who are commonly seen by practicing SLPs, primarily in medical settings.

Improvements in computers during the last two decades have significantly enhanced our ability to study aspects of human anatomy and physiology otherwise inaccessible (e.g., deep structures of living brains) and to consider sophisticated experimental questions (e.g., the temporal course of neural function and the nature of individual differences). Thus, in many ways these techniques have placed us on the threshold of the first century of human neuroscience.

Neuroscience is significant in the process of life care planning because it allows life care planners to obtain the critical, and now more measurable, information to make projections about disability related to the communication disorders, as well as provides thoughtful input into the long-term medical, educational, clinical, rehabilitative, psychosocial, recreational, vocational, and technology needs of the individuals. Access to neuroscientific information also mandates that the life care planner carefully identify the SLP in the life care planning process, to ensure that the SLP demonstrates the knowledge and skills necessary to provide irrefutable information that will stand up under scrutiny of other team members in the life care planning process, as well as from other medical, legal, and funding sources.

This chapter will discuss the role of the SLP and the advanced areas of training and preparation needed to demonstrate the level of knowledge and skills in communication sciences and disorders necessary in life care planning. Qualifications and credentials of an SLP are reviewed (ASHA, 1989), along with the assessment process and funding and economic considerations that impact the area of speech-language pathology (ASHA, 1991). Neurolitigation considerations for the SLP expert are discussed in the second half of the chapter. The whole concept of taking a role in the life care planning process is a new consideration for the SLP, who will provide an integral part in the development of the life care plan for individuals with communication or swallowing deficits. The credibility and complexity of communication disorders are just beginning to be recognized, as well as the impact that deficits in communication disorders has on multiple parts of the life care plan. If the life care planner recognizes that an individual has a communication deficit, the SLP may furnish information in the areas of cognitive communication, vocational, educational, aids to independent living, psychosocial, speech, language, swallowing, medical complications, and future medical planning.

Person-First Language

Students as well as professionals in speech-language pathology (and audiology) must keep in mind that the problems individuals experience do not define who they are. People are not their problems; problems are something people experience. Therefore, as clinicians and researchers we follow the "client/person first" conventions as closely as possible; in other words, we refer to "a boy with an articulation disorder," "a girl with a hearing impairment," "a woman with a voice disorder," and so on. Professionally, we avoid phrases such as "he's an articulation client," "she's hearing impaired," "she's a voice case," and so on, because the wording implies that the person's problem is his or her identity. It is easy to slip into the habit of referring to the problem that the person has rather than to the person who has a problem. We need to learn early and maintain our vigilance to always use person-first language.

The Role of the SLP in Life Care Planning

The purpose of a life care plan is to identify the comprehensive and individualized needs of a person as they relate to a disability or chronic illness with relevant associated cost considerations. These needs are the operational components of a life care planning process. They should never be compromised or manipulated. The costs assigned to these needs are determined by the geographical consumer rate for the identified services and equipment. The costs can be developed through understanding the range of available funding streams, creative and innovative ways of negotiating, available resources, and the cost projection analyses that accompany such planning.

The SLP must be well-grounded in the theory of normal development in all ages, in any previous learning or developmental problems affecting the individual, and in the current status of the individual and must be able to predict future functioning of the individual. Many times SLPs will practice in the treatment of either the pediatric or the adult population. This frequently precludes the SLP from being able to look backward or beyond to make accurate recommendations about future functioning needs.

It is always useful for the SLP, who is consulting in the life care planning process, to be able to actively engage in the clinical treatment of individuals and their families. This enhances the SLP's credibility, because the SLP should have realistic estimates of current needs and prognostic predictions. However, it is also imperative that the consulting SLP have a fluid understanding of the current literature and research that directly or indirectly impacts the area of communication sciences and disorders. This includes knowledge of the most current assessment procedures, state-of-the-art assistive technology, trends in pharmacology and medical care, and possible needs in the areas of residential and geriatric care (American Speech-Language-Hearing Association, 2015).

Qualifications and Credentials of an SLP for Life Care Planning Purposes

The generally accepted national standard for practice in speech-language pathology (communication sciences and disorders) is the American Speech-Language-Hearing Association (ASHA) certificate of clinical competence in speech-language pathology (CCC-SLP). The ASHA CCC-SLP requires a master's degree in speech-language pathology, completion of a one-year clinical fellowship, and successful passage of the national examination. For states with licensure, the legal right to practice will vary with the individual licensing acts. Most licensure laws were modeled after the ASHA CCC standard (ASHA, 2014). Licensure, unlike certification, is mandatory for those states that regulate the practice of audiology and speech-language pathology. In many states, licensure requirements parallel those of ASHA certification. Furthermore, ASHA certification will satisfy many of the requirements of state licensure when one applies for reciprocity. Table 9.1 shows the states with

Table 9.1 State Licensure for SLPs and Audiologists

Alabama	Kentucky	Ohio
Alaska	Louisiana	Oklahoma
Arizona	Maine	Oregon
Arkansas	Massachusetts	Pennsylvania
California	Michigan[a]	Rhode Island
Colorado[a]	Minnesota	South Carolina
Connecticut	Mississippi	South Dakota[a]
Delaware	Missouri	Tennessee
District of Columbia	Montana	Texas
Florida	Nebraska	Utah
Georgia	Nevada	Vermont
Hawaii	New Hampshire	Virginia
Idaho	New Jersey	Washington
Illinois	New Mexico	West Virginia
Indiana	New York	Wisconsin
Iowa	North Carolina	
Kansas	North Dakota	

[a] Does *not* regulate the profession of speech-language pathology.

licensure of SLPs and audiologists. See Chapter 10 on the Role of the Audiologist in this text for additional information on audiology licensure.

Speech-language pathologists and audiologists must hold both national and state credentials. State credentials differ from state to state. Often, the state education agency requirements do not equate to the national standard, requiring only a bachelor's degree and education certification in a state to practice. Twenty states require school-based audiologists and SLPs to be licensed (Alabama, California, Florida, Georgia, Hawaii, Illinois, Kansas, Maryland, Michigan, Missouri, Montana, Nevada, New York, North Carolina, North Dakota, Oregon, South Dakota, Texas, Virginia, and Wyoming) (ASHA, 2018). SLPs with specific interests may hold additional certifications determined by societies and organizations in a particular area, such as the Rehabilitation Engineering and Assistive Technology Society of North America (also known as RESNA) or the special interest groups of ASHA. The special interest groups within ASHA are listed in Table 9.2.

Codes of ethics for all organizations in which an individual holds membership must be acknowledged and followed. Ethics is defined as "the study of standards of conduct and moral judgment and the system or code of morals of a particular profession" (ASHA, 2015). When applied to a field or professional area, such as augmentative communication, or a profession, such as audiology or speech-language pathology, the ethical conduct of practitioners is embodied both in a code (or canon) of ethics and in standards of practice. SLPs and audiologists must comply with the code of ethics for their discipline. The code of ethics for a discipline is typically developed by the professional association serving it. The ASHA code of ethics sets forth the fundamental principles and rules considered essential to the preservation of the highest standards of integrity and ethical conduct to which members of the profession of speech-language pathology and audiology are bound. All professional activity must be consistent with the code of ethics. The Principle of Ethics II, Rule B, especially important in the area of assistive technology, states "individuals shall engage in only those aspects of the profession that are within their competence, considering their level of education and training" (ASHA, 2015).

Table 9.2 ASHA Special Interest Groups (SIGs)

1. Language learning and education
2. Neurophysiology and neurogenic speech and language disorders
3. Voice and voice disorders
4. Fluency and fluency disorders
5. Speech science and orofacial disorders
6. Hearing and hearing disorders: research and diagnostics
7. Aural rehabilitation and its instrumentation
8. Hearing conservation and occupational audiology
9. Hearing and hearing disorders
10. Issues in higher education
11. Administration and supervision
12. Augmentative and alternative communication
13. Swallowing and swallowing disorders (dysphagia)
14. Communication disorders and sciences in culturally and linguistically diverse populations
15. Gerontology
16. School-based issues
17. Global issues in communication sciences and related disorders
18. Telepractice
19. Speech science

When funding is available, third-party intermediaries in most instances require the ASHA CCC and licensure. The national certification standards are generally tied to the ASHA CCC for both funding by third-party intermediaries and for service delivery. On the other hand, other certifications in existence, such as the education agency certification, traditionally do not equate to the CCC. If you are not familiar with an individual and his or her credentials, it is wise to contact ASHA and the state licensing board to determine his or her credentials. It is also important to note that licensing laws usually relate to direct patient assessment and treatment in the state where the service is provided, but do not address review of records or expert testimony. The national certification is a generic certification whereby the individual has met the minimum entry-level requirements across a broad spectrum of knowledge areas in communication sciences and disorders. When funding is available, third-party intermediaries use as a guideline the requirements for service delivery established by Medicare and Medicaid (i.e., ASHA CCC-SLP) and, where applicable, a current state license.

SLPs who have the expertise to provide information in their area must also understand and participate in transdisciplinary integrated assessment and treatment models; have knowledge of funding streams and creative funding; be knowledgeable about state and federal policies, laws, and changes in these laws and policies; and be knowledgeable about collaborative sources and how to build them. They must also be able to provide clear, concise, understandable documentation that is written in a defensible but understandable format with functional milestones and goals available. For a complete communication assessment and many of the services related to delivery of care for individuals exhibiting communication and swallowing difficulties described in this chapter, it is advisable that the consulting SLP hold a doctoral degree with emphasis in the areas of assistive technology. (See Appendixes 9.1 and 9.2 at the end of the chapter for an outline of relevant information.)

There are key areas relevant to the professions of SLP and audiology that have current state legislative and regulatory actions. States have enacted legislation or adopted regulations in many of these areas of licensure and scope of practice, health care and insurance, and education. Licensure and scope of practice revisions have occurred in 2016 in 20 states, to include the addition of music therapy, military licensure for spouses, ABA licensure, and board antitrust licensure. In health care and insurance, seven states have included insurance coverage for autism (Kansas, Kentucky, New York, North Carolina, Ohio, Oklahoma, Pennsylvania), four states included hearing aid coverage for a tax credit (Louisiana, Massachusetts, New Jersey, and New York), with many states including telemedicine in their laws. Many states have made changes in their laws to reflect Medicaid changes, insurance coverage for SLP services, and universal health care/EHB inclusions. State licensure laws have included educational components including early intervention/EHDI/EPSDT (Early Hearing Detection and Intervention/Early and Periodic Screening, Diagnostic, and Treatment), dyslexia, special education services, teacher certification requirements, salary supplement/loan forgiveness, and language acquisition.

SLP Training and Preparation

The competent SLP has received preparation in the following areas, as they relate to human communication, swallowing, and development across the life span:

- Theories and processes of normal development and aging, including motor, cognitive, social-emotional, and communication
- Physiology of speech production and swallowing, including respiration, phonation, articulation, resonance, and the vocal/aerodigestive tract

- Embryological, genetic factors in development, including the development of craniofacial structures and the nervous system
- Anatomic structures, neuroanatomy, and neurophysiology supporting speech, language, hearing, swallowing, and respiration
- Organic etiologies of disorders of communication and swallowing
- Psychological and psychosocial influences on communication and swallowing
- Neurolinguistic, linguistic, cultural, and social influences on communication
- Theories of speech perception and production, language development, and cognition
- Ethics related to diagnosis, treatment, and professional conduct

Interprofessional Education and Interprofessional Practice (IPE and IPP)

The American Speech-Language-Hearing Association (ASHA) represents more than 182,000 members and affiliates who are audiologists, speech-language pathologists, speech, language, and hearing scientists, audiology and speech-language pathology support personnel, and students. ASHA affiliates with the following organizations that promote interprofessional practice (IPP) and interprofessional education (IPE): The National Academy of Medicine (NAM) Global Forum on Innovation in Health Professional Education (November 2012–present), Interprofessional Collaborative (IPC; 2006–present), and the World Health Organization (WHO).

The evolution of health care reform is creating a different landscape. As part of this evolution, ASHA established a 10-year (2015–2025) strategic objective to advance interprofessional education and collaborative practice (IPE/IPP), to collaborate among health professions within the framework of IPE/IPP, to support outcomes measurement to advance service delivery, and to promote SLPs and audiologists as leaders in communication health and health literacy.

As interprofessional education expands, academic programs and practice settings are adopting models that prepare future clinicians for patient-centered collaborative practice, such as:

- Case-based simulations
- Case presentations
- Clinical practice
- Course work
- Evidence-based practice
- Grand rounds
- Interdisciplinary seminars
- Journal groups
- Leadership training—Leadership Education in Neurodevelopmental and Related Disabilities (LEND)
- Learning communities
- Problem-based learning
- Professional issues colloquia
- Research projects
- Service learning
- Basic computer theory and systems applications, including frequently used software and input and output devices, as they relate to evaluation and treatment of language, cognitive communication, augmentative and alternative communication (AAC), swallowing, voice disorders (see Table 9.3), and central auditory processing disorders.

Academic programs in audiology and speech-language pathology are represented in more than 300 U.S. colleges and universities offering undergraduate through PhD education. More than 40 percent of all audiology and speech-language pathology degree programs are housed in colleges of allied health.

Interpersonal Communication, Human Learning, Counseling Theories and Practices, and Family Systems and Systems Theory

The SLP who is consulting on a life care plan should demonstrate an advanced knowledge and understanding of health care and educational facility practices; the common diseases and conditions affecting human communication, swallowing, and development across the life span; and medical, educational, surgical, and behavioral treatment as they relate to communication disorders, including knowledge of:

- Medical terminology
- Physicians' orders, confidentiality, legal issues in medical practices, and information and data systems management
- Elements of the physical examination and vital sign monitors
- Medical and laboratory tests and their purposes
- Medical record documentation practices

Table 9.3 Voice Disorders Addressed by the SLP

Functional	*Neurological*	*Organic*
Diplophonia	Ataxic dysarthria	Cancer
Falsetto	Essential tremor	Congenital abnormalities
Functional aphonia	Guillain-Barré syndrome	Contact ulcers
Functional dysphonia	Hyperkinetic (spasmodic dysphonia, essential tremor)	Endocrine changes
Muscle tension dysphonia	Hypokinetic (Parkinson's disease)	Granuloma
Nodules	Lower motor neuron (LMN)	Hemangioma
Phonation breaks	Mixed (amyotrophic lateral sclerosis, traumatic brain injury [TBI], multiple sclerosis)	Hyperkeratosis
Pitch breaks	Myasthenia gravis	Infectious laryngitis
Polyps	Resonance disturbance	Laryngectomy
Reinke's edema	Spasmodic dysphonia	Leukoplakia
Traumatic laryngitis	Spastic dysarthria	Papilloma
Ventricular dysphonia	Unilateral dysarthria	Pubertal changes
Vocal cord thickening	Upper motor neuron (UMN) Vocal fold paralysis	Sulcus vocalis Webbing

- Pharmacologic factors affecting communication and cognitive processes, development, and behavior
- Assistive Technology (AT), Augmentative and Alternative Communication (AAC) approaches, and the range of bioengineering adaptations used in medical settings
- Concepts of quality control and risk management
- Concepts in medical setting environmental safety (such as universal precautions, procedures, and infection control principles; radiation exposure precautions; and the Safe Medical Devices Act)
- Team processes
- Performance improvement processes
- Theories, concepts, and practices in outcomes measures
- Theories and concepts related to the impact of psychosocial and spiritual needs and the individual's cultural values on health care services
- Voice and laryngeal health and disorders
- Respiratory functions, tracheostomy tubes, and respiratory support requirements
- Neuroanatomy, neuropathology, and the neurophysiological support of swallowing, speech, language, and related cognitive abilities (Table 9.4), and the effects of diseases and disorders of the nervous system
- Concepts in human nutrition and hydration needs and their disorders
- Methods and interpretations in neuroimaging and other forms of anatomic imaging
- Esophageal, oropharyngeal, laryngeal, and neurologic tumors
- Concepts in neuropsychology and psychiatric and psychosocial disorders
- Common medical conditions
- Educational terminology
- Federal mandates related to education
- Broad understanding of curricula and literacy
- Educational philosophy of state education agencies
- Medical and surgical management of communication and swallowing

The SLP should be able to demonstrate advanced skills and abilities in diagnostics, treatment, and service delivery. The SLP should be able to review medical records and conduct succinct

Table 9.4 Language versus Cognition

Language	*Cognition*
Phonology	Attention
Morphology	Memory
Lexicon	Orientation
Syntax	Organizing
Semantics	Planning
	Reasoning
	Problem solving

Note: This table lists the areas of language and cognition the SLP assesses and treats.

clinical case histories and interviews to gather relevant information related to communication and swallowing, and to select and administer appropriate diagnostic tools and procedures and treatment for communication and swallowing disorders that are functionally relevant, family centered, culturally sensitive, and theoretically grounded.

The SLP should be able to:

- Obtain a representative sample and describe articulation and voice production in meaningful, accurate, and reliable terminology that addresses intelligibility and the audio-perceptual judgments of quality, tension, pitch, loudness, variability, steadiness, oral and nasal resonance, and severity of the disorder.
- Interpret a range of acoustic and physiologic measures of voice production (see Table 9.3).
- Understand acquired communication disorders to include aphasia, apraxia, dysarthria, traumatic brain injury, locked-in syndrome, and progressive deteriorating central and peripheral nervous system diseases.
- Demonstrate skills in instrumental assessments (acoustic, aerodynamic, electroglottographic, electromyographic, manometric, and ultrasonic measures).
- Apply techniques that ensure validity of signal processing, analysis routines, and elimination of task or signal artifacts.
- Understand assessment and treatment of autism spectrum disorders and pervasive developmental disorders.
- Use one or more techniques for imaging the larynx, vocal tract, and nasopharynx (flexible/rigid endoscopy, ultrasonography, or stroboscopy).
- Select and implement training and treatment procedures appropriate for speech prostheses and orthotics (tracheoesophageal puncture prosthesis, electrolarynges, speaking trachs and one-way valves, palatal lifts, voice amplifiers, voice output communication aids, obturators, and palatal augmentation prostheses).
- Conduct an oropharyngeal swallow examination accurately identifying abnormal structures and functions; identify symptoms, medical conditions, and medications pertinent to dysphagia; interpret and document examination findings; use instrumental techniques for screening and diagnosis of oropharyngeal dysphagia and for biofeedback in dysphagia management.
- Conduct reliable and accurate modified barium swallow procedures following a standard protocol that includes identification of structural abnormalities; swallowing motility disorders; presence, time, and etiology of aspiration; and appropriate treatment techniques (posture, maneuvers, bolus modification).
- Determine patient management decisions regarding oral/nonoral intake, diet, risk precautions, candidacy for intervention, and treatment strategies.
- Select and appropriately apply aided and unaided communication, including both linguistic and nonlinguistic modes and methods.

In December 1995, Jean-Dominique Bauby, the 43-year-old editor of the French magazine *ELLE* (published in many languages), suffered from a severe stroke in his brain stem that left him permanently paralyzed from head to toe, although his mind was intact—a victim of locked-in syndrome. Where once he had been renowned for his gregariousness and wit, Bauby now found himself imprisoned in an inert body, able to communicate only by blinking his left eye. It is remarkable that in doing so he was able to compose an eloquent memoir, which was published two days before his death in 1996 and went on to become an international bestseller. Bauby was able to accomplish this time-consuming and tedious task through the help of an assistant from his publisher. For each letter of every word of the 132-page book, the assistant would begin with the letter A and proceed through the alphabet until she reached the correct letter, at which time Bauby would make his only possible response, the blink of his left eye, to indicate that was the letter he wanted. In this manner he dictated his memoir, *The Diving Bell and the Butterfly* (adapted from Bauby, 1996/Rizzo, 1999).

Table 9.5 Physical and Communication Impairments That May Need AAC or AT

Developmental disabilities such as cerebral palsy, Down syndrome
Autism spectrum disorders and pervasive developmental disorders
Childhood apraxia of speech
Aphasia
Apraxia
Dysarthria
Traumatic brain injuries (closed and open)
Locked-in syndrome
Progressive deteriorating central and peripheral nervous system diseases (Parkinson's disease, ALS, multiple sclerosis, Guillain-Barré syndrome, dementias, and Alzheimer's)

- Locate and access assistive technology (AT), services, and funding sources.
- Work effectively with interpreters and translators and use assistive listening devices when needed for patient care.
- Communicate findings and treatment plans in a manner that is fitting and consistent with health care facility procedures.
- Counsel and educate patients and families and work within family systems to elicit participation in the treatment plan and work as a member of a health educational care team. (See also Table 9.5 for a description of the types of physical and communication impairments that may need AAC or AT evaluation by a SLP.)

The SLP will need to consider all of the following categories, regardless of the age of the individual, in the development of information for the life care plan: an oral and pharyngeal swallowing (dysphagia) assessment to include modified barium swallows, videostroboscopy evaluation, prostodontic intervention, and palatal prostheses; cognitive communication information; auditory processing information to include central auditory processing, augmentative communication assessment information, AT assessment information, voice and vocal information including videostroboscopy, and Botox assessment information; oral peripheral motor information; hearing acuity information; assistive listening device; and cochlear implant information.

The critical information obtained from a thorough communication sciences and disorders assessment must

Jenny Craig, the well-known cofounder of weight-loss centers, had a bizarre accident in 1995. She was watching television while sitting on a couch with no headrest. She fell asleep and her head fell forward with her chin on her chest. A loud noise from the TV startled her and her head jerked up, causing the mandible to snap over her maxilla. She had to pry her teeth apart and began to speak with a lisp as a result of trying to keep her lower teeth from hitting her upper teeth. She immediately saw her dentist, who referred her to a temporal mandibular joint (TMJ) specialist who told her that she had dislocated her jaw. The TMJ specialist recommended she try dental appliances, none of which helped. Her speech problem became worse and chronic. She was diagnosed with focal dystonia of the mandible (involuntary muscle contractions that induce abnormal movements and postures caused by the trauma of the sudden jerking of her mandible). She received Botox injections in her cheeks, which had no beneficial effect on her speech. Three years after the accident, she saw a reconstructive surgeon who specialized in cleft lip and palate and was able to repair some of the damaged muscle tissue that had been caused by the years of abnormal mandibular movements. In addition, the surgeon was the first person to recommend speech therapy. Craig began working with an SLP 5 days a week, 1 hour per day plus speech exercises in between appointments. Although her speech is not the same as it had been before the unusual accident, Craig is thankful she can communicate with people (Rizzo, 1999).

be considered within all the parameters of the life care plan itself. In other words, any and all areas that are impacted by deficits in communication and swallowing must be addressed with recommendations, if deemed appropriate by the evaluating SLP. These parameters include projected evaluation, projected therapeutic modalities, diagnostic testing and educational assessment, mobility (including accessories and maintenance of mobility technology), aids for independent functioning, orthotics and prosthetics, home furnishing and accessories, pharmacology needs, home/facility care, future medical care, transportation, health and strength maintenance, architectural renovations, potential complications, orthopedic equipment needs, vocational/educational planning, AT in the areas of sensory deficits, cognitive challenges, and communication disorders (including hearing and processing difficulties needing assistive listening devices). (See Appendix 9.2 at the end of the chapter for an outline.)

Research in Communication Sciences and Disorders

Research in the field of speech-language pathology (and audiology) is getting increased attention over the past several years. Trending research includes looking at children with specific language impairments, increased use of technology to treat individuals with communication impairments, the use of brain reading techniques to identify neural representations of social thoughts, possibly establishing the first biological based diagnostic tool to detect autism, the increased risk to individuals with traumatic brain injuries to develop neurodegenerative diseases, ways to prevent noise-induced hearing loss, the use of innovative prostheses, and new tests and treatments for communication disorders by using new drugs and new diagnostic procedures. Today, research and developments in this field are based on application and patient needs and funded accordingly. Health economy considerations will play a major role in all new speech and language pathology and audiology developments in the field of communication sciences and disorders in the future. Life care planners need to be current and knowledgeable about the trial research, as well as the emerging research and the application to patient treatment in the field of communication sciences and disorders in order to uphold the responsibility to the life plan recipients of providing the best and most current life care plan possible as the template for treatment, future needs, and economic planning for the individual. The research in communication sciences and disorders changes daily, the outcomes improve the services of speech-language pathologists and audiologists, and the patients' communication disorders outcomes improve as a result. Life care planners are encouraged to improve their understanding of the field of communication sciences and disorders and to critically assess the information they include in their life care plan to assure that they are offering the best plan available for individuals with communication disorders. This author encourages all readers to promote this concept as they develop their future life care plans. It is important for life care planners to understand the roles, responsibilities, certifications, and credentials, and to be able to critically evaluate the skills and knowledge the speech-language pathologists (and audiologists) bring to the development of the life care plan. Life care planners are challenged to be aware of emerging research in the areas of communication sciences and disorders so they can determine if there are technologies or procedures that will enhance the delivery of services in the present or in the future for the recipient of the life care plan.

Two key areas of research in Communication Sciences and Disorders are laryngeal imaging and biofeedback for acquired apraxia of speech, both of which warrant some comments.

Laryngeal Imaging

Speech-language pathologists use oral or nasal endoscopic laryngeal imaging to peer at the vocal cords as they vibrate. Cameras capable of recording laryngeal vocal fold vibration at a rate of 2,000 frames per second by means of high-speed digital imaging (HSDI) are now commercially available, prompting an increasing amount of published normative data regarding vocal fold vibratory characteristics using this method. As a result, the ability to identify pathologic vocal fold function using HSDI is receiving increased attention in the attempt to distinguish abnormal from normal function. Since the 1960s, videostroboscopy has been the primary method used to evaluate vocal fold vibration and is the clinical criterion standard for laryngeal imaging. However, a major limiting factor of this imaging method is that the slow-motion image seen with videostroboscopy is actually a composite image averaged over several vibratory cycles rather than a real time image. In addition, the clinical use of videostroboscopy is limited because it relies on periodic vocal fold vibration and a stable phonation frequency to activate the strobe light—conditions that are not always present in disordered voices. Patients with aperiodic vocal fold vibration, characterized clinically as a hoarse or rough vocal quality, cannot undergo adequate assessment using videostroboscopy because the strobe is able to illuminate only a single frequency of vibration at a time and cannot track aperiodic vibrations.

High-speed digital imaging of the larynx is not subject to the limitations of videostroboscopy because it uses a conventional rigid endoscope to record images of the larynx at a rate of 2,000 images per second, irrespective of vibratory frequency (Kendall, 2009). This allows imaging of aperiodic vibration. In addition, HSDI can visualize vocal onset and offset, which occurs too quickly to be captured by videostroboscopy and where significant aperiodicity occurs as a normal phenomenon (Kiritani et al., 1993). Improvements are noted in this technology which keeps getting smarter and sharper by most standards. Studies analyzing the application of HSDI in the clinical setting are beginning to emerge. High-speed digital imaging analysis of the glottal area and the amplitude of vibration for each vocal fold has been applied to the evaluation of unilateral vocal fold paralysis before and after medialization (Kiritani et al., 1993). Another area in which HSDI has great potential is in the assessment of vocal tremor and in the differentiation of spasmodic dysphonia from muscle tension dysphonia. This disorder produces the acoustic characteristics of tremor and breaks in phonation, and videostroboscopy cannot capture the aperiodic vibratory pattern in these patients. High-speed digital imaging is being applied to assist with quantification of vocal tremor, which previously has been very difficult.

Videostroboscopy has continued to be the mainstay of clinical laryngeal imaging since the 1980s and basic stroboscopy technology is now being coupled with high definition video sensors to significantly improve image quality and, through increased spatial resolution, potentially enhance assessment of vocal fold tissue health and function. Videostroboscopy has limitations that other developing technologies are addressing. New high-speed/high-resolution digital video cameras with unprecedented increases in light sensitivity and frame rates are capturing vocal cord actions that cannot be seen with videostroboscopy alone. These actions include true cycle to cycle details of vocal fold vibration, as well as nonperiodic phenomena associated with more severe types of dysphonia, voice breaks, and the beginning and end of voiced sounds. Researchers also are working to develop better tools to parse the huge amount of data collected during high-speed imaging.

While current clinical laryngeal imaging uses endoscopes capable of providing only uncalibrated two-dimensional views of the vocal folds' surfaces, researchers are developing new laser-based technologies such as depth-kymography, which shows precise size calibration of endoscopic images and tracks the important vertical displacement of vocal fold vibration. Another laser-based approach, dynamic optical coherence tomography, can capture dynamic cross-sectional images of vibrating vocal fold tissue to illustrate more clearly how disorders or medical treatments, such as Botox injections, affect its functioning (Kobler et al., 2010).

HSDI offers benefits over standard videostroboscopy in the analysis of aperiodic vocal fold motion and will likely develop as an important adjunct to videostroboscopy in the evaluation of voice disorders. This technology is still in the early stages of clinical application. As the knowledge base with this form of laryngeal analysis expands, our ability to evaluate and treat patients with dysphonia will improve.

Implications for Life Care Plans

High-speed digital imaging will illustrate more clearly how disorders or medical treatments such as Botox injections can affect the functioning of vocal fold tissue. This in turn will improve typical treatments, length of treatment, and long-term outcomes in individuals with medical vocal pathology. Life care planners need to be knowledgeable about neuropathology and need to be able to discern if more intense specific imaging can give improved diagnostic information to develop a more accurate life care plan and thus a more refined financial picture of the client's medical and rehabilitation needs.

Biofeedback for Acquired Apraxia of Speech

Research has shown that biofeedback will help people with acquired apraxia of speech to improve their motor planning abilities. Acquired apraxia of speech is a motor speech disorder in which the messages from the brain to the mouth are disrupted and the person cannot move his or her lips or tongue to the right place to say sounds correctly, even though the muscles are not weak. The severity of apraxia depends on the nature of the brain damage, and apraxia can occur in conjunction with dysarthria (muscle weakness affecting speech production) or aphasia (language difficulties related to neurological damage). Apraxia is known as acquired apraxia of speech, verbal apraxia, and dyspraxia. Electropalatography (EPG) appears to be a promising treatment tool for people with this disorder (Kuruvilla et al., 2008).

The EPG is a tool that displays and records tongue contact with the palate during speech production. The speaker wears a pseudopalate, a custom-made acrylic plate that looks like a dental retainer and is embedded with electrodes. The pseudopalate fits tightly against the upper palate and sends electronic signals of tongue to palate contacts to an external processor and then to a laptop or desktop computer. With advances in technology, the goal is for the system to become wireless. As we go to press, there are patents pending for wireless EPGs (Ghovanloo & Block, 2014). One example is the wireless real-time tongue tracking for speech impairment diagnosis, speech therapy with audiovisual biofeedback, and silent speech interfaces. (*Patent Applicant*: Georgia Tech Research Corporation, Pub. No.: US 2014/0342324 A1, Nov 20, 2014.)

Through EPG, a speech-language pathologist can display, record, and store the timing and location of tongue-to-palate contacts, and also provide visual biofeedback to the speaker. With a split screen, the system can display the contact patterns of two people—the patient and clinician—and the patient can try to emulate the clinician's patterns for treatment targets. Treatment targets (words, phrases, or sentences) can vary in length based on a patient's treatment goals with no limit to the length of recorded speech production. The clinician or patient can review recorded productions in real time, slow motion, or stop motion, and can print out views of tongue-to-palate contact or save them to a file (Cahill et al., 2005).

The science of EPG has been used to treat a number of speech disorders including those associated with cleft palate, hearing impairment, and developmental articulatory errors, but only a few case studies have used EPG to treat people with acquired apraxia of speech or with various dysarthrias or other motor speech disorders. The potential to give people with these disorders additional information about articulation, however, makes it a promising treatment, because it provides visual and tactile feedback for therapy targets, especially for speech sounds that are less visible.

The following reviews of three studies using EPG are provided for additional information and clarification of the use of EPG. Readers may refer to the full articles for additional details. (See full article citations in the References.)

The first review is from the Motor Speech Research Unit, Division of Speech Pathology, The University of Queensland, Brisbane, Queensland, Australia (Kuruvilla et al., 2008). The aim of the investigation was to compare EPG-derived spatial and timing measures between a group of 11 dysarthric individuals post-severe traumatic brain injury (TBI) and 10 age- and sex-matched neurologically nonimpaired individuals. Participants of the TBI group were diagnosed with dysarthria ranging from mild to moderate to severe dysarthria. Each participant from the TBI and comparison group was fitted with a custom-made artificial acrylic palate that recorded lingual palatal contact during target consonant production in sentence- and syllable-repetition tasks at a habitual rate and loudness level. Analysis of temporal parameters between the comparison and TBI groups revealed prolonged durations of the various phases of consonant production, which were attributed to articulatory slowness, impaired speech motor control, impaired accuracy, and impaired coordination of articulatory movements in the dysarthric speakers post-TBI. For the spatial measurements, quantitative analysis, as well as visual inspection of the tongue-to-palate contact diagrams, indicated spatial aberrations in dysarthric speech post-TBI. Both the spatial and temporal aberrations may have at least partially caused the perceptual judgment of articulatory impairments in the dysarthric speakers.

The second study is from the Developmental Cognitive Neuroscience Unit, UCL Institute of Child Health in the United Kingdom (Morgan et al., 2007). Dysarthria with severe articulatory impairment is a common and debilitating sequelae following severe TBI and the present study investigated the effectiveness of EPG in treating the articulatory component of dysarthria post-TBI. In the study, the articulatory component of dysarthria post-TBI was treated once per week with EPG over a 10-week period in three adolescents (aged 14 years, 10 months to 15 years, 1 month). Perceptual (articulation, intelligibility) and EPG (spatial, durational) assessments were conducted pre- and post-treatment to determine outcome.

Perceptual improvement was noted for phoneme precision and length and spatial EPG measures confirmed increased precision of phoneme production. However, no clear pattern of change for phoneme duration occurred. Intelligibility increased at word and sentence level, with little change reported in everyday speech intelligibility (Kuruvilla et al., 2008).

This preliminary study indicates that EPG treatment may be effective for improving speech at the isolated phoneme, word, or sentence level of articulation. These preliminary results are encouraging, and the study is the first to report speech changes post-treatment in participants with severe TBI and persistent dysarthria (Kuruvilla et al., 2008). Further research is required, however, in order to understand the regenerative capacity of articulatory function post-brain injury and to determine optimal treatment parameters for achieving generalization of therapy to everyday connected speech.

The third source of information is from the Division of Speech Pathology, School of Health and Rehabilitation Sciences, The University of Queensland, St. Lucia, Queensland, Australia (Cahill et al., 2005). The purpose of the investigation was to assess the articulatory function of a group of children with TBI, using both perceptual and instrumental techniques. The performance of 24 children with TBI was assessed on a battery of perceptual (Frenchay Dysarthria Assessment,

Assessment of Intelligibility of Dysarthric Speech, and speech sample analysis) and instrumental (lip and tongue pressure transduction systems) assessments and compared with that of 24 nonneurologically impaired children matched for age and sex (Cahill et al., 2005).

Perceptual assessment identified consonant and vowel imprecision, increased length of phonemes, and over-all reduction in speech intelligibility, while instrumental assessment revealed significant impairment in lip and tongue function in the TBI group, with rate and pressure in repetitive lip and tongue tasks particularly impaired. Significant negative correlations were identified between the degree of deviance of perceptual articulatory features and decreased function on many nonspeech measures of lip function, as well as maximum tongue pressure and fine force tongue control at 20 percent of maximum tongue pressure. Additionally, subclinical articulatory deficits were identified in the children with TBI who were nondysarthric. The results of the instrumental assessment of lip and tongue function in this study support the finding of substantial articulatory dysfunction in this group of children following TBI (Cahill et al., 2005). Hence, remediation of articulatory function should be a therapeutic priority in these children.

The EPG, an innovative computer-based tool for assessing and treating speech motor difficulties, enables the speaker to "see" the placement of his or her tongue during speech and to attempt to correct any lingual palatal errors. This visual supplementation of auditory feedback offers potential therapeutic benefits for individuals with intellectual disabilities, hearing impairments, or following TBI, and for individuals who are attempting to stabilize their speech sound production during a progressive neurological disease process. Many of these individuals show relative strengths in visual versus auditory and simultaneous versus sequential processing. The EPG also provides speech-language pathologists with an objective measure of articulatory ability.

Implications for Life Care Plans

In spite of early aiding and speech therapy intervention, many school-aged children and adolescents with severe-to-profound hearing impairments have unintelligible speech. The development of their speech production skills can be compromised by difficulties amplifying differing speech sounds in the environment, as well as clearly seeing various tongue and mouth movements that distinguish speech sounds. The use of EPG as a treatment model in speech-language pathology will shorten treatment goals, improve the accuracy of the direct treatment, and reduce the financial impact in the long run. This is the forefront of using technology to impact traditional speech-language pathology treatment that can be incorporated into the patient's life care plan as applicable.

Terminology in the Field of Communication Sciences and Disorders

The importance of terminology relative to our communication with other professionals and the general public, as well as the very special needs of international and transdisciplinary communication and development, has become increasingly apparent. In addition to improved consistency in the use of terms, there is the need to carefully examine what meanings the developing jargon may have to other individuals who rely primarily on a dictionary and common sense. Although many people in the field may know what is meant by a given term, others may not share the same meaning. Some terms used by people in one country may not easily translate into other languages. Even more apparent, with the diversity of people in the world today, care must be exercised to consider multiple interpretations of a term, sometimes affected by the perspective of one's culture.

Because of the transdisciplinary nature of the medical-legal-clinical world, there are also problems of various disciplines using other jargon to describe essentially the same phenomenon, act, or characteristic. These problems reflect the need for an emerging field like life care planning to develop an internally consistent and logical terminology that will facilitate the international and transdisciplinary development of the field. It is important to actively educate individuals on the life care planning team concerning specific terminology that defines and describes areas of assessment and treatment within the field of communication sciences and disorders. Refer to Appendix 9.13 for a list of communication sciences and disorders (both audiology and speech-language pathology acronyms).

The SLP Review of Records and Intake

The SLP must perform his own case intake, consisting of talking with the referral source, determining the time frames needed to complete testing, arranging the financial and billing agreements, and arranging for a release of all pertinent information. Additional testing needed may be identified at this time or during the initial interview arrangements.

The SLP will then review a copy of the medical records to include:

- Nursing notes
- Doctor's orders
- Other services' reports
- Educational information
- Vocational information
- Day-in-the-life videos
- Other relevant documentation, depending on the etiology and diagnosis

A thorough assessment battery is then administered, gathering information from the spouse, family, or other relatives, including the clients themselves. This step may also include the opportunity for the SLP to consult and interview other team members whose information may have a bearing on final recommendations of the SLP. At this time, if additional medical, clinical, vocational, or educational information or evaluations are needed, requests for these additional information-gathering steps should be submitted to the referral source. A letter may be composed outlining the correct questions with supporting data to ensure that the SLP has the opportunity to solicit the needed information.

At the completion of the assessment, the SLP must be able to provide a written report, documenting the test results, observations, and conclusions with clear recommendations. These recommendations must be detailed to include a projection of future care costs, frequency of service or treatment, duration, base cost, source of information, and recognized vendors or manufacturers, current prices, collaborative sources, and categories of information. It is recommended that the consulting SLP be knowledgeable about the local sources and costs of these recommendations, either through direct contact with suppliers or through catalog and desktop/computerized research. Recommendations from the SLP should be discussed with the client and family, treatment team members, and other life care team members if they directly impact the final recommendations and the cost analysis of the plan by the economist. Any coordination and agreement needed between team members including the economist should occur at this time. A draft of the communication sciences and disorders assessment and recommendations report should be written and distributed to the life care planner for review relative to the accuracy and completeness of the information. The SLP must be able to explain, from a life care planning perspective, the reasons and rationales that are relative to their recommendations. These must be lifelong recommendations and objectives, developed in an integrated format. Once the document is correct and complete, a final draft should be compiled and distributed to the life care planner and the referral source. It should be determined, by these two parties, whether the written documentation should be sent to other internal life care planning team members, including the family and client, and to external individuals.

Assessment Process

There are four methods of gathering and interpreting quantitative and qualitative information about the client that should be used in the communication sciences and disorders assessment process by the SLP. These four measures are a collection of the initial database, interview procedures, clinical assessment, and formal assessment procedures (Dunn & Dunn, 1991). Often more than one method is used to gather information about the same aspect of a client's skills and abilities, the context, the activity, or the use of technology or equipment. Information collected should include the reason and need for referral, medical diagnosis, and educational and vocational background information. This information is collected during the referral and intake phase, and its purpose is to provide preliminary data for planning the assessment. The interview takes place during the identification phase as a means of gathering information regarding the consumer and her needs. It is important that the consumer, family members, rehabilitation or education professionals, and other care providers be interviewed.

Formal assessment procedures are administered in a prescribed way and have set methods of scoring and interpretation. Therefore, they can be duplicated and analyzed. They may or may not be standardized. Clinical assessment techniques involve skilled observation of the consumer and are used throughout the assessment process. These techniques may be structured so that a series of steps is followed to determine specific skills, or they may be intentionally left unstructured to see what takes place. Observation can be done during a simulated task in a clinic setting or in a context familiar to the consumer such as a classroom or workplace. Differential diagnosis is an ongoing and essential component of the assessment process and one that requires an advanced level of understanding and perspective about the trauma or injury.

Pediatric and Adolescent Assessments

Evaluating children (pediatric and adolescent) presents complex and challenging issues, complicated by the catastrophic nature of the disease, disability, or trauma and frequently challenged by the almost insurmountable task of planning a child's life. For these reasons, it is critical to make accurate and thorough projections and careful analysis of the disability, educate team members and caregivers about the pediatric disabilities, and develop a differential diagnostic therapeutic approach to service delivery to the child. The list of pediatric and adolescent considerations in the communication sciences and disorders assessment is lengthy, detailed, and can be complex. It is important to disclose that the list is not all-inclusive, because changes occur as research and science enhance the process. Readers should see Appendix 9.14 for a basic speech and language checklist for birth to 24 months.

There are areas that warrant consideration when performing a communication evaluation for a pediatric or adolescent individual that are not considered, or at least not in the same detail, when evaluating an adult. Chronological age and pre-trauma development are used as the normal benchmarks against which to measure the disability issues. Routine medical needs must be addressed to the pediatric specialists who would provide the information that impacts a child's communication development. These include pediatric physiatry, otolaryngology, pediatric neurology, developmental medicine, audiology, dental/orthodontic, prosthodontist, and pediatric neuro-ophthalmology and ophthalmology. It should be noted here that there is a trend in the medical specialty fields to identify specialists who work solely with adolescents. Additional cognitive and educational information is gathered from the following sources:

- Educational consultants to private and public educational programs
- Personal caregivers and attendants
- Pediatric neuropsychological assessment
- Occupational and physical therapy
- Vision and hearing specialists
- Evaluators of driving
- Programs for the development of social and pragmatic skills
- Prevocational and vocational training programs

One area receiving an increased amount of attention at this time is autism. Autism (autistic disorders) is within the broader diagnostic category of autism spectrum disorder (ASD). Other diagnoses in the category include Asperger's syndrome, pervasive developmental disorder (PDD) (sometimes referred to as PDD-NOS), and childhood disintegrative disorder. These disorders occur in males approximately four times more often than in females. In earlier years, autism affected one in 500 children; however, with the explosive increase in the United States (and apparently in other countries), whether because of better diagnoses or actual increases in cases, it is now estimated that one in 150 children ages 10 and younger are classified as having some form of ASD (Bishop, 1989; Gillberg, 1991; Tonge, 2002; Owens, 2004). SLPs are aggressively involved in treating children and adolescents with ASD.

Federal Mandates and Policies

The SLP, as an outcome of the assessment results, frequently provides AT or augmentative and alternative communication (AAC) recommendations. AT is defined as any technology used to enable individuals to perform tasks that are difficult or impossible due to disabilities (Lloyd et al., 1997). AAC is defined as the supplement or replacement of natural speech or writing using aided or unaided symbols, and the field is referred to as the clinical/educational practice to improve the communication skills of individuals with little or no functional speech (Lloyd et al., 1997). It is important to be knowledgeable about the laws and policies that support the use of AT or AAC. The list of federal mandates that relate to the use of AT, the development of AT services (evaluation and therapy), and the integration of AT devices and services into medicine, education, independent living, and vocational arenas is lengthy. The partial list of mandates as shown in Table 9.6 continues to change (and improve) and is not considered to be inclusive. It is included to give readers an idea of the growing list of political directives that acknowledge the consumer's need for AT devices and services.

Industrial advancements and competition have driven the recent development of AT devices, but the development of services and service delivery in the United States has been influenced significantly by federal legislation. Over the last 40 years, the federal government has enacted a series of bills and initiatives requiring federal agencies, states, and private industry to support the

Table 9.6 Federal Mandates

Federal Mandates
Section 504 of the Rehabilitation Act of 1973
Rehabilitation Act of 1973, Reauthorization and Amendments of 1993 and 1998
Individuals with Disabilities Education Act (IDEA), PL 101-476
Technology-Related Assistance for Individuals with Disabilities Act of 1988, PL 100-407
Technology-Related Assistance for Individuals with Disabilities Act Amendments, PL 103-218
Americans with Disabilities Act (ADA) of 1990, PL 101-336
Goals 2000: Educate America Act, PL 103-85
Improving America's Schools Act, PL 103-382
Telecommunications Act of 1996, PL 104-104
Telecommunications for the Disabled Act of 1982
Telecommunications Accessibility Enhancement Act of 1988
Rehabilitation Act, Section 508
Decoder Circuitry Act

employment of people with disabilities. Milestones over the 40 years include the following most recent legislation.

The Rehabilitation Act of 1973 mandates reasonable accommodation in federally funded employment and higher education for AT and services. This act has established several important principles upon which subsequent legislation has been based. These include *reasonable accommodations* in employment and in secondary education. The act mandates that employers and institutions of higher education receiving federal funds seek to accommodate the needs of employees and students who have disabilities. It specifically prohibited discrimination in employment or admission to academic programs solely on the basis of a handicapping condition. Sections 503 (educational institutions) and 504 (employers receiving federal funds) of this act describe both reasonable accommodations and *least restrictive environment* (LRE), a term relating to the degree of modification in a job or academic program that is acceptable. Many of the efforts to achieve accommodations in the least restrictive environment involved the use of assistive technologies.

The Education for All Handicapped Children Act (EHA) of 1975 extends reasonable accommodations for students from ages 5 to 21, providing a Free Appropriate Public Education (FAPE). This act initiated procedures to ensure that each public school system identifies and provides all children with disabilities with an education. States were also mandated to establish procedures for enforcement. AT plays a more significant role in gaining access to educational programs. The act created the Individual Education Plan (IEP) to be made for all students with disabilities. This act, also known as PL 94-142, established the right of all children to a free and appropriate education, regardless of handicapping condition. When PL 94-142 passed, children with disabilities who were not in school programs or those who were but who were not receiving services began Individual Education Plans (IEPs) with measurable goals, AT, and services. Lack of local services or lack of funding was not a reason to deny services. The impact of this law has been far-reaching. Devices ranging from sensory aids (visual and auditory) to augmentative communication devices to specialized computers have been utilized to provide access to educational programs for children with disabilities. Several additional acts leading up to PL 94-142 gave the foundation for the passage of this act.

The passage of the Elementary and Secondary Education Act (PL 89-10) in 1965 to improve quality of education for individuals and the passage of Elementary and Secondary Education Amendments for Children with Handicaps (PL 89-313) established the foundation for future legislation dealing with children with handicaps. The zero-reject principle is the principle developed out of EHA, stating that all children, regardless of the severity of their disability, have a right to special education services. These services are provided by the local education agency (LEA) in the LRE. The Handicapped Infants and Toddlers Act of 1986 extended the preceding act to children ages five and under, expanding emphasis on educationally related AT.

Assistive technology (AT) includes both devices and services. The Individuals with Disabilities Education Act (IDEA) (reauthorized in 2004) defines an AT device as any item, piece of equipment, or product system, whether acquired commercially off the shelf, modified, or customized, that is used to increase, maintain, or improve functional capabilities of individuals with disabilities. Devices can replace a missing limb, help prevent the worsening of a condition, improve physical functioning, increase a person's capacity to learn, or strengthen a physical or other weakness. AT services support people with disabilities or their caregivers to help them select, acquire, or use AT devices. Such services also include functional evaluations, training on or demonstration of devices, and purchasing or leasing devices. (See Appendix 9.9 for a list of online AT resources and Appendix 9.16 for an AT Resource Directory.) Specifically, AT services include the following:

- Evaluating the needs of an individual with a disability, including a functional evaluation of the individual in the individual's customary environment
- Purchasing, leasing, or otherwise providing for the acquisition of AT devices by individuals with disabilities
- Selecting, designing, fitting, customizing, adapting, applying, maintaining, repairing, or replacing of AT services
- Coordinating and using other therapies, interventions, or services with AT devices, such as those associated with existing education and rehabilitation plans and programs
- Training or technical assistance for an individual with disabilities or family of an individual with disabilities
- Training or technical assistance for professionals (including individuals providing education and rehabilitation services), employers, or other individuals who provide services to, employ, or are otherwise substantially involved in the major life functions of individuals with disabilities

Gleason Act

In 2015, Steve Gleason, former NFL standout athlete for the New Orleans Saints, redefined what it means to be a hero. Diagnosed with ALS (Amyotrophic Lateral Sclerosis, or Lou Gehrig's disease) in 2011, Steve's mind is unaffected by the disease, but he can no longer move any part of his body—except his eyes. He communicates his thoughts to the world through technology operated by his eye movements, in much the same way as did physicist Stephen Hawking. In 2014, Medicare took steps to restrict access to this technology, known as Speech Generating Devices (SGDs). Medicare's action was unacceptable to Steve and others who need communication devices after experiencing ALS, strokes, traumatic brain injury, cerebral palsy, Parkinson's, spinal cord injuries, chemical accidents, and many other types of injuries, accidents, and other complex neurological conditions.

Using the very technology Medicare stopped covering in many care settings last year, Steve first used his Team Gleason Foundation (www.teamgleason.org) to ensure that everyone who needed a

SGD had one. Team Gleason became the safety net for many people that Medicare denied. Steve called on Congress to stop Medicare's restrictive policies on behalf of thousands of SGD users. He engaged members of Congress from his home town district (in Eastern Washington) and his adopted home town state (Louisiana). Motivated by Steve's passion and tenacity, Senator David Vitter (R-LA), Congressman Steve Scalise (R-LA), and Congresswoman Cathy McMorris Rodgers (R-WA) introduced legislation named for Steve. The Steve Gleason Act ensures that Medicare will pay for SGDs, and it allows people to keep SGDs for as long as they need them, regardless of the care setting they find themselves in (hospital, skilled nursing or long-term care facility, or hospice). It also provides coverage for accessories needed to allow the SGDs to work effectively.

After the Steve Gleason Act was introduced in February 2015, Steve relentlessly led the charge toward passage, engaging his huge social media following and partnering with many other advocacy groups, including the Center for Medicare Advocacy (www.medicareadvocacy.org). The U.S. Senate passed the Steve Gleason Act unanimously on April 22, 2015. By contrast, S. 984, the bill number assigned to the Gleason Act in the Senate, changes the capped rental provision. In the original text, the change from capped rental was permanent. There was a start date, but no end date. The Gleason Act that passed the Senate offers capped rental relief only for 3 years: *between October 1, 2015 to October 1, 2018*. Then, absent additional action by Congress, capped rental is reinstated.

The Steve Gleason Act of 2015 does not address all of the coverage problems with SGDs. Medicare is in the process of revising a National Coverage Determination (NCD) that addresses coverage for an SGD that has the capability of other-than-speech functioning. This is sometimes referred to as "unlocking" the device for phone, Internet, texting, word processing, and other capabilities. In December 2014, Medicare received over 2,000 comments on this NCD process. The Center has offered to review Medicare's recommendations on the NCD.

The groundswell of support for SGD coverage, and for the people who use SGDs, has become apparent, encouraging the Medicare agency and Congress to seek ways to combat the loss of coverage. It has taken a great deal of effort and thousands of voices to bring attention to, and action for, those who need SGDs. That, and leaders such as Steve Gleason, who fights the good coverage fight while using an SGD himself. It is very fitting that this act bears his name.

AT can help people learn, compete in the work environment, achieve independence, or improve quality of life. Although the use of AT is not an end in itself, it is part of an ongoing therapeutic process to improve functional capabilities.

Examples of ATs

- *Aids for Daily Living*: Self-help aids for use in activities such as eating, bathing, cooking, dressing, toileting, home maintenance, and so on. Examples include modified eating utensils, adapted books, pencil holders, page turners, dressing aids, and adapted personal hygiene aids.
- *Aids for the Hearing Impaired*: Aids for specific populations including assistive listening devices (infrared, FM loop systems), hearing aids, TTYs, visual and tactile alerting systems, and so on.
- *Aids for the Vision Impaired*: Aids for specific populations including magnifiers, Braille or speech output devices, large-print screens, closed-circuit television for magnifying documents, and so on.
- *Augmentative and Alternative Communication (AAC)*: Electronic and nonelectronic devices that help persons with speech and/or hearing disabilities communicate: communication boards, speech synthesizers, modified typewriters, head pointers, and text-to-voice software (Venkatagiri, 1996). (See Appendix 9.18 for a list of AAC organizations.)

- *Computer Access Aids*: Headsticks, light pointers, modified or alternate keyboards, switches activated by pressure, sound or voice, touch screens, special software, and voice-to-text software that enable persons with disabilities to use a computer. This category includes speech recognition software.
- *Environmental Controls*: Electronic systems that help people control various appliances, switches for telephone, TV, or other appliances activated by pressure, eyebrows, or breath.
- *Home/Workplace Modifications*: Structural adaptations that remove or reduce physical barriers: ramps, lifts, bathroom changes, automatic door openers, and expanded doorways.
- *Mobility Aids*: Devices that help people move within their environments: electric or manual wheelchairs, modifications of vehicles for travel, scooters, crutches, canes, and walkers.
- *Prosthetics and Orthotics*: Replacement or augmentation of body parts with artificial limbs or other orthotic aids such as splints or braces. There are also prosthetics to assist with cognitive limitations or deficits, including audiotapes or pagers (that function as prompts or reminders).
- *Recreation*: Devices to enable participation in sports, social, and cultural events. Examples include audio description for movies, adaptive controls for video games, adaptive fishing rods, cuffs for grasping paddles or racquets, and seating systems for boats.
- *Seating and Positioning*: Adapted seating, cushions, standing tables, positioning belts, braces, cushions and wedges to maintain posture, and devices that provide body support to help people perform a range of daily tasks.
- *Service Animals*: The ADA defines a service animal as any guide dog (for visually impaired and blind individuals), signal dog (for hearing-impaired or deaf individuals), or other animal individually trained to provide assistance to an individual with a disability.
- *Vehicle Modifications*: Adaptive driving aids, hand controls, wheelchair and other lifts, modified vans, or other motor vehicles used for personal transportation.

The 1986 amendment to the Rehabilitation Act of 1973 required all states to include provision for AT services in the rehabilitation plans of the state vocational rehab agencies. Section 508 mandates equal access to electronic office equipment for all federal employees. The Technology-Related Assistance for Individuals with Disabilities Act (Tech Act) of 1988 mandates consumer-driven AT services and system changes in the states. This act created the development of the Tech Act programs throughout the country. The act was reauthorized in 1994. This legislation authorized funds for states to establish and implement a consumer-responsive, statewide program of technology-related assistance for individuals with disabilities, including identification of barriers to administering this assistance. Table 9.7 lists the priorities for the continuation of Tech Act activities and Appendix 9.15 lists the State Assistive Technology Programs.

The Americans with Disabilities Act (ADA) (PL 101-336) of 1990 (reauthorized in 2002) prohibits discrimination based on disability in employment, transportation, and telecommunications. The ADA furthers the goal of full participation of people with disabilities by giving civil rights protection to individuals with disabilities that are like those provided to individuals on the basis of race, sex, national origin, and religion. It guarantees equal opportunity for individuals with disabilities in employment, public accommodations, transportation, state and local government services, and telecommunications. President George H. W. Bush signed the ADA into law on July 26, 1990. Copies of the full Americans with Disabilities Act of 1990 may be obtained at no cost from the U.S. Subcommittee on Disability Policy, 113 Hart, Senate Office Building, Washington, DC 20510. The ADA Private Transportation hotline is 800-949-4232.

The IDEA of 1991 (Public Law 105-17 and the reauthorization of PL 94-142), which became the Individuals with Disabilities Improvement Act (IDIA) of 2003, mandates that all local educational

Table 9.7 Tech Act Priorities

To promote public awareness of AT at the national level
To provide training and education about AT on a national basis for stakeholders, including other national social service and business organizations, members of the insurance and health care industry, and public office holders/policy makers
To develop positions on a full range of national AT- and disability-related issues and to share these positions with other organizations or policy makers, as needed, to ensure that the views of the states and territories and their consumers with regard to AT service delivery are adequately represented
To provide a forum for exchanging information and promoting the system change accomplishments and activities of the Tech Act projects
To identify the need and opportunities for the development of nationally conducted activities to increase access to AT
To develop and promote a national agenda

agencies provide AT devices and services to benefit students with disabilities. The IDEA mandate includes that local educational agencies be responsible for providing AT devices and services if these are required as part of the child's educational or related services or as a supplementary aid or service. AT devices are identified in the IDEA as "any item, piece of equipment or product system, whether acquired commercially off the shelf, modified, or customized, that is used to increase, maintain, or improve the functional capabilities of children with disabilities" (Section 300.5). The IDIA was also aligned with the No Child Left Behind (NCLB) Act of 2001. Refer to www.asha.org for additional information on IDEA, IDIA, and NCLB.

The definition of an AT device, as provided in the IDEA, is very broad and gives IEP teams the flexibility that they need to make decisions about appropriate AT devices for individual students. AT includes a range of low and high technology, hardware and software, and technology solutions that are generally considered instructional technology tools if they have been identified as educationally necessary and documented in the student's IEP. The need for AT is determined by the student's IEP committee as *educationally* necessary. AT service is any service that directly assists a child with a disability in the selection, acquisition, and use of an AT device. The term includes:

1. The evaluation of the needs of a child with a disability, including a functional evaluation of the child in the child's customary environment;
2. Purchasing, leasing, or otherwise providing for the acquisition of AT devices by children with disabilities;
3. Selecting, designing, fitting, customizing, adapting, applying, retaining, repairing, or replacing AT devices;
4. Coordinating and using other therapies, interventions, or services with AT devices, such as those associated with existing education and rehabilitation plans and programs;
5. Training and technical assistance for a child with a disability or, if appropriate, that child's family; and
6. Training or technical assistance for professionals (including individuals or rehabilitation services), employers, or other individuals who provide services to employ or are otherwise substantially involved in the major life functions of children with disabilities (Section 300.6).

The rules and regulations for special education in each state may also address the provision of assistive devices and services in various sections of the state's educational policy and regulations, including the definition of assistive devices, the definition of service, within what parts of the IEP AT may be included (related services, supplemental aids and services, etc.), whether AT is needed to provide the student a FAPE, whether an AT assessment is needed, if AT is needed for the student to participate in local or state testing, and whether the technology is needed in a nonschool setting.

The reauthorization of the Rehabilitation Act of 1973 (1992, 1997) mandates rehabilitation technology to be a primary benefit to be included in the rehabilitation plan for the state rehabilitation agencies. The rehab plan was required to include how AT will be used in the rehabilitation process of each individual client. In 1992, Congress passed the reauthorization of the Rehabilitation Act of 1973. This legislation (PL 102-569 in 1992 and PL 105-17 in 1997) makes the rehabilitation act consistent with the principles of self-determination of the ADA, and it is more consumer-responsive than the original version. Rehabilitation technology is defined in this law to include rehabilitation engineering and AT devices and services. Under this legislation each state must specify how AT devices and services or work site assessments are to be provided. The individualized written rehabilitation plan (IWRP, but now referred to as the Individual Work Plan, or IWP) must include the provisions of rehabilitation technology services to assist in the implementation of intermediate and long-term objectives, and rehabilitation technology is exempt from what are termed comparable benefits funding considerations. The latter concept means that vocational rehabilitation monies are considered to be the first source of funding for purchase of AT regardless of whether the individual has other funding sources. Also included within the mandate of this legislation was the continuation of rehabilitation engineering research centers, which focus on one or more core areas of research and development.

The Ticket to Work and Work Incentive Improvement Act of 1999 provides consumer choices for the provision of vocational rehabilitation and job training and other support services. The Ticket to Work and Work Incentive Improvement Act of 1999 has a number of incentives that can be offered to benefit recipients to help them reintegrate into the workplace. Agencies that provide employment training and job placement to people with disabilities will receive a fixed portion of that person's prospective Social Security case benefit when the individual goes back to work and in the first few years during the individual's employment.

The New Freedom Initiative (February 2001) increases funding for research and development of AT resources nationwide. Although not legislation, this initiative also promotes full access to the community for people with disabilities through expanded transportation options, educational opportunities, and greater integration into the workforce. Readers should refer to Appendix 9.4 for funding terminology information.

SLPs (and audiologists) must address the unique privacy concerns, both ethical and regulatory, that confront individuals who rely on AT and the SLPs and other practitioners who provide them with services (Blackstone et al., 2002). The Health Insurance Portability and Accountability Act of 1996 (HIPAA) was created by Congress to provide guidelines for the protection of health care information and to establish standard formats for the electronic transmission of clinical data such as claims, referrals, explanation of benefits (EOB), remittance advices (RAs), and others. Although there are nine separate elements to the HIPAA legislation, the Department of Health and Human Services (DHHS) has thus far promulgated three in the form of final regulatory rules, the privacy rule and the transaction and code set rules, and the security of health care data as they are generated and stored by providers and others who have access to this protected information.

The privacy rule of HIPAA is intended as a federal floor to protect the privacy of individually identifiable health information contained in a patient's medical record. The protected information includes a patient's name, address, Social Security number, financial data, or any other identifying information in addition to the medical record itself. The rule creates substantial new compliance issues for covered entities, which include virtually all health care providers, health plans, health information clearinghouses, and those business associates who engage directly or through contractual arrangements with any of those. It also covers paper files containing this protected information that is not yet in electronic form. In short, it covers all information, including both hard and soft files. The compliance date for the privacy rule was April 14, 2003. Substantial civil and criminal penalties, up to and including jail time, can be assessed for noncompliance.

The final HIPAA privacy rule covers all individually identifiable health care information in any form, electronic or nonelectronic, that is held or transmitted by a covered entity such as a health care provider, a third-party payer, or any of their business associates who come into contact with these data. Under HIPAA, there are legal penalties for covered entities that receive or use unauthorized information intentionally. SLPs, by transmitting personal health information (PHI) in electronic form, are regulated by HIPAA. The following points about HIPAA and AT should be followed to remain compliant.

SLPs should consider assistive devices that facilitate the security of PHI by providing essential design features, vocabulary, and training that emphasize the rights to privacy and informed consent of individuals who rely on assistive devices, strategies, and techniques. The SLP is responsible for making sure the PHI is not openly accessible. New devices offer both text and audio-data logging. These logs potentially put the user at risk if they are available to others. All AAC users should receive a copy of the provider's Notice of Privacy Practices. The Notice of Privacy Practices explains how the provider will use the individual's PHI and outlines the provider's confidentiality program. SLPs should educate themselves on HIPAA regulations, should conduct a gap analysis of their practice policies and procedures, and should undertake a compliance implementation program. The privacy and safety of individuals using communication boards and AAC devices should be considered when including personal information (name, address, phone number, religion, political affiliation, etc.). Remember that not all AT users understand the privacy issues, either. Eavesdropping, communication partners speaking loudly to interpret the message, and people reading what is on the screen are all potential violations of privacy. AT users need training to learn to protect their privacy and need help selecting vocabulary such as "Please do not read my display." AT users also need training to coordinate their speech output to conform to public expectations of conversations, help to lower the volume of their device, password protection and encryption of the message buffer and data logging system in the AT device to protect the user's content, and privacy/confidentiality training for their communication partners. See http://www.asha.org/practice/reimbursement/hipaa/default/ (ASHA, 2016) for additional HIPAA information.

Speech-to-Speech Relay System

Background

Speech-to-speech (STS) is one form of Telecommunications Relay Service (TRS). TRS is a service that allows persons with hearing and speech disabilities to access the telephone system to place and receive telephone calls. STS enables persons with a speech disability to make telephone calls using their own voice (or an assistive voice device). Like all forms of TRS, STS uses specially trained operators—called communications assistants (CAs)—to relay the conversation back and forth between the person with the speech disability and the other party to the call. STS CAs are specially trained in understanding a variety of speech disorders, which enables them to repeat what the caller says in a manner that makes the caller's words clear and understandable to the called party.

Who Uses STS?

Often people with speech disabilities cannot communicate by telephone because the parties they are calling cannot understand their speech. People with cerebral palsy, multiple sclerosis, muscular dystrophy, and Parkinson's disease, and those who are coping with limitations from a stroke or traumatic brain injury, may have speech disabilities. People who stutter or have had a laryngectomy may also have difficulty being understood. In general, anyone with a speech disability or anyone who wishes to call someone with a speech disability can use STS.

Using STS

A special phone is not needed for STS. You simply call the relay center by dialing 711, and indicate you wish to make an STS call. You are then connected to an STS CA who will repeat your spoken words, making the spoken words clear to the other party. Persons with speech disabilities may also receive STS calls.

Alternatives

Persons with speech disabilities may use a TTY to make a TRS call, but many such people have some type of physical limitation that makes typing into a text input device difficult. STS offers an alternative to a TTY or other text input device when the only other option would be not to communicate via telephone at all. Some STS providers also offer STS service for Spanish-to-Spanish callers.

Mandatory Minimum Standards for STS

The FCC imposes mandatory minimum standards on providers of all forms of TRS, such as ensuring user confidentiality, making service available 24 hours a day, 7 days a week, and answering 85 percent of calls within 10 seconds. The FCC also imposes certain additional requirements on STS providers. For example, STS CAs must remain with a call for a minimum of 15 minutes. In addition:

- An STS CA may, at the request of the user, retain information from a particular call in order to facilitate the completion of consecutive calls. The user may ask the TRS CA to retain such information, or the CA may ask the user if she wants the CA to repeat the same information during subsequent calls. The STS CA may retain the information only for as long as it takes to complete the subsequent calls.
- STS providers must offer STS users the option to maintain at the relay center a list of names and telephone numbers that the STS user commonly calls. When the STS user requests one of these names, the CA must repeat the name and state the telephone number to the STS user. This information must be transferred to any new STS provider.

For further information on the TRS mandatory minimum standards, go to www.fcc.gov/cgb/consumerfacts/trs.html.

Filing a Complaint with the FCC

If you have a problem with STS Relay Service, first try to resolve it with the provider. If you are unable to resolve it directly, you can file a complaint with the FCC. There is no charge for filing a complaint. You can file your complaint using the online complaint Form 2000C found on the FCC website at www.fcc.gov/cgb/complaints.html. You can also file your complaint with the FCC's Consumer Center by e-mailing fccinfo@fcc.gov, calling 1-888-CALL-FCC (1-888-225-5322) voice or 1-888-TELL-FCC (1-888-835-5322) TTY, faxing 1-866-418-0232, or writing to: Federal Communications Commission, Consumer & Governmental Affairs Bureau, Consumer Inquiries and Complaints Division, 445 12th Street SW, Washington, DC 20554.

Manufacturers' Roles

Manufacturers' roles in AT are often disputed and discussed. The responsibility of the manufacturer/vendor/representative varies depending on the expertise of the AT team and the expertise of the SLP. Devices are designed into a prototype device to convert it to a version that can be fabricated in small quantities and tested with potential users. Testing of this production prototype is commonly referred to as *alpha testing* and is normally conducted as an in-house function by the manufacturers. Once the device appears to be functioning properly, several additional replicas are fabricated. During this development stage, the manufacturer is able to determine potential problems that may develop during the manufacturing phase and the prototypes can be evaluated more extensively by several individuals, usually clinicians and consumers simultaneously (beta testing). This accomplishes the identification of potential problems in the product, evaluation of product documentation to ensure that it is clear and useful, and evaluation of the product with a variety of individuals with disabilities to identify the target population as accurately as possible. Manufacturing then occurs, by which a working prototype of the AAC device is converted into a device that is then produced. For a list of vendors, please refer to Appendix 9.5 and Appendix 9.15, which contain a wealth of AAC and AT resources. Appendix 9.6 shows selected AAC websites.

Funding and Economic Issues

There are a variety of financing and funding options (see Appendix 9.3 for some examples) for services and technology needs that a qualified SLP could recommend for support in the life care planning process. It is the consulting SLP's responsibility to understand where and how to access this information on collateral funding sources. These include public programs such as maternal and child health, education, vocational rehabilitation, developmental disability programs, Department of Veterans Affairs programs, and Older Americans Act programs. There are alternative funding sources such as loans, libraries, foundations, and charitable organizations, as well as understanding options under the U.S. tax code, and the issues of civil rights, universal access, and telecommunications. A recommended outline for a funding request is shown in Appendix 9.17.

Information on current initiatives and emerging promising best practices related to the funding and acquisition of technology and services is also available and should be considered in the development of the life care plan for the areas of speech-language pathology and AT. Knowledge of policy and funding information (Appendix 9.4) adds credibility and strength to this portion of the life care planning process. Frequently, recommended technology and services in the areas of communication sciences and disorders/speech-language pathology are costly and require a lengthier and more complex plan of treatment than some other areas of the plan. If the consultant in this area can show an ability to understand and develop funding options and plans, the success of this portion of the plan is strengthened. The SLP who is involved in the life care planning process must have a current and accurate analysis of the marketplace with regard to the cost of services and technology or other goods needed in his portion of recommendations in the life care process. This also directly relates to potential policy changes in health care and education that may directly affect specific recommendations in the areas of communication sciences and disorders and current funding terminology (Appendix 9.4).

Medical Coding

Medical coding is useful to life care planners and SLPs (Table 9.9) for documentation and billing purposes. *Current Procedural Terminology*, 4th Edition (CPT), is a systematic listing and coding of procedures and services performed by physicians, based upon the procedure being consistent with contemporary medical practice and being performed by many physicians in clinical practice in multiple locations. Each procedure is identified with a 5-digit CPT code. International Classification of Diseases-10-Clinical Modification (ICD-10-CM) is an indexing of medical information by disease and operations. V codes are codes within the ICD-10-CM classification system that may be used in any health care setting. V codes may be used as either a first listed (principal diagnosis code in the inpatient setting) or secondary code, depending on the circumstances of the encounter. V codes indicate a reason for an encounter and are not procedure codes. A corresponding procedure code must accompany a V code to describe the procedure performed. Readers should refer to the American Medical Association's bookstore website (www.amabook-store.com) for current manuals or software with up-to-date listings of all CPT, ICD-10 codes, and V codes. Table 9.8 lists the newest ICD-10-CM SLP codes in 2016. Table 9.9 lists all the speech-language pathology CPT codes as of time of publication. Table 9.10 offer example life care plan entries with costs. The Model Superbill for SLPs (Appendix 9.12) (ASHA, 2016) at the end of this chapter is another point of reference for SLP medical coding.

Readers should refer to the AMA CPT Code Manual (2016) and the ASHA website (www.asha.org) for clarification of the AAC codes or for further information on any of the speech, language, and hearing codes. Medical codes are always subject to updating and changes, so clinicians should stay current with medical coding terminology (Table 9.11). Secondly, readers need to remember that there are Level II HCPCS national codes for speech-generating and non-Speech Generating Devices (Medicare terminology for an AAC device), called E codes. The device codes (Level II HCPCS E codes) are specifically for devices, accessories, and software. The AAC CPT codes are for evaluation and treatment services. Readers will also find a wealth of resources in Appendix 9.7 (Toll-Free Phone Numbers and Hotlines), Appendix 9.8 (Internet Resources), Appendix 9.10 (International Sites), and Appendix 9.11 (Periodicals and Newsletters).

Neurolitigation

Following the development of the complete plan by the life care planner, it is possible that the plan will become part of neurolitigation. Success in neurolitigation frequently depends on the quality and quantity of expert evidence, which directly relates to the presentation of the life care plan, especially during medical malpractice cases and traumatic brain injury and spinal cord injury cases. Courts may admit the life care plan into evidence and rely on those plans as the predicate for compensatory damage awards when a well-qualified rehabilitation specialist prepares those plans. Included should be a list of treatment interventions that are reasonable and necessary and that show the real need for the individual to incur the expenses noted in the plan, and accurate, reasonable, and conservative costs for future care. SLPs participating in the life care planning process need to appreciate these requirements and understand their possible role in neurolitigation. It is possible that the consulting

Table 9.8 Comprehensive List of SLP CPT Codes (2016)

Swallowing Function		
92526	Treatment of swallowing dysfunction and/or oral function for feeding	_______
92610	Evaluation of swallowing function	
92611	Motion fluoroscopic evaluation of swallowing function	
92612	Flexible fiber-optic endoscopic evaluation of swallowing	
92613	with physician interpretation and report	
92614	Flexible fiber-optic endoscopic evaluation laryngeal sensory testing by line or video recording	_______
92615	With physician interpretation and report	
92616	Flexible fiber-optic endoscopic evaluation of swallowing and laryngeal sensory testing	_______
92617	With physician interpretation and report	
Speech and Language		
92507	Treatment of speech, language, voice, communication, and/or auditory processing disorder, individual	_______
92508	Group, two or more individuals	
97532	Development of cognitive skills to improve attention, memory, problem solving, direct one-on-one patient contact by the provider; each 15 minutes	_______
97533	Sensory integrative techniques to enhance sensory processing and promote adaptive responses to environmental demands; each 15 minutes	_______
92511	Nasopharyngoscopy w/ endoscope	_______
92520	Laryngeal function studies	
92521	Evaluation of speech fluency (e.g., stuttering, cluttering)	
92522	Evaluation of speech sound production (e.g,. articulation, phonological process, apraxia, dysarthria)	
92523	Evaluation of speech sound production (e.g., articulation, phonological processes, apraxia, dysarthria) with evaluation of language comprehension and expression. (e.g., receptive and expressive language)	
92524	Behavioral and qualitative analysis of voice and resonance	
92626	Evaluation of auditory rehabilitation status, first hour	_______
92627	Each additional 15 minutes	

(Continued)

Table 9.8 (Continued) Comprehensive List of SLP CPT Codes (2016)

92630	Auditory rehabilitation; prelingual hearing loss	
92633	Auditory rehabilitation; postlingual hearing loss	
96105	Assessment of aphasia with interpretation and report, per hour	________
96110	Developmental testing; limited, w/interpretation and report	________
96111	Extended, with interpretation and report, per hour	
96125	Standardized cognitive performance testing (e.g., Ross Information Processing Assessment) per hour of a qualified health care professional's time, both face-to-face time administering tests to the patient and time interpreting these test results and preparing the report	________
31575	Laryngoscopy; flexible fiber-optic; diagnostic	
31579	Laryngoscopy; flexible or rigid fiber-optic, with stroboscopy	
Augmentative and Alternative Communication		
92597	Evaluation for use/fitting of voice prosthetic device to supplement oral speech	________
92605	Evaluation for prescription of non-speech-generating augmentative and alternative communication device, first hour	________
92618	Each additional 30 minutes	
92606	Therapeutic service(s) for the use of non-speech-generating augmentative and alternative communication device, including programming and modification	________
92607	Evaluation for prescription for speech-generating augmentative and alternative communication device; face-to-face with the patient; evaluation, first hour	________
92608	Evaluation for speech device; each additional 30 minutes	
92609	Therapeutic services for the use of Speech Generating Device, including programming and modification	________
V5336	Repair/modification of AAC device (excluding adaptive hearing aid)	________
Other Procedures		
92700	Unlisted otorhinolaryngological service or procedure	
98966	• Telephone assessment and management service provided by a qualified nonphysician health care professional to an established patient, parent, or guardian not originating from a related assessment and management service provided within the previous 7 days nor leading to an assessment and management service provided within the next 24 hours or soonest available appointment • 5–10 minutes of medical discussion	

(*Continued*)

Table 9.8 (Continued) Comprehensive List of SLP CPT Codes (2016)

98967	11–20 minutes of medical discussion	
98968	21–30 minutes of medical discussion	
98969	Online assessment and management service provided by a qualified nonphysician health care professional to an established patient, guardian, or health care provider not originating from a related assessment and management service provided within the previous 7 days, using the Internet or similar electronic communication network	
99366	Medical team conference with interdisciplinary team of health care professionals, face-to-face with patient and/or family, 30 minutes or more; participation by nonphysician qualified health care professional	
99368	Medical team conference with interdisciplinary team of health care professionals, patient and/or family not present, 30 minutes or more; participation by nonphysician qualified health care professional	

Table 9.9 New 2016 ICD-10-CM SLP Codes

Other Developmental Disorders of Speech and Language
F80.82 Social pragmatic communication disorder (Excludes1: Asperger's syndrome [F84.5], autistic disorder [F84.0])
ASHA Note: The "Excludes1" note means that F80.82 may not be reported in conjunction with F84.5 or F84.0
Sequelae of Cerebrovascular Disease
Cognitive Deficits Following Nontraumatic Subarachnoid Hemorrhage
I69.010 Attention and concentration deficit following nontraumatic subarachnoid hemorrhage
I69.011 Memory deficit following nontraumatic subarachnoid hemorrhage
I69.012 Visuospatial deficit and spatial neglect following nontraumatic subarachnoid hemorrhage
I69.013 Psychomotor deficit following nontraumatic subarachnoid hemorrhage
I69.014 Frontal lobe and executive function deficit following nontraumatic subarachnoid hemorrhage
I69.015 Cognitive social or emotional deficit following nontraumatic subarachnoid hemorrhage
I69.018 Other symptoms and signs involving cognitive functions following nontraumatic subarachnoid hemorrhage
I69.019 Unspecified symptoms and signs involving cognitive functions following nontraumatic subarachnoid hemorrhage

(*Continued*)

Table 9.9 (Continued) New 2016 ICD-10-CM SLP Codes

Cognitive Deficits Following Nontraumatic Intracerebral Hemorrhage
I69.110 Attention and concentration deficit following nontraumatic intracerebral hemorrhage
I69.111 Memory deficit following nontraumatic intracerebral hemorrhage
I69.112 Visuospatial deficit and spatial neglect following nontraumatic intracerebral hemorrhage
I69.113 Psychomotor deficit following nontraumatic intracerebral hemorrhage
I69.114 Frontal lobe and executive function deficit following nontraumatic intracerebral hemorrhage
I69.115 Cognitive social or emotional deficit following nontraumatic intracerebral hemorrhage
I69.118 Other symptoms and signs involving cognitive functions following nontraumatic intracerebral hemorrhage
I69.119 Unspecified symptoms and signs involving cognitive functions following nontraumatic intracerebral hemorrhage
Cognitive Deficits Following Other Nontraumatic Intracranial Hemorrhage
I69.210 Attention and concentration deficit following other nontraumatic intracranial hemorrhage
I69.211 Memory deficit following other nontraumatic intracranial hemorrhage
I69.212 Visuospatial deficit and spatial neglect following other nontraumatic intracranial hemorrhage
I69.213 Psychomotor deficit following other nontraumatic intracranial hemorrhage
I69.214 Frontal lobe and executive function deficit following other nontraumatic intracranial hemorrhage
I69.215 Cognitive social or emotional deficit following other nontraumatic intracranial hemorrhage
I69.218 Other symptoms and signs involving cognitive functions following other nontraumatic intracranial hemorrhage
I69.219 Unspecified symptoms and signs involving cognitive functions following other nontraumatic intracranial hemorrhage
Cognitive Deficits Following Cerebral Infarction
I69.310 Attention and concentration deficit following cerebral infarction
I69.311 Memory deficit following cerebral infarction
I69.312 Visuospatial deficit and spatial neglect following cerebral infarction
I69.313 Psychomotor deficit following cerebral infarction

(*Continued*)

Table 9.9 (Continued) New 2016 ICD-10-CM SLP Codes

I69.314 Frontal lobe and executive function deficit following cerebral infarction
I69.315 Cognitive social or emotional deficit following cerebral infarction
I69.318 Other symptoms and signs involving cognitive functions following cerebral infarction
I69.319 Unspecified symptoms and signs involving cognitive functions following cerebral infarction
Cognitive Deficits Following Other Cerebrovascular Disease
I69.810 Attention and concentration deficit following other cerebrovascular disease
I69.811 Memory deficit following other cerebrovascular disease
I69.812 Visuospatial deficit and spatial neglect following other cerebrovascular disease
I69.813 Psychomotor deficit following other cerebrovascular disease
I69.814 Frontal lobe and executive function deficit following other cerebrovascular disease
I69.815 Cognitive social or emotional deficit following other cerebrovascular disease
I69.818 Other symptoms and signs involving cognitive functions following other cerebrovascular disease
I69.819 Unspecified symptoms and signs involving cognitive functions following other cerebrovascular disease
Cognitive Deficits Following Unspecified Cerebrovascular Disease
I69.910 Attention and concentration deficit following unspecified cerebrovascular disease
I69.911 Memory deficit following unspecified cerebrovascular disease
I69.912 Visuospatial deficit and spatial neglect following unspecified cerebrovascular disease
I69.913 Psychomotor deficit following unspecified cerebrovascular disease
I69.914 Frontal lobe and executive function deficit following unspecified cerebrovascular disease
I69.915 Cognitive social or emotional deficit following unspecified cerebrovascular disease
I69.918 Other symptoms and signs involving cognitive functions following unspecified cerebrovascular disease
I69.919 Unspecified symptoms and signs involving cognitive functions following unspecified cerebrovascular disease
Revised ICD-10-CM Codes
Specific Developmental Disorders of Speech and Language
No change **F80.0** Phonological disorder *Add* Speech-sound disorder
Pervasive Developmental Disorders

(Continued)

Table 9.9 (Continued) New 2016 ICD-10-CM SLP Codes

No change **F84.0** Autistic disorder *Add* Autism spectrum disorder
No change **F88** Other disorders of psychological development *No change* Developmental agnosia *Add* Global developmental delay *Add* Other specified neurodevelopmental disorder
No change **F89** Unspecified disorder of psychological development *Add* Neurodevelopmental disorder NOS

Note: These revisions do not change the intent of the codes but add new language to include descriptive information or examples related to disorders captured under each code.

SLP will have to give testimony in a deposition concerning his or her area within the life care plan or may be considered as an expert witness if the case goes to trial. The SLP will be responsible for answering questions and explaining his or her portions of the life care plan.

Regardless of particular knowledge, skills, experience, training, or education, the expert who is able to clearly articulate his or her opinions and conclusions, who understands the dynamics of the litigation process, and who comports with commonsense techniques for presenting testimony is the expert the attorney wishes to use to advance the client's cause. Obviously, the expert must be both professional and knowledgeable in demeanor and appearance, must be familiar with the various types of rehabilitation programs and therapeutic services available, must possess an in-depth knowledge of the current literature, and understand and be able to explain intervention strategies employed at all levels of treatment. Being able to explain the complexities involved in extremely specialized fields of expertise, without appearing to condescend to lay jurors, is particularly important.

The following is a list of general considerations that SLPs who function as experts for the purpose of explaining their part of the life care planning process should espouse. The chapter author considered whether to leave this section in at time of revision but based on input from life care planners and SLPs who may review this prior to deposition or trial, she decided to include it.

1. Tell the truth. Then you will not have to remember what you said.
2. Phrase your answers with care. Be conscious of what they will look like in black and white.
3. Answer only the question asked; do not volunteer information.
4. Do not answer a question that you do not understand. It is not up to you to educate the examiner, and if he/she misuses words common in your profession, do not explain distinctions or ask questions as to what he/she means; it is up to him/her to formulate an intelligible question.
5. Do not guess, speculate, or assume anything. You only know what you have seen or heard; there is a difference between what you know and whether you have information concerning a particular subject.
6. Do not be positive about a subject unless you are; it is no crime to fail to remember or to be vague if that is the truth.
7. Do not adopt the examiner's phraseology or conclusions. If the question contains a false assumption ("Isn't it true that all communication tests are conducted in this manner?") or terms that are not precisely correct ("So you *frequently* performed this treatment for this patient?"), point out the language you do not wish to accept and stick to the facts. Beware of

Table 9.10 Example Life Care Plan Entries

Recommendation	*Medical Needs*	*Dates*	*Frequency*	*Expected Cost*
	Swallow study with fiber endoscopy	2008–2010	Every 6 months through 2010, then optional depending on complications and need.	$250
	Swallow study with MBS	2009–2028	Yearly for life.	$450
	Otolaryngology	2008–life	Yearly for life, more if additional respiratory complications occur.	$400
	Nutrition consult	2008–life	Yearly for life because of the traumatic injury. Nutrition is a crucial part of the lifelong plan.	$150
	Audiological evaluation	2008–life	Yearly for life expectancy, because of the traumatic injury and later aging.	$820
	Optional: pulmonology	Only if complications	Unknown	Unknown
Home and Accessories				
	Environmental control unit	2008–life expectancy	Replace every 5 years.	$1,200 plus $100 per year maintenance and updates
AT Equipment and Supplies				
	Augmentative and alternative communication	2008–life expectancy	Replace or upgrade every 5 years for life. Initial AAC device may need to be basic, but the system will either have to increase in complexity with the client's recovery or be replaced with a new device of increasing complexity.	Initially, $1,500, later at $5,000

(*Continued*)

Table 9.10 (Continued) Example Life Care Plan Entries

	Wheelchair mount and latching system for AAC	2008–life expectancy	When power chair is replaced but at 5 years as a maximum replacement time.	$1,500
	Computer, desktop, and printer	2008–life expectancy	For integration of the AAC device, to increase communication and therapy options initially, later for independent living purposes.	$2,500
	Assisted listening device to include earphone, speaker's microphone	2008–2018	For auditory processing in therapy and in the community, enhancing listening ability and minimizing "noise" in the environment.	$800
	MyoTrac 2 biofeedback portable unit for swallowing and motor speech	2008–2012	For biofeedback of swallowing, motor speech in therapy.	$1,600 every 5 years (with 1-year warranty), pack of 10 sensors $65 (replace one every 3 years)
	Low-technology and no-technology assistive devices for communication and cognition	2008–life expectancy	For quick communication (basic AAC devices) for attention, to communicate immediate needs quickly.	$200 per year
	Memory aids	2008–life expectancy	Initially will start with low-tech device such as a card, simple voice output, then progress to an electronic calendar and organizer.	$200 per year
	Adapted phone for AAC	2009	One time only, but upgrades in the technology will be needed.	Phone: $500 with upgrades at $200 every 5 years

(Continued)

Table 9.10 (Continued) Example Life Care Plan Entries

	Work/study station (electronic)	2008–2037	Update every 5 years, needs to be electronic with the necessary adapted equipment.	$8,000 for initial, then $1,000 every 5 years for electronic upgrade and $300 per year for maintenance of the electronics on the desk.
Speech Pathology Services				
	Assessment to include swallowing, cognition, speech (motor), auditory processing, and reading/writing	2008–life expectancy	Yearly assessment (reassessment) until 2013, then every 5 years for life.	$1,000–$1,500 per year
	Assessment for augmentative communication system and additional AT	2008–life expectancy	Yearly reassessment until 2013, then every 5 years for life. Note: the SLP evaluation and the AT evaluation may be combined, completed by one person; however, the expected cost should then be combined (i.e., $2,000–$3,000) yearly, etc.	$1,000–$1,500
	SLP therapy	2008–2016, then dependent upon the reevaluation every 5 years	First year: 5 hours per week. Second year: 3 hours per week. Third year: 2 hours per week. Fourth/fifth years: 1 hour per week if progress continues without further complications (illnesses, other accidents, etc.).	$175 per hour

(*Continued*)

Table 9.10 (Continued) Example Life Care Plan Entries

	SLP (AT/AAC) technology training	2008–2016, then dependent upon the AT reevaluation and the AT devices	First year: 5 hours per week. Second year: 3 hours per week. Third year: 2 hours per week. Fourth/fifth years: 1 hour per week if progress continues without further complications (illnesses, other accidents, etc.). Will need 2 hours per week for 4 weeks every 5 years if new technology is introduced and/or when aging issues complicate the use of the technology (typically at age 50 and 70 for someone with a disability).	$175 per hour
Vocational program and independent living program		2012–2037	Job training, and/or independent living training.	No additional cost
Rehabilitation engineering: tech support and home/ transportation access		2028–2047	Technology support, home modifications as needed, transportation modifications as needed. First year: 10 hours per month; second year: 4 hours per quarter (16 hours for the year); third/fourth/ fifth years: 10 hours per year. Every year after 2013, 5 hours as needed.	$100 per hour

questions that start with "Isn't it fair to say" or that attempt to paraphrase or summarize your previous testimony on a particular point.

8. Do not explain the manner in which you reached your answer, because such tactics invariably involve facts other than those concerning what you have been asked.
9. Do not testify concerning a document that is an exhibit until you have read it over thoroughly. Do not discuss documents that are not exhibits unless specifically asked about them, and then do not be positive about their content unless you are certain of your answer. Make no assumptions about documents.
10. Never get upset, explain, or argue with the examiner. You are liable to say things that are not correct, and in any event, it is not your duty to help him/her in this task.
11. If an objection to a question is made by counsel who retained you, listen very carefully, as it may provide information as to some underlying snare.
12. Avoid small talk, levity, ethnic or derogatory slurs of any kind, and even the mildest obscenity. Better to come across as formal than as a not serious or offensive person.
13. If at any time during the deposition you realize you previously said something that was a mistake or incorrect, correct the error as soon as possible. Do not waive your right to read and sign a deposition. Should a realization of an error arrive after the deposition has been completed, you should make such correction on the errata sheet that will be supplied to you at the time you are asked to sign off on the deposition as transcribed.

Presentation of testimony by selected members of the rehabilitation team in litigation can be of immense benefit to counsel, the court, and lay jurors in furthering the understanding of costs associated with present and future needs and care and treatment, and in providing a framework on which an insurer or jury can justify a substantial settlement or award. One's abilities to be effective in this regard are aided by a clear understanding of one's role as an expert witness and the ability to interact with others and clearly articulate one's specialized knowledge in the areas at issue, placed in the context of a full understanding of the dynamics of the litigation process and an awareness of the techniques of proper presentation.

Hot Topics in Speech-Language Pathology Update

The following is a list of hot topics in the field of speech-language pathology/communication disorders. These topics will continue to develop over the next several years, affecting recommendations in life care plans. Life care planners are encouraged to monitor these topics and to be assured that they are always on the cutting edge of this information as they develop strong well-written and well-researched life care plans.

- Development of assessment and treatment guidelines for autism spectrum disorders
- Development of assessment and treatment guidelines for central auditory processing disorders
- Development of specific treatment guidelines in neurological treatment of communication disorders (e.g., cognitive communication, aphasia, apraxia, dysarthria, and dementia)
- Development of research in gastroesophageal reflux disease (GERD)
- Efficacy and evidence-based studies to determine what treatments are effective
- Development of a stronger presence with funding streams and sources
- Improving treatment outcomes with all areas of treatment
- Development of instrumentation to improve diagnostic and treatment measures (fiber endoscopy, e-stimulation, cervical auscultation, deep pharyngeal stimulation)

- Increased inclusion as a member of medical surgical teams for management of head and neck issues (e.g., laryngectomies, palatal surgeries, vocal cord surgeries) and brain surgeries (e.g., removal of tumors, control postcerebral vascular accidents, seizure controls)
- Increased research and treatment of progressive neurological diseases such as Parkinson's, dementia, Alzheimer's, and multiple sclerosis
- Increased research participation with neurotrophic cortical electrode implantation
- Increased research with speech-language treatment post-cochlear implants
- Research with pharmacological therapeutic interventions to improve communication in patients with communication disorders
- Use of Vital Stimulation to correct swallowing problems
- Collaborative surgical and prosthetic intervention for craniofacial anomalies
- Telepractice

With the increased awareness and concern about individuals with blast-related and other brain injuries, ASHA members need comprehensive knowledge and practical skills to provide optimal services. To assist professionals working in rehabilitation settings, the Joint Committee on Interprofessional Relations Between the American Speech-Language-Hearing Association (ASHA) and the American Psychological Association's (APA) Division 40 (Clinical Neuropsychology) has developed resources now available to ASHA members. Speech-language pathology and neuropsychology are two of the professions involved in the assessment and treatment of children and adults with cognitive-communication and language disorders resulting from congenital or acquired brain impairment. Since its inception, the committee has produced several documents to assist professionals engaged in brain injury rehabilitation. Policy documents are accessible at ASHA Practice Policy (www.asha.org).

Case Study

The client, Sam Hall, age 22, sustained a brain injury following a motor vehicle accident. His traumatic brain injury (TBI) resulted in physical and mental deficits that required AT. A complete series of tests were administered, including cognitive and oral–motor (results will not be included in this brief example) assessments as appropriate, and the client clearly appeared capable of participation in speech and language therapy, as well as swallowing therapy and therapy to address his AT needs. The partial Life Care Plan shown in the following was part of a comprehensive life care plan; however, only the appropriate topics for the SLP are included.

Conclusion

The opportunity to participate in the life care planning process should not be taken lightly. It has been one of the most rewarding parts of the profession of speech-language pathology for this author. It requires professionals who are respected among their peers for their hard work, diligent study, research, data collection and use, expert testimony, and even ability to explain their results and information in written form. Standards must be placed on what the industry expects from its consultants when the consultants provide strong, useful assessments and recommendations. It is time for life care planners to set a level of accountability, responsibility, and recognition for the consultants that they use to develop the communication and swallowing areas of the life care plan, and it is time for SLPs to empower themselves for this process.

Appendices

Appendix 9.1 Communication Sciences and Disorders/SLP Assessment Process

1. *Who* is a qualified SLP for life care planning purposes?
   A. Training, licensure, certification, and practice settings
   B. Ability to network
   C. Integrated transdisciplinary model
   D. Knowledge of funding streams and creative funding
   E. Knowledge of state and federal policy, laws, and procedures
   F. Knowledge of the development of collaborative sources

2. *What* will a qualified SLP need?
   A. Review of all pertinent medical, vocational, educational, pharmacological, and sociological information
   B. Differences between a staff speech-language pathology evaluation and the type of data needed to support a life care plan and to support the medical-legal challenges
   C. Time needed to complete a communication sciences and disorders assessment
   D. Understanding of related professional information and how it impacts and affects the speech-language information and plans
   E. An ability to understand future trends and their application to the life care plan

3. *Components* of a communication disorders assessment
   A. Oral and pharyngeal swallowing (dysphagia) assessment to include modified barium swallows, videostroboscopy evaluations, prostodontic intervention, and palatal prostheses
   B. Cognitive communication information
   C. Audiological information to include central auditory processing information
   D. Augmentative communication assessment information
   E. AT (assistive technology) assessment information
   F. Voice (to include videostroboscopy, Botox assessment information, etc.)
   G. Oral peripheral motor information
   H. Hearing acuity information
   I. Assistive listening device or cochlear implant information

4. *Written* documentation prepared in a defensible but understandable plan with functional milestones and goals
   A. Ability to determine lifelong goals and functional outcomes
   B. Ability to understand how to develop services and technology needs over time
   C. Ability to explain how decisions within other areas of the life care plan will impact assessment, treatment, and technology needs within the communication sciences and disorders part of the plan
   D. Ability to explain present data in terms of future impact

Appendix 9.2 Communication Sciences and Disorders: Checklist for Life Care Planning

1. Does the funding source understand the purpose and usefulness of a complete evaluation from an SLP?
2. Check qualifications, credentials, and areas of expertise of the SLP you have selected to provide the information.
3. Does the SLP understand the concepts of the life care planning process and how the information provided by him will be used?
4. Is the SLP aware of the professional content areas within communication sciences and disorders that must be included/considered in the report to the life care planner?
A. Expressive language
B. Receptive language
C. Cognitive communication
D. Oral and pharyngeal dysphagia
E. Augmentative communication
F. AT (assistive technology)
G. Hearing and auditory processing as it relates to communication
H. Voice and voicing aspects
I. Fluency and rate
5. Can the SLP provide the results in a timely manner that meets deadlines?
6. Has the SLP been provided access to all available and necessary records, including medical, educational, vocational, and specialized testing?
7. Are the client and family available for a thorough test battery? Are there access restrictions?
8. Once information is gathered, is the SLP able to provide thorough written documentation with clear recommendations?
9. Have the questions in the following areas been considered during the communication sciences and disorders assessment?
Evaluations/Assessments
___ Have all the necessary assessments in the areas of communication sciences and disorders (language, speech, swallowing, augmentative communication, AT, hearing, central auditory processing, videostroboscopy, modified barium swallow studies) been considered?
___ When will reassessments be scheduled?
___ At what ages or levels of functioning will these reassessments (or additional assessments) be considered?

(*Continued*)

Appendix 9.2 (Continued) Communication Sciences and Disorders: Checklist for Life Care Planning

Therapy
___ How will necessary therapies be identified?
___ How will collaborative sources be used?
AT
___ How will technology recommendations for augmentative communication be integrated with other AT recommendations or other AT that is already present?
___ Consider the use of low and high technology to include wheelchairs, environmental controls, vision equipment, hearing aids, computers, adaptive aids, and assistive listening systems.
___ Have maintenance schedules, maintenance contracts, extended warranties, and replacement schedules been considered?
___ What is the range of AT that is needed?
___ Have the following been considered: computers, means of access, size of screens, assisted listening, low-technology communication needs, high-technology communication needs, memory aids, swallowing program equipment, necessary software, ancillary battery power, systems to integrate augmentative communication with computers for complete system development, adapted phones, variety of synthetic and digitized voices, amount of memory needed in computerized systems, and positional items for mounting and portability?
Home Furnishing/Accessories
___ How will AT within the existing home and environment be included?
___ Have probable versus potential environmental changes been considered?
Drug Supplies and Needs
___ Is there a need for medications for saliva control?
___ Have all pharmacological interventions been recommended for motor control (ataxia, tremors, etc.), for memory enhancement, for seizure control?
___ Have potential side effects of drugs or pharmacological intervention plans been considered in relationship to all areas of communication, swallowing, or auditory processing? These drug recommendations directly impact treatment recommendations and must be aggressively considered in the plan.
Future Medical Care
___ What annual evaluations will be needed?
___ What specialties will need to repeat the evaluations for specific treatment needs and recommendations?

(*Continued*)

Appendix 9.2 (Continued) Communication Sciences and Disorders: Checklist for Life Care Planning

Potential Complications
___ What complications could potentially occur as a result of poor treatment or no treatment in the areas where recommendations have been made?
___ What complications in speech, language, swallowing, communication, cognitive communication, oral–motor, hearing, and processing could occur with this etiology during the life span?
Vocational Planning
___ How will communication, hearing, and language/speech recommendations, as well as augmentative communication and AT recommendations, integrate with vocational plans and needs at this time and in the future?
Educational Planning
___ How will communication, hearing, and language/speech recommendations as well as augmentative communication and AT recommendations, integrate with educational plans and needs at this time and in the future?
___ What systems and equipment are available within educational programs (primary, secondary, and postsecondary)?
___ Is the software appropriate for cognitive needs and projections in the future?
___ Have specialized camps, summer training programs, specialized preschools, and specialized short-term programs for upgrading and improvement, as well as further training needs in the future, been considered?
___10. Is the SLP able to explain from a life care planning perspective the reasons and rationales relative to the recommendations?
___11. Does the SLP understand how to develop lifelong recommendations and objectives? An integrated plan?
___12. Is the SLP able to give detailed specifications in the written documentation that allow the life care planner the ability to develop life care plan specifics (i.e., vendors, dates, current prices, specific individuals, collaborative sources, and categories of information)?
___13. Once the draft of the life care plan is complete, is the SLP furnished a draft for careful review relative to the accuracy and completeness of the information?
___14. Is the SLP aware that the data collection and analysis (evaluation) information may be presented to an insurance carrier, in testimony through deposition, or at a trial?

Appendix 9.3 Funding and Financing

Public Programs
Medicaid and Medicare
Required and optional services
Intermediate care facilities for persons who are mentally disabled (ICFs/MR)
Early and Periodic Screening, Diagnosis, and Treatment (EPSDT)
Section 2176 Home- and Community-Based (HCB) waivers
Community-supported living arrangements
Maternal and child health
Maternal and child health block grant
Children with special health care needs
Special Projects of Regional and National Significance (SPRANS)
Education
Individuals with Disabilities Education Act (IDEA) State Grants (Part B)
IDEA: Programs for Infants and Toddlers with Disabilities and Their Families (Part H)
State-operated programs (89–313)
Vocational education
Head start
Vocational rehabilitation
State grants
Supported employment
Independent living (Parts A, B, and C)
Social Security benefits
Title II: Social Security Disability Insurance (SSDI)
Title XVI: Supplemental Security Income (SSI)
Work incentive programs
Developmental disability programs
Department of Veterans Affairs programs
Older Americans Act programs
Alternative Financing
Revolving loan fund

(*Continued*)

Appendix 9.3 (Continued) Funding and Financing

Lending library
Discount program
Low-interest loans
Private foundations
Service clubs
Special state appropriations
State bond issues
Employee accommodations program
Equipment loan program
Corporate-sponsored loans
Charitable organizations
Funding Options through Private Insurance
Health insurance
Workers' compensation
Casualty insurance
Disability insurance
Funding Options through the U.S. Tax Code
Medical care expense deduction
Business deductions
Employee business deductions
ADA credit for small business
Credit for architectural and transportation barrier removal
Targeted jobs tax credit
Charitable contributions deduction

Appendix 9.4 Funding Glossary

Access: Generally refers to an individual's ability to obtain public or private health insurance coverage. Also used to indicate an individual's ability to easily obtain health services. That ability may be affected by restrictions on enrollees' distance from health care, waiting time to receive services, or individual's capability to communicate with providers, as well as to comprehend and carry out treatment instructions. Access may also be impacted by restrictions imposed on the physicians' choice of treatment options and various cost-containment strategies.
Accountable health plans (AHPs): Under leading health reform proposals, vertically integrated organizations of providers and insurers that offer a standard benefit package approved at the national level by Congress and a federal board or commission. AHPs would be certified by the states and would be required to publish reports on their prices, patient satisfaction, and health outcomes. These health plans would fully integrate the financial, managerial, clinical, and preventive aspects of health care. Accountable health plans are also referred to as certified health plans, alliance health plans, accountable health partnerships, and qualified health plans under current reform bills.
Actual acquisition cost: The pharmacist's net payment made to purchase a drug product, after taking into account such items as purchasing allowances, discounts, rebates, and the like.
Actual charge: The amount a physician or other provider actually bills a patient for a particular medical service, procedure, or supply in a specific instance. The actual charge may differ from the usual, customary, prevailing, or reasonable charge.
Acute care: Medical care for health problems or illnesses that are short-term or intense in nature.
Administrative costs: The costs assumed by a managed care plan for administrative services such as claims processing, billing, and overhead costs.
Adverse selection: Among applicants for a given group or individual program, the tendency for those with an impaired health status, or who are prone to higher than average utilization of benefits, to be enrolled in disproportionate numbers and lower deductible plans. See also *community rating*.
Aged: For purposes of Medicare enrollment, persons 65 years of age or over are considered to be aged. Medicaid eligibility is determined on the basis of financial need for people who meet Supplemental Security Income eligibility criteria (aged, blind, or disabled individuals) and Aid to Families with Dependent Children criteria (adults and children). Eligibility determinations are made for an entire economic unit or case (sometimes a family) based on whether one member of a case meets the criteria. For example, an aged case could consist of a 66-year-old male and his 63-year-old wife. In contrast, a disabled enrollee could be over 65 years of age.
Agency for Health Care Policy and Research (AHCPR): The agency of the Public Health Service responsible for enhancing the quality, appropriateness, and effectiveness of health care services.
Allied health professionals: Nonphysician health workers, including, but not limited to, nurses, pharmacists, respiratory therapists, phlebotomists, pulmonary therapists, occupational therapists, recreational physical therapists, lab technicians, social workers, and dental hygienists.

(*Continued*)

Appendix 9.4 (Continued) Funding Glossary

All-payer system: A reimbursement setup where all insurers reimburse providers using the same accounting system.
Alternative delivery system: A phrase that describes nontraditional health insurance programs that finance and provide health care to members. These include health maintenance organizations (HMOs) and preferred provider organizations (PPOs).
Ambulatory care: Health care services provided on an outpatient basis. No overnight stay in the hospital is required. The services of ambulatory care centers, hospital outpatient departments, physicians' offices, and home health care services fall under this heading.
Ambulatory surgery: Any minor surgical procedures that can be performed at any type of medical facility on an outpatient basis—not requiring an overnight stay.
Claim: The formal demand by the insured to collect reimbursement for a loss covered under an insurance policy.
Claims Clearinghouse System: System that allows electronic claims submission through a single source.
Claims review: The method by which an enrollee's health care service claims are reviewed before reimbursement is made. The purpose of this monitoring system is to validate the medical appropriateness of the provided services and to be sure the cost of the service is not excessive.
Clearinghouse capability: A company's ability to submit electronic and paper claims to several third-party payers.
Clinical indicator: A tool used to monitor and evaluate care to assure desirable outcomes and to explain or prevent undesirable outcomes.
Clinical Practice Guidelines: Guidelines that specify the appropriate course(s) of treatment for specified health conditions.
Closed-panel HMO: Employment system in which physicians staffing an HMO are employed solely by the HMO.
Coinsurance: A cost-sharing requirement under a health insurance policy that provides that the insured will assume a portion or percentage of the costs of covered services. After the deductible is paid, this provision forces the subscriber to pay for a certain percentage of any remaining medical bills—usually 20 percent.
Community rating: A method health insurers use to determine the premium costs for a group it is planning to insure. Under this system, the insurer bases the premiums on the average health care costs of the community, not the age, sex, occupation, or health of individual subscribers.
Competitive Medical Plan (CMP): An organization defined by the federal Medicare program that provides enrolled members with physician, hospital, and laboratory services on a capitation basis. These services are provided primarily by physicians who are under contract, employed by, or partners in the CMP. A CMP has fewer restrictions imposed than a federally qualified health maintenance organization but may be a state-licensed HMO.

(*Continued*)

Appendix 9.4 (Continued) Funding Glossary

Comprehensive Major Medical Coverage: A form of health insurance that combines the coverage of basic medical expense contracts and specialized medical care contracts into one comprehensive plan. These plans have both a deductible and coinsurance.
Consolidated Omnibus Reconciliation Act (COBRA): Federal law enacted in 1985. It permits an employee who has been terminated or has a reduction in work hours to continue his or her health insurance coverage for a period of up to 18 months. This law also covers the employee's dependents.
Continuous Quality Improvement (CQI): A quality model that incorporates statistical tools to analyze processes and improvement in quality of care.
Contract: An agreement by which the insurer agrees to provide insurance benefits, to protect against losses, and to provide a written statement outlining the insurance provisions. The insured agrees to pay the insurer a set fee, called a premium, and other considerations.
Contributory: A general term that describes any employee insurance plan where the employee pays part of the premium.
Copayment: Copayments are a type of cost-sharing under Medicaid whereby insured or covered persons pay a specified flat amount per unit of service or unit of time, and the insurer pays the rest of the cost.
Cost-per-case limits: Reimbursement limits imposed by the government on each Medicare admission to hospitals.
Cost sharing: The general set of financing arrangements whereby the consumer must pay out of pocket to receive care, either at the time of initiating care or during the provision of health care services, or both. Cost sharing can also occur when an insured pays a portion of the monthly premium for health care insurance.
Cost shifting: A practice by health insurers to increase premiums for one group of businesses to offset costs from another line of business, like Medicare and Medicaid recipients.
Exclusivity clause: A part of a contract that prohibits physicians from contracting with more than one health maintenance organization or preferred provider organization.
Expenditures: Under Medicaid, expenditures refer to an amount paid out by a state agency for the covered medical expenses of eligible participants.
Experience rating: A system where an insurance company evaluates the risk of an individual or group by looking at the applicant's health history.
Extended care: Long-term care, ranging from routine assistance for daily activities to sophisticated medical and nursing care for those needing it. The care, covered under certain insurance policies, can be provided in homes, daycare centers, or other facilities.
Family planning services: Family planning services are any medically approved means, including diagnosis, treatment, drugs, supplies and devices, and related counseling that are furnished or prescribed by or under the supervision of a physician for individuals of childbearing age for purposes of enabling such individuals freely to determine the number or spacing of their children.

(*Continued*)

Appendix 9.4 (Continued) Funding Glossary

Federally qualified HMOs: HMOs that meet certain federally stipulated provisions aimed at protecting consumers, for example, providing a broad range of basic health services, assuring financial solvency, and monitoring the quality of care. HMOs must apply to the federal government for qualification. The process is administered by the Office of Prepaid Health Care of the Health Care Financing Administration (HCFA), Department of Health and Human Services (DHHS).
Fee-for-service: The traditional way of billing for health care services. Under this system, there is a separate charge for each patient visit and the service provided.
First-dollar coverage: Health policies that pay all medical expenses up to a predetermined limit, without a deductible charge.
Fiscal agent: A fiscal agent is a contractor that processes or pays vendor claims on behalf of the Medicaid agency.
Fiscal intermediary: The agent (e.g., Blue Cross or an insurance company) that has contracted with providers of service to process claims for reimbursement under health care coverage. In addition to handling financial matters, it may perform other functions such as providing consultative services or serving as a center for communicating with providers and making audits of providers' records.
Fiscal year: Any 12-month period for which annual accounts are kept. The federal government's fiscal year extends from October 1 to the following September 30.
Fixed fee: An established fee schedule for pharmacy services allowed by certain government and private third-party programs in lieu of cost-of-doing-business markups.
Formulary: A list of selected pharmaceuticals and their appropriate dosages felt to be the most useful and cost-effective for patient care. Organizations often develop a formulary under the aegis of a pharmacy and therapeutics (P&T) committee. In HMOs, physicians are often required to prescribe from the formulary.
Freedom of Choice: Legislation restricting or eliminating the right of insurers to narrow the subscribers' selection of providers in return for a price discount.
Freestanding hospital: Any hospital that is not affiliated with a multihospital system.
Gatekeeper: A component of an independent practice association HMO that requires a subscriber to see a primary physician and get the physician's approval before seeing a specialist about a medical condition.
Generic substitution: Substituting a generic version of a branded off-patent pharmaceutical for the branded product when the latter is prescribed. Some HMOs and Medicaid programs mandate generic substitution. Mandatory generic substitution within the Medicare program is currently being debated in Congress.
Global budget: A budget that would determine the total amount of money that a geographic area could spend each year for health care. Under a global budget, providers and hospitals receive predetermined payments. As an enforcement mechanism for staying within budget, providers and hospitals will not receive additional funding if their costs exceed their budgeted payments.

(*Continued*)

Appendix 9.4 (Continued) Funding Glossary

Infant mortality rate: Deaths in the first year of life per 1,000 births. The U.S. rate in 2015 was 5.9 deaths per 1,000 live births (CDC, 2018). According to the U.S. General Accounting Office, 50 percent of these deaths are due to lifestyle factors, 20 percent due to environmental factors, 20 percent due to biological factors, and 10 percent due to inadequate health care.
Inpatient hospital services: Inpatient hospital services are items and services furnished to an inpatient of a hospital by the hospital, including bed and board, nursing and related services, diagnostic and therapeutic services, and medical or surgical services.
Intensive care: Skilled nursing services prescribed by a physician, delivered with the guidance of a registered nurse. Scope of care is provided to individuals with serious medical conditions that persist for long periods of time.
Intermediate care facility: An intermediate care facility is an institution furnishing health-related care and services to individuals who do not require the degree of care provided by hospitals or skilled nursing facilities as defined under Title XIX (Medicaid) of the Social Security Act.
Job-lock: The inability of an individual to change employers for fear of losing health coverage, particularly if the employee or a dependent has a preexisting condition.
Laboratory and radiological services: Professional and technical laboratory and radiological services ordered by a licensed practitioner, provided in an office or similar facility (other than a hospital outpatient department or clinic) or by a qualified lab.
Legend drug: A drug product that cannot be dispensed legally without a prescription.
Long-term care: Continuous health care delivered by a hospital or other health care institution to a patient for 30 days or more.
Magnetic resonance imaging (MRI): State-of-the-art machine used as a diagnostic tool, using magnetic waves to produce comprehensive pictures of the anatomy.
Managed care: A term coined originally to refer to the prepaid health care sector, for example, HMOs and CMPs, where care is provided under a fixed budget and costs are managed. Increasingly, the term is being used by many analysts to include PPOs and even forms of indemnity insurance coverage that incorporate preadmission certification and other utilization controls.
Maximum allowable cost, or reasonable cost range: A maximum cost is fixed for which the pharmacist can be reimbursed for selected products, as identified in a formulary.
Medicaid: A government program that covers medical expenses for the poor and certain other classes of uninsured people, established by Title XIX of the Social Security Act. Each state administers its own program. Medicaid is funded by both the state and federal governments.
Medicaid buy-in: A provision in certain health reform proposals whereby the uninsured would be allowed to purchase Medicaid coverage by paying premiums on a sliding scale based on income.
Medicaid Management Information System: Federally developed guidelines for computer system design to achieve national standardization of Medicaid claims processing, payment, review, and reporting for all health care claims.

(*Continued*)

Appendix 9.4 (Continued) Funding Glossary

Medically needy: Under Medicaid, medically needy cases are aged, blind, or disabled individuals or families and children who are otherwise eligible for Medicaid and whose income resources are above the limits for eligibility as categorically needy but are within limits set under the Medicaid state plan.
Medical Savings Accounts (MSAs): An account into which individuals can contribute a limited amount to cover medical costs or to buy insurance. Contributions to the accounts are sometimes tax deductible. MSAs are often cited as an incentive to limit health spending. Also called *medical IRAs*.
Practice variation: An assessment of the patterns of a practitioner's practice to determine if the practitioner provides care that is significantly different from others with similar practices. If there is a significant difference, the practitioner's practice is analyzed to determine the reasons for the variation and whether that practitioner's practice patterns should be modified.
Preferred Provider Organization (PPO): Type of health insurance program where a limited group of physicians and hospitals provide a broad range of medical care for a predetermined fee. Patients using the group providers usually have their health care expenses covered in full. Those covered under the PPO who do not use the preferred providers for care usually have to pay for a portion of their medical expenses.
Prepaid Group Practice Plans: Organized medical groups of essentially full-time physicians in appropriate specialties, as well as other professional and sub-professional personnel, who, for regular compensation, undertake to provide comprehensive care to an enrolled population for premium payments that are made in advance by the consumer or their employers.
Prescribed drugs: Prescribed drugs are drugs dispensed by a licensed pharmacist on the prescription of a practitioner licensed by law to administer such drugs, and drugs dispensed by a licensed practitioner to his own patients. This item does not include a practitioner's drug charges that are not separable from his other charges, or drugs covered by a hospital's bill.
Preventative care programs: Often called wellness programs, these programs use exercise and health education and promotion as vehicles to keep people healthy and good insurance risks.
Primary care: General medical care that typically deals with common injuries and illness.
Prior authorization: The approval a provider must obtain from an insurer or other entity before performing certain procedures using certain medical products or admitting a patient electively in order for the service to be covered under the plan.
Prospective financing: Financing for health care services based on prices or budgets determined prior to the delivery of service. Payments can be per unit of service, per member, or per time period. In all its forms prospective financing differs from cost-based reimbursement, under which a provider is paid for costs incurred.
Prospective Payment Assessment Commission (ProPAC): A 15-member commission, appointed by the director of the Office of Technology Assessment, that makes recommendations to the secretary of the Department of Health and Human Services on various aspects of the diagnosis-related group system of Medicare reimbursement.

(*Continued*)

Appendix 9.4 (Continued) Funding Glossary

Providers: Physicians, hospitals, and other health care organizations that treat individuals for illness and injuries.
Rate setting: A form of financing under which hospitals or nursing homes are paid prices that are prospectively determined, generally by a state agency. Prospectively determined prices may be paid by all payers for all covered services, as in all payer systems, or by only some payers. The unit of payment can be service, patient, or time period. See also *prospective financing*.
Rational drug therapy: Prescribing the right drug for the right patient, at the right time, in the right amounts, and with due consideration for relative costs.
Reasonable charge: In processing claims for supplementary medical insurance benefits, carriers use HCFA guidelines to establish the reasonable charge for services rendered. The reasonable charge is the lowest of the actual charge billed by the physician or supplier, the charge the physician or supplier customarily bills her patients for the same services, and the prevailing charge that most physicians or suppliers in that locality bill for the same service. Increases in the physicians' prevailing charge levels are recognized only to the extent justified by an index reflecting changes in the costs of practice and in general earnings.
State plan: The Medicaid state plan is a comprehensive written commitment by a Medicaid agency to administer or supervise the administration of a Medicaid program in accordance with federal requirements.
Stop loss: That point at which a third party has reinsurance to protect against the overly large single claim or the excessively high aggregate claim during a given period of time. Large employers, who are self-insured, may also purchase reinsurance for stop-loss purposes.
Supplemental Security Income (SSI): SSI is a program of income support for low-income aged, blind, and/or disabled persons established by Title XVI of the Social Security Act.
Therapeutic substitution: A practice entailing a pharmacist's dispensing a drug felt to be therapeutically equivalent to the drug prescribed by a physician without obtaining permission from the prescribing physician. Generally, the P&T committee of an HMO will formally approve therapeutic substitutions that it feels are permissible, and only those so designated can be made by the pharmacist dispensing for the HMO.
Third-party administrator: Individual or company that contracts with employers who want to self-insure the health of their employees. They develop and coordinate self-insurance programs, process and pay the claims, and may help locate stop-loss insurance for the employer. They also can analyze the effectiveness of the program and trace the patterns of those using the benefits.
Third-party liability: Under Medicaid, third-party liability exists if there is any entity (i.e., other government programs or insurance) that is or may be liable to pay all or part of the medical cost or injury, disease, or disability of an applicant or recipient of Medicaid.
Total Quality Management (TQM): See *Continuous Quality Improvement*.
Universal access: The availability of affordable public or private insurance coverage for every U.S. citizen or legal resident. There is no guarantee, however, that all individuals will actually choose to, or have the funds to, purchase coverage. See also *universal coverage*.

(*Continued*)

Appendix 9.4 (Continued) Funding Glossary

Universal coverage: The guaranteed provision of at least basic health care services to every U.S. citizen or legal resident. See also *universal access*.
Usual, customary, and reasonable charges: Method of reimbursement used under Medicaid by which state Medicaid programs set reimbursement rates using the Medicare method or a fee schedule, whichever is lower.
Utilization review: A tool used by providers, health care organizations, and insurance companies to influence the use of health care resources with the objective of containing costs.
Vendor: A medical vendor is an institution, agency, organization, or individual practitioner that provides health or medical services.
Vendor payments: In welfare programs, direct payments are made by the state to such providers as physicians, pharmacists, and health care institutions rather than to the welfare recipient himself.
Waiver: A rider or clause in a health insurance contract excluding an insurer's liability for some sort of preexisting illness or injury. Also refers to a plan amendment, such as an HCFA waiver or plan modification.
Waivers (Section 1115 or 1915(b)): Section 1115 of the Social Security Act grants the secretary of Health and Human Services broad authority to waive certain laws relating to Medicaid for the purpose of conducting pilot, experimental, or demonstration projects. Section 1115 demonstration waivers allow states to change provisions of their Medicaid programs, including eligibility requirements, the scope of services available, the freedom to choose a provider, a provider's choice to participate in a plan, the method of reimbursing providers, and the statewide application of the program. Projects typically run 3 to 5 years. States cannot change the federal Medicaid assistance percentage through a waiver.

Appendix 9.5 Vendor List

Ablenet, Inc. 1081 Tenth Ave. SE Minneapolis, MN 55414-1312 Telephone: 800-322-0956 Website: www.ablenetinc.com	Assistive Technology, Inc. 7 Wells Ave., Newton, MA 02459 Website: www.assistivetech.com
Adaptivation 55 East Long Lake Rd. Mailstop PMB-337 Troy, MI 48098 Telephone: 248-594-6997 Website: www.adaptivation.com	Enabling Devices/Toys for Special Children 385 Warburton Ave., Hastings-on-Hudson, NY 10706 Telephone: 800-832-8697 Website: www. tobiidynavox.com
Applied Human Factors, Inc. P.O. Box 228 Helotes, TX 78023 Telephone: 888-243-0098 Website: www.ahf-net.com	Enkidu Research, Inc. 247 Pine Hill Rd., Spencerport, NY 14559 Telephone: 518-431-1200

(*Continued*)

Appendix 9.5 (Continued) Vendor List

Hearit, LLC 8346 North Mammoth Dr., Tucson, AZ 85743-1046 Telephone: 800-298-7184 Website: www.hearitllc.com	Toby Churchill, LTD. 20 Panton St., Cambridge, CB2 1HP United Kingdom Telephone: 01954-281-210 Website: www.toby-churchill.com
Madentec, LTD 9935-29A Ave., Edmonton, Alberta T6N 1A9 Canada Telephone: 888-686-4868 Website: www.madentec.com	Tobii Dyanavox Systems, LLC 2100 Wharton, Suite 400, Pittsburgh, PA 15203-1942 Telephone: 800-793-9227 Website: www.tobiidynavox.com
Mayer-Johnson, Inc. P.O. Box 1579 Solana Beach, CA 92075-7579 Telephone: 800-588-4548 Website: www.mayer-johnson.com	Turning Point Therapy & Technology Inc. P.O. Box 310751, New Braunfels, TX 78131-0751 Telephone: 877-608-9812 Website: www.turningpointtechnology.com
Prentke Romich Company 1022 Heyl Rd., Wooster, OH 44691-9744 Telephone: 330-262-1984 Website: www.prentrom.com	Words+, Inc. 1220 West Ave. J, Lancaster, CA 93534-2902 Telephone: 800-869-8521 Website: www.words-plus.com
Tash, Inc. 3512 Mayland Court, Richmond, VA 23233 Telephone: 202-540-9020 Website: www.tash.org	Zygo Industries, Inc P.O. Box 1008, Portland, OR 97207-1008 Telephone: 510-493-0997 Website: www.zygo-usa.com

Appendix 9.6 Selected AAC Websites

Communication Aid Manufacturers
1. AbleNet *www.ablenetinc.com* AbleNet produces a variety of communication aids, switches, and other adaptive devices. It will loan a package of equipment with an accompanying training script for in-service training. The website offers links for the products catalog, AAC news, frequently asked questions, and other AAC-related websites.
2. Adaptivation *www.adaptivation.com* Adaptivation distributes AT to persons with disabilities. Adaptivation products include the Chipper, Voice Pal, and many other related devices and the accessories that go with them. The website includes links for its products catalog, domestic and foreign dealers, upcoming workshops, and other AAC-related websites.

(*Continued*)

Appendix 9.6 (Continued) Selected AAC Websites

3. Adaptive Switch Laboratories, Inc. *www.asl-inc.com* Adaptive Switch Laboratories, Inc. is a company that makes and sells a variety of switches and mounting kits. Its products are compatible with a variety of wheelchairs. Product catalogs and price lists can be found on its website. The ASL website also includes information about educational seminars and leasing programs.
4. AMDi *www.amdi.net* AMDi designs electronic devices for governmental, industrial, and commercial customers. Some of its products include the Tech/Speak, Tech/Talk, and Tech/Four. Its website provides the products catalog and price list.
5. Assistive Technology, Inc. *www.assistivetech.com* Assistive Technology, Inc. is the manufacturer of the Gemini AAC device and universally accessible Macintosh computer, suited to a range of input methods. Assistive Technology also produces LINK, a talking keyboard. The website includes links to its products catalog and upcoming tradeshows and conferences.
6. Communication Devices, Inc. *www.commdevices.com* Communication Devices, Inc. is the manufacturer of the Holly.com line of augmentative communication devices. This website also has links to other AAC websites.
7. Electronic Speech Enhancement, Inc. *www.speachenhancer.com* The entrepreneurs at Electronic Speech Enhancement, Inc. developed a technology called speech enhancement to combat the challenge of making speech clearer, not just louder. The ESE website includes links for its products and its ordering process.
8. Enabling Devices *www.enablingdevices.com* Enabling Devices, a division of Toys for Special Education, Inc., is dedicated to providing affordable learning and assistive devices for the physically challenged. The website for Enabling Devices includes links to its products catalog and an online shopping option. This website also includes links to many other related websites.
9. The Great Talking Box Company *www.synapseadaptive.com* The Great Talking Box Company distributes affordable communication devices such as EasyTalk, DifiCom 2000, and e-talk, along with accessories. The Great Talking Box Company website has other useful information such as trade show and sales information.
10. Gus Communications, Inc. *www.gusinc.com* Some of the products offered by Gus Communication, Inc. include a software package that is compatible with any Windows-based personal computer. The Gus Communications, Inc. website includes links for its products, ordering, and demos of its products that can be downloaded onto any IBM-compatible computer.

(*Continued*)

Appendix 9.6 (Continued) Selected AAC Websites

11. IntelliTools *www.intelllitools.com for classroom software* IntelliTools develops and markets computer products for special education. The company's mission is to help children with educational challenges (physical and cognitive) and optimize their social and academic participation and success. Products by IntelliTools include Creativity Tools, Curriculum Resources, and SwitchIt! software. Along with information about its products, the IntelliTools website also includes links for tutorials and training, technical support, product demos, and links to other AAC-related websites.
12. LC Technologies, Inc. *www.eyegaze.com* LC Technologies, Inc. is a company that manufactures the Eyegaze Communication System, a system that "empowers people to communicate with the world by only the movement of their eyes." Its website includes product brochures and prices. In addition, it also provides papers and presentations by individuals who have used or worked with Eyegaze Communication Systems.
13. Luminaud, Inc. *www.luminaud.com* Luminaud, Inc. is a manufacturer and supplier of a wide range of electronic speech equipment and tracheostomy products. Some of its products include Minivox, Chattervox, and other voice amplification products. Its website includes its products catalog and price lists and links to other AAC-related websites.
14. Madentec *www.madentec.com* Madentec is a company that distributes products such as the computer enhancer Tracker 2000, a head-pointer access system. In addition, it sells a variety of electronic aids for environmental control. The Madentec website also includes frequently asked questions and links that provide games to play using Tracker 2000.
15. Mayer-Johnson, Inc. *www.mayer-johnson.com* Mayer-Johnson, Inc. offers products for special needs and education. Products by Mayer-Johnson, Inc. include Picture Communication Symbols, BoardMaker software Picture Communication Symbols,* and many other AAC-related devices and materials. Its website includes links to other AAC websites and the products catalog, as well as upcoming conferences and tech support for the Mayer-Johnson line of products. *Picture Communication Symbols (PCS) are copyright © 1981–2000, Mayer-Johnson, Inc. All rights reserved.
16. Prentke Romich Company *www.prentrom.com* The Prentke Romich Company (PRC) produces a number of devices that take advantage of Minspeak semantic compaction. This vocabulary system features more than 4,000 vocabulary words available on a single overlay. Prentke Romich Company has a variety of training options, including video conferencing and web-based modules. The PRC website offers links to its products catalog, product representatives, training seminars, and conferences, as well as a link to other AAC-related websites.

(*Continued*)

Appendix 9.6 (Continued) Selected AAC Websites

17. RJ Cooper & Associates *www.rjcooper.com* RJ Cooper & Associates makes products for persons with special needs, including special software and hardware adaptations. RJ Cooper & Associates also sells a variety of switches and related devices, including the Big Baby Switch especially designed for babies. Its website includes a single-switch arcade game that can be downloaded to a computer, as well as links to its TechWeek vacation, lectures, and workshops.
18. Saltillo Corporation *www.saltillo.com* Saltillo Corporation is a company that distributes communication products for nonspeaking individuals. Its products are designed to be easy to use by the communicator and his/her support staff. The Saltillo Corporation website contains details and purchasing information about ChatBox and its accessories, among other AAC devices. The website also contains helpful technical support, distributor locations, and its rental policies.
19. Slater Software, Inc. *www.slatersoftware.com* Slater Software, Inc. is the producer of the Picture It, Pixreader, and Pixwriter software packages that teach literacy skills to children with special needs. Its website includes descriptions of products along with Adaptive Plays and Interactive Books. It also includes a link to the products catalog.
20. Synergy *www.speakwithus.com* Synergy is a company that makes AAC/computer systems and a wide range of software and adaptive inputs. Synergy offers an AAC/functional computer system for both Macintosh and IBM-compatible computers. Its website includes links for funding assistance, frequently asked questions, and upcoming workshops and lectures.
21. Tash, Inc. *www.tash.org* Tash, Inc. is the manufacturer of a variety of switches, adaptive devices, and mounting devices. Its website offers online shopping and the option of requesting a catalog.
22. Words+, Inc. *www.words-plus.com* Words+, Inc. is a company dedicated to improving the quality of life for people with disabilities. Its products include computer software, the Freedom 2000, and the Message Mate line of products. The Words+, Inc. website includes links for its products catalog, upcoming workshops, and links to other AAC-related websites.
23. ZYGO Industries, Inc. *www.zygo-usa.com* ZYGO Industries, Inc. is the manufacturer of the Macaw family of digitized AAC systems. ZYGO Industries, Inc. also manufactures a variety of other AT devices. It has a CD-ROM and videotape that contains samples of its products. Its website includes links to its products catalog and a link to information about funding for AT.

(*Continued*)

Appendix 9.6 (Continued) Selected AAC Websites

AAC Associations
24. American Speech-Language-Hearing Association (ASHA) *www.asha.org* Home page for Special Interest Division 12 (AAC). Available once you register at the ASHA website: www.asha.org/speech/disabilities/disabilities.cfm. This page is user-friendly and available to the public. It is a good reference for those beginning to learn about AAC. This page provides general information about AAC, including information about putting together an AAC team and selecting a device.
25. International Society for Augmentative and Alternative Communication (ISAAC) *www.isaac-online.org* ISAAC is an international organization devoted to advancing augmentative and alternative communication (AAC). The mission of ISAAC is to improve communication and the quality of life for people with severe communication impairments. ISAAC does this by facilitating information exchange and focusing attention on work in the field. The ISAAC website provides links to AAC resources, publications, events, and conferences.
26. U.S. Society for Augmentative and Alternative Communication (USSAAC) *www.ussaac.org* USSAAC is a national chapter of ISAAC devoted to advancing augmentative and alternative communication (AAC) in the United States. The mission is to improve communication and the quality of life for people with severe communication impairments by facilitating information exchange through its conferences and a quarterly newsletter titled *Speak UP!*
Education Sites
27. The AAC-RERC (Augmentative and Alternative Communication—Rehabilitation Engineering Research Center on Communication Enhancement) *www.aac-rerc.psu.edu* The AAC-RERC is dedicated to assisting individuals who use AAC by advancing and promoting AAC technologies and supporting individuals that use, manufacture, and recommend them. The AAC-RERC is funded by the National Institute on Disability and Rehabilitation Research (NIDRR, Grant H133E980026). The website includes current information on Medicare funding policies, research on improving AAC technologies for young children, and links to vendor websites and university AAC sites.
28. AAC at Penn State *www.aac-rerc.psu.edu* The website describes current research in AAC, including some on improving AAC technology for young children. It also describes research programs directed toward improving clinical practice and enhancing outcomes for individuals who use AAC. Penn State is also a partner in the AAC-RERC (Augmentative and Alternative Communication—Rehabilitation Engineering Research Center on Communication Enhancement; see #27).
29. California State University–Northridge CSUN (2018) Scholarworks.csun.edu/handle/10211.3/202980 The *Journal on Technology & Persons with Disabilities* published by the CSUN Center on Disabilities gathers the best papers from the Annual International Technology and Persons with Disabilities Conferences, otherwise referred to as the CSUN conferences.

(*Continued*)

Appendix 9.6 (Continued) Selected AAC Websites

30. Closing the Gap *www.closingthegap.com* This website includes product information on new hardware and software and current issues involving AT and AAC. It also has links to newsletter articles and how to subscribe to the bimonthly newsletter.
31. Communication Aids for Language and Learning (CALL) Centre, University of Edinburgh *http://callcentre.education.ed.ac.uk* The CALL Centre is a Scottish National Resource and Research Centre located within the University of Edinburgh's Department of Equity Studies and Special Education, in the Faculty of Education.
32. Trace Research and Development Center *www.trace.umd.edu* This website provides information on all types of AT, including AAC. The comprehensive nature of the site provides students with the broad perspective they will need to work effectively with clients who require technology beyond a communication device. The front page is organized into four headings: New and Highlighted Items, Designing a More Useable World, Cooperative Electronic Library (Co-Net), and Publications and Media Catalog. The last two sections relate to AAC most directly. Co-Net includes information on products, people, and services; publications and media; and also text documents. For the most up-to-date product information, the website directs the user to the ABLEDATA website (see #35).
33. The University of Nebraska–Lincoln AAC website *www.cehs.unl.edu/aac* The University of Nebraska–Lincoln (UNL) AAC website contains academic and clinical training information, as well as vendor information for people working with AAC. It also provides a variety of links to AAC and other speech-language pathology sites.
Other AAC Resources
34. AAC Intervention.com *www.aacintervention.com* AAC Intervention.com is a website that sells products to aid in making overlays for early intervention with AAC. It also provides helpful information on how to begin using AAC with a nonspeaking child. This website has some unique features such as local and national presentation/conference dates and tips of the month.
35. ABLEDATA *www.abledata.com* ABLEDATA is a federally funded project whose primary mission is to provide information on AT and rehabilitation equipment available from domestic and international sources to consumers, organizations, professionals, and caregivers within the United States. Its website includes links for resource centers, product information, and other AAC-related websites.
36. Augmentative Communication, Inc. *www.augcominc.com* Augmentative Communication, Inc. publishes *Alternatively Speaking* (*AS*) and *Augmentative Communication News* (*CAN*), newsletters that together provide the latest information on hot topics in the field, discussion of vital issues for AAC stakeholders, and news from the AAC community. The Augmentative Communication, Inc. website also provides links for presentations, articles in the publications, and other AAC-related websites.

(*Continued*)

Appendix 9.6 (Continued) Selected AAC Websites

Additional Resources
Additional resources can be obtained by • Checking references and appendices in the four original texts cited and the other publications cited (e.g., the Lloyd et al. text has extensive appendices on developers, manufacturers, vendors, and associations as of 1997). • Checking websites with the typical cautions used when one browses websites. • Subscribing to the ASHA SID 12 newsletter in particular and specific volumes, including *Augmentative and Alternative Communication Newsletter*, June 2001, Vol. 10, No. 2, pp. 32–33 (an issue devoted to a bibliography of AAC books, chapters, and journals). • Subscribing to ISAAC's official journal—*Augmentative and Alternative Communication.* The previous information is reprinted with permission from the American Speech-Language-Hearing Association and Special Interest Division 12, Augmentative and Alternative Communication.
Additional Links to Other AAC-Related Sites
AAC-RERC *www.aac-rerc.psu.edu* AAC-RERC is the Rehabilitation Engineering Research Center on Communication Enhancement. This is one of a network of RERCs funded by the National Institute on Disability and Rehabilitation Research (NIDRR) of the U.S. Department of Education.
ABLEDATA *www.abledata.com* ABLEDATA is a federally funded project whose primary mission is to provide information on AT and rehabilitation equipment available from domestic and international sources to consumers, organizations, professionals, and caregivers within the United States.
ACOLUG *www.temple.edu* ACOLUG is a listserv created to exchange ideas, information, and experiences on augmentative communication by people from all over the world. By using e-mail, people who use augmentative communication and their friends and families discuss issues related to augmentative communication, such as equipment, funding, learning techniques, and supports. Anyone can join, and there is no cost.
Apraxia-Kids *www.apraxiakids.org* The Apraxia-Kids Internet Resources provides comprehensive information regarding Childhood Apraxia of Speech. The site, which is appropriate for both families and professionals, includes expert articles on diagnosis, treatment, AAC, related disabilities, an e-mail discussion list, a monthly online newsletter, message boards, and resource listings. Additionally, there is a research section with the latest news on apraxia research.

(*Continued*)

Appendix 9.6 (Continued) Selected AAC Websites

ASHA *www.asha.org* ASHA is the American Speech-Language-Hearing Association. ASHA is the professional organization of SLPs and audiologists. SLPs are the primary service providers for people who rely on AAC and are generally the best resource on an AAC team for addressing language issues. ASHA has a special interest division, SID-12, that addresses AAC.
ATIA *www.atia.org* ATIA is the Assistive Technology Industry Association. ATIA organizes an annual conference on AT.
Augmentative Communication, Inc. *www.augcominc.com* *Augmentative Communication News* and *Alternatively Speaking* provide the latest information on hot topics in the field, discussion of vital issues for AAC stakeholders, and news from the AAC community.
C.H.E.R.A.B. *www.cherabfoundation.org* The Communication Help, Education, Research, Apraxia Base Foundation websites are for anyone who cares for a child that has delayed speech, a speech disorder, is a late talker, etc., as well as for those who care for a child that has received a diagnosis of apraxia.
Childhood Apraxia of Speech Association of North America (CASANA) *www.apraxia-kids.org* The Childhood Apraxia of Speech Association is a not-for-profit organization whose mission is to strengthen the support systems in the lives of children with apraxia so that each child is afforded his best opportunity to develop speech.
CSUN *www.csun.edu/cod* California State University–Northridge (CSUN) Center on Disabilities organizes the annual Conference on Technology and Persons with Disabilities. CSUN also offers the Assistive Technology Applications Certificate Program.
CTG *http://closingthegap.com* Closing the Gap organized an annual conference on computer technology for people with disabilities and publishes a newsletter.
ISAAC *www.isaac-online.org* ISAAC is the International Society for Augmentative and Alternative Communication. Membership is open to anyone interested in AAC. ISAAC activities include a biennial conference and sponsorship of *AAC Journal*. Many ISAAC national chapters address more local interests.

(*Continued*)

Appendix 9.6 (Continued) Selected AAC Websites

PEC *www.soutaac.org* The Pittsburgh Employment Conference for Augmented Communicators is the largest gathering in the world of people who rely on AAC. Topics of interest to employment-age individuals are addressed at the annual conference.
RESNA *www.resna.org* RESNA (Rehabilitation and Assistive Technology Society of North America) is an interdisciplinary association of people with a common interest in technology and disability. Its purpose is to improve the potential of people with disabilities to achieve their goals through the use of technology. It serves that purpose by promoting research, development, education, advocacy, and the provision of technology and by supporting the people engaged in these activities. RESNA was founded in 1979 as a not-for-profit organization. There are currently over 1600 individual and 150 organizational members.
USSAAC *www.ussaac.org* USSAAC (U.S. Society for Augmentative and Alternative Communication) is the U.S. chapter of ISAAC.
WheelchairNet *www.wheelchairnet.org* WheelchairNet is a community for people who have a common interest in (or in some cases a passion for) wheelchair technology and its improvement and successful application. WheelchairNet is a virtual community—a community that exists only in cyberspace. WheelchairNet is operated by the RERC on Wheeled Mobility at the University of Pittsburgh.

Appendix 9.7 Toll-Free Phone Numbers and Hotlines

AMC Cancer Information Line 800-525-3777
American Association on Mental Retardation 800-424-3688
American Council of the Blind 800-424-8666
American Diabetes Association, Inc. 800-342-2383
American Foundation for the Blind 800-232-3044

(*Continued*)

Appendix 9.7 (Continued) Toll-Free Phone Numbers and Hotlines

American Liver Foundation 800-465-4837
American Paralysis Association 800-225-0292
American Parkinson Disease Association 800-223-2732
American Speech-Language-Hearing Association 800-638-8255
American Spinal Cord Injury 804-565-6396
American Trauma Society 800-556-7890
Arthritis Foundation 800-283-7800
Arc of the United States 800-433-5255
AT&T National Special Needs Center 800-772-3140
Beginnings 800-541-4327
Better Hearing Institute Hearing Helpline 800-EAR-WELL
Blind Children's Center 323-664-2153
BOSMA Enterprises 866-602-6762
The Candlelighters Childhood Cancer Foundation 702-737-1919
Captioned Films for the Deaf 800-237-6213
Center for Special Education Technology c/o Council for Exceptional Children 888-232-7733
Consumer Product Safety Commission 800-638-2772
Cornelia deLange Syndrome Foundation 800-753-2357

(*Continued*)

Appendix 9.7 (Continued) Toll-Free Phone Numbers and Hotlines

Dial a Hearing Screening Test 800-222-3277
Disabilities AT&T, National Special Needs Center 800-233-1222 800-833-3232
Dyslexia Society, Orton 800-222-3123
Easter Seal Society 800-221-6827
Educators Publishing Service, Inc. Specific Language Disabilities (Dyslexia) 800-225-5750
Epilepsy Foundation of America 800-332-1000
ERIC Clearinghouse on Adult Career and Vocational Education 800-538-3742
Family Support Network 714-447-3301
Federal Hill-Burton Free Care Program 888-275-4772
Federal Internal Revenue Service 800-829-1040
Financial Aid for Education Available from the Federal Government 800-333-INFO
Georgia Assistive Technology Project (Atlanta) 800-497-8665 (Warm Springs) 800-578-8665
Georgia Relay Center 800-255-0135 (Voice to TT) 800-255-0056 (TT to Voice)
Guide Dog Foundation for the Blind 800-548-4337
Handicapped Travel Divisions, National Tour Assoc. 800-682-8886
Brain Injury Association of America 800-444-6443
Health Resource Center 877-222-VETS

(Continued)

Appendix 9.7 (Continued) Toll-Free Phone Numbers and Hotlines

Hearing Helpline 800-521-5247
Hearing Information Center, Senior Hearing Aids 800-622-3277
Higher Education and Adult Training of People with Handicaps (HEATH Resource Center) 800-54-HEATH
Huntington's Disease Society of America 800-345-4372
IBM National Center for Person with Disabilities 800-426-2133
International Shriners Headquarters 800-237-5055
Job Accommodations Network (JAN) 800-526-7234
John Tracy Clinic on Deafness 213-748-5481
Juvenile Diabetes Foundation Hotline 213-748-5481
Kidney Foundation, National 800-622-9010
Kidney Fund, National 800-638-8299
The Lighthouse National Center for Vision and Aging 855-653-2273
Lupus Foundation of America 202-349-1155
Medicare, Hotline 800-633-4227
Medigap, U.S. Department of Health and Human Services 877-696-6775
Muscular Dystrophy Association 800-572-1717
Muscular Sclerosis, Georgia Regional Office 800-344-4867
National AIDS Hotline 800-232-4636

(*Continued*)

Appendix 9.7 (Continued) Toll-Free Phone Numbers and Hotlines

National Alliance for the Mentally Ill (NAMI) 800-950-NAMI
National Association for Parents of the Visually Impaired 800-562-6265
National Association for Rehabilitation Facilities 888-427-7722
National Association for Sickle Cell Disease, Inc. 800-421-8453
National Cancer Institute Information Service 800-4-CANCER
National Center for Sight 702-20HAPPY
National Committee for Citizens in Education 800-NETWORK
National Council on Aging 571-527-3900
National Cystic Fibrosis Foundation 800-344-4823
National Down Syndrome Congress 800-232-6372
National Down Syndrome Society 800-221-4602
National Eye Care Project Helpline 800-222-EYES
National Headache Foundation 888-NHF-5552
National Hearing Aid Society Hearing Aid Hotline 800-521-5247
National Information Center for Children and Youth with Disabilities (NICHCY) 800-695-0285
National Information Clearinghouse for Infants with Disabilities and Life-Threatening Conditions 800-922-9234, ext. 201
National Information System Vietnam Vets/Children 888-820-1756

(*Continued*)

Appendix 9.7 (Continued) Toll-Free Phone Numbers and Hotlines

National Insurance Consumer Hotline 800-200-7710
National Library Service for Blind & Physically Handicapped 800-424-8567
National Multiple Sclerosis Society 800-344-4867
National Organization for Rare Disorders (NORD) 800-999-6673
National Organization on Disability 646-505-1191
National Parkinson Foundation 800-4PD-INFO
National Rehabilitation Information Center (NARIC) 800-346-2742
National Retinitis Pigmentosa Foundation 800-683-5555
National Reye's Syndrome Foundation 800-233-7393
National Sexually Transmitted Diseases Hotline 800-232-4636
National Spinal Cord Injury Association 800-962-9629
National Stroke Association 800-787-6537
National Tuberous Sclerosis Association 800-225-6872
North American Riding for the Handicapped Assoc., Inc. 800-369-7433
Occupational Hearing Service 800-222-EARS
Orton Dyslexia Society 800-222-3123
Parkinson's Disease Foundation, Inc. 800-457-6676
Practitioner's Reporting System 800-767-6732

(*Continued*)

Appendix 9.7 (Continued) Toll-Free Phone Numbers and Hotlines

Rural Health Information Hub 800-270-1898/888-268-2743
Tele-Consumer Hotline 800-323-1124
TRIPOD GRAPEVINE, Service for Hearing Impaired 800-352-8888
United Cerebral Palsy Association 800-872-5827
U.S. Department of Veteran Affairs www.va.gov
INFORMATION ON 1-800 NUMBERS 800-555-1212

Appendix 9.8 Internet Resources

Adaptive Solutions Assistive Technology Tracker www.adaptive-sol.com
Alexander Graham Bell Association for the Deaf www.agbell.org
Alliance for Technology Access www.ataccess.org
ALS Association www.alsa.org
American Association on Intellectual and Developmental Disabilities https://aaidd.org/
American Foundation for the Blind, Technology Center www.afb.org
American Medical Association www.ama-assn.org
American Physical Therapy Association www.apta.org
American Speech-Language-Hearing Association www.asha.org

(*Continued*)

Appendix 9.8 (Continued) Internet Resources

Assistive Technology, Inc. www.assistive-tech.com
Assistive Technology Tracker www.adaptive-sol.com
Audible, Inc. www.audible.com
Augmentative Communication On-Line User Group (ACOLUG) (must join, members only) Go to https://listserv.temple.edu/cgi-bin/wa?A0=ACOLUG and click on the third link "join or leave the list" and then follow the instructions provided.
Brain Actuated Technologies, Inc. www.brainfingers.com
California Relay Service 800-735-2929 http://ddtp.cpuc.ca.gov/default1.aspx?id=1482
California State University–Northridge, Center on Disabilities www.csun.edu/cod/
Center for International Rehabilitation Research Information and Exchange (CIRRIE) http://cirrie.buffalo.edu
Centers for Disease Control and Prevention www.cdc.gov
Council for Exceptional Children www.cec.sped.org
Council for Licensure Enforcement and Regulation (CLEAR) www.clearhq.org
Cyberlink Interface www.brainfingers.com
Department of Veterans Affairs www.va.gov
Design to Learn www.designtolearn.com
Doug Dodgen and Associates AAC Feature Match Software www.dougdodgen.com
Dragon Dictate Systems www.dragonsys.com
Eisenhower National Clearinghouse for Math and Science Education ww.Goenc.org

(Continued)

Appendix 9.8 (Continued) Internet Resources

Equal Access to Software and Information (EASI) www.easi.cc/
Food and Drug Administration www.fda.gov
Guillain-Barre Fact Sheet https://www.ninds.nih.gov/Disorders/Patient-Caregiver-Education/Fact-Sheets/ Guillain-Barr%C3%A9-Syndrome-Fact-Sheet
Harris Communications 15159 Technology Dr. Eden Prairie, MN 55344-2277 https://www.harriscomm.com/
Health Care Financing Administration www.hcfa.gov
HMS School for Children with Cerebral Palsy Philadelphia, PA www.hmsschool.org
Human Factors and Ergonomics Society (HFES) HFES is one of the major professional organizations for practitioners and researchers in ergonomics and human factors. http://hfes.org
Institute of Medicine www.nas.edu/iom
International Society for Augmentative and Alternative Communication (ISAAC) www.isaac-online.org
Internet Disability Resources Mary Barros-Baily and Dawn Boyd Ahab Press, Inc. 2 Gannett Dr., Suite 200 White Plains, NY 10604-3404 E-mail: AHAB4@aol.com http://www.icdri.org/
ISAAC www.isaac-online.org
Krown Manufacturing, Inc. www.krownmfg.com
Kurzweil Applied Intelligence www.kurzweiltech.com/kai.html
LifeSpan Access Profile Don Johnston Company www.donjohnston.com

(*Continued*)

Appendix 9.8 (Continued) Internet Resources

Madentec www.madentec.com
Muscular Dystrophy Association (MDA) www.mda.org
National Easter Seal Society www.easterseals.org
National Federation of the Blind (NFB) www.nfb.org
National Institutes of Health www.nih.gov
National Organization for Competency Assurance (NOCA) www.noca.org
National Organization on Disability www.nod.org
United Spinal Association www.spinalcord.org
National Technical Institute for the Deaf www.ntid.rit.edu
Oklahoma Able Tech www.okstate.edu/wellness/at-home.htm
Pittsburgh Employment Conference (PEC) SHOUT@agi.net
Prentke Romich Company (PRC) www.prentrom.com
Quality Indicators for Assistive Technology Services www.giat.org
Rehabilitation Engineering and Assistive Technology Society of North America (RESNA) RESNA is an interdisciplinary association of people with a common interest in technology and disability. This association promotes research, development, education, advocacy, and the provision of technology. www.resna.org
Social Security Disability Administration Disability Information www.ssa.gov
Speech to Speech www.speechtospeech.org
Texas Commission for the Blind www.dars.state.tx.us

(*Continued*)

Appendix 9.8 (Continued) Internet Resources

The Arc (of the United States) www.thearc.org
Trace Research and Development Center www.trace.umd.edu/
Turning Point Technologies 877-608-9812 http://www.talkingmyway.com/contact.asp
United Cerebral Palsy, Funding for Assistive Technology www.ucp.org/resources/assistive-technology
United Way of America home page www.unitedway.org
University of Nebraska–Lincoln AAC Vendors Information http://aac.unl.edu/
University of Washington Speech and Hearing Sciences Department UW AugComm https://depts.washington.edu/sphsc This site has been established as part of the UW Tele-Collaboration Project to provide information and resources for professionals and community members with an interest in AAC.
Greater Detroit Agency for the Blind and Visually Impaired Technology Information and Resources Services www.gdabvi.org
U.S. government site for Medicare information www.medicare.gov
USSAAC (U.S. Chapter of ISAAC) USAAC@aol.com https://www.ussaac.org/
Wisconsin Assistive Technology Initiative http://aac-rerc.com http://wati.org
World Health Organization www.who.ch
Wynd Communications www.Purplevrs.com
YAACK (Augmentative Communication Connecting Young Kids http://cehs.unl.edu/aac/connecting-young-kids-yaack/

Appendix 9.9 Online Assistive Technology Resources

Ability Hub
AbilityHub.com's purpose is to help users find information on adaptive equipment and alternative methods available for accessing computers. Ability Hub's founder is Dan Gilman, a certified ATP (assistive technology practitioner) with RESNA.
ABLEDATA
A national database of information on more than 17,000 products that are currently available for people with disabilities.
Access Board
An independent federal agency. Contains information on Section 508 of the Rehabilitation Act, as amended requiring that electronic and information technology developed, procured, maintained, or used by the federal government be accessible to people with disabilities. In 1998, the board established an Electronic and Information Technology Access Advisory Committee (EITAAC) to help the board develop standards under Section 508.
Accessible Website Design Resources
Connects to a Government Services Administration (GSA) site with links to several organizations with "how-tos" on designing websites for accessibility for people with disabilities, including a link to "Top Ten Mistakes in Web Design."
Alliance for Technology Access
Provides location information for the Alliance for Technology Access regional centers. The Alliance assists individuals with disabilities in accessing technology, mainly through computer resources.
Apple's Disability Solutions
Information on computer access solutions for individuals with disabilities.
Assistive Technology Funding and Systems Change Project (ATFSCP)
AT funding and systems change information.
AT Quick Reference Series
This TechConnections resource provides quick reference guides for work-related accommodations, such as Voice Input Systems, accessible calculators, mouse alternatives, one-handed keyboards, and other assistive technologies.
AZtech, Inc.
Information on transforming inventions into products for individuals with disabilities.
Breaking New Ground Resource Center
Provides information and resources on AT for agricultural workers and agricultural worksites. In 1990, the Outreach Center of Breaking New Ground became a part of the USDA AgrAbility program.

(*Continued*)

Appendix 9.9 (Continued) Online Assistive Technology Resources

Center for Information Technology Accommodation (CITA)
Legislation and policies on information systems accessibility, including the Assistive Technology Act of 1998.
Closing the Gap
Closing the Gap's role is to provide information on microcomputer materials and practices that can help enrich the lives of persons with special needs.
Consortium for Citizens with Disabilities (CCD)
CCD is a working coalition of more than 100 national consumer, advocacy, provider, and professional organizations working together with and on behalf of the 54 million children and adults with disabilities and their families living in the United States. The CCD has several task forces on various disability issues, such as employment and training, developmental disabilities, health, Social Security, long-term services and supports, telecommunications and technology, rights, etc.
Cornucopia of Disability Information (CODI)
A wealth of information relating to disabilities, including topics such as aging, statistics, computing, centers for independent living, and universal design. This site is based at the State University of New York–Buffalo.
CPB/WGBH National Center for Accessible Media
"Making Educational Software Accessible: Design Guidelines, Including Math and Science Solutions." These guidelines represent an ambitious initiative to capture access challenges and solutions and present them in a format specifically designed to educate and assist educational software developers. The detailed guidelines and solutions specific to math and science are unique to this document. This work is the result of a 3-year project funded by the National Science Foundation's Program for Persons with Disabilities. The CPB/WGBH National Center for Accessible Media developed this document with input from a distinguished board of advisors with expertise in accessible design, AT, and the education of students with disabilities.
DISABILITY Resources on the Internet
This site was created and is maintained by Jim Lubin, a person with quadriplegia.
Do-It Internet Resources
Resources are listed in many categories, including general resources, education, technology, legal, social, and political issues.
EPVA Assistive Technology
The Eastern Paralyzed Veterans Association (EPVA) launched a website for AT in 2002. Available at this site are product reviews on wheelchairs and cushions and a tech guide on driving aids, transfer devices, and exercise equipment.
Equal Access to Software and Information (EASI)
EASI is part of the Teaching, Learning, and Technology Group, an affiliate of the American Association of Higher Education. EASI's mission is to promote the same access to information and resources for people with disabilities as everyone else.

(*Continued*)

Appendix 9.9 (Continued) Online Assistive Technology Resources

Federal Communications Commission (FCC)
Contains the Telecommunications Act of 1996 and links to FCC's Disabilities Issues Task Force that contain press releases and reports that affect telecommunications and technology issues for people with disabilities.
IBM Special Needs Solutions
Information on IBM computer access solutions for persons with disabilities.
International Center for Disability Resources on the Internet
The center will collect and present best practices in areas related to disability and accessibility issues. The center will collect disability-related Internet resources, including resources that may be helpful to the disability community.
Job Accommodation Network (JAN)
A service of the U.S. Department of Labor's President's Committee on Employment of People with Disabilities, JAN provides information about job accommodation and the employability of people with functional limitations. Publishes quarterly reports on the number of cases handled by information and ADA-related concerns, among many other outcome data statistics.
Learning Disabilities OnLine
Interactive guide to learning disabilities for parents, teachers, and children.
National Clearing House of Rehabilitation Training Materials (NCHRTM)
Download AT-related documents from this site. Sample titles include "Assistive Technology: Practical Intervention Strategies"; "ADA: Train the Trainer Program"; and "Reasonable Accommodations in the Workplace."
National Rehabilitation Information Center (NARIC)
NARIC is a library and information center on disability and rehabilitation. More than 50,000 National Institute on Disability and Rehabilitation Research (NIDRR)-funded, other federal agency, and private disability-related publications are held and abstracted by NARIC in its REHABDATA database, searchable online.
National Institute on Disability and Rehabilitation Research (NIDRR)
NIDRR, part of the U.S. Department of Education, manages and funds more than 300 projects on disability and rehabilitation research, including 56 state and U.S. territory AT projects and several Rehabilitation Engineering Research Centers.
On a Roll—Talk Radio
Talk Radio focusing on life and disability news, updated daily. While at the site, check out the RealAudio archives of this award-winning radio talk show.
One-Hand Typing
Information on free downloads, how-to manuals, therapists, and more.

(Continued)

Appendix 9.9 (Continued) Online Assistive Technology Resources

TeamRehab Report
A monthly magazine for professionals in rehabilitation technology and services.
Trace Research & Development Center
The Trace Center conducts research aimed at improving technology that can benefit individuals with disabilities by making it more accessible in four main areas: communication, control, computer access, and next-generation communication information and transaction systems.
West Virginia Rehabilitation Research and Training Center (WVRRTC)
Information resources on vocational rehabilitation, including links to the Job Accommodation Network and Project Enable.
WheelchairNet
WheelchairNet is a continuously developing resource for a broad community of people who are interested in wheelchairs: consumers, clinicians, manufacturers, researchers, funders. It contains resources for lifestyle, wheelchair technology and research developments, discussions, products, industry product standards, funding, services, etc.
World Wide Web Consortium (W3C)
The W3C, an international industry consortium, was founded in October 1994 to lead the World Wide Web to its full potential by developing common protocols that promote its evolution and ensure its operability. The W3C also includes the World Accessibility Initiative, which provides guidelines on website accessibility.

Appendix 9.10 International Sites

AAATE
www.fernuni-hagden.de/FTB/AAATE.html
ARATA
www.iinet.net.au/~sharano/arata
International Center for Disability Resources on the Internet
The center will collect and present best practices in areas related to disability and accessibility issues. The center will collect disability-related Internet resources, including resources that may be helpful to the disability community.
Untangling the Web: Where Do I Go for Disability Information?
Lists websites in many categories, including general information resources, disability legislation, employment resources, and more.
Yuri Rubinsky Insight Foundation: webABLE!
Contains an accessibility database that provides links to an extensive list of Internet resources related to disability and accessibility. Resources include mailing lists, websites, and newsgroups.

Appendix 9.11 Periodicals and Newsletters

ABLEDATA, 8455 Colesville Rd., Suite 935, Silver Springs, MD 20910; Telephone: 800-227-0216.
Alternatively Speaking, Augmentative Communication, Inc., 1 Surf Way, Suite 237, Monterey, CA 93940.
Augmentative Communication News, Augmentative Communication, Inc., 1 Surf Way, Suite 237, Monterey, CA 93940; newsletter.
The Bumpy Gazette, Repro-Tronics, Inc., 75 Carver Ave., Westwood, NJ 07675; Telephone: 800-948-8453; Website: www.reprotronics.com
Closing the Gap Resource Directory, P.O. Box 68, Henderson, MN 56044; Telephone: 612-248-3294.
Conn SENSE Bulletin, Special Education Center, Technology Lab, The University of Connecticut, U-64, Room 227, 249 Glenbrook Rd., Storrs, CT 06269-2064; Telephone: 203-486-0172.
The ISAAC Bulletin, 49 The Donway West, Suite 308, Toronto, ON M3C 3M9, Canada; Telephone: 905-850-6848; Website: www.isaac-online.org.
REACH/Rehabilitation Engineering Associates, Telephone: 800-485-5040; newsletter.
SpeakUp!, c/o Beatrice Bruno, P.O. Box 21418, Sarasota, FL 34276; www.ussaac.org
Spotlight on AAC, Prentke Romich Company, Inc., 1022 Heyl Rd., Wooster, OH 44691; Telephone: 800-262-1984, ext. 440.
Technology Resource Directory, Susan Mack, Exceptional Parent, 1170 Commonwealth Ave., 3rd Floor, Boston, MA 02134-9942.
Voices, Hear Our Voices, Newsletter Department, 1660 L St. NW, Suite 700, Washington, DC 20036; Telephone: 205-930-9025.
WorkTech, Seaside Education Associates, Inc., P.O. Box 6341, Lincoln Center, MA 01773; newsletter.

Appendix 9.12 Model Superbill for Speech-Language Pathology

The following is a model of a superbill that could be used by a speech-language pathology practice when billing private health plans. This sample is not meant to dictate which services should or should not be listed on the bill. Most billable codes are from the American Medical Association (AMA) Current Procedural Terminology (CPT), © 2016. Prosthetic and durable medical equipment codes, such as Speech Generating Device codes, are published by the Centers for Medicaid and Medicare (CMS) as Healthcare Common Procedure Codes.

The superbill is a standard form that health plans use to process claims. For the professional rendering services, it provides a time-efficient means to document services, fees, codes, and other information required by insurance companies (i.e., certification and licensure). The patient uses this form to file for health plan payment.

Note: *This is only a model; therefore, some procedures, codes, or other pertinent information may not be found on the following model. For a complete list of CPT and ICD-10 code, the ASHA Health Plan Coding & Claims Guide is available through ASHA's Billing & Reimbursement website or by calling ASHA's Product Sales at 1-888-498-6699.*

Appendix 9.12 (Continued) Model Superbill for Speech-Language Pathology

Model Speech-Language Pathology Superbill

PATIENT: INSURED:
REFERRING PHYSICIAN: ADDRESS:
FILE: ____________ INSURANCE PLAN #: ____________
DATE: ____________ INSURANCE PLAN #: ____________
DATE INITIAL SYMPTOM:________ DATE FIRST CONSULTATION: ____________
PLACE OF SERVICE:________HOME:________OFFICE________OTHER ________

DIAGNOSIS:

Primary (Speech-language pathology)____________ ICD-9 code ____________
Secondary (Medical)____________ ICD-9 code ____________

SERVICES:

CPT	**Procedure**	**Charge**
Swallowing Function		
92526	Treatment of swallowing dysfunction and/or oral function for feeding	______
92610	Evaluation of swallowing function	______
92611	Motion fluoroscopic evaluation of swallowing function	______
92612	Flexible fiber-optic endoscopic evaluation of swallowing;	______
92613	with physician interpretation and report	______
92614	Flexible fiber-optic endoscopic evaluation laryngeal sensory testing by line or video recording;	______
92615	with physician interpretation and report	______
92616	Flexible fiber-optic endoscopic evaluation of swallowing and laryngeal sensory testing;	______
92617	with physician interpretation and report	______
Speech and Language		
92507	Treatment of speech, language, voice, communication, and/or auditory processing disorder, individual	______
92508	Group, two or more individuals	______
97532	Development of cognitive skills to improve attention, memory, problem solving, direct one-on-one patient contact by the provider; each 15 minutes	______
97533	Sensory integrative techniques to enhance sensory processing and promote adaptive responses to environmental demands; each 15 minutes	______
92511	Nasopharyngoscopy w/endoscope	______

(*Continued*)

Appendix 9.12 (Continued) Model Superbill for Speech-Language Pathology

92520	Laryngeal function studies	______
92521	Evaluation of speech fluency (e.g., stuttering, cluttering)	______
92522	Evaluation of speech sound production (e.g., articulation, phonological process, apraxia, dysarthria)	______
92523	Evaluation of speech sound production (e.g., articulation, phonological processes, apraxia, dysarthria) with evaluation of language comprehension and expression. (e.g., receptive and expressive language).	______
92524	Behavioral and qualitative analysis of voice and resonance	______
92626	Evaluation of auditory rehabilitation status, first hour	
92627	each additional 15 minutes	
92630	Auditory rehabilitation; prelingual hearing loss	
92633	Auditory rehabilitation; postlingual hearing loss	______
96105	Assessment of aphasia with interpretation and report, per hour	______
96110	Developmental testing; limited, w/interpretation and report	______
96111	Extended, with interpretation and report, per hour	
96125	Standardized cognitive performance testing (e.g., Ross Information Processing Assessment) per hour of a qualified health care professional's time, both face-to-face time administering tests to the patient and time interpreting these test results and preparing the report	______
31575	Laryngoscopy; flexible fiber-optic; diagnostic	
31579	Laryngoscopy; flexible or rigid fiber-optic, with stroboscopy	
Augmentative and Alternative Communication		
92597	Evaluation for use/fitting of voice prosthetic device to supplement oral speech	______
92605	Evaluation for prescription of non-speech-generating augmentative and alternative communication device, first hour	______
92618	Each additional 30 minutes	______
92606	Therapeutic service(s) for the use of non-speech-generating augmentative and alternative communication device, including programming and modification	______
92607	Evaluation for prescription for speech-generating augmentative and alternative communication device; face-to-face with the patient; evaluation, first hour	______

(Continued)

Appendix 9.12 (Continued) Model Superbill for Speech-Language Pathology

92608	Evaluation for speech device; each additional 30 minutes	
92609	Therapeutic services for the use of Speech Generating Device, including programming and modification	______
V5336	Repair/modification of AAC device (excluding adaptive hearing aid)	______
Other Procedures		
92700	Unlisted otorhinolaryngological service or procedure	
98966	Telephone assessment and management service provided by a qualified nonphysician health care professional to an established patient, parent, or guardian not originating from a related assessment and management service provided within the previous 7 days nor leading to an assessment and management service provided within the next 24 hours or soonest available appointment. 5–10 minutes of medical discussion	
98967	11–20 minutes of medical discussion	
98968	21–30 minutes of medical discussion	
98969	Online assessment and management service provided by a qualified nonphysician health care professional to an established patient, guardian, or health care provider not originating from a related assessment and management service provided within the previous 7 days, using the Internet or similar electronic communication network.	
99366	Medical team conference with interdisciplinary team of health care professionals, face-to-face with patient and/or family, 30 minutes or more; participation by nonphysician qualified health care professional.	
99368	Medical team conference with interdisciplinary team of health care professionals, patient and/or family not present, 30 minutes or more; participation by nonphysician qualified health care professional.	
	TOTAL CHARGES	______
I HEREBY AUTHORIZE DIRECT PAYMENT OF BENEFITS TO SPEECH SERVICES, INC. *SIGNATURE:* ____________________		
I HEREBY AUTHORIZE IRENE SMITH, M.A.-CCC-SLP TO RELEASE ANY INFORMATION ACQUIRED IN THE COURSE OF TREATMENT. *SIGNATURE:* ____________________		

(*Continued*)

Appendix 9.12 (Continued) Model Superbill for Speech-Language Pathology

IRENE SMITH, MA, CCC-SLP SPEECH SERVICES, INC. 555 ANYWHERE ROAD ANYWHERE, CA 55555 (555) 555-5555		
SS #000-00-0000	**Tax ID #00-00000**	**California License #0000**
Speech-Language Pathology		
White copy: Office	Canary copy: Insurance	Pink Copy: Patient

Appendix 9.13 Key Acronyms and Phrases Used in Communication Sciences and Disorders

AAA	American Academy of Audiology
AAS	American Auditory Society
ABD	All but dissertation
ACPCA	American Cleft Palate Craniofacial Association
ADA	Americans with Disabilities Act
AIC	Asian Indian Caucus
ANCDS	Academy of Neurological Communication Disorders and Sciences
APA	American Psychological Association
API	Asian Pacific Islander
ARO	Association for Research in Otolaryngology
ASA	Acoustical Society of America
ASHA	American Speech-Language-Hearing Association
ASHF	American Speech-Language-Hearing Foundation
ASL	American Sign Language
AuD	Doctorate of audiology
BA	Bachelor of arts
BBS	Bachelor of health sciences
BHSM	Better Hearing and Speech Month

(*Continued*)

Appendix 9.13 (Continued) Key Acronyms and Phrases Used in Communication Sciences and Disorders

BS	Bachelor of sciences
CAOHC	Council for Accreditation in Occupational Hearing Conversation
CAPCSD	Council for Academic Programs in Communications Sciences and Disorders
CCC	Certificate of clinical competence
CEU	Continuing education unit
CF	Clinical fellowship
CLD	Culturally and linguistically different
CSD	Communication sciences and disorders
CV	Curriculum vitae
DIVISIONS	Special interest divisions
EB	Executive board
EC	Executive council
FAFSA	Free Application for Federal Student Aid
GPA	Grade point average
GSF	Graduate school fair
GUR	General university requirement
IDEA	Individuals with Disabilities Education Act
IEP	Individual Education Plan
IRB	Institutional Review Board
LC	Legislative council
LSA	Linguistic Society of America
MA	Master of arts
MS	Master of science
NAFDA	National Association of Future Doctors of Audiology
NAPP	National Association of Preprofessional Programs
NBASLH	National Black Association for Speech–Language Pathology and Hearing
NBGSA	National Black Graduate Student Association, Inc.
NESPA	National Examination in Speech-Language Pathology and Audiology
NIH	National Institute of Health

(*Continued*)

Appendix 9.13 (Continued) Key Acronyms and Phrases Used in Communication Sciences and Disorders

NSF	National Science Foundation
NSSLHA	National Student Speech–Language–Hearing Association
OT	Occupational therapist *or* occupational therapy
PAC	Political action committee
PET	Positron emission topography
PhD	Doctor of philosophy
PT	Physical therapist *or* physical therapy
Quals	Qualifying examinations
RC	Regional counselor
SHS	Speech, language, and hearing scientist
SLP	Speech-language pathologist
SLP-A	Speech-language pathology assistant

Appendix 9.14 How Do I Know If My Child Is Reaching the Milestones?

Birth to 5 months	Yes	No
Reacts to loud sounds.		
Turns head toward a sound source.		
Watches your face when you speak.		
Vocalizes pleasure and displeasure sounds (laughs, giggles, cries, or fusses).		
Makes noise when talked to.		
6 to 11 months		
Understands "no-no."		
Babbles (says "ba-ba-ba" or "ma-ma-ma").		
Tries to communicate by actions or gestures.		
Tries to repeat your sounds.		
12 to 17 months		
Attends to a book or toy for about 2 minutes.		
Follows simple directions accompanied by gestures.		
Answers simple directions nonverbally.		

(*Continued*)

Appendix 9.14 (Continued) How Do I Know If My Child Is Reaching the Milestones?

Points to objects, pictures, and family members.		
Says two or three words to label a person or object (pronunciation may not be clear).		
Tries to imitate simple words.		
18 to 23 months		
Enjoys being read to.		
Follows simple commands without gestures.		
Points to simple body parts such as "nose."		
Understands simple verbs such as "eat," "sleep."		
Correctly pronounces most vowels and n, m, p, b, words. Also begins to use other speech sounds.		
Says 8 to 10 words (pronunciation may still be unclear).		
Asks for common foods by name.		
Makes animal sounds such as "moo."		
Starts to combine words such as "more milk."		
Begins to use pronouns such as "mine."		

Appendix 9.15 State AT Programs

Names of the State	*Websites*
ALABAMA Alabama Statewide Technology Access and Response Project (STAR) System for Alabamians with Disabilities	www.rehab.alabama.org
ALASKA Alaska Assistive Technology Program	www.labor.state.ak.us/at/index.htm
AMERICAN SAMOA American Samoa Assistive Technology Service Projects (ASATS)	
ARIZONA Arizona Technology Access Program (AZTAP)	www.nau.edu/ihd/aztap
ARKANSAS Arkansas Increasing Capabilities Access Network (ICAN)	www.ar-ican.org
CALIFORNIA California Assistive Technology System (CATS)	www.dor.ca.gov/at

(*Continued*)

Appendix 9.15 (Continued) State AT Programs

COLORADO Colorado Assistive Technology Project	ucdenver.edu/academics/colleges/engineering/research/assitivetechnologypartners/pages/
CONNECTICUT Connective Assistive Technology Project	www.cttechact.com
DELAWARE Delaware Assistive Technology Initiative (DATI)	www.dati.org
DISTRICT OF COLUMBIA University Legal Service AT Program for the District of Columbia (ULS/ATP)	www.atpdc.org
FLORIDA Florida Alliance for Assistive Services and Technology (FAAST)	www.faast.org
GEORGIA Georgia Tools for Life	www.gaftl.com
GUAM Guam System for Assistive Technology (GSAT)	www.gsatcedders.org
HAWAII Assistive Technology Resource Centers of Hawaii (ATRC)	www.atrc.org
IDAHO Idaho Assistive Technology Project	www.idahoat.org
ILLINOIS Illinois Assistive Technology Project	www.iltech.org
INDIANA Assistive Technology Through Action in Indiana ATTAIN, Inc.	www.attaininc.org
IOWA Iowa Program for Assistive Technology (IPAT)	www.iowaat.org
KANSAS Assistive Technology for Kansans Project	www.atk.ku.edu
KENTUCKY Kentucky Assistive Technology Service Network (KATS)	www.katsnet.org
LOUISIANA Louisiana Assistive Technology Access Network (LATAN)	www.latan.org
MAINE Maine Consumer Information and Technology Training Exchange (Maine CITE)	www.mainecite.org

(Continued)

Appendix 9.15 (Continued) State AT Programs

MARIANA ISLANDS Commonwealth of the Northern Mariana Islands Assistive Technology Project	http://www.icdri.org/legal/nmarianaATP.htm
MARYLAND Maryland Technology Assistive Program (MD TAP)	www.mdtap.org
MASSACHUSETTS Massachusetts Assistive Technology Partnership (MATP)	www.matp.org
MICHIGAN Michigan Assistive Technology Project	www.copower.org/assisstive-tech
MINNESOTA Minnesota STAR Program	www.mn.gov/admin/star
MISSISSIPPI Mississippi Start Project	www.msprojectstart.org
MISSOURI Missouri Assistive Technology	www.at.mo.gov
MONTANA MonTech Program	www.montech.ruralinstitute.umt.edu
NEBRASKA Nebraska Assistive Technology Partnership	www.atd.ne.gov
NEVADA Nevada Assistive Technology Collaborative	adds.nv.gov/programs/physical/ATforIL/Nevada_assitive_technologyg_(NATC)/
NEW HAMPSHIRE New Hampshire Technology Partnership Project	www.iod.unh.edu/projects/technology_policy.html
NEW JERSEY Assistive Technology Advocacy Center (ATAC) of NJ P&A	www.drnj.org
NEW MEXICO New Mexico Technology Assistance Program	www.tapgcd.state.nm.us
NEW YORK New York State TRAID Project	justicecenter.ny.gov/services-support/assistive-technology-triad
NORTH CAROLINA North Carolina Assistive Technology Program	www.ncatp.org
NORTH DAKOTA North Dakota Interagency Program for Assistive Technology (IPAT)	www.ndipat.org
OHIO Assistive Technology of Ohio	www.atohio.engineering.osu.edu

(*Continued*)

Appendix 9.15 (Continued) State AT Programs

OKLAHOMA Oklahoma ABLE Tech	www.ok.gov/abletech
OREGON Oregon Technology Access for Life Needs Project (TALN)	www.accesstechnologiesinc.org
PENNSYLVANIA Pennsylvania's Initiative on Assistive Technology (PIAT)	disabilities.temple.edu
PUERTO RICO Puerto Rico Assistive Technology Project	www.pratp.upr.edu
RHODE ISLAND Rhode Island Assistive Technology Access Partnership (ATAP)	www.techaccess-ri.org
SOUTH CAROLINA South Carolina Assistive Technology Project	www.scatp.med.sc.edu
SOUTH DAKOTA South Dakota DakotaLink	https://www.dakotalink.net
TENNESSEE Tennessee Technology Access Project (TTAP)	http://www.icdri.org/legal/ TennesseeATP.htm
TEXAS Texas Assistive Technology Partnership	techaccess.edb.utexas.edu
UTAH Utah Assistive Technology Program	www.uatpat.org
VERMONT Vermont Assistive Technology Project	www.atp.vermont.gov
VIRGINIA RESNA Technical Assistance Project Virginia Assistive Technology System(VATS)	www.resna.org www.vats.org
WASHINGTON Washington Assistive Technology Alliance (WATS)	www.watap.org
WEST VIRGINIA West Virginia Assistive Technology System (WVATS)	www.wvats.cedwvu.org
WISCONSIN Wisconsin Assistive Technology Program (WisTech)	www.dhs.wisconsin.gov/ disabilities/wistech.htm
WYOMING Wyoming's New Options in Technology Project (WYNOT)	www.uwyo.edu/wind/watr

Appendix 9.16 AT Resource Directory

Producers' Names	*Websites*
2SimpleUSA Inc.	www.2simple.com
ABA Materials	www.helpingtogrow.com
Abasoft Corporation	
Ability Research, Inc.	www.abilityresearch.com
AbleLink Technologies, Inc.	www.ablelinktech.com
AbleNet, Inc.	www.ablenetinc.com
Academic Communication Associates, Inc.	www.acadcom.com
Academic Software, Inc.	www.acsw.com
Academic Therapy Publications	www.AcademicTherapy.com
Accelerations Educational Software	www.DTTrainer.com
Accessible Book Collection	www.accessiblebookcollection.Org
Acoustic Magic, Inc.	www.Acousticmagic.com
Advanced Multimedia Devices, Inc.	www.amdi.net
AGS Publishing	www.pearsonschool.com
Ai Squared	www.aisquared.com
Altimate Medical Inc.	www.easystand.com
American Printing House for the Blind (APH)	www.aph.org
American Thermoform Corporation	www.Americanthermoform.com
Apple Computer, Inc.	www.apple.com
Applied Human Factors, Inc.	www.ahf-net.com
Arrow Educational Products, Inc.	www.arrowinc.com
Artic Technologies International, Inc.	www.artitech.com
Artificial Language Laboratory	www.msu.edu/~artlang/
Assistive Technology, Inc.	www.assistivetech.com
AssistiveWare	www.assistiveware.com
AT KidSystems, Inc.	www.atkidsystems.com
ATbyMJM	www.atbymjm.com
Atlanta Area School for the Deaf	www.aasdweb.com/cats
Attainment Company, Inc.	www.attainmentcompany.com

(*Continued*)

Appendix 9.16 (Continued) AT Resource Directory

Attention Getters	www.sanfordskills.com
AudioEye	www.audioeye.com
Avocent Corporation	www.emersonnetworkpower.com
B Able To, Inc.	www.bableto.com
Baby Bumblebee	www.babybumblebee.com
Beyond Sight, Inc.	www.beyondsight.com
Bigkeys Company	www.bigkeys.com
Biolink Computer Research and Development, Ltd.	www.visionaware.com
Blista-Brailletec	www.brailletec.de
Bodelin Technologies	www.theproscope.com
Bookshare.org/Bentech Initiative	www.bookshare.org
Braille Books Dot Com	www.BrailleBooks.com
Brain Actuated Technologies, Inc.	www.brainfingers.com
BrainTrain, Inc.	www.braintrain.com
Break Boundaries	www.breakboundaries.com
BrightEye Technology	www.brighteye.com
Bytes of Learning, Inc.	www.bytesoflearning.com
CaluScribe	www.tcnj.edu/~technj/2010/calcuscribe.htm
CameraMouse, Inc.	www.cameramouse.com
CAST	www.cast.org
CataLaw, Inc.	www.myskeletonkey.com
Chester Creek Technologies	www.chestercreektech.com
Cirque Corporation	www.cirque.com
CJT Enterprises, Inc.	www.cjt-yes.com
Clarity	www.clarityusa.com
Clear View Innovations	www.clearviewinnovations.com
CLEARVUE & SVE	www.smavideo.com
Click and Go Interactive, Inc.	www.golocalinteractive.com
CO-Sign Communications	www.deafsign.com

(*Continued*)

Appendix 9.16 (Continued) AT Resource Directory

Cognitive Concepts, Inc.	www.earobics.com
Colligo Corp.	www.colligo.com
Comfort Keyboard Co., Inc.	www.comfortkeyboard.com
Compu-Teach	www.compu-teach.com
Compusult Limited	www.hear-it.com
Computer Application Specialties Company	www.braille2000.com
Computerade Products	www.computerade.com
Contour Design	www.contourdesign.com
Core Learning, Ltd.	www.core-learning.com
CPC-Computer Prompting Captioning Co.	www.cpcweb.com
CreateAbility Concepts, Inc.	www.createabilityinc.com
Creative Communicating	www.creativecommunicating.com
Creative Vision Technologies, Inc.	www.neotechnologies.co.in
Crick Software, Inc.	www.cricksoft.com
Curriculum Associates, Inc.	www.curriculumassociates.com
Custom Solutions	www.customsolutions.us
Daedalus Technologies, Inc.	www.daessy.com
Dainoff Designs, Inc.	www.bookandcopyholders.com
Dancing Dots Braille Music Technology	www.DancingDots.com
Dasher Project, University of Cambridge	www.inference.phy.cam.ac.uk/ dasher/
Data Impact Software	www.dataimpactssol.com
DataCal Enterprises	www.datacal.com
DBH Adaptive Technology	www.usatechguide.org
Design Science, Inc.	www.dessci.com
DisabilitySoft.com	www.attendantmanager.com
Dolphin Computer Access, Inc.	www.dolphinusa.com
Don Johnston, Inc.	www.donjohnston.com
Duxbury Systems, Inc.	www.duxburysystems.com
DynaVox Technologies	www.dynavoxtech.com

(Continued)

Appendix 9.16 (Continued) AT Resource Directory

e-Speaking	www.e-speaking.com
Easter Seals New Brunswick	www.easterseals.nb.ca
EasyChair Workstation Div, Mack Bailey Enterprises	www.easychairworkstation.com
Edcon Publishing Group	www.edconpublishing.com
Educational Activities Software	www.edact.com
EKEG Electronics Co. Ltd.	www.abledata.com
EloTouchSystems, Inc	www.elotouch.com
En-Vision America, Inc.	www.envisionamerica.com
Enabling Devices, Toys for Special Children	www.enablingdevices.com
Enabling Technologies Company	www.brailler.com
Enhanced Vision	www.enhancedvision.com
ErgoQuest, Inc.	www.ergoquest.com
Extensions for Independence	www.semel.ucla.edu
EyeTech Digital Systems, Inc.	www.eyetechds.com
FableVision	www.fablevision.com
Freedom Scientific, Inc., Blind/Low-Vision Group	www.FreedomScientific.com
Freedom Scientific, Learning Systems Group	www.freedomscientific.com/lsg
Freedom Vision	www.freedomvisionsurgery.com
FrogPad, Inc.	www.frogpad.com
G.G. Electronics Ltd.	www.ggelectronics.com
GAMCO Educational Software	www.gamco.com
Giving Greetings	www.givinggreetings.com
Golden Child Resources	www.goldenchildresources.com
GPK, Inc.	www.gpk.com
GTCO Cal Comp, Inc.	www.gtcocalcomp.com
Gus Communications, Inc.	www.gusinc.com
GW Micro, Inc.	www.gwmicro.com
H.K. EyeCan Ltd.	www.eyecan.ca
Harcourt Assessment, Inc.	www.PsychCorp.com
Harkle	www.harkle.com

(Continued)

Appendix 9.16 (Continued) AT Resource Directory

Harmonic Vision, Inc.	www.harmonicvision.com
Headsprout	www.headsprout.com
HEC Reading Horizons	www.readinghorizons.com
Horizon Wimba	www.horizonwimba.com
HumanWare	www.humanware.com
Hunter Digital, Ltd.	www.hunterdigitalmarketing.com
Hypersoft-netSRL	www.knowledgemanager.us
IBM Accessibility Center	www.ibm.com/able
In Touch Systems	www.magicwandkeyboard.com
INCAP GmbH	www.incap.de
Inclusive TLC	www.inclusiveTLC.com
Independent Concepts, Inc.	www.colny.org
Independent Living Aids, Inc.	www.independentliving.com
Infinity Station	www.InfinityStation.com
Infogrip, Inc.	infogrip.com
Ingenuity Works	www.ingenuityworks.com
Innovation Management Group, Inc.	www.imgpresents.com
Innovative Communication Programming	www.elr.com.au
Innovative Rehabilitation Technology, Inc.	www.irti.net
Inspiration Software, Inc.	www.inspiration.com
IntelliTools, Inc.	www.interconweb.com
Interactive Therapeutics, Inc.	www.interactivetherapy.com
Interest-Driven Learning, Inc.	www.drpeet.com
iTech Consulting "Early Works"	www.earlyworkseducation.net.au
Jeff Stewart's Teaching Tools	
Judy Lynn Software, Inc.	www.judylynn.com
JWor Enterprises, Inc.	www.jwor.com
Kensington Technology Group	www.kensington.com
KEYTEC, Inc.	www.magictouch.com
KidAccess, Inc.	www.kidaccess.com

(Continued)

Appendix 9.16 (Continued) AT Resource Directory

KidzMouse, Inc.	www.kidzmouse.com
Kinesis Corporation	www.kinesis.com
Kurzweil Educational Systems, Inc.	www.kurzweiledu.com
KY Enterprises	www.quadcontrol.com
LAB Resources	www.lab-resources.net
Laidback We R, Inc.	www.laptop-laidback.com
Laureate Learning Systems, Inc.	www.LaureateLearning.com
LaZee Tek	www.lazeetek.com
LC Technologies/Eyegaze Systems	www.eyegaze.com
LeapFrog School House	www.LeapFrogSchoolHouse.com
Learning in Motion	www.learn.motion.com
Learning Upgrade, LLC	www.learningupgrade.com
Leithauser Research	www.leithauserresearch.com
Lekotek of Georgia, Inc.	www.lekotekga.org
Lexia Learning System, Inc.	www.lexialearning.com
Life Science Associates	www.lifesciassoc.home.pipeline.com
LightSPEED Technologies, Inc.	www.lightspeed-tek.com
Lingraphicare	www.aphasia.com
LocuTour Multimedia	www.locutour.com
Lucid Research, Ltd.	www.lucid-research.com
Luidia, Inc.	www.e-beam.com
Luminaud, Inc.	www.luminaud.com
MAB Assistive Technologies	www.nchpad.org
MacSpeech, Inc.	www.macspeech.com
Madentec Limited	www.madentec.com
Magitek.com, LLC	www.magitek.com
MagniSight	www.magnisight.com
Marblesoft	www.marblesoft.com
Mariner Software	www.marinersoftware.com
MarvelSoft Enterprises, Inc.	www.marvelsoft.com

(Continued)

Appendix 9.16 (Continued) AT Resource Directory

Matias Corporation	www.half-qwerty.com
Maxess Products, Ltd.	www.maxessproducts.co.uk
Mayer-Johnson, LLC	www.mayer-johnson.com
Med Labs, Inc.	www.medlabsinc.com
Merit Software	www.meritsoftware.com
Metroplex Voice Computing	www.mathtalk.com
Milliken Publishing Company	www.millikenpub.com
MindPlay	www.mindplay.com
MOBIUS Corporation	www.mobius-llc.com
Model Me Kids	www.modelmckids.com
Namco, Ltd.	www.namco.com
NanoPac, Inc.	www.nanopac.com
National Federation of the Blind (NFB)	www.nfb.org
NaturalPoint, Inc.	www.naturalpoint.com
Neil Squire Foundation	www.neilsquire.ca
Neuropsychonline	www.neuropyschonline.com
NeuroScience Publishers	www.neuroscience.cnter.com
Next Generation Technologies, Inc.	www.ngtvoice.com
Nordic Software, Inc.	www.nordicsoftware.com
Nuance Communications, Inc. (formally Scansoft)	www.nuance.com
NXi Communications, Inc.	www.nextalk.com
Optelec U.S., Inc.	www.optelec.com
Opus Technologies	www.opustec.com
Origin Instruments, Co.	www.orin.com
P.I. Engineering, Inc.	www.piengineering.com
Prentke Romich Co.	www.prentrom.com
PRO-ED	www.proedinc.com
Quillsoft, Ltd.	www.wordq.com
QuizWorks Company	www.quizworks.com
Read Naturally	www.readnaturally.com

(*Continued*)

Appendix 9.16 (Continued) AT Resource Directory

ReadPlease Corporation	www.readplease.com
Rehabilitation Technology Services	www.vdbvi.org/rehabtech.htm
RehabTool.com	www.rehabtool.com
Renaissance Learning, Inc. (formerly Humanities Software)	www.renlearn.com
Rifton Equipment-Community Products, LLC	www.rifton.com
RJ Cooper and Associates	www.rjcooper.com
Rogers Center for Learning	www.rogerscenter.com
RVB Systems Group	lwww.barcode-solutions.com
SAJE Technology	www.saje-tech.com
Saltillo Corporation	www.saltillo.com
SaylCan	www.sayican.com
See It Right! Corporation	www.seeitright.com
Silver Lining Multimedia, Inc.	www.silverliningmm.com
Slater Software, Inc.	www.slatersoftware.com
Smarthome	www.smarthome.com
Social Skill Builder, Inc.	www.socialskillbuilder.com
SoftDawn Software	www.typeonehand.com
SoftTouch, Inc.	www.softtouch.com
Span-America Medical systems, Inc.	www.spanamerica.com
Spark-Space	www.spark-space.com
Special Communications	www.specialcommunications.com
Steck-Vaughn/Harcourt Achieve	www.harcourtachieve.com
Stepware, Inc.	www.acereader.com
Street Electrical Manufacturing Company, LLC	www.quadjoy.com
Sunburst Technology	www.sunburst.com
Switch in Time	www.switchintime.com
Synapse Adaptive	www.synapse-ada.com
Talking Fingers Inc.	www.talkingfingers.com
TalkingMyWay	turningpointtechnology.com

(*Continued*)

Appendix 9.16 (Continued) AT Resource Directory

TalkingThermostats.com	www.talkingthermostats.com
TASH International, Inc.	www.tash.org
Taylor Associates	www.readingplus.com
Teaching Made Easier, LLC	www.TeachingMadeEasier.com
Telex Communications, Inc.	www.telex.com
Teltronics	www.teltronic.com
Terrapin Software	www.terrapinlogo.com
Texthelp Systems, Inc.	www.telex.com
Textware Solutions Division of JDI Technology, Inc.	www.textware.com
The Conover Company	www.conovercompany.com
The Great Talking Box Company	www.greattalkingbox.com
The School Board Co., Inc.	www.sbci.org
Thinking Publications	www.ThinkingPublications.com
Tiger DRS, Inc.	www.drspeech.com
Tobii Technology	www.tobii.com
Tom Snyder Productions	www.tomsnyder.com
Trinity Software	www.trinitysoft.net
TrueTip, LLC	www.truetip.com
Turning Point Therapy and Technology, Inc.	www.turningpointtechnology.com
Ultratec, Inc.	www.ultratec.com
Unique Logic & Technology	www.playattention.com
Valpar International Corporation	www.valparint.com
Vcom3D, Inc.	www.vcom3d.com
ViewPlus Technologies, Inc.	www.viewplus.com
Vision Management Consulting, LLC	www.visionplanet.com
Vision Technology, Inc.	www.visiontechnology.com
VisionCue, LLC	www.visioncue.com
Viziflex Seels	www.viziflex.com
Vocational Research Institute	www.vri.org
Voicewave Technology, Inc.	www.SpeechEnhancer.com

(*Continued*)

Appendix 9.16 (Continued) AT Resource Directory

VORT Corporation	www.vort.com
WestTest Engineering Corporation	www.westest.com
Widgit Software	www.widgit.com
Wizcom Technologies	www.wicomtech.com
Woodbine House	www.woodbinehouse.com
Words+, Inc.	www.words-plus.com
Workable Solutions	www.workablesolutions
Zero2000 Software	www.zero2000.com
ZYGO Industries, Inc.	www.zygo-usa.com

Appendix 9.17 Outline for Funding Request

1. Demographic Information

   Patient's name, date of birth, medical diagnosis, date of onset, patient's contact information, physician's contact information, SLP contact information, patient's primary support contact information, and date of SLP evaluation.

2. Current Communication Impairment

   a. Impairment and Severity
   This section should explicitly demonstrate how the medical condition results in severe expressive speech impairment. Include ICD-9 codes as appropriate. Describe the impairment severity, as well as the type of communication disorder (dysarthria, aphasia, apraxia, aphonia).

   b. Anticipated Course of Impairment
   This section should demonstrate the current status and the expected course of the speech impairment as it relates to the underlying disease/condition. Staging scales may be used.

3. Comprehensive Assessment

   a. Hearing Status
   This section should explicitly provide information about the person's hearing status as it relates to a SGD and accessories. If the hearing ability is not an issue, it should be stated. Include information about the communication partners, information about acuity, localization, understanding of natural speech, and understanding specific SGDs.

   b. Vision Status
   This section should explicitly provide information about the person's visual status as it relates to using a SGD and accessories. If the person's vision is not an issue, it should be stated. Describe the vision using an SGD, including acuity, visual fields, lighting needs, angle of view, contrast, color, detail, and spacing.

(*Continued*)

Appendix 9.17 (Continued) Outline for Funding Request

c. Physical Status
This section should provide information about the person's physical skills and abilities as they relate to using an SGD and accessories. The report should state that the patient possesses the physical abilities to effectively use an SGD and required accessories to communicate. Describe pertinent considerations such as motor skills, ambulatory status, positioning needed, how scanning will occur if needed, selection options, and if accommodations may assist with physical access.

d. Language Skills
This section should explicitly provide information about the person's language skills and abilities as they relate to using an SGD and accessories. Describe the level of linguistic impairments (mild to severe language impairment), performance on any language assessment (e.g., BDAE, WAB, picture descriptions), competency or ability to develop skills (e.g., form, content, use), type of symbol use that will be required, or whether a combination of different types of symbols.

e. Cognitive Skills
This section should explicitly provide information about the person's cognitive skills and abilities as they relate to the use of an SGD and accessories. If cognitive/linguistic abilities are not an issue, it should be stated. Discuss the level of cognitive impairment, if significant impairment, how it relates to a person's need for an SGD, describe a person's attention and problem-solving skills as they relate to, enhance, or develop daily, functional communication skills.

4. Daily Communication Needs

a. Specific Daily Functional Communication Needs
This section should list the person's daily functional communication needs in areas described. Supplement the categories by considering daily communication situations, environments, partners, and specific messages. Include specific daily communication needs that may encourage increased independence, such as access to telephone.

b. Ability to Meet Communication Needs with Non-SGD Treatment Approaches
This section should document why the patient is unable to fulfill daily functional communication needs using natural speech (or speech aids) and non-SGD treatment approaches including a statement that states that daily functional communication needs cannot be met using natural communication methods or low-tech/no-tech AAC techniques because of_________(specific). Discuss communication prognosis without an SGD, the individual's ability to use strategies and natural modes of daily communication, why high-tech instead of low-tech strategies, show explicitly what other forms have been considered and ruled out, and mention issues related to communication partners and caregivers.

5. Functional Communication Goals

This section should state the daily functional communication treatment goals that will be met using an SGD. This is a very important section. Functional goals are key to demonstrating the need for ongoing treatment. They are also key to demonstrating positive outcomes with SGD use and why a particular SGD will benefit the individual and enable her to achieve functional communication goals. SLPs should prepare immediate-term, short- to mid-term, and long-term functional goals. Include a timetable.

(*Continued*)

Appendix 9.17 (Continued) Outline for Funding Request

6. Rationale for Device Selection

This section will explain why certain device features are required based on the person's skills and abilities as described in the daily communication needs. This section provides data that lead first to the selection of a specific device code and, second, to a specific device within that code, as well as specific accessories. At this point, SLPs work with rehab engineers, physical therapists, occupational therapists, and use AAC devices with simulations or clinical trials.

a. General Features of Recommended SGD and Accessories

Direct selection, scanning, and encoding access techniques are considered, as are message characteristics and features (type of symbols, storage capacity, vocabulary expansion, and rate enhancement). Output features to include voice output, visual display, and feedback and other features such as portability (size and weight, transportation requirements) and battery time required are other considerations.

7. Recommended Device and Accessory Codes

The coverage limitations and issues related to whether a manufacturer/supplier will accept assignment need to be considered, with reference to the SGD category chart.

8. Description of Equipment and Procedures Used During Any Demonstrations of the Recommended SGD and Any Other SGDs and Accessories

Evidence that the individual participated in the assessment process needs to be noted with some prediction of outcomes with the use of the SGD device.

9. SGD and Accessories Recommended

At this point, the individual's ability to achieve his functional communication goals requires the acquisition and use of the (name of the device) and (name the specific accessories) needs to be noted. The identified SGD should represent the clinically most appropriate device for (name of beneficiary). Specific SGD and accessories are listed in this section as well as why they enable the individual to achieve functional communication goals.

10. Patient and Family Support of the SGD

Discuss participation of the family/caregivers/client and state they agree to the selected SGD equipment and its use for daily communication.

11. Physician Involvement Statement

Confirmation that the treating physician (name, address, phone number) on _____ (date) saw the report and concurred with it, thus writing a prescription for the recommended SGD and accessories (date the report was forwarded to the physician should be before the date of the prescription).

12. Treatment Plan

Frequency of therapy, functional goals with dates, type of treatment (individual versus group), follow-up recommendations, projected frequency of reassessment, and possible examples of a treatment plan.

(Continued)

Appendix 9.17 (Continued) Outline for Funding Request

13. Functional Benefit of Upgrade This section is required only if the SLP is requesting an upgrade of equipment. The features or capabilities of the upgrade recommendations are included, plus additional communication goals that can be achieved with the upgraded equipment and the importance of the patient's ability to complete these communication goals.
14. SLP Assurance of Financial Independence and Signature The statement confirming that the SLP performing this assessment is not an employee of and does not have a financial relationship with the supplier of an SGD. This disclaimer statement, the SLP's name, ASHA certification number, and state license number complete the report.

Appendix 9.18 AAC Organizations

Names of Organizations	*Websites*
AAC Institute	www.aacinstitute.org
Alexander Graham Bell Association for the Deaf	www.agbell.org
American Foundation for the Blind, Technology Center	www.afb.org
American Occupational Therapy Association (AOTA)	www.aota.org
American Physical Therapy Association (APTA)	www.apta.org
American Printing House for the Blind (APH)	www.aph.org
American Speech-Language- Hearing Association (ASHA)	www.asha.org
Apple Computer, Inc.	www.apple.com
Artificial Language Laboratory	www.msu.edu/~artlang/
Autism Society of America	www.autism-society.org
CAST, Inc.	www.cast.org
Center for Assistive Technology & Environmental Access (CATEA)	www.catea.org
Center for Best Practices in Early Childhood	www.wiu.edu/thecenter
Center on Disabilities California State University, Northridge (CSUN)	www.csun.edu/cod
Cerebral Palsy Foundation of Kansas, Inc.	www.cprf.org
Closing the Gap, Inc.	www.closingthegap.com
Council for Exceptional Children (CEC)	www.cec.sped.org
DO-IT (Disabilities Opportunities, Internetworking & Technology)	www.washington.edu/doit

(*Continued*)

Appendix 9.18 (Continued) AAC Organizations

Easter Seals, Inc.	www.easter-seals.org
IBM Independence Series Information Center	
Independent Living Research Utilization Program	www.ilru.org
Infinitec, Inc.	www.infinitec.org
International Dyslexia Association	www.interdys.org
International Society for Augmentative and Alternative Communication (ISAAC)	www.isaac-online.org
Irlen Institute	www.irlen.com
Job Accommodation Network (JAN)	www.askjan.org
LD Resources	www.ldresources.com
Learning Disabilities Association of America (LDA)	www.ldaamerica.org
Minnesota Governor's Council on Development Disabilities	www.mn.gov/mcddc
National Center to Improve Practice (NCIP)	www.edc.org
National Council on Disability	www.ncd.gov
National Federation of the Blind (NFB)	www.nfb.org
National Information Center for Children and Youth with Disabilities (NICHCY)	www.nichcy.org
National Institute for Rehabilitation Engineering (NIRE)	www.angelfire.com/nj/nire2/
National Lekotek Center	www.lekotek.org
National Technical Institute for the Deaf/Rochester Institute of Technology	www.rit.edu/NTID
Publications & Information Dissemination	www.clerccenter.gallaudet.edu
Sensory Access Foundation	www.sensoryaccess.com
TASH (Association for Persons with Severe Handicaps)	www.tash.org
Technology and Media (TAM)	www.cec.sped.org
The Arc of the United States	www.thearc.org
Trace Research and Development Center	www.trace.wisc.edu
Trafford Center for Technology and Learning Disabilities	www.frostig.org
United Cerebral Palsy Associations, Inc. (UCPA)	www.ucp.org
United States Society for Augmentative & Alternative Communication (USSAAC)	www.ussaac.org

References

American Medical Association. 2016. *Current Procedural Terminology CPT 2016.* http://www.asha.org/practice/reimbursement/coding/

American Speech-Language-Hearing Association. 1989. Competencies for SLPs providing services in augmentative communication. *American Speech-Language-Hearing Association, 31*, 61–64, 107–110.

American Speech-Language-Hearing Association. 1991. Augmentative and alternative communication. *American Speech-Language-Hearing Association, 33*, 8–12.

American Speech-Language-Hearing Association. 2014. https://www.asha.org/certification/2014-speech-language-pathology-certification-standards/

American Speech-Language-Hearing Association. 2015. *Code of Ethics[Ethics].* www.asha.org/policy.

American Speech-Language-Hearing Association. 2016. (HIPAA) http://www.asha.org/practice/reimbursement/hipaa/default/

American Speech-Language-Hearing Association. 2016. Scope of practice in speech-language pathology [Scope of Practice]. www.asha.org/policy.

American Speech-Language-Hearing Association. 2018. https://www.asha.org/uploadedFiles/State-Teacher-Requirements-Licensing-Trends-SLP.pdf

Bhatnagar, S. 2012. *Neuroscience for the Study of Communicative Disorders* (3rd ed.) Baltimore, MD: Wolters Kluwer/Lippincott Williams & Wilkins.

Bishop, D. V. M. 1989. Autism, Asperger's Syndrome and semantic-pragmatic disorder: Where are the boundaries? *British Journal of Disorders of Communication, 24*, 107–121.

Blackstone, S., Higgenbotham, J., & Williams, A. 2002. Privacy in the information age. *The ASHA Leader, 7*, 12 13.

Cahill, L. M., Murdoch, B. E., & Theodoros, D. G. 2005. Articulatory function following traumatic brain injury in childhood: a perceptual and instrumental analysis. *Brain Injury, 19*(1), 41–58. Informa Healthcare.

CDC. 2018 https://www.cdc.gov/reproductivehealth/maternalinfanthealth/infantmortality.htm

Dunn, L., & Dunn, L. 1991. *Peabody Picture Vocabulary Test (Rev. ed.).* Circle Pines, MN: American Guidance Service.

Ghovanloo, M., & Block, J. 2014. Wireless real-time tongue tracking for speech impairment diagnosis, speech therapy with audiovisual biofeedback, and silent speech interfaces. US Patent US14281794. Retrieved April 24, 2018 from https://patents.google.com/patent/US9911358B2/en

Gillberg, C. 1991. Clinical and neurobiological aspects of Asperger syndrome in six family studies. In U. Frith (Ed.), *Autism and Asperger Syndrome* (pp. 122–146). Cambridge, UK: Cambridge University Press.

Kendall, K. A. 2009. High speed laryngeal imaging compared with videostroboscopy in healthy subjects. *Arch Otolaryngology Head Neck Surgery, 135*(3), 274–281.

Kiritani, S., Hirose, H., & Imagawa, H. 1993. High-speed digital image-analysis of vocal cord vibration in diplophonia. *Speech Communication, 13*(1–2), 23–32.

Kobler, J. B., Chang, E. W., Zeitels, S. M., & Seok-Hyun, Y. 2010. Dynamic imaging of vocal fold oscillation with four-dimensional optical coherence tomography. *Laryngoscope, 120*(7), 1354–1362.

Kuruvilla, M. S., Murdoch, B. E., & Goozee, J. V. 2008. Electropalatographic (EPB) assessment of tongue-to-palate contacts in dysarthric speakers following TBI. *Clinical Linguist and Phonetics, 22*(9), 703–725. Informa Healthcare.

Lloyd, L., Fuller, D., & Arvidson, H. 1997. *Augmentative and Alternative Communication: A Handbook of Principles and Practices.* Boston, MA: Allyn & Bacon.

Morgan, A., Liegeois, F., & Occomore, L. 2007. Electropalatography treatment for articulation impairment in children with dysarthria post-traumatic brain injury. *Brain Injury, 21*(11), 1183–93. Informa Healthcare.

Owens, Jr. R. E., 2004. *Language Development: An Introduction* (5th ed.) Needham Heights, MA: Allyn & Bacon.

Rizzo, M. Painful silence (May 3, 1999). People.com Retrieved April 27, 2018 from http://people.com/archive/painful-silence-vol-51-no-16/

Tonge, B. J. 2002. Autism, autistic spectrum and the need for a better definition. *The Medical Journal of Australia, 176*(9), 412.

Venkatagiri, H. 1996. The quality of digitized and synthesized speech: What clinicians should know. *American Journal of Speech-Language Pathology, A Journal of Clinical Practice, 5*, 24–28.

Chapter 10

The Role of the Audiologist in Life Care Planning

William D. Mustain and Carolyn Wiles Higdon

Contents

Introduction 256
Audiological Evaluation Procedures 258
  Clinical Process for Audiological Evaluation 259
  External Ear Canal Examination and Cerumen Management 259
  Pure Tone Audiometry 259
  Speech Audiometry 261
  Acoustic Immittance/Impedance 262
Pediatric Audiological Assessment 264
  Nonbehavioral Hearing Assessment Techniques 264
  Otoacoustic Emissions (OAEs) 264
  Auditory Evoked Response (AER) 264
  Identification of Hearing Loss in the Newborn 265
  High Risk Registry 265
  Universal Newborn Hearing Screening 266
Causes of Hearing Loss 267
  Perinatal Causes of Hearing Loss 268
  Postnatal Causes of Hearing Loss 268
  Pressure-Equalizing (PE) Tubes 269
Multicultural Considerations 270
  Neurophysiologic Intraoperative Monitoring 271
  Balance (Vestibular) System Assessment 272
Ototoxic Drug Therapy (Audiological Management) 273
Impact of Hearing Loss 274
  Impact on Communication 274
  Impact on Physical Functioning 274
  Impact on Cognitive Functioning 275

Impact on Quality of Life.....275
Impact on Mental Health.....275
Audiological (Aural) Rehabilitation Assessment.....275
Audiological (Aural) Rehabilitation Management.....276
Audiological (Re)habilitation for Children.....277
Assistive Listening Devices (ALDs).....278
Hearing Aid Selection and Fitting.....281
Styles of Hearing Aids.....282
Types of Hearing Aids.....282
Special Features for Hearing Aids.....283
Implantable Hearing Devices.....284
Cochlear Implants.....284
Cochlear Implant Centers.....285
The Clinical Process.....285
Brain Stem Implants.....286
Bone Anchored Hearing Devices.....286
Auditory Processing Disorders Assessment (as Performed by an Audiologist).....286
APDs Management (as Performed by an Audiologist).....288
Tinnitus Management.....288
American Speech-Language-Hearing Association (ASHA) Audiology Scope of Practice.....289
Credentials Held by Audiologists.....291
Referral Considerations.....292
Types of Hearing Loss.....292
Assessment Procedures.....292
Mode of Presentation.....293
Test Battery.....293
Outcomes of Audiology Services.....293
How to Communicate with People Who Are Hard of Hearing.....294
How to Communicate with People Who Are Deaf.....295
First Aid for Hearing Aids.....295
Symptom Solution.....296
Causes, Tests, and Remedies.....296
Behaviors of Children at Risk for Auditory Disorders.....297
Conditions Associated with Hearing Loss.....298
Costs Related to Amplification.....298
Funding Issues Related to Audiological Services.....299
Types of Counseling.....299
Example Case.....301
Conclusion.....303
Appendices.....304
References.....313

Introduction

Audiology, an autonomous profession that encompasses both health care and educational professional areas of practice, is the study of hearing, balance, and related disorders. The audiologist is the independent hearing health care professional who provides comprehensive diagnostic and habilitative/rehabilitative services for all areas of auditory, balance, and related disorders. These services are provided to individuals across the entire age span from birth through adulthood, which is in concert with the goals of a life care plan; to individuals from diverse language, ethnic, cultural, and socioeconomic backgrounds; and to individuals who have multiple disabilities. Within life care planning, the audiologist should be involved in pediatric and adult rehabilitation efforts when clients experience decreased hearing sensitivity, auditory processing problems, auditory neuropathy (auditory dys-synchrony), or balance problems. Clients may experience auditory or balance deficits due to genetic or natural aging factors, ear disease, physical trauma, brain injury, environmental noise exposure, or reactions to medications that are toxic to the auditory or balance system.

Life care planners seeking information on current audiology preferred practices, technical papers, position statements, reimbursement codes, standards, and certification and licensure (Appendix 10.1 at the end of this chapter) will find the American Speech-Language-Hearing Association (ASHA) web portal (https://www.asha.org/public/) the most comprehensive site for peer-reviewed documentation of practice issues and current reimbursement codes. The ASHA Code of Ethics (ASHA, 2016), Scope of Practice in Audiology (ASHA, 2004a); Preferred Practice Patterns for the Profession of Audiology (ASHA, 2006); Joint Audiology Committee on Clinical Practice (1999); Statements and Algorithms (ASHA, 1999); and current billing and reimbursement documents will be of significant interest to life care planners seeking best practices information and quality hearing health care for their clients. The information is also available on the ASHA web portal.

Services provided by audiologists include the ability to:

- Test for and diagnose hearing and balance disorders
- Select, fit, and dispense hearing aids and assistive devices
- Provide audiological/aural (re)habilitation services
- Educate consumers and professionals on prevention of hearing loss
- Participate in hearing conservation programs to help prevent workplace-related and recreational hearing loss
- Consult for federal, state, and local agencies in reducing community noise
- Conduct research

Audiology services are available in the following work settings:

- Colleges and universities
- Public and private schools
- Hospitals
- Community-based hearing and speech centers
- State and local health departments
- Private practices
- Rehabilitation centers
- Nursing care facilities
- Industry
- State and federal governmental agencies
- Military

Audiology can be categorized by either the setting in which one practices or the population one serves. Bess and Humes (1995) identified the following specialty areas in which audiologists generally practice (see Figure 10.1). The *pediatric audiologist* concentrates on the audiological management of children of all ages. The pediatric audiologist is often employed in a children's hospital or a health care facility primarily serving children. The *medical audiologist* works with patients of all ages and

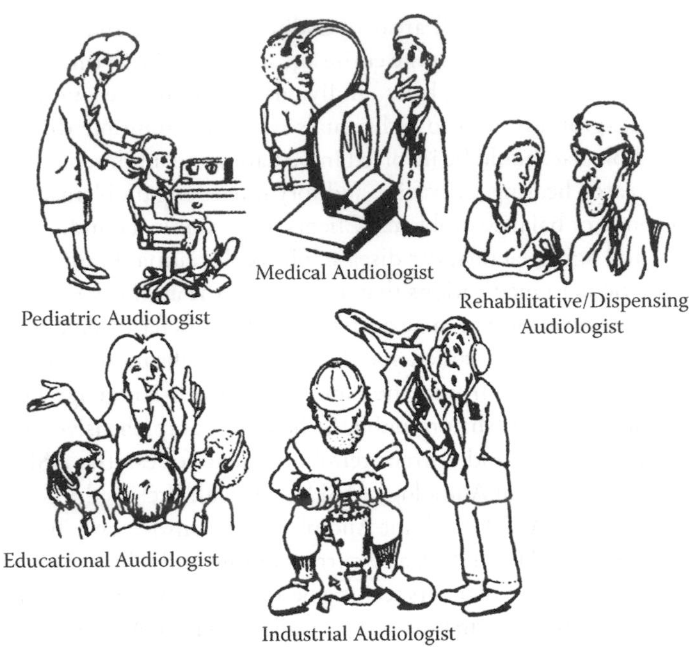

Figure 10.1 Audiology specialties. (From Bess, F. & Humes, L., *Audiology: The Fundamentals*, 2nd Edition, p. 7, Baltimore, MD: Williams & Williams, 1995. With permission.)

is more concerned with establishing the site and cause of a hearing or balance problem. Medical audiologists are typically employed in hospitals as part of either a hearing and speech department or a department of otolaryngology (i.e., ear, nose, and throat). Some audiologists who work in a medical environment perform intraoperative monitoring, which involves monitoring central and peripheral nerve function during surgical procedures. The *rehabilitative/dispensing audiologist* focuses on the management of children or adults with hearing impairment. Rehabilitative audiologists are often in private practice and may specialize in the direct dispensing of hearing aids in addition to offering other audiological rehabilitation services. Rehabilitative audiologists are also employed by a variety of health care facilities (e.g., hospitals and nursing homes). The *industrial audiologist* provides consultative hearing conservation services to companies whose workers are exposed to high noise levels. The industrial audiologist may be in private practice or work on a part-time basis. The *forensic audiologist* serves as an expert witness in legal issues related to hearing and balance. The forensic audiologist may serve as an expert witness for the plaintiff or defense in compensation cases and may also serve as a consultant in community or environmental noise issues. Finally, the *educational audiologist* serves children in the schools and is employed or contracted by the educational system. Many audiologists, not just those in academic environments, engage in basic and applied research that is not only essential to understanding human auditory function but also necessary in order to develop testing materials and procedures and improved amplification systems.

Audiological Evaluation Procedures

When referring a patient to an audiologist for evaluation, one may expect certain procedures to be conducted to quantify and qualify hearing loss on the basis of responses to acoustic stimuli and to screen for other associated communication disorders. These procedures include a pure tone hearing test (ASHA, 2004a), speech audiometry (ASHA, 1988), and acoustic immittance (ASHA, 1991) procedures accomplished in accordance with American National Standards Institute standards (ANSI, 1981, 1986, 1987, 1999a, 1999b, 2010) and under Centers for Disease Control (CDC) standard health care precautions guidelines (CDC, 1988; U.S. Department of Labor, 1998). Of course, these audiological procedures may be modified depending on the age or level of cooperation of the patient.

Clinical Process for Audiological Evaluation

The clinical process for audiological evaluation includes the following (ASHA, 1999):

- Case history
- Otoscopic examination of the external ear canal
- Cerumen management, if necessary
- Pure tone threshold testing by air conduction and bone conduction with appropriate masking
- Speech threshold testing with appropriate masking
- Word recognition (speech discrimination) testing with appropriate masking
- Acoustic immittance testing (tympanometry, static compliance, and acoustic reflex measures)
- Other procedures, which include, but are not limited to, otoacoustic emissions screening, speech and language screening, communication inventories, and screening for APDs and other related auditory disorders

External Ear Canal Examination and Cerumen Management

Otoscopic examination of the external ear canal is performed to identify cerumen (ear wax) which may preclude obtaining valid and reliable assessment results and, the removal of which may improve auditory sensitivity. Established procedures include the following (Roeser & Crandell, 1991; ASHA, 1992a; Ballachandra & Peers, 1992):

- Mechanical removal
- Irrigation
- Suction

It should be noted that in some states, cerumen management is not within the scope of practice of audiologists. Reimbursement for the service varies by state and region and also from third-party payers.

Pure Tone Audiometry

Pure tone audiometry is performed to determine if hearing is normal or impaired. An audiologist, using a calibrated electronic device, called an audiometer, and standardized procedures, measures hearing sensitivity. The individual being tested initially wears earphones and the audiologist presents tones of varying frequencies and intensities to each ear. When the individual hears the tone, they respond by raising their hand or pressing a response button. The lowest intensity level at which the tone is heard two out of three times is called threshold. This process is then repeated with the individual wearing a bone vibrator placed on the mastoid bone. When thresholds using earphones are outside the normal range, a comparison with the bone vibrator thresholds will indicate which part of the auditory system is responsible for the hearing loss.

The audiogram is a graphic representation of hearing sensitivity. It shows an individual's threshold for tones of different frequencies. Frequency, measured in hertz (Hz), is plotted along the abscissa and intensity, measured in decibels (dB), is plotted along the ordinate. Thresholds for the left ear are plotted with an *X* and thresholds for the right ear are plotted with a *0*. Normal hearing is considered to be between –10 and +20 dB HL. Hearing level (HL) is the number of decibels relative to normal hearing, which is 0 dB HL on the audiogram. The audiogram shown in Figure 10.2 indicates normal hearing in the left ear and a hearing loss in the right ear. The area enclosed by the two wavy lines is called the speech banana. This area represents the frequencies and intensities of spoken English and assists the audiologist in explaining how a given hearing loss may affect a person's ability to understand speech. In the example audiogram, the person will not be able to hear speech sounds above 1,000 Hz in the right ear because his/her thresholds are out of the speech banana. Were this person to have this degree of hearing loss in both ears, he may be expected to have difficulty understanding high-frequency speech sounds such as *s*, *f*, *th*, *p*, *t*, *k*, *sh*, and *ch*, for example. In addition, he may be expected to have considerable difficulty understanding conversational speech in the presence of background noise, such as in a cafeteria. Figure 10.3 shows the frequency of various speech sounds, as well as the intensity of some common environmental sounds.

Audiograms indicate presence of a hearing loss and also the type and degree of loss. There are three types of hearing loss directly associated with the peripheral auditory mechanism:

1. Conductive (a problem in the outer or middle ear)
2. Sensorineural (a problem in the inner ear or the eighth cranial nerve, which carries the auditory signals to the brain)
3. Mixed conductive and sensorineural loss

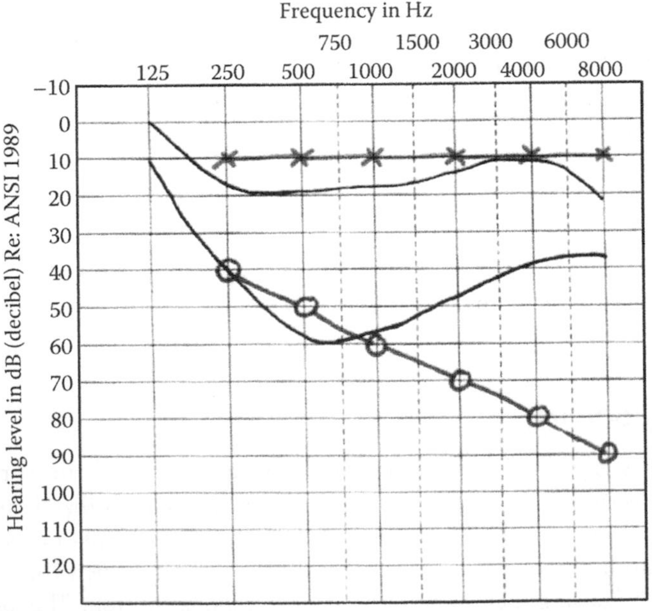

Figure 10.2 Audiogram.

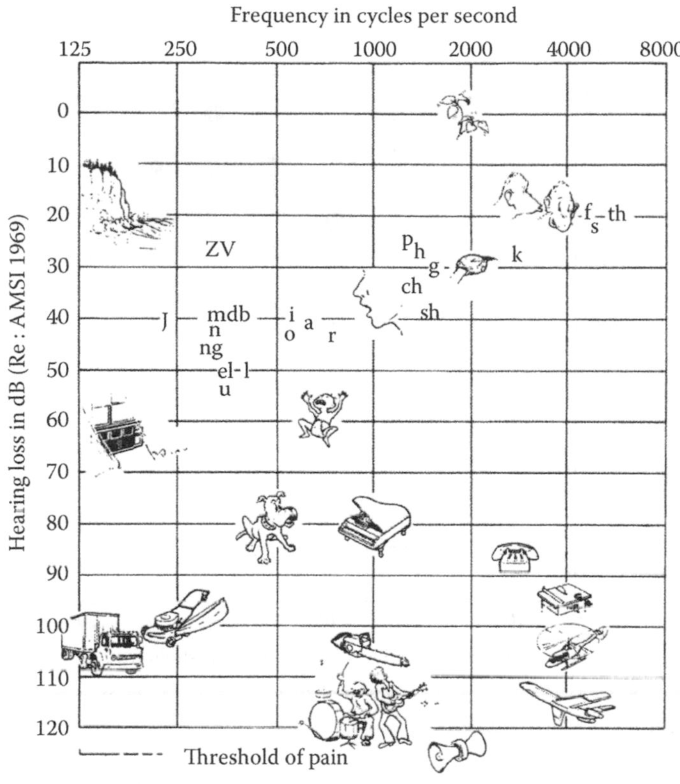

Figure 10.3 Frequency spectrum of familiar sounds plotted on a standard audiogram. (From Northern, J., & Downs, M., *Hearing in Children*, 4th Edition, p. 17, Baltimore, MD: Williams & Williams, 1991. With permission.)

As mentioned earlier, comparison of earphone (air conduction) and bone vibrator (bone conduction) hearing provides the necessary information for determination of type of hearing loss. Other nonperipheral auditory deficits may include auditory processing disorders and an auditory neuropathy (auditory dys-synchrony).

Speech Audiometry

Audiological assessment also includes speech audiometry. The audiologist evaluates how well a person can hear and understand speech. Speech audiometry consists of speech threshold and word recognition (understanding) or speech discrimination testing. Speech threshold testing determines how soft a speech sound a person can recognize, whereas word recognition testing tells the audiologist what percentage of conversational speech is correctly understood at a particular intensity level. One method of obtaining a word recognition/speech discrimination score is called the articulation gain function (Figure 10.4) (or performance intensity/phonetic balance function). This method helps assure that the patient's maximum score possible will be identified.

Most people understand conversational speech maximally at approximately 40 dB above their speech threshold. The evaluator starts by presenting the speech level at 40 dB above the patient's

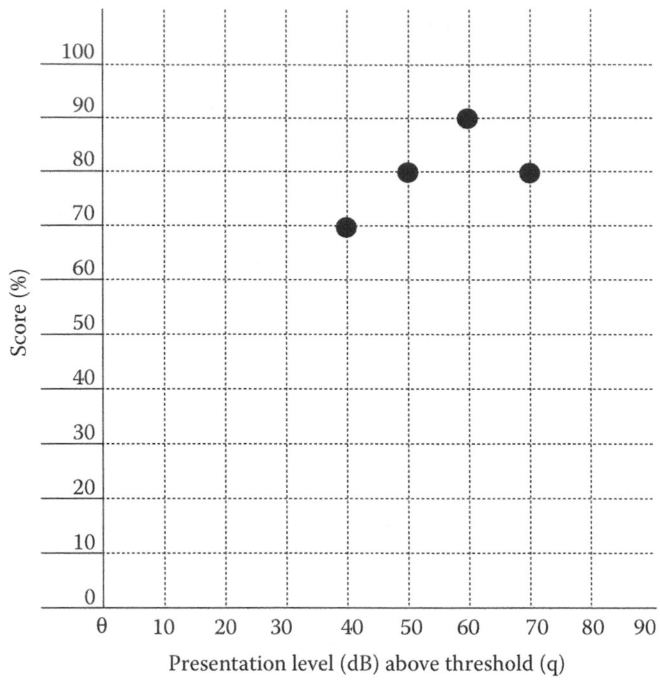

Figure 10.4 Articulation gain function.

speech threshold and reading a list of 50 single-syllable words with the person instructed to repeat back each word.

The percentage correct score at 40 dB above a person's threshold is then plotted. If 100 percent correct is not achieved, the test is repeated using a similar list of words at 50 dB above the person's threshold, and that score is plotted. This procedure is repeated until the person's best score is obtained. The score in the example graph indicates that the person will understand approximately 90 percent of speech that is 60 dB above threshold.

Acoustic Immittance/Impedance

Acoustic immittance, sometimes referred to as acoustic impedance, measures the mobility of the middle ear system. The middle ear is basically a vibratory system consisting of the eardrum and the three middle ear bones: the malleus, incus, and stapes. The middle ear is responsible for taking acoustic energy (sound) and transferring it via mechanical energy from the outer ear to the fluids in the inner ear. The functioning of the middle ear affects the way people hear. Tympanometry is a measure of the mobility of the middle ear (compliance) as a function of middle ear pressure, measured in da pascals (daPa). The results are displayed on a graph called a tympanogram (Figure 10.5), and interpretation of these results can help indicate the site of the lesion or the part of the auditory system causing a hearing loss (ASHA, 1991).

An electroacoustic immittance meter is used to measure the middle ear function. A plug is inserted into the ear canal, and the instrument takes the measurements and graphs the information.

Tympanograms can be classified into five types based on the peak pressure and where, in terms of pressure, the peak occurs. Although tympanometry does not provide direct evidence of hearing loss, abnormal results are often associated with a temporary or conductive type hearing loss.

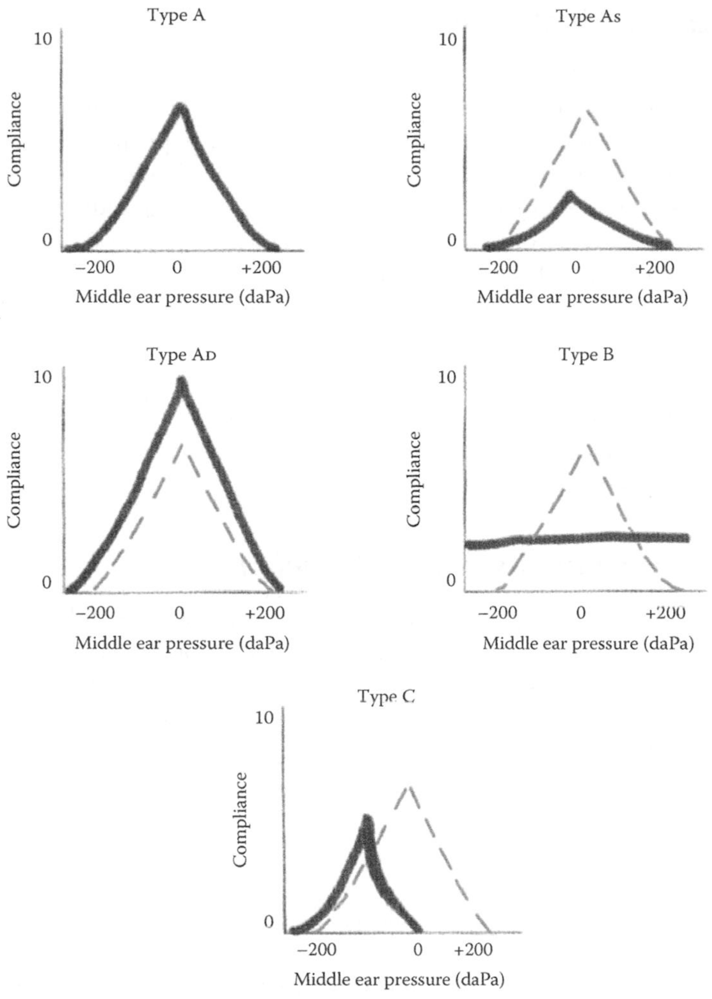

Figure 10.5 Tympanograms.

Type	*Description*	*Possible Pathology*
Type A	Middle ear pressure is between +100 and 150 daPa. Compliance is normal.	Normal function
Type A_s	Middle ear pressure is normal. Compliance is reduced.	Otosclerosis
Type A_d	Middle ear pressure is normal. Compliance is increased.	Disarticulation
Type B	Middle ear pressure cannot be measured. Compliance is reduced.	Middle ear effusion Eardrum perforation
Type C	Middle ear pressure is negative. Compliance may be normal or reduced.	Eustachian tube dysfunction

Pediatric Audiological Assessment

Audiological assessment of infants and young children (under 5 years of age) (ASHA, 2006) and other individuals with developmental delay may preclude the use of standard adult audiological assessment procedures. Valid assessment of hearing in this population typically requires an audiologist skilled in pediatric assessment and may involve multiple office visits. The assessment may include one or more assessment tools (acoustic immittance measures, audiological (re)habilitation and education needs assessment, otoacoustic emissions [OAE], electrophysiological assessment, and developmentally appropriate behavioral procedures).

Behavioral testing measures make use of operant conditioning and include the following:

- Visual Reinforcement Audiometry (VRA)
- Conditioned Play Audiometry
- Tangible Reinforcement Operant Conditioning Audiometry (TROCA)
- Behavioral Observation Audiometry (BOA)

Nonbehavioral Hearing Assessment Techniques

The behavioral assessment techniques listed previously are usually successful with developmentally normal infants and young children, beginning at age 6 to 7 months. However, when behavioral testing fails to confirm hearing status, several nonbehavioral assessment procedures are available. These "objective techniques" measure various physiological aspects of normal auditory function which are associated with normal hearing. They require no active participation from the individual being assessed and can often be recorded during sleep or if necessary under sedation.

Otoacoustic Emissions (OAEs)

OAEs are acoustic signals generated by the inner ear of healthy ears in normal-hearing individuals. The acoustic signals are by-products of the activity of the outer hair cells in the cochlea. The clinical significance is that they are evidence of a vital sensory process arising in the cochlea, and OAEs only occur in a normal cochlea with normal hearing.

The OAE evaluation is relatively quick (approximately 5 min. per ear) and is noninvasive. A soft rubber tip is inserted in the ear canal and a series of comfortably loud tones or clicks are presented. No response is necessary from the patient; he only needs to sit quietly while the test is being conducted. OAEs can be completed at any age from shortly after birth to above 90.

In addition to applications for pediatric hearing assessment, OAEs are powerful diagnostic tools that assist audiologists in ruling out unusual auditory disorders, where there are unexplained differences in hearing between two ears, when a sudden hearing loss occurs, in medical-legal cases, and in cases of questionable validity of hearing test results.

Auditory Evoked Response (AER)

An AER assessment describes the clinical status of the auditory neural pathway and associated sensory elements, and assists in differential diagnosis and in estimating threshold sensitivity. The assessment may also be conducted with patients who are difficult to test by conventional behavioral methods and for the purposes of site of lesion identification or in resolution of conflicting data (ASHA, 2003).

Patients are prepared for the assessment by placement of recording electrodes on the head, and they wear earphones for introduction of stimuli. The AER procedures may include the following:

- Electrocochleography (ECochG)
- Auditory brain stem response (ABR)
- Auditory middle latency response (AMLR)
- Auditory late (long latency) response (ALR)
- P300 response
- Mismatched negativity (MMN) response

The AER of greatest value in nonbehavioral hearing assessment is the auditory brain stem response (ABR). This procedure can provide physiological evidence of audibility for frequency specific stimuli and effectively rule out significant hearing loss. It forms the basis for universal newborn hearing screening, which will be discussed later in this chapter.

Identification of Hearing Loss in the Newborn

Hearing loss significant enough to affect the understanding of speech creates a potential handicap and adversely affects quality of life, regardless of age of onset. However, hearing loss present at birth or occurring during the newborn period has even greater implications. Normal hearing, particularly during the first 3 years of life, is essential to the development of speech and language. Children affected with congenital or newborn hearing loss may lose their ability to acquire fundamental speech, language, cognition, and social skills required for later schooling and success in society. Therefore, early identification and intervention for newborn hearing loss has been a priority for audiologists for decades. However, the fact that newborns show little behavioral responses to sound made early identification of hearing loss in this population particularly challenging.

High Risk Registry

In the 1960s–1970s, most organized attempts at identification of newborn hearing loss relied on the use of a High Risk Registry. Newborns identified by the birth hospital as being "at risk" for congenital hearing loss, based on prenatal events or family history were referred for audiological follow-up. Prenatal events refer to adverse effects on the cochlea during embryological and fetal development, resulting in congenital hearing loss. Development of the external, middle, and inner ear takes place between the fourth and eighth weeks of gestation. Some infants have hereditary factors that put them at risk for hearing loss. Genetic abnormalities such as a variety of sensorimotor impairments; difficulty with balance and coordination; mental retardation; musculoskeletal anomalies; thyroid disorders; abnormal skin pigmentation; visual disorders; cleft palate; and skull, facial, and external ear deformities may accompany the hearing loss. Combinations of these various disorders are referred to as syndromes, and a combination of genetic and in utero environmental factors is referred to as multifactorial genetic consideration.

Teratogens are environmental agents that result in malformations and anomalies of specific organs and systems that are undergoing rapid development in the embryo or fetus. Exposure to teratogens may result in major congenital anomalies. Some of these teratogens and infectious diseases are drugs (alcohol, cocaine, cigarette smoke), congenital HIV and AIDS, rubella, cytomegalovirus (CMV), herpes simplex-type virus, toxoplasmosis, congenital syphilis, and thalidomide (the most

Table 10.1 Risk Factors for Hearing Loss in Infants and Young Children

Risk Factors
Family history of childhood hearing loss
Congenital infections (TORCH)[a]
Craniofacial anomalies
Low birth weight (less than 3.5 lbs or 1.6 Kg)
Hyperbilirubinemia requiring blood exchange
Bacterial meningitis
Asphyxia
Ototoxic medication
Mechanical ventilation of more than 10 days
Syndromes that include hearing loss

[a] TORCH is an acronym describing congenital perinatal infections, including toxoplasmosis, other infections (like syphilis), rubella, CMV, and herpes simplex

notorious teratogen in history). Table 10.1 summarizes categories of risk factors for hearing loss in infants and young children.

Universal Newborn Hearing Screening

By the 1980s, it had become apparent that many newborns with congenital hearing loss had no apparent prenatal risk factors for hearing loss and were therefore not being identified as requiring audiological follow-up. This is because a high percentage of congenital hearing loss is genetically based.

In 1988, the Maternal and Child Health Bureau, a division of the U.S. Health Resources and Services Administration (HRSA), funded several research projects to test the feasibility of screening newborns for hearing loss before hospital discharge. Two of these projects, in Rhode Island and Hawaii, led to the implementation of the first statewide newborn hearing screening programs.

By the early 1990s, advances in screening technology using nonbehavioral hearing assessment technologies, such as OAEs and AER, led many professional organizations to call for hearing screening at birth (Joint Committee on Infant Hearing, 1994). In 2000, the Joint Committee on Infant Hearing (JCIH) endorsed universal newborn hearing screening through an integrated, interdisciplinary system of Early Hearing Detection and Intervention (EHDI) programs operating at the state level. That same year congress approved federal funding for EHDI programs, as well as authorized HRSA to develop newborn hearing screening and follow-up services, the Centers for Disease Control and Prevention (CDC) to develop data and tracking systems, and the National Institute for Deafness and Communicative Disorders to support research in EHDI. By 2005, every state had implemented newborn hearing screening, and as of 2012 over 95 percent of all newborns in the United States were being screened for hearing loss before hospital discharge (CDC, 2015).

Although the vast majority of newborns in the United States receive hearing screening before hospital discharge, problems remain in assuring a proper diagnosis for screening failures and in the provision of appropriate and timely intervention to those diagnosed with hearing loss. According to recent CDC data, between 25 and 35 percent of newborn screening failures are "lost to follow-up,"

Table 10.2 Birth to 24 Months: Red Flags

Birth to 28 days
1. An illness or condition requiring admission of 48 hours or greater to a neonatal intensive care unit (NICU).
2. Stigmata or other findings associated with a syndrome known to include sensorineural or conductive hearing loss.
3. Family history of permanent childhood sensorineural hearing loss.
4. Craniofacial anomalies, including morphological anomalies of the pinna and ear canal.
5. In utero infection such as cytomegalovirus, herpes, toxoplasmosis, or rubella.
29 days to 24 months
All of the above, plus the following:
1. Parent or caregiver concern regarding hearing, speech, language, developmental delay, or a combination of these.
2. Postnatal infections associated with sensorineural hearing loss, including bacterial meningitis.
3. Recurrent or persistent otitis media with effusion for at least 3 months.
4. Neonatal indicators—specifically, hyperbilirubinemia at a serum level requiring blood exchange transfusion, persistent pulmonary hypertension of the newborn associated with mechanical ventilation, and conditions requiring the use of extracorporal membrane oxygenation.
5. Syndromes associated with progressive hearing loss such as neurofibromatosis, osteoporosis, and Usher's syndrome.
6. Neurodegenerative disorders such as Hunter's syndrome, kyphosis, gargoylism, or sensorimotor neuropathies such as Friedreich's ataxia and Charcot-Marie-Tooth syndrome.
7. Recurrent or persistent otitis media with effusion for at least 3 months.
8. Head trauma.

either because they do not receive the indicated post-screening diagnosis and intervention services, or services provided are not tracked effectively. Also, certain conditions can make a newborn at risk for late onset hearing loss (see Table 10.2). An infant with any of these "red flags" should receive audiological follow-up, even if they pass the newborn hearing screening (JCIH, 2000).

Causes of Hearing Loss

Hearing loss can occur at any age, from birth through adulthood. Causative factors include genetics, systemic diseases and infections, vascular events, tumors, localized and generalized trauma, and environmental toxins. These factors can affect one or more of the components of the auditory system (outer/middle ear, inner ear, or central nervous system). The resulting hearing loss can vary in terms of degree, prognosis for recovery and response to intervention depending on the age of onset, and the components of the auditory system affected.

Perinatal Causes of Hearing Loss

Perinatal causes of hearing loss are those that occur during the birth process. Infants who must be admitted to neonatal intensive care units (NICUs) are 20 times more likely to have hearing problems than infants in normal newborn nurseries (Simmons et al., 1980). Hearing loss in infants who were in NICUs is often associated with the identifiable disorders that caused the need for the NICU or treatment for the disorders. Respiratory distress syndrome (RDS/hyaline membrane disease) is the most common respiratory disease in premature infants. Infants with RDS receive treatment by invasive procedures such as intubation and suctioning, putting them at an additional risk of infections. If infants become septic (generalized infection), general treatment is with antibiotics with potential ototoxic properties, placing them at a higher risk for hearing loss.

Congenital heart disease (CHD) is among the most common birth defects, affecting as many as 1 in 100 newborns (Fogle, 2008), and may exhibit cyanosis, respiratory distress, congestive heart failure, or a combination of these. In addition, these infants frequently exhibit failure-to-thrive and feeding problems. CHD is often associated with syndromes such as growth deficiencies, mental retardation, Down syndrome, and external ear anomalies. Again, ototoxic drugs may be needed to fight the infections.

Central nervous system disorders may have hearing loss as one component of the disorder, including cerebral hemorrhage, hydrocephalus, hypoxic encephalopathy, and neonatal seizures. Any individual who experiences hypoxia may have compromised neurological status and hearing abilities.

Postnatal Causes of Hearing Loss

Postnatal causes of cochlear hearing loss are factors occurring after birth. These include bacterial meningitis, measles, mumps, chicken pox, influenza, and viral pneumonia. Most viral-producing hearing losses are bilateral, except for mumps. The body's natural reaction to infection is elevation of temperature; however, when fever becomes excessive, cellular damage can occur, including cells of the cochlea. Treatments may warrant ototoxic antibiotics. Diabetes mellitus and kidney disease have been implicated in sensorineural hearing loss, as have head traumas, which cause both neurological disorders and hearing loss (Fogle, 2008). As noted previously, Table 10.1 lists some of the risk factors for hearing loss in infants and young children.

In older children (and adults), one of the most preventable is noise-induced hearing loss. Most people will have reduced hearing as they grow older (especially after the age of 60); however, there are things individuals can do to try to preserve their hearing. Noise-induced hearing loss, once called "blacksmith's deafness" from the continual clanging of metal on metal, dates back hundreds of years. During World War II, it received much more attention because of the heavy artillery used in the war. Acoustic trauma from a single exposure may cause permanent hearing loss. Gradual hearing loss from repeated exposure to excessive sound can damage or destroy the delicate hair cells in the cochlea. Hearing conservation programs and hearing research programs (ASHA, 2006) have developed public education campaigns to alert people, especially adolescents and teenagers, to the damage caused to hearing with loud music. Wearing ear plugs or ear muffs to help block the loud sounds or music, limiting the time of an iPod session with breaks to allow your hearing to rest, and keeping the volume reduced are just a few suggestions included in a hearing conservation program. Table 10.3 shows the

Table 10.3 Decibel Levels of Common Sounds

Decibels	*Sound*
130+	Jet takeoff, gunfire (pain threshold)
120+	Rock concert speaker sound, sandblasting, thunderclap, fireworks, pneumatic drill
110+	Dance club, snowmobile, powerboats, hammering metal
90+	Subway trains, motorcycle, workshop tools, lawn mower
80+	Heavy city traffic, factory noise, vacuum cleaner, garbage disposal, Niagara Falls
70+	Dog barking, noisy restaurant, busy traffic
60+	Ringing telephone, baby crying, alarm clock 2 feet away
50+	Quiet automobile 10 feet away
40+	Everyday conversation
30+	Quiet street at night with no traffic
20+	Whispered conversation
10+	Soft rustle of leaves, birds singing, dripping water faucet
0	Just audible sound

Source: Adapted from Northern, J. L. & Downs, M. P. *Hearing in Children* (5th Edition). Baltimore, MD: Lippincott Williams & Wilkins, 2002; Van Bereijk, W., Pierce, J., & David, E., *Science*, 131, 219–220, 1960; American Industrial Hygiene Association, 2007.

readers the decibel levels of some of the most common environmental sounds, and Table 10.4 lists the decibel levels of some musical instruments, as well as some types of music. Table 10.5 shows the noise exposure of sound in decibels for certain periods of time that may create hearing risk.

Pressure-Equalizing (PE) Tubes

Many infants and children have repeated ear infections requiring pressure-equalizing (PE) tubes. The surgical procedure is called a myringotomy, performed with a small surgical incision into the tympanic membrane to relieve pressure and release fluid or pus from the middle ear. A small suction device may be inserted through the incision to delicately suction out the fluid and pus. Antibiotics are given before and continued afterward to manage infection (Mosby, 2006).

Following the myringotomy and cleaning of the middle ear, the otolaryngologist may insert a PE tube through the incision in the tympanic membrane. The tube is plastic, tiny, and hollow with a flange on each end that prevents the tube from falling into the middle ear or falling out of the tympanic membrane prematurely. The tube allows direct ventilation of the middle ear and functions as an artificial Eustachian tube to maintain normal middle ear pressure. The tube may remain in place from several weeks to several months, after which time it extrudes (pushes out) naturally into the external auditory canal, usually without the child noticing. Newer-designed tubes may remain in place indefinitely.

Table 10.4 Decibel Levels of Musical Instruments

Decibels	*Instruments*
60–70	Normal piano practice
70	Fortissimo singers 3 feet away
75–85	Chamber music in small auditorium
84–111	Flute
85–114	Trombone
106	Timpani and bass drum rolls
120–137	Symphonic music peak
150	Rock music peak

Source: Adapted from HeadWize, www.headwise.com/articles/hearing_art.htm.

Table 10.5 OSHA Regulations 1910.95—Occupational Noise Exposure (Adapted)

Decibels	*Time*
90	8 hours
92	6 hours
95	4 hours
97	3 hours
100	2 hours
102	1.5 hours
105	1 hour
110	0.5 hour
115	0.25 hour or less

Note: When two or more periods of noise exposure occur, the combined effect should be considered rather than the individual effect of each. Exposure to impulse or impact noise should not exceed 140 dB peak sound pressure level.

Multicultural Considerations

The Gallaudet Research Institute has conducted an Annual Survey of Deaf and Hard-of-Hearing Children and Youth for more than 30 years. The survey represents the largest database of information on deaf and hard-of-hearing children in the United States (if not the world).

For more than 10 years, prematurity, heredity, and meningitis have been identified as the three primary causes of hearing loss across all racial and ethnic groups (Holden-Pitt & Diaz, 1998).

Over the years, there have been a disproportionate number of African American and Hispanic children who are born premature or develop meningitis. Research (Van Naarden & Decoufle, 1999) seems to show that African American children weighing less than 2500 grams (5.5 pounds) had much higher rates of hearing impairment than their Caucasian peers. In addition, the prevalence rates of hearing impairment for normal birth weight and borderline normal birth weight were higher for both male and female African American children than for Caucasian male and female children.

Differences have been found in the incidence of otitis media among racial groups, with American Indians and Alaskan Eskimos having the highest and African Americans having the lowest (National Center for Health Statistics, 1994). The differences may be attributed to the variations in structure and function of the Eustachian tubes among the various racial groups (Doyle, 1977; Spivey & Hirschhorn, 1977; Beery, Doyle, & Cantekin, 1980).

Differences in rates of hearing loss based on gender and race have been found in industrial noise-exposed populations. White males show the greatest effects of noise on auditory thresholds, followed by black males, white females, and then black females (Jerger et al., 1986). La Ferriere et al. (1974) found that in addition to more melanin (responsible for tissue pigmentation) content in the skin and eyes, individuals with darker skin have more melanin in their inner ear. The temporary threshold shift in hearing was inversely related to the skin pigmentation: the least pigmented subjects showed the greatest temporary threshold shift, and the most pigmented subjects showed the least shift (Barrenas & Lindgren, 1990). The hypothesis is that melanin in the inner ear may, in some unknown way, protect the ear from excessive noise. The National Center for Health Statistics (1994) and the National Institute of Deafness and Communication Disorders (2002) found that as hearing acuity declines with advancing age (presbycusis), white females have better hearing than white males, and both black males and females hear better than white male and female individuals. There is no explanation for these differences until further research can be done.

Socioeconomic status also plays a role in the incidence of hearing loss. In general, individuals with lower incomes (below $20,000 per year, i.e., "low-lower" income level) and less education (no high school diploma) are more likely to have a hearing loss than individuals with higher income (more than $50,000 per year, i.e., "low-middle" income level) and a high school diploma (National Council on Aging, 1999).

Neurophysiologic Intraoperative Monitoring

Neurophysiologic intraoperative monitoring involves continuous direct or indirect measurement and interpretation of myogenic and neural responses to intraoperative events or modality-specific, controlled stimulation in the course of surgery on or in the vicinity of those structures. The important aspect of intraoperative monitoring is the online moment-to-moment correlation between the changes in neurophysiologic responses and intraoperative events.

The principal objectives of neurophysiologic intraoperative monitoring are (1) to avoid intraoperative injury to neural structures, (2) to facilitate specific stages of the surgical procedure, (3) to reduce the risk of permanent postoperative neurological injury, and (4) to assist the surgeon in identifying specific neural structures (ASHA, 1992b).

Although neurophysiologic intraoperative monitoring is within the scope of practice of audiology, it requires knowledge and skills not routinely acquired during the academic preparation of most audiologists. Audiologists may acquire board certification through the American Audiology Board of Intraoperative Monitoring.

Balance (Vestibular) System Assessment

The clinical assessment process may include some or all of the following:

- *Electronystagmography (ENG):* Surface electrodes are placed around the eyes in order to record vestibular initiated eye movements (nystagmus), in particular the vestibular ocular reflex (VOR). These electrodes record changes in the electrical potential between the cornea and the retina, which are used to measure eye movement. Subtests of the ENG battery include tests of coordinated eye movement (saccadic eye movement, smooth pursuit eye movement, and optokinetic-induced eye movement) and tests for the presence of nystagmus under a variety of conditions (horizontal and vertical gaze, static head and body position change, and rapid position change). A physical stimulus, usually cool and warm water or air, is also presented to each in order to generate a VOR and determine the relative strength of response from each ear (bithermal caloric test).
- *Videonystagmography (VNG):* Most clinical vestibular laboratories no longer use surface electrode recording of eye movement, but rather employ newer, computerized, video-based recording techniques. The patient wears goggles that house an infrared camera. This camera sends a real-time video recording of the eyes to a computer where eye movement analysis is performed. This technology provides a more precise measurement of eye movement and also allows video storage for later analysis, consultation with colleagues, and teaching purposes. The subtests for VNG are the same as those for ENG assessment.
- *Rotary Chair:* Video technology is used to record eye movements in response to computer-controlled chair rotation around the Earth's vertical axis. This rotation provides stimulation of the vestibular system and produces a VOR, which is computer analyzed with regard to gain, phase, and symmetry.
- *Computerized Dynamic Posturography (CDP):* Postural stability can be assessed under simulated real-life conditions using dynamic force plate technology. The patient stands on a pressure-sensitive force plate, which measures lateral and vertical forces. This can be used to quantify postural sway under static and dynamic conditions. The Sensory Organization Test (SOT) isolates the principal components of balance (vestibular, visual, and somatosensory) and analyzes the patient's ability to use each alone and in combination in order to maintain standing posture. The Motor Control Test (MCT) evaluates a patient's ability to react to unpredictable surface perturbations (up, down, backward, and forward). CDP is helpful in evaluating patients with complaints of unsteadiness and disequilibrium, neurological or orthopedically compromised patients, or symptomatic patients with negative or equivocal findings on VNG/ENG assessment. It can also be used as a quantitative method for evaluating the efficacy of vestibular rehabilitation.
- *Vestibular-Evoked Myogenic Potentials (VEMPS):* Until recently, procedures for evaluating the vestibular system have focused on the semicircular canals, the part of the balance system which detects angular movement. There were no procedures to assess the otolithic system, which detects linear movement. In the early 1990s several research groups demonstrated a sound evoked modification in the activity of contracted muscles in the neck. This myogenic evoked potential has been shown to originate from the otolithic system and now enjoys widespread

use as a vestibular assessment tool. This same response can be recorded from the muscles around the eyes and is called the ocular vestibular evoked myogenic potential or OVEMP.

- *Video Head Impulse Test (VHIT):* The newest addition to the vestibular test battery is the VHIT. This procedure assesses eye movements produced by rapid head thrusts. It makes use of video-based recording and allows evaluation of all six semicircular canals, as opposed to the caloric test which only evaluates the horizontal canal. The addition of the VEMP and VHIT to the traditional vestibular test battery now allows assessment of the entire balance system.

Ototoxic Drug Therapy (Audiological Management)

Any drug with the potential to cause toxic reactions to structures of the inner ear, including the cochlea, vestibule, semicircular canals, and otoliths, is considered ototoxic (Govaerts et al., 1990). Drug-induced damage affecting the auditory and vestibular systems can be called, respectively, cochleotoxicity and vestibulotoxicity. Over 200 drugs have been labeled ototoxic (see list in Lien et al., 1983; Rybak, 1986; Govaerts et al., 1990). Different ototoxic drugs can cause either permanent or temporary structural damage of varying degree and reversibility (Brummett, 1980; Bendush, 1982). The actual frequency of occurrence of cochleotoxicity associated with specific drugs is unclear because of inconsistencies in reported data (Powell et al., 1983; Kopelman et al., 1988; Pasic & Dobie, 1991).

Permanent hearing loss or balance disorders caused by ototoxic drugs can have serious vocational, educational, and social consequences. These effects may be minimized or even prevented if the ototoxic process is detected early in treatment.

Although the role and responsibility for designing and implementing an auditory monitoring program for ototoxicity rest with the audiologist, the implementation and continuation of such a program require a collaborative effort between the audiologist, physician, and other medical center personnel. The relationship between ototoxicity and drug administration parameters such as dosage, duration of treatment, and serum concentration is highly variable (Barza & Lauermann, 1978; Schentag, 1980; Fausti et al., 1992, 1993). An attending physician, therefore, cannot rely solely on dosage or serum concentration to predict the risk of ototoxicity. The prospective assessment of hearing function remains the only reliable method for detecting the presence of cochleotoxicity prior to symptomatic hearing loss. Evidence suggests that high-frequency audiometry is the method of choice for the earliest detection of ototoxic hearing loss (Laukli & Mair, 1985; Fausti et al., 1990; Frank, 1990; Frank & Dreisbach, 1991; Valente et al., 1992).

The basic ototoxicity monitoring program requires the following (ASHA, 1994):

- Specific criteria for identification of toxicity
- Timely identification of at-risk patients
- Pretreatment counseling regarding potential cochleotoxic effects
- Valid baseline measures (pretreatment or early in treatment)
- Monitoring evaluations at sufficient intervals to document progression of hearing loss or fluctuation in sensitivity
- Follow-up evaluations to determine post-treatment effects

If ototoxic hearing loss results in a communication deficit, the audiologist will recommend audiological rehabilitation (including amplification if necessary), assistive listening devices, speech reading, and so on. Audiological rehabilitation management should begin as soon as possible after the hearing loss is identified.

Impact of Hearing Loss

Life care planners and other individuals should be aware of the impact that hearing loss, and particularly untreated hearing loss, can have. Hearing loss affects people differently, depending on the degree and type of loss, their personality type, the demands of their individual hearing environment and the type of intervention they receive. But there is almost always some negative impact associated with a hearing loss. This includes not only effects on the ability to communicate with others, but often more wide-ranging consequences, impacting physical functioning, quality of life, cognitive functioning and even mental health.

Impact on Communication

Generally, the effects of a conductive (outer or middle ear) hearing loss, which cannot be medically remediated, can be effectively eliminated by making sound louder. In a conductive hearing loss the inner ear is normal, so amplifying sound provides functionally normal hearing, in the same way that eyeglasses provide normal vision for most visual problems. It must be cautioned that young children commonly experience conductive hearing loss due to ear and upper respiratory infections. Although these episodes are usually self-limiting or respond to medical intervention when necessary, some children persist with conductive hearing loss, which may affect their speech and language development. These children should be referred to an audiologist as well as a speech-language pathologist.

An individual with a sensorineural (inner ear) hearing loss, however, can be expected to experience some degree of difficulty *understanding* speech, particularly when the listening environment is less than ideal. This means that when a person with a sensorineural hearing loss is greater than three to four feet from the source of the sound or when there is noise in the background (there almost always is *some* noise in the background), that person will likely misunderstand some of what is being said. This is because the pattern of hearing with a sensorineural hearing loss is typically worse in the high frequencies or pitches and better in the low frequencies or pitches. In order to understand speech clearly, we must hear all the pitches equally well. The vowels are generally low in pitch (and loud) compared to consonants, which are high in pitch (and soft). Also, damage to sensory cells and nerve fibers create more than just loudness loss. There are varying degrees of distortion present in the damaged ear that cannot be overcome by simply raising the volume.

A properly fitted hearing aid can be extremely beneficial. However, it is important for all to recognize that even with appropriate amplification, individuals with sensorineural hearing loss will still frequently have difficulty understanding what is being said, particularly with noise in the background.

Impact on Physical Functioning

Recent research studies have examined the potential functional consequences of hearing loss (Lin & Ferrucci, 2012, Jiam et al., 2016). Hearing loss has been shown to be associated with increased fall risk in the elderly. Since the peripheral organs for hearing and balance share space in the cochlear, diseases affecting one may affect the other. Hearing loss has been shown to affect spatial orientation and postural stability in the elderly and may contribute to an increased fall risk (Viljanen et al.,

2009). When people have trouble hearing, they have to spend more energy to understand what is coming from their ears. Older people also have less functional reserve that they can allocate to this task. As a result, they can have trouble dealing with a separate but simultaneous task, such as walking or dealing with a sudden obstacle (Ferrucci & Studenski, 2011). Several studies suggest that hearing aid use may improve postural stability and by inference may reduce risk of falls (Lacerda et al., 2012; Rumalla et al., 2015).

Impact on Cognitive Functioning

Accumulating research evidence points to a link between age related hearing loss and cognitive decline (Waye & Johnsrude, 2015). Several possible mechanisms have been offered. The information-degradation hypothesis suggests that higher level cognitive processes suffer when more mental resources are used in order to deal with impaired perception, such as hearing loss. The sensory-deprivation hypothesis implies these perceptual changes may cause permanent cognitive declines through neuroplastic changes as a result of long-term sensory deprivation. These changes may disadvantage general cognition in favor of processes supporting speech perception (Lin et al., 2013).

Impact on Quality of Life

Hearing loss has also been associated with social isolation and poor perceived quality of life. Weinstein and Ventry (1982) found that people who were socially isolated had a greater self-perceived hearing disability, worse auditory processing difficulties, and poorer hearing. The people who were most subjectively and most objectively isolated were the ones with the worst-measured hearing, the greatest self-perceived hearing disability, and the most challenges in auditory processing. A more recent study analyzed results of 50 studies in the literature which compared quality of life of the hearing impaired and non-hearing impaired (Ciorba et al., 2012). For non-hearing impaired individuals, 68 percent rated their quality of life as excellent as compared to only 39 percent of the individuals with hearing loss.

Impact on Mental Health

The literature shows a relationship between hearing loss and depression. A 2010 meta-analysis reviewed the results of 31 studies published between 1997 and 2007 in order to determine the association between chronic disease and depression in old age (Chang-Quan et al., 2010). Seven of these studies compared poor hearing with good hearing individuals. Results showed that poor hearing is an important risk factor for depression. In a study from Canada, MacDonald (2011) found a strong relationship between self-reported hearing problems and depression. Saito et al. (2010), in a study conducted in Japan, found that the odds of depressive symptoms were high in people with self-reported hearing disability as compared to those without hearing disability. Gopinath et al. (2012) also found an independent association between hearing disability and the presence of depressive symptoms.

Audiological (Aural) Rehabilitation Assessment

Audiological rehabilitation assessment evaluates and describes the receptive and expressive communication skills of individuals with a hearing loss or related hearing disorders. Individuals of all ages are assessed on the basis of results from the audiological assessment, hearing aid or assistive system/device assessment, fitting, or orientation; sensory aid assessment; and assessment of communication needs or preferences.

The assessment includes an evaluation of the impact of the loss of hearing on the individual and his/her family/caregiver. The assessment may result in the development of a culturally appropriate audiological rehabilitation management plan, including, when appropriate (ASHA, 2006):

- Fitting and dispensing recommendations, and educating the consumer and family/caregivers in the use of and adjustment to sensory aids, hearing assistive devices, alerting systems, and captioning devices
- Counseling relating to psychosocial aspects of hearing loss and processes to enhance communication competence
- Skills training and consultation concerning environmental modifications to facilitate development of receptive and expressive communication
- Evaluation and modification of the audiological management plan

Audiological (Aural) Rehabilitation Management

Audiological rehabilitation is provided to persons of all ages who have any degree or type of hearing loss on the basis of the results of the audiological rehabilitation assessment. Audiological rehabilitation facilitates receptive and expressive communication of individuals with a hearing loss or related hearing disorders, and results in achievement of improved, altered, augmented, or compensated communication processes. Performance in both clinical and natural environments is considered. The family/caregiver plays an integral part in the rehabilitation process.

Short- and long-term functional communication goals and specific objectives are determined from assessment and direct the framework for treatment. They are reviewed periodically to determine continued relevance and appropriateness.

When it comes to dealing with hearing loss, some think that simply obtaining hearing aids or other listening devices is the rehabilitation. Audiological rehabilitation, however, is a much broader concept. It focuses on reducing difficulties related to hearing loss and listening. The overall goal is to maximize communication success in everyday environments and situations.

Audiological rehabilitation services may include the following:

- Learning how to listen
- Learning how hearing loss affects speech
- Learning skills in speech reading (lip reading, facial expression, gestures, body language)
- Building confidence in handling communication situations
- Learning what to do when you do not get the message
- Learning how to use your hearing aids or cochlear implant
- Learning about different kinds of technology to improve communication
- Learning how to advocate for yourself
- Learning what your rights are under various laws
- Promoting family and caregiver understanding and support of your needs
- Learning how you can make it easier for your family to communicate with you

Audiologists and speech-language pathologists often collaborate in delivering aural rehabilitation services. Depending on the patient's particular need, one or the other professionals may take a lead.

For example, the audiologist:

- Would be responsible for fitting and dispensing hearing aids, sensory aids, and assistive listening devices, and training you how to use them
- Can provide counseling about your hearing loss and processes to enhance communication
- Can provide skills training concerning environmental modifications to facilitate development of receptive and expressive communication
- Can conduct aural rehabilitation assessment and design a management plan

The speech-language pathologist:

- Would be responsible for evaluating receptive and expressive communication skills and providing services to develop or improve receptive and expressive communication
- Can provide treatment focusing on comprehension of language in oral, signed, or written modes
- Can provide treatment dealing with speech and voice production
- Can provide treatment such as auditory training and speech reading
- Can provide training in communication strategies (https://www.asha.org/Practice-Portal/Professional-Issues/Aural-Rehabilitation-for-Adults/)

Audiological (Re)habilitation for Children

Specific services for children depend on individual needs as dictated by the current age of the child, the age of onset of the hearing loss, the age at which the hearing loss was discovered, the severity of the hearing loss, the type of hearing loss, the extent of hearing loss, and the age at which amplification was introduced. The audiological rehabilitation plan is also influenced by the communication mode the child is using. Examples of communication modes are speaking/listening/looking, cued speech, manually coded English, total communication, auditory-oral, auditory-verbal, and American Sign Language.

The most debilitating consequence of onset of hearing loss in childhood is its disruption in learning speech and language. The combination of early detection of hearing loss and early use of amplification has been shown to have a dramatically positive effect on the language acquisition abilities of a child with hearing loss. In fact, infants identified with a hearing loss by 6 months can be expected to attain language development on a par with hearing peers if appropriately managed.

Audiological habilitation/rehabilitation services for children typically involve the following in addition to selection and fitting of appropriate amplification:

- *Training in auditory perception.* This includes activities to increase awareness of sound, identify sounds, tell the difference between sounds (sound discrimination), and attach meaning to sounds. Ultimately, this training increases the child's ability to distinguish one word from another using any remaining hearing. Auditory perception also includes developing skills in hearing with hearing aids and assistive listening devices and in how to handle easy and difficult listening situations.
- *Using visual cues.* This goes beyond distinguishing sounds and words on the lips. It involves using all kinds of visual cues that give meaning to a message such as the speaker's facial expression, body language, and the context and environment in which the communication is taking place.

- *Improving speech.* This involves skill development in production of speech sounds (by themselves, in words, and in conversation), voice quality, speaking rate, breath control, loudness, and speech rhythms.
- *Developing language.* This involves developing language understanding (reception) and language usage (expression) according to developmental expectations. It is a complex process involving concepts, vocabulary, world knowledge, use in different social situations, narrative skills, expression through writing, understanding rules of grammar, and so on.
- *Managing communication.* This involves the child's understanding the hearing loss, developing assertiveness skills to use in different listening situations, handling communication breakdowns, and modifying situations to make communication easier.
- *Managing hearing aids and assistive listening devices.* Because children are fitted with hearing aids at young ages, early care and adjustment are done by family members or caregivers. It is important for children to participate in hearing aid care and management as much as possible. As they grow and develop, the goal is for their own adjustment, cleaning, and troubleshooting of the hearing aid and, ultimately, taking over responsibility for making appointments with service providers.

Services for children occur in the contexts of early intervention (ages birth to 3) and school services (ages 3–21) through the Individuals with Disabilities Education Act (IDEA). In early intervention, an individualized family service plan (IFSP) is developed and may include audiology services, speech-language pathology services, the services of teachers of the deaf and hard-of-hearing, and the services of other professionals as needed. When the child turns three, an individualized education program (IEP) is developed. The services provided are designed to maximize the child's success in the general education environment. Again, the IEP may specify audiology services, speech-language pathology services, and the services of teachers of the deaf and hard-of-hearing. Each professional has a role to play in the child's educational achievement and success.

Assistive Listening Devices (ALDs)

An ALD is any type of device that can help a person function better in day-to-day communication situations. An ALD can be used with or without hearing aids to overcome the negative effects of *distance* (sound fades as distance increases, or speech may become unintelligible for someone with a hearing impairment), *background noise* (classrooms and meeting areas tend to be noisy, and noise can come from within the room, such as heating and cooling, or from outside the room, such as hallways and traffic), and *poor room acoustics* (reverberation: sound waves reflect off walls and hit other walls repeatedly, and multiple reflection/reverberation disrupts speech understanding by causing echoes). So even though a patient has a hearing aid, assistive listening devices can offer greater ease of hearing (and therefore reduced stress and fatigue) in many day-to-day communication situations (https://www.asha.org/public/hearing/Hearing-Assistive-Technology/).

Examples of ALDs include the following:

- *Personal frequency-modulated (FM) systems* are like a miniature radio station operating on special frequencies assigned by the Federal Communications Commission. The personal FM system consists of a transmitter microphone used by the speaker and a receiver used by you, the listener. The receiver transmits the sound to your hearing aid either through direct audio input or through a looped cord worn around your neck. A personal FM system does not require any wire so mobility is greatly enhanced. FM systems/auditory trainers have been standard equipment for children with hearing loss in educational settings for many years. Audiologists are the uniquely qualified professionals to select, evaluate, fit, and dispense FM systems. Before selecting an FM system for personal use, it is necessary to assess auditory capacity and the current level of auditory and communication function and to identify other factors related to device use. The issue of potential damage to the auditory mechanism should be considered when fitting any assistive listening device. This is of special concern when considering the fitting of a self-contained FM system to a person with near-normal hearing, mild hearing loss, or fluctuating hearing loss (ASHA, 2002). All amplification equipment is subject to failure; therefore, daily monitoring is required (Bess, 1988). Periodic comprehensive monitoring of the FM system by the audiologist includes electroacoustic analysis, probe microphone measurements, and other in-depth troubleshooting measures. In addition, the periodic assessments of hearing and of performance with the FM device are necessary to monitor stability of hearing, appropriate device settings, function, and degree of benefit. The evaluations should be performed at least annually for adults and children 5 years of age and older. For children under 5 years of age and for individuals with fluctuating or conductive hearing loss, the follow-up evaluations should be much more frequent.

If a self-contained FM system is going to be used, decisions must be made relative to the gain, frequency response, input/output functions, and saturation sound pressure level requirements for the individual listener. During the preselection process, assessments may include, but are not limited to, audiological assessment, observation of auditory performance in representative settings, consultation with the user or others knowledgeable about the user's performance, questionnaires and scales, hands-on demonstration, and a trial period. Other factors to be considered in the preselection process include the following (ASHA, 2002):

- The person's ability to wear, adjust, and manage the device
- Support available in the educational setting (e.g., in-service to teachers, classmates)
- Acceptance of the device
- Appropriate situations and settings for use
- Time schedule for use
- Compatibility with personal hearing aids and other audio sources (such as cell phones), as well as options for coupling
- Individual device characteristics and accessories
- External source interference (e.g., pagers, radio stations, computers, etc.)
- Cost and accessibility
- Legislative mandates

Personal FM systems are useful in a variety of situations such as listening to a travel guide, in a classroom lecture, in a restaurant, in a sales meeting, to a book review, in nursing homes, in senior centers, and so on. Personal FM systems are also especially useful for children with auditory processing disorders (or ADD/ADHD) who are distracted by classroom noise or other background noise. The teacher wears the microphone, taking the sound of her voice directly into the child's ears.

FM systems are also used in theaters, places of worship, museums, public meeting places, corporate conference rooms, convention centers, and other large areas for gathering. In this situation, the microphone/transmitter is built into the overall sound system. Patients are provided with an FM receiver that can connect to their hearing aid or to a headset.

- *Infrared systems* are often used in the home with TV sets. They, like the FM system, are also used in large-area settings like theaters. Sound is transmitted using infrared light waves. The TV is set at a volume comfortable for family members. The infrared system transmitter transmits the TV signal to the receiver, which can be adjusted to a desired volume. Thus, TV watching as a family becomes pleasurable for all. It is not blaring for family members with normal hearing.
- *Induction loop systems* are most common in large-group areas. They can also be purchased for individual use. An induction loop wire is permanently installed (perhaps under a carpet) and connects to a microphone used by a speaker. (In the case of individual systems, a wire loop is laid on the floor around the listener and the speaker.) The person talking into the microphone creates a current in the wire that makes an electromagnetic field in the room. When the patient switches his/her hearing aid to the T (telecoil/telephone) setting, the hearing aid telecoil picks up the electromagnetic signal and the patient can adjust its volume through the hearing aid.
- *One-to-one communicators* are sometimes used in a restaurant, a nursing home, or when riding in a car, when the patient wants to be able to easily hear one person. Or perhaps she is delivering a lecture or running a meeting and a person in the audience has a question. The person with the question is given a microphone to speak into. The sound is amplified and delivered directly into the speaker's hearing aid (or headset if she does not have a hearing aid), and the speaker can adjust the volume to her comfort level. When using the one-to-one communicator, the speaker does not have to shout, private conversations can remain private, and, when in a car, her eyes can remain on the road.
- *Personal sound amplification products or PSAPs* are a relatively new category of assistive listening devices. A PSAP is an electronic device that is worn behind the ear or inside the ear. Although it looks similar to a hearing aid it is not considered a hearing aid and is intended to provide amplification to help normal hearing individuals in unfavorable listening situations. PSAPs are not intended to compensate for hearing loss and are not regulated by the FDA. These devices are readily available online and over the counter, and often sell for considerably less than conventional hearing aids. However, they generally amplify all sound and lack the programing flexibility of hearing aids. PSAPs may be good for individuals with mild hearing loss and for those who need amplification but are not ready to commit to purchasing hearing aids.
- There are many other assistive listening devices such as telephone amplifying devices for cordless, cell, digital, and wired phones; amplified answering machines; amplified telephones with different frequency responses; paging systems; computers; wake-up alarms; and so on.
- There are also *alerting devices* that signal when a sound occurs. For example, there are doorbell, knock-at-the-door, or phone-alerting devices; fire alarm/smoke alarm devices; baby-cry devices or room-to-room sound alerting systems; vibrating clock alarms; vibrating paging systems; vibrating watch alarms; and so on. Many use strobe light or conventional light to alert; others use vibrating systems to alert.
- There are other assistive listening devices such as closed captioning, a device for an individual with a hearing impairment used to provide written text to match spoken words on a TV program (Fogle, 2008). A telephone text (TTY) transmits text messages through the telephone line. A telecommunication device (TDD) has a visual display of typed messages

over the phone, available also for printed messages. Text messaging through the cellular phone is easy, convenient, and gaining in popularity.

Hearing Aid Selection and Fitting

Myth: Hearing aids restore hearing to normal just as an eyeglass prescription can restore vision to 20/20.

Fact: Hearing aids do not restore hearing to normal. Just as eyeglasses do not cure vision problems, hearing aids do not cure hearing loss. Like eyeglasses, hearing aids provide benefit and improvement. They can improve hearing and listening abilities, and they can substantially improve quality of life.

Any individual who subjectively reports and audiometrically demonstrates hearing loss of a degree that interferes with communication should be considered for fitting with amplification. The clinical process is initially the same as that for a basic audiological assessment. The complete audiological assessment and needs assessment is necessary to initiate a treatment plan that may include amplification. The process of the hearing aid selection in conjunction with determination of the treatment plan is necessary prior to initiating the selection regimen. The Food and Drug Administration (FDA) regulates the conditions for sale of medical devices, including hearing aids, and requires a recent medical clearance by a licensed physician prior to purchase of a hearing aid. The medical clearance can be waived if the prospective hearing aid user is over 18 years of age.

Prior to hearing aid selection and fitting the patient must be counseled regarding the potential benefits and limitations associated with personal amplification. The fitting of a personal amplification system and verification of its appropriateness for the communication needs of the patient, family, and caregiver are necessary requisites. There must be validation of the benefit to and satisfaction of the patient, family, and caregiver. In many cases it is necessary to demonstrate a support system is in place to assist in maximizing the use and maintenance of the personal amplification system. The clinical decision-making process is based on professional judgment and individual patient characteristics that may significantly influence the nature and course of the selection and fitting process. The process may vary by audiologist and may vary based on the patient needs, cooperation, comprehension, and process setting. The following procedures require the completion of an audiological assessment within the prior 6 months. (Most audiologists will require their own assessment at the time of the hearing aid selection process.)

The audiological clinical process may include, but is not necessarily limited to, the following (AJA, 1998, ASHA, 1999) (the components are not designed to be all-inclusive):

- Recent history of auditory function
- Appropriate physical examination (e.g., otoscopy)
- Cerumen (ear wax) management
- Suprathreshold loudness measurements
- Ear impressions
- Hearing aid selection procedure
- Hearing aid performance verification in 2 cc coupler and in the real ear for quality control
- Individual or group orientation to amplification
- Unaided/aided communication inventory

- Individual or group hearing aid follow-up
- Qualitative assessment of amplification
- Measurement of satisfaction and benefit
- Unaided and aided speech recognition measures

Hearing aids differ in design, size, the amount of amplification, ease of handling, volume control, and the availability of special features. But they do have similar components, which include:

- A microphone to pick up sound
- Amplifier circuitry to make the sound louder
- A receiver (miniature loudspeaker) to deliver the amplified sound into the ear
- Batteries to power the electronic parts

Some hearing aids also require ear molds (earpieces) to direct the flow of sound into the ear. These ear molds are most often custom made and may require periodic replacement.

Styles of Hearing Aids

In-the-canal (ITC) and *completely-in-the-canal* (CIC) aids are contained in a tiny case that fits partly or completely into the ear canal. They are the smallest aids available and offer cosmetic and some listening advantages.

All parts of *in-the-ear* (ITE) aids are contained in a shell that fills in the outer part of the ear. These aids are larger than canal aids and, for some people, may be easier to handle than smaller aids.

All parts of *behind-the-ear* (BTE) aids are contained in a small plastic case that rests behind the ear; the case is connected to an ear mold by a piece of clear tubing. This style is often chosen for young children for safety and growth reasons.

Contralateral Routing of Signal (CROS) hearing aids are used for patients with one unaidable ear, due to the severity of loss, and one normal hearing ear on the contralateral side. A microphone is placed at the ear level of the "bad" side and the signal picked up by this microphone is "routed" (either through hardwire or an FM transmitter) to the receiver in the ear level hearing aid on the "good" or normal ear. If the better ear also has a hearing loss, the arrangement is called BICROS, indicating that a microphone and an amplifier are also placed on the side of the better ear.

Types of Hearing Aids

Regardless of the style, hearing aids can also be differentiated by the type of technology or circuitry used. In the early days, hearing aid technology involved vacuum tubes and large, heavy batteries. Today, microchips, computerization, and digitized sound processing are used in hearing aid design.

- *Conventional analog hearing aids* are designed with a particular frequency response based on your audiogram. The audiologist tells the manufacturer what settings to install. Although there are some adjustments, the aid essentially amplifies all sounds (speech and noise) in the same way. This technology is the least expensive, and it can be appropriate for many different types of hearing loss.
- *Analog programmable hearing aids* have a microchip that allows the aid to have settings programmed for different listening environments such as quiet conversation in your home,

noisy situations like a restaurant, or large areas like a theater. The audiologist uses a computer to program the hearing aid for different listening situations depending on the individual hearing loss profile, speech understanding, and range of tolerance for louder sounds.

- Some aids can store several programs. As the listening environment changes, a wearer can change the hearing aid settings by pushing a button on the hearing aid or by using a remote control to switch channels. The aid can be reprogrammed by the audiologist if hearing or hearing needs change. These aids are more expensive than conventional analog hearing aids, but generally have a longer life span and may provide better hearing in different listening situations.
- *Digital programmable hearing aids* have all the features of analog programmable aids but use digitized sound processing to convert sound waves into digital signals. A computer chip in the aid analyzes the signals of your environment to determine if the sound is noise or speech and then makes modifications to provide a clear, amplified distortion-free signal. Digital hearing aids are usually self-adjusting. The digital processing allows for more flexibility in programming the aid so that the sound it transmits matches a specific pattern of hearing loss. This digital technology is the most expensive, but it allows for improvement in programmability, greater precision in fitting, management of loudness discomfort, control of acoustic feedback (whistling sounds), and noise reduction.

Special Features for Hearing Aids

Many hearing aids have optional features that can be built in to assist in different communication situations. Some options are

- *Directional microphone.* Some hearing aids have a switch to activate a directional microphone that responds to sound coming from a specific direction, as occurs in a face-to-face conversation. A patient can switch from the normal nondirectional (omnidirectional) setting, which picks up sound almost equally from any direction, to focus on a sound coming from in front. When the directional microphone is activated, sound coming from behind is reduced.
- *Telephone switch.* Some hearing aids are made with an induction coil inside. You can switch from the normal microphone "on" setting to a "T" setting to hear better on the telephone. (All wired telephones produced today must be hearing aid compatible.) In the T setting, environment sounds are eliminated, and the patient only picks up sound from the telephone. Furthermore, the person can talk without the hearing aid "whistling" because the microphone of the hearing aid is turned off.
- The T setting can also be used in theaters, auditoriums, houses of worship, and so on, that have induction loop or FM installations. The sound of the talker, who can be a distance away, is amplified significantly more than any background noises. Some hearing aids have a combination M (microphone)/T (telephone) switch so that while listening with an induction loop, the wearers can still hear nearby conversation.
- *Direct audio input.* Some hearing aids have a direct-audio-input capability that allows them to plug in a remote microphone or an FM assistive listening system, connect directly to a TV, or connect with other devices such as a computer, CD player, tape player, radio, and so on (https://www.asha.org/public/hearing/Features-Available-in-Hearing-Aids/).

Advances in digital signal processing in recent years have paved the way for digital hearing aids to become the standard of current audiological practice. The current emphasis for research and development is on specific features such as directional technology and digital noise reduction to maximize speech understanding and sound quality. The introduction of digital noise reduction (DNR) has provided greater ease of listening for many hearing-impaired individuals based on subjective measures. The challenge remains to develop algorithms that separate speech from noise. Notable technological developments are also being made in the field of implantable hearing devices.

Implantable Hearing Devices

For the vast majority of hearing impaired individuals successful aural rehabilitation includes the fitting of a personal hearing aid of a type previously described. However, for a small segment of the hearing impaired population, the degree of hearing loss and/or the presence of certain ear anomalies may preclude the use of a traditional hearing aid. For these individuals an implantable hearing device such as a cochlear implant, a brain stem implant, or a bone anchored hearing device may be indicated.

Cochlear Implants

For profound hearing loss, conventional hearing aids may not have sufficient gain to make sound audible. In these cases electrical stimulation of the auditory nerve by electrodes implanted in the cochlear can produce sound awareness. With time and training this can lead to speech understanding.

Cochlear implants have external (outside) and internal (surgically implanted) parts. The *external parts* include a microphone, a speech processor, and a transmitter. The *microphone* looks like a behind-the-ear hearing aid. It picks up sounds—just like a hearing aid microphone does—and sends them to the speech processor. The *speech processor* may be housed, with the microphone, behind the ear, or it may be a small box worn in a chest pocket. The speech processor is a computer that analyzes and digitizes the sound signals and sends them to a transmitter worn on the head just behind the ear. The *transmitter* sends the coded signals to an implanted receiver just under the skin.

The *internal (implanted) parts* include a receiver and electrodes. The *receiver* is just under the skin behind the ear. The receiver takes the coded electrical signals from the transmitter and delivers them to the array of electrodes that have been surgically inserted into the cochlea. The *electrodes* stimulate the fibers of the auditory nerve, and sound sensations are perceived (https://www.asha.org/public/hearing/Cochlear-Implant/).

As of December 2012, approximately 324,200 registered devices have been implanted worldwide. In the United States, roughly 58,000 devices have been implanted in adults and 38,000 in children (NIDCD, 2016). Cochlear implants may be indicated for individuals who are profoundly hearing impaired or deaf due to genetic factors, ototoxic drugs, meningitis, rubella, and head trauma. A criterion for candidacy (Table 10.6) primarily requires that the auditory nerve must not be destroyed. General guidelines include the following:

- Be at least one year of age (with anticipation of even younger in near future).
- Have severe to profound bilateral sensorineural deafness.
- Demonstrate no significant benefit from traditional amplification.
- Have strong family support.
- Have no medical contraindications to surgery.

Table 10.6 Cochlear Implant Candidacy Criteria

Young children: 12 months to 2 years
Profound sensorineural hearing loss (nerve deafness) in both ears
Lack of progress in development of auditory skill with hearing aid or other amplification
High motivation and realistic expectations from family
Other medical conditions, if present, do not interfere with cochlear implant procedure
Children: 2–17 years
Severe-to-profound sensorineural hearing loss (nerve deafness) in both ears
Receive little or no benefit from hearing aids
Lack of progress in the development of auditory skills
High motivation and realistic expectations from family
Adults: 18 years and over
Severe to profound sensorineural hearing loss in both ears
Receive little or no useful benefit from hearing aids
Qualified candidates are those scoring, with a hearing aid, 50 percent or less on sentence recognition tests in the ear to be implanted and 60 percent or less in the nonimplanted ear or bilaterally.

Source: From Cochlear Nucleus website (http://www.cochlearamericas.com).

- For children, have a supportive school system.
- For adults, have appropriate expectations.
- Have the ability to pay for the device and services—the total cost of an implant in 2008 was more than $60,000 and, in 2017, can be as much as $100,000 (see http://www.entnet.org/content/cochlearimplants), not including replacements (see example case in the following). However, some insurance companies and Medicare/Medicaid may pay (see https://www.cochlear.com/us/home/take-the-next-step/insurance-resource-center).

Cochlear Implant Centers

There are various cochlear implant centers around the country. Teams of professionals work together with adults and children from start to finish. Team members include an audiologist, otologist/surgeon, medical specialists as needed, psychologist, counselors, and speech-language pathologists. They work with potential candidates and their families to determine candidacy for an implant, perform the surgery, and provide follow-up care both through the center and through local agencies or school districts near the cochlear implant recipient.

The Clinical Process

Once a person is referred to the cochlear implant center, extensive testing is done to determine if the person is a suitable candidate. This evaluation usually includes extensive audiological testing, psychological testing, examination and tests performed by the surgeon, X-rays, magnetic resonance images, physical examination, and counseling to assure suitability and motivation to participate in the process. It is important that the candidate understands what the implant will and will not do and the commitment required for care and follow-up services.

Once the decision is made to go ahead, the surgery is done. Sometimes it involves an overnight stay in the hospital, and sometimes it is done on an outpatient basis.

About four to six weeks after surgery, the person returns to the center to be fitted with the microphone and speech processor and to activate and program (called *mapping*) the implant. The initial fitting process is done over several days and may include additional visits over several months, because as each electrode in the cochlea is activated, it must be adjusted and programmed into the speech processor. As the person develops skill in using the implant, further adjustments and reprogramming are required. Once the optimum program is obtained, fewer visits are required. Usually there are annual visits to the center for checkups.

Both children and adults are involved in extensive rehabilitation services from an audiologist, speech-language pathologist, teachers, and counselors as they learn to listen, improve speech, use speech reading, and handle communication. They are taught how to use the implant and how to respond to the sounds they are receiving. If one has heard before, sounds through the cochlear implant may seem unnatural at first. If a person has never heard, they must be taught what the sounds are.

Brain Stem Implants

If the cochlear is congenitally absent or severely damaged by disease, or if the auditory nerve is damaged during surgery to remove a tumor, a cochlear implant is of no value. In these rare cases of profound deafness, an auditory brain stem implant may be indicated. The auditory brain stem implant uses technology similar to that of the cochlear implant, but instead of electrical stimulation being used to stimulate the cochlea, it is used to stimulate the brain stem.

Bone Anchored Hearing Devices

Bone anchored devices are used to help people with chronic ear infections, congenital external auditory canal atresia, and single sided deafness who cannot benefit from conventional hearing aids. The system is surgically implanted and allows sound to be conducted through the bone rather than via the middle ear—a process known as direct bone conduction. The bone anchored device consists of three parts: a titanium implant, an external abutment, and a sound processor. The system works by enhancing natural bone transmission as a pathway for sound to travel to the inner ear, bypassing the external auditory canal and middle ear. The titanium implant is placed during a short surgical procedure and over time naturally integrates with the skull bone. For hearing, the sound processor transmits sound vibrations through the external abutment to the titanium implant. The vibrating implant sets up vibrations within the skull and inner ear that finally stimulate the nerve fibers of the inner ear, allowing hearing.

Auditory Processing Disorders Assessment (as Performed by an Audiologist)

Auditory processing disorders (APDs) is the current terminology for what was referred to in earlier literature as central auditory processing disorders (CAPDs). With current research and improved diagnostic tools, we now know that not all APDs can be related to a central origin. An APD assessment helps to define the functional status of the central auditory nervous system (CANS) and central auditory processes.

The assessment is indicated for individuals of all ages who have symptoms or complaints of hearing difficulty with documented normal peripheral auditory function, have a central nervous system (CNS) disorder potentially affecting the central auditory system, or have learning problems possibly related to the auditory difficulties. The APD assessment requires a team approach and is to be conducted with other audiological, speech, and language tests, as well as neuropsychological tests, to evaluate the overall communication behavior, including spoken language processing and production, and educational achievement of the individual (ASHA, 1999).

ASHA (1996) in the *American Journal of Audiology* defined (central) APDs as a problem in one or more of six areas:

1. Sound localization and lateralization (knowing where in space a sound source is located)
2. Auditory discrimination (usually with reference to speech, but the ability to tell that one sound is different from another)
3. Auditory pattern recognition (musical rhythms are one example of an auditory pattern)
4. Temporal aspects of audition (auditory processing relies on making fine discriminations of timing changes in auditory input, especially differences in timing by the way input comes through one ear as opposed to the other)
5. Auditory performance decrements with competing acoustic signals (listening in noise)
6. Auditory performance decrements with degraded acoustic signals (listening to sounds that are muffled, missing information, or for some reason not clear—the best example is trying to listen to speech taking place on the other side of a wall; the wall filters or blocks out certain parts of the speech signal, but a typical listener can often understand the conversation)

The interpretation of results is derived for multiple tests; there is no single test to determine the presence of an APD. The APD battery of tests may involve a series of appointments over a period of time. The test results will be measured against age-appropriate norms and knowledge of the CANS in normal and disordered states. The procedures in an APD battery should be viewed as separate entities for purposes of service delivery and reimbursement.

The clinical process is as follows:

- Appropriate communication, medical, and educational history is taken.
- Assessment is typically part of an interdisciplinary (audiology and speech-language pathology) approach.
- Assessment of peripheral hearing sensitivity to assure normal hearing sensitivity.
- Patient is prepared for behavioral and electrophysiological assessment of the CANS.
- Types of central auditory behavioral tests include:
  - Tests of temporal processes
  - Tests of dichotic listening
  - Low redundancy monaural speech tests
  - Tests of binaural interaction
- Central auditory electrophysiological tests include:
  - Auditory brain stem response (ABR)
  - Middle latency evoked response (MLR)
  - N1 and P2 (late potentials) responses (P300)
  - Mismatched negativity (MMN)

- Middle ear reflex
- Crossed suppression of otoacoustic emissions

APDs Management (as Performed by an Audiologist)

The comprehensive rehabilitation and management of APDs may include interventions directed to acoustic signal enhancement, improvement of language and cognitive capacities, skills development, use of compensatory strategies, employment of listening strategies, and improvement of the listening environment (ASHA, 1990, 1996). Management (treatment) is conducted to improve auditory processing, listening, spoken language processing, and the overall communication process. Improvements in auditory processing and listening can benefit learning and daily living activities.

APD management is recommended when there is a likelihood of improving communication behavior in any age group. Any individual who is documented to have an APD after completion of the APD test battery, and who is impaired or compromised on the basis of the results, is a candidate for management (treatment). Generalization of skills and strategies is enhanced by extending practice to the natural environment through collaboration among key professionals (ASHA, 1999).

The clinical process may be, but is not limited to, the following (ASHA, 1999):

- A treatment plan is formulated based on the patient's complaints, symptoms, history, central auditory test results, and functional performance deficits.
- Treatment may be conducted in an interdisciplinary (audiology and speech-language pathology) and interdisciplinary manner.
- The treatment plan should incorporate several major approaches:
  - Auditory training and stimulation
  - Communication and educational strategies
  - Metalinguistic and metacognitive skills and strategies
  - Assistive listening devices
  - Acoustic enhancement and environmental modifications of the listening environment

Tinnitus Management

Tinnitus, more commonly spoken of as ringing in the ear or head noise, has been experienced by almost everyone at one time or another. It is defined as the perception of sound in the head when no external sound is present. In addition to ringing, head noises have been described as hissing, roaring, pulsing, whooshing, chirping, whistling, and clicking. Ringing and head noises can occur in one ear or both ears and can be perceived to be occurring inside or outside the ear. Tinnitus can accompany hearing loss. It can exist independent of a hearing loss.

Tinnitus cannot be measured objectively. Rather, the audiologist relies on information provided in describing the tinnitus. The audiologist will ask questions like:

- Which ear is involved? Right? Left? Both?
- Is the ringing constant? Do you notice it more at certain times of the day?
- Can you describe the sound or the ringing?
- Does the sound have a pitch to it? High pitch? Low pitch?

- How loud does it seem? Does it seem loud or soft?
- Does the sound change or fluctuate?
- Do you notice conditions that make the tinnitus worse (e.g., when drinking caffeinated beverages, when taking particular medicines, or after exposure to noise)?
- Does the tinnitus affect your sleep? Your work? Your ability to concentrate?
- How annoying is it? Extremely so? Not terribly bothersome?

Knowing the cause of tinnitus is a relief, instead of having to live with the uncertainty of the condition. When tinnitus is demystified, stress level (which can make tinnitus worse) is frequently reduced, and there is a feeling of greater control.

The most effective treatment for tinnitus is to eliminate the underlying cause. Because tinnitus can be a symptom of a treatable medical condition, medical or surgical treatment can take place to correct the tinnitus.

Unfortunately, in many cases the cause of tinnitus cannot be identified, or medical or surgical treatment is not the appropriate course of action. In these cases, the tinnitus itself may need to be treated.

Drug therapy, vitamin therapy, biofeedback, hypnosis, electrical stimulation, relaxation therapy, counseling, habituation therapies, and tinnitus maskers are among many forms of management available. Audiologists and otolaryngologists routinely collaborate in identifying the cause and providing treatment. A treatment that is useful and successful for one person may not be appropriate for another.

Nonmedical management of tinnitus has traditionally involved masking or covering up the patient's internally produced head noises with externally generated sound. This can take the form of enhanced environmental sound provided by traditional hearing aids, since most patients with handicapping tinnitus also have hearing loss. If there is no hearing loss, or if hearing aid use is not appropriate, a tinnitus instrument, similar in appearance to a hearing aid, can be used to provide a masking sound. The particulars of the masking sound used will vary according to information provided by the patient, such as the loudness, pitch, and quality of the tinnitus. Treatment protocols for tinnitus involve habituation to rather than covering up of the tinnitus. This is known as Tinnitus Retraining Therapy (Jastreboff, 1996). This treatment approach involves directive counseling designed to remove negative associations attached to the tinnitus. Sound therapy is also used, but not to cover up the tinnitus. Instead an emotionally neutral sound, such as white noise, is paired with the tinnitus in order to facilitate habituation. Tinnitus Retraining Therapy takes 12–18 months, but its proponents cite significant relief from annoying tinnitus in over 80 percent of patients treated (Jastreboff, 1996).

The scope of practice of audiologists is described in the following and should demonstrate the breadth and depth of knowledge and skill audiologists possess.

American Speech-Language-Hearing Association (ASHA) Audiology Scope of Practice

The practice of audiology includes the following (ASHA, 2004a):

- Activities that identify, assess, diagnose, manage, and interpret test results related to disorders of human hearing, balance, and other neural systems

- Otoscopic examination and external ear canal management for removal of cerumen in order to evaluate hearing or balance, make ear impressions, fit hearing protection or prosthetic devices, and monitor the continuous use of hearing aids
- Conducting an interpretation of behavioral, electroacoustic, or electrophysiological methods used to assess hearing, balance, and neural system function
- Evaluation and management of children and adults with central APDs
- Supervision and conducting of newborn hearing screening programs
- Measurement and interpretation of sensory and motor-evoked potentials, electromyography, and other electrodiagnostic tests for purposes of neurophysiologic intraoperative monitoring and cranial nerve assessment
- Provision of hearing care by selecting, evaluating, fitting, facilitating adjustment to, and dispensing prosthetic devices for hearing loss, including hearing aids, sensory aids, hearing assistive devices, alerting and telecommunication systems, and captioning devices
- Assessment of candidacy of persons with hearing loss for cochlear implants and provision of fitting, programming, and audiological rehabilitation to optimize device use
- Provision of audiological rehabilitation, including speech reading, communication management, language development, auditory skill development, and counseling for psychosocial adjustment to hearing loss for persons with hearing loss and their families and caregivers
- Consultation with educators as members of interdisciplinary teams about communication management, educational implications of hearing loss, educational programming, classroom acoustics, and large-area amplification systems for children with hearing loss
- Prevention of hearing loss and conservation of hearing function by designing, implementing, and coordinating occupational, school, and community hearing conservation and identification programs
- Consultation and provision of rehabilitation to persons with balance disorders using habituation, exercise therapy, and balance retraining
- Designing and conducting basic and applied audiological research to increase the knowledge base, to develop new methods and programs, and to determine the efficacy of assessment and treatment paradigms; dissemination of research findings to other professionals and to the public
- Education and administration in audiology graduate and professional education programs
- Measurement of functional outcomes, consumer satisfaction, effectiveness, efficiency, and cost–benefit of practices and programs to maintain and improve the quality of audiological services
- Administration and supervision of professional and technical personnel who provide support functions to the practice of audiology
- Screening of speech-language, use of sign language (e.g., American Sign Language and cued speech), and other factors affecting communication function for the purposes of an audiological evaluation or initial identification of individuals with other communication disorders
- Consultation about accessibility for persons with hearing loss in public and private buildings, programs, and services
- Assessment and nonmedical management of tinnitus using biofeedback, masking, hearing aids, education, and counseling
- Consultation to individuals, public and private agencies, and governmental bodies, or as an expert witness regarding legal interpretations of audiology findings, effects of hearing loss and balance system disorders, and relevant noise-related considerations

- Case management and service as a liaison for the consumer, family, and agencies in order to monitor audiological status and management and to make recommendations about educational and vocational programming
- Consultation with industry on the development of products and instrumentation related to the measurement and management of auditory or balance function
- Participation in the development of professional and technical standards

Credentials Held by Audiologists

As health professionals concerned with the welfare of the patients they serve, audiologists must possess certain credentials to practice audiology. These credentials signify a specific level of education and competence that serve to protect consumers. Certification and licensure are the two most common credentials possessed by audiologists. Table 10.7 delineates the characteristics of certification and licensure.

Table 10.7 Characteristics of Certification and Licensure

Purpose	Grants recognition to practitioners who have met certain qualifications	Protects the public's life, health, safety, or economic well-being
Function	Restricts the use of the designated title to individuals who choose to meet the qualifications	Restricts scope of practice so that it is illegal for unlicensed individuals to provide the services
Qualifications	Formal education, experience, personal characteristics, and completion of examination	May piggyback on qualifications required for certification
Establishment of Regulations	Developed and approved by members of the association	Developed by regulatory body and approved according to the state's Administrative Procedure Act
Provider	Usually a private association	State agency
Status	Voluntary	Mandatory
Penalties for Violation	Rescind membership Rescind certification	Admonishment License revocation Monetary fine Restrictions on practice Incarceration License suspension
Continuing Education	Certifying entity may sponsor continuing education opportunities for members; may be required for recertification	May be required for licensees to renew

Source: ASHA State Policy Division 10/10/95-aew.

In order to be certified by ASHA and licensed/registered/certified by a particular state regulatory board or agency to practice audiology, one must possess a doctoral degree earned from an accredited college or university audiology graduate (doctoral) program (note: this requirement is relatively new, so one may encounter audiologists who do not possess doctoral degrees). College and university graduate audiology programs seek accreditation from the Council on Academic Accreditation of the American Speech-Language-Hearing Association. This ensures that graduates of these programs are eligible for the certificate of clinical competence (CCC) issued by the Council for Clinical Certification of ASHA. The U.S. Department of Education and the Council on Recognition of Postsecondary Accreditation have approved ASHA as a credentialing agency. The standard on which the certificate of clinical competence in audiology (CCC-A) is based has served as the foundation for most states' licensing laws. ASHA's national certification standards have undergone costly scientific tests of validity (ASHA, 2004b). ASHA-certified audiologists possess specific knowledge and competencies and must pass a national examination as well as maintain currency through continuing education.

Additionally, most states require audiologists to be licensed, registered, or certified in order to practice audiology in that particular state. Each state's licensing or regulatory board has specific educational and competency requirements, which are assessed through examination. Renewal of state credentials usually requires maintenance of currency through continuing education.

Referral Considerations

Referrals to audiologists can be made directly by contacting the office, center, hospital, or facility in which the audiologist is employed. ASHA, at (800) 638-8255, the American Academy of Audiology, at (703) 790-8466, or a state speech-language-hearing association can provide the names of audiologists practicing in specific geographic areas. ASHA maintains a referral source (PROSERV) on its consumer website at www.asha.org.

It is important and helpful to be aware of the types of test procedures and terminology used by audiologists. This will assist the case manager in making appropriate referrals and in conversing knowledgeably with the audiologist. The following are some of the test procedures and terminology used by audiologists.

Types of Hearing Loss

Conductive: Abnormalities of the outer or middle ear
Sensorineural: Abnormalities of the inner ear
Mixed: Combination of conductive and sensorineural
Central: Abnormalities of the central auditory nervous system

Assessment Procedures

Behavioral Observation Audiometry (BOA): Controlled observation of responses (i.e., changes in behavior such as quieting, arousal from sleep, eye shift, eye widening, eyebrow raising, body movement, and head turn) to acoustic stimuli

Visual Reinforcement Audiometry (VRA): Reinforcement with lighted toys when the child turns toward the sound source

Conditioned Play Audiometry (CPA): Conditioning the child to respond to the stimuli through game playing

Conventional Audiometry: Hand-raising or button-pushing response to stimuli
Auditory Evoked Potentials (AEPs): Measurement of changes in electrical activity of the auditory nervous system in response to acoustic stimuli
Otoacoustic Emissions (OAEs): Measurement of sound generated by motion of the outer hair cells
(Central) Auditory Processing Disorder (APD) Evaluation: Assessment of the central auditory system's ability to process complex auditory stimuli.

Mode of Presentation

Sound Field: Testing via loudspeakers; does not allow a unilateral or asymmetrical hearing loss to be ruled out
Air Conduction: Testing via earphones; allows each ear to be evaluated in isolation
Bone Conduction: Testing via a bone vibrator; directly stimulates better cochlea function

Test Battery

Frequency-Specific Information: Absolute versus minimum response
Speech Awareness Threshold (SAT): Lowest intensity level at which there is awareness of speech
Speech Reception Threshold (SRT): Lowest intensity level at which a spondee word can be repeated 50 percent of the time
Word Recognition Ability: Percentage of monosyllabic words repeated correctly when presented at a comfortable listening level
Tympanometry: Measurement of the mobility of the tympanic membrane/middle ear system as a function of varying degrees of air pressure in the external ear canal

a. *Static Compliance:* Mobility of the tympanic membrane/middle ear system
b. *Equivalent Volume:* Ear canal volume

Acoustic Reflex Measurements: Observation of the contraction of the muscles of the middle ear in response to loud sounds

Outcomes of Audiology Services

Outcomes of audiology services may be measured to determine treatment effectiveness, efficiency, cost–benefit analysis, and consumer satisfaction. Specific outcome data may assist consumers to make decisions about audiology service delivery. The following list describes the types of outcomes that consumers may expect to receive from an audiologist:

- Interpretation of otoscopic examination for appropriate management or referral
- Identification of populations and individuals with or at risk for hearing loss or related auditory disorders:
  - With normal hearing or no related auditory disorders
  - With communication disorders associated with hearing loss
  - With or at risk of balance disorders, and tinnitus
- Professional interpretation of the results of audiological findings
- Referrals to other professions, agencies, or consumer organizations

- Counseling for personal adjustment and discussion of the effects of hearing loss and the potential benefits to be gained from audiological rehabilitation and sensory aids, including hearing and tactile aids, hearing assistive devices, cochlear implants, captioning devices, and signal/warning devices
- Counseling regarding the effects of balance system dysfunction
- Selection, monitoring, dispensing, and maintenance of hearing aids and large-area amplification systems
- Development of culturally appropriate, audiological, rehabilitative management plans, including, when appropriate:
  - Fitting and dispensing recommendations, and educating the consumer and family/caregivers in the use of and adjustment to sensory aids, hearing assistive devices, alerting systems, and captioning devices
  - Counseling relating to psychosocial aspects of hearing loss and processes to enhance communication competence
  - Skills training and consultation concerning environmental modifications to facilitate development of receptive and expressive communication
  - Evaluation and modification of the audiological management plan
- Preparation of a report summarizing findings, interpretation, recommendations, and audiological management plan
- Consultation in development of an individualized education program (IEP) for school-age children or an individualized family service plan (IFSP) for children from birth to 36 months of age
- Provision of in-service programs for personnel and advising school districts in planning educational programs and accessibility for students with hearing loss
- Planning, development, implementation, and evaluation of hearing conservation programs

How to Communicate with People Who Are Hard of Hearing

The following suggestions are examples of effective strategies for communicating with individuals with hearing impairment:

- *Positioning*
  - Be sure the light, whether natural or artificial, falls on your face. Do not stand with the sun to your back or in front of a window.
  - If you are aware that the hard-of-hearing person has a better ear, stand or sit on that side.
  - Avoid background noise to the extent possible.
- *Method*
  - Get the person's attention before you start talking. You may need to touch the person to attract attention.
  - Speak to the hard-of-hearing person from an ideal distance of 3 to 6 feet in face-to-face visual contact.
  - Speak as clearly as possible in a natural way.
  - Speak more slowly to the hard-of-hearing person. Pausing between sentences will assist the listener.
  - Do not shout. Shouting often results in distortion of speech and it displays a negative visual signal to the listener. Do not drop your voice at the end of the sentence.

  - If the person does not understand what you said, rephrase it.
  - When changing the subject, indicate the new topic with a word or two or a phrase.
- *Physical*
  - Do not obscure your mouth with your hands. Do not chew or smoke while talking.
  - Facial expressions and lip movements are important clues to the hard-of-hearing person. Feelings are more often expressed by nonverbal communication than through words.
- *Attitude*
  - Do not become impatient.
  - Stay positive and relaxed.
  - Never talk about a hard-of-hearing person in his/her presence. Talk *to* them, not *about* them.
  - Ask what you can do to facilitate communication.

How to Communicate with People Who Are Deaf

The following is a list of suggestions for communicating with someone who is deaf:

- DO be facially expressive when communicating.
- DO NOT break eye contact when communicating with people who are deaf. Lack of eye contact is considered rude when communicating with a visually oriented person.
- DO get the attention of a person who is deaf by tapping the shoulder.
- DO NOT take offense at direct questions regarding qualifications or personal life. Direct questions between one person who is deaf and another person who is deaf are culturally quite common and can spill over into interactions with hearing people with no attempt to be rude.
- DO be conscious of hearing-loss terminology. Within the culture of the deaf, the norm is profound deafness and a mild hearing loss may mean "hard of hearing" to the person who is deaf.
- While a person who is deaf is signing, DO NOT touch their hands.
- DO define individuals who are deaf by their abilities, rather than their disabilities.
- DO NOT talk with another hearing person in the presence of a person who is deaf without signing or ensuring a clear line of sight for speech reading. Just as those with acquired hearing loss may be suspicious when they do not understand what others are saying, so may individuals who are deaf. Use sign language, written communication, or ensure that the individual who is deaf can speech read (lip read) what is said.
- DO attempt to use sign language with an individual who is deaf. Any attempt is appreciated, but if you are not fluent, the services of an interpreter should be obtained.
- DO NOT use the term *oral* as it implies oral ideologies (oralists). Rather, use the term *spoken English* or *spoken communication*. Similarly, *communication training* may be preferred to *aural rehabilitation* because the former implies improvements in aspects of communication, such as written communication, that are not aurally based.

First Aid for Hearing Aids

The following are some suggestions for troubleshooting minor hearing aid difficulties. If the problem is not resolved, the hearing aid may require factory repair and should be returned to an audiologist or hearing instrument specialist (preferably the same who dispensed the aid).

Symptom Solution

Hearing aid dead:

- Assure aid is turned on
- Assure battery is inserted correctly
- Try new battery
- Clean battery contacts with pencil eraser
- Assure earmold not clogged with wax (BTE aid)
- Assure receiver port not clogged with wax (ITE aid)

Hearing aid weak:

- Replace battery
- Clean receiver port (ITE aid)
- Clean earmold tip
- Assure microphone port not occluded (ITE aid)

Hearing aid distorted:

- Replace battery
- Clean receiver port (ITE aid)

Hearing aid whistles:

- Assure tight fit of earmold (BTE) or ITE aid
- Assure ear canal is free of cerumen

Causes, Tests, and Remedies

1. *Cause:* Dead or rundown battery. *Test:* Substitute new battery. *Remedy:* Replace worn-out battery.
2. *Cause:* Battery reversed in holder so that positive end is where negative end should be. *Test:* Examine. *Remedy:* Insert battery correctly.
3. *Cause:* Poor contacts at cord receptacle of battery holder due to dirty pins or springs. *Test:* With hearing aid turned on, wiggle plugs in receptacles and withdraw and reinsert each plug and the battery. *Remedy:* Rub accessible contacts briskly with lead pencil eraser, then wipe with clean cloth moistened with dry-cleaning liquid. Inaccessible contacts usually can be cleaned with a broom straw dipped in cleaning fluid.
4. *Cause:* Internal break or near-break inside receiver cord. *Test:* While listening, flex all parts of cords by running fingers along entire length and wiggle cords at terminals. Intermittent or raspy sounds indicate broken wires. *Remedy:* Replace cords with new ones. Worn ones cannot be repaired satisfactorily.
5. *Cause:* Plugs not fully or firmly inserted in receptacles. *Test:* While listening, withdraw and firmly reinsert each plug in turn. *Remedy:* Insert correctly.

6. *Cause:* Ear tip not properly seated in ear. *Test:* With the fingers, press the receiver firmly into the ear and twist back and forth slightly to make sure that the ear tip is properly positioned. *Remedy:* Position correctly.
7. *Cause:* Ear tip plugged with wax or with drop of water from cleaning. *Test:* Examine ear tip visually and blow through it to determine whether passage is open. *Remedy:* Disconnect ear tip from receiver, then wash ear tip in lukewarm water and soap, using pipe cleaner or long-bristle brush to reach down into the canal. Rinse with clear water and dry. A dry pipe cleaner may be used to dry out the canal; blowing through the canal will remove surplus water.
8. *Cause:* Insufficient pressure of bone receiver on mastoid. *Test:* While listening, press the bone receiver more tightly against the head with the fingers. *Remedy:* Bend the receiver headband to provide greater pressure. Your audiologist who is more skilled in maintaining conformation with the head preferably does this.
9. *Cause:* Receiver close to wall or other sound-reflecting surfaces. *Test:* Examine. *Remedy:* Avoid sitting with the fitted side of the head near a wall or other surfaces. Such surfaces tend to reflect the sound from the receiver so that it is more readily picked up by the microphone, thus causing whistling.
10. *Cause:* Microphone worn too close to receiver. *Test:* Try moving instrument to provide wider separation between it and the receiver. *Remedy:* Avoid wearing microphone and receiver on same side of body or close together.
11. *Cause:* Plastic tubing not firmly seated at hearing aid or ear tip ends, or tubing so sharply bent as to block the passage of sound through it. *Test:* Examine and check for tightness at ends. *Remedy:* Push tubing ends firmly onto nubs. See that there is no kink or sharp bend. Replace the tubing if necessary.

Behaviors of Children at Risk for Auditory Disorders

Certain characteristic behaviors by children should alert parents and teachers to be concerned about their hearing. Some of the signs are:

- Often misunderstands what is said
- Constantly requests that information be repeated
- Has difficulty following oral instructions
- Gives inconsistent responses to auditory stimuli
- Turns up the volume of the television, radio, or stereo
- Gives slow or delayed response to verbal stimuli
- Has poor auditory attention
- Has poor auditory memory (span and sequence)
- Is easily distracted
- Has difficulty listening in the presence of background noise
- Has poor receptive and expressive language
- Has difficulty with phonics and speech sound discrimination
- Learns poorly through the auditory channel
- Has reading, spelling, and other learning problems
- Exhibits behavior problems
- Says "Huh?" or "What?" frequently

Conditions Associated with Hearing Loss

Some common indicators associated with hearing loss include:

- Family history of hearing loss
- In utero infection (e.g., cytomegalovirus, rubella, syphilis, or toxoplasmosis)
- Craniofacial anomalies, including those with morphological abnormalities of the pinna and ear canal
- Birth weight less than 1,500 grams (3.3 pounds)
- Hyperbilirubinemia at a serum level requiring exchange transfusion
- Ototoxic medications, including, but not limited to, chemotherapeutic agents, or aminoglycosides used in multiple courses or in combination with loop diuretics
- Bacterial meningitis and other infections associated with sensorineural hearing loss
- Severe depression at birth with Apgar scores of 0–4 at 1 min. or 0–6 at 5 min.
- Prolonged mechanical ventilation 5 days or longer (e.g., persistent pulmonary hypertension)
- Stigmata or other findings associated with a syndrome known to include a sensorineural or conductive hearing loss
- Parent/caregiver concern regarding hearing, speech, language, or developmental delay
- Head trauma associated with loss of consciousness or skull fracture
- Recurrent or persistent otitis media with effusion for at least 3 months
- Neurofibromatosis type II and neurodegenerative disorders
- Anatomic deformities and other disorders, which affect Eustachian tube, function

Costs Related to Amplification

The cost of hearing aids varies from approximately $500 to $2,500 per instrument depending upon type and options. A single behind-the-ear instrument may be as little as $500, while a digital instrument will typically cost $2,100 to $2,500. Middle ear implantable instruments may run $25,000, plus $5,000 per year for technical support. Many patients with disabilities may need manufacturer support to ensure they are capable of operating the volume control and other instrument options. Digital hearing aids often have an external control much like a television remote control. Care must be given to ensure appropriate fitting and follow-up services. Pitfalls that must be avoided are indiscriminate fitting of patients with amplification not appropriate for their loss and insufficient follow-up and audiological/aural rehabilitation.

- A hearing aid should be effective for 3 to 5 years before *replacement* is necessary. It is wise to purchase replacement and repair warranties.
- A standard factory *warranty* will be 1 to 2 years.
- *Battery costs* may vary depending on the severity of the hearing loss and the power required of the hearing aid. A package of six batteries will cost $4 to $5. The average life expectancy for a battery is approximately 10 days to 2 weeks when the instrument is worn during waking hours. If an instrument is out of warranty, the cost of repair is approximately $150 to include a one-year warranty.

Children under 21 are entitled to mandatory hearing services, including hearing aids, under Medicaid. Hearing aid coverage for adults is optional and varies from state to state. A list of state Medicaid office contacts can be found at https://www.medicaid.gov/about-us/contact-us/index.html.

Although Medicare does not pay for hearing devices in fee-for-service plans, hearing aids may be covered by Medicare+Choice plans, such as health maintenance organizations. The Centers for Medicare and Medicaid Services (CMS) clarified in 2001 that Medicare carriers should pay for diagnostic audiological tests regardless of a hearing aid recommendation.

Funding Issues Related to Audiological Services

Obviously, people with the financial resources to pay privately for these devices and services will be able to obtain what they need. However, most rely upon alternative funding, and specific issues are mentioned in the following:

- *Medicaid*: States must cover hearing aids for children through the Early and Periodic Screening, Diagnosis, and Treatment Program. Coverage for adults is optional and rarely included in a state plan.
- *Medicare*: Medicare does not cover hearing aids or tests related to hearing aids. Social health maintenance organizations (SHMOs) are part of a demonstration project that includes some long-term care. All SHMOs cover hearing aids. As HMOs enter the Medicare market, many are providing partial coverage of hearing aids. For example, the Medicare HMO might cover $500 of a hearing aid. Some states and regional third-party payers allow balance billing—check in your state and with your dispensing audiologist.
- *Private Health Plans:* Most do not cover hearing aids unless there is a labor union contract such as the United Automobile Workers (UAW), which covers the costs related to one hearing aid every 3 years. The benefit is not limited to automobile workers but is found in many contracts negotiated by the UAW. Another example of a union contract is the California Public Employees Retirement System, which offers a hearing benefit to retirees enrolled in Medicare managed care plans. Some private plans such as Blue Cross and Blue Shield may cover a hearing aid if the need is related to an accident or illness.

Please refer to the Audiology Superbill (Appendix 10.4) for current procedural codes and V codes.

Types of Counseling

Counseling individuals with hearing loss or those who are deaf, as well as counseling family members, work associates, and friends of the individuals depends on the type of counseling needed at a specific time. Several types of counseling, the definition of the type of counseling, and the proposed outcomes are listed in Table 10.8. Successful counseling requires skill as well as knowledge about the individual type of hearing loss and is most successful when done by a qualified audiologist.

Table 10.8 Types of Counseling

Type of Counseling	*Definitions*	*Outcomes*
Informational	To provide education.	For the person and family to understand hearing loss, to be knowledgeable about appropriate technology, and to increase their willingness to participate in aural rehabilitation.
Rational Acceptance	For individuals to learn ways to manage their hearing losses and their communication difficulties.	For the individual to optimally use communication strategies, to structure the listening environment to maximize communication, to increase willingness to participate in aural rehabilitation.
Adjustment	To help individuals work through their negative feelings about their hearing loss and increase their sense of self-worth.	For the individual to begin viewing the hearing impairment as separate from self-concept and self-image, and to improve both of these, and to become more willing to participate in aural rehabilitation.
Psychosocial	To facilitate emotional adjustment in the context of the aural rehabilitation plan. Usually small groups with communication partners are encouraged to attend.	Self-acceptance, increased self-confidence, and more effective communication strategies.
Assertiveness Training	Incorporated into the aural rehabilitation sessions, to learn the differences among aggressive behavior, which involves the violation of other people's rights; passive behavior, which involves allowing others to violate their rights; and assertive behavior, in which individuals protect their rights without violating those of other people (Hull, 2001). Also, teaching individuals how to anticipate communication situations in advance and figure out ways to minimize difficulties.	Emphasis is on language and choice of words, and consequences of behaviors. Learning to anticipate in communication situations and to learn repair strategies that may help the individual with a hearing loss (so that the individual may request one of the repair strategies).

Example Case

Following is an example *portion* of a plan for a 6-year-old child, with a severe sensorineural hearing loss due to meningitis at the age of one, who met the criteria for a cochlear implant. His parents were very bright based on educational achievements and testing. Both were employed by the school system. The child and an older sibling were both judged to be intellectually gifted.

Area	*Recommendation*	*Dates*	*Frequency*	*Expected Cost*
Medical/ Surgery	Cochlear implant device[a]	2008	Replacement 1x in life	$40,000
	Overnight hospital stay	2008	1x	$925
	Surgeon fees	2008	1x	Included in the device cost
	Audiologist fees	2008	1x for the implant itself	Included in the device cost
Assessment/ Therapy	Speech pathology	2008 to 2033	Intensive speech perception training and additional language and speech therapy for the first 5 years, then weekly until age 22	Provided by school system under IDEA for school year, 5x/ week for 5 years. If private pay during summer months, expected cost at $150 per hour
Area	*Recommendation*	*Dates*	*Frequency*	*Expected Cost*
	Audiology for programming, mapping, adjustments, general maintenance, tuning[b]	2008 to life	Seen after the first 4–6 weeks for calibration, then seen monthly for the year, then yearly recheck, unless complications	$150 per hour
	ENT	2008 to life	First 4–6 weeks, seen weekly, then monthly for the first year, then yearly thereafter for life unless complications	$300 per visit
Assistive Technology	TTY (text phone); SuperPrinter 4425 recommended (includes printer, auto answer, ring, and flasher)[c]	2008 to life	Every 10 years	$500 (includes 1-year warranty)

(*Continued*)

	TTY paper refill (3 pack of 2.5 inch thermal paper)	2008 to life	Every 3 months or as needed depending on the use	$16 per year (estimate)
	TTY batteries (6)	2008 to life	Yearly or more depending on use	$20 for a pack of two
	Sonic Alert or Silent Call Alerting System, including receiver, transmitters, and rechargeable battery	2008 to life	Sonic Alert: 1x only. Silent Call: every 10 years	Sonic Alert: $260 with 1-year warranty. Silent Call: $540 with vibrating unit and 2-year warranty
	Door knock signaler with light	2008 to life	Every 10 years	$65 for package
	Portable smoke detector	2008 to life	Every 10 years	$175
	Allowance for batteries, light bulbs, etc.	2008 to life	Batteries: monthly. >Bulbs: yearly depending on use	$50 per year (estimate)
	Baby cry alerter (assumes child)	Estimate 2032	1x (assumes child)	Sonic Alert: $40 (may also be used as smoke detector)
	Replacement cords and batteries for implant device	$1,000 to life	Every 3 months for two cords at $10 each. One time per year for 2 pack batteries at $10 per year	$90 per year
Area	*Recommendation*	*Dates*	*Frequency*	*Expected Cost*
	Replacement headset	2010 (after 3-year warranty to life)	Project 3–4 upgrades over life	$500 every 3 years
	Upgrade external processor	2023	1x	$6,000
	Silent Call or Sleep Alert charger unit	2008	Every 10 years.	$110
	Service contract for external speech processor and headset (internal device has a 99-year warranty)	2008 to life	Every 2 years	$750 for 2 years (after 3-year manufacturer warranty expires)

(*Continued*)

Education	Public school	2008 to 2022	School year.	$0 provided under IDEA.
Interpreter		2008 to life	6 hours/day, 5 days/wk, August to June until 2022, then 2–4 hours/wk average to life	$0 for school hours until age 18 (2022), then $25 per hour for medical, dental, contracts, legal, and other noneducation-related activities
Counseling	Parents	2008	1 hr/wk	$150 per hr
	Child/adult	2008 to 2010, then weekly until age 18, then as needed to life	2x per week from 2008 to 2010. Weekly to 2022. As needed	$0 with school counselor. $150 per hour privately. $0 should be paid by vocational rehabilitation

[a] No provision for technology advances.

[b] Economist to determine present value.

[c] TTY unit uses regular phone lines; however, units are unable to distinguish between incoming TTY call or voice calls. A separate phone line dedicated to TTY calls may be appropriate. Cost for additional phone line installation is estimated between $100 and $110 plus monthly charge of $35. Does not include long-distance charges that are usually higher due to length of time to transmit written words rather than spoken words. Cost cannot be projected. Internet access cost is $25/month.

Conclusion

In many life care plans, audiological services can be a critical component. In personal injury litigation, common sequelae from head trauma can destroy or reduce hearing, disrupt balance, and produce serious ringing in the ears (tinnitus). In medical illness, malpractice, or mistakes, the audiologist is commonly an important member for diagnosis and treatment of hearing dysfunction. Of particular interest is the role the audiologist can play with regard to children. Hearing deficits can seriously hamper educational achievement resulting in poor social adjustment and a poor vocational outlook. Indeed, many deaf children are initially termed as "mentally retarded," or more appropriately, diagnosed as a person with an intellectual disability, and do not receive services during critical developmental periods. This chapter assists the life care planner by providing information related to the roles and responsibilities of the audiologist and provides resources for information, services, and products to assist the hearing impaired.

Appendices

Appendix 10.1 State Requirements for Audiologists (2008)

Thirty states permit audiologists to dispense hearing aids under an audiology license by virtue of amending the hearing aid dealers' licensure law, the audiology licensure law, or both.

Alabama	Mississippi
Alaska	New Mexico**
Arkansas	New York
Colorado	Oklahoma
Connecticut*	Ohio
Florida	Rhode Island
Georgia	South Carolina
Idaho	South Dakota
Illinois	Tennessee
Indiana	Texas*
Louisiana	Utah
Massachusetts	Vermont
Maryland	Washington
Michigan	West Virginia
Minnesota	Wisconsin
*Certain conditions apply. **Audiologists must obtain an endorsement to dispense hearing aids.	

The following 20 states and the District of Columbia require audiologists to hold HAD (Hearing Aid Dispenser) licensure to dispense hearing aids.

Arizona	Nebraska
California	Nevada
Delaware	New Hampshire
District of Columbia	New Jersey
Hawaii	North Carolina
Iowa	North Dakota
Kansas	Oregon
Kentucky	Pennsylvania
Maine	Virginia
Missouri	Wyoming
Montana	

Appendix 10.2 Degree of Hearing Loss

Hearing Level	*Hearing Ability*
Normal (–10–10 dB)	Can hear speech normally
Minimal (10–25 dB)	Has difficulty hearing faint speech in a noisy place
Mild (25–40 dB)	Has difficulty hearing faint or distance speech, even in a quiet environment
Moderate (40–55 dB)	Hears conversational speech only at a close distance
Moderately severe (55–70 dB)	Hears loud conversational speech
Severe (70–90 dB)	Cannot hear conversational speech
Profound (>90 dB)	May hear loud sounds; hearing is not the primary communication channel

Appendix 10.3 Resources

Harc Mercantile Kalamazoo, MI 800-438-4272 (V) 800-413-5245 (TTY) www.harcmercantile.com	MVM Technical Corporation 1 Union Square West, Room 210 New York, NY 10003 212-741-1967 www.perceptions4people.org
Harris Communications Eden Prairie, MN 800-825-6758 (V) 800-825-9187 (TTY) www.harriscomm.com	Soundbytes New York, NY 800-667-1777 www.soundbytes.com
Hear-More, Inc. Farmingdale, NY 800-881-4327 (V/TTY) www.hearmore.com	United TTY Sales Olney, MD 866-889-4872 www.UnitedTTY.com
Hitec Burr Ridge, IL 800-288-8303 www.hitec.com	Weitbrecht Communications Santa Monica, CA 800-233-9130 (V/TTY) www.weitbrecht.com
Some Other Distributors of Assistive Listening Devices	
Audio Enhancement www.audioenhancement.com	Centrum Sound https://www.centrumsound.com/Assistive_Listening_Devices.html

(*Continued*)

Appendix 10.3 (Continued) Resources

<table>
<tr><td>Hear You Are, Inc.
Stanhope, NJ
201-347-7662 (V)
201-347-7662 (F)
hearyouare@aol.com</td><td>Radio Shack
www.radioshack.com (2018, website is still active)</td></tr>
<tr><td>Heidico
Reno, NV
702-324-7104 (V/TTY/F)
https://abledata.acl.gov/organizations/heidico-inc</td><td>Sound Associates
www.soundassociates.com</td></tr>
<tr><td>Hello Direct
www.hello-direct.com</td><td>Sound Remedy
New York, NY
212-242-1036 (V/F)
https://abledata.acl.gov/organizations/sound-remedy-inc</td></tr>
<tr><td colspan="2">There are also many centers across the country where individuals can examine the types of assistive listening devices available in order to determine which products to purchase. To locate an assistive device demonstration center in your area, call the American Speech-Language-Hearing Association's Action Center at 800-638-8255, e-mail actioncenter@asha.org, or call Self Help for Hard of Hearing People, Inc. (SHHH) at 301-657-2248 (voice) or 301-657-2249 (TTY).</td></tr>
<tr><td colspan="2">Selected Resources for Information, Services, and Products Information</td></tr>
<tr><td>Alexander Graham Bell Association for the Deaf
3417 Volta Place, NW
Washington, DC 20007
202-337-5220 (V/TTY)</td><td>American Athletic Association for the Deaf
3607 Washington Blvd., #4
Ogden, UT 84403
801-393-5710 (V)
801-393-7916 (TTY)</td></tr>
<tr><td>American Academy of Audiology
11730 Plaza America Dr., Suite 300
Reston, VA 20190
703-790-8466</td><td>American Speech-Language-Hearing Association
2200 Research Blvd.
Rockville, MD 20850
Members: 800-498-2071
Nonmember: 800-638-8255
Fax: 301-296-8580</td></tr>
<tr><td>American Association for the Deaf-Blind
814 Thayer Ave., Room 302
Silver Spring, MD 20910
301-588-6545 (V/TTY)</td><td>Helen Keller National Center for Deaf-Blind Youths and Adults
111 Middle Neck Rd.
Sands Point, NY 11050
516-944-8900 (V)
516-944-8637 (TTY)</td></tr>
<tr><td>American Association for Deaf Children
10th and Tahlequah Streets
Sulfur, OK 73086
800-942-ASDC</td><td>National Association for the Deaf
814 Thayer Ave., Room 302
Silver Spring, MD 20910
301-587-1788 (V)
301-587-1789 (TTY)</td></tr>
</table>

(Continued)

Appendix 10.3 (Continued) Resources

National Information Center on Deafness Gallaudet University 800 Florida Ave. NE Washington, DC 20002	*General Products* LS&S Group P.O. Box 6783 Northbrook, IL 60065 800-317-8533 E-mail: lssgrp@aol.com
Products/Services Canines Paws with a Cause 1235 100th St. SE Byron Center, MI 49315 800-253-PAWS	NFSS Communications 8120 Fenton St. Silver Spring, MD 20910 888-589-6671 (V) 888-589-6670 (TTY)
Cochlear Implant Cochlear Corporation Suite 200 61 Inverness Dr. East Englewood, CO 80112 800-523-5798	Potomac Technology One Church St., Suite 402 Rockville, MD 20850 301-762-4005 (V) 301-762-0851 (TTY)
Interpreters Registry of Interpreters for the Deaf 9719 Colesville Rd., Suite 310 Silver Spring, MD 20910 301-608-0050 (V/TTY)	*Tactile Aids* Audiological Engineering Corporation 35 Medford St. Somerville, MA 02143 800-283-4601 (V) 800-955-7204 (TTY)
General Products HARC Mercantile, LTD. 1111 West Centre Ave. P.O. Box 3055 Kalamazoo, MI 49003 800-445-9968 (V) 800-413-5245 (TTY)	

Appendix 10.4 Model Superbill for Audiology

The following is a model of a superbill that could be used by an audiology practice when billing private health plans. This sample is not meant to dictate which services should or should not be listed on the bill. Most billable codes are from the American Medical Association (AMA) Current Procedural Terminology (CPT). Prosthetic and durable medical equipment codes, such as hearing aid codes, are published by the Centers for Medicaid and Medicare (CMS) as the Healthcare Common Procedure Code System (HCPCS). The superbill is a standard form that health plans use to process claims. For the professional who is rendering services, it provides a time-efficient means to document services, fees, codes, and other information required by insurance companies (i.e., certification and licensure). The patient uses this form to file for health plan payment.

(*Continued*)

Appendix 10.4 (Continued) Model Superbill for Audiology

Note: This is only a model, therefore some procedures, codes, or other pertinent information may not be found on the following model. A complete list of audiology related codes is available in Coding & Billing for Audiology and Speech-Language Pathology. This product can be purchased through ASHA's Billing & Reimbursement website or by calling ASHA's Product Sales at 1-888-498-6699.

MODEL AUDIOLOGY SUPERBILL

Patient Name:______________________ Date of Birth:______________________
File:______________________ Insurance Plan:______________________
Date:______________________ Insurance Plan#:______________________

Procedure	CPT	Fee
Audiological Assessment Procedures		
Screening test, pure tone, air only	92551	________
Pure tone audiometry (threshold); air only	92552	________
Pure tone audiometry; air and bone	92553	________
Speech audiometry; threshold	92555	________
Speech audiometry with speech recognition	92556	________
Comprehensive audiometry threshold evaluation and speech recognition	92557	________
Audiometric testing of groups	92559	________
Bekesy audiometry; screening	92560	________
Bekesy audiometry; diagnostic	92561	________
Loudness balance test, alternate binaural or monaural	92562	________
Tone decay test	92563	________
Short increment sensitivity index (SISI)	92564	________
Stenger test, pure tone	92565	________
Tympanometry (impedance testing)	92567	________
Acoustic reflex testing (threshold)	92568	________
Acoustic reflex decay test	92570	________
Filtered speech test	92571	________
Staggered spondaic word test	92572	________
Sensorineural activity test	92575	________
Synthetic sentence test	92576	________

(*Continued*)

Appendix 10.4 (Continued) Model Superbill for Audiology

Stenger test, speech	92577	________
Visual reinforcement audiometry (VRA)	92579	________
Conditioning play audiometry	92582	________
Select picture audiometry	92583	________
Electrocochleography	92584	________
Auditory Evoked Potentials, comprehensive	92585	________
Auditory Evoked Potentials, limited	92586	________
Evoked otoacoustics emissions, limited	92587	________
Evoked otoacoustics emissions, comprehensive	92588	________
Evaluation of central auditory function, with report; initial 60 minutes	92620	________
Each additional 15 minutes	92621	________
Assessment of tinnitus (includes pitch and loudness matching	92625	________
Hearing Aid Assessment and Fitting Procedures		
Hearing aid exam and selection; monaural	92590	________
Hearing aid exam and selection; binaural	92591	________
Hearing aid check; monaural	92592	________
Hearing aid check; binaural	92593	________
Electroacoustic evaluation for hearing aid; monaural	92594	________
Electroacoustic evaluation for hearing aid; binaural	92595	________
Ear protector attenuation measurements	92596	________
Balance System Assessment Procedures		
Spontaneous nystagmus, including gaze	92531	________
Positional nystagmus	92532	________
Caloric vestibular test, each irrigation (binaural, bithermal stimulation constitutes four tests)	92533	________
Optokinetic nystagmus	92534	________
Caloric vestibular test, bilateral; bithermal (total of four irrigations)	92537	
Caloric vestibular test, bilateral; monothermal (total of two irrigations)	92538	
Spontaneous nystagmus test, including gaze and fixation nystagmus, with recording	92541	________

(Continued)

Appendix 10.4 (Continued) Model Superbill for Audiology

Positional nystagmus test, minimum of four positions	92542	________
Optokinetic nystagmus test, bidirectional, foveal or peripheral stimulation, with recording	92544	________
Oscillating tracking test, with recording	92545	________
Sinusoidal vertical axis rotational testing	92546	________
Use of vertical electrodes in any or all of the above tests	92547	________
Computerized dynamic posturography	92548	________
Vestibular and Balance Rehabilitation Services		________
Canalith repositioning procedure	95992	________
Cerumen Management Services		
Removal of impacted cerumen, one or both ears Auditory Implant Services	69210	________
Auditory Implant Services Cochlear implant follow-up exam < 7 years of age	92601	________
Reprogram cochlear implant < 7 years of age	92602	________
Cochlear implant follow-up exam > 7 years of age	92603	________
Reprogram cochlear implant > 7 years of age	92604	________
Diagnostic analysis with programming of auditory brain stem implant, per hour	92640	________
Habilitative and Rehabilitative Services		
Evaluation of speech, language, voice, communication, and/or auditory processing	92506	________
Treatment of speech, language, voice, communication, and/or auditory processing disorder; individual	92507	________
Group, two or more individuals	92508	________
Evaluation of auditory rehabilitation status, first hour	92626	________
Evaluation of auditory rehabilitation status, each additional 15 minutes	92627	________
Auditory rehabilitation; prelingual hearing loss	92630	________
Auditory rehabilitation; postlingual hearing loss	92633	________
Hearing Aids (HCPCS Level II Codes)		
Assessment for hearing aid	V5010	________

(Continued)

Appendix 10.4 (Continued) Model Superbill for Audiology

Fitting/orientation/checking of hearing aid	V5011	________
Repair/modification of hearing aid	V5014	________
Conformity evaluation	V5020	________
Hearing aid, monaural, body worn air conduction	V5030	________
Hearing aid, monaural, bone conduction	V5040	________
Hearing aid, monaural, in the ear	V5050	________
Hearing aid, monaural, behind the ear	V5060	________
Glasses, air conduction	V5070	________
Glasses, bone conduction	V5080	________
Dispensing fee, unspecified hearing aid	V5090	________
Hearing aid, bilateral, body worn	V5100	________
Dispensing fee, bilateral	V5110	________
Binaural, body	V5120	________
Binaural, in the ear	V5130	________
Binaural, behind the ear	V5140	________
Binaural, glasses	V5150	________
Dispensing fee, binaural	V5160	________
Hearing aid, CROS, in the ear	V5170	________
Hearing aid, CROS, behind the ear	V5180	________
Hearing aid, CROS, glasses	V5190	________
Dispensing fee, CROS	V5200	________
Hearing aid, BICROS, in the ear	V5210	________
Hearing aid, BICROS, behind the ear	V5220	________
Hearing aid, BICROS, glasses	V5230	________
Dispensing fee, BICROS	V5240	________
Dispensing fee, monaural hearing aid	V5241	________
Hearing aid, analog, monaural, CIC (completely in the ear canal)	V5242	________
Hearing aid, analog, monaural, ITC (in the canal)	V5243	________
Hearing aid, digitally programmable analog, monaural, CIC	V5244	________

(*Continued*)

Appendix 10.4 (Continued) Model Superbill for Audiology

Hearing aid, digitally programmable analog, monaural, ITC	V5245	________
Hearing aid, digitally programmable analog, monaural, ITE (in the ear)	V5246	________
Hearing aid, digitally programmable analog, monaural, BTE	V5247	________
Hearing aid, analog, binaural, CIC	V5248	________
Hearing aid, analog, binaural, ITC	V5249	________
Hearing aid, digitally programmable analog, binaural, CIC	V5250	________
Hearing aid, digitally programmable analog, binaural, ITC	V5251	________
Hearing aid, digitally programmable, binaural, ITE	V5252	________
Hearing aid, digitally programmable, binaural, BTE	V5253	________
Hearing aid, digital, monaural, CIC	V5254	________
Hearing aid, digital, monaural, ITC	V5255	________
Hearing aid, digital, monaural, ITE	V5256	________
Hearing aid, digital, monaural, BTE	V5257	________
Hearing aid, digital, binaural, CIC	V5258	________
Hearing aid, digital, binaural, ITC	V5259	________
Hearing aid, digital, binaural, ITE	V5260	________
Hearing aid, digital, binaural, BTE	V5261	________
Hearing aid, disposable, any type, monaural	V5262	________
Hearing aid, disposable, any type, binaural	V5263	________
Earmold/insert, not disposable, any type	V5264	________
Earmold/insert, disposable, any type	V5265	________
Battery for use in hearing device	V5266	________
Hearing aid supplies/accessories	V5267	________
Assistive listening device, telephone amplifier, any type	V5268	________
Assistive listening device, alerting, any type	V5269	________
Assistive listening device, television amplifier, any type	V5270	________
Assistive listening device, television caption decoder	V5271	________
Assistive listening device, TDD	V5272	________
Assistive listening device, for use with cochlear implant	V5273	________

(*Continued*)

Appendix 10.4 (Continued) Model Superbill for Audiology

Assistive learning device not otherwise specified	V5274	__________
Ear impression, each	V5275	__________
Hearing service, miscellaneous	V5299	__________
Other Procedures		
Otorhinolaryngological service or procedure	92700	__________

Steven Smith, AuD, CCC-Aud
Audiology & Hearing Center, Inc.
999 Anywhere Street
Rockville, MD 00000
Federal ID #00-00000 (999) 999-9999

Audiological Diagnosis:______________________________

ICD-9 Code: ______________________________

Hearing Aid/Earmold Defect: ______________________________

Previous Balance: $__________**Today's Fee: $**__________**Total Due: $**__________

Amount Paid: $__________**Balance: $**__________

Today's Payment Paid By Cash__________

Check/Credit card__________

White copy: Office Canary copy: Insurance Pink copy: Patient

References

American Industrial Hygiene Association. 2007. www.aiha.org/Content/AccessInfo/consumer/ProtectYourselffromNoiseInducedHearingLoss.htm.

American National Standards Institute. 1981. *Reference Equivalent Threshold Force Levels for Audiometric Bone Vibrators*. New York, NY: Acoustical Society of America.

American National Standards Institute. 1986. *Artificial Head Bone for the Calibration of Audiometer Bone Vibrators*. New York, NY: Acoustical Society of America.

American National Standards Institute. 1987. *Specifications for Instruments to Measure Aural Acoustic Impedance and Admittance (ANSI S3.39-1987)*. New York, NY: Acoustical Society of America.

American National Standards Institute. 1999a. *Maximum Permissible Ambient Noise Levels for Audiometric Test Rooms ANSI S3.1-1999. (R2013)* New York, NY: Acoustical Society of America.

American National Standards Institute. 1999b. *Method for Manual Pure-Tone Audiometry ANSI S3.21 2004 (R12009)*. New York, NY: Acoustical Society of America.

American National Standards Institute. 2010. *Specifications for Audiometers ANSI S3.6 199-2010*. New York, NY: Acoustical Society of America.

American Speech-Language-Hearing Association. 1988. Guidelines for determining threshold level for speech. *ASHA*, 30, 85–89.

American Speech-Language-Hearing Association. 1990. Audiological assessment of central auditory processing: An annotated bibliography. *ASHA*, 32, 13–30.

American Speech-Language-Hearing Association. 1991. Acoustic immittance: A bibliography. *ASHA*, 33, 1–44.

American Speech-Language-Hearing Association. 1992a. External auditory canal examination and cerumen management. [Guidelines, Knowledge and Skills, Position Statement]. Available from www.asha.org/policy.

American Speech-Language-Hearing Association. 1992b. Neurophysiologic intraoperative monitoring. [Position Statement]. Available from www.asha.org/policy.

American Speech-Language-Hearing Association. 1994. Guidelines for the audiologic management of individuals receiving cochleotoxic drug therapy. *ASHA*, 36, 11–19.

American Speech-Language-Hearing Association. 1996. Central auditory processing: Current status of research and implications for clinical practice. *American Journal of Audiology*, 5, 41–54.

American Speech-Language-Hearing Association. 1999. Joint audiology committee clinical practice statements and algorithms. [Guidelines]. Available at www.asha.org/policy.

American Speech-Language-Hearing Association. 2002. Guidelines for fitting and monitoring FM systems. *ASHA Desk Reference*, 2, 151–172.

American Speech-Language-Hearing Association. 2003. Guidelines: Competencies in auditory evoked potential measurement and clinical applications. [Knowledge and Skills]. Available at www.asha.org/policy.

American Speech-Language-Hearing Association. 2004a. Scope of practice in audiology. [Scope of Practice]. Available at www.asha.org/policy.

American Speech-Language-Hearing Association. 2004b. Guidelines for fitting and monitoring FM systems. Retrieved April 15, 2008, from http://asha.org/hearing/gen_audiology.cfm.

American Speech-Language-Hearing Association. 2006. Preferred practice patterns for the practice of audiology. Available at www.asha.org/policy/.

American Speech-Language-Hearing Association. 2016. Code of ethics. Available at www.asha.org/policy/.

Ballachandra, B. B., & Peers, C. J. 1992. Cerumen management: Instruments and procedures. *ASHA*, 32, 43–46.

Barrenas, M., & Lindgren, F. 1990. The influence of inner ear melanin on susceptibility to TTS in humans. *Scandinavian Audiology*, 19, 97–102.

Barza, M., & Lauermann, M. 1978. Why monitor serum levels of gentamicin? *Clinical Pharmacokinetics*, 3, 202–215.

Beery, Q., Doyle, W., & Cantekin, E. 1980. Eustachian tube function in an American Indian population. *Annals of Otology, Rhinology, and Laryngology*, 89, 28–33.

Bendush, C. L. 1982. Ototoxicity: Clinical considerations and comparative information. In A. Whelton and H. C. Neu (Eds.), *The Aminoglycosides: Microbiology, Clinical Use and Toxicology*. New York, NY: Marcel Dekker.

Bess, F. H. (Ed.). 1988. *Hearing Impairment in Children*. Parkton, MD: York Press.

Bess, F. H., & Humes, L. E. 1995. *Audiology: The Fundamentals*. Baltimore, MD: Williams & Wilkins.

Brummett, R. E. 1980. Drug-induced ototoxicity. *Drugs*, 19, 412–428.

Centers for Disease Control. 1988. Universal Precautions for the Prevention of Transmission of HIV, HBV, and Other Bloodborne Pathogens in Health Care Settings, 37, 24.

Centers for Disease Control. 2015. Progress in identifying infants with hearing loss–United States, 2006–2012. *Morbidity and Mortality Weekly Reports*, 64(13), 351–356.

Chang-Quan, H. et al. 2010. Chronic diseases and risk for depression in old age: a meta-analysis of published literature. *Ageing Research Reviews*, 9(2), 131–141.

Ciorba, A. et al. 2012. The impact of hearing loss on the quality of life of elderly adults. *Clinical Interventions in Ageing*, 7, 159–163.

Doyle, W. J. 1977. A function-anatomic description of Eustachian tube vector relations in four ethnic populations–an osteologic study. *Unpublished doctoral dissertation*. University of Pittsburgh, PA.

Fausti, S. A., Frey, R. H., Henry, J. A., Knutsen, J. M., & Olson, D. J. 1990. Reliability and validity of high frequency (8–20 kHz) thresholds obtained on a computer based audiometer as compared to a documented laboratory system. *Journal of the American Academy of Audiology*, 1, 162–170.

Fausti, S. A., Henry, J. A., Schaffer, H. I., Olson, D. J., Frey, R. H., & Bagby, B. C. 1993. High frequency monitoring for early detection of cisplatin ototoxicity. *Archives of Otolaryngology-Head and Neck Surgery*, 119, 661–668.

Fausti, S. A., Henry, J. A., Schaffer, H. I., Olson, D. J., Frey, R. H., & McDonald, W. J. 1992. High frequency audiometric monitoring for early detection of aminoglycoside ototoxicity. *Journal of Infectious Diseases*, 165, 1026–1032.

Ferrucci, L., & S. Studenski. 2011. Clinical problems of aging. In D. L. Longo, A. Fauci, D. Kasper, S. Hauser, J. L. Jameson and J. Loscalzo (Eds.), *Harrison's Principles of Internal Medicine*. New York, NY: McGraw-Hill.

Fogle, P. 2008. *Foundations of Communication Sciences & Disorders*. Clifton Park, NY: Thomson Delmar Learning.

Frank, T. 1990. High frequency hearing thresholds in young adults using a commercially available audiometer. *Ear and Hearing*, 11, 450–454.

Frank, R., & Dreisbach, L. E. 1991. Repeatability of high frequency thresholds. *Ear and Hearing*, 12, 294–295.

Gopinath, B. et al. 2012. Hearing-impaired adults are at increased risk of experiencing emotional distress and social engagement restrictions five years later. *Age and Ageing* 41(5):618–623.

Govaerts, P. J., Claes, J., Van De Heyning, P. H., Jorens, P. G., Marquet, J., & De Broe, M. E. 1990. Aminoglycoside-induced ototoxicity. *Toxicology Letters*, 52, 227–251.

Holden-Pitt, L., & Diaz, A. 1998. Thirty years of the Annual Survey of Deaf and Hard-of-Hearing Children & Youth: A glance over the decades. *American Annals of the Deaf*, 143, 73–76.

Jastreboff, P. J. 1996. Clinical implications of the neurophysiological model of tinnitus. In G. Reich and J. Vernon (Eds.), *Proceedings of the Fifth International Tinnitus Seminar 1995*. Portland, OR: American Tinnitus Association, pp. 500–507.

Jerger, J., Jerger, S., Pepe, D., & Miller, R. 1986. Race difference in susceptibility to noise-induced haring loss. *American Journal of Otology*, 7, 425–429.

Jiam, N. et al. 2016. Hearing loss and falls: A systematic review and meta-analysis, Laryngoscope, Version of Record online: 24 MAR 2016.

Joint Audiology Committee on Clinical Practice. 1999. *Clinical Practice Statements and Algorithms*. Rockville, MD: American Speech-Language-Hearing Association.

Joint Committee on Infant Hearing. 1994. Position statement. *ASHA*, 36, 38–41.

Joint Committee on Infant Hearing. 2000, August. Joint Committee on Infant Hearing 2000 position statement: Principles and guideline for early detection and intervention programs. *Pediatrics*, 106, 809–810.

Kopelman, J., Budnick, A. S., Sessions, R. B., Kramer, M. B., & Wong, G. Y. 1988. Ototoxicity of high dose cisplatin by bolus administration in patients with advanced cancers and normal hearing. *Laryngoscope*, 98, 858–864.

Lacerda, C. et al. 2012. Effects of hearing aids in the balance, quality of life and fear to fall in elderly people with sensorineural hearing loss. *International Archieves of Otorhinolaryngology*, 16(2), 156–162.

La Ferriere, K., Kaufman-Arenberg, I., Hawkins, J., & Johnson, L. 1974. Melanocytes of the vestibular labyrinth and the relationship to microvasculature. *Annals of Otology, Rhinology, and Laryngology*, 83, 685–694.

Laukli, E., & Mair, L. W. S. 1985. High frequency audiometry: Normative studies and preliminary experiences. *Scandinavian Audiology*, 14, 151–158.

Lien, E. J., Lipsett, L. R., & Lien, L. L. 1983. Structure side effect sorting of drugs. VI. Ototoxicities. *Journal of Clinical and Hospital Pharmacy*, 8, 15–33.

Lin, F. & Ferrucci, L. 2012. Hearing loss and falls among older adults in the United States. *Archives of Internal Medicine*, 172(4), 369–371.

Lin, F. et al. 2013. Hearing loss and cognitive decline in older adults. *JAMA Internal Medicine*, 173(4), 293–299.

MacDonald, M. 2011. The association between degree of hearing loss and depression in older adults. *Master's thesis*. University of British Columbia, Vancouver.

Mosby. 2006. *Mosby's Dictionary of Medicine, Nursing, & Health Professions* (7th Edition). St. Louis, MO: Mosby Elsevier.

National Center for Health Statistics. 1994. Prevalence and characteristics of persons with hearing trouble. United States, 1990–1991. *Vital and Health Statistics*, 10, 1–8.

National Council on Aging. 1999. *The Consequences of Untreated Hearing Loss in Older Persons*. Washington, DC: National Council on Aging.
National Institute of Deafness and Communication Disorders. 2002. *Report of the Ad hoc Committee on Epidemiology and Statistics in Communication*. Bethesda, MD: National Institutes of Health.
Northern, J. L., & Downs, M. P. 2002. *Hearing in Children* (5th ed.). Baltimore, MD: Lippincott Williams & Wilkins.
Pasic, T. R., & Dobie, R. A. 1991. Cis-platinum ototoxicity in children. *The Laryngoscope*, 101, 985–991.
Powell, S. H., Thompson, W. L., & Luthe, M. A. 1983. Once daily vs. continuous aminoglycoside dosing: Efficacy and toxicity in animal and clinical studies of gentamicin, netilmicin, and tobromycin. *Journal of Infectious Diseases*, 147, 918–932.
Roeser, R., & Crandell, C. 1991. The audiologist's responsibility in cerumen management. *ASHA*, 33, 51–53.
Rumalla, K. et al. 2015. The effect of hearing aids on postural stability. *The Laryngoscope*, 125, 720–723.
Rybak, L. P. 1986. Drug ototoxicity. *Annual Review of Pharmacology and Toxicology*, 26, 79–99.
Saito, H. et al. 2010. Hearing handicap predicts the development of depressive symptoms after 3 years in older community-dwelling Japanese. *Journal of the American Geriatrics Society*, 58(1), 93–97.
Schentag, J. J. 1980. Aminoglycosides. In W. E. Evans, J. J. Schentag and W. J. Jusko (Eds.), *Applied Pharmacokinetics: Principles of Therapeutic Drug Monitoring*. San Francisco, CA: Applied Therapeutics.
Simmons, F. B., McFarland, W. H., & Jones, F. R. 1980. Patterns of deafness in newborns. *Laryngoscope*, 90, 448–453.
Spivey, G. H., & Hirschhorn, N. 1977. A migrant study of adopted Apache children. *Johns Hopkins Medical Journal*, 140, 43–46.
U.S. Department of Labor. 1998, September 9. Occupational Exposure to Bloodborne Pathogens: Request for Information. Occupational Safety and Health Administration, Docket H370A.
Valente, M. L., Gulledge-Potts, M., Valente, M., French-St. George, J., & Goebel, J. 1992. High frequency thresholds: Sound suite versus hospital room. *Journal of the American Academy of Audiology*, 3, 287–294.
Van Bereijk, W., Pierce, J., & David, E. 1960. Waves and the ear. *Science*, 131, 219–220.
Van Naarden, K., & Decoufle, P. 1999. Relative and attributable risks for moderate to profound bilateral sensorineural hearing impairment associated with lower birth weight children 3 to 10 years old. *Pediatrics*, 104, 905–910.
Viljanen, A. et al. 2009. Hearing acuity as a predictor of walking difficulties in older women. *Journal of the American Geriatric Society*, 57, 1532–5415.
Wayne, R. & Johnsrude, I. 2015. A review of causal mechanisms underlying the link between age-related hearing loss and cognitive decline. *Ageing Research Reviews*, 23, 154–166.
Weinstein, B. & Ventry, I. 1982. Hearing impairment and social isolation in the elderly. *Journal of Speech, Language, and Hearing Research*, 25(4), 593–599.

Chapter 11

The Role of the Economist in Life Care Planning

Everett G. Dillman

Contents

Introduction....317
Categories of Costs....318
  Medical Services....318
  Medical Commodities....319
  Nonmedical Services....319
  Nonmedical Commodities....319
What Should Be Included....319
  Marginal Costs....321
  Value of the Items....325
Delivery Period and Amount....327
Actual or Average Annual....330
Economy of Effort....330
Total Lifetime Values....331
Complications....331
Affordable Care Act....331
Conclusion....332
References....332

Introduction

An economist is frequently called upon to compute the present value of future medical and care costs set forth in a life care plan prepared by a specialist. Although the economist generally will have little or no input in the development of the plan, the economist does have an interest in how the plan is structured and what it contains. This chapter examines the content of life care plans from the point of view of an economist and identifies some areas of potential concern.

The structure of the life care plan, including what elements are covered, will differ to some extent from author to author. Experience has shown, however, that there are a number of consistent patterns that emerge, some of which will cause difficulty for economic analysis (Dillman, 1987, 1988). The areas of concern from an economic point of view include:

1. Cost categories
2. Items that should be included
3. Timing of the items
4. The use of a range or annual averages of costs
5. Emphasis placed on trivial items

Each of these elements will be discussed in more detail.

Categories of Costs

In making the economic evaluation, the economist must consider the fact that the costs of the various items included in the plan will not remain static over time but can be expected to increase with inflation. The historical rates of increase will differ depending on the particular item, as the prices of some things tend to increase faster than others. For instance, the inflation of doctors' fees and hospital costs has historically been much greater than the inflation for such items as bandages, hospital beds, and other commodities.

In considering future inflation, the economist may look at the past inflation of the type of good being evaluated or may look at various studies which project inflation. Although it may be possible to develop data series for many individualized items, the economic analysis may place the items into the broad classifications of medical services, nonmedical services, medical commodities, and nonmedical commodities. There are limited historical data for most of the more detailed cost classifications such as doctors' fees. Some economists use the limited time series data or rely on various forecasts which are considered reliable while other economists are not comfortable with a limited time series thus use broader classifications. Which data series to use in computing present value is a matter for the economist and not the life care planner and thus will not be covered in this discussion.

Two of the categories, medical services and medical commodities, are subsets of the Consumer Price Index (CPI) and are defined by the Bureau of Labor Statistics (www.bls.gov/cpi/cpifact4.htm). These definitions as well as those for the other two categories follow.

Medical Services

This category involves professional and hospital services. Included are payments for physicians, dentists, and other professionals such as optometrists, ophthalmologists, opticians, psychologists, chiropractors, nurse practitioners, and therapists. The category of hospital services includes nursing home care. Hospital services for inpatients, such as pharmacy, laboratory tests, radiology, short-stay units, ambulatory surgery, physical therapy, and emergency room fees billed by the hospital, also fall into this category. Additionally, this category includes fees paid to individuals or agencies for the personal care of invalids, elderly, or convalescents in the home including food preparation, bathing, light housekeeping, and other services.

Medical Commodities

The medical commodities classification includes the following:

- *Prescription drugs and medical supplies.* This includes all drugs and medical supplies dispensed by prescriptions. Also included are all prescription-dispensed over-the-counter drugs, that is, those drugs that are obtained over the counter but are prescribed by the doctor and dispensed by the pharmacist.
- *Internal and respiratory over-the-counter drugs.* This includes all nonprescription medication taken by swallowing or inhaling, as well as suppositories or enemas.
- *Topicals and dressings.* Includes all nonprescription medicines and dressings used externally.
- *Medical equipment for general use.* Includes nonprescription medical equipment not worn or not used for supporting the body. Included in this group are nonprescription male and female contraceptives. Whirlpools and vaporizers are also included.
- *Supportive and convalescent medical equipment.* This category includes all supportive and convalescent medical equipment and auxiliaries to such equipment. Also included are prostheses, crutches, wheelchairs, and associated accessories.
- *Hearing aids.* Includes all types of hearing aids and the cost of testing and fitting of the hearing aid.

Nonmedical Services

The nonmedical services category is concerned with all personal services that are not included in medical services. Examples would include services such as housecleaning, home maintenance, lawn care, and auto repair. Some services that are medically related will fall into this group, such as wheelchair repair and maintenance of a van wheelchair lift. Nonprofessional attendant care (when not provided through a health care provider) can be classified as a nonmedical service.

Since the long-term inflation rate of nonmedical services is less than that for medical services, when there is doubt as to the correct classification, the conservative approach would be to place the service item in the nonmedical services category.

Nonmedical Commodities

The nonmedical commodities category includes all the commodity (i.e., not services) items that do not fall under medical commodities. Such items might be specialty foods, housing, and alterations to housing, automobiles, games, bedding, and computers.

The historical inflation rates of each of these categories are given by the appropriate subseries of the CPI, or, in the case of nonmedical services, the average increase in hourly wages in the private nonagricultural economy. These are shown in Tables 11.1 through 11.6.

What Should Be Included

The life care plan, in personal injury litigation, should include all medical and care items (both services and commodities) that will be, or should be, incurred because of the incident in question. Which specific items to include is usually not a question for the economist. The economist must

Table 11.1 Consumer Price Index for Medical Components: All Urban Consumers

Year	*All Items CPI 1982–1984 = 100.0*	*Medical Care 1982–1984 = 100.0*
1980	82.4	
1981	90.9	
1982	96.5	
1983	99.6	
1984	103.9	106.8
1985	107.6	113.5
1986	109.6	122.0
1987	113.6	130.1
1988	118.3	138.6
1989	124.0	149.3
1990	130.7	162.8
1991	136.2	177.0
1992	140.3	190.1
1993	144.5	201.4
1994	148.2	211.0
1995	152.4	220.5
1996	156.9	228.2
1997	160.5	234.6
1998	163.0	242.1
1999	166.6	250.6
2000	172.2	260.8
2001	177.1	272.8
2002	179.9	285.6
2003	184.0	297.1
2004	188.9	310.1
2005	195.3	323.2
2006	201.6	336.2

(Continued)

Table 11.1 (Continued) Consumer Price Index for Medical Components: All Urban Consumers

Year	*All Items CPI 1982–1984 = 100.0*	*Medical Care 1982–1984 = 100.0*
2007	207.3	351.1
2008	215.3	364.1
2009	214.5	375.6
2010	218.1	388.4
2011	224.9	400.3
2012	229.6	414.9
2013	233.0	425.1
2014	236.7	435.3
2015	237.0	446.8
2016	240.0	463.7
2017	245.1	475.3

Source: U.S. Department of Labor, Bureau of Labor Statistics.

make sure that only marginal costs are considered, that is, those items that normally would not be purchased from earnings absent the injuries. This, of course, would not apply if earning capacity is not an element of damages.

In addition, the value of the items or services should be evaluated even if provided at no cost by family members, significant others, or some other collateral source. Each of these concepts will be briefly discussed.

Marginal Costs

A marginal cost, as it pertains to a life care plan in personal injury litigation, can be defined as an additional or extra cost that is incurred because, and only because, of the injury in question. For instance, the entire cost of a new car (every 3 years or so) would generally *not* be considered a marginal cost. The individual would normally need transportation even if not injured. Under normal circumstances the transportation would have been paid for out of the individual's earning capacity, which is, of course, usually another element of potential damage. What would be appropriate, however, is the additional cost required by the nature of the limitations. A van rather than a regular car might be necessary to transport a client in a wheelchair. If so, the additional cost of a van instead of a regular car would be appropriate. Any special modifications such as a lift or special controls would also qualify as a marginal cost. To obtain the marginal cost, one would subtract the cost of a normal item, such as a compact car, from the cost of the recommended item.*

* Some economists are reluctant to make this deduction but will compute the present value if the reduced value is included in the life care plan. Some economists become annoyed if the life care planner tells the economist what he/she should do with a statement such as, "… the economist should reduce the cost of the van by the cost of a standard sedan…"

Table 11.2 Consumer Price Index for Medical Commodities: All Urban Consumers

Year	*Medical Commodities 1982–1984 = 100.0*	*Prescription Drugs 1982–1984 = 100.0*	*Nonprescription Drugs December 2009 = 100*	*Medical Equipment and Supplies December 2009 = 100*
1980	75.4	72.5		
1981	83.7	80.8		
1982	92.3	90.2		
1983	100.2	100.1		
1984	107.5	109.7		
1985	115.2	120.1		
1986	122.8	130.4		
1987	131.0	140.8		
1988	139.9	152.0		
1989	150.8	165.2		
1990	163.4	181.7		
1991	176.8	199.7		
1992	188.1	214.7		
1993	195.0	223.0		
1994	200.7	230.6		
1995	204.5	235.0		
1996	210.4	242.9		
1997	215.3	249.3		
1998	221.8	258.6		
1999	230.7	273.4		
2000	238.1	285.4		
2001	247.6	300.9		
2002	256.4	316.5		
2003	262.8	326.3		
2004	269.3	337.1		
2005	276.0	349.0		
2006	285.9	363.9		

(*Continued*)

Table 11.2 (Continued) Consumer Price Index for Medical Commodities: All Urban Consumers

Year	*Medical Commodities 1982–1984 = 100.0*	*Prescription Drugs 1982–1984 = 100.0*	*Nonprescription Drugs December 2009 = 100*	*Medical Equipment and Supplies December 2009 = 100*
2007	290.0	369.2		
2008	296.0	378.3		
2009	305.1	391.1		
2010	314.7	407.8	100.0	99.1
2011	324.1	425.0	98.6	99.3
2012	333.6	440.1	99.3	100.6
2013	335.1	442.6	99.4	101.0
2014	343.4	458.3	98.5	100.5
2015	354.6	479.3	97.8	99.7
2016	366.8	502.5	96.6	99.3
2017	377.0	519.6	97.4	99.6

For the initial cost of a vehicle, the life care planner should not include the value of any trade-in. The value of a trade-in is an asset owned by the individual. The value of the vehicle to be traded in is no different than a down payment taken from savings. The measure is how much more does the new vehicle cost, given the requirements necessitated by the injury, than the type of vehicle that normally would have been purchased by the injured party. For instance, assume an individual owned a sedan with a trade-in value of $2,000. A new similar sedan could be purchased for $15,000, without trade-in, or $13,000 with trade-in. However, the nature of the injury is such that a van with lift is necessary at a cost of $25,000. The marginal cost would be $25,000 minus $15,000, or $10,000. The trade-in is completely irrelevant. However, trade-ins of vehicles purchased through the life care plan should be considered. That is, if a new van is needed every 5 years at a current value of $25,000 and the van initially purchased has a trade in value of $5,000 after 5 years of use, the marginal cost, which should be included in the plan would be $25,000 less $5,000, or $20,000.

The same concept holds true for equity received in the sale of a home necessitated by the purchase of new facilities that will be necessary to accommodate the injuries. Only the additional cost should be included in the life care plan. That cost can be estimated by the difference between the market price of the old home and that of the new one. Any equity held in the old home is irrelevant.

The case of a renter is somewhat different. If the life care plan includes the cost of the recommended facility as well as the rent currently paid, the economist can compute an inputted value to the stream of rental payments. That is, the economist can estimate the value of the rented home and thus determine the marginal cost of the recommended facility.

Items such as television sets, radios, and books are often set forth in life care plans. In some cases, the inclusion of such items may be justified because of the specifics of the case, but often the items are duplications of what the individual would normally have purchased without the injury

Table 11.3 Consumer Price Index for Medical Services: All Urban Consumers

Year	*Medical Care Services 1982–1984 = 100.0*	*Professional Medical Services 1982–1984 = 100.0*	*Physician's Services 1982–1984 = 100.0*	*Dental Services 1984–1986 = 100.0*	*Eye Care 1982–1984 = 100.0*	*Other Professional Services December 1986 = 100.0*
1980	74.8		76.5	78.9		
1981	82.8		84.9	86.5		
1982	92.6		92.9	93.1		
1983	100.7		100.1	99.4		
1984	106.7	107.0	107.0	107.5		
1985	113.2	113.5	113.3	114.2		
1986	121.9	120.8	121.5	120.6		
1987	130.0	128.8	130.4	128.8	103.5	102.4
1988	138.3	137.5	139.8	137.5	108.7	108.3
1989	148.9	146.4	150.1	146.1	112.4	114.2
1990	162.7	156.1	160.8	155.8	117.3	120.2
1991	177.1	165.7	170.5	167.4	121.9	126.6
1992	190.5	175.8	181.2	178.7	127.0	131.7
1993	202.9	184.7	191.3	188.1	130.4	135.9
1994	213.4	192.5	199.8	197.1	133.0	141.3
1995	224.2	201.0	208.8	206.8	137.0	143.9
1996	232.4	208.3	216.4	216.5	139.3	146.6
1997	239.1	215.4	222.9	226.6	141.5	151.8
1998	246.8	222.2	229.5	236.2	144.1	155.4
1999	255.1	229.2	236.0	247.2	145.5	158.7
2000	266.0	237.7	244.7	258.5	149.7	161.9
2001	278.8	246.5	253.6	269.0	154.5	167.3
2002	292.9	253.9	260.6	281.0	155.5	171.8
2003	306.0	261.2	267.7	292.5	155.9	177.1
2004	321.3	271.5	278.3	306.9	159.3	181.9
2005	336.7	281.7	287.5	324.0	163.2	186.8

(Continued)

Table 11.3 (Continued) Consumer Price Index for Medical Services: All Urban Consumers

Year	*Medical Care Services 1982–1984 = 100.0*	*Professional Medical Services 1982–1984 = 100.0*	*Physician's Services 1982–1984 = 100.0*	*Dental Services 1984–1986 = 100.0*	*Eye Care 1982–1984 = 100.0*	*Other Professional Services December 1986 = 100.0*
2006	350.6	289.3	291.9	340.9	168.1	192.2
2007	369.3	300.8	303.2	358.4	171.6	197.4
2008	384.9	311.0	311.3	376.9	174.1	205.5
2009	397.3	319.4	320.8	388.1	175.5	209.8
2010	411.2	328.2	331.3	398.8	176.7	214.4
2011	423.8	335.7	340.3	408.0	178.3	217.4
2012	440.3	342.0	347.3	417.5	179.9	219.6
2013	454.0	349.5	354.2	431.8	180.8	223.3
2014	464.8	355.2	359.1	441.0	183.9	226.4
2015	476.2	361.5	366.1	452.2	184.0	228.2
2016	494.8	371.5	378.1	465.0	187.0	231.0
2017	506.8	375.1	380.1	472.6	187.3	236.6

and therefore are not a marginal cost and should not be a part of the plan. Marginal costs, however, may be included in the rare case where no compensation for lost earning capacity is included in the total damage estimate.

Value of the Items

Care must be taken to include the type and extent of all additional commodities and services necessitated by the injury, even if these have been, or are expected to be, provided without direct out-of-pocket cost to the client. For example, an injured party may require 24-hour, 7-days-a-week attendant care, which has been provided in the past by family members. Even if the family members are able and willing to continue to provide the services, from an economic point of view the value of the services should be estimated and included as a part of the life care plan. In economics, this is called the *opportunity cost* (Dillman, 1988).

The concept of marginal cost may also come into play when assigning a value to some of the services provided. That is, some of the services provided by the family member would have been provided even without the injury and consequently should not be double counted. For instance, if the injured party is a young child who requires constant care, only the additional care necessitated by the injury should be considered. The normal and customary care a mother and other family members would provide the child should not be considered an additional cost necessitated by the injury.

Table 11.4 Consumer Price Index for Hospital Services: All Urban Consumers

Year	*Hospital and Related Services 1982–1984 = 100.0*	*Hospital Services December 1986 = 100.0*	*Nursing Homes and Adult Day Services December 1996 = 100*	*Care of Invalids and Elderly at Home December 2005 = 100*
1988	143.9			
1989	160.5			
1990	178.0			
1991	196.1			
1992	214.0			
1993	231.9			
1994	245.6			
1995	257.8			
1996	269.5			
1997	278.4	101.7	102.3	
1998	287.5	105.0	107.1	
1999	299.5	109.3	111.6	
2000	317.3	115.9	117.0	
2001	338.3	123.6	121.8	
2002	367.8	134.7	127.9	
2003	394.8	144.7	135.2	
2004	417.9	153.4	140.4	
2005	439.9	161.6	145.0	
2006	468.1	172.1	151.0	101.8
2007	498.9	183.6	159.6	103.2
2008	534.0	197.2	165.3	107.9
2009	567.9	210.7	171.6	109.9
2010	607.7	227.2	177.0	111.3
2011	641.5	241.2	182.2	113.1
2012	672.1	253.6	188.8	114.5

(*Continued*)

Table 11.4 (Continued) Consumer Price Index for Hospital Services: All Urban Consumers

Year	*Hospital and Related Services 1982–1984 = 100.0*	*Hospital Services December 1986 = 100.0*	*Nursing Homes and Adult Day Services December 1996 = 100*	*Care of Invalids and Elderly at Home December 2005 = 100*
2013	701.3	265.4	194.5	115.1
2014	733.8	278.8	200.1	116.7
2015	761.9	290.1	206.4	117.9
2016	795.1	303.3	213.7	120.6
2017	831.7	318.2	220.3	119.6

In some life care plans an attendant or aide is priced at the going market rate, as if one were to directly hire and become the employer. In other plans, the service is considered to be provided by a home care provider. If the direct-hire approach is to be recommended, consideration must be given to the following:

- The hourly wage must be at least the federal minimum wage.
- The employer (i.e., the client) will be responsible for the withholding and payment of all Social Security taxes. Arrangements must be made for the filing of all reports in a timely fashion.
- Provision must be made for vacations, sickness, or other unavailability of the employee.
- The client will be responsible for hiring and training. The turnover of such employees can be expected to be very high.

The administrative tasks necessary when an employee is used may prove too burdensome for the client, who is, after all, injured or at least in need of assistance. Although family members may assume the responsibility for these administrative matters, it is not incumbent upon them to do so. In most cases, the preferred treatment would be to assume that attendant costs would be provided by a home care agency. (*Editors' note*: For a detailed explanation of costs associated with private hire, see Thomas & Kitchen, 1996, Private hire: The real costs, *Inside Life Care Planning* 1: 1, 3–5.)

Delivery Period and Amount

In computing the present value of the life care plan, the economist must know the timing of each cost element as well as the length of time the element will be needed. There are two separate considerations concerning the delivery period: *when* the element will be needed (including replacements) and for *how long* it will be needed.

When something is needed the life care planner must be specific as to initial cost as well as the duration. Care must be taken that the timing does not overlap that is, a statement such as "ages 5 through 18" overlaps with the duration "18 through 25." The entry should state from age 5 through 18, then age 19 through 25, and so on.

Table 11.5 Historical Hourly Earnings for Nonagricultural Wage and Salary Employees, 1947–2001

Year	*Hourly Wages*	*Year*	*Hourly Wages*
1980	6.85	1999	13.49
1981	7.44	2000	14.02
1982	7.87	2001	14.54
1983	8.20	2002	14.97
1984	8.49	2003	15.37
1985	8.74	2004	15.69
1986	8.93	2005	16.13
1987	9.14	2006	16.76
1988	9.44	2007	17.42
1989	9.80	2008	18.06
1990	10.20	2009	18.61
1991	10.52	2010	19.05
1992	10.77	2011	19.44
1993	11.05	2012	19.74
1994	11.34	2013	20.13
1995	11.65	2014	20.61
1996	12.04	2015	21.03
1997	12.51	2016	21.54
1998	13.01	2017	22.05

Source: Economic Report of the President 2018.

The life care planner should attempt to be as specific as possible as to exactly when a procedure or item will be required. Estimates such as "when needed" or "as required" are often seen in life care plans but cannot be evaluated by the economist.

Statements such as "two operations will be required over lifetime" are less precise than the economist would prefer but can be used and evaluated. In such a case, the economist may make the estimate by assuming that the procedures will occur at equal time intervals over the life expectancy. As an alternative, the economist may total the costs for all like procedures and divide by the number of years of life expectancy to give an annual amortized cost. This would represent the average annual cost for the procedures. If the delivery times are given as a range (e.g., every 3 to 5 years), the economist may space the delivery at the mean (e.g., 4 years) or, again, compute an annual average. Using an average per year is slightly less accurate than using given amounts in specific years, however. However, in many cases, the exact timing will not be known by the life care planner.

Table 11.6 Average Annual Increases for Medical and Care Costs

Cost Category	*Data Series*	*Average Annual Rate of Increase (1980–2007)*
Medical services	Medical care services	
	CPI	5.31
Medical commodities	Medical care commodities	
	CPI	4.45
Nonmedical services	Average hourly earnings	3.21
Nonmedical commodities	All items (CPI)	2.99

Source: Tables 11.1 through 11.5.

Statements such as "an operation will be needed within the next 10 years" are very imprecise but still may be evaluated by the economist. The most conservative evaluation would place the timing at the beginning of the period if the inflation rate is expected to exceed the discount rate, or at the end of the period if the interest rate is expected to exceed inflation. A compromise evaluation may be made by timing the procedure at the midpoint of the stated duration or by averaging the cost over this period and using an annual average.

The duration of the delivery period is also a very important consideration. The life care plan should note when the element is to start (usually identified by age or year) and when it is to end. Statements such as "these costs will continue until he reaches adulthood" provides the economist with imprecise information.

Care must be exercised in assigning a range of values to the items (as opposed to a range of delivery times). Ranges in values may occur for two reasons. If the item is identical from two different vendors, the lowest cost should be the only one included. *Identical,* however, refers both to the characteristics of the item as well as its availability. If there is some difference in the characteristics that is not identical, only the preferred one should be recommended. It is incumbent upon the life care planner to make that recommendation; the economist cannot do so.

In other words, ranges in values should not, in most cases, be included in the plan even if the source for the values presents a range, but rather the mean of the values should be presented. However, there is one instance, long-term care, where the presentation of a range of values would be appropriate. In some cases, long-term care may be provided by a health care facility. On the other hand, provision for care, at least for some period, may be made in a home setting among loved ones. This cost of around-the-clock home care, may be significantly higher than the facility cost. However, the intangible values of being with and around loved ones is something that should be presented to the finder of fact, which is a jury in most litigated cases.

A life care plan frequently includes items such as wheelchairs, hospital beds, or other medical equipment that may have to be replaced periodically. In some cases, some trade-in value may be present. If so, the life care plan should only include the out-of-pocket cost of the replacement equipment. This pertains only to equipment initially purchased through funds provided by the life care plan and not to a residual value of things already owned by the individual as was discussed concerning purchase of a vehicle.

Some equipment items may have been purchased prior to funding the life care plan. In such a case, this expense would have been included in past damages and should not be included in the life care plan, which provides for future medical and care needs.

Life care plans often include costs of institutional care where, of course, food and lodging are provided by the facility and thus are included in the cost. Economists differ as to whether the "normal" per diem costs of this food and lodging should be an offset against the total cost. The argument for such an offset is that these expenditures would be made anyway and paid for out of earning capacity. The argument against such a deduction is that the type and quality of lodging and food are not the same as the individual would otherwise expect. In any event, the decision whether to deduct should be left to the economist.

Many of the elements identified in the life care plan will be delivered over the life expectancy of the injured party. The question may arise as to what is the life expectancy of the client given the medical condition. A change to the life expectancies set forth in the typical mortality table is not an economic determination but rather a medical one. The economist should be made aware of any modifications to a normal life expectancy made by a specialist. It should be emphasized that the client's life expectancy should be based on the assumption of quality care, as set forth in the life care plan. For this reason, data from studies of the mortality rates of patients with like conditions but who did not have the advantages of quality care should not be used, uncritically, as evidence of a changed life expectancy for the client.

Actual or Average Annual

The costs of the various items may be stated in terms of a specific value in one or more years or may be stated in terms of an average cost per year. For instance, assume a medical item costs $12,000 and will have to be replaced every 4 years. The life care planner may opt to average the expenditures as $3,000 per year. The present value of items listed in these two ways will differ slightly because of the math involved. If the initial costs and the replacement periods are known exactly, then analyzing the data based on a specific amount in a given year will be slightly more accurate than using the average per year. The problem in most cases, however, is that both the initial costs and the length of the replacement periods are estimates, averages, or ranges. When this is the case, little accuracy will be lost by allocating the costs on an average basis.

Economy of Effort

A comprehensive life care plan will contain a large number of items, some of which cost little and some of which cost a great deal. Experience has shown that most of the costs are concentrated in just a relatively few items, usually those elements associated with care, such as the costs of doctors, hospitals, nurses, LPNs, or attendants. The total value of the commodity items generally represents only a small proportion of the total costs.

Many life care plans set forth trivial commodity items in minute detail. Some go as far as to estimate the number of additional boxes of facial tissue that will be used annually. On the other hand, the same plan may set forth two or more care options that differ by many thousands (or even hundreds of thousands) of dollars per year. In many cases, the care options will be assigned a cost, but detailed discussion as to the relative benefits of each option will not be given. The reader of the plan will have little or no idea of the relative advantages or disadvantages of the various care options.

The life care plan would be strengthened if the major research, development, and discussion were concentrated on needs that make the greatest impact on total costs. That is, the important items should be emphasized. In many cases, even if the marginal costs of the trivial items (such as facial tissue) were eliminated from the analysis, there would be little difference in the final total cost of the life care plan.

Total Lifetime Values

The only important total cost, over the life expectancy, that needs to be considered in a life care plan is the total present value. This is the number the jury will be asked to consider to provide for the lifetime medical and care needs of the client. Present value considers the rates of price inflation as well as the earning power of money (i.e., interest).

When a life care planner gives a total lifetime value of the recommended items by adding all of the items over life expectancy, the results may be confusing and even misleading. If such a total is intended to represent present value, the implicit assumption is that inflation and interest will cancel out. Unless the economist uses the total offset discounting method, the present value calculation will always differ from the lifetime total. These differences will often confuse the jury since they will be presented with two values for the total, that is, one provided by the life care planner and the other by the economist. Although, this may be clarified in trial it still may be confusing.

Total lifetime values for individual categories within the life care plan, such as medications or physician services, is a good way for the economist to check his or her work. That is, the economist must enter the amount given in the life care plan in "today's value" before computing present value. As a check the economist may compare the totals given in the life care plan with his/her totals.

Complications

Life care plans frequently enumerate complications that may arise during the individual's life. However, complications that only rise to the level of "potential" do not meet the criterion of "probable" as defined in the legal sense. That is, the chance of a complication occurring should be at least over 50 percent to be included. From a purely statistical point of view, any potential complication could be evaluated if the probability of it occurring were known, but unless that probability exceeded 50 percent it would, in all likelihood, not be allowed into evidence.* This, of course, is not intended to be a legal opinion.

Affordable Care Act

The Affordable Care Act may affect the life care planner's work and, thus, the economist's present value calculations (Field et al., 2015; Congdon-Hohman & Matheson, 2013). (*Editors' note*: At the time of this publication, the future of the Affordable Care Act was in flux.) First, the act requires insurance companies to accept clients regardless of pre-existing medical conditions. It might be argued, then, that the damage suffered by the injured party should be zero since the act also

* A probability is nothing more than the number of times something occurs to the number of times it could possibly occur. For instance, if a lung transplant is needed in one out of four cases, the probability of it happening is 1 divided by 4, 1/4, or 25 percent.

requires everyone, with a few exceptions, to have insurance. However, this would not be the case if the jurisdiction allowed subrogation. Subrogation is the right of the third party provider, that is the insurance company, to recover payment they made on the policy holders behalf. Whether subrogation is allowed may depend on the legal jurisdiction, that is Federal versus various State Courts. Also, many, if not most, insurance plans will not cover certain items, such as long-term care, which may make up a significant portion of many life care plans. The details of which items are covered and which are not, is a matter for the life care planner. The role of the economist is to compute the present value of the items included in the life care plan, not to determine which items to include nor the cost of the various elements. Of course, many forensic economists are familiar with what is and what is not to be included in the analysis in a specific jurisdiction because of prior experiences. If a conflict is thought to exist it should be incumbent upon the economist to attempt to resolve it through consultation with the life care planner.

Conclusion

When an economist is called upon to compute the present value of the future medical and care costs set forth in a life care plan prepared by a specialist, the economist must rely on the accuracy of data, including the need, the dollar values, the timing, and the duration. Since the life care plan is the foundation for the economic analysis, the economist has an interest in how the plan is presented.

References

Congdon-Hohman, J., & Matheson, V. 2013. Potential Effects of the Affordable Care Act on the Award of Life Care Expenses. *Journal of Forensic Economics*, *24*(2), 153–160.

Dillman, E. 1987. The Necessary Economic and Vocational Interface in Personal Injury Cases. *Journal of Private Sector Rehabilitation*, *2*, 121–142.

Dillman, E. 1988. *Economic Damages and Discounting Methods*. Athens, GA: Elliott & Fitzpatrick.

Field, T., Johnson, C., Choppa, A., & Fountaine, J. 2015. The Collateral Source Rule and the Affordable Care Act: Implications for Life Care Planning and Economic Damage. *Journal of Life Care Planning*, *13*(3), 3–16.

SELECTED DISABILITIES: TOPICS AND ISSUES

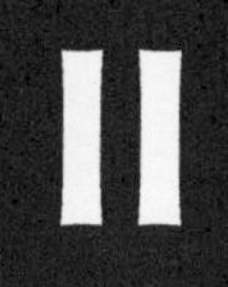

Chapter 12

Life Care Planning for the Amputee

Robert H. Meier, III

Contents

Introduction 336
Phases of Amputation Rehabilitation 337
Preoperative 338
Amputation Surgery and Reconstruction Phase 338
Acute Postoperative Phase 339
Preprosthetic Phase 340
Prosthetic Fabrication 340
Prosthetic Training 340
Community Reintegration 341
Vocational Rehabilitation 342
Follow-Up 342
Demographics of Limb Amputation 343
Phantom and Residual Limb Pain 344
Levels of Limb Amputation 344
Prosthetic Prescription 345
Partial Hand 346
Wrist Disarticulation/Below Elbow (Transradial) 347
Elbow Disarticulation/Above Elbow (Transhumeral) 348
Shoulder Disarticulation 348
Partial/Hindfoot 349
Below Knee (Transtibial) 349
Knee Disarticulation/Above Knee (Transfemoral) 349
Hip Disarticulation 350
Prosthetic Complications 350
Prosthetic Costs 350
Prosthetic Replacement 351

Aging with an Amputation 351
Newer Surgeries for the Limb Amputee 352
Life Care Planning with the Physiatrist 352
Potential Complications 354
Case Example 355
Life Care Plan Narrative for Mr. AK Amputee 356
Projected Rehabilitation Program 356
Projected Evaluations 357
Projected Therapeutic Modalities 357
Diagnostic Testing 357
Wheelchair Needs 357
Wheelchair Accessories and Maintenance 357
Aids for Independent Function 357
Orthotics/Prosthetics 358
Home Furnishings and Accessories 358
Drug/Supply Needs 358
Home/Facility Care 358
Future Medical Care—Routine 358
Transportation 358
Health and Strength Maintenance 359
Architectural Renovations 359
Potential Complications 359
Vocational/Educational Plan 359
Future Medical Care—Aggressive Treatment 359
Orthopedic Equipment Needs 359
Conclusion 364
References 364

Introduction

The physiatrist has been trained in the team approach to provide rehabilitative care to persons with simple and complex disabilities. The physiatrist should serve as an ally with the life care planner in determining the ideal outcome of rehabilitative care over the lifespan. In addition, if the physiatrist has been the care provider throughout the active rehabilitation treatment phase, he or she also will have insights into the psychosocial issues of the person with the disability that will enhance the life care plan. The physiatrist can also medically case manage the variety of health professionals and treatments that are necessary, especially in cases of catastrophic disability. The physiatrist is an excellent resource to provide rehabilitative care and determine appropriate equipment costs and how appropriate they may be since a physician is usually required to order any equipment.

For the person with an amputation, the physiatrist should have the ability to provide meaningful information for the life care plan, especially in the following areas:

1. Point of maximum medical improvement
2. Life expectancy
3. Expected functional outcomes
4. Costs of prosthetic devices
5. Frequency of prosthetic replacement

6. Quantity and types of rehabilitation services and their costs
7. Adaptive equipment needs and costs
8. Architectural modifications for function
9. Attendant care hours and level of service
10. Psychosocial needs
11. Vocational and avocational expectations and modifications
12. Work restrictions
13. Future medical needs, potential medical problems, and their treatment options
14. Future surgical needs

If the local physiatrist is unable to provide useful life care planning information, there is a network of specialized physiatrists who have years of experience in working with the rehabilitation of specific areas of disability. These specialists can be located through the life care planner network. They should have extensive experience in providing health care for a person with an amputation, representing the level(s) specific for a particular case. The physiatrist can be of great service to the life care planner in indicating the appropriate level of functional outcome to be achieved and the future needs for the amputee.

Phases of Amputation Rehabilitation

The loss of a body part is an emotionally traumatic experience. Yet most persons who sustain an amputation can look forward to a fulfilling life of meaningful function using contemporary prosthetic designs. The emotional outcomes are often more important than whether a prosthesis has been supplied or particular functional goals have been achieved. Sometimes, the rehabilitation model is so focused on the prosthesis and their required outcomes for payment, that the amputee and his/her wishes are overlooked. The key to successful prosthetic rehabilitation is having an understanding of the desired functional outcome and the rehabilitative process necessary for achieving that outcome, including the idealized psychosocial outcomes desired. In addition, the physiatrist should provide a time framework for the achievement of the ideal outcome. The physiatrist can also outline the most cost efficient array of rehabilitative services to achieve the desired rehabilitation goals.

To understand the rehabilitative process for a person with an amputation, it is best to consider the following phases of amputation rehabilitation. At all times, it should be kept in mind that amputation rehabilitation is a process and ideally requires more than just making and applying a prosthesis appropriate for the level of amputation. It should be a coordinated rehabilitation effort with clearly stated goals and timelines. In addition, it is an ongoing process since the amputation is a permanent disability and will require knowledgeable rehabilitation ministrations throughout the lifespan. These phases, while somewhat artificial, do interweave and flow from one to the next. By knowing the phase of the amputation rehabilitative process, the life care planner can identify the issues to be considered in each phase and assist the amputee toward the next phase. The hallmarks of each phase can be used to determine if the amputee is successfully moving through the phases or is delayed in a phase. Being delayed in a phase of rehabilitative care can detract from the best functional or psychosocial outcome and can also add to the costs of health care. In addition, a huge part of rehabilitation in today's health care environment with shorter hospital stays has to be amputee education. If a thorough education program cannot be achieved with a short inpatient stay, then this education must be included in any outpatient program. Amputee education regarding prosthetics, stump care, regular ongoing exercise, prosthetic advances, and functional options are often not taught by the physiatrist, the surgeon, the therapist, or the prosthetist. However, this comprehensive amputation education will enable the amputee to remain free of future unnecessary health care visits. This education is a part of today's emphasis on amputee empowerment so that the amputee can control their future health care and prosthetic needs.

The phases for amputation rehabilitation staging and the setting in which they are usually accomplished in today's health systems are:

OUTPATIENT
1. Preoperative

INPATIENT
2. Surgical
3. Acute postsurgical (some inpatient and some outpatient)

OUTPATIENT
4. Preprosthetic
5. Prosthetic prescription and fabrication
6. Prosthetic training
7. Community reentry
8. Vocational/Avocational
9. Follow-up

Hallmarks of each phase have been assigned to measure the progress of the person with an amputation from one phase to the next (Table 12.1). There is usually some overlap from one phase to the next and the person may move more quickly through one phase than another (Meier, 1994). The focus throughout all these phases is on the needs and desires of the amputee. The person's ability to adapt to an altered body image and in some cases, an altered lifestyle, is essential for achieving the idealized outcome. Paying attention to and providing service for their psychosocial well-being is paramount to successful rehabilitative outcomes.

The earlier attention is paid to emotional adaptation to the amputation, the more likely desired goals can be achieved and the patient can begin to feel "whole" again with restored prior levels of function, decision making, and feelings of control. Providing this control earlier in the rehabilitation process can result in fewer issues with pain, depression, and anxiety since the person has regained control over his/her life despite losing a body part. These phases are conceptual but do help the team with a framework of where the amputee is in their progress and where they are headed. It is very helpful during the acute phases of rehabilitation to know what the desired end points will be and how to provide a treatment framework in how to achieve these desired endpoints.

Preoperative

On a few occasions, the patient is delayed in the decision for an amputation. This is an ideal time for the rehabilitation team to assess and begin a treatment plan focusing on function of the remaining extremities. This is also an appropriate time to practice preventive care to maintain full range of motion and strength in the proximal limb muscles of the side to be amputated and also in the intact limb. An aerobic conditioning program should be provided during this phase since this type of exercise will hasten the postoperative functional recovery, especially in the use of a leg or arm prosthesis.

Amputation Surgery and Reconstruction Phase

Amputation surgery should proceed as a reconstructive surgery that will provide a residual limb with the best function, whether or not a prosthesis is likely to be prescribed. A reconstructive

Table 12.1 Medical and Rehabilitation Progression of Amputation

	Phase	*Hallmarks*
1.	Preoperative	Assess body condition, patient education; discuss surgical level, postoperative rehabilitation, and prosthetic plans
2.	Amputation surgery	Length, myoplastic closure, soft tissue coverage, nerve reconstruction handling, rigid dressing
3.	Acute postoperative	Wound healing, pain control, proximal body motion, emotional support
4.	Preprosthetic	Shaping and shrinking amputation stump, increasing muscle strength, restoring patient locus of control
5.	Prosthetic fabrication	Team consensus on prosthetic prescription, experienced prosthetic fabrication
6.	Prosthetic training	Increase wearing of prosthesis, mobility, and ADL skills
7.	Community reintegration	Resume roles in family and community activities; regain emotional equilibrium and healthy coping strategies; pursue recreational activities
8.	Vocational rehabilitation	Assess and plan vocational activities for future. May need further education, training, or job modification
9.	Follow-up	Provide lifelong prosthetic, functional, medical, and emotional support; provide regular assessment of functional level and prosthetic problem solving

philosophy of amputation is best accomplished by a surgeon who has performed a number of amputations and understands contemporary prosthetic options and ideal functional outcomes.

In some cases, further reconstructive surgery for the residual limb will be necessary in order to achieve the best prosthetic function and the ideal outcomes following prosthetic fitting. This type of surgery may include both plastic and orthopedic surgery in order to improve the bony elements of the residual limb or to enhance the quality of soft tissue coverage. The costs of this surgical reconstruction would need to be included in the life care plan. Recently introduced in the United States but not available in all locations is a procedure called "osseous integration." This will be explained later in this text but is likely to become a standard practice in the United States within the next 5–10 years. Including this surgery as a possibility in the life care plan should be strongly considered, in addition to the type of prosthetic replacement required for functional restoration.

Acute Postoperative Phase

This is a time for wound healing and pain control. Usually, there is wound care necessary until the sutures are removed. The rehabilitation focus is on the remaining limbs and instructing the amputee in preventive exercise for the amputated limb and the intact limbs. Psychosocial support is essential during this period of loss for the individual.

Preprosthetic Phase

This period is usually accomplished on an outpatient basis. Once the sutures are removed, attention is paid to shaping and shrinking the residual limb in preparation for prosthetic casting. This is a good time to educate the amputee and the family regarding the prosthetic options available, and to develop and review the rehabilitation plan, if it has not previously been accomplished. At this time careful therapeutic attention should be paid to aerobic conditioning and strength training. Emotional stresses that surround change in body image, function, family roles, and income should be anticipated. Empowering the amputee to view him- or herself as a healthy individual and regaining control of his/her life are important components of this phase.

Prosthetic Fabrication

At this phase, the team, including the amputee, should decide on a prosthetic prescription that best meets the person's needs and desires (Meier & Heckman, 2014). More and more, the prosthetic prescription is also dependent on what a third-party payer will sponsor. It is preferable that a prosthetist who is experienced in fitting the specific level of amputation be used to fabricate the prosthesis. The time framework from prosthetic casting until final fitting of the prosthesis should be presented to the amputee and the rehabilitation team for planning purposes.

Prosthetic prescription is often determined by the prosthetist with little input from other team members, including the patient. There is a great new array of prosthetic componentry with sophisticated technology required for fabrication and training to achieve the best outcomes. However, this newer technology is usually more expensive than the pre-existing components with little to no research to demonstrate when it is most appropriate to use. In addition, there is meager research to indicate whether it is cost effective or efficacious to utilize in the prosthetic prescription. Just because it is newer technology, it is not always better than existing technology.

As a general rule, assuming good wound healing has occurred, the lower limb amputee should be fitted within eight weeks of amputation and the arm amputee fitted within four to six weeks of amputation surgery. If the upper limb amputee is delayed in fitting, their chances of using a prosthesis for bimanual activities decreases significantly. They become accustomed to performing activities in a one-handed manner and, therefore, do not find the prosthesis to be of much assistance in performing their daily activities.

Prosthetic Training

This phase is most often accomplished in an outpatient therapy setting with therapists who have trained many amputees with similar levels of amputation and similar types of prosthetic components. It is important that the therapist has worked with the types of prosthetic components included in the prosthesis. Due to today's prosthetic technology changing so quickly, it is important that the treating therapist keep abreast of the latest componentry and understand the biomechanics of each component. This phase should continue until the expected level of functional outcome has been achieved. The length of treatment time will vary depending on the level of amputation, the amputee's health, level of function prior to the amputation, associated injuries, and medical problems. The rehabilitation team should proceed with gradual prosthetic wearing and functional training with the goal of achieving the idealized functional outcomes listed in Tables 12.2 through 12.4. The rehabilitation treatment plan should focus on the level of function necessary for community reintegration, as well as vocational and avocational outcomes.

Table 12.2 Functional Expectations for the Below-Knee Amputee

1.	Wears the prosthesis during all waking hours
2.	Walks on level and uneven surfaces
3.	Climbs stairs step over step
4.	Drives a car (if desired)
5.	Can fall safely and arise from the floor
6.	Can run (if cardiovascular status permits)
7.	Can hop without the prosthesis
8.	Participates in avocational interests
9.	Has returned to same or modified work
10.	Does not use any gait aid
11.	Performs aerobic conditioning exercise (if cardiovascular system permits)
12.	Knows how to inspect skin of the amputated and nonamputated legs and foot
13.	Knows how to change stump socks to accommodate for soft tissue changes
14.	Knows how to buy a correctly fitting shoe for the remaining foot
15.	Independent in ADL
16.	Understands the necessity of follow-up

An aside is warranted at this point of the discussion. It is more and more difficult to find therapists, both OT and PT, who are trained or have experience using these new components. For a comprehensive and appropriate life care plan, it may be important to include the cost of sending the amputee to a Center of Excellence (COE) which has vast experience in rehabilitation, specifically for persons with all levels of amputation. Therefore, the LCP may need to include costs of transportation to the COE, per diem expenses, and account for the frequency of this type of visit.

It should be noted that some amputees choose to not wear a prosthesis and function quite well. Many of these non-prosthetic wearing amputees develop a meaningful quality of life that suits them. A prosthesis may not always be appropriate to include in a life care plan.

Community Reintegration

The person with the amputation should begin to resume his/her role in the family and the community as quickly as possible following the amputation. Prosthetic training can assist with community reintegration by restoring meaningful function. A psychologist or social worker should assist the amputee in developing productive social interactions with their family, friends, peers, and other persons in their community. This reintegration demonstrates a positive emotional adaptive process from the amputee with the motivation to achieve an optimal quality of life. There are some amputees who, for whatever their individual reasons, have not developed a positive emotional adjustment and do not relate a positive quality of life. This maladaptation is more frequently seen in persons who have chronic pain that has not been adequately addressed or who have been depressed or anxious without appropriate counseling.

Table 12.3 Functional Expectations for the Above-Knee Amputee

(Greater energy expenditure than for below-knee prosthetic use)	
1.	Wears the prosthesis during all waking hours
2.	Walks on level and uneven surfaces
3.	Climbs stairs step over step (some may do one step at a time)
4.	Drives a car (if desired)
5.	Can fall safely and arise from the floor
6.	Can hop without the prosthesis
7.	Participates in avocational interests
8.	Has returned to same or modified work
9.	Does not use any gait aid (some may need a cane)
10.	Performs aerobic conditioning exercise (if cardiovascular system permits)
11.	Knows how to inspect skin of the amputated and nonamputated legs and foot
12.	Knows how to buy a correctly fitting shoe for the remaining foot
13.	Independent in ADL
14.	Understands the necessity of follow-up
15.	A few can run with high-level training

Vocational Rehabilitation

The physiatrist should be closely involved during this phase of amputee rehabilitation, as he or she is most knowledgeable in the expected level of prosthetic use in a variety of vocational settings. The physiatrist is also best suited to place the work restrictions in relationship to the level of amputation and functional outcome. Working as a team, the case manager, the physiatrist, the therapist, the prosthetist, and the vocational rehabilitation specialist can provide an excellent support system for the amputee and enhance their successful return to the workplace. Return to gainful employment will often require work hardening, proper physical conditioning, further education or re-training, a modified worksite, a program to ease back into the worksite, adaptive equipment and emotional preparation for return to work. Again, this is best managed with a coordinated effort from the amputation rehabilitation team and not just by thrusting the injured worker back to full time work without the proper preparation to assure success. This additional provision of services should be spelled out in the life care plan.

Generally, it is ill advised to provide a vocational prognosis until the person has achieved maximum functional outcome with or without use of a prosthesis.

Follow-Up

In order to ensure the most appropriate level of prosthetic function, prevent prosthetic problems, and address emotional adjustment to amputation, a regular and periodic program of rehabilitation

Table 12.4 Functional Expectations for the Above- and Below-Elbow Amputee

1.	Independent in donning and doffing the prosthesis
2.	Independent in Activities of Daily Living
3.	Can write legibly with remaining hand
4.	Has successfully switched dominance (if necessary)
5.	Drives (if desired)
6.	Has returned to work (same or modified job)
7.	Can tie laces with one hand or with the remaining hand and the prosthesis
8.	Uses a button hook easily
9.	Has prepared a meal in the kitchen
10.	Has been shown adaptive equipment for the kitchen and ADL
11.	Has performed carpentry and automotive maintenance (if desired)
12.	Wears prosthesis during all waking hours
13.	Uses the prosthesis for bimanual activities
14.	Understands the necessity of follow-up

follow-up should be provided for the amputee. Once the ideal level of function has been achieved and the amputee is wearing a definitive prosthesis, the person should be seen in regular follow-up on an annual or every-other-year basis. This schedule permits measurement of the functional outcomes of amputation rehabilitation. It also serves to enhance the education of the amputee regarding preventive care and further prosthetic needs.

Restoration of meaningful function, body compensation, and emotional adaptation to an amputation take a significant time from the amputation until the patient is well stabilized. In the person with a unilateral leg amputation, without significant comorbid factors or bilateral limb loss, the process of amputation and its rehabilitation will generally take the majority of 12–18 months in most patients. Certainly prosthetic fitting and training take less than the twelve to eighteen months but the true return to a full life cannot be hurried and the achievement of Maximum Medical Improvement (MMI) falls within this 12–18-month framework. In the person with a unilateral arm amputation, this process of rehabilitation to achieve MMI is more likely to occur in 6 to 9 months from the onset of the amputation. Of course, if there are significant comorbid factors or there is bilateral limb loss, achieving MMI may take a longer period of time.

Demographics of Limb Amputation

Amputation of the leg is more common than amputation of the arm and occurs in a 3:1 ratio (Meier, 2014). The leg amputee is usually a person in the sixth or seventh decade of life who sustains the amputation because of occlusive arterial vascular disease. Often this person also has associated diabetes mellitus. In addition to the vascular disease in the legs, there is often accompanying arterial disease in the coronary and cerebral arteries. With associated diabetes, the complications can include peripheral neuropathy, renal disease, and diminished eyesight. All of these comorbid factors can diminish the functional outcomes expected from prosthetic rehabilitation.

The arm amputee is usually a young person who has sustained a work-related injury. The amputation most frequently involves the right arm and most often results in a below-elbow (transradial) amputation of the dominant arm. The arm amputee, unlike the leg amputee, can function independently with the use of one arm. Full-time functional prosthetic use in the arm amputee is less likely to occur than in the leg amputee.

Phantom and Residual Limb Pain

This phenomenon occurs in most patients immediately following the amputation surgery and usually subsides during the first 4–6 months after the amputation. In only a few amputees does phantom limb or residual limb pain become so problematic that it interferes with the quality of life. Phantom and residual limb pain should not be treated with opioid medications other than during the acute postoperative period. Today, a variety of medications can be used to alleviate this pain. Popular at this time are: pregabalin (Lyrica), gabapentin (Neurontin), dexromethorphan, tricyclic antidepressants, and carbamazepine (Davis, 1993). These medications affect the way the body processes pain messages in the peripheral and central nervous systems. Other physical modalities have been utilized but have met with varied success depending on the individual amputee. If the phantom pain interferes greatly with the quality of life and/or prosthetic function, an amputee pain specialist should be consulted. Often, pain in the amputee is related to the level of anxiety, depression, and altered sleep that is present. Post-Traumatic Stress Disorder (PTSD) is often present and may contribute to the level of perceived pain. Problematic pain in the amputee must be approached using emotional counseling and not just medications or modalities. The other item to consider including in the life care plan is a smoking cessation program, if the amputee is a chronic smoker. It is not reasonable to have a pain treatment program if the amputee is still smoking. Stopping smoking should be the first component of any pain treatment program.

Pain in the residual limb should be differentiated from phantom pain. Often, residual limb pain is caused by a poorly fitting prosthesis and can be alleviated with socket modifications. Residual limb pain may also be caused by the development of a neuroma from a peripheral nerve that was severed at the time of the amputation. There are a variety of conservative and surgical methods to attempt to decrease the pain from a neuroma (Sherman, Sherman, & Gail, 1980).

On a few occasions, neuromodulation through the use of peripheral nerve or central neural stimulation is warranted. This surgery should be provided by a team that has experience in evaluating and treating a number of limb amputees.

Levels of Limb Amputation

In general, the longer the length of the residual limb, the better the prosthetic function that can be expected. In the leg, amputation below the knee (transtibial) provides for lower energy expenditure than the use of an above-knee (transfemoral) prosthesis. Salvaging the leg at a below-knee level is now the goal of leg amputation surgery in the United States (Moore & Malone, 1989). Disarticulation levels for the arm and leg have certain relative contraindications and should be carefully considered on an individual basis. Full thickness skin and soft tissue coverage are also helpful in achieving ideal prosthetic functional outcomes. However, with the new gel liner interfaces, scarred skin and poor soft tissue coverage can be dealt with in a more satisfactory manner than in the past.

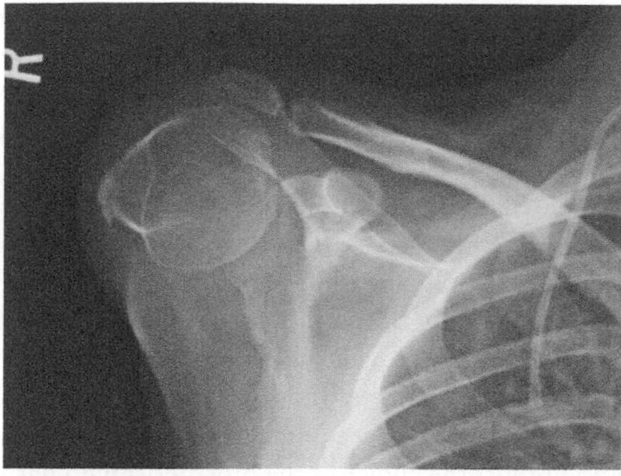

Figure 12.1 X-ray showing extremely short above-elbow amputation post-electrical burn with nothing remaining other than the humeral head.

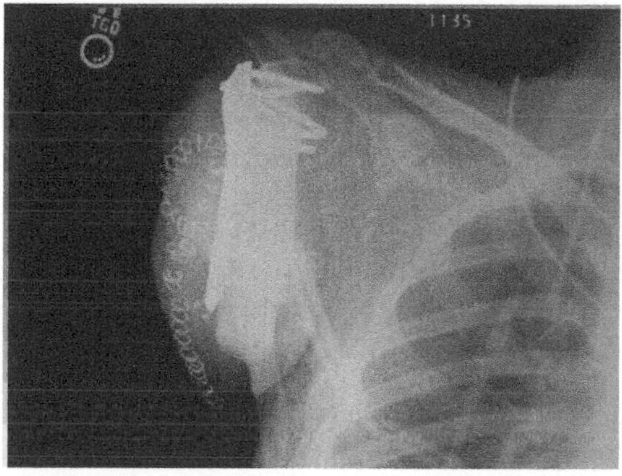

Figure 12.2 X-ray showing same arm with lengthening using allograft bone plated into the residual humeral head. A pedicle graft of latissimus dorsi muscle and overlying soft tissue were used to cover the added bone length. Amputee is now able to wear and use an above-elbow prosthesis.

In today's reconstructive surgery for the amputee, very short residual limbs can be lengthened using bone allograft or Ilizarov techniques. In addition, poor scar and soft tissue coverage can be replaced with full thickness skin and overlying muscle using a pedicle or free flap tissue transfer. Other types of surgery are now being provided for better residual limb management and will be discussed later in this text (see Figures 12.1 and 12.2).

Prosthetic Prescription

There has been an explosion of available prosthetic components in the past ten years and it is hard to keep up with the constant barrage of new options for the amputee. Most of the new components have added to the expense of the prosthesis without scientific demonstration that they have enhanced the functional outcome. Many of the new components are lighter weight and therefore more comfortable to wear. New prosthetic foot designs have added the ability to run and jump, whereas these desired functions were not previously possible with the older component designs (Esquenazi & Torres, 1991). The use of electric components for the arm amputee has not been universally applied in the United States. This technology remains less frequently prescribed than the conventional body-powered designs. The prices of prostheses, especially those using the new socket designs and components, have risen dramatically. A high tech above-knee prosthesis frequently will cost between $20,000 to $140,000, while an above-elbow myoelectric arm can cost $50,000 to $240,000. With costs at these levels, it is imperative that the amputee be treated in a comprehensive interdisciplinary center of amputation rehabilitative excellence. New microprocessor components are flooding the market providing more prosthetic options. However, there is little scientific evidence that they provide measurable improvement over other tried and true components. Using new technology can be sexy but may not improve the overall quality of life or enhanced function so one must be careful in recommending them. Component choice must still be a team decision process and not just the choice of the prosthetist who has potential motivation for financial gain from the prescription of more expensive technology. A proper life care plan includes a prosthetic device and components that have been approved by a physician with knowledge of contemporary prosthetic componentry and training.

The usual components required for a prosthetic leg include the socket, a foot/ankle complex, and a means of suspension. Of course, for the above-knee prosthesis, a knee component is also prescribed.

For the arm amputee, there is a socket that fits onto the residual limb and for the below-elbow amputee, a wrist joint, a terminal device, and a suspension system are required elements of the prescription. Terminal devices can be a hook or a hand (Sears, 1991). The hand can be passive or it can move. For the above-elbow amputee, an elbow joint is prescribed. In considering the arm prosthetic prescription, the team needs to consider the three basic prosthetic designs available. They are a passive prosthesis that provides mainly cosmetic restoration, one that is cable controlled by body power, or one that has electric moving parts. A comparison of these types of arm prostheses is presented in Table 12.5 (Esquenazi, Leonard, Meier, et al., 1989). There are some incredible newer arm component technologies available today. However, when providing the "latest and greatest bionic" arm technology there are a number of things to consider. Will there be a nearby prosthetic lab to evaluate malfunction and provide repair? Is the added weight of the new technology well tolerated by the arm amputee? Is there a therapist who understands the new componentry and can train the amputee to achieve the best and most appropriate outcome when using the arm/hand?

Partial Hand

This level of amputation can be handled in several ways. Many partial hand amputees choose to not wear any prosthetic restoration. However, if cosmesis is desired, a cosmetic glove can be fabricated. This is usually made from a mold taken of the residual hand. A custom-made silicone glove that is hand-colored can provide excellent cosmesis and is reasonably durable. However, if it is worn at work, a protective glove should be worn. Another manner to prosthetically handle this level is to make an opposition bar that can provide improved prehension between the prosthetic bar and the residual moving parts of the hand. If the thumb has been amputated, an excellent prosthetic thumb can be fabricated. The functional and cosmetic results from this prosthesis often decrease the need for surgical reconstruction of the amputated thumb.

There are now some excellent powered partial hand prostheses available that can provide meaningful function for the part of the hand that has been lost. Individual fingers can be replaced that move for function (Figures 12.3 and 12.4).

Table 12.5 Advantages and Disadvantages of Various Upper-Limb Prostheses

Type	*Pros*	*Cons*
Cosmetic (passive)	Most lightweight	High cost if custom made
	Best cosmesis	Least functional
	Least harnessing	Low-cost gloves stain easily
Body powered	Moderate cost	Most body movement to operate
	Moderately lightweight	Most harnessing
	Most durable	Least satisfactory appearance
	Highest sensory feedback	
Externally powered (myoelectric and switch control)	Moderate or no harnessing	Heaviest
	Least body movement to operate	Most expensive
	Moderate cosmesis	Most maintenance
	More function-proximal levels	Limited sensory feedback
Hybrid (cable elbow/electric TD)	All cable excursion to elbow	Electric TD weights forearm (harder to lift)
	Increased TD pinch	Good for elbow disarticulation (or long above elbow)
Hybrid (electric elbow/cable TD)	All cable excursion to TD	Least cosmesis
	Low effort to position TD	Lower pinch force for TD
	Low maintenance TD	

Source: Adapted from Esquenazi, A., Leonard, J. A., & Meier, R. H. 1989. Prosthetics. *Archives of Physical Medicine Rehabilitation*, *70*(suppl.), 207.

Wrist Disarticulation/Below Elbow (Transradial)

The below-elbow prosthesis is usually composed of a double-walled plastic laminate socket that fits intimately over the residual limb. A locking, quick-change wrist unit is commonly prescribed through which the terminal device is attached to the forearm shell. This wrist unit permits ease of change of various terminal devices and locks the terminal device in a position of function when handling heavier objects. For most people who will return to heavy-duty work, a body-powered prosthesis will be useful. For the business or white collar worker, a myoelectric or a passive cosmetic prosthesis may be preferable (Meier & Atkins, 2004).

Newer hands with isolated finger motion (I-Limb, Michaelangelo, and Bebionic) are now commercially available for myoelectric control, and they permit individual finger motion with articulation of the usual finger joints. These technologies have added significantly to the cost of a hand or arm prosthesis so current pricing should be provided by a prosthetic laboratory that

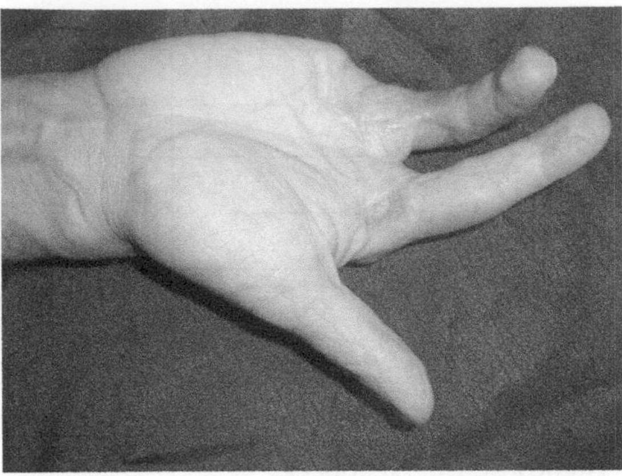

Figure 12.3 Traumatic amputations of the ring and little fingers with cosmetic deformity.

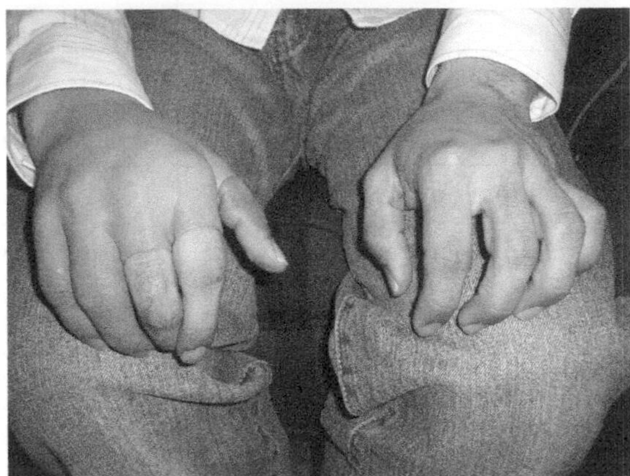

Figure 12.4 Finger amputations shown in Figure 12.3 now covered with a passive cosmetic glove replacing the ring and little fingers that permits use of the residual thumb, index, and long digits.

specializes in upper limb prosthetic fabrication. In addition, learning to use this new technology may require additional travel and therapy expense since not all local therapists have training knowledge, and the amputee may need to travel to an upper extremity center of excellence in order to assure the best fitting and outcomes (Figure 12.5).

Elbow Disarticulation/Above Elbow (Transhumeral)

The prosthetic options at this level of restoration are body-powered or electric control. The electric prosthesis is many times the expense of the body-powered arm. For a very short above-elbow level of amputation, an electric prosthesis may be the only functional restoration that is reasonable.

Shoulder Disarticulation

This level can be fitted with a lighter weight endoskeletal design with a passive elbow joint and a moving terminal device. At this proximal level of amputation, an electric prosthesis will permit more functional motion of the component parts. However, it is heavier to wear and much more costly.

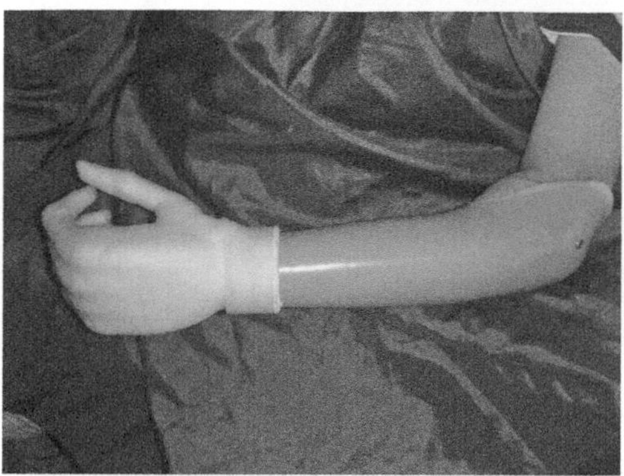

Figure 12.5 "I-Hand" without coverage of a cosmetic glove. Individual fingers move using myoelectric signals.

Partial/Hindfoot

Often this level of amputation can be fitted with a full-length insole with toe filler that fits inside the shoe. This insole can usually be interchanged between various shoes. The bottom of the shoe may need to be modified to provide a more normal gait pattern.

Below Knee (Transtibial)

The prosthesis that is currently used for this level of amputation was popularized in the mid-1950s. It is called a patellar tendon bearing (PTB) design. It was originally designed to place superincumbent body weight on the remaining anatomic landmarks that were pressure tolerant. It relieves pressure from the pressure-intolerant areas of the residual stump. For this level, the prosthetic prescription includes the design of the prosthetic socket, a foot/ankle complex, and a means of suspending the prosthesis on the residual leg. A current popular suspension design is called the triple "S" system or the silicone suction suspension. A silicone sleeve is worn against the skin and a knurled pin extends from the distal end. This pin locks inside a coupling in the distal end of the prosthetic socket. The silicone sleeve provides additional padding to the inside of the socket against the skin. Other types of gel liners are in vogue today and have made prosthetic leg wearing more comfortable. These liners reduce the number of skin problems seen with prosthetic wear and function.

Microprocessor foot/ankle technology is now available; examples are the BiOM foot in addition to products made by Ossur. They add weight, cost, and increased maintenance to a prosthetic leg so their advantages may not overcome their disadvantages. Their application should again become a team decision, and there are trial periods where they can be used for a short time to get the amputee's opinion of their function for that individual.

Knee Disarticulation/Above Knee (Transfemoral)

The contemporary socket design for the above-knee amputee has changed in the 1980s and 1990s (Leonard & Meier, 1993). There are a number of designs available but the one in greatest use is a narrow mediolateral, ischial containment design. New socket designs also include thermoplastic inner liners that have improved the comfort of prosthetic wearing. Gel liners are also available for this level of amputation. A variety of knee units are available that provide differing degrees of knee stability and cosmesis with gait.

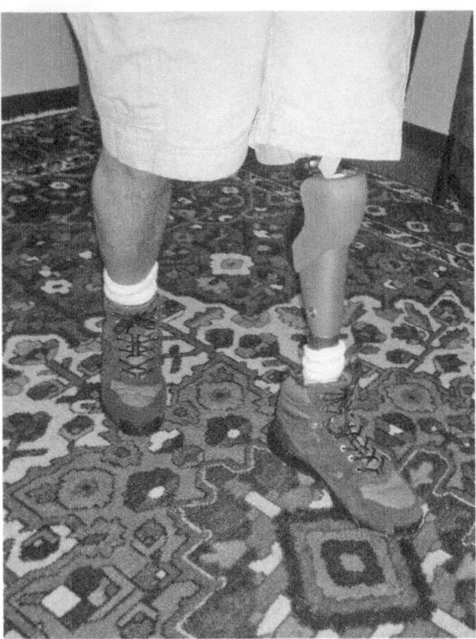

Figure 12.6 One example of the several microprocessor knee units for above-knee amputation prosthetic restoration. This example is a "C leg" manufactured by Otto Bock.

Today, a "computerized" knee unit is available and is, in most cases, the preferred design for use. Some amputees find they have to think less about walking to ensure knee stability with one of these knee units. Also, the knee is less likely to bend causing a fall than some of the prior knee units that were totally controlled by the amputees themselves. These computerized knees are significantly more expensive than their passive counterparts. Some of these units have also made it possible for the above-knee amputee to go up and down steps using a step-over-step pattern (Figure 12.6).

Hip Disarticulation

This is a difficult level to fit comfortably and to have the amputee walk successfully with the prosthesis. This level of amputation should be handled by a prosthetist who makes ten or more of this type of prosthesis a year. More importantly, for best success, this amputee should have their rehabilitation in a center that has trained a number of amputees to wear this type of prosthesis with good results.

Prosthetic Complications

A well-fitted prosthesis is in intimate contact with the skin of the residual limb. There are shearing forces applied to the skin in arm and leg prostheses. In the leg amputee, there are also direct pressures applied from the prosthesis to the skin of the residual leg. These forces can create skin pressure problems. These issues are usually addressed with prosthetic socket modifications or the use of gel-skin interfaces. A differing socket design may also be necessary to change the forces applied to the skin.

Prosthetic Costs

Because of the high cost of prosthetics, a team of experienced amputee rehabilitation specialists should develop a prescription. To have the prosthetist develop the prescription in a vacuum is almost a conflict of interest and should be avoided.

When assembling the prosthetic costs of the life care plan, it is essential that the life care planner understand what estimate the prosthetist is providing. There are at least three ways of pricing a prosthesis. There is a usual and customary cost of a prosthesis. This cost would be the full, non-discounted, non-Medicare allowable cost that usually will have significant mark-up built into the numbers provided from the prosthetic laboratory. Almost never is this price paid to the prosthetist for the final prosthetic device. The more appropriate number to use for prosthetic costs is the Medicare allowable reimbursement. This is the usual amount at which a prosthesis will be paid. Some managed care and insurance providers will discount from the Medicare allowable fee schedule or will provide an add-on amount that will be a specific percentage above the Medicare allowable reimbursement schedule.

Also, if the life care planner is obtaining price quotations from a variety of prosthetic facilities, it is imperative that the same "L" codes be utilized when comparing the various pieces of the prosthesis. The "L" code is the Medicare system of providing specific numbers for specific prosthetic components. If specific "L" codes are not used in obtaining the variety of quotes, it will be like comparing apples and oranges. However, it may be of benefit to obtain a variety of prosthetic price quotes and provide a range in the life care plan using a high estimate, a low estimate, and the median price. Prosthetic pricing does vary from laboratory to laboratory for the exact same prosthesis. Prosthetic price quotes also can vary dramatically from one region of the United States to another geographic region.

The life care planner should be expected to support each of the major "L" codes included in the prosthetic prescription. This would likely include the major components of the prescription. A way to do this would be to explain the major components in the life care plan. Also, the life care planner should be certain to indicate why the physician who generated the prescription had included those particular components. This should provide the basis for prosthetic costs that have been increasing with this new technology.

Prosthetic Replacement

Within the first 2 years following the amputation, several socket changes are usually necessary to accommodate the rapid soft tissue changes that occur. These changes improve the prosthetic fit and comfort of wearing. Usually after this time, a prosthesis should last the amputee from 3 to 5 years before a replacement prosthesis is prescribed. Certainly, the level of activity in using the prosthesis will affect the frequency with which these replacements are needed. Modifications to the prosthesis are usually needed once every 6 months on average. An estimate for routine prosthetic maintenance should be obtained from a prosthetic facility but on average, it is estimated that 10 percent of the original cost of the prosthesis be provided once the warranty of the prosthesis has expired.

As the amputee ages, especially with a leg amputation, and becomes less active, the time between prosthetic replacements can be reasonably increased by a year or so than the average replacement times of 3 to 5 years. Also, the use of alternative mobility may come into play usually at age 65 and above. So, at this point in time, a motorized scooter may enter the life care plan, or a Stairglide may be placed in the home for safe stair negotiation.

Complete replacement of a leg prosthesis is generally felt to be essential for the active prosthetic wearer every 3 to 5 years. This provides a mean of 4 years between new prosthetic fabrication.

For the conventional, body-powered arm prosthetic user, the same replacement schedule is provided as for the leg. For the electric arm prosthesis, the replacement schedule increases to every 7 years.

Aging with an Amputation

As the amputee matures and reaches age 60–65, it is expected that prosthetic use decreases. This decreased use should increase the length of time between essential prosthetic replacement.

It is likely that an average replacement for a new prosthesis would occur every 5 years instead of the previously recommended 4 years. Also, the use of alternative mobility may come into play usually at age 65 and above. So, at this point in time, a motorized scooter may enter the life care plan, or a Stairglide may be placed in the home for safe stair negotiation. As functional use of the prosthesis decreases, it should also be expected that additional assistance for essential household function should be provided in the life care plan. This sort of assistance would include outdoor home maintenance and yard work, heavier housework, or items such as bed making, laundry, housecleaning, mopping, vacuuming, and so on. Also, the incidence of low back pain in the more mature amputee has been found in about 75 percent of lower limb amputees. This pain is generally secondary to biomechanical issues but should be evaluated and treated on a regular basis.

Also, aging with a disability research has shown the onset of additional disabling changes in body systems within 20–30 years from the onset of the initial disability. In the amputee, issues of overuse and biomechanical stress and strain do occur over years of altered biomechanics. Often, changes are seen in the extremity opposite to the amputated one and also in the more proximal body segments which take additional stress and strain to compensate for the amputation.

Newer Surgeries for the Limb Amputee

Within the past 20 years, newer surgeries have been developed to enhance function and comfort for the amputee. These procedures will be listed individually since they have differing purposes:

1. *Osseous Integration*—Perhaps the single most important development for the limb amputation has been popularized by Brannemark originally in Sweden. This surgery provides for direct skeletal attachment of the prosthesis following the implantation of a metal coupler in the bone of the residual limb. This attachment eliminates the need for a prosthetic socket covering the fleshy part of the residual arm or leg so there is no pressure on the soft tissues as was present in the custom made sockets in past use.
2. *Targeted Muscle Reinnervation*—A procedure where the peripheral nerves that are not in use because there are no distal muscles for it to innervate is rerouted. It then re-grows into other muscles present in the limb that remains (Kuiken et al. 2009). This provides additional sites for muscle signal using a myoelectric component. In addition, some amputees have noted a significant decrease in pain that had been present before this surgery was performed.
3. *Bone Allograft*—Using cadaver bone, additional bone length can be added to the residual bone length and then covered with a composite soft tissue graft. This procedure can add 3 to 6 inches of new length to a shorter residual limb. This provides added level arm for powering the prosthesis.
4. *Ertl Osteoplasty*—This procedure is most commonly utilized for a below knee (transtibial) amputation. A bony bridge between the distal tibia and fibula is created and heals with the formation of new bone. This procedure often creates a more squared off distal design of the stump. It is felt to stabilize the loose fibula which otherwise can move a great deal in the stump and cause discomfort with prosthetic wear. In addition, with a stable bony structure it may make comfortable prosthetic fit more readily achieved and prevent marked distal stump atrophy or shape change.

Life Care Planning with the Physiatrist

There are three differing scenarios for physiatric involvement with life care planning. The best scenario is when the physiatrist to be involved with the life care plan has been the treating physiatrist throughout the individual's rehabilitation process. In this scenario, the physiatrist has become quite involved with developing and facilitating the amputee's rehabilitation treatment goals and plan. Having worked with the amputee through the phases of amputation rehabilitation, this physiatrist can give the most useful prognostic information for the life care plan. The physiatrist will have a clear picture of the amputee's psychosocial support system and their needs and desires, as well as the amputee's preamputation lifestyle and how likely it will be to achieve the desired quality of life post-amputation.

Another scenario is the physiatrist who has been asked to participate in a life care plan but has never been involved with the amputee's rehabilitation program. This physiatrist should evaluate the individual to provide meaningful information for a life care plan. Often, this requires a visit from the amputee to the physiatrist for a thorough assessment. This may be accomplished over a one- to several-day period of time, depending on the complexity of the case. Almost always, this evaluation will be performed during an outpatient visit. The evaluation usually includes the physiatric assessment and visits with an occupational therapist, a physical therapist, a psychologist, and a prosthetist. Other rehabilitation professionals and consultants may be included in this evaluation depending on other areas of disability or comorbid factors that are present. The product of this evaluation should be a report that provides all the information that a life care planner will find useful in developing the final plan. For this reason, it is essential that the life care planner pose all of the important questions they wish the physician to address before the evaluation process begins.

The evaluation process by the physiatrist should include the following elements that are clearly delineated during the evaluation and the physiatrist's opinions that are to be included in the life care document.

These items should include:

1. History
2. Past medical history
3. Review of systems including thorough assessment of pain *and sexual function*
4. Medications
5. Psychosocial history
6. Activity status—before the amputation and at the time of the evaluation
7. Vocational history
8. Avocational history
9. Prosthetic history
10. Adaptive equipment used
11. Achievement of maximum medical improvement
12. Future needs
    a. Prosthetic
    b. Emotional
    c. Rehabilitative
    d. Medical
    e. Surgical
    f. Equipment
    g. Architectural modifications
    h. Attendant care
    i. Vocational options
    j. Follow-up plan
    k. Health maintenance and preventive care
13. Specifically stated goals obtained from the amputee for their future life

A third manner for physiatric involvement in life care planning is the "curbside consultation." In this instance, the physiatrist does not have the advantage of evaluating the amputee in a personal visit but instead reviews the case records and provides input into the life care plan based on the physiatrist's experience with similar patients. This manner of physiatric involvement can be very useful to the life care planner in helping to assure that important life care planning issues for a person with an amputation are not overlooked and that the life care plan is as complete as possible.

Potential Complications

Potential complications are dependent on the reason for the amputation (trauma, electrocution, diabetes, cancer, cardiovascular disease, etc.), fit of prosthesis (if one is used), work demands, living environment, quality of medical treatment, and other factors. However, common considerations include (Weed & Sluis, 1990):

1. Some of the most common complications are psychological. In many cases, psychological counseling will be provided while the client is an inpatient and may be continued following discharge from acute care. If psychological counseling is offered, the costs for this should be placed on the Projected Therapeutic Modalities page. In one example case, the client experienced significant depression, was hospitalized for suicidal ideation, and had undergone a significant amount of psychological counseling following discharge. In this case, the family unit fell apart and a number of family counseling issues were raised.
2. In the event of amputations where the client wears a prosthesis, one would expect the probability of occasional skin breakdown. In one case, the client suffered amputations as a result of an electrocution injury. In this situation, the skin loses its integrity due to the burn. The client may require surgical intervention in order to repair skin breakdown.
3. Bone spurs occasionally become a problem and may require surgery.
4. Phantom pain or sensations are very common, at least during acute recovery, and may need some sort of treatment.
5. Other complications include osteoarthritis, which may be experienced in the knees and lower back, as well as back pain that may be experienced due to an abnormal gait. Fit of the prostheses is of paramount importance to avoid these kinds of complications. In addition to proper fit, specific gait training to educate the client as to proper body mechanics will be important.
6. Another often overlooked complication has to do with weight gain. Weight gain affects the fit of the prostheses, requiring either adjustment or a complete refabrication of the socket.
7. Complicated recoveries from other injuries may be a result of the inability of the client to manage self-care during periods of injury or illness. For example, an individual who is a triple amputee (bilateral below knee and dominant arm at the shoulder) may be unable to take care of himself for even bowel and bladder care or other survival needs should he injure his other arm.
8. Knee problems when not wearing the prosthesis is often a complication for bilateral below-knee amputees. It is sometimes much easier to avoid the time it takes to put on a prosthesis by simply walking on one's knees in order to get around the house, such as going to the bathroom at night or trying to get out of the house in case of an emergency. After years of using this method to move around, it is not uncommon for clients to experience knee problems.
9. While working in hot environments or having to exert considerable effort to walk or engage in physical activity with a prosthesis, sweating can become an irritating problem. Prostheses

tend to feel heavy and awkward and will require an approximate 10 percent increase in energy for a single below-knee amputation and much more energy expenditure with multiple amputations (Friedmann, 1981). It does not take an educated observer to understand that a bilateral above-knee amputee will expend considerable energy simply getting from one place to another. In fact, many amputees may prefer to use a wheelchair to do things quicker. In addition, an upper-extremity amputee, such as a shoulder disarticulation, requires the addition of a mechanical arm or a Utah arm, which also requires considerable effort. This may result in excessive sweating and irritation as well. In addition, working in a hot environment, such as outdoors in the summertime in the south or in a boiler room indoors, may become intolerable.

10. Neuromas are also fairly frequent and can be quite irritating if the prosthesis impacts on the area where the neuroma resides. Often surgery is the treatment of choice.
11. Overuse syndromes are now seen for the amputee who leads an active lifestyle and usually involve the remaining, intact extremity. For the arm amputee, a common issue would be the development of carpal tunnel syndrome from repetitive use of the hand and wrist which is compensation for the loss of the hand and arm from the other side. Another commonly seen arm issue is earlier degenerative joint disease or impingement at the shoulder of the intact arm. Again this comes from increased stress and strain on the joints of the intact arm.

Case Example

Mr. AK Amputee is a 35-year-old man who, as a commercial truck driver, was severely injured in a head-on collision while driving his 18-wheel truck carrying a heavy load of steel. He was urgently taken to a Level 1 trauma-designated hospital in Houston, Texas. His life was salvaged despite nearly severing his right leg above the knee. Significant attempts to save the right leg were successful after eight surgeries. However, 12 months after his injury, the hardware in his right leg became infected with methicillin resistant staphylococcus aureus (MRSA) and threatened his life. It was decided to perform a mid-femoral amputation. Following the amputation, he healed primarily but was significantly deconditioned. He was prepared and fitted for an above-knee prosthesis with input from a full array of rehabilitation health professionals.

Mr. AK Amputee has been married and in a stable relationship for 10 years. He and his wife have two children ages 6 and 8. He has a high school diploma and has periodic pain well-controlled with an occasional nonsteroidal tablet. He does have Type II diabetes that is controlled with oral medication. He is otherwise healthy with no other complaints. Before the amputation, he was active in his community through his children's school activities. He enjoyed swimming and playing golf on weekends. He wants to return to these activities. He and his family live in a ranch style home with all major living areas on one floor.

He has been told he cannot return to work. He is concerned about future vocational options and whether his education will be enough to become employed again.

After completing the life care plan tables, it is useful to provide supportive explanation for each line contained in the life care plan. This explanation can be supported by a professional recommendation, literature citation, or standard of practice. If an item is recommended by a health care professional, that name should be listed on that same line. It is helpful to indicate the first draft is not for distribution until discussed with the appropriate parties and any questions have been answered.

Life Care Plan Narrative for Mr. AK Amputee

The narrative below is an attempt to explain the recommended items in the Life Care Plan (LCP) charts. I will list my reasons for suggesting the items listed. The recommendations made in the LCP are based on the assumption that this person will elect to wear and use a prosthetic leg for the above-knee level of amputation. Some persons with above-knee amputations do not do this and instead opt to use a wheelchair for their mobility. Some items in the LCP may have been recommended by other persons. In these cases, a thorough explanation of why this item is essential should be made.

The other important component to include in a life care plan is what the idealized outcome should be for function, future health needs, anticipated equipment needs, pain control, and emotional well-being. Potential life complications should also be projected and any costs associated with that health care.

An above-knee amputee without other comorbidities should be expected to achieve the following functions:

1. Ambulation with prosthesis on all surfaces
2. No gait aids
3. Independent in donning and doffing prosthesis
4. Standing up to two continuous hours
5. Walking up to two continuous hours
6. Get up from kneeling
7. Return to recreational activities (hunting, fishing, golfing, jogging, skiing), if performed prior to amputation
8. Return to previous work
9. Comfortable with falling techniques
10. Perform cardiovascular conditioning program safely
11. Drive
12. Shop
13. Perform housework, gardening, home maintenance
14. Independent in Activities of Daily Living (ADL)
15. Know how to purchase correct footwear
16. Can inspect skin and nails for remaining foot
17. Ascend and descend stairs one step at a time usually
18. Can run (if patient desires and has adequate cardiopulmonary reserve)

The ability to perform all of these functions often requires a coordinated team effort of various health professionals who have had significant experience in working with other persons with above-knee amputation and have followed those persons back into the community with full function. Usually, this team will be facilitated by a physiatrist or orthopedic surgeon with significant amputation experience.

Projected Rehabilitation Program

These rehabilitation modalities are recommended for Mr. AK Amputee in order to take him through the adaptive process of leg amputation and prosthetic restoration to maximum function with an artificial leg. This process normally takes some 12–18 months from the time of the amputation. Returning to work and successful integration into the workplace may take a bit longer. This program does not just focus on use of a prosthetic leg but pays close attention to the issues of pain, emotional well-being, weight control, recreation, and integration back into the family and his community. It should involve more than a surgeon, a prosthetist, and the amputee.

Projected Evaluations

It is anticipated that with his weight and an above-knee amputation, he will develop low back pain at age 65 that will require ongoing conservative orthopedic back care. This treatment is usually nonsurgical.

Projected Therapeutic Modalities

He will also require periodic evaluations and therapy from occupational therapy, physical therapy, and psychology as his prosthesis needs maintenance and replacement. New componentry and changes in his own anatomy require periodic and regular follow-up with these therapists. Often physical therapy is useful when a new prosthesis is fabricated, often every 3 to 5 years since the fit. New components take a period of accommodation before achieving ideal function.

Diagnostic Testing

I do anticipate the need for periodic MRI studies of his low back related to the low back pain that I anticipate will have an onset about age 65.

Wheelchair Needs

An ultra lightweight manual wheelchair is often used when he does not wear his prosthesis or needs to go long distances beyond his capability to use the prosthesis for walking. A wheelchair cushion should also be provided and replaced once every 3 years.

Wheelchair Accessories and Maintenance

He needs an allowance for regular and periodic wheelchair maintenance. This equates to 10 percent of the original cost of the wheelchair that is required every 2 years for the 7-year life of the wheelchair.

Aids for Independent Function

He should have a shower commode chair that can be used in the shower for safety reasons. The replacement schedule is listed.

Orthotics/Prosthetics

With the transfemoral (above-knee) level of amputation, he will require a contemporary design of above-knee prosthesis. The price for this will vary depending on the prosthetic components that are prescribed and also on the prosthetic laboratory that makes the prosthesis. A cost range should be provided by the prosthetic laboratory but, at times, it may be helpful to know the price range from other prosthetic laboratories or elsewhere in the United States. The price of the prosthesis will vary depending on the components used which are usually designated by "L" codes used for Medicare pricing. Routine prosthetic maintenance is recommended and costs 10 percent annually of the base price of the prosthesis. This maintenance cost is incurred once the warranty of the prosthesis has expired, generally at the end of the first year following fabrication.

Gel liners that are used to pad the skin are replaced on an annual basis and stump socks must be used as the size of the amputated leg and soft tissues change in shape and volume. These socks also need to be replaced annually.

Often, a custom-made foot insole orthotic is appropriate for the remaining foot. This is an attempt to distribute weight more evenly over the plantar aspect of the remaining foot. Hopefully, this will maintain skin and bone architecture through the remainder of life. This is especially important if the amputee has diabetes.

Home Furnishings and Accessories

This will vary depending on the amputee but most often few items are required following the amputation.

Drug/Supply Needs

This depends on what may be prescribed because of the amputation. It most likely will be pain medication, at least for a short period of time. Most amputees should not complain of long term pain issues.

Home/Facility Care

It is anticipated that he should have assistance with the heavier housework and with outside home maintenance. I do not assume that a spouse is available for providing assistance. I therefore always include some home assistance in order to try to avoid excess wear and tear on the remaining body parts which are essential for future functioning.

Future Medical Care—Routine

See under Potential Complications. Future medical care may be related to comorbid diagnoses such as diabetes mellitus, peripheral arterial disease, or cardiac abnormalities.

Transportation

He will need to drive an automatic transmission motor vehicle and it could be outfitted with a left-footed accelerator, if a right-leg amputee.

Health and Strength Maintenance

He should regularly participate in an exercise program to maintain his cardiopulmonary status essential for leg prosthetic use. A YMCA or similar health club would be excellent for this type of aerobic conditioning. Swimming is also an excellent exercise regimen for a person with an above-knee amputation.

It should be assumed that function will change as he ages and therefore prosthetic replacement may be less frequent. Thus, he might need a 3-year replacement schedule between ages 35–65 but then with less strenuous activity, replacement would go to every 5 years.

Often, the socket will need more frequent replacement than all of the lower prosthetic leg components (knee, foot/ankle). A new socket is often desirable every 2 years while the entire leg replacement is less frequent, every 3 to 5 years.

Architectural Renovations

He may need to have a bathroom modified for functional safety. Occasionally, a walk-in shower is desirable but not essential for safe bathing activity. Some multi-level homes benefit from the addition of a Stairglide if climbing stairs is difficult. Bathroom modifications for wheelchair access may also be desirable.

Potential Complications

He is likely to develop a minor skin infection from time to time with prosthetic wear and use. This infection should be easily treated with not wearing the prosthesis for a few days and the use of oral antibiotics. Crutches are necessary for this period of time.

Low back pain is an expected complication for him to develop at age 65. This should be managed conservatively by an orthopedic back specialist and may require medication to decrease the pain. He may also need periodic MRI evaluation of his spine.

Vocational/Educational Plan

Because he has been out of work for so long, I believe that he will need a formal vocational assessment and a vocational plan to be developed. I also believe he will benefit from formal job coaching as he returns to work in order to enhance the likelihood he will be successful in the chosen occupation and that the ergonomics of the workplace fit his disability needs.

Future Medical Care—Aggressive Treatment

This is unlikely unless medical issues develope related to the cause of the amputation and may complicate future prosthetic function.

Orthopedic Equipment Needs

He should have ergonomically designed crutches available for use on a periodic basis.

These items listed in the LCP more probably than not will return Mr. AK Amputee to his most full function and to assure the best quality of life in his future.

Robert H. Meier, III, MD Director Amputee Services of America NAME: **Mr. AK Amputee** DOB: 09/15/1982 DOI: 11/12/2015 AGE: 35 yrs. REPORT DATE: 12/16/2017			
FUTURE CARE PLAN			
For purposes of this plan, the following initials are placed in parentheses according to their respective recommendations: *(XYZ) = Dr. XYZ, physician*			
Routine Future Medical Care—Physician Only			
Recommendation (by whom)	**Frequency and Duration**	**Purpose**	**Expected Cost**
Amputation Rehabilitation Physician—PM&R	Every 2 yrs. after initial rehabilitation program is completed	Assess prosthetic function, fit, maintenance, and quality of life	$325
Orthopedic Surgeon	Every 2 yrs.	Assess issues related to prior fractures, bone surgery, and low back issues	$325
Projected Evaluations—Nonphysician (Include all allied health evals)			
Recommendation (by whom)	**Year Initiated/ Suspended**	**Frequency/Duration**	**Expected Cost**
Physical Therapy	2020	1 visit every 3 yrs. with new prosthesis	$350 for eval and $175 for therapy visits
Psychology	2022	Every 5 yrs. for 5 visits	$225/visit for assessment of coping skills, parenting, emotional adaptation to life changes, and disabilities
Occupational Therapy	2020	Every 3 yrs.	$350 for evaluation of ADL skills and need for adaptive equipment

(Continued)

Projected Therapeutic Modalities			
Recommendation (by whom)	**Year Initiated/ Suspended**	**Frequency/Duration**	**Expected Cost**
Physical Therapy	2020	4 visits every 3 yrs. with new prosthesis	$175 for therapy visits
Diagnostic Testing/Educational Assessment			
Recommendation (by whom)	**Year Initiated/ Suspended**	**Frequency/Duration**	**Expected Cost**
Potentially consider for future work			
Assistive Technology			
Recommendation (by whom)	**Year Initiated**	**Frequency**	**Expected Cost**
Consider if usual for employment			
Wheelchair Needs			
Recommendation (by whom)	**Year Purchased**	**Replacement Schedule**	**Expected Cost**
Ultra-lightweight wheelchair	2017	Every 7 yrs. until age 65 then every 5 yrs.	$2,800
Powered scooter	Age 65 or 2055	Every 5 yrs.	$3,500
Wheelchair Maintenance and Accessories			
Recommendation (by whom)	**Year Purchased**	**Replacement Schedule**	**Expected Cost**
Annual maintenance	2017	Annual	$280
Annual scooter maintenance	2055	Annual	$350
Battery replacement	2058	Every 3 yrs.	
Independent Aids for Functioning			
Recommendation (by whom)	**Year Purchased**	**Replacement Schedule**	**Expected Cost**
Commode chair	2017	Every 7 years	$246 (no wheels) to $1001 (with wheels)
Prosthetics			
Recommendation (by whom)	**Year Purchased**	**Replacement Schedule**	**Expected Cost**
Above knee prosthesis for general duty	2017	Every 3 yrs. until age 65 then every 5 yrs. for life	Per prosthetic laboratory

(*Continued*)

Socket replacement	2019	Every 1½ yrs. until age 65 then every 2½ yrs. for life	Per prosthetic laboratory
Above-knee prosthesis for high performance activities such as running, golf, etc.			Per prosthetic laboratory
Possible water leg for showering, water sports, or beach activities			Per prosthetic laboratory
Home Furnishings and Equipment			
Recommendation (by whom)	**Year Purchased**	**Replacement**	**Expected Cost**
Depending on home design			Potentially use VA housing allowance for modification
Health and Strength Maintenance (Leisure Time Activities)			
Recommendation (by whom)	**Year of Purchase**	**Replacement Schedule**	**Expected Cost**
Gym Membership til age 72	2017	Annual membership fee	
Transportation			
Recommendation (by whom)	**Year Purchased**	**Replacement Schedule**	**Expected Cost**
None unless vehicle is to be modified			
Drug Needs Drug needs and costs are representative of the client's current need and may change from time to time.			
Recommendation (by whom)	**Purpose**	**Cost per Unit**	**Cost per Year**
None at present			
Supply Needs Supply needs and costs are representative of the client's current need and may change from time to time.			
Recommendation (by whom)	**Purpose**	**Cost per Unit**	**Cost per Year**
Prosthetic liners	Cushion fit of prosthetic socket	$1,600/pr with annual replacement	$1600

(Continued)

Vocational/Educational Plan			
Recommendation (by whom)	**Initiated/ Suspended**	**Purpose**	**Expected Cost**
Depends on whether plan is to include potential for return to work?			Depends on what potential there may be for useful employment

Architectural Considerations
Consider whether VA allowance is to be used.

Home/Facility Care			
Recommendation (by whom)	**Initiated/ Suspended**	**Hours/Shifts/Days**	**Expected Cost**
Homemaking assistance	2017 until 2056	4 hrs. three times a week for heavier duty housework	$20/hr. to include Social Security, health insurance, etc.
Homemaking assistance	2056 until 2066	6 hrs. three times a week for heavier housework	Same
Homemaking assistance	2066 for lifetime	4 hrs./day every day	Assistance with ADL, all housework and shopping

Future Medical Care, Surgical Intervention, Aggressive Treatment			
Recommendation (by whom)	**Year Initiated/ Suspended**	**Frequency**	**Expected Cost**
Because of Mr. AK Amputee's extensive bony injuries and multiple surgeries, I am anticipating the following medical problems to be more likely than not: 1. Total hip replacement 2. Low back pain 3. Degenerative joint disease in arm, legs, and lower back			Chances are that he will require regular and ongoing medical and orthopedic assessments for long term medical problems. I also expect he will require a total hip replacement, nonsurgical low back treatments, multiple pain, and arthritis medications.

(*Continued*)

Potential Complications *Potential complications are included for information only.* *No frequency or duration of complications is available.*
He is likely to develop a minor skin infection from time to time with prosthetic wear and use. This infection should be easily treated with not wearing the prosthesis for a few days and the use of oral antibiotics. Crutches are necessary for this period of time. Lower back pain is an expected complication for him to develop at age 65. This should be managed conservatively by an orthopedic back specialist and may require medication to decrease the pain. He may also need periodic MRI evaluation of his spine.

At the conclusion, a Life Care Planning Narrative is useful to explain every line item of recommended service or equipment as it relates to the individual for whom the care plan is developed.

Conclusion

The physiatrist should play a valuable role in assisting in the development of the life care plan for the person who has sustained an amputation. An emphasis should be placed on the amputee achieving the ideal level of function with an appropriate rehabilitation program. Just providing a prosthesis is not the same as providing an integrated rehabilitation program that includes a prosthesis. The emphasis should be placed on the amputee's needs and desires. Measuring the functional outcome, the success of community reintegration, and the individual's emotional adaptation to the changes in their life are important in developing an accurate life care plan. The physiatrist should serve as an invaluable collaborator with the life care planner in order to develop the most accurate and comprehensive life care plan.

Amputation rehabilitation and prosthetic options are changing so quickly today, it is important that the life care planner use rehabilitation professionals who have access to the most current information and practices. The annual quantity of particular levels of amputation and prosthetic services should be a known component when using a source of clinical information. An example could be: if the prosthetist does not fit at least 25 of a particular level of amputation per year, that prosthetist is not particularly experienced to render an opinion. The same could be said for any other rehabilitation team professional whether it be surgeon, physician, or therapist. The number 25 is plucked from the air since perhaps treating 10 would be sufficient. The point for the life care planner is to assess how many amputees of a particular level the person providing the information for the LCP does actually treat in a year's time and which they might use when queried in a deposition or on a witness stand. It is also essential that the person providing input to the LCP is current in their understanding of contemporary amputation techniques and amputee rehabilitation practices.

References

Davis, R. 1993. Phantom sensation, phantom pain and stump pain. *Archives of Physical Medicine Rehabilitation*, *74*(70), 79–84.

Esquenazi, A., Leonard, J. A., & Meier, R. H. 1989. Prosthetics. *Archives of Physical Medicine Rehabilitation*, *70*(suppl.), 207.

Esquenazi, A., & Torres, M. M. 1991. In L. W. Friedmann (Ed.), *Physical Medicine and Rehabilitation Clinics of North America*. Philadelphia, PA: W.B. Saunders.

Friedmann, L. 1981. Amputation. In W. Stolov & M. Clowers (Eds.), *Handbook of Severe Disability*. Washington, DC: U.S. Department of Education, Rehabilitation Services Administration, 169–188.

Kuiken, T. A., Li, G., & Lock, B. A. et al. 2009. Targeted muscle reinnervation for real-time myoelectric control of multifunction artificial arms. *JAMA*, *301*(6), 619–28.

Leonard, J. A., & Meier, R. H. 1993. Upper and lower extremity prosthetics. In J. A. DeLisa (Ed.), *Rehabilitation Medicine: Principles and Practices*. Philadelphia, PA: J.B. Lippincott, pp. 507–525.

Meier, R. H. 1994. Upper limb amputee rehabilitation. In A. Esquenazi (Ed.), *Prosthetics: State of the Art Reviews*. Philadelphia, PA: Hanley & Belfus, pp. 165–185.

Meier, R. H. 2014. Amputee Rehabilitation. *Physical Medicine and Rehabilitation Clinics of North America. Clinics Review Series*. Philadelphia: Elsevier 25:1.

Meier, R. H., & Atkins, D. J. 2004. *Functional Restoration of Adults and Children with Upper Extremity Amputation*. New York, NY: Demos Medical Publishing.

Meier, R. H. & Heckman, J. T. 2014. Principles of contemporary rehabilitation of the amputee. *Phys Med Rehabil Clin N Am*, *25*, 29–33.

Moore, W. S., & Malone, J. M. (Eds.). 1989. *Lower Extremity Amputation*. Philadelphia, PA: W.B. Saunders.

Sears, H. H. 1991. Approaches to prescription of body-powered and myoelectric prosthetics. In L. W. Friedmann (Ed.), *Prosthetics: Physical Medicine and Rehabilitation Clinics of North America*. Philadelphia, PA: W.B. Saunders, pp. 361–371.

Sherman, R. A., Sherman, C. J., & Gail, N. A. 1980. Survey of current phantom limb treatment in the United States. *Pain*, *8*, 85–99.

Weed, R., & Sluis, A. 1990. *Life Care Plans for the Amputee: A Step by Step Guide*. Boca Raton, FL: CRC Press.

Chapter 13

Life Care Planning for Acquired Brain Injury

David L. Ripley and Roger O. Weed

Contents

Introduction.......... 368
Definitions.......... 368
Epidemiology.......... 369
Costs.......... 369
Etiology.......... 370
Anatomy of the Brain.......... 370
    Coverings.......... 370
    Cerebral Cortex.......... 370
    Midbrain.......... 372
    Brain Stem.......... 372
    Cerebellum.......... 372
Brain Injury Classification.......... 372
Initial Treatment.......... 374
Rehabilitation Care.......... 376
Medical Complications.......... 376
    Cranial Complications.......... 377
    Endocrine Disorders.......... 377
    Pulmonary Complications.......... 377
    Cardiovascular Complications.......... 377
    Neurological Complications.......... 378
    Gastrointestinal Complications.......... 378
    Genitourinary Complications.......... 378
    Musculoskeletal Complications.......... 378
    Cognitive Problems.......... 379
Recovery from TBI.......... 379
Long-Term Impairments.......... 380
Community Reintegration.......... 381

Vocational Rehabilitation 382
Case Study 384
Conclusion 395
References 395

Introduction

Traumatic brain injury (TBI) is one of the leading causes of neurological impairment in the United States and in 2004 accounted for over 1.4 million visits to the emergency room each year with 50,000 deaths, 235,000 admissions to the hospital, and 1.1 million being treated and released (Centers for Disease Control, National Center for Injury Prevention and Control, 1999; Centers for Disease Control and Prevention, 2008a). Further, the Centers for Disease Control (CDC) in 2008 estimated that approximately 5.3 million Americans have a lifelong need for care. Acquired brain injury (ABI) is the leading cause of neurological impairment for individuals between the ages of 16 and 30 years of age. ABI technically includes brain injury as a result of cerebrovascular disease (or stroke), but for the purposes of this chapter, the focus will predominately be on brain injury of traumatic etiology (Kraus et al., 1984).

Creating an appropriate life care plan for an individual with ABI can be a formidable challenge. The brain, as the neurological control center for the body, affects almost every aspect of physiological functioning. Injury to the brain therefore can affect almost every function (Rosenthal, 1990; Kraus, 1991; Kaufman et al., 1993; Macciocchi et al., 1993; Piek, 1995). Practitioners in the field of brain injury rehabilitation must be prepared to deal with problems in essentially every organ system in the body, as well as a variety of cognitive and behavioral problems (Wood, 1987; Uomoto & Brockway, 1992).

Because the majority of people who sustain a brain injury are young at the time of their injury, it is difficult in many circumstances to estimate lifetime earning capacity and needs (Wehman et al., 1988; Stapleton et al., 1989; Corthell, 1993; Dikmen et al., 1994; Goodall et al., 1994; Ip et al., 1995; Horn & Zasler, 1996; Zasler, 1997). Additionally, as acute trauma management and medical and rehabilitation care improve, the survival of patients with these injuries will continue to increase (High et al., 1996; Kreutzer et al., 2001). The result is that many more people survive with increasingly complex medical and rehabilitation problems (Centers for Disease Control and Prevention, 2008b). Due to the variability in recovery following TBI, life care planners are often forced to develop, in a sense, multiple care plans to accommodate the different potential outcomes that may occur in a single individual.

Definitions

Due to a variety of descriptions used by medical professionals throughout the years, and the problems this caused with communication, the American Congress of Rehabilitation Medicine (ACRM) in 1993 proposed a uniform nomenclature for brain injury. The following definitions are part of the ACRM's recommendations (American Congress of Rehabilitation Medicine Head Injury Interdisciplinary Special Interest Group, 1993):

- *Acquired brain injury*: Injury to the brain that occurs after the brain has developed; may be due to trauma, surgery, intracranial bleeding, ischemia, or tumor.
- *Traumatic brain injury*: Injury to the brain caused by trauma. One form of acquired brain injury.

- *Coma*: Specific diagnostic term indicating lack of arousability, including loss of sleep–wake cycles on EEG, and lack of meaningful interaction/response to the environment.
- *Vegetative state*: Patients who have no meaningful response to the environment after their eyes are open.
- *Persistent vegetative state*: A vegetative state that persists longer than 3 months, or 1 year if due to trauma.
- *Locked-in syndrome*: A condition in which patients are awake, capable of communication, aware of their environment, but unable to move or speak.
- *Minimally responsive*: Patients who are no longer comatose or vegetative but remain severely disabled (used for patients who are demonstrating inconsistent responses to stimuli yet have some meaningful interaction with the environment).

Epidemiology

The U.S. Centers for Disease Control and Prevention (2008a) have determined that the annual combined total incidence for TBI is estimated to be 102 cases per 100,000 people. It is useful to break down the incidence of TBI based on injury severity. Various methods of rating injury severity are used and will be discussed later in the chapter. However, the incidence when breaking down by injury severity is 14 per 100,000 for severe TBI, 15 per 100,000 for moderate TBI, and 131 per 100,000 for mild TBI.

There are several factors associated with a higher risk for TBI. Males are more than twice as likely as females to sustain a TBI (Centers for Disease Control and Prevention, 2008b). Additionally, patients with brain injury tend to be from lower socioeconomic groups, have a history of substance use or abuse, and have a history of engaging in risky behaviors (Centers for Disease Control and Prevention, 1997). Additionally, brain-injured patients are more likely to live in an urban area. Alcohol is frequently involved in accidents resulting in brain injury and is considered to be the most common preventable cause of TBI. Education about safety, such as wearing seatbelts and bicycle helmets, and not driving while intoxicated, seems to have contributed to a slight decline in the incidence of hospitalization following TBI in recent years.

Brain injury generally follows a *bimodal* distribution with respect to age. The largest peak is in late adolescence and early adulthood, when individuals are more likely to engage in high-risk activities. The later peak begins for individuals older than age 65, when falls become more common. Because the largest peak occurrence is in the period of time from late adolescence to early adulthood, life care planning for this group is particularly challenging, as lifelong concerns must be taken into consideration, including aging and aging issues, education, vocational rehabilitation, and community reintegration. Age may also be correlated with outcomes, as older individuals (over age 65) tend to have a slower recovery and worse outcomes following brain injury.

Costs

The costs associated with treating TBI are estimated to be $48.3 billion annually. Costs associated with hospitalization were estimated to be $60 billion in 2000, the most current data available (Finkelstein, Corso, Miller, & Associates, 2006, as cited by the Centers for Disease Control and Prevention, 2008a; Brown et al., 2008).

Review of model systems data for 2007 reveals that the average cost for inpatient treatment of a case of TBI was approximately $154,000 (Traumatic Brain Injury Model Systems, 2008; also see http://www.cdc.gov/traumaticbraininjury/get_the_facts.html). This estimate was based on the cost for acute hospital care and acute inpatient rehabilitation and does not include rehabilitation efforts (which were reported to be an additional $56,901 after the patient has left the hospital); it also does not include physicians' fees.

Etiology

Traumatic brain injuries can occur as a result of a number of causes. From 2006 to 2010, falls were the leading cause of TBI, accounting for 40 percent of all TBIs in the United States that resulted in an emergency department (ED) visit, hospitalization, or death. Falls disproportionately affect the elderly and very young (Cipolle et al., 2014). Unintentional blunt trauma is the second leading cause, followed by motor vehicle crashes. Over the last several years, TBI as a result of motor vehicle crashes has decreased in the United States, possibly as a result of updated safety mechanisms. Assaults are the fourth most common cause overall and represent a disproportionately large cause of TBI in urban areas (Centers for Disease Control and Prevention, 2008b; Traumatic Brain Injury Model Systems, 2008).

Anatomy of the Brain

Coverings

The brain is protected by a number of layers of differing tissue. A layer of skin is the outermost covering, followed by a layer of connective tissue and muscle. The bony calvarium, or skull, provides the greatest protection of the brain. Fractures of the skull are present in a number of brain injuries and are generally associated with a more severe injury. Under the skull are three distinct layers that provide the direct cover of the brain. The outermost, thickest layer is called the *dura mater* and is attached to the inner layer of the skull in many places. Underneath this layer is the *arachnoid mater*, which derives its name from its similarity in appearance to a spider web. The arachnoid mater follows the surface of the brain closely, but does not follow the surface down deep into the crevices, or *sulci*, on the surface of the brain. The innermost layer of covering is called the *pia mater*, and this layer does follow the brain into the sulci.

Cerebral Cortex

The outer surface of the brain is called the cerebral cortex. There are many convolutions of the surface of the brain, which serve to increase the surface area of the outside of the brain. The bulges are referred to as *gyri*, and the involutions are referred to as *sulci*. The origination of neural messages to the rest of the body, for the most part, occurs on the surface of the brain. In most cases, seizure activity also originates at the level of the cortex.

The cortex of the brain is divided into lobes that represent areas of specific functioning (see Figure 13.1). The *frontal lobe* is responsible for higher cognitive processes, such as planning, organization, and problem solving. It is also the part of the brain responsible for control of impulsive and instinctual behavior (Grafman et al., 1996). Last, the origination of motor activity occurs in the most posterior portion of the frontal lobe.

The *parietal lobe* is predominately concerned with the registration of sensory information, particularly the ability to sense when something has touched the skin. Other types of sensory information are processed in this area, and the parietal lobe gives us the ability to orient objects in space, follow a map, and appreciate music. Individuals with injury to the parietal lobe will often exhibit *neglect*, or lack of awareness of part of their own body.

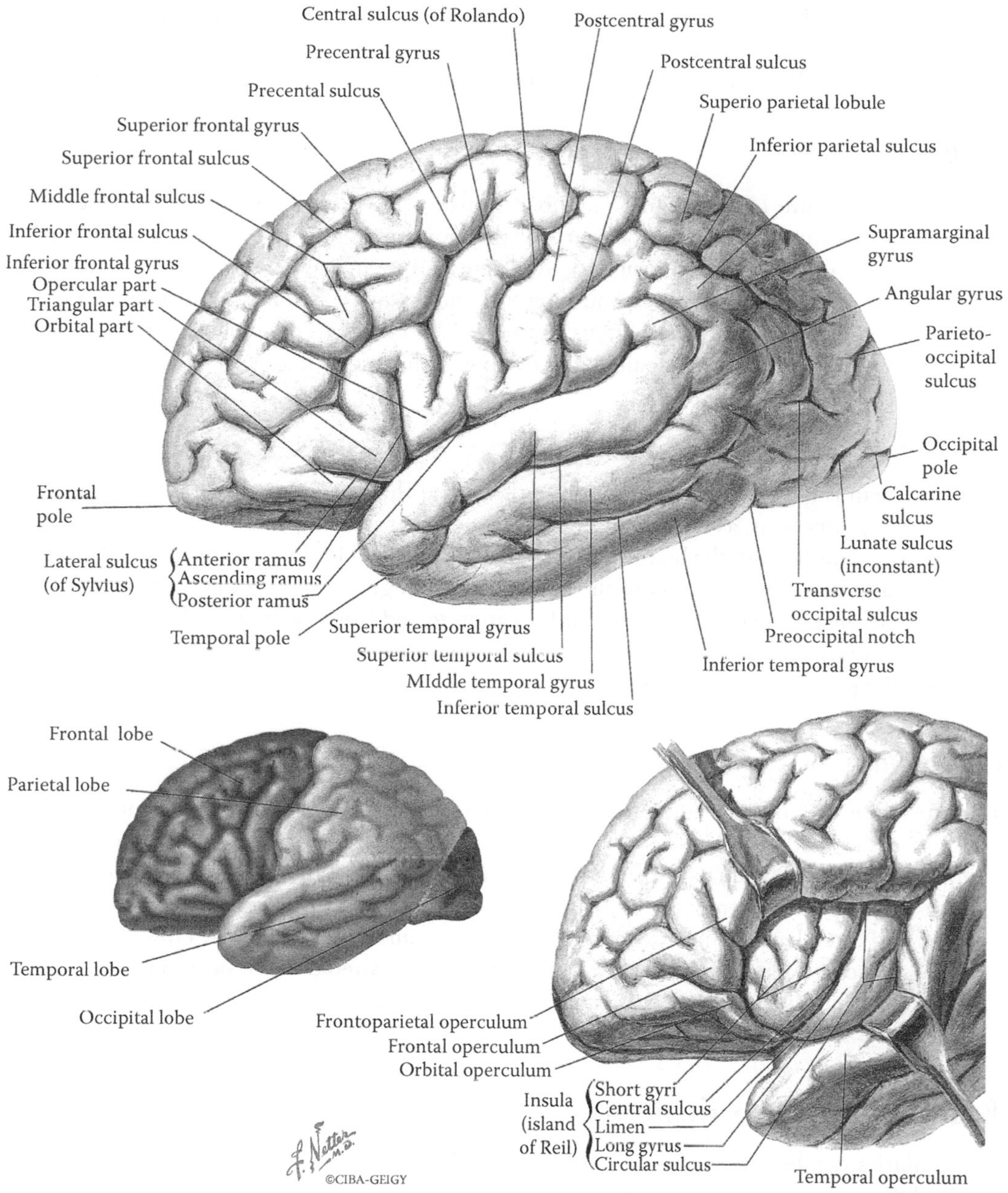

Figure 13.1 Cerebrum, lateral views. (From Netter, F.H. *Atlas of Human Anatomy*, 2nd ed. Icon Learning Systems, 1997. With permission.)

The *temporal lobes* are located on the sides of the brain. These lobes are critical in the registration of auditory information and are critical in the understanding and formulation of language. The inner portion of the temporal lobes also contains structures that are responsible for memory formation, as well as the origination of emotions. Individuals with seizures most frequently have injury to their temporal lobe.

The *occipital lobe* is located on the most posterior aspect of the brain. Visual information is registered and processed here. Individuals with injury to this area may have *cortical blindness*, which is an inability to see because of failure of the brain to recognize the neural signals sent from the eyes.

Midbrain

The midbrain (Figure 13.2) contains a number of structures whose predominant activities are to receive signals transmitted from other parts of the brain or from elsewhere in the body, and to modify the signal before transmitting it on to where it ultimately will register. Structures within the midbrain help to control movement, interpret sensory information, and also help with such activities as controlling our level of consciousness. Patients who are comatose or who are in a persistent vegetative state have impaired functioning in the midbrain.

Brain Stem

The brain stem is the most inferior portion of the brain. This part of the brain is critical for basic life-sustaining functions, as it is responsible for regulating breathing and heart rates. Most of the cranial nerves exit here, so the brain stem is intimately involved in the transmission and reception of sensory and motor information of the head, such as tongue movement, facial movement, and sensation. Because all sensory and motor information to and from the body and brain must travel through the brain stem, even a very small area of injury to the brain stem can have devastating effects on the person with the injury.

Cerebellum

The cerebellum is an area of the brain that facilitates coordinated motor movements. There are extensive neural pathways between the cerebellum and other areas of the brain concerned with motor movement. Individuals with injury to the cerebellum exhibit *ataxia*, or lack of control of smooth coordinated movements. Interestingly, patients with ataxia often have no problems with strength and often have the muscle strength to carry out any activity you ask. However, they lack an ability to control their limbs' movements, such that it is often difficult or impossible for them to perform basic activities like picking up a glass or walking.

Brain Injury Classification

Brain injuries can be classified by a number of methods (Marshall et al., 1992; Teasdale et al., 1992). ABIs are generally classified as traumatic, anoxic/hypoxic-ischemic, vascular, or other. Anoxic or hypoxic-ischemic brain injuries occur when areas of the brain do not receive enough oxygen. This is frequently the cause of secondary injury after a traumatic injury, but may also occur independently of trauma. The most frequent cause of hypoxic-ischemic brain injury is secondary to myocardial infarction or heart failure. During resuscitative efforts for a heart attack, the brain may be deprived of oxygen for several minutes. Vascular brain injuries, commonly called strokes, most commonly occur as a result of thromboembolic phenomena. However, other types of vascular brain injuries include aneurysms, arteriovenous malformation, and spontaneous intracranial hemorrhages. Finally, injury to the brain may occur as a result of viral or bacterial infections, metabolic derangements, or tumors.

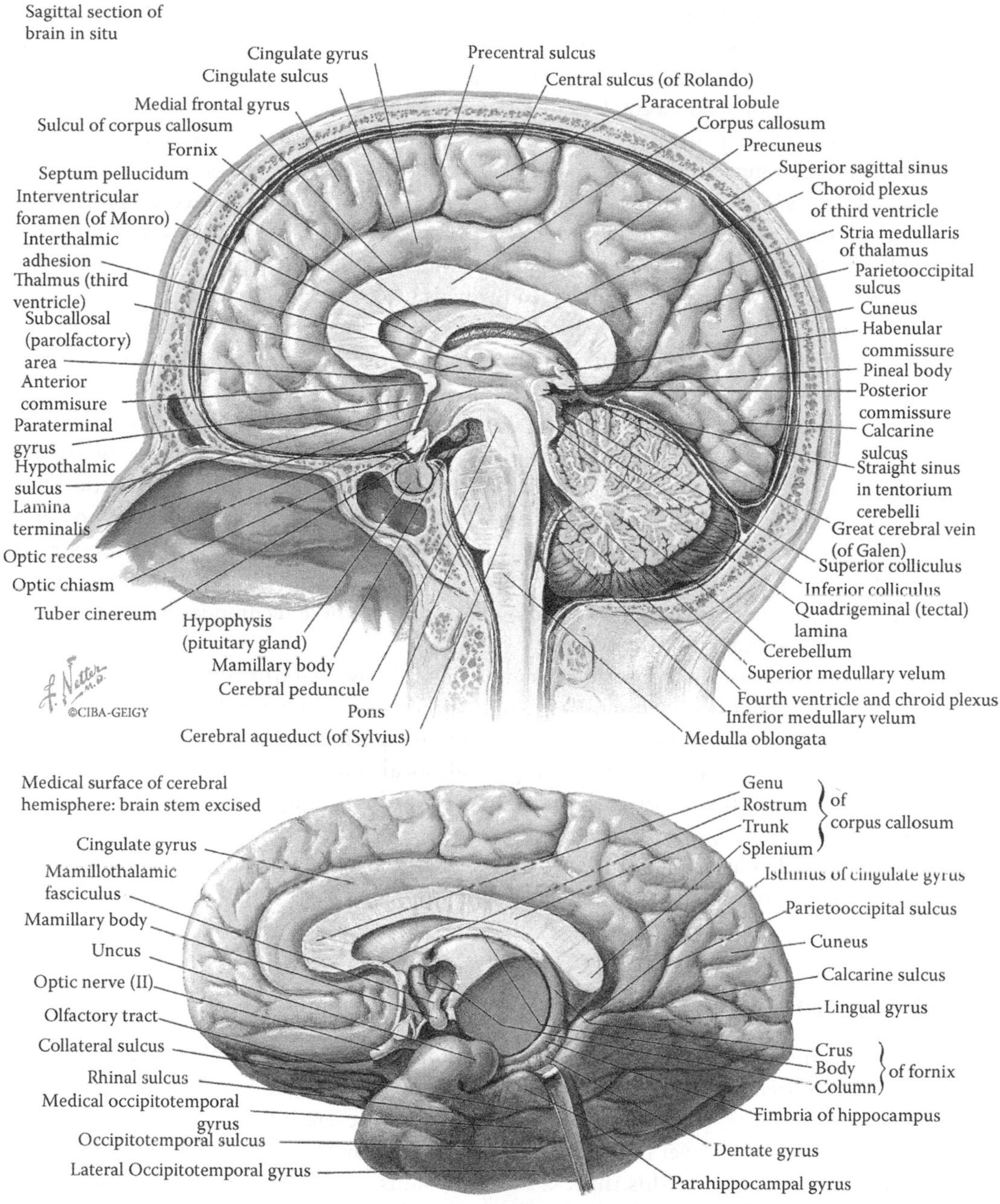

Figure 13.2 Cerebrum, medial views. (From Netter, F.H. *Atlas of Human Anatomy*, 2nd ed. Icon Learning Systems, 1997. With permission.)

Traumatic brain injuries, the broadest category of ABI, may be further subdivided a number of ways. One of the most basic methods of subcategorization is to divide them between *open* or *closed*. Open injuries are those injuries in which there is disruption of the scalp and skull, creating the possibility that the brain may be contaminated by material from the outside environment. Penetrating brain injuries are a type of open injury, in which a foreign body (such as a bullet) passes through the skull and outer coverings of the brain into the brain tissue itself. Closed head injuries are those in which the skull remains intact and the brain is not exposed to the outside environment, although significant injury may occur from the impact of the brain against the inner part of the skull, or from shearing of axons secondary to rotational forces.

Medical professionals caring for survivors of brain injury will also classify the injuries based on severity. The most common, widely utilized method of classification is the *Glasgow Coma Scale,* a method that classifies injuries based on clinical presentation (see Table 13.1). A medical professional will rate the patient's response in three separate areas: eye opening, motor response, and verbal response. The scale gives scores for each of the areas, which are summed to give a total score that can be used to rank the severity of the injury. Individuals who score 3 to 8 are said to have a severe injury, from 9 to 12 a moderate injury, and from 13 to 15 a mild injury. This information may be useful to predict the outcome and likelihood of long-term impairments (Clifton et al., 1993; Zafonte et al., 1996; Teasdale et al., 1998).

Other methods of rating injury severity are available but not as widely utilized. One alternative method of injury classification uses duration of *post-traumatic amnesia* as the best method of predicting outcomes following TBI (Zafonte et al., 1997). Other methods of classification have tried to use radiographic findings, such as location and size of lesions on computed tomography (CT) or magnetic resonance imaging (MRI) (Teasdale et al., 1992). Newer MRI techniques are now available which have greater sensitivity to injured brain tissue and greater clinical correlation with functional status (Gerber et al., 2004). However, none of these techniques have yet become consistently integrated into clinical practice.

Another broad categorization of brain injury is to divide between *diffuse* and *focal* brain injuries. Diffuse injuries are generally due to shearing injury of the axons and generally occur across broad areas of the brain. Focal injuries occur with trauma to one specific region of the brain. These two types of injury may occur concomitantly. In general, focal injuries result in shorter periods of unconsciousness than diffuse injuries. Individuals with diffuse injury, sometimes referred to as diffuse axonal injury (DAI), may have prolonged periods of unconsciousness from several days to weeks. In general, individuals with DAI have a prolonged recovery period compared to those with focal injuries (Bontke & Boake, 1991; Berker, 1996).

Initial Treatment

When a patient presents to the emergency room following TBI, the initial activities focus on life preservation. Often, concomitant injuries preclude addressing the brain injuries until later in the course of treatment. However, for those patients with severe injuries, the initial protocols involve rating the patient's level of arousal using the Glasgow Coma Scale, and some form of neuroradiographic imaging. At this time, CT scan remains the preferred type of image, due to the faster speed with which images can be obtained and the fact that the types of injury that require emergency surgical intervention show much more readily on CT than MRI. However, MRI techniques are more sensitive to intracranial injury (Levin, 1992; Marshall et al., 1992; Rappaport et al., 1992; Piek, 1995; Horn & Zasler, 1996; Gerber et al., 2004).

Once the patient is stabilized, a more detailed assessment of the injury will occur, and further treatment may be recommended. For severe injuries, assessment by a neurosurgeon will usually occur. If there is evidence of specific, severe types of bleeding or increased pressure inside the head, surgery will be performed to evacuate the blood or alleviate the pressure. Sometimes an intracranial pressure monitor will be placed to accurately measure the pressure inside the brain.

Table 13.1 The Glasgow Coma Scale

Patient's Response		*Score*
Eye opening		
	Spontaneously	4
	To voice	3
	To painful stimulus	2
	No eye opening	1
Motor		
	Follows commands	6
	Localizes to pain	5
	Withdraws from pain	4
	Flexor response	3
	Extensor response	2
	No motor response	1
Verbal		
	Oriented	5
	Converses but disoriented	4
	Inappropriate words	3
	Incomprehensible verbal utterances	2
	Not vocalizing	1
Total		
	(Sum of score from each of three areas)	(3–15)
	Injury classification:	
	Severe	3–8
	Moderate	9–12
	Mild	13–15

Note: A score with a T (e.g., 8T) means the patient was intubated for airway purposes and may be unable to fully respond.

Patients frequently require assistance with basic life functions. They may be placed on a mechanical ventilator to help them breathe. For prolonged management, sometimes a tracheotomy is performed to facilitate prolonged ventilator support. Additionally, for patients that are unconscious for prolonged periods of time, or have prolonged difficulty with swallowing, a feeding tube may be surgically introduced. Many patients with severe injury have sustained injuries to other parts of their body as well. Surgical attention is often necessary during the early hospitalization to address fractures, damaged internal organs, internal bleeding, and other medical concerns.

Rehabilitation Care

While patients are still in the hospital, physical and occupational therapy referrals should occur to maintain joint range of motion and strength and to begin working on activities of self-care. The more severely injured patients should be referred to a rehabilitation facility following their acute hospitalization to begin the work of trying to be restored to their highest level of functioning. An assessment by a physiatrist, a medical doctor with training in physical medicine and rehabilitation (PM&R), is important during this phase to facilitate the coordination of services and medical treatment to promote the best outcome following TBI (Rosenthal, 1990; Almli & Finger, 1992; Bontke et al., 1993; Berker, 1996; Semlyen et al., 1998).

Patients will often require further medical and rehabilitation care after medical issues are stabilized (Cope, 1995). Rehabilitation services may be provided in a number of different settings. The most appropriate level of care depends on the nature of the concomitant medical issues, as well as the level of functioning of the patient (Evans & Ruff 1992; Mazmanian et al., 1993; Hall & Cope, 1995; Schmidt, 1997). The most common level of rehabilitation care is in an *inpatient rehabilitation facility* (IRF), where patients receive 3 or more hours of therapy a day from several different therapy disciplines (i.e., physical therapy, occupational therapy, speech therapy), as well as ongoing medical attention, usually by a physician who specializes in Physical Medicine and Rehabilitation (PM&R) (Malec & Basford, 1996). Some IRFs have programs specifically tailored for the rehabilitation of individuals with brain Injury. These centers often provide greater expertise in the care of individuals with traumatic brain injury.

Once patients are medically stable and safe to be managed at home, therapy efforts transition to an outpatient setting. *Rehabilitation day programs* are therapy programs designed for individuals who still need therapy from several different disciplines in a team format, but no longer need as close medical attention as individuals in the acute inpatient setting. Some individuals will not need the interdisciplinary model of therapy, but only require therapy from one or two disciplines; then single-service outpatient therapy is indicated. In some cases, if medical issues prohibit active participation in therapy, patients may be sent to other settings, such as Long Term Acute Care Hospitals (LTACHs) or Skilled Nursing Facilities (SNFs). In these settings, rehabilitation services may be provided, but generally not to the extent and intensity of that provided in Inpatient Rehabilitation Facilities, and generally not with the same level of Medical and Rehabilitation oversight.

Medical Complications

An adept life care planner who works with survivors of brain injury must be aware of the potential medical complications that arise following brain injury and their impact on recovery, long-term function, and reintegration in the community. As the brain is the control center for all neurological processes in the body, injury to the brain can result in complications to almost every organ system. It is beyond the scope of this chapter to discuss all complications, although there are several common complications that we will describe (Kraus et al., 1984; Corrigan & Mysiw, 1988; Bigler, 1989; Bloomfield, 1989; Russell-Jones & Shorvon, 1989; Kraus, 1991; Uomoto &

Brockway, 1992; Bontke et al., 1993; Jorge et al., 1993; Katz & Alexander, 1994; Kaufman et al., 1993; Piek, 1995; Cifu et al., 1996a).

Cranial Complications

Injury to the cranial nerves frequently occurs following TBI. As a result, patients may have difficulty with basic sensory functions, such as vision, hearing, smell, and taste. Facial paresis is frequently seen, with resultant difficulty in oromotor functions, as in speaking, resultant dizziness, and balance disorders. This by itself may lead to problems with standing, walking, and transfers. It is very common for the olfactory nerve, the cranial nerve that controls sense of smell, to be damaged due to its structure, sometimes resulting in problems with eating and appetite. Fractures of the temporal bone, a part of the skull, can result in disruption of the cranial nerve associated with hearing, resulting in hearing impairment.

Many patients will have significant difficulty with vision problems following brain injury. Problems may range from inability to see objects in certain parts of the field of vision (sometimes referred to as a field cut) to blurry or double vision. This may be due to injury to the visual pathways within the brain, to injury to the nerves that control eye movements, or to injury to the eye itself. An evaluation by a neuro-ophthalmologist, a physician with training in neurological disorders that affect vision, is sometimes very helpful.

Endocrine Disorders

Endocrinology is the study of hormones and their function. Many hormones are regulated or secreted by the pituitary gland, a structure at the base of the brain. The pituitary can frequently be damaged during injury to the brain due to its location and structure. Common endocrine disorders following brain injury include syndrome of inappropriate diuretic hormone (SIADH), growth hormone deficiency, and irregularities of gonadal steroid production, and thyroid dysfunction. Endocrinopathies are much more evident in women, because menstrual irregularities, as a result of altered pituitary-gonadal axis functioning, may persist for a year or longer after brain injury. This may also be a source of problems with infertility following injury.

Pulmonary Complications

Patients with severe TBI frequently have respiratory failure as sequelae of the initial trauma. As a result, patients often require mechanical ventilation with a breathing machine (ventilator). Sometimes physicians must perform a tracheotomy, or a surgically created hole, to allow the patient to breathe and to help prevent complications from prolonged ventilator management. Patients who are immobile for prolonged periods of time are at a higher risk for developing pneumonia. A pulmonary embolus, or a blood clot that lodges in the blood vessels of the lungs, is also a potential complication of prolonged immobility.

Cardiovascular Complications

Direct effects of brain injury on the cardiovascular system are infrequent. However, immobility may lead to secondary complications over time. The most common is the formation of deep vein thromboses (DVTs) or blood clots in the veins. These clots can be potentially life threatening, as they can break free and lodge in the lung vessels causing a pulmonary embolus, as noted previously. DVTs may also result in post-phlebitic syndrome, or a painful condition of inflammation of the veins. Another complication that may lead to cardiovascular injury is called central storming, in which abnormally high levels of stimulant hormones are released into the bloodstream, resulting in fevers, high heart rates, and high blood pressure. This phenomenon can result in heart injury to people who are susceptible.

Neurological Complications

Typical neurological problems include weakness, sensory deficits, and the previously mentioned cranial nerve problems. Individuals who have had a brain injury are at increased risk for developing seizures. The presence of a penetrating brain injury, skull fracture, or significant amounts of subarachnoid blood increases the risk for seizures. The upper motor neuron syndrome is possibly the most frequently seen neurological complication after all forms of brain injury, with its constellation of symptoms of weakness, spasticity, and increased reflexes. Spasticity is a velocity-dependent increase in motor tone that is seen frequently following injury to motor nerves in the central nervous system. This is such a profound problem after brain injury that it will be discussed in detail later in the chapter. Additionally, cognitive and behavioral problems are frequent neurological complications and will also be discussed in more detail later.

Gastrointestinal Complications

Patients frequently exhibit dysphagia, or impairment in the ability to swallow, as a result of weakness of the pharyngeal muscles. Often, patients require the placement of a feeding tube to prevent aspiration of food and to allow for feeding while the pharyngeal muscles remain weak. Additional gastrointestinal problems may include incontinence secondary to neurological impairment of the muscles controlling bowel function or alternatively from cognitive impairment. Constipation is frequently seen due to the same alteration in neurological functioning of the bladder, or often due to medications.

Genitourinary Complications

Neurological control of the bladder may be impaired, resulting in incontinence. However, most cases of incontinence following brain injury are a result of disinhibition instead of true neurological impairment. Patients with neurological impairment of bladder function may retain urine, which can lead to other problems, including frequent infections of the urinary tract, infection of the kidneys, and renal and bladder stones. Sexual dysfunction may also be an issue, although, again, these problems are predominately behavioral as opposed to physiological impairment of sexual functioning. Frequently, sexual inhibition may occur as a result of altered body image due to impairments such as weakness, spasticity, or changes in physical appearance due to the injury, although more frequently, patients become sexually disinhibited due to injury to the areas of the brain responsible for control of impulsive behavior (Kreuter et al., 1998). Sexual functioning is an area that is frequently overlooked by medical professionals. In women, infertility may occur secondary to the endocrine changes mentioned earlier (Ripley et al., 2008).

Musculoskeletal Complications

Musculoskeletal complications are very common following brain injury. Injury to the motor nerves in the brain may result in the upper motor neuron syndrome, which consists of the constellation of symptoms of spasticity, weakness, and hyperreflexia. Areas of weakness can vary depending on where the injury is located in the brain. Due to the brain's structural organization, injury on one side of the brain results in weakness on the opposite side of the body. Additionally, the weak side is frequently associated with spasticity. If unchecked, spasticity and immobility may ultimately result in *contractures*, which is tightening of the soft tissues and shortening of tendons around a joint resulting in a reduction in the patient's mobility. As a result of associated trauma, patients with brain injuries also frequently have associated fractures, peripheral nerve injuries, or soft tissue injury that can also make rehabilitation difficult. An interesting musculoskeletal problem that sometimes occurs following TBI is *heterotopic ossification*, a condition in which bone is formed inappropriately in soft tissue areas. This problem, if left untreated, can result in ankylosis, or fusion of a joint, such that moving it is impossible. Extremity pain may also be a problem, due to inherent injury to the extremity or from neurological damage to the sensory pathways.

Cognitive Problems

Injury to the brain can result in any number of changes in mental function, including changes in personality. The specific changes, of course, depend on the specific structures damaged. Very commonly, brain-injured patients experience problems with memory, attention, and arousal, as well as difficulties with language and communication (Seel et al., 1997). Even patients who experience a relatively good recovery will often have subtle cognitive deficits that make returning to work or living independently difficult. A list of potential cognitive problems after TBI can be found in Table 13.2 (Groswasser & Stern, 1998).

Recovery from TBI

Recovery from brain injury is a highly variable process. Severely injured patients recover *in general* along a set of stages, classified as the Rancho Los Amigos Scale of Cognitive Functioning (see Table 13.3). Patients do not always progress through each stage in a stepwise fashion; some patients may skip one or more stages. This scale has its greatest usefulness in communicating with other team members about the condition of the patient, although at times it is helpful for family members, particularly when patients are in an agitated state. Some families find it somewhat comforting to know that the agitated state is part of a normal recovery process following TBI.

Most sources indicate that full neurological recovery of the brain following a severe injury takes approximately one year. Although this is a good estimate for most patients, there are certainly exceptions, and some patients have demonstrated significant recovery even after one

Table 13.2 Potential Cognitive Problems after TBI

Apathy	Impulsivity	Irritability	Aggression
Depression	Lability	Silliness	Denial
Forgetfulness	Memory problems	Bizarre ideation	Slovenliness
Anxiety	Sexual problems	Substance abuse	Spatial neglect
Anasognosia	Attention deficit	Fatigue	Social problems

Table 13.3 Rancho Los Amigos Scale of Cognitive Functioning: Variable Outcomes Dependent on Nature and Severity of Injury

I	No response: Unresponsive to any stimulus.
II	Generalized response: Limited, inconsistent, non-purposeful responses, often to pain only.
III	Localized response: Purposeful responses; may follow simple commands; may focus on presented object.
IV	Confused, agitated: Heightened state of activity; confusion, disorientation, aggressive behavior.
V	Confused, inappropriate, non-agitated: Appears alert; responds to commands; distractible; does not concentrate on task.
VI	Confused, appropriate: Good directed behavior, needs cuing; can relearn old skills; serious memory problems; some awareness of self and others.
VII	Automatic, appropriate: Robot-like appropriate behavior, minimal confusion; shallow recall, poor insight into condition; initiates tasks, but needs structure; poor judgment, problem-solving and planning skills.
VIII	Purposeful, appropriate: Alert, oriented; recalls and integrates past events; learns new activities and can continue without supervision; independent in home and living skills; capable of driving; defects in stress tolerance, judgment, abstract reasoning persist; many functions at reduced levels in society.

year. Researchers are learning more about the process of neuroplasticity and factors affecting better outcomes (Ginsberg et al., 1997; Pike & Hamm, 1997).

Long-Term Impairments

Impairments following brain injury may include almost any complication imaginable. However, there are certain impairments that occur with such regularity after TBI that they warrant special mention. These impairments are the main issues that cause long-term problems after brain injury. Any life care plan for a patient who is traumatically severely injured should be sure to address these particular issues.

- *Weakness*: Injury to the motor cortex or motor pathways may lead to weakness. Severe enough injury will result in paralysis. Weakness is usually the biggest factor affecting a person's ability to perform activities of self-care, such as dressing, grooming, and feeding. It may also impair an individual's ability to walk and move about and, in extreme cases, may lead to the necessity of assistance with transfers.
- *Spasticity*: Spasticity, defined as "velocity-dependent increase in motor tone," as mentioned earlier in the chapter, often remains a huge obstacle to independence after a brain injury. Spasticity is manifested clinically as an involuntary "tightening" of the muscles, resulting in difficulty moving a joint through normal range of motion. Spasticity is often associated with weakness and further complicates the patient's ability to move and perform activities of self-care. Furthermore, severe spasticity places the patient at risk for a number of other complications, such as contractures and skin breakdown. Much of the medical treatment following TBI centers around the prevention

and treatment of spasticity. A number of medical interventions in the treatment of spasticity have become available in recent years. Aside from oral medications and therapeutic interventions such as splinting, casting, bracing, and range-of-motion exercises, patients are frequently treated with a variety of injections for spasticity. These may include nerve blocks using ethanol or phenol or, more commonly now, botulinum toxin injections. A newer treatment device, the intrathecal pump, may be surgically implanted to provide a higher concentration of medicine for spasticity directly at the level of the spinal cord, where it is most effective. The advantage to this technique is that it allows greater control over the administration of medicine, while avoiding many of the side effects associated with oral administration of medication. This treatment is not for everyone, however, and should be discussed with the patient's doctor. Finally, various surgical techniques may be used, usually as last-resort efforts, for treatment of spasticity. These include various tendon-lengthening procedures, rhizotomy, or cordotomy.

- *Behavioral problems*: Although other issues may be more of a focus of medical treatment, it is often behavioral issues that prevent successful community reintegration and return to gainful employment. Patients may have low frustration tolerance, impaired judgment, and, in many cases, emotional lability or frank aggression that hinder successful rehabilitation outcomes. Behavioral problems are usually addressed on a number of levels, including psychological counseling, behavior modification plans, medications, and, in worst cases, inpatient neurobehavioral treatment programs.
- *Cognitive*: Several studies have examined the frequency of patients' complaints following TBI. The most common complaint in all studies is problems with memory. Areas of the brain associated with memory formation are particularly susceptible to injury following trauma, due to their proximity to bony protuberances inside the skull. Additionally, these structures are particularly susceptible to anoxic injury as well, which can occur secondarily following trauma. Deficits in attention, motivation, and sensory input can also secondarily result in memory problems.
- *Aging*: As noted in the vocational category that follows, aging with a brain injury can result in a faster than average decline physically, as well as cognitively. Reduced physical skills and judgment can also result in additional injury as time passes. Indeed, once a person has experienced a brain injury, he or she is much more likely to have a second injury than people without a brain injury. Also, for some mild to moderately brain-injured clients, social isolation and awareness of deficits eventually erode the hope and optimism that occur while progress is being made, and behavior and emotional problems may arise several years after the original insult. These problems are not as much related to aging as to the passage of time and the slow realization that they will never achieve their pre-injury levels and may be unable to enjoy normal social and love relationships (Trudel & Purdum, 1998).

Community Reintegration

Successful return to the community remains a significant challenge given all of the potential barriers a patient may face due to the impairments sustained as a result of the injury (Berens, 2008; Smith-Knapp et al., 1996; Wall et al., 1998). With changes in personality, and behavioral problems, interpersonal relationships often become difficult. Many patients require ongoing supervision for safety reasons, which interferes with social activities. Driving a motor vehicle is a significant concern, and a formal driving evaluation should be performed by a therapist trained to look for the specific problems that may interfere with safe driving.

An additional issue frequently seen is the return to recreational activities. A high percentage of brain injury patients engaged in high-risk activities prior to their injury (Chesnut et al., 1993). In fact, it is often engagement in high-risk activities that led to the brain injury in the first place. It is extremely important that individuals protect themselves against a second injury, particularly while the brain is healing. The *second impact syndrome*, in which a person healing from one injury is exposed to a second injury, may result in exponentially worse or even fatal outcomes, even with a relatively minor second injury. It is therefore extremely important that the patient be restricted from engaging in activities that may place him or her at risk for another injury. A therapeutic recreation specialist may be helpful in identifying and developing appropriate leisure interests after brain injury as well as helping develop techniques to pursue those interests when physical and cognitive impairments make them difficult. In addition, substance abuse may adversely affect recovery and ultimate outcome, further complicating the vocational and life care planning needs (Corrigan, 1995).

Vocational Rehabilitation

Return to gainful employment after brain injury remains a significant challenge (Dikmen et al., 1994; Goodall et al., 1994; Ip et al., 1995; Wehman et al., 1988, 1993; Stapleton et al., 1989; Cifu et al., 1997; Zasler, 1997). Most studies indicate that following a brain injury, approximately one-quarter to one-third of individuals return to work within a 1- to 2-year period following the injury (Traumatic Brain Injury National Data and Statistical Center, 2004). Even with milder brain injuries, work-related issues often become the major problem due to significant problems with interpersonal relationships and behavioral changes (Baker, 1990; Chwalisz, 1992; DePompei & Williams, 1994). Most TBIs occur in individuals between the ages of 16 and 30, a time in most people's lives when education is being completed and career goals established. For those who have completed their education, the cognitive problems often prohibit the use of previously gained knowledge. Additionally, memory problems may make further education or training impossible, in the worst cases.

It is strongly recommended that individuals undergo a neuropsychological evaluation to determine their capacity for education and work (Weed, 1996, 1998; Macciochi et al., 1998). A proper, thorough neuropsychological evaluation will give information about how the patient learns and processes information, and will help the vocational rehabilitation counselor in establishing appropriate return-to-work goals (also see Table 13.4 for a checklist of questions to the neuropsychologist, which, although also included in the vocational chapter of this book, appears relevant enough to include in this chapter). Many clients, in fact, are unable to return to competitive employment due to their impairments, or need significant support and assistance to do so. Many patients have no difficulty obtaining employment, but have a great deal of trouble maintaining employment. Research regarding employment suggests that the most difficult to place long term are people with mental illness and brain injury.

In order to adequately assess the vocational and life planning needs of a person with a brain injury, it is recommended that, as clinical judgment dictates, other allied health professionals be considered. The occupational therapist may be an appropriate referral for an assessment for seating and positioning, adaptive aids, and other vocationally related issues. For some clients, Activities of Daily Living training, including household safety, would be included. The speech and language pathologist will be instrumental in determining augmentative communications and assistive technology for clients with more severe injuries, as well as in providing an assessment of receptive and expressive speech and language. They also often offer cognitive remediation strategies. A physical therapist is often the most appropriate referral to determine the client's true physical capabilities by compiling a functional capacity assessment (or physical capacity assessment) that is more detailed than most physicians can report. For the young adult or pediatric case, an

Table 13.4 Neuropsychologist Questions

In addition to the standard evaluation report, add the following as appropriate:	
1.	Please describe, in layman's terms, the injury to the brain.
2.	Please describe the effects of the accident on the client's ability to function.
3.	Please provide an opinion to the following topics: a. Intelligence level (include pre- vs. post-incident if able)? b. Personality style with regard to the workplace and home? c. Stamina level? d. Functional limitations and assets? e. Ability for education/training? f. Vocational implications—style of learning? g. Level of insight into present functioning? h. Ability to compensate for deficits? i. Ability to initiate action? j. Memory impairments (short-term, long-term, auditory, visual, etc.)? k. Ability to identify and correct errors? l. Recommendations for compensation strategies? m. Need for companion or attendant care?
4.	What is the proposed treatment plan? a. Counseling (individual and family)? b. Cognitive therapy? c. Reevaluations? d. Referral to others (e.g., physicians)? e. Other?
5.	How much and how long (include cost per session or hour and reevaluations)?

Source: Roger O. Weed, with acknowledgment to Robert Frasier for some content.

educational consultant can be very important to maximize the client's educational potential. Under the Individuals with Disabilities Education Act (IDEA), the public school system is responsible for providing specialized services to children with disabilities. However, many of these clients are unserved for a variety of reasons. One reason is that the client has not been adequately assessed in order to identify deficits that would meet the criteria for specialized education. Another reason is that the client may meet the definition, but the school's funding is inadequate and the school will fail to provide appropriate support. Educational consultants who are familiar with the rules often can negotiate the appropriate education protocol.

Several methods of vocational assistance have been developed, including sheltered workshops and supported employment. The supported employment model involves a job coach who spends time with the patient at the worksite and assists with training the patient for the job, accommodations of the workspace if necessary, and helping with problems that may occur if needed. Much of the support involves educating the employer about the nature of brain injury (McMahon & Shaw, 1991; Wehman et al., 1993).

In addition, the effects of aging with a brain injury may affect work life expectancy (Weed, 1998). Data reveal that many clients with a brain injury cognitively or physically deteriorate at a faster rate and appear years older than their chronological age; it is not uncommon for clients to depart from work (i.e., retire early) at an age younger than that of most able-bodied workers. Reduced physical skills from the initial injury mean the person has less of a reserve than the average person, so as he or she ages, he or she may reach the threshold of dependence at an earlier age. There also may be an increased risk of Alzheimer's disease at an earlier age, leading to loss of independence earlier than with the average person (Chandra et al., 1989; Gedye et al., 1989; Rosenthal, 1990; Cifu et al., 1996b; Thompson et al., 1997). For example, it may be appropriate to phase out work and phase in a day program or volunteer activities by the time the client is in his or her fifties. The decline in work life can also be a result of moving from full-time to part-time work, as well as earlier retirement.

Case Study

A 32-year-old client was riding a motorcycle that was hit by a car. At the time of the interview, 3 years post-injury, he stated that he did not remember the incident or anything a couple of weeks prior to the incident. Following the incident, his first consistent memory is approximately 2 to 3 months later. He was treated for 2 months in an acute care hospital and then for 5 months in a brain injury rehabilitation hospital. The client was diagnosed with severe TBI with physical and cognitive deficits, including ventriculoperitoneal shunt and orthopedic injuries requiring extensive care.

Neuropsychological testing results concluded that the client had sustained a very severe TBI. Testing revealed reduced intellectual capacity of one standard deviation, perhaps slightly more, below pre-injury levels. His primary deficit is in visual/motor problem solving. He is able to sight read beyond a high school level. He has significant deficits in mathematical calculations, with overall performance at a level much lower than expected given his pre-injury educational level. No anomia was noted, and he is able to mildly retrieve words without perseveration or intrusive errors. He has significant difficulty with fine motor coordination, with reduced range in the left upper extremity. He has significantly improved executive function from prior testing, which is the most promising part of the overall evaluation, although he continues to exhibit occasions of temper outbursts. He has moderately to severely impaired short-term memory, especially with verbal short-term memory given the absence of consolidation of information. He has a positive affect, although he has times of unhappiness/frustration, and is basically functioning in a more adaptive manner.

He has a young daughter and must be supervised when with her. His wife is supportive and has quit work to be his caregiver. He must have someone available for assistance with judgment, safety, food preparation, and financial commitments. Work is not a reasonable goal, although volunteer activities part-time would be therapeutic.

LIFE CARE PLAN
Note: For purposes of this plan, the following initials are placed in parentheses according to their respective recommendations: JP = Jeffrey Preston, MD, physiatrist MC = Michael Cathy, MD, psychiatrist RH = Robert Hampton, MD, ophthalmologist IR = Ian Raston, MD, hand surgeon WW = William White, MD, internist AP = Amy Passy, PT, physical therapist JH = John Hurry, PsyD, neuropsychologist RW = Roger Weed, PhD, life care planner

(Continued)

Routine Future Medical Care—Physician Only			
Recommendation (by whom)	*Initiated/ Duration*	*Purpose*	*Expected Cost*
Physiatrist (JP) X-rays: left hip, knee, or shoulder (JP) Head CT scan (JP) Head MRI (JP) EEG (JP)	4 times/year to life expectancy 3 times/year to life expectancy 1 time/year to life expectancy Every 5 years to life, 1 time/year to life expectancy	Monitor overall rehabilitation program and prevent/reduce complications, etc. Monitor development of expected degenerative joint disease Assess integrity of shunt Monitor structural changes to brain. Assess brain wave activity due to high risk for seizures	$276–$320/year at $69–$80/visit (see Note 1) Range: $609–$1,365/year at $203–$455 each, 3 times/year to life. CT scan: $2,173–$2,296/year to life. MRI: $3,016–$4,370 every 5 years to life EEG: $854/year to life
Note 1: Cost for physiatrist does not include one-time new patient evaluation at $100 to $150 required by one physiatrist. *Note 2:* Costs for X-rays, CT scan, MRI, and EEG include both diagnostic study and physician interpretation fee. Cost range for MRI depends on whether the study is done with or without contrast. If done with contrast, an additional fee for the contrast dye will incur.			
Neurologist (JP)	2 times/year to life expectancy	Monitor neurological status	$148–$460/year at $74–$115/visit
Orthopedic surgeon (JP)	2 times/year to life expectancy	Monitor orthopedic status and development of expected degenerative joint disease	New patient: $180, 1 time only Follow-up: $120–$160/ year to life at $60–$80/ visit
Note: See also expected future left knee and hip replacement surgery recommended by Dr. Preston.			
Neuro-ophthalmologist (RH)	2 times/year to life expectancy	Monitor visual impairments	$160/year at $80/ visit
Note: Economist to deduct cost of routine ophthalmology or optometry follow-up since it is recommended for the general population.			

(*Continued*)

Psychiatrist (MC)	4–6 times/year for 2–3 years, then 2–3 times/ year to life expectancy	Medication management	$288–$432/year for 2–3 years, then $144–$216/year to life at 72/visit
Hand surgeon (IR)	1 time/year to life expectancy	Monitor left-hand problems related to neurological disorder	$60/year to life expectancy
Internist (WW)	4 times/year to life expectancy	General medical care and treatment	$424/year at $106/ visit
Note 1: The internist reports the client is expected to require more frequent visits and at a higher level per visit than typically expected of the general population. Visits included in the plan are *over and above* recommendations for the general population. *Note 2:* The client also may need evaluation and follow-up by specialists, including neurosurgeon, urologist, and others as needed depending on complications and at the discretion of his treating physicians. See also Potential Complications.			
Projected Evaluations—Nonphysician (Include all allied health evaluations)			
Recommendation (by whom)	*Dates*	*Frequency/Duration*	*Expected Cost*
Physical therapy evaluation to assess gait changes (JP)	2001 to life expectancy	1 time/year to life expectancy	$200–$250/year to life expectancy
Note 1: According to the records, the client was discharged from physical therapy in April 2001 and transitioned to a home exercise program. The therapist recommended physical therapy reevaluation in 3 to 4 months to determine maintenance of his function and carryover of skills. *Note 2:* See also Health and Strength Maintenance for ongoing fitness program.			
Occupational therapy evaluation to evaluate for and monitor adaptive equipment needs (JP)	2001 to life expectancy	1 time/year to life expectancy	$300–$350/year to life expectancy
Note: According to the physiatrist, speech therapy does not appear to be indicated for the client and no recommendations are made for yearly speech evaluations or therapy to monitor his status and provide recommendations depending on needs.			
Home accessibility evaluation by qualified occupational therapist (RW)	2001	1 time only	$200 (average) for in-home occupational therapy evaluation with recommendations

(*Continued*)

Note: Although the client's home generally appears appropriate for him at this time, a home accessibility evaluation is reasonable and appropriate to evaluate the home and make recommendations for additional modifications to ensure the client maintains his highest level of independence and function in his home, especially given an expected further decline in physical functioning as he ages.			
Projected Therapeutic Modalities			
Recommendation (by whom)	*Year Initiated*	*Frequency/Duration*	*Expected Cost*
Physical therapy to develop, monitor, and supervise fitness program and home exercise program (JP)	2001	4 times/year to life expectancy	$988/year to life for four 1-hour sessions/year at $247/session
Note: See also Health and Strength Maintenance for ongoing fitness program.			
Neuropsychologist consultation for coping strategies, adjustment issues, cognitive remediation, and behavior management strategies (JH)	2001	4–6 times/year to life expectancy	$392–$840/year to life at $98–$140 (depends on length of visit)
Note 1: It is likely the client also will need counseling episodically throughout his lifetime, especially during transitional times in his life (i.e., mid-30s, middle age, elderly, etc.), as well as during life-changing events that may occur (i.e., birth of second child, expected in January 2004, etc.). Frequency and duration of counseling are unknown, and no additional cost is included in plan totals. *Note 2:* The client's wife/family also may need counseling as needed throughout their life expectancy depending on circumstances. The neuropsychologist states he is available to the client and wife as needed, typically for telephonic intervention related to various issues/questions that arise, at no additional cost to the client. The physiatrist also states the client's family/wife may need counseling intervention at some time in the future.			
Case manager experienced in working with clients with a brain injury to problem solve, coordinate care, client advocate, etc. (RW)	2001	2 hours/month (average) to life expectancy	$1,800–$2,136/year (average) to life expectancy at $75–$89/hour (does not include mileage to appointments and to meet with client)

(*Continued*)

Financial planner/consultant (JH)	2001 to life expectancy	2 hours/month (average)	$1,920–$2,499/year (average) to life expectancy at $80–$100/hour (estimate)
Note: The client requires assistance and oversight with legal and business contracts, budgeting, financial planning, major decision making, and other money management decisions. Although his wife currently performs these activities, it is recommended a financial consultant, independent from the family, be utilized.			
Diagnostic Testing/Educational Assessment			
Recommendation (by whom)	*Year Initiated*	*Frequency/Duration*	*Expected Cost*
Neuropsychology evaluations (JH)	2020–2025 (50–55 years of age), then repeat 5 years later	2 times over course of lifetime	$1,200–$1,600 total at $600–$800/ evaluation
Wheeled Mobility Needs, Accessories, and Maintenance			
Recommendation (by whom)	*Year Purchased*	*Replacement Schedule*	*Expected Cost*
Power scooter (JP), Scooter maintenance (RW)	2001 to life expectancy 2002	Scooter: Every 5 years (average) Batteries: 1 time/ year (average) to life expectancy 1 time/ year after warranty expires	Scooter: $2,700–$2,900 every 5 years average. Batteries (2): $180/ year at $89.95 each. Maintenance: $100/ year (average estimate)
Note 1: The physiatrist recommends a power scooter for prolonged mobility assistance and extended outings in the community. See also scooter lift for vehicle in the following sections. *Note 2:* The client states (and records confirm) that he previously used a manual wheelchair for mobility assistance and no longer requires the chair. For purposes of future care planning, it is presumed the wheelchair is available in the home for his use in the future, if needed, and no cost for replacement is included in plan totals.			
Home Furnishings/Aids for Independent Function			
Recommendation (by whom)	*Year Purchased*	*Replacement Schedule*	*Expected Cost*
Shower/tub bench with back (JP)	2001 (already has)	Every 5 years (average) to life expectancy	$48.95–$59.95 every 5 years (average) to life expectancy

(*Continued*)

Elevated toilet seat (JP)	1997 (already has)	N/A; see note	N/A; see note
Note: The client states he no longer uses this item; however, for purposes of future care planning, it is presumed the elevated toilet seat is available in the home for his future use, if needed, and no cost for replacement is included in plan totals.			
Allowance for daily planner/ scheduler, memory book and other compensatory tools, handheld shower, cordless phone, etc. (JH, RW)	2001 (already has some items)	1 time/year allowance to life expectancy	$50/year (average) to life expectancy
Orthotics/Prosthetics			
Recommendation (by whom)	*Year Purchased*	*Replacement Schedule*	*Expected Cost*
Custom left ankle, foot orthosis (AFO) (JP)	2015 or 2020 (age 45 or 50)	Every 2–3 years (average) to life expectancy	$600–$1,000 every 2–3 years (average) to life (includes measuring, molding, casting, fittings, and adjustments)
Note 1: The physiatrist states the client also may benefit from custom insoles or orthopedic footwear due to his altered gait; however, no information is available regarding specific type or kind of orthopedic supply and no additional cost is included in plan totals. See Potential Complications. *Note 2:* The orthotist suggests replacement every 1 to 2 years (average) depending on wear and tear, maintenance, and need or changes in the client's mobility and musculoskeletal structure.			
Orthopedic Equipment Needs			
Recommendation (by whom)	*Year Purchased*	*Replacement Schedule*	*Expected Cost*
Cane with offset handle (JP, WW)	2001 (already has)	Every 10 years (average) to life expectancy	$20–$25 every 10 years (average) to life expectancy
Standard folding walker (JP, WW)	2000 (already has)	Every 10 years (average) to life expectancy	$70–$85 every 10 years (average) to life expectancy
Note 1: The client currently uses a cane with offset handle for mobility assistance primarily in the community. The physiatrist recommends both a cane and walker be available to him throughout his life expectancy. If a rolling walker is needed, cost is $200 to $270 each. *Note 2:* The physiatrist also recommends a power scooter for long-distance outings in the community (see scooter).			

(*Continued*)

Drug Needs			
Drug needs and costs are representative of the client's current need and may change from time to time.			
Recommendation (by whom)	*Purpose*	*Cost per Month*	*Cost per Year*
Clonazepam (Klonopin), 0.5 mg, 2 times/day (MC) Oxybutynin (Ditropan), 5 mg, 3 times/day (WW)	Seizure prevention Bladder control and management Reduce	\$21.12–\$43.59 for 60 tablets/month, \$17.11–\$25.79 for 90 tablets/month, \$34.27–\$42.59 for	\$257–\$530/year to life expectancy, \$208–\$314/year to life expectancy, \$730–\$907/year to life expectancy
Zanaflex, 4 mg, 1/2 tablet in A.M., 1/2 tablet at noon, 1 tablet at bedtime (1 1/2 tablets/day) (WW) Baclofen, 20 mg, 3 times/day (WW) Propranolol LA (Inderal), 60 mg, 2 times/day (WW)	spasticity/ataxia. Reduce spasticity/ataxia. Reduce spasticity/ataxia	30 tablets/month, \$25.92–\$47.69 for 90 tablets/month, \$47–\$61.79 for 60 tablets/month	\$315–\$580/year to life expectancy, \$572–\$752/year to life expectancy
Note: According to the physiatrist, the client is expected to require these or similar medications throughout his life expectancy. The internist also states medications are expected to be needed throughout his lifetime.			
Supply Needs			
Supply needs and costs are representative of the client's current need and may change from time to time.			
Recommendation (by whom)	*Purpose*	*Replacement Schedule*	*Cost per Year*
Prism glasses (RH)	Reduce double vision	Expect replacement every 1–2 years (average)	\$283 for frames and lenses every 1–2 years (average) to life expectancy
Note 1: According to the ophthalmologist, the client's vision impairment as related to the brain injury is expected to remain the same over his lifetime. He states there will probably be no new problems with his vision assuming no additional or further ocular trauma occurs. See also Potential Complications. *Note 2:* The client states he does not use other supplies related to injuries received in the incident.			

(*Continued*)

Home/Facility Care			
Recommendation (by whom)	*Year Initiated/ Suspended*	*Hours/Shifts/Days of Attendance or Care*	*Expected Cost*
Competent companion for assistance, safety, and supervision in the home (JP, JH) Child care assistance (JP, JH)	2001	10–12 hours/day, 7 days/week, 365 days/ year to life expectancy. As needed	$35,953–$65,700/ year to life expectancy at $9.85–$15/hour. Defer to economist for loss of child care services
Note 1: The client's wife currently performs the function of a live-in caregiver. *Note 2:* Of the nine home health agencies contacted in the client's local area, only one agency offered a live-in caregiver and the service currently was not available due to staffing shortages and difficulty in hiring and retaining live-ins. When and if available, live-in at the one agency is $139.20/day. *Note 3:* The neuropsychologist states the client does not require overnight *awake* care and should be able to summon emergency assistance if needed.			
Note 4: Both the neuropsychologist and physiatrist state the client is expected to have difficulty with child-raising activities with his 2-year-old daughter and his expected second child in January 2004 and requires child care assistance. Economic value of time that a father normally spends in child-rearing and child-raising activities and that which is lost due to the client's injury are deferred to the economist. *Note 5:* The cost of in-home care may be reduced through negotiation with the home health agency for long-term contract, private hire, or if family or friends assume some of the care.			
Yard care and interior/ exterior home maintenance and repairs (per interview)	2001	N/A	Defer to economist as part of loss of household services
Note: The client's home is in obvious need of repair due to injury caused by maneuvering the wheelchair in the home (i.e., injury to doorways, flooring, walls, etc.). The client states he is unable to do the repairs and is unable to paint or do other interior/exterior home maintenance tasks since the injury.			
Transportation			
Recommendation (by whom)	*Year Purchased*	*Replacement*	*Expected Cost*
Cellular telephone for emergency communication (RW)	2000 (already has)	Every 5 years (estimate)	N/A (had pre-injury)
Scooter lift for vehicle (RW)	2001 or when scooter purchased; see scooter	Every 5–7 years (average) to life expectancy or at time of vehicle replacement	$2,500 every 5–7 years (average) for hoist arm scooter lift

(Continued)

Note: Although the client received satisfactory scores in the behind-the-wheel adapted driving evaluation in July 2001, the neuropsychologist opines that driving is not recommended due to judgment impairments and slow processing that impair his ability to act quickly or in emergencies.			
Health and Strength Maintenance (Leisure Time Activities)			
Recommendation (by whom)	*Year of Purchase or Attendance*	*Replacement or Attendance Schedule*	*Expected Cost*
Fitness program: Option 1 Gym membership (JP) Option 2 Home exercise equipment to include treadmill, parallel bars, and multi-station exercise machine	2001 to life expectancy	N/A; already has equipment; plan for 2-time replacements (estimate) over his lifetime	N/A; no additional cost over general population 2011: $3,000 (estimate) 2021: $3,000 (estimate)
Note 1: The physiatrist recommends a physical conditioning/exercise program under the supervision of a physical therapist to monitor and oversee/supervise fitness program. See also physical therapy for recommended four times/year physical therapist supervision. *Note 2:* The physical therapist suggests a recumbent stationary bicycle also may be useful for the client.			
Membership to National Brain Injury Association and local support groups/ networking (RW)	2001 to life expectancy	Yearly membership	$35/year to life expectancy
Vocational/Educational Plan			
Recommendation (by whom)	*Year Initiated/ Suspended*	*Purpose*	*Expected Cost*
Computer with monitor, printer, Internet access, software package, and other features (RW)	1-time-only replacement estimated in 2002 (approximately 4 years after purchase of current computer in 1998)	Increase independence for educational and recreational activity	$2,000 (average) for 1-time-only replacement in approximately 2002
Note 1: Dr. Preston states in his deposition that a personal computer is medically indicated for the client to include possible access for environmental control unit (ECU) or adaptive devices integration in the future. *Note 2:* A one-time-only replacement cost for computer and related equipment/supplies is included in plan. Replacement after that is presumed to be consistent with use of a personal computer by the general population.			

(*Continued*)

Note: The client has no competitive vocational potential. Volunteer activity is a best option for him to increase his sense of productivity and self-worth, and provide a sense of purpose. If professional services are required in the future to develop or cultivate an alternate volunteer program for the client, expect 20 to 40 hours for vocational counseling and related services, including vocational evaluation, labor market research, job site analysis, etc., at $75 to $89/hour. However, costs for these services are not included in the plan.			
Architectural Considerations			
(List considerations for home accessibility and modifications.) The client currently lives with his wife and 2-year-old daughter in a ranch-style house that has been modified to accommodate him and generally appears appropriate for his current needs. A ramp has been constructed to the back door, which is the entrance the client uses to enter and exit the home, and grab bars have been installed in the bathroom. The front entrance has steps leading to the front door, although no handrail is available and the client demonstrates he generally is able to ascend and descend the stairs with difficulty in a modified fashion and with altered gait.			
The client requires a one-story home with accessibility features and minimal, if any, stairs. If stairs, he requires handrails. See also home accessibility evaluation for one-time-only evaluation to assure the home is accessible both now and for the future as he ages and experiences an expected reduction in his physical capabilities.			
Future Medical Care, Surgical Intervention, Aggressive Treatment			
Recommendation (by whom)	*Year Initiated*	*Frequency*	*Expected Cost**
Eye muscle surgery (RH)	2002–2003 (age 32–33)	1 time only, if successful	$5,000 (approximate)
Left total knee replacement (JP) Left knee revision (JP)	2020 (age 50) Approximately 2030–2032 and every 10–12 years (average) thereafter to life expectancy	Initial knee replacement in 2020, then every 10–12 years (average) knee revision to life expectancy	Replacement in approximately 2020: $30,948, 1st revision: $35,608, 2nd revision: $34,378
Left total hip replacement (JP) Left hip revision (JP)	2020 (age 50) Approximately 2030–2032 and every 10–12 years (average) thereafter to life expectancy	Initial hip replacement in 2020, then every 10–12 years (average) hip revision to life expectancy	Replacement in approximately 2020: $31,568, 1st revision: $39,811, 2nd revision: $37,479
*Expected cost for knee and hip replacement/revision includes surgeon fee and average hospital charges and does not include surgeon assistant fee, if applicable, anesthesiologist fee, or subacute or rehab unit stay. One case of a client similar in age to this client with diagnosis of degenerative joint disease required total knee replacement at a cost of $40,733, inclusive.			

(*Continued*)

Note 1: The physiatrist states he expects the client to require joint replacement in both left hip and left knee due to altered gait and increased wear and tear on his lower-extremity joints, as well as expected degenerative joint disease. He states the severity of the degenerative joint disease depends on maintenance of the client's weight and overall health and fitness. *Note 2:* According to one orthopedic surgeon who performs knee and hip replacement surgeries, knee and hip prostheses last on average 10 to 12 years (based on geriatric population); however, the client may require more frequent revision due to his young age at time of projected initial replacement and expected increased activity level (more so than geriatric activity level). See also Potential Complications. *Note 3:* For purposes of future care planning and based on the physiatrist's recommendation for initial hip and knee joint replacement at approximately age 50, presume two hip and knee revisions over the client's lifetime at approximately age 60 to 62 and age 72 to 74. *Note 4:* The orthopedic surgeon states joint revision surgeries are more difficult than the initial replacement surgery and each subsequent revision is more difficult than the previous one. Recovery also tends to take longer. However, no additional cost for extended recovery is included in plan totals for revision surgeries.			
Note 5: Pain medication is expected to be needed following each joint revision surgery, as well as probable anti-inflammatory medication. Exact kind, dose, and duration of medication are unknown and no additional cost for medications is included in plan totals. *Note 6:* Orthopedic visits following joint replacement/revision generally include one post-op visit (at no cost) plus three other visits at 3, 6, and 12 months post-replacement/post-revision at $60 to $80/visit. Routine follow-up also includes AP and lateral X-rays of hip at $174.25/X-ray and knee at $261.25/X-ray at each post-op visit. Additional medical needs following joint replacement/revision likely include postoperative physical therapy and probable long-term need for cane or walker for mobility assistance. Aqua therapy also may be indicated following joint replacement/revision.			
Ventriculoperitoneal (VP), shunt revision (JP)	Approximately 2011 (15 years after initial shunt placement)	1 time only, assuming no complications	Neurosurgeon evaluation: $286 Revision surgery: $28,927
Note 1: The client was released from the care of his neurosurgeon in February 1998 to be followed by the physiatrist and return as needed if there were complications with his shunt or changes in his neurologic status. The physiatrist states it is probable the client will require at least one shunt revision over his lifetime due to expected complications. *Note 2:* Expected cost for VP shunt revision includes surgeon fee and hospital charges only and does not include diagnostic studies that may be needed such as abdominal X-rays or head CT scan, or anesthesiology charges. See head CT scan, which may be used for diagnostic purposes at time of shunt revision.			
Potential Complications			
Note: Potential complications are included for information only. No frequency or duration of complications is available. No costs are included in the plan.			

(*Continued*)

Neurologic problems, including increased risk for seizures, shunt complications, increased spasticity that is expected to get worse over time, etc., which require aggressive treatment (including Botox injections), diagnostic tests, and prescription medication. Psychological difficulties, including poor adjustment to disability, anger, aggression, irritability, depression, poor social behavior, increased social isolation, increased risk for suicide if not getting adequate care, etc., which could require medication and psychotherapy or hospitalization to treat. The psychiatrist states the client is at higher risk for affective symptoms. Additionally, the neuropsychologist states an anger management program may be an option in the future. Increased risk for early onset of dementia due to the effect of TBI and the aging process, as well as more prone to earlier onset of memory problems and overall decline in cognitive abilities associated with aging. Increased risk for falls and additional injuries (i.e., bone fractures, secondary brain injury, etc.) due to spasticity, impulsivity, poor balance, and reduced physical abilities. The physiatrist states there is a very high probability of the client experiencing falls with resultant fractures. The neuropsychologist states a second brain injury would be devastating and the client would not recover to the extent he has recovered from the primary brain injury.
Musculoskeletal and mobility problems due to altered gait. May require custom orthopedic footwear and insoles. May also experience additional hand problems, depending on his neurological status, that require surgical correction. May require more frequent hip or knee revisions than normally expected or have longer than expected recovery following joint revisions. Urology problems if Ditropan medication becomes ineffective and urology services are needed, including evaluation, diagnostic studies, other medications, surgery, etc. Visual problems, including additional or further ocular trauma or need for other aggressive treatment/surgery to correct or improve his double vision caused by left trochlear nerve palsy and partial oculomotor palsy. More extensive or expensive medical care and equipment than expected. Adverse reaction to long-term use of medication(s).

Conclusion

Thousands of our citizens experience a brain injury each year. The more knowledgeable one is about this specialized industry, the better equipped one is to obtain effective treatment while controlling costs and complications. Life care plans can effectively help ask the right questions and guide the individual, family, and funding source through the complex maze of rehabilitation and long-term care. Effective vocational rehabilitation can help integrate the person back into the community, perhaps as an employed, productive individual. In order to accomplish these monumental tasks, numerous professionals and family members must work together in a collaborative fashion to achieve common goals.

References

Almli, C. R., & Finger, S. 1992. Brain injury and recovery of function: Theories and mechanisms of functional reorganization. *Journal of Head Trauma Rehabilitation*, *7*, 70–77.

American Congress of Rehabilitation Medicine Head Injury Interdisciplinary Special Interest Group. 1993. Definition of mild traumatic brain injury. *Journal of Head Trauma Rehabilitation*, *8*, 86–87.

Baker, J. E. 1990. Family adaptation when one member has a head injury. *Journal of Neuroscience Nursing*, *22*, 232–237.

Berens, D. E. 2008. The ABI Clubhouse Outcomes Measurement Tool: Instrument development and pilot study. Unpublished manuscript.

Berker, E. 1996. Diagnosis, physiology, pathology and rehabilitation of traumatic brain injuries. *International Journal of Neuroscience*, *85*, 95–220.

Bigler, E. D. 1989. Behavioural and cognitive changes in traumatic brain injury: A spouse's perspective. *Brain Injury*, *3*, 73–78.

Bloomfield, E. L. 1989. Extracerebral complications of head injury. *Critical Care Clinics*, *5*, 881–892.

Bontke, C. F., & Boake, C. 1991. Traumatic brain injury rehabilitation. *Neurosurgery Clinics of North America*, *2*, 473–482.

Bontke, C. F., Lehmkuhl, L. D., Englander, J., Mann, N., Ragnarsson, K.T., Zasler, N. D. et al. 1993. Medical complications and associated injuries of persons treated in the traumatic brain injury model systems programs. *Journal of Head Trauma Rehabilitation*, *8*, 34–46.

Brown, A., Elovic, E., Kothari, S., Flanagan, S., & Kwasnica, C. 2008. Congenital and acquired brain injury. 1. Epidemiology, pathophysiology, prognostication, innovative treatments and prevention. *Archive of Physical Medicine and Rehabilitation*, *89*, S3–S8.

Centers for Disease Control and Prevention (CDC). 1997. Sports-related recurrent brain injuries--United States. *MMWR Morbidity and Mortality Weekly Report*, *46*(10), 224–227.

Centers for Disease Control and Prevention. 2008a. How many people have TBI? Retrieved June 7, 2008, from www.cdc.gov/ncipc/tbi/TBI.htm.

Centers for Disease Control and Prevention. 2008b. Facts about TBI. Retrieved June 7, 2008, from www.cdc.gov/ncipc/tbi/FactSheets/Facts_About_TBI.pdf.

Centers for Disease Control, National Center for Injury Prevention and Control. 1999. *Traumatic Brain Injury in the United States: A Report to Congress*. Atlanta, GA: Author.

Chandra, V., Kokmen, E., Schoenberg, B. S., & Beard, C. M. 1989. Head trauma with loss of consciousness as a risk factor for Alzheimer's disease. *Neurology*, *39*, 1576–1578.

Chesnut, R. M., Marshall, L. F., Klauber, M. R., Blunt, B. A., Baldwin, N., Eisenberg, H. M. et al. 1993. The role of secondary brain injury in determining outcome from severe head injury. *Journal of Trauma*, *34*, 216–222.

Chwalisz, K. 1992. Perceived stress and caregiver burden after brain injury: A theoretical integration. *Rehabilitation Psychology*, *37*, 189–203.

Cifu, D. X., Kaelin, D. L., & Wall, B. E. 1996a. Deep venous thrombosis: Incidence on admission to a brain injury rehabilitation program. *Archives of Physical Medicine and Rehabilitation*, *77*, 1182–1185.

Cifu, D. X., Keyser-Marcus, L., Lopez, E., Wehman, P., Kreutzer, J. S., Englander, J. et al. 1997. Acute predictors of successful return to work 1 year after traumatic brain injury: A multicenter analysis. *Archives of Physical Medicine and Rehabilitation*, *78*, 125–131.

Cifu, D. X., Kreutzer, J. S., Marwitz, J. H., Rosenthal, M., Englander, J., & High, W. 1996b. Functional outcomes of older adults with traumatic brain injury: A prospective, multicenter analysis. *Archives of Physical Medicine and Rehabilitation*, *77*, 883–888.

Cipolle M. D., Geffe K., Getchell J., Reed J. F.3rd, Fulda G., Sugarman M., & Tinkoff G. H. 2014. Long-term outcome in elderly patients after operation for traumatic intracranial hemorrhage. *Delaware Medical Journal*, *86*(8), 237–244.

Clifton, G. L., Kreutzer, J. S., Choi, S. C., Devany, C. W., Eisenberg, H. M., Foulkes, M. A. et al. 1993. Relationship between Glasgow Outcome Scale and neuropsychological measures after brain injury. *Neurosurgery*, *33*, 34–38.

Cope, D. N. 1995. The effectiveness of traumatic brain injury rehabilitation: A review. *Brain Injury*, *9*, 649–670.

Corrigan, J. D. 1995. Substance abuse as a mediating factor in outcome from traumatic brain injury. *Archives of Physical Medicine and Rehabilitation*, *76*, 302–309.

Corrigan, J. D., & Mysiw, W. J. 1988. Agitation following traumatic head injury: Equivocal evidence for a discrete stage of cognitive recovery. *Archives of Physical Medicine and Rehabilitation, 69*, 487–492.

Corthell, D. W. 1993. *Employment Outcomes for Persons with Acquired Brain Injury*. Washington, DC: Research and Training Center WU-SMW, National Institute on Disability and Rehabilitation and Research.

DePompei, R., & Williams, J. 1994. Working with families after TBI: A family-centered approach. *Topics in Language Disorders, 15*, 68–81.

Dikmen, S. S., Temkin, N. R., Machamer, J. E., Holubkov, A. L., Fraser, R. T., & Winn, H. R. 1994. Employment following traumatic head injuries. *Archives of Neurology, 51*, 177–186.

Evans, R. W., & Ruff, R. M. 1992. Outcome and value: A perspective on rehabilitation outcomes achieved in acquired brain injury. *Journal of Head Trauma Rehabilitation, 7*, 24–36.

Gedye, A., Beattie, B. L., Tuokko, H., Horton, A., & Korsarek, E. 1989. Severe head injury hastens age of onset of Alzheimer's disease. *Journal of the American Geriatrics Society, 37*, 970–973.

Gerber, D. J., Weintraub, A. H., Cusick, C. P., Ricci, P. E., & Whiteneck, G. G. 2004. Magnetic resonance imaging of traumatic brain injury: Relationship of T2*SE and T2GE to clinical severity and outcome. *Brain Injury Rehabilitation, 18*, 1083–1097.

Ginsberg, M. D., Zhao, W., Back, T., Belayev, L., Stagliano, N., Dietrich, W. D. et al. 1997. Three-dimensional autoradiographic image-processing strategies for the study of brain injury and plasticity. *Advances in Neurology, 73*, 239–250.

Goodall, P., Lawyer, H. L., & Wehman, P. 1994. Vocational rehabilitation and traumatic brain injury: A legislative and public policy perspective. *Journal of Head Trauma Rehabilitation, 9*, 61–81.

Grafman, J., Schwab, K., Warden, D., Pridgen, A., Brown, H. R., & Salazar, A. M. 1996. Frontal lobe injuries, violence, and aggression: A report of the Vietnam Head Injury Study. *Neurology, 46*, 1231–1238.

Groswasser, Z., & Stern, M. J. 1998. A psychodynamic model of behavior after acute central nervous system damage. *Journal of Head Trauma Rehabilitation, 13*, 69–79.

Hall, K. M., & Cope, D. N. 1995. The benefit of rehabilitation in traumatic brain injury: A literature review. *Journal of Head Trauma Rehabilitation, 10*, 1–13.

High, W. M., Hall, K. M., Rosenthal, M., Mann, N., Zafonte, R., Cifu, D. X. et al. 1996. Factors affecting hospital length of stay and charges following traumatic brain injury. *Journal of Head Trauma Rehabilitation, 11*, 85–96.

Horn, L. J., & Zasler, N. D. 1996. *Medical Rehabilitation of Traumatic Brain Injury*. Philadelphia, PA: Hanley & Belfus.

Ip, R. Y., Dornan, J., & Schentag, C. 1995. Traumatic brain injury: Factors predicting return to work or school. *Brain Injury, 9*, 517–532.

Jorge, R. E., Robinson, R. G., Starkstein, S. E., & Arndt, S. V. 1993. Depression and anxiety following traumatic brain injury. *Journal of Neuropsychiatry and Clinical Neuroscience, 5*, 369–374.

Katz, D. I., & Alexander, M. P. 1994. Traumatic brain injury: Predicting course of recovery and outcome for patients admitted to rehabilitation. *Archives of Neurology, 51*, 661–670.

Kaufman, H. H., Timberlake, G., Voelker, J., & Pait, T. G. 1993. Medical complications of head injury. *Medical Clinics in North America, 77*, 43–60.

Kraus, J. F. 1991. Epidemiologic features of injuries to the central nervous system. In D. W. Anderson (Ed.), *Neuroepidemiology: A Tribute to Bruce Schoenberg* (pp. 333–357). Boca Raton, FL: CRC Press.

Kraus, J. F., Black, M. A., Hessol, N., Ley, P., Rokaw, W., Sullivan, C. et al. 1984. The incidence of acute brain injury and serious impairment in a defined population. *American Journal of Epidemiology, 119*, 186–201.

Kreuter, M., Dahllof, A. G., Gudjonsson, G., Sullivan, M., & Siosteen, A. 1998. Sexual adjustment and its predictors after traumatic brain injury. *Brain Injury, 12*, 349–368.

Kreutzer, J., Kowlakowski, S., Ripley, D., Cifu, D., Rosenthal, M., Bushnik, T. et al. 2001. Charges and lengths of stay for acute and inpatient rehabilitation treatment of traumatic brain injury 1990–1996. *Brain Injury, 15*, 763–774.

Levin, H. S. 1992. Head injury and its rehabilitation. *Current Opinion in Neurology and Neurosurgery, 5*, 673–676.

Macciocchi, S. N., Littlefield, L. M., & Diamond, P. T. 1998. Neuropsychological assessment and functional capacity. *Neurorehabilitation, 11*, 67–74.

Macciocchi, S. N., Reid, D. B., & Barth, J. T. 1993. Disability following head injury. *Current Opinion in Neurology, 6*, 773–777.

Malec, J. F., & Basford, J. S. 1996. Postacute brain injury rehabilitation. *Archives of Physical Medicine and Rehabilitation, 77*, 198–207.

Marshall, L. F., Marshall, S. B., Klauber, M. R., Van Berkum, C. M., Eisenberg, H., Jane, J. A. et al. 1992. The diagnosis of head injury requires a classification based on computed axial tomography. *Journal of Neurotrauma, 1*, S287–S292.

Mazmanian, P. E., Kreutzer, J. S., Devany, C. W., & Martin, K. O. 1993. A survey of accredited and other rehabilitation facilities: Education, training and cognitive rehabilitation in brain-injury programmes. *Brain Injury, 7*, 319–331.

McMahon, B., & Shaw, L. 1991. *Work Worth Doing*. Orlando, FL: PMD Press.

Piek, J. 1995. Medical complications in severe head injury. *New Horizons, 3*, 534–538.

Pike, B. R., & Hamm, R. J. 1997. Activating the posttraumatic cholinergic system for the treatment of cognitive impairment following traumatic brain injury. *Pharmacology, Biochemistry and Behavior, 57*, 785–791.

Rappaport, M., Dougherty, A. M., & Kelting, D. L. 1992. Evaluation of coma and vegetative states. *Archives of Physical Medicine and Rehabilitation, 73*, 628–634.

Ripley D. L., Harrison-Felix C., Sendroy-Terrill M., Cusick C.P., Dannels-McClure A., & Morey C. 2008. The impact of female reproductive function on outcomes after traumatic brain injury. *Archives of Physical Medicine and Rehabilitation, 89*(6), 1090–1096. doi:10.1016/j.apmr.2007.10.038.

Rosenthal, M. 1990. *Rehabilitation of the adult and child with traumatic brain injury* (2nd ed.). Philadelphia, PA: Davis.

Russell-Jones, D. L., & Shorvon, S. D. 1989. The frequency and consequences of head injury in epileptic seizures. *Journal of Neurology, Neurosurgery and Psychiatry, 52*, 659–662.

Schmidt, N. D. 1997. Outcome-oriented rehabilitation: A response to managed care. *Journal of Head Trauma Rehabilitation, 12*, 44–50.

Seel, R. T., Kreutzer, J. S., & Sander, A. M. 1997. Concordance of patients' and family members' ratings of neurobehavioral functioning after traumatic brain injury. *Archives of Physical Medicine and Rehabilitation, 78*, 1254–1259.

Semlyen, J. K., Summers, S. J., & Barnes, M. P. 1998. Traumatic brain injury: Efficacy of multidisciplinary rehabilitation. *Archives of Physical Medicine and Rehabilitation, 79*, 678–683.

Smith-Knapp, K., Corrigan, J. D., & Arnett, J. A. 1996. Predicting functional independence from neuropsychological tests following traumatic brain injury. *Brain Injury, 10*, 651–661.

Stapleton, M., Parente, R., & Bennett, P. 1989. Job coaching traumatically brain injured individuals: Lessons learned. *Cognitive Rehabilitation, 7*, 18–21.

Teasdale, G. M., Pettigrew, L. E., Wilson, J. T., Murray, G., & Jennett, B. 1998. Analyzing outcome of treatment of severe head injury: A review and update on advancing the use of the Glasgow Outcome Scale. *Journal of Neurotrauma, 15*, 587–597.

Teasdale, G., Teasdale, E., & Hadley, D. 1992. Computed tomographic and magnetic resonance imaging classification of head injury. *Journal of Neurotrauma, 1*, S249–S257.

Thompson, J. D., Schellenberg, G. D., & Larson, E. B. 1997. Head injury and risk of Alzheimer's disease by apolipoprotein E genotype. *American Journal of Epidemiology, 146*, 373–384.

Traumatic Brain Injury Model Systems. 2008. Traumatic Brain Injury Facts and Figures. Retrieved June 7, 2008, from www.tbindsc.org/200820TBIMS20Slide%20Presentation.pdf.

Traumatic Brain Injury National Data and Statistical Center. 2004. The traumatic brain injury model systems of care. Retrieved February 18, 2008, from www.tbindsc.org.

Trudel, T., & Purdum, C. 1998. Aging with a brain injury, long term issues. *The Rehabilitation Professional*, 6, 37–41.

Uomoto, J. M., & Brockway, J. A. 1992. Anger management training for brain injured patients and their family members. *Archives of Physical Medicine and Rehabilitation, 73*, 674–679.

Wall, J. R., Rosenthal, M., & Niemczura, J. G. 1998. Community-based training after acquired brain injury: Preliminary findings. *Brain Injury, 12*, 215–224.

Weed, R. 1996. Life care planning and earnings capacity analysis for brain injured clients involved in personal injury litigation utilizing the RAPEL method. *Journal of Neurorehabilitation, 7*, 119–135.

Weed, R. 1998. Aging with a brain injury: The effects on life care plans and vocational opinions. *The Rehabilitation Professional, 6*, 30–34.

Wehman, P., Kregel, J., Sherron, P., Nguyen, S., Kreutzer, J., Fry, R. et al. 1993. Critical factors associated with the successful supported employment placement of patients with severe traumatic brain injury. *Brain Injury, 7*, 31–44.

Wehman, P., Kreutzer, J., Wood, W., & Morton, M. V. 1988. Supported work model for persons with traumatic brain injury: Toward job placement and retention. Special issue: Traumatic brain injury. *Rehabilitation Counseling Bulletin, 31*, 298–312.

Wood, R. L. 1987. *Brain Injury Rehabilitation: A Neurobehavioural Approach*. London: Croom Helm.

Zafonte, R. D., Hammond, F. M., Mann, N. R., Wood, D. L., Black, K. L., & Millis, S. R. 1996. Relationship between Glasgow Coma Scale and functional outcome. *American Journal of Physical Medicine and Rehabilitation, 75*, 364–369.

Zafonte, R. D., Mann, N. R., Millis, S. R., Black, K. L., Wood, D. L., & Hammond, F. 1997. Posttraumatic amnesia: Its relation to functional outcome. *Archives of Physical Medicine and Rehabilitation, 78*, 1103–1106.

Zasler, N. D. 1997. The role of medical rehabilitation in vocational reentry. *Journal of Head Trauma Rehabilitation, 12*, 42–56.

Chapter 14

Life Care Planning for the Burn Patient

Ruth B. Rimmer and Kevin N. Foster

Contents

Introduction 402
Burn Injury Prevalence 403
Classification of Burns 404
Majors Problems Associated with Burn Injury 405
Role of the Skin 405
Common Surgical Procedures 406
Reconstruction 407
Pressure Garments and Splints 407
Prosthetics 407
Nutritional Issues 408
Rehabilitation 408
Massage Therapy 408
Outpatient Services 409
Pediatric Life Care Plans 409
Psychological Issues 409
Vocational Rehabilitation 410
Complications 411
Burn Injury: Damage Assessment Checklist 423
Sample Life Care Plan for John Doe 426
Narrative Summary 426
Introduction 426
Burn Injury 427
Injury Event 428
Personal Interviews with John Doe and Jane Doe 430
Face and Neck 432
Upper Extremities and Shoulders 432

Forearms, Elbows, and Wrists........ 432
Web Space Releases........ 432
Legs—Thighs and Calves........ 433
Ankles and Feet........ 433
Laser Therapy........ 433
Skin Cancer........ 433
Pressure Garments........ 433
Massage Therapy........ 434
Psycho/Social Issues........ 435
Psychiatric Care—Psychiatric Evaluations........ 435
Psychiatry........ 435
Individual Psychotherapy........ 435
Couples Therapy........ 436
Family Therapy........ 436
Transportation........ 436
Adaptive Sports Excursion........ 436
Health and Strength Maintenance........ 436
Case Management........ 437
Supplies........ 437
Medication........ 437
Respite Care........ 437
Personal Attendant and Home Care........ 437
Conclusion........ 438
Burn Care Resources........ 438
Books........ 438
Resources for Family Members of Burn Survivors........ 439
Journals........ 439
Burn Survivor Websites........ 439
References........ 439

Introduction

A well-documented and thorough life care plan plays an important role in the long-term recovery of a burn-injured individual. Serious burns cause a significant interruption of the patient's life, including physical, social, emotional, and financial stability. Therefore, it is vitally important that the life care plan for the burn patient is holistic and addresses concerns regarding the client's medical, emotional, social, and financial needs and well-being. It should be noted that the patient's family is also significantly impacted by the burn event.

Burn care has evolved dramatically over the past 25 years. Acute burn care has improved greatly and has resulted in dramatically higher survival rates (Brusselaers et al., 2005). Persons, especially children, with a large percentage of total body surface area burns (% TBSA) survive routinely (Sheridan et al., 2000). While it is encouraging that mortality has declined, an individual's survival of serious burn injury often results in lifelong challenges and complications for both the burn patient and their family. Recovery often necessitates post-acute care rehabilitation, for ongoing reconstructive surgeries with accompanying therapies, home health care, and the need for assistance with psychological, social, educational, financial, and vocational rehabilitation issues. A well-thought-out and comprehensive life care plan can provide the survivor and the family with a vital road map that will assist them in navigating the long and arduous road to recovery.

Burn care is a highly specialized field of medicine. The burn care team is multidisciplinary and is made up of an extensive array of medical professionals. A burn injury is complex and complicated from both a physical and a psychological standpoint, and survivors benefit from a multifaceted team approach to their care (Demling, 1995).

In the acute hospital setting, the patient is cared for by a team of burn care professionals, which includes burn surgeons, physician's assistants, nurses, burn techs, physical and occupational therapists, nutritionists, respiratory therapists, psychologists, social workers, and case managers. Patients often require additional care from specialists such as plastic/reconstructive surgeons, hand surgeons, cardiologists, neurologists, psychiatrists, and speech therapists. The acute medical care setting for burn patients is labor intensive, and the care is expensive. It takes tremendous effort on the part of the entire burn care team, as well as an immense effort on the part of the patient and the patient's family for basic survival to occur (Herndon & Blakeney, 2007). Rehabilitation begins in the hospital and is often extended in a specialized rehabilitation facility after discharge from the acute burn care setting for weeks or even months.

Life care planners and medical case managers should be familiar with the prevalence, etiology, and pathophysiology of burn injuries. Over the past two decades there has been a notable reduction in the total number of burn injuries in the United States; however, every year approximately 486,000 persons in the United States continue to require medical attention for their burn injuries (American Burn Association, 2016). It is estimated that approximately 40,000 of those injured will be hospitalized and that approximately 3,275 individuals will die from their burns (American Burn Association, 2016). Survival is predicated on a number of factors including age, severity of the burn, comorbid trauma, inhalation injury, and premorbid health conditions. Burn patients between the ages of 5 and 20 are among those most likely to have a favorable outcome. Infants and patients over 70 have marked increase for morbidity and mortality (Saffle et al., 1995).

The severity of the burn is determined by a number of factors including the size of the burn injury, the need for skin grafting, and the presence or absence of an inhalation injury. The larger the percentage of TBSA (total body surface area) burned, the less favorable the outcome is likely to be. The depth of the burn, including the degree of the burn, also influences the ultimate outcome, with deeper burns resulting in a less favorable prognosis and the need for the patient to receive skin grafts. Inhalation injury is another factor, which often contributes to poorer outcomes. Burns may present with other trauma, which can also complicate survival and future care needs. Premorbid medical conditions can also have a negative influence on the patient's outcome (Hartford and Kealy, 2007). All of these details are important to consider when developing the life care plan or managing a burn case; therefore, a thorough review of the patient's medical records and familiarity with the patient's medical history are imperative.

Burn Injury Prevalence

The risk of being burned, as well as the etiology of the burn, is related to a person's age, type of employment, economic status, type of recreational activities in which one engages, and location of residence. Although the specific number of burn injuries in the United States is unknown, individuals suffer from far more minor than major burns. It is estimated that only 3% to 4% of burn-injured persons reporting to emergency rooms are admitted or transferred to a burn center/unit. However, burn injuries are still a significant problem and an expensive injury. According to the Centers for Disease Control and Prevention (CDC), burns and fires are the third leading cause of death in the home. They are also the third leading cause of death in children (National Safety Council, 2013). The economic cost of burn injury is high with hospital bills for severe burns ranging from many thousands to millions of dollars for one patient. Ongoing reconstruction and rehabilitation are also costly, which is another reason why an accurate life care plan is so important.

While burns can be caused in a variety of ways, the most prevalent cause of burn injuries requiring admission to the hospital are fire/flame, scalds (most common in young children and the elderly), and chemical, electrical, and radiation burns. Flame and scald burns account for the vast majority or approximately 43% of all reported cases. Scald burns account for the second most common cause at 36% (American Burn Association, 2016). The arms and hands, head and neck, and lower extremities are the areas of the body most likely to sustain burns. Of nonfatal burns, 45% involve the hand and arm, 25% involve the neck and head, and 16% result in burns to the leg and foot (Pruitt et al., 2007). The face, limbs, hands, and feet are vital to both physical and social function, and burns to these body parts, especially scarring across the joints, can be disfiguring as well as disabling (Demling & LaLonde, 1989).

Classification of Burns

The treatment of burns is often determined by the classification of the injury. Burn injuries are typically classified by etiology, depth of the burn (layers), location of the burn, and the percentage of total body surface area burned (% TBSA). Burn depth, which refers to the layers that have been damaged, is classified as superficial (first degree), superficial partial thickness (second degree), deep partial thickness (second degree), full thickness (third degree), and deep full thickness (fourth degree). Physicians will often defer the classification of a burn injury for several days, in order to correctly determine the true depth of the burn.

- *Superficial (first degree) burns* involve only the superficial epidermis and usually require 3 to 7 days for healing with no scarring.
- *Superficial partial-thickness (second degree) burns* involve the epidermis and the dermis excluding hair follicles, sweat glands, and sebaceous glands and should heal in less than 21 days with minimal scarring.
- *Deep partial-thickness (also second-degree) burns* involve the epidermis and most of the dermis, requiring more than 21 days for healing, and may develop severe hypertrophic scarring.
- *Full-thickness (third degree) burns* result in total destruction of the skin, both epidermis and dermis and hypodermis, and may involve additional tissue. Full-thickness burns of any significant size require skin grafting.
- *Deep full-thickness (fourth degree) burns* involve fat, nerve endings, muscle, and/or bone and are usually a result of prolonged contact with heat or an electrical injury and may require flap coverage or amputation (Fisher & Helm, 1984).

Burns are also categorized by the percentage of TBSA involved. It is customary to establish the percentage of partial- and full-thickness burns separately. The American Burn Association (ABA) classifies burn injuries as mild, moderate, and major. Moderate and major burns require hospitalization.

- Minor burns are those that involve less than 15% TBSA and are partial thickness. In the elderly and pediatric populations 10%–20% full thickness is considered minor unless the eyes, ears, face, hands, or perineum are burned.
- Moderate burns include a total body surface area of 15%–25% (10%–20% for pediatric patients less than age 10 or adults over age 40) without regard to the depth and 2%–10% full-thickness burns unless the eyes, ears, face, or perineum are burned.

- Major burns include those partial-thickness burns that cover more than 25% of the body (20% for children and adults less than the age of 40) or those full-thickness burns that cover more than 10% of the total body surface area, as well as all burns to the face, eyes, ears, feet, and perineum. Burns sustained from electricity or lightning or those involving inhalation injury are also considered major. Burns with comorbid trauma and all burns that present with premorbid illness or are in the very young or the elderly are also labeled as major burns (Hartford & Kealy, 2007).

Majors Problems Associated with Burn Injury

Role of the Skin

The skin plays a major role in sustaining life since it makes up the largest organ system of the body. The main functions of the skin are:

- Protective barrier
- Regulates body temperature
- Fluid conservation
- Receives environmental stimuli
- Excretory gland
- Absorbs vitamin D
- Determines identity

Human skin is made up of several layers: the epidermis (10%), which is the outer layer, and the dermis (90%), which is the inner layer. The average thickness of adult skin is one to two millimeters. The top layer contains cells that determine skin color and make up the protective layer of skin. The dermis is found beneath the epidermis. The dermis contains connective tissue, capillaries, collagen, and elastic fibers. This layer supplies structure and nutrition to the epidermis, provides elasticity of the skin, and contains the hair follicles and excretory glands including the sweat and sebaceous glands. There are sensory nerve endings found throughout the skin; therefore, deeper burns may cause permanent changes in a person's capacity to sense pain, touch, and temperature (Cromes & Helm, 1993).

When both layers of the skin, the epidermis and dermis, are destroyed, the patient loses hair follicles and sweat and sebaceous glands. A layer of fat and connective tissue is found under the dermis, and muscle, bone, and tendons are beneath this layer. Sensory nerve endings are distributed throughout the skin and subcutaneous layer. Therefore, burn injury, depending on the depth, may result in a permanent change in the burn victim's capacity to sense pain, touch, and temperature (Fisher & Helm, 1984).

Wound care is a key component of acute and rehabilitative burn care. Wounds must be maintained in a manner that facilitates and at the very least does not impede re-epithelialization of the skin. This includes care designed to minimize infection, remove dead tissue, reduce heat loss, and prevent further tissue loss. A typical approach to wound care involves cleaning the wound and debriding it twice daily. Donor site dressings must also be changed once or twice a day. Wound care is extremely painful for the patient. If reconstructive surgery is a future recommendation for a patient, a provision for home health care will likely be necessary.

A variety of musculoskeletal complications often accompany burn survival (Schneider & Qu, 2011). These may include scar contractures, bone loss, heterotopic ossification (HO), scoliosis, and arthritis. Other issues affecting the rehabilitation of burn-injured individuals are impairment from muscle mass loss, scar contractures, HO, amputations, nervous system injury, and psychological problems, all of which present significant challenges for recovery from burns. Hypertrophic scarring and contractures, especially those involving the joints, mouth, and neck, can cause long-term functional problems. Scarring and hypertrophic ossification may lead to limited range of motion or joint fusion, and much like amputations may result in decreased function and the inability to engage in normal activity. It is important to document these types of problems in the life care plan as early identification and treatment of these types of problems should be considered as treatment goals in the recovery phase (Schneider & Qu, 2011).

Patients who survived severe burns (TBSA of >30%) were found to have weak muscles for many years after the initial trauma (St-Pierre et al., 1998). This is likely due to an incomplete recovery from the burns. The need exits for long-term musculoskeletal assessments in burn patients because their loss of lean body mass has a negative effect on rehabilitation and compromises a successful community reintegration (Edelman et al., 2003). Other problems revealed by the study included joint pain, sleep disruption, fatigue, shortness of breath, heat and cold sensitivity, body image, and sexuality issues. Additionally, a disproportionate number of burn survivors have also been found to be physically unfit when compared to non-burned adults (Ganio, 2015). Therefore, an exercise program designed to contribute to the long-term rehabilitation of the client and other interventions to address common complications of burn injury should be included in the life care plan recommendations.

Common Surgical Procedures

There are a number of common surgical procedures in burn care. If the burn injury is circumferential, the skin can become very tight and stiff and stop the blood flow to the areas below the burn. An escharotomy, a cut made down through the burned skin (the eschar), may be performed. A faciotomy, which is a deeper cut into the tissue below the skin (facia), may also be performed, in order to expose the muscle. Medical records will document these procedures.

Grafting is a surgical procedure that involves the transplantation of skin. Grafting becomes necessary when the patient has burns that will not heal spontaneously. There are several types of skin grafts. The first is an autograft, which is created when the individual's own skin is taken from an unharmed part of the body (donor site) and placed over the burned area.

If the burned area is not ready for an autograft, a temporary skin covering may be used, allograft (homograft) or a xenograft (pigskin). This thin temporary covering is placed over the wound and allows for better pain control and provides a barrier to infection. These temporary grafts stick to the skin, but will be removed when the area is ready for a permanent skin graft (autograft). Skin grafts may take after the first surgery but sometimes they fail and the patient must be returned to the operating room, possibly several times, until all of the dead, burned skin has been removed (debrided or excised). A dermal replacement may also be used because it provides an outstanding barrier for infection, is easy to apply, and adheres well to lesions. It can be very costly, so be sure to inquire if dermal replacement will be necessary for any reconstructive surgeries (Khosh, 2008).

Tissue expansion with scar excision and tissue advancement is another procedure used to improve appearance and function. It has become a major reconstructive modality over the past three decades and increasingly more popular in burn reconstruction. Tissue expansion has many advantages because the existing scarring can be excised and the new expanded skin advanced to cover the wound. The end result is a great match in color and texture. It is a complicated 3 to 4 month process for the patient, but can provide very effective results.

It is important to note the number and type of surgeries the burn patient has undergone in the narrative portion of the life care plan. It helps to illustrate just how burdensome and difficult the patient's acute care stay was.

Reconstruction

A seriously burned patient, especially a child, may need a great deal of post-acute care reconstructive surgery. The purpose of burn reconstruction is to provide the patient with function, comfort, and improved appearance. In children, reconstruction may also be done to allow for growth. The burn patient is likely to have a lifelong relationship with a reconstructive surgeon (Barret, 2004).

It is customary for definitive correction of burn scars to be postponed for at least a year or more. Scars mature over time, and some scars through the use of pressure garments and splints may not need surgical correction. Scar contractures can be uncomfortable as well as unsightly. They may also impede function. It is important for life care planners to inquire as to which reconstruction procedures will be necessary and how often it is probable that they will be repeated over the life span. It is especially important to address those scar contractures that are present over joints, and skeletal deformities also need to be considered.

Once the surgery has been performed, the patient will likely need home health care, physical or occupational therapy, and pressure garments. These items are all important to the long-term success of any reconstructive surgery. The surgeries may also need to be repeated multiple times over the life span, especially when the burn is sustained in childhood or adolescence.

Pressure Garments and Splints

Burn injuries that destroy dermis also cause elimination of the normal pressure that these layers of skin provide. Absent this pressure, hypertrophic scars can form, causing deformities and impairment of function. Pressure garments help to prevent and control the formation of hypertrophic scars by applying counter pressure to the wounded area. They also aid in reducing the effects of hypertrophic scarring, itching, and increased circulation to the area (Linares et al., 1972). Pressure garments are fitted by a specialist, usually prior to discharge from acute care.

Pressure garments can play a vital role in the proper healing of wounds and reduce the effects of scarring, but for the garments to perform their job properly, they need to fit tightly and be in good condition. Patients often wear their garments for anywhere from 12 to 24 months after initial discharge. They must typically be worn 23 hours per day. Therefore, patients are prescribed two sets with each fitting so that they may have one to wear and one to wash. Patients will often be fitted for new garments after reconstruction procedures.

Positioning is also very important for the burn patient. Patients are often sent home with splints. They are also often ordered after reconstruction. The life care planner should inquire into the need and frequency of both garments and splints when discussing projected surgeries.

Prosthetics

A very severe burn, a fourth-degree or circumferential third-degree burn, may result in an amputation. This may involve a digit, hand, limb, or even a nose or ears. A prosthetist or orthotist can provide information regarding the cost, replacement schedule, and need for other accessories for the patient. An anaplastologist, an individual who has the ability to create and customize highly individualized prosthetics for the face, can be consulted for information regarding prosthetic eyes, ear, noses, fingers, and so on. It is important to consider any additional physical or occupational therapy that will be needed with prosthetic/orthotic usage.

Nutritional Issues

Burn injuries affect the body's metabolic rate, and burn patients suffer from post-traumatic hypercatabolism. This well-known phenomenon causes the breakdown of tissue and exhausts the body's energy stores. The magnitude of the problem is defined by the total body surface area and severity of the burns. Glucose uptake is compromised, cholesterol and lipoprotein concentrations are decreased, and protein catabolism causes patients to lose protein content. The increased metabolism is amplified by pain, anxiety, hypovolemia, and infection, as well as loss of body heat (Gallal & Yousef, 2002). Burn patients' nutritional needs are of key importance, and patients are often given enteral feedings with a high caloric content to promote healing. Supplements are often prescribed after discharge from acute care, as well as after reconstructive procedures to insure proper healing. Significant weight gain after a severe burn injury can also be a problem. A weight loss program should be considered as part of the life care plan if the client has experienced this complication.

Rehabilitation

Patient-specific rehabilitation services begin immediately during acute burn injury care and continue after, often long after, the patient is discharged from their initial hospitalization. The literature suggests that recovery from a major burn may take several years to return a patient to a satisfactory level of function (Brown et al., 2004; Warden & Warner, 2007). The depth and location of the burn are key factors in determining the type and goals of immediate and aggressive therapeutic intervention. The preservation of function and mobility are the short-term goals of rehabilitation. Long-term goals involve returning the patient to independence through the ability to perform Activities of Daily Living, compensation for functional loss, management of scars and pain, and reintegration into the home and community (Serghiou et al., 2007).

It is important to remember that discharge from the hospital does not mean that the patient is restored to good health. A burn patient's wounds have been covered, but they may have to return to the hospital for additional surgeries and will likely have orders for outpatient physical therapy and/or occupational therapy, burn clinic visits, pain management, psychological care, as well as the need for pressure garment fittings. Ongoing wound care, as mentioned previously, is also a facet of the rehabilitative phase of burn recovery.

Rehabilitation should begin immediately so that the scars do not mature and cause more severe contractions and limitations, which can increase complications, diminish function, and result in additional treatment and a greater cost of care. Burn scar maturation can vary from 6 to 18 months and longer. During this period, it is important to mobilize the burn area to decrease the likelihood of contractures, deformities, and hypertrophic scarring. Once scar maturation has occurred, correction of most deformities and cosmetic abnormalities involves costly surgical procedures with physical/occupational therapy, home health care, and burn clinic or doctor office follow-up in order for functional gains to be maintained (Cromes & Helm, 1993).

Massage Therapy

Scar massage has been found to be beneficial to burn patients and provides several important functions, including the promotion of collagen, the remodeling of scars, decreased itching, decreased anger, and decreased anxiety while providing moisture and pliability to the burned areas and donor sites (Field et al., 1998; Cho et al., 2014). It can also be a positive source of therapeutic touch. It should be considered after scar revision surgery and for ongoing pain, chronic itching, and scar management.

Persistent, post-burn itching is estimated to affect about 87% of all patients and can persist for many years after the initial burn injury (Gabriel, 2009; see http://www.utsouthwestern.org/rehabilitation).

Outpatient Services

Over 75% of the 40,000 patients who are hospitalized annually for their burn injuries are admitted to the 125 hospitals that have burn centers or units (National Hospital Discharge Survey, 2003). Many of these specialized care centers are regional in nature. Therefore, patients must sometimes relocate, temporarily, to a burn center in order to receive ongoing and appropriate outpatient burn and rehabilitation care (Hartford and Kealy, 2007).

A comprehensive burn rehabilitation course may require as much as 6 hours of therapeutic intervention per day, 5 days per week. The frequency usually decreases gradually to three times per week and eventually to two times per week. The patient often requires attendant care from a family member or health care provider for dressing changes, exercise routines, and Activities of Daily Living. A severely burn-injured individual may have need of assistance for weeks or even months. If parents, spouses, or other family members are providing attendant care or transportation, an estimate of compensation for their time and effort should be considered for inclusion in the life care plan.

Physician follow-up visits are needed approximately every one to two weeks in the initial outpatient stage, with frequency decreasing to once or twice per month, as long as the patient is on physical therapy or occupational therapy treatment, and for the first few weeks after treatment is stopped. Treatment typically lasts for anywhere from 12 to 16 weeks. To make sure the patient is maintaining function after therapy has stopped, typical physician follow-up should continue but gradually decrease to once every 3 months for 12 to 18 months, then biannually for another 12 to 18 months, then annual visits, unless unforeseen complications arise. However, the number of weeks or months and the actual physician follow-up plan is always specific to the patient; therefore, a physician should make the actual recommendation.

Pediatric Life Care Plans

Life care plans for severely burn-injured children can be very complicated. Pediatric patients often need multiple reconstructive surgeries as they grow. Children may have cognitive problems due to trauma and/or inhalation injury, and there will be great demand placed on their parents and family in order to support them in their need for ongoing care. Educational needs also should be considered. Summer burn camp is a rehabilitation program that can bring great benefits to a burn-surviving child and should be considered for inclusion in the life care of a pediatric burn-survivor. The World Burn Congress, an annual rehabilitative event sponsored by the Phoenix Society, can also be beneficial for children and their families and can be extremely helpful for adult burn survivors and their families as well.

Psychological Issues

Psychological adjustment to a severe burn injury can often be profound (Smith et al., 2006). A significant number of burn-injured patients will suffer from post-traumatic stress disorder and experience intrusive memories related to the event during the acute care phase (Ehde et al., 1999). Depression and anxiety on the part of the patient and/or the family may also occur. Psychological intervention may have begun in the burn center during the acute care stage of hospitalization, if it was available. However, not all burn centers or units have psychological services available as a regular part of their care protocol.

The medical chart should be reviewed to ascertain what psychological problems may have arisen during inpatient care and what psychiatric or psychological services, if any, were delivered. Supportive services and crisis management care are often offered to patient's families in the burn center; however, as basic survival becomes the major goal during the initial phase of hospitalization, psychological matters may not have been addressed, or may have been addressed inadequately.

Acute stress disorder may be diagnosed during acute hospitalization. Post-traumatic stress disorder, a complication which longitudinal studies have found to affect up to 45% of adults who were hospitalized for their burn injury one year post-burn and nearly a third of burn patients within 2 years of their burn, cannot be diagnosed until at least 30 days after the initial traumatic event (Perry et al., 1992; Weichman et al., 2001). Therefore, it is important to address psychological issues of both the patient and the family, not only during the inpatient stay, but after discharge from the burn center or burn unit as well.

Many burn-injured patients persist with periods of fear and anxiety (Rimmer et al., 2014). These symptoms often recur when the patient has to return to the hospital for reconstructive surgeries. Adults may express their anxiety through physical symptoms such as palpitations, perspiration, nausea, and shaking. Children may become clingy or fearful, cry often, have headaches and stomachaches, or become disruptive and angry. The psychological impact of a burn injury has become a major focus of burn care. "Health care professionals are increasingly recognizing that they cannot neglect the psychological and social dimensions both for patients and their families. Research has shown that patients and clients who receive psychosocial support as part of their rehabilitation are more likely to adjust positively to living with a disfigurement" (Partridge, 2008).

A psychosocial survey should be performed for the patient. As mentioned earlier, the patient and the patient's family may have been unable to address psychological and social issues such as post-traumatic stress disorder, financial pressures, or depression before discharge from acute care. They may be experiencing new problems at home such as sleep disturbance, anxiety, sexual concerns, body image problems, itching, identity issues, inability to return to work or school, and unresolved pain issues. If the patient or the family expresses concerns regarding any or all of these matters, there should be an evaluation by a psychologist or psychiatrist. A neuropsychology evaluation, used to examine brain function and possible impairments, is often recommended for severely burned pediatric patients and may be ideal for any burn patient who has experienced an inhalation injury or trauma to the head concomitant with the burn injury.

Life care planners should make inquiries regarding any currently prescribed psychotropic drugs and the length of need for such medications. If medication is needed on an ongoing basis through life expectancy, it is likely that the patient will need ongoing visits with a psychiatrist. Consideration should be made for immediate psychological intervention if problems are occurring, as well as for the need for ongoing psychological care during major life shifts and periods of reconstructive surgery. Play therapy for children, individual therapy for adolescents and adults, and couples and family counseling for spouses, parents, and siblings should be considered as well because a serious burn injury takes a toll on the entire family unit.

Vocational Rehabilitation

There is limited literature available on the details surrounding return to work following a serious burn injury. One study revealed that the majority of burn survivors do return to work within 2 years with an average of 17 weeks off the job (Brych et al., 2001). However, there are a number of reported factors that tend to impede return to work. The most common risk factors associated with longer durations of work absence following serious injury and found to increase the unlikelihood of returning to work include the patient's admission to intensive care units, a lengthy hospitalization, and a low education level. These are not unusual circumstances for individuals who have sustained severe burn injuries.

Other factors impeding return to work, which are related directly to burn injury, include total body surface area, length of hospitalization, thickness of burns, number of surgeries, age, presence of hand burns, reduced endurance, alcohol or drug dependence, and prior psychological or psychiatric problems. The longer the time lapse since the burn injury, the higher the likelihood of returning to work. Positive factors for likelihood of returning to work include pre-employment status, age, good coping skills, and higher level of education. However, having more full-thickness burn injuries was associated with a lower likelihood of returning to work (Dyster-Aas et al., 2007).

Several studies have shown that burn patients who are able to return to work report more satisfaction and a better overall quality of life than those who remain unemployed. Therefore, vocational rehabilitation issues should be taken into consideration during the early part of outpatient rehabilitation. Employers should be contacted on a regular basis to keep them updated on the status of the patient, in order to encourage a good relationship, and to diminish the patient's fears that former employment will be lost. A comprehensive job description can be utilized to determine therapy needs in order to assist the patient in maintaining job skills. Part-time employment or light duty should be discussed in order to diminish financial stress and to avoid establishing a pattern of dependency (Weed & Berens, 2005).

A majority of burn patients are able to return to work but they are often unable to return to the job they had prior to their burn injury (Brych et al., 2001). If job modifications or return to the same type of employment is unlikely, vocational evaluation and training should be considered as soon as the patient is healthy enough to begin. Research from the University of Washington revealed that only 37% of survivors, 2 years out from their injury, had gone back to the same job, and to the same employer without accommodation. Almost 50% had received disability, not gone back to work, or had some degree of employment interruption (Brych et al., 2001).

Those individuals who have been deemed permanently impaired may benefit from the assistance of a knowledgeable rehabilitation counselor (a board certified rehabilitation counselor/CRC is preferred) who has the necessary background to conduct an assessment of the person's physical, cognitive, and emotional functioning levels. A vocational evaluation by a qualified vocational evaluator may be justified. A psychological assessment and functional capacity evaluation should also be considered.

A burn patient's ability to return to work is highly individualized. The infirmity can range from no loss of function to living with an amputation and the need to adjust to a prosthesis. Life care planners are often confronted with electrical burns, which may have resulted in amputation, cognitive and emotional impairment, and vision problems. One study, which involved patients who had endured amputation from electrical burns and had been cared for at a burn center of excellence, reported a superior return-to-work rate than people with disabilities in general (Weed & Atkins, 2004). Productivity is a highly valued personal characteristic; therefore, helping clients with their return to work or assisting them in finding a new vocation or different form of recreation can be most helpful.

Complications

Complications after burn injury can be extensive and wide-reaching. They may affect any or many body systems (Warden & Warner, 2007). It is important to ask the treating physician what the potential complications are for a particular patient. Chart 14.1 includes common complications associated with burn injury. They have been divided by body systems with recommendations for intervention, and the likely frequency and duration of treatment, and surgical options. The list includes the most significant and usual burn injury-related complications. The most common treatment options are also included.

Chart 14.1 Complications Commonly Associated with Burn Injury

Complication	*Location*	*Clinical Presentation*	*Diagnosis*	*Nonsurgical Options*	*Surgical Options*	*Additional Comments*
Skin Complications						
Nonhealing wounds: acute	Can occur anywhere on burned, grafted, or donor site skin. Most often in poorly vascularized areas, areas under tension, or areas of contact or friction.	Open, painful, wounds, often with bleeding or exudate	Clinical exam	Debridement of devitalized tissue and local wound care with a plethora of wound care products; improved nutrition; treatment of infections (which may not be clinically obvious); hyperbaric oxygen therapy (unproven)	Primary wound closure; partial-thickness skin grafting; full-thickness skin grafting; soft tissue rotation or flaps	Wound care is an art, not a science: what works for one patient may not work for another. A key element is patience. Assume wound closure of about 1 cm per month of therapy.
Nonhealing wounds: chronic	As previous entry; often associated with infections such as MRSA or vascular insufficiency.	As in previous entry; nonhealing or lack of progression over weeks or months; breakdown of a previously healed wound	Clinical exam; wound culture; noninvasive vascular studies	As in previous entry; antibiotics; good nutrition is key	As in previous entry	As in previous entry
Skin blistering	May occur anywhere; most often seen in freshly healed wound or donor sites.	Superficial, pink, moist painful open wounds on a site that had been previously healed	Patient history; clinical exam	Local wound care with a variety of wound care products	Rarely requires split-thickness skin grafting	Usually heals with conservative care

(*Continued*)

Chart 14.1 (Continued) Complications Commonly Associated with Burn Injury

Complication	*Location*	*Clinical Presentation*	*Diagnosis*	*Nonsurgical Options*	*Surgical Options*	*Additional Comments*
Pigmentation changes	Can occur anywhere; most often seen in grafted skin especially on the face and head; may be seen in healed burns; rarely seen in healed donor sites.	Skin that is darker (more common) or lighter (less common) than normal	Clinical examination	Makeup: can be difficult to locate and expensive to use	Tattooing and other pigmentation procedures; most only partially correct the abnormality	Pigmentation changes evolve over 6 to 24 months; it is important to wait until the wounds are completely stable
Hypertrophic scars	Can occur anywhere; most often seen in grafted areas, but common in healed burns also; rarely seen in donor sites' deeper burns, burns that were open for a longer period of time, or burns that were infected tend to form worse hypertrophic scars. More common in persons with greater skin pigmentation.	Thick, red, or purple, hard, nonpliable, raised scars; often itchy and/or painful	Clinical exam	Custom-fitted compression garments reduce and improve almost all of the symptoms associated with hypertrophic scars; silicone sheeting under the compression garment often is synergistic; custom plastic masks may be effective for face scars; garments must be worn 23½ hours per day to be truly effective; a variety of topical medications may improve symptoms: aloe, diphenhydramine lotion, aspirin cream, calcium channel blocker cream, ketamine lotion, and many others; some systemic medications may help: antihistamines, nonsteroidal anti-inflammatory drugs, and others; other therapy such as massage, ultrasound, etc., may be useful in selected cases	Scar excisions with primary closure; sequential excision and closure of a scar; excision and grafting; excision and soft tissue coverage following skin expansion	Wait for scars to mature to a stable point, usually 6 to 24 months after closure. This is the hardest part of burn care: waiting for the scars to mature. The most important factor in scar formation is genetics: some people are born to be good healers, and others are born to be scar formers.

(Continued)

Chart 14.1 (Continued) Complications Commonly Associated with Burn Injury

Complication	*Location*	*Clinical Presentation*	*Diagnosis*	*Nonsurgical Options*	*Surgical Options*	*Additional Comments*
Keloids	As in previous entry	As in previous entry; tend to form in persons with high levels of skin pigmentation	Clinical examination	As in previous entry; steroid injection and/or radiation therapy may be useful	As in previous entry	Often recur following excision, regardless of treatment.
Painful scars	Can occur anywhere. More common on extremities than on torso or head.	Painful scars, most sensitive to touch, heat, or cold; often make sleep difficult; can be unpredictable in extent and manifestation of pain; typically burning, may be sharp	Clinical examination of scar: palpation, and range of motion	As previously, for hypertrophic scars; desensitization and neuropathic pain medications may be useful (neurontin, amitriptyline)	Scar excision may be helpful, but usually only temporarily, if at all, effective; surgery should be avoided if at all possible	This complication is very difficult to manage. Complete resolution is unusual; most patients have residual pain for many years.
Wound contracture	Can occur anywhere that has been burned; usually seen with deep burns that have healed or been grafted. Most common: neck, axilla, hands, elbow, knees.	Skin tightness, especially with extension, decreased range of motion, and decreased functionality	Clinical examination, and range of motion measurements	Aggressive physical or occupational therapy to prevent and treat; splinting in position of function; serious contractures may require serial splinting in progressive extension or flexion; massage, ultrasound may be useful adjuncts	Generally depend upon therapy to prevent and treat; persistent contractures that interfere with function can be released surgically, with local soft tissue transfer or skin grafting	Wait until scar is mature and physical therapy and occupational therapy have been maximized before considering surgery. Therapy is very important after surgical release.

(*Continued*)

Chart 14.1 (Continued) Complications Commonly Associated with Burn Injury

Complication	*Location*	*Clinical Presentation*	*Diagnosis*	*Nonsurgical Options*	*Surgical Options*	*Additional Comments*
Microstomia (small mouth)	Mouth	Face, lip, and neck burns, typically; neck and chest burn wound contracture can pull down on the lip, also	Clinical exam, mouth opening measurements	Prevention with a microstomia appliance; as in previous entry for hypertrophic scars; aggressive occupational therapy	Can be released surgically; usually quite successful	Prevention is key. A microstomia appliance must be worn at all times to effectively prevent or treat.
Ectropion (contraction of scar tissue of the eyelid or eversion of the eyelid caused by contraction of facial skin)	Occurs with deep facial burns or burns to the eye area; usually becomes obvious during acute hospitalization.	Inability to close the eyes, thereby causing corneal damage due to drying	Clinical exam, ophthalmology consult	Therapy, including scar massage and stretching	Daily therapy until problem resolves	Surgical intervention for release and skin grafting is usually indicated.

(*Continued*)

Chart 14.1 (Continued) Complications Commonly Associated with Burn Injury

Complication	*Location*	*Clinical Presentation*	*Diagnosis*	*Nonsurgical Options*	*Surgical Options*	*Additional Comments*
Skin infection	Can occur anywhere. May result from infection of ingrown hairs, ingrown glandular secretions, clogged pores, poor vascularization. Often caused by streptococcus or staphylococcus (including MRSA).	Skin redness, pain, erythema, swelling; may see pustules (especially with MRSA) or frank pus; may be subclinical	Skin examination and wound culture	Local wound care, pus drainage, debridement of devitalized tissue, removal of foreign body (staple or suture)	May require aggressive debridement, drainage, excision in the operating room	Don't forget to look for infections that are not obvious in wounds that are not healing.
Fingernail loss	Occurs with deep hand burns.	May see fingernail loss without regrowth, deformed nails, jagged nails	Clinical exam	Meticulous nail trimming and cleansing; massage	Can use toenails for reconstructive and cosmetic procedures	Often overlooked in a patient with other major burns.
Hair follicle loss	Usually full-thickness burn to scalp with follicle destruction.	Permanent hair loss and poor cosmesis	Clinical exam	Creative hair dressing, wigs, hairpieces, hats, glasses; no effective medications	Reconstruction with tissue expansion in nearby hair-bearing area with subsequent wound excision and soft tissue transfer	Scalp hair loss is recalcitrant; often requires multiple procedures. Eyebrows can be reconstructed with hair transfers or tattooing.

(Continued)

Chart 14.1 (Continued) Complications Commonly Associated with Burn Injury

Complication	*Location*	*Clinical Presentation*	*Diagnosis*	*Nonsurgical Options*	*Surgical Options*	*Additional Comments*
Ingrown hairs	Occurs on hair-bearing areas of the body that have been burned and grafted.	Pain, itching, irritation, infection	Clinical examination	Local wound care, drainage of pus, topical antibiotics; may require systemic antibiotics	Surgical excision of the offending hair; may require reconstruction or skin grafting	Tends to occur on face and upper extremities in men.
Loss of sebaceous and/or sweat glands	Almost always associated with deep burns that have been grafted; may occur in deep healed burns.	Dry, scaly, itching skin; skin may be cracked or fissured	Clinical examination	Local wound care with lubrication creams/lotions/ointments	No effective surgery	Requires life-long treatment, typically.
Loss of or decreased skin innervation	Almost always associated with deep burns that have been grafted; may occur in deep healed burns.	Loss of sensation to fine touch, temperature, vibration	Sensory testing	Reassurance of patient; wait for function to return; compression garments, silicone, massage may all help; avoid irritation, trauma; padded clothing	No effective surgery	Requires life-long treatment, typically.
Marjolin's ulcer (squamous cell carcinoma)	Typically develops in a healed or grafted burn that is chronically open; typically occurs 10–30 years after injury.	Nonhealing wound with associated mass or growth	Wound biopsy	Nothing	Radical excision; possible adjuvant therapy	Relatively rare; occurs in far less than 1% of patients.

(*Continued*)

Chart 14.1 (Continued) Complications Commonly Associated with Burn Injury

Complication	*Location*	*Clinical Presentation*	*Diagnosis*	*Nonsurgical Options*	*Surgical Options*	*Additional Comments*
Eye and Ear Complications						
Eyelid contracture	Burned upper or lower lids.	Inability to close eyes; dry eyes; frequent tearing	Ophthalmologic examination	Tarsorrhaphy sutures	Reconstruction with full-thickness skin grafts	Prevention is key.
Ectropion (eversion of the eyelid caused by contraction of facial skin)	Usually occurs on upper or lower lid after serious facial burn.	Pain, irritation, tearing, bleeding, inability to close eye	Clinical examination	Massage and passive stretching may help	Excision and grafting is usually required	Usually occurs acutely during initial hospitalization; difficult to prevent.
Cataract	Occurs following electrical injury.	Deteriorating visual acuity	Ophthalmologic examination	Usually none	Often requires operative intervention	Screening eye examination should be done on all patients with electrical injury.
Loss of ear cartilage	Full-thickness burn to ear.	Loss of normal anatomic appearance and contour of ear	Clinical examination	Massage and passive stretching may help minimally	Usually requires bone graft and skin grafting; occasionally requires soft tissue transfer	Cosmetic deformity primarily; hearing usually not affected.

(*Continued*)

Chart 14.1 (Continued) Complications Commonly Associated with Burn Injury

Complication	*Location*	*Clinical Presentation*	*Diagnosis*	*Nonsurgical Options*	*Surgical Options*	*Additional Comments*
Lung and Heart Complications						
Tracheal stenosis	Tracheal narrowing as a result of prolonged intubation.	Difficulty breathing; poor exercise tolerance; stridor	Clinical examination; bronchoscopy, laryngoscopy computerized tomography	Dilation	Usually requires surgical correction	Usually present at time of discharge from initial hospitalization.
Pulmonary insufficiency	Results from inhalation injury (toxic effect of breathing products of combustion); may be exacerbated by pulmonary infections while hospitalized.	Poor exercise tolerance; easy fatiguability; frequent pulmonary infections; cough	Clinical examination; pulmonary function testing; bronchoscopy	Exercise; bronchodilators	None	May not manifest until years after initial injury; usually present to some degree at time of discharge from initial hospitalization.
Cardiac dysrhythmias, cardiac dysfunction, coronary artery disease	Occurs following electrical injury.	Chest pain, shortness of breath, poor exercise tolerance	Clinical examination, ECG, echocardiogram; Holter monitor	Exercise, diet, medications	Usually none; may rarely require coronary artery bypass grafting	Very rare complication seen only after electrical injury.

(*Continued*)

Chart 14.1 (Continued) Complications Commonly Associated with Burn Injury

Complication	*Location*	*Clinical Presentation*	*Diagnosis*	*Nonsurgical Options*	*Surgical Options*	*Additional Comments*
Neurologic Complications						
Neuroma	Nerve or nerve ending that becomes hypersensitive following a burn; usually the result of the nerve or nerve ending getting caught up in the inflammatory process.	Specific hypersensitive or painful and/or tender area usually on an extremity; may be hypersensitive to hot or cold or both	Clinical examination	Compression garments, silicone, topical analgesics, massage, ultrasound	May require surgical excision	Tends not to respond completely regardless of treatment modality.
Reflexive Sympathetic Dystrophy (RSD)	Idiosyncratic pain syndrome that is poorly defined; usually occurs following serious burn; more common in extremities, especially lower extremity.	Hypersensitive, painful, stiff, inflammatory skin; intolerance of cold or heat or both; may see redness and swelling; exam may be completely normal	Clinical examination	Compression garments, aggressive occupational or physical therapy; ganglion block may be helpful; a variety of medications have been used	Usually none	Difficult to diagnose—typically a diagnosis of exclusion; very difficult to treat successfully.

(*Continued*)

Chart 14.1 (Continued) Complications Commonly Associated with Burn Injury

Complication	*Location*	*Clinical Presentation*	*Diagnosis*	*Nonsurgical Options*	*Surgical Options*	*Additional Comments*
Musculoskeletal Complications						
Heterotrophic ossification	Usually seen in large joints of burned extremities; elbow is the most commonly involved joint.	Decreased range of motion; usually diagnosed by occupational therapists	Clinical examination; X-ray; bone scan	Passive and active range of motion to prevent and treat; dynamic and passive splints or casting; continuous passive range-of-motion devices	Excision and removal of heterotopic bone; postoperative therapy is very important	Difficult to treat conservatively in severe cases; usually requires surgery.
Joint subluxation	Typically seen in the small joint in hands, fingers, feet, and toes on burned extremities.	Obvious deformity; decreased function and decreased range of motion	Clinical examination and X-rays	Prevention with range of motion and strengthening, splinting	Surgical release and reconstruction	Wait until scar is mature to surgically correct.
Boutonniere deformity of finger	Dorsal aspect of burn hands involving extensor tendon.	Obvious deformity; decreased function and decreased range of motion	Clinical examination and X-rays	Prevention with range of motion and strengthening, splinting	Surgical release and reconstruction	
Swan neck deformity of finger	Contracture of hand muscles and tendons.	Obvious deformity; decreased function and decreased range of motion	Clinical examination and X-rays	Prevention with range of motion and strengthening, splinting	Surgical release and reconstruction	

(Continued)

Chart 14.1 (Continued) Complications Commonly Associated with Burn Injury

Complication	*Location*	*Clinical Presentation*	*Diagnosis*	*Nonsurgical Options*	*Surgical Options*	*Additional Comments*
Mallet finger deformity	Deep burns to the dorsum or back of hand: involves extensor tendons.	Obvious deformity; decreased function and decreased range of motion; inability to extend the distal interphalangeal joint of finger	Clinical examination and X-rays	Prevention with range of motion and strengthening, splinting	Surgical release and reconstruction with tendon repair	
Exposed tendons	Deep burns, usually of hands or feet.	Obviously exposed tendons with decreased function	Clinical examination	Local wound care; protection of tendon from desiccation	Soft tissue transfer and reconstruction	Usually requires surgery; may use skin substitutes.
Shortened extremity	Burn scars on extremities prevent normal bone growth.	Obviously shortened extremity with decreased function	Clinical examination	Aggressive physical and occupational therapy	May require reconstruction for severe limitation of function	Usually requires wound contracture release simultaneously.
Limb amputation	Full-thickness burns of extremities; often with compartment syndrome and/or vascular insufficiency.	Obvious loss of extremity	None	Preoperative planning, if possible; immediate postoperative prosthesis if possible; maintenance of joint above amputation in neutral position; stump care; strengthening and balance training	Stump may require revision for chronic wound and/or poor soft tissue padding	Involvement of patient and family in care vital to success.

Burn Injury: Damage Assessment Checklist

Serious burn injuries are considered catastrophic injuries. There is usually significant cost associated with the recovery and rehabilitation of the burn patient, which can necessitate lifelong care. Pediatric burn patients often require extensive reconstruction and rehabilitation, especially during but not limited to their growth and developmental years. A burn injury impacts the entire family system, so it is important to consider the family's needs as well.

Patients may need a variety of physicians to care for them including but not limited to plastic reconstructive surgeons, physiatrists, orthopedic surgeons, pediatric intensivists, cardiologists, internists, pulmonologists, and psychiatrists for lifelong care.

Allied health care, including psychological, physical, occupational, and vocational therapies, as well as the need for case management are important items to consider. In-home assistance, respite care, home maintenance and cleaning services, and assisted living in advanced years are also often a necessity.

Patients often have an ongoing need for pain medications, moisturizers, pressure garments, prosthetics and orthotics, splints, special makeup, and other supplies. Transportation and mobility assistance, as well as exercise for optimum function should also be considered.

The following checklist can be utilized when meeting with care providers and considering future care needs.

Burn Life Care Plan Checklist

Annual Evaluations ______________

Physicians/Surgeons ______________

____

____

____

Primary Care ______________

Surgeries Related to Growth or Aging:

Contracture Releases ______________

Dermabrasion ______________

Hand Surgeries ______________

Hypertrophic Scarring ______________

Heterotrophic Ossification ______________

Tissue Expansion ______________

Scar Excision ______________

Emergency Room Visits ______________

Physical Discomfort:

Pain Control ______________

Itching ______________

- Skin Breakdown ______________
- Range-of-Motion Issues ______________
- Sleep Problems ______________

Aesthetic Issues:

- Eyebrows ______________
- Nipples ______________
- Fingernails ______________
- Eyelashes ______________
- Special Makeup ______________
- Breast Implants ______________
- Special Bra ______________
- Breast Prosthesis ______________

Pressure Garments:

- Face Mask ______________
- Arms ______________
- Trunk ______________
- Back ______________
- Legs ______________
- Hands/Gloves ______________
- Zippers ______________
- Silicone Sheeting ______________

Splinting ______________

Occupational Therapy Needs ______________

Physical Therapy Needs ______________

Speech Therapy Needs ______________

Massage Therapy ______________

- Lotions ______________

Dressing Change Materials ______________

Sun Protection Needs:

- Sunscreen ______________
- Special UV-Protective Clothing ______________

Nutritional Needs ________________

Case Management ________________

Psychological Interventions:

- Psychiatry ________________
- Play Therapy ________________
- Neuropsychological Testing ________________
- Family Therapy ________________
- Individual Psychotherapy ________________
- Support Group ________________
- Burn Camp ________________
- World Burn Congress ________________
- Hypnosis ________________

Educational Needs:

- Private School ________________
- Tutoring ________________
- IEP Assistance ________________

Vocational Needs:

- Job Training ________________
- Vocational Counseling ________________
- Work Hardening ________________
- Workplace Reintegration ________________

Recreational Issues:

- Recreation Therapy ________________

Home Care:

- Home Health ________________
- Respite Care for Parents/Spouse ________________
- Aids to Daily Living ________________
- Assisted Living Needs ________________
- Housekeeping ________________
- Handyman ________________

Mobility:

Wheelchair ______________

Scooter ______________

Walker ______________

Prosthetics ______________

Pulmonary Issues:

Pulmonologist ______________

Breathing Treatments ______________

Humidifier ______________

Dressing Change Materials ______________

Pain Medications ______________

Other Medications ______________

Conservatorship ______________

Sample Life Care Plan for John Doe

Narrative Summary

Introduction

Mr. Attorney has requested that a life care plan be provided for John Doe as it pertains to the severe 62% third degree, total body surface area burn injuries that he sustained in a home explosion on XX/XX/2014. This life care plan will assist in determining John's long-term needs, as they relate to his significant burn injuries. This document will outline a plan of care with the projected burn injury-related costs that John Doe is likely to incur over his lifetime. The goal is to develop a personalized life care plan that will help to maintain John's medical stability, sustain or increase his functional status and quality of life, and assist in the prevention of further injury-related complications.

This life care plan report will consist of two parts, a narrative section and a table segment. The narrative will include a summary of the available medical records, health care provider interviews, and details from two personal interviews with John Doe, his wife Jane, and this life care planner.

The second section of the life care plan will be presented in table form and will provide, in detail, the future injury-related projected care needs, costs, rationale, and recommenders of such care. This will include an itemized listing of likely future medical care expenses, with likely procedures/hospitalizations/surgeries, evaluations, therapies, diagnostic testing, medications, home care, transportation, and health and strength maintenance, and finally, it will outline potential complications. Costs will be broken down into annual and onetime expenses.

All prices quoted in this life care plan are present year and are calculated for a 12-month period. This plan will need to be reevaluated if the client becomes medically unstable, has a significant change in functional status and/or his condition changes due to the burn disease process.

DEMOGRAPHIC INFORMATION:
Client Name: John Doe Injury Date: XX/XX/2014
Address: City:
Phone: (757) XXX-XXXX Birth Date: 9/22/XXXX
Gender: Male Ethnicity: Caucasian
Education: High School Graduate
U. S. Citizen: Yes Marital Status—Married—15 years
Glasses: No Dominant Hand: Right
Current Employment:
Family: Wife—Jane, 1 son—Jack—age—9, 1 daughter—Susie– age—7

Foundation for Report
In-Patient Medical Records................Burn Center Medical Center, Anytown, USA
In-Patient Medical Records.........Physical Rehabilitation Center
Outpatient Records Rehabilitation.......................—Anytown, USA
Consultation—Dr. Surgeon, Burn Surgeon/Plastic Surgeon
Consultation—Dr. Surgeon, Burn/Plastic Surgeon
Email Consultation—2/24/2014- Dr. Surgeon
Phone Consultation—Dr.—Treating Psychiatrist—14/06/2013
Hanger Prosthetics—14/15/2013
Burn Center Medical Center Billing
Personal Interview with This Life Care Planner—John and Jane Doe

Medical Records and Reports Reviewed:
Burn Center Health System..........Medical Records
Best Rehabilitation Hospital..........................Billing Records
Ms. Surgeon, MD, Plastic/Burn Surgeon................Billing Records
Physical and Occupational Therapy ....Medical Records
Physical and Occupational Therapy..............Billing Records

Summary: John Doe, a 32-year-old, Caucasian male, who sustained severe burns to 62% of his body at the age of 26. Specifically, he sustained deep burns to his neck, scalp, ears, both his upper and lower extremities, flanks, as well as his bilateral hands, ankles, and feet.

Burn Injury

John Doe suffered multiple third degree burns to 62% of his body. Many unburned areas of his body were harvested as donor sites for the multiple skin graft surgeries that he underwent. Normal skin was harvested to provide cover for the extensive third- and deep second-degree burns to his arms, scalp, forehead, buttocks, and legs. Therefore, damage to his skin far exceeds the 62% that was originally burned. A third-degree burn results in serious disruption of normal skin and creates the subsequent need for skin grafting. The harvesting of a skin graft from the individual's unburned skin often results in additional significant scarring as the body tries to diminish and "fix" the burn wounds. The hypertrophic scarring that now covers much of John's body impedes his function and physical activity level. It has also diminished his body's ability to regulate its temperature.

Injury Event

John Doe reports that he was burned at home on XX/XX/2014 when an explosion severely injured him. John Doe was rushed to Burn Center Medical Center in Anytown, State, by helicopter. He arrived lying on his abdomen. This was because of the severe back pain he was experiencing due to deep and extensive burns. He also complained of pain to his bilateral hands and his lower extremities.

Burn Center, Anytown, USA
Problems documented during John's burn care hospitalization:
Primary Diagnosis: Full-thickness skin loss due to third-degree burns
Secondary Diagnosis:

1. 62% of body burned; 62% third degree
2. Acute kidney failure
3. Methicilin susceptible pneumonia due to staphylococcus aureus
4. Nutritional marasmus (severe malnutrition)
5. Hyperosmolality and/or hypernatremia—electrolyte problem—a rise in serum sodium
6. Full-thickness skin loss due to burn (third degree), multiple sites
7. Hypotension (low blood pressure)
8. Neutropenia (abnormally low white blood cell count)
9. Acute respiratory failure
10. Bacteremia (viable bacteria in the blood stream)
11. Acute post-hemorrhagic anemia (anemia from bleeding)
12. Ventilator associated pneumonia
13. Full-thickness skin loss due to burn (third degree, not otherwise specified), abdomen
14. Full-thickness skin loss due to burn (third degree), hands
15. Thrombocytopenia (abnormally low amount of platelets)
16. Abnormal glucose (blood sugar level)
17. Constipation
18. Bacterial infection due to gram-negative bacteria
19. Leukocytosis (high white blood cell count)
20. Burns multiple sites (except with eye) of face/head/neck
21. Essential hypertension (high blood pressure with no identifiable cause)

Surgical and Invasive Procedure Details—John Doe was taken to the operating room **24 times** for the following procedures:

BURN CENTER—Surgical and Invasive Procedures
XX/19/2014– Burn Center Burn Center
Discharge Diagnosis

- 62% total body surface area burns
- Acute blood loss with anemia that resolved

Consults during Burn Admission

- Plastic surgery
- Physical therapy
- Occupational therapy
- Nutrition
- Psychology

Burn Center—Surgical and Invasive Procedures

Procedure	*Provider*	*Date*
Excisional debridement of wound/infection/burn	Surgeon, MD	XX/XX/14
Temporary tracheostomy	Surgeon, MD	XX/XX/14
Continuous invasive mechanical ventilation for 84 consecutive days	Surgeon, MD	XX/07/14
Homograft to skin	Surgeon, MD	XX/19/14
Excisional debridement of wound/infection/burn	Surgeon, MD	XX/12/14
Excisional debridement of wound/infection/burn	Surgeon, MD	XX/15/14
Excisional debridement of wound/infection/burn	Surgeon, MD	XX/16/14
Skin graft	Surgeon, MD	XX/19/14
Skin graft	Surgeon, MD	XX/19/14
Skin graft	Surgeon, MD	XX/22/14
Homograft to skin	Surgeon, MD	XX/22/14
Excisional debridement of wound/infection/burn	Surgeon, MD	XX/26/14
Homograft to skin	Surgeon, MD	XX/26/14
Skin graft	Surgeon, MD	05/03/14
Homograft to skin	Surgeon, MD	05/03/14
Skin graft	Surgeon, MD	05/13/14
Homograft to skin	Surgeon, MD	05/13/14
Excisional debridement of wound/infection/burn	Surgeon, MD	05/31/14
Venous catheterization	Surgeon, MD	XX/03/14
Arterial catheterization	Surgeon, MD	XX/03/14
Bronchoscopy	Surgeon, MD	XX/07/14
Incision of skin and subcutaneous tissue	Surgeon, MD	XX/03/14
Non-excisional debridement of wound/infection/burn	Surgeon, MD	XX/19/14
Enteral infusion of concentrated nutritional substances	Surgeon, MD	XX/03/14
Transfusion of packed blood cells	Surgeon, MD	XX/13/14
Non-excisional debridement of wound/infection/burn	Surgeon, MD	XX/22/14
Non-excisional debridement of wound/infection/burn	Surgeon, MD	XX/26/14

(*Continued*)

Non-excisional debridement of wound/infection/burn	Surgeon, MD	XX/29/14
Non-excisional debridement of wound/infection/burn	Surgeon, MD	05/03/14
Non-excisional debridement of wound/infection/burn	Surgeon, MD	05/06/14
Non-excisional debridement of wound/infection/burn	Surgeon, MD	05/13/14
Hydrotherapy	Surgeon, MD	05/29/14
Non-excisional debridement of wound/infection/burn	Surgeon, MD	05/29/14
Non-excisional debridement of wound/infection/burn	Surgeon, MD	05/31/14

Upon discharge from the Burn Center, John Doe was transferred and admitted to Best Rehabilitation Hospital on XX/19/2014 for complex rehabilitation. He remained there for daily comprehensive inpatient rehabilitation until XX/10/2014.

John Doe returned to his home in Springfield, State after being discharged from Best Rehabilitation Hospital. John Doe shared that he continued to receive physical/occupational therapy two to three times per week for more than a year after his discharge from rehab. He needed extensive therapy in order to regain many functions including retaining the ability to put his shoes and socks on his feet.

Personal Interviews with John Doe and Jane Doe

August 09, 2015 in Springfield, State & January XX/XX/2016 in Springfield, State.

The purpose of this interview was to ascertain to what extent John's multiple injuries are interfering with his ability to manage his Activities of Daily Living.

Current Status and Disabling Problems: John Doe continues to suffer from physical and emotional problems related to his severe burn injuries. He remains highly anxious, has ongoing pain and itching, frequent headaches, sensitivity to hot and cold weather, dry skin, swelling of his hands and feet, fatigue, and decreased endurance and sleep disruption. He reports experiencing ongoing body image issues. He reported that he no longer recognizes his own body.

John Doe also reported severe sleep problems and intermittent nightmares. He has been unable to return to his former job due to physical restraints. He acknowledged that he continues to feel depressed and anxious much of the time. John Doe shared that his relationship with his wife, Jane, has been strained due to his discomfort with having to lean on her so much, and so often. He said she has been a constant support for him, but his role as husband, father, and head of the family has been compromised due to his lack of independence. His sex life has also been negatively affected since sustaining his injuries and disfigurement. John has been unable to continue with many of his other customary activities, especially sports, hunting, and fishing, due to his extensive arm and leg burns, and the resulting physical limitations he continues to experience. Again, this is especially problematic due to his scar contractures and resulting disabilities which have caused significant physical and emotional challenges for him.

Burn and trauma injuries are complex and place a great deal of stress on the body's major organs. The skin is the largest organ of the body and when it is severely damaged by third-degree burns, it causes physiologic and metabolic disruption of the entire body. Burns have been documented as the most injurious insult the human body can endure. The injuries John Doe sustained were unexpected, and therefore created a crisis situation for him. John, his wife Jane, his parents, and his children, have all experienced emotional and psychological distress because of his extensive burns.

Medical History: John Doe reported enjoying good health before his injuries.

Family History: John Doe was born and raised in State by his mother and father, John and Joy Doe. His parents are both living, and he reports that they are both healthy. He also has a brother, age 42, who is also healthy. John Doe has been married to his wife, Jane, for 15 years and has a 7-year-old son, Johnny, and a 4-year-old daughter, Jill.

Social History: He was happy and felt fulfilled with close family relationships and good friends prior to the explosion. He was active in sports, hunting, and fishing, and was happy with his marriage and his children. John Doe shared that he loved his former job and is distressed because his doctor says it is highly likely that he will be unable to return to it due to the physical demands of his prior job.

Educational History: John Doe graduated from Anytown High School. Upon graduation he went directly to work into the plumbing business with his father. His wife Jane has a degree in accounting and was working as a CPA at the time of the explosion. She left her job to be with him throughout his lengthy hospitalization.

Employment History: John Doe started his career with Anytown Plumbing after graduating from high school.

Hobbies: John Doe loved going hunting and fishing in the past. He has been unable to engage in these activities since sustaining his physically limiting burn injuries.

Current Social Activities: John Doe reports that his social life is quite different now. He is uncomfortable going out in public and can no longer do many of the things he enjoyed doing prior to XX/XX/2014. He can't be out in the sun for any extended period of time. This has greatly limited his activity. He reports being sensitive to both the heat and the cold and laments being unable to even spend the day at the beach with his family, one of his favorite former pastimes.

Appearance Issues: John, since sustaining his burns, reports that he feels self-conscious about his body and wears long sleeve shirts and pants at all times because of his extensive scarring. He did try wearing short sleeve shirts in the summer, due to the heat, but felt uncomfortable when people looked at his scars. He shared that it is easier to stay at home, rather than have he and his family subjected to people's comments and stares. His fatigue and pain also make it difficult for him to enjoy the activities he did in the past. John Doe always took good care of his body and tried to maintain a healthy physique. His physician, Dr. Surgeon, shared that his sound physical condition, prior to the burns, is probably the reason he survived. Physical fitness, prior to sustaining his burns was a top priority, and he said that he has not yet begun to adjust to the changes in his body; either his appearance and his diminished physical function. John Doe finds himself trying to hide his hands when he is outside of his home.

John Doe should continue to undergo psychological intervention to assist him in accepting the permanent, disfiguring changes to his arms, abdomen, neck, torso, hands, feet, and legs. He will benefit greatly from professional psychological/social interventions, in order to better cope with the unwanted stares and questions he gets from both acquaintances and strangers. The following recommended procedures will help to decrease his itching, increase his range of motion, soften his scars, and reduce his pain; however, John's body will never look like it did prior to the fire.

"Sample Surgical Interventions"
Burn Reconstructive Surgery Consult
The Surgeon MD,—Burn Surgeon
Burn Center Burn Center
XX/15/2016

Dr. Surgeon reports that John Doe will likely require multiple surgical interventions, in order to improve the range of motion and function of his body.

He will require inpatient and outpatient occupational and physical therapy, home health care, outpatient therapy, laser surgery, medication, psychological intervention, pressure garments, splinting, and personal assistance. Much of the scarring on his body cannot be improved upon, and much of the scarring from his skin grafts will likely be permanent in nature.

The following reconstructive surgeries have been recommended by Dr. Surgeon. The likely costs of these procedures can be found in the life care plan tables. Dr. Surgeon has also recommended allied health care related to the surgeries in the form of home health for dressing changes and occupational therapy post-operatively. He has also recommended the number of hospital days associated with future operations. John Doe will need to be fitted for pressure garments and splinting after many of the surgeries.

Face and Neck

John Doe burned his face, scalp, and neck and has sensitivity in the residual scarring especially on his neck and scalp. Laser surgery is recommended for these areas.

Upper Extremities and Shoulders

John Doe has significant scarring to both of his upper arms. His shoulders have unburned skin and this skin will be harvested during future surgeries to "fix" other severely scarred areas of his body. Dr. Surgeon will place tissue expanders under the unburned skin to correct the upper arm scarring. This will be done to improve function, diminish pain, and improve cosmesis. This intensive reconstruction will require a one-night inpatient surgical placement of a tissue expander in the shoulder area under general anesthesia. This type of surgery is challenging, as this is an uncomfortable location for expander placement, but necessary for effective correction. After the initial surgery, John Doe will return to the burn clinic, every week for between 7 and 10 weeks to have the expanders filled with saline solution. When the expanded skin is ready, John Doe will be taken to the operating room, again, as an inpatient. The expanders will be removed and the new tissue and flap will be advanced to the area where the old scarring was excised. He will be hospitalized for 4 to 7 days after the second procedure and will need daily home health for dressing changes for a month, with occupational therapy two times a week for 4 to 6 months. Each arm will be done separately. The entire process will take approximately 4 months.

Forearms, Elbows, and Wrists

He has a great deal of disfiguring and limiting scarring with hyper-pigmentation on both his forearms and wrists. Both forearms are heavily scarred and the scars are impeding full use and range of motion of his arms and hands. The scars are also painful and itchy. His surgeon will excise the scars, then apply skin grafts. Each arm will be operated on separately. This will be an inpatient procedure with a 4- to 7-day hospital stay. He will need a month of outpatient wound care and 6 months of occupational therapy post-surgery.

Web Space Releases

John Doe will need web space release surgery between all of the fingers on his bilateral hands. This will necessitate two separate surgeries (each hand will be done separately), under general anesthesia, for web spaces one, two, three, and four. These surgeries will be performed inpatient with a five-night hospital stay and a month of daily dressing changes at home, two visits to the plastic surgeon's office, and 6 to 12 months of outpatient occupational therapy. Dr. Surgeon said it is likely that the web space releases will need to be repeated every 10 to 12 years through life expectancy. He will need a hand splint and pressure glove after each surgery.

Legs—Thighs and Calves

The lower extremities present with extensive skin grafts, hyperpigmentation, and hypertrophic scarring. John Doe will likely need tangential excision of the hypertrophic scarring on the upper thighs with re-grafting. Both the front and back sides of each leg are heavily scarred. He will go to the operating room to have the scarring excised and have a skin substitute placed over the wound. He will then return to the operating room, three weeks later, for skin grafting to this area. Each thigh will be operated on separately. This lengthy process will include inpatient hospitalization, post-operative home health, post-operative therapy, pressure garments and splints.

Ankles and Feet

John Doe will also need ankle and foot contracture releases and skin grafting bilaterally to improve function and range of motion. Currently, John Doe is unable to bend his ankles far enough to put his feet in a pair of work boots. He has very little unscarred skin on his body; therefore Dr. Surgeon said that a dermal substitute will be used for this procedure. This process will require a 21-day hospital stay with use of a wound vac between surgeries. A second operation will then be performed to cover the skin substitute with an autograft (skin graft) and the two surgeries will require 21 days in the hospital with four weeks of outpatient wound care. Physical therapy would be required two times a week for up to 12 months. This process will likely need to be repeated on each ankle and foot every 10 to 15 years through his life expectancy to allow for range of motion and function.

The costs associated with all surgeries are listed in the life care plan tables. It should be noted that any surgical complications or infections could result in significantly higher medical costs for John Doe over his lifetime.

Laser Therapy

John Doe has a great deal of residual scarring from both his burns and donor sites. Dr. Surgeon has recommended laser therapy/surgery for John. Laser is a painful procedure; therefore, it is recommended that the laser procedures be performed under general anesthesia in an outpatient operating room. These surgeries will be performed on an outpatient basis. Recommendations are for John Doe to undergo six to eight sessions of laser therapy, after the recommended hand surgeries. See tables for pricing.

Skin Cancer

All burned areas and donor sites are at increased risk of skin cancer and must be protected by sunscreen daily.

Pressure Garments

John Doe will need to be fitted for pressure garments and gloves following his reconstruction surgeries. Although the garments can be uncomfortable, especially during the summer months, they help to flatten scars, increase blood supply, and decrease itching. They are typically worn for 10 to 12 months after each procedure. He should wear TED hose, through life expectancy, due to his history of deep vein thrombosis and the daily swelling of his lower legs.

Massage Therapy

John Doe will benefit from ongoing scar massage therapy. It is recommended that he have massage 44 to 48 times per year through life expectancy. Research has revealed that massage therapy can be an effective adjunct for improving function, reducing pain, diminishing itching, improving skin integrity, and helping burn patients to improve and maintain range of motion.

Ongoing Medical Needs
Burn Recovery Consult
Dr. Surgeon—1/27/2016
Burn/Plastic Surgeon
Burn Center Burn Center

The following are the ongoing medical evaluations and allied health services that John Doe will likely need according to Dr. Surgeon, his treating physician.

Burn Surgeon/Plastic Surgeon: John Doe should have an annual evaluation with a burn surgeon in order to monitor his burns, scars, and any potential complications which may arise through life expectancy.

Dermatologist: An annual visit should occur due to his heightened risk for skin cancer, through life expectancy.

Occupational Therapist: He should have an evaluation, once a year, through life expectancy. It is recommended 12 visits every 2 years to assist John Doe with management of Activities of Daily Living (ADLs), function and range of motion with hands, wrists, and arms.

Audiologist: He should have his hearing evaluated post-explosion.

Dietary Evaluation: John Doe has gained a significant amount of weight since sustaining his burn injuries. His doctor said that he has to lose weight before surgery and will need to maintain his weight during the years of his major reconstruction. A weight loss program is recommended.

Physiatrist: He should have an evaluation and two to three visits annually with a physiatrist for pain management and functional issues through life expectancy.

Physical Therapist: He should have an evaluation once a year through life expectancy, as well as 12 visits per year from age 55 through life expectancy. He will need therapy to improve range of motion, balance, and function. He will be having ongoing physical therapy after recommended surgeries.

Pain Specialist: John Doe continues to see a pain specialist and should be evaluated annually for pain issues. He should have access to three additional visits, per year, for pain management through life expectancy.

Sleep Study: John Doe continues to have major problems with sleeping. Dr. X recommended a sleep study, but it has not be approved as of yet. Due to the long term sleep issues of many burn patients, it is recommended that John Doe have access to a sleep study every 5 years through life expectancy.

Potential Complications: The aging process is accelerated in those with disabilities and causes them to age more quickly than the normal population. Skin breakdown, osteoporosis, arthritis, restricted range of motion, anxiety and depression, and the potential for vascular and immune problems can negatively affect burn patients as they age. John Doe is already experiencing compromised usage of his arms, wrists, and has ongoing problems with his legs and knees. John Doe will be forever saddled with many of these problems and will likely need much assistance with daily living activities in his advanced age. In summary, the life care planner should consider potential complications of arthritis, skin breakdown, major depression, systemic infection, surgical complications, osteoporosis, ongoing sexual dysfunction, chronic pain, range of motion, function issues, and dementia.

Psycho/Social Issues

Individuals, such as John, who always enjoyed a normal physical appearance with good physical function who suddenly find themselves disfigured with physical limitations after a severe burn injury, are often extremely distressed. In reality, after such a disfiguring and physically limiting injury the individual must recreate themselves. They have to discover new ways of navigating the world from both a physical and emotional standpoint. Accomplishing tasks and social interactions that were once "easy" become uncomfortable and challenging. The individual must create a new identity and find different ways to complete physical tasks; both are arduous and complicated undertakings. Suffering a serious burn and trauma injury creates a need for lifelong medical intervention and creates an ongoing significant disruption of one's vocational and leisure lifestyle.

Psychiatric Care—Psychiatric Evaluations

Psychiatry

John Doe relayed experiencing many symptoms common for persons suffering from post-traumatic stress disorder. This is a psychological anxiety disorder that is triggered by a traumatic event, such as the explosion and fire he experienced, in addition to the ongoing trauma of John's burns and the loss of the vocation he loved. A psychiatric evaluation, every year until 2024, and then every 1 to 2 years through life expectancy, is recommended in order to monitor his well-being and address any medications he may need. He will also need to see a family physician XX times per year through life expectancy to monitor the psychotropic drugs prescribed for his post-traumatic stress disorder symptoms.

John Doe is currently seeing Dr. X. At this time, he is seeing the doctor every 2 months. Once he has become stabilized, he should have four visits per year, over the following 5 years with Dr. X. After that, it is likely that John Doe can be followed by a primary care physician for monitoring of his psychotropic medications. However, he should still be assessed by a psychiatrist every 2 years through life expectancy, to ensure that he is receiving proper care and medication.

Individual Psychotherapy

Psychological and social adjustment is key to helping move individuals from the status of burn victim to burn survivor. Therefore, it is recommended that John Doe continue to attend psychotherapy. Therapy can help him to improve his coping skills, address his grief, and help him deal with the struggle of adjusting to his physical and emotional challenges. He will benefit from 24 visits per year over the next 4 years due to his diagnosis of post-traumatic stress disorder (PTSD) and depression. It is then recommended that he have access to 16 visits every year for the following XX to 10 years when he will likely be undergoing the majority of his reconstructive surgeries. He should then have access to one to XX visits every XX years through life expectancy. It will be important for him to have access to therapy across the lifespan as aging with a disability and/or pain greatly increases the risk of depression and anxiety in the elderly.

Couples Therapy

John Doe shared that his wife and children have been seriously affected by his injuries. The burden of his injuries has impacted them in many ways. His daughter, Jill, just a toddler when he was injured, was frightened by his appearance when he came home from the hospital. The stress of dealing with the many changes in the couple's lives and responsibilities at home has been monumental in scope. His wife has had to take on significantly more responsibilities and John feels like he is unable to fulfill his duties of husband and father.

Therapy sessions are recommended for John Doe and his wife, Jane, six to eight times per year as they learn to live with the many changes in their lives. They also expressed some concern with their sexual relationship and intimacy issues. Good family/social support and acceptance are key elements of successful burn survival. More sessions would be beneficial, but much of their time will be taken up due to medical/surgical/therapy sessions.

Family Therapy

It is recommended that John Doe and his family engage in therapy, 12 sessions every 2 years, over the next 12 years. Parenting children with a chronically ill parent is difficult at best, and John Doe has already expressed being impatient and frustrated with his children. This is not an unusual response from an individual dealing with chronic pain and sleep problems. It is also very hard for children to watch their parents suffer. Burn injury is a family affair and reintegration into the family after an acute burn care hospitalization can be quite difficult. Therefore, therapy to help everyone cope is recommended.

Transportation

An allowance for mileage has been made in the life care plan tables for John Doe and his wife for travel to Anytown for surgeries and medical appointments. An allotment for a scooter for extended outings has also been made, as John Doe is having trouble with balance and with standing for any extended period of time.

Adaptive Sports Excursion

He should have the opportunity to attend this type of activity, annually, for the next 15 years. The purpose of this type of program is to enhance the quality of life of people with disabilities through exceptional outdoor adventure activities. Such programs empower participants in their daily lives and have a positive enduring effect on self-efficacy, health, independence, and overall well-being.

Health and Strength Maintenance

Dr. Surgeon also recommends that John Doe be involved in an organized exercise program now and in the future for weight control, flexibility, endurance, strengthening, and for overall physical and mental well-being. A membership at the local gym, combined with a personal trainer to manage his health and strength program is recommended to help him stay as fit as possible and perform his exercise as safely as possible.

Case Management

Case management should be provided for John, as he will benefit from assistance in navigating his way through the surgical (plastic and reconstruction), rehabilitation, psychological, and vocational therapies he will need over his lifetime. Dr. Surgeon and this life care planner concur that he will need a case manager who can provide consistent and knowledgeable long-term burn case management over his lifespan, as this responsibility should not be delegated to his wife. We recommend that he have access to case management 36 to 40 hours per year through age 55, and then 12 to 16 hours, per year, through life expectancy.

Supplies

John Doe will require supplies for ongoing hydration of his scars, sun protective clothing, and dressing change materials. The supplies he will likely need are listed in the life care plan tables.

Medication

Pain, itching, and anxiety are often ongoing problems for burn-injured persons. These issues can continue for many years after the initial burn injury. John Doe reports that he is still highly anxious and experiences pain on a daily basis. The medications that he is likely to need, post-operatively and in the future, are listed and priced in the life care plan tables.

Respite Care

It is recommended that 104 hours of respite relief (2 hours per week) per year and 100 hours of childcare should be provided for John Doe and his wife, Jane, annually. This should be made available for the next 15 years as they plan to have additional children. John Doe will likely be hospitalized for reconstructive surgery many times over the next 10 to 15 years, and Jane will not only need respite from caring for him, but a provision for childcare when she needs to accompany him to future surgeries, doctor visits, and therapies.

Personal Attendant and Home Care

John Doe should receive weekly assistance with cleaning, cooking, home management, skin care, and stretching. He should have access to personal assistance for lotion application, scar massage, grooming, and light housekeeping for 15 hours per week, from now through age 50. From age 50 through 69, this allowance should be increased to 24 hours per week, as individuals with major trauma to their bodies age more rapidly than uninjured persons. From age 70 to life expectancy, he should have 96 hours of care available. It is also recommended that he receive ongoing interior and exterior maintenance assistance and lawn care due to serious limitations of his arms, wrists, and legs, his limited stamina, and his inability to regulate his body temperature effectively. These responsibilities should not continue to be relegated to his wife or family. (An allowance for the "normal cost of living" which would be incurred by John Doe for a one-bedroom apartment has been subtracted from the cost of assisted living care.)

John Doe withstood the initial impact of serious, disfiguring, disabling, and life-changing burn injuries. He will continue to be tested with future surgeries, social reaction to his burn scars, grief of loss, relationship, body image, and sexuality issues, as well as the emotional and physical pain and limitations associated with being burned and being different. He will need strong ongoing support from those around him in order to survive this ordeal.

The goal of this life care plan is to provide the necessary care that will maintain/increase John Doe's medical stability, quality of life and to anticipate and prevent potential complications. The plan provides for medical and surgical care, evaluations, therapies, diagnostic testing, medications, supplies, mobility equipment, home care, transportation needs, and other services to promote and maintain independence and to prevent complications. This plan should be reevaluated/modified if complications develop and/or as progressive aging alters John's medical condition and functional status. All of these recommendations along with the likely costs of care and the recommender of included future care, are outlined within the life care plan tables.

Conclusion

Major burn injury is associated with deformity, extreme emotional and physical pain, financial hardship, and extensive rehabilitation. Recovery from a major burn can take a lifetime. Life care planners and case managers can help the patient and the patient's family navigate the rocky road of recovery by insuring that the care they receive will help to improve function and diminish complications over the patient's life span.

The fight for survival begins during the acute care phase but extends long after discharge from the hospital. The patient must continue to follow through with ongoing therapies, proper usage of splints and pressure garments, and ongoing exercise programs, and receive the necessary psychological and physical care associated with his or her burn injuries for maximum recovery. Allowing patients to have some measure of control of appropriate options (dressing change schedule, treatment schedule, etc.) can assist them in reducing their anxiety and help them to become more independent in their care.

The rehabilitation process for a burn patient can be overwhelming not only to the patient but to family and friends as well. The importance of addressing their psychosocial needs is paramount and is a very important component of the rehabilitation process. It will allow for a smoother transition to home, school, the workplace, and more successful reentry into the community at large (Helm & Cromes, 1995). By and large, burn rehabilitation is multifaceted, costly, and time consuming. It takes great courage and endurance on the part of the client and the client's support system to persevere. A thorough life care plan, coupled with effective case management, can help to decrease the complications associated with burn injuries and increase the likelihood of an ongoing yet successful recovery.

Burn Care Resources

Books

Total Burn Care, 5th Edition (2017)
Edited by David N. Herndon, MD
Published by Saunders Elsevier

Principles and Practices of Burn Surgery (2005)
Juan P. Barret-Nerin, MD and David N. Herndon, MD
Published by Marcel Dekker, Inc., ISBN: 0824754530

Burn Care (1999)
Steven E. Wolf, MD and David N. Herndon, MD
Published by Landes Bioscience, Georgetown, Texas 78626, ISBN: 1–57059–526–7

Burn Unit: Saving Lives after the Flames (Hardcover)
Barbara Ravage

Journeys through Hell: Stories of Burn Survivors' Reconstruction of Self and Identity
Dennis J. Stouffer, ISBN: 084767892X

Rising from the Flames: The Experience of the Severely Burned
Albert Howard Carter, Jane A. Petro, Albert Howard Carter, III
ISBN: 0812215176

Severe Burns: A Family Guide to Medical and Emotional Recovery
Andrew M. Munster. The Baltimore Regional Burn Center
ISBN: 0801846536

Resources for Family Members of Burn Survivors

Sundara, D. 2011. A review of issues and concerns of family members of adult burn survivors. *Journal of Burn Care and Research*, 32, 349–357.

Rea, S., Lim, J., Falder, S., & Wood, F. 2008. Use of the Internet by burn patients, their families and friends. Burns, 34, 345–349.

Blakeney, P. E., Rosenberg, L., Rosenberg, R., & Faber A. W. 2008. Psychosocial care of persons with severe burns. *Burns*, 34, 433.

Phillips, C., Fussel, A., & Rumsey, N. 2007. Considerations for psychosocial support following burn injury—A family perspective. *Burns*, 33, 986–994.

Sproul, J. L., Malloy, S., & Abriam-Yago, K. 2009. Perceived sources of support of adult burn survivors. *Journal of Burn Care & Research*, 30, 975–992.

Journals

- *Journal of Burn Care & Research*: https://academic.oup.com/jbcr
- *Journal of Burns & Wounds*: www.burnsjournal.com
- *Burns*: Elsevier.com

Burn Survivor Websites

- Burn Survivors Online (www.burnsurvivorsonline.com)
- Phoenix Society for Burn Survivors (www.phoenix-society.org/community/)
- Burn Surviviors around the World (http://www.burnsurvivorsttw.org)

References

American Burn Association, 2016. Accessed October 21, 2017. http://ameriburn.org/who-we-are/media/burn-incidence-fact-sheet.

Barret, J. P. 2004. *ABC of Burns: Burns Reconstruction*. Retrieved July 25, 2008, from www.bmj.com/cgi/reprint/329/7460/274.pdf.

Brown, M., Helm, P., & Weed, R. 2004. Life care planning for the burn patient. In R. Weed (Ed.), *Life Care Planning and Case Management Handbook* (2nd ed., pp. 351–380). Boca Raton, FL: CRC Press.

Brusselaers, N., Hoste, E. A., Monstrey, S., Colpaert, K. E., De Waele, J. J., Vandewoude, K. H. et al. 2005. Outcome and changes over time in survival following severe burns from 1985 to 2004. *Intensive Care Medicine, 31*, 1648–1653.

Brych, S., Engrav, L., Rivara, F., Ptacek, J., Lezotte, D., & Esselman, P. 2001. Time off work and return to work after burns: Systematic review of the literature and a large two-center series. *Journal of Burn Care & Rehabilitation, 22*, 401–405.

Cho, Y. S., Jeon, J. H. et al. 2014. The effect of burn rehabilitation massage therapy on hypertrophic scar after burn: A randomized controlled trial. *Burns, 8*, 1513–1520.

Cromes, G. H., Jr., & Helm, P. A. 1993. Burns. In M. Eisenberg, R. Glueckauf, & H. Zaretsky (Eds.). *Medical Aspects of Disability* (pp. 92–104). New York, NY: Springer Publishing Company.

Demling, R. H. 1995. The advantage of the burn team approach. *Journal of Burn Care & Rehabilitation, 16*, 569–572.

Demling, R. H., & LaLonde, I. C. 1989. *Burn Trauma*. New York, NY: Thieme Medical Publishers.

Dyster-Aas, J., Kildal, M., & Willebrand, M. 2007. Return to work and health-related quality of life after burn injury. *Journal of Rehabilitation Medicine, 39*, 49–55.

Edelman L. S., McNaught T., Chan G. M., & Morris S. E. 2003 Sustained bone mineral density changes after burn injury. *J Surg Res, 114*, 172–8.

Ehde, D. M., Patterson, D. R., Weichman, S. A., & Wilson, L. G. 1999. Post-traumatic stress symptoms and distress following acute burn injury. *Burns, 25*, 587–592.

Field, T., Peck, M., Krugman, S., Tuchel, T., Schanberg, S., Kuhn, C. et al. 1998. Burn injuries benefit from massage therapy. *Journal of Burn Care and Rehabilitation, 19*, 242–244.

Fisher, S. V., & Helm, P. A. 1984. *Comprehensive Rehabilitation of Burns*. Baltimore, MD: Williams & Wilkins.

Gabriel, V. 2009. Evidence-based review for the treatment of post-burn pruritus. *Journal of Burn Care & Research*, 30(1), 55–61. https://doi.org/10.1097/BCR.0b013e318191fd95.

Gallal, A. R. S., & Yousef, S. M. 2002. Our experience in the nutritional support of burn patients. *Annals of Burns and Fire Disasters, XV*, 1–6.

Ganio, M. S. et al. 2015. Aerobic fitness is disproportionately low in adult burn survivors years after injury. *Journal of Burn Care & Research, 36*(4), 513–519.

Hartford, C. E., & Kealy, G. P. 2007. Care of outpatient burns. In D. Herndon (Ed.), *Total Burn Care* (3rd ed., p. 69). New York, NY: Saunders, Elsevier, pp. 3274–3278.

Helm, P. A., & Cromes, G. H. Jr. 1995. Burn injury rehabilitation. In The National Rehabilitation Hospital Research Center (Ed.), *The State-of-the-Science in Medical Rehabilitation* (pp. IV1–IV22). Falls Church, VA: Birch & Davis Associates.

Herndon, D., & Blakeney, P. 2007. Teamwork for total burn care: Achievements, directions and hopes. In D. Herndon (Ed.), *Total Burn Care* (3rd ed., pp. 11–15). New York, NY: Saunders, Elsevier.

Khosh, M. M. 2008. *Skin Grafts, Full-Thickness*. Retrieved August 2, 2008, from www.emedicine.com/ent/topic48.htm.

Linares, H. A., Kischer, C. W., Dobrkovsky, M., & Larson, D. L. 1972. The histiotypic organization of the hypertrophic scar in humans. *Journal of Investigative Dermatology, 59*, 323–331.

National Hospital Discharge Survey. 2003. *Annual Summary with Detailed Diagnosis and Procedure Data Series 13*. Retrieved July 24, 2008, from www.cdc.gov/nchs/about/major/hdasd/listpubs.htm.

National Safety Council Report on Injuries in America. 2003. *Injury Facts® Data, 2004*. Itasca, IL: National Safety Council.

Partridge, J. 2008. *Changing Faces*. Retrieved June 16, 2008, from www.changingfaces.org.uk/Health-Care-Professionals.

Perry, S., Difede, J., Musngi, G., Frances, A., & Jacobsberg, L. 1992. Predictors of posttraumatic stress disorder after burn injury. *American Journal of Psychiatry, 149*, 931–935.

Pruitt, B., Goodwin, C., & Mason, A. 2007. Epidemiological, demographic and outcome characteristics of burn injury. In D. Herndon, *Total Burn Care* (3rd ed., pp. 14–32). New York, NY: Saunders, Elsevier.

Rimmer, R. B., Bay, C. R. et al. 2014. Burn-injured youth may be at increased risk for long-term anxiety. *Journal of Burn Care & Rehabilitation, 35*, 154–161.

Saffle, J., Davis, B., & Williams, P. 1995. Recent outcomes in the treatment of burn injury: Burn association patient registry. *Journal of Burn Care Rehabilitation, 16*, 219–230.

Schneider J. C., & Qu H. D. 2011. Neurologic and musculoskeletal complications of burn injuries. *Phys Med Rehabil Clin N Am, 22*, 261–75, vi.

Serghiou, M. A., Ott, S., Farmer, S., Morgan, D., Gibson, P., & Suman, O. E. 2007. Comprehensive rehabilitation of the burn patient. In D. Herndon (Ed.), *Total Burn Care* (3rd ed., p. 620). New York, NY: Saunders, Elsevier.

Sheridan, R. L. et al. 2000. Current expectations for survival in pediatric burns. *Archives of Pediatrics & Adolescent Medicine, 154*(3), 245–249.

Smith, J. S., Smith, K. R., Rainey, S. L., & DelGiorno, J. 2006. The psychology of burn care. *Journal of Trauma Nursing, 13*, 105–106.

St-Pierre D. M., Choinière M., Forget R., & Garrel D. R. 1998 Muscle strength in individuals with healed burns. *Arch Phys Med Rehabil, 79*, 155–61.

Warden, G. D., & Warner, P. M. 2007. Functional sequelae and disability assessment. In D. Herndon (Ed.), *Total Burn Care* (3rd ed., p. 782). New York, NY: Saunders, Elsevier.

Weed, R., & Atkins, D. 2004. Return to work issues for persons with upper extremity amputation. In D. Atkins and R. Meier (Eds.), *Functional Restoration of Adults and Children with Upper Extremity Amputation* (pp. 337–351). New York, NY: Demos Publishing.

Weed, R. O., & Berens, D. E. 2005. Basics of burn injury: Implications for case management and life care planning. *Lippincott's Case Management, 10*, 22–29.

Weichman, S. A., Ptacek, J. T., Patterson, D. R., Gibran, N. S., Engrav, L. E., & Heimbach, D. M. 2001. Clinical research award: Rates, trends, and severity of depression following burn injuries. *Journal of Burn Care and Rehabilitation, 22*, 417–424.

Chapter 15

Life Care Planning for Depressive Disorders, Obsessive-Compulsive Disorder, and Schizophrenia

Nicole M. Wolf

Contents

Introduction 444
Major Depressive Disorder (MDD) 445
Epidemiology and Course of Illness 445
Symptoms 445
Treatment 446
Pharmacotherapy 446
Psychotherapeutic Interventions 446
Vocational Impact of MDD 447
Reasonable Accommodations 447
Costs of MDD 447
Bipolar Disorder 447
Epidemiology and Course of Illness 448
Symptoms 448
Mania 449
Hypomania 449
Depressive Episode 449
Mixed Episode 449
Treatment 450
Pharmacotherapy 450
Psychotherapeutic Interventions 451
Vocational Impact of Bipolar Disorder 452

Reasonable Accommodations....452
Costs of Bipolar Disorder....452
Obsessive-Compulsive Disorder (OCD)....452
Epidemiology and Course of Illness....453
Symptoms....453
Treatment....453
Pharmacotherapy....454
Psychotherapeutic Interventions....454
Vocational Impact of OCD....455
Reasonable Accommodations....455
Costs of OCD....455
Schizophrenia....455
Epidemiology and Course of Illness....456
Symptoms....456
Positive Symptoms....456
Negative Symptoms....457
Associated Symptoms or Features....457
Treatment Phases of Schizophrenia....457
Treatment Refractory Schizophrenia....458
Pharmacotherapy....458
Vocational Impact of Schizophrenia....460
Functional Limitations and Reasonable Accommodations....460
Vocational Programs....460
Costs of Schizophrenia....461
Case Study....461
Conclusion....464
References....464

Introduction

The impact of mental illness on the cost of health care and productivity has been largely underestimated. The Center for Behavioral Health Statistics and Quality (CBHSQ) reports mental illness affects about one in five adults or about 18.1 percent of Americans ages 18 and older (CBHSQ, 2015). It is estimated that 43.6 million American adults have a mental illness. Furthermore, an estimated 9.8 million adults or 4.2 percent of the American population has a serious mental illness resulting in significant impairments in daily functioning (CBHSQ, 2015). Neuropsychiatric disorders are the leading cause of disability in the United States (U.S. Burden of Disease Collaborators, 2013). Psychiatric illness programs have not traditionally used life care planners. However, life care planning for mental illness can be considered an untapped market since the disease is lifelong and requires reasonably predictable care (Hilligoss, 2003). The prediction of expected care can be summarized in a life care plan (Weed, 1999; Weed & Field, 2001). In order to provide an accurate life care plan, it is important to consider the complexity of mental illness, including symptoms, treatment, and impact on functioning. The following sections provide an overview of major depressive disorder, bipolar disorder, obsessive-compulsive disorder, and schizophrenia. At the end of the chapter, implications for life care planning are considered, including a checklist to help create the life care plan and an example of a life care plan for an individual with schizophrenia.

Major Depressive Disorder (MDD)

Major depressive disorder is the second leading cause of disability worldwide (Ferrari et al., 2013). In 2014, an estimated 6.6 percent of adults (15.7 million people) had at least one major depressive episode in the past year. Of this group, 4.3 percent or 10.2 million adults were considered to have significant impairments due to depression (CBHSQ, 2015). In any given year, it is estimated that 18.1 percent of the adult U.S. population have a mood disorder and 6.7 percent have major depressive disorder specifically (Kessler et al., 2005a). The term *mood disorders* typically includes major depressive disorder (MDD), persistent depressive disorder (previously known as dysthymia), and bipolar disorder (see the section on Bipolar Disorder).

Epidemiology and Course of Illness

The Epidemiologic Catchment Area (ECA) study sponsored by the National Institutes of Health estimated, in adults, the 1-month prevalence of MDD at 2.2 percent and a lifetime prevalence of 5.8 percent (Robins & Reiger, 1991). More recent studies have found higher lifetime prevalence rates. Kessler et al. (2005b) reported that MDD had a lifetime prevalence rate of 16.6 percent, which was higher than all other DSM-IV disorders. Another large epidemiological study reported a lifetime prevalence rate of 13.25 percent (Hasin et al., 2005). A major depressive episode often occurs after an individual experiences a severe psychosocial stressor such as divorce or the death of a loved one. MDD can occur at any age, but the average age of onset is in the late twenties. The disorder may develop suddenly or take days or weeks to become clinically diagnostic. The duration of MDD is varied, and time to recovery can vary from a few months to a year or more (APA, 2013). Some individuals will later develop bipolar disorder after experiencing a hypomanic or manic episode. It is estimated that 50 to 85 percent of individuals with MDD will have another episode (Mueller et al., 1999). Risk factors for relapse include age of onset, the severity of the first episode, the number of episodes, family history of psychopathology, comorbid substance abuse, anxiety disorders, negative cognition styles, and stressful life events (Burcusa & Iacono, 2007). It is important to note that some people will have residual symptoms after an episode of depression resolves. The most common residual symptoms are anxiety, core mood symptoms, insomnia, and somatic symptoms (Romera et al., 2013).

Symptoms

MDD is characterized by one or more major depressive episodes, with an absence of any hypomanic, manic, or mixed episodes. The fundamental feature of a major depressive episode is a persistent depressed mood that lasts at least two weeks or loss of interest or pleasure in almost all activities. Other symptoms of a major depressive episode include changes in sleep, appetite, weight, or psychomotor activity; lack of energy; feeling guilty or worthless; decreased ability to focus, think, or make decisions; and thoughts of death or suicidal thoughts, plans, or attempts (APA, 2013). At least five of these symptoms must be present and last for at least two weeks in order to meet the criteria of a major depressive episode. MDD can manifest a wide range of impairments, from mild to severe. In severe episodes, individuals with MDD can have psychotic symptoms, characterized by the presence of delusions (false, irrational beliefs) and hallucinations. Another severe manifestation of MDD is the presence of catatonic features, where there is a severe change in motor movements and behavior (e.g., an individual may remain motionless, engage in bizarre postures, or become mute) (APA, 2013).

Treatment

The American Psychiatric Association has established treatment guidelines for MDD (APA, 2010). Treatment is conceptualized into three phases: (1) the acute phase, during which the goal is to induce remission and a return to baseline functioning; (2) the continuation phase, during which the goal is to preserve remission; and (3) the maintenance phase, during which the goal is to prevent future episodes. Both pharmacotherapy and psychotherapeutic interventions are used to meet these goals. Treatment recommendations will vary based on the severity and characteristics of the depressive episodes and response to treatment.

Pharmacotherapy

Antidepressants

Antidepressant medications are utilized during all phases of treatment. Commonly prescribed antidepressants include selective serotonin reuptake inhibitors (SSRIs), serotonin norepinephrine reuptake inhibitors (SNRIs), mirtazapine, and bupropion. Older agents such as tricyclics and monoamine oxidase inhibitors (MAOIs) may also be prescribed, most often when individuals fail first-line treatments. SSRIs include fluoxetine, fluvoxamine, sertraline, paroxetine, escitalopram, and citalopram. Common side effects of SSRIs include gastrointestinal distress, insomnia/agitation, sexual side effects, headaches, extrapyramidal side effects, effects on weight, falls, serotonin syndrome, and discontinuation syndrome (APA, 2010). SNRIs include venlafaxine, duloxetine, desvenlafaxine, and levomilnacipran. Common side effects of SNRIs include nausea, decreased appetite, headache, gastrointestinal distress, dizziness, dose-related hypertension, and discontinuation syndrome (Keller et al., 2007; APA, 2010). Tricyclic agents include amitriptyline, clomipramine, doxepin, and imipramine. Common side effects of tricyclics include cardiovascular and anticholinergic effects, weight gain, sedation, myoclonus, seizures, and falls (APA, 2010). MAOIs include phenelzine, tranylcypromine, and selegiline. Individuals taking MAOIs must avoid certain foods and beverages such as aged cheese and meats, fava beans, and red wine because a serious, life-threatening interaction (hypertensive crisis) may occur (Pies, 1998). Common side effects of MAOIs include cardiovascular effects, weight gain, sexual side effects, headaches, insomnia, and sedation (APA, 2010).

Adjunctive Medications

If an individual does not have an adequate response to antidepressant medications, other agents such as another antidepressant from a different class, mood stabilizers, and antipsychotics may be added in hopes of greater efficacy. There is evidence that adding bupriopion, mirtazapine, or venlafaxine to an SSRI is an effective strategy (Trivedi et al., 2006). Lithium has demonstrated efficacy in up to 50 percent of individuals who do not respond to antidepressant therapy alone (Price et al., 1986). There is evidence that augmenting with an antipsychotic is also effective (Shelton et al., 2001; Papakostas et al., 2007). Last, electroconvulsive therapy (ECT) may be considered in moderate to severe depression, depression with psychotic or catatonic features, treatment refractory depression, and for suicidality. A meta-analytic review of ECT reports that it was more effective than all other pharmacologic treatments (Pagnin et al., 2004). This study did not include lithium or antipsychotics.

Psychotherapeutic Interventions

Types of therapy that have demonstrated efficacy in treating depression include cognitive-behavioral therapy, interpersonal psychotherapy, psychodynamic therapy, and problem-solving therapy (APA,

2010). Individuals with MDD often have marital and family issues, so therapy with the spouse or family may be helpful. Group therapy may also be beneficial to individuals with MDD. Depression-focused psychotherapy alone is recommended for people with mild to moderate depression and women who are pregnant, trying to become pregnant, or breastfeeding. For moderate to severe depression, psychotherapy plus antidepressant treatment is recommended (APA, 2010).

Vocational Impact of MDD

Loss of interest in work activities, decreased motivation, poor initiative, lack of drive, changes in appetite, insomnia, fatigue, psychomotor agitation or retardation, negative thinking, and decreased ability to focus and concentrate can have a profound negative impact on work performance and work relationships (Fischler & Booth, 1999; Steadman & Taskila, 2015). These symptoms can make it difficult to learn new skills. Individuals with MDD may have irritability that negatively affects relationships with coworkers. They may be overly sensitive to criticism and have difficulty coping with others. The symptoms of MDD can make it difficult for an individual to stay on task or complete a project. Stress tolerance is decreased in MDD; therefore, a high-stress, fast-paced work environment may be inappropriate.

Reasonable Accommodations

Accommodations for an individual with MDD will depend on the severity of symptoms. It is important to offer flexibility in scheduling to allow for appointments for medication management or therapy. A quiet workstation away from distractions may improve attention and focus. A predictable routine can help minimize stress and maintain stamina. Hourly goals can help with maintaining work pace. Working in a team may decrease feelings of loneliness. Last, new information or new job skills may require extra instruction and additional time to learn. Providing written instructions can help to improve accuracy and aid in retention.

Costs of MDD

Major depressive disorder is a costly illness in terms of both direct costs (e.g., hospitalizations, doctor's visits, medications) and indirect costs (e.g., missed work, reduced productivity, quality of life). The annual cost of MDD in 2010 was estimated at $210.5 billion. Of this total, 45 percent was attributable to direct costs, 5 percent to suicide-related costs, and 50 percent to workplace costs (Greenberg et al., 2015). In regards to treatment costs, outpatient and inpatient medical services accounted for 15 to 18 percent of direct cost and pharmacy costs were 13 percent (Greenberg et al., 2015). The American College of Occupational and Environmental Medicine (ACOEM) reports that MDD has been shown to be equivalent to coronary heart disease in terms of reduced productivity (2012). It is estimated that people with MDD function at an even lower rate than people with hypertension, diabetes, or arthritis (ACOEM, 2002). A large meta-analysis did not find evidence of cost-effectiveness differences between SSRIs, with the exception of escitalopram or of SSRIs versus TCAs (Pan et al., 2012).

Bipolar Disorder

Clinical classifications on bipolar disorder first appeared around the turn of the century, when Emil Kraepelin divided psychotic disorders into two major categories: manic-depressive insanity and dementia praecox (Wyatt, 2001). These terms are the predecessors of bipolar disorder and schizophrenia, respectively. Bipolar disorder can be classified as bipolar I, bipolar II, and bipolar disorder not otherwise specified. Individuals with bipolar I have experienced at least one episode of mania, while individuals with bipolar II have not. Instead, they experience a milder form of mania termed *hypomania*. Both of these mood states will be further explained in the symptoms section. Unless otherwise stated in the text, in the following sections the term *bipolar disorder* refers to bipolar I.

Epidemiology and Course of Illness

The Epidemiologic Catchment Area study estimated the prevalence of bipolar I and bipolar II disorders in the adult population at 0.8 percent and 0.5 percent, respectively (Robins & Reiger, 1991). In any given year, about 2.6 percent of the population or about 5.7 million American adults have bipolar disorder (Kessler et al., 2005a). The ECA study reports the mean age of onset at 21 years of age (Robins & Reiger, 1991). Disturbingly, it is estimated that almost 70 percent of individuals with bipolar disorder who seek help are misdiagnosed, commonly with unipolar depression (Hirschfeld et al., 2003). There are generally an equal number of men and women affected with bipolar disorder, although their course of illness may be different. Women with bipolar disorder have higher rates of rapid cycling moods, mixed states, alcohol use disorder, depressive symptoms, and lifetime eating disorders (APA, 2013). Bipolar disorder is likely a result of a genetic predisposition combined with environmental influences, including stressful events (Rush, 2003).

Bipolar disorder can have a devastating impact on quality of life. When left untreated, an individual may experience 10 or more episodes of mania and depression over a lifetime (Goodwin & Jamison, 1990). As many as 30 to 60 percent of individuals with bipolar disorder experience interpersonal and occupational impairments (Sanchez-Moreno et al., 2009). The divorce rates among these individuals are two to three times higher than those of the general population (Manning et al., 1997). The ECA study found that individuals with bipolar disorder were the most likely of all of the mentally ill groups to have a history of previous suicide attempts. In fact, 25 to 60 percent of all individuals with bipolar disorder will attempt suicide at least once in their lifetime, and 18.9 percent succeed (Robins & Reiger, 1991). The lifetime suicide risk of people with bipolar disorder is 15 times higher than the general population (APA, 2013).

The course of illness in most individuals is chronic, often with alternating periods of depression and mania. Symptoms typically reduce for a period of time between these episodes; however, some individuals continue to have residual mood symptoms (Marangell et al., 2009). About 10 to 15 percent of individuals with bipolar disorder have rapid cycling, which is defined as four or more episodes of mania, mixed mania, hypomania, or depression occurring in a 12-month period (Bowden, 1996).

Symptoms

Symptoms associated with bipolar disorder include mania, hypomania, depressive, and mixed states. Psychotic features may occur with all of these states except hypomania. Psychotic features are defined as a break with reality characterized by delusions and hallucinations. The DSM-V (APA, 2013) criteria for each of these mood states are detailed in the following section.

Mania

The characteristics of mania include the following:

- Mood disturbance for at least one week: Abnormal and persistently elevated, expansive, or irritable mood
- Pressured speech: Talkative, with pressure to keep talking, difficult to interrupt
- Distractibility: Sifficulty maintaining attention, distracted by irrelevant information or stimuli
- Flight of ideas: Racing thoughts, frequently changing subjects
- Inflated self-esteem or grandiosity: An exaggerated sense of self-importance or of one's status, accomplishments, wealth, talents, or beauty
- Decreased need for sleep: Sleeps very little or not at all, may deny need for sleep
- Excessive involvement with high-risk activities (e.g., gambling, sexual activity with strangers, or lavish spending of money)
- Increase in goal-directed activity or psychomotor agitation

Hypomania

Hypomania and mania share some of the same characteristics. Hypomania typically has milder symptoms; however, functioning is still impacted. The symptoms are not severe enough to cause significant vocational or social impairment or to warrant hospitalization. Additionally, psychotic features are never present during a hypomanic episode (APA, 2013).

Depressive Episode

To meet the criteria for a depressive episode, five or more symptoms must be present during a two week period and at least one of the symptoms is either depressed mood or loss of interest/pleasure. The criteria for a depressive episode are as follows:

- Depressed mood occurring most of the day for at least 2 weeks
- Significantly reduced interest or pleasure in all or almost all activities occurring most of the day
- Significant weight loss or weight gain or change in appetite
- Insomnia or hypersomnia
- Psychomotor agitation or retardation that is observable by others
- Feelings of worthlessness or excessive/inappropriate guilt, which may take on a delusional quality
- Fatigue or lack of energy
- Decreased ability to think or focus or make decisions
- Recurrent thoughts of death and/or suicidal ideation, plan, or attempt

Mixed Episode

A mixed episode occurs when the criteria for both a manic and depressive episode are met at the same time nearly every day for at least one week (APA, 2013). A mixed episode causes severe impairment and may lead to hospitalization. During a mixed state, it is common to have agitation, difficulty sleeping, significant changes in appetite, psychosis, and suicidal thoughts.

Treatment

The APA *Practice Guidelines for the Treatment of Patients with Bipolar Disorder* provide the following treatment guidelines and goals (APA, 2002):

- Perform a thorough diagnostic evaluation.
- Evaluate the safety of the patient and others and determine a treatment setting.
- Establish and maintain a therapeutic alliance.
- Monitor the patient's psychiatric status.
- Provide psychoeducation about bipolar disorder.
- Enhance treatment compliance.
- Promote regular patterns of activity and sleep.
- Anticipate stressors.
- Identify new episodes early.
- Minimize functional impairments.

To achieve these goals, a combination of pharmacologic and psychotherapeutic interventions is required.

Pharmacotherapy

Medications are used to treat acute manic symptoms, alleviate depression, and prevent future episodes. Common categories of drugs that are used to treat bipolar disorder include mood stabilizers/anticonvulsants, antipsychotics, and adjunctive agents. While lithium has been the most commonly prescribed medication for the treatment of bipolar disorder for decades, the use of other mood stabilizers and atypical antipsychotics as first-line treatments has become increasingly common due to their perceived greater tolerability and mounting evidence of efficacy.

Lithium

Lithium has been the mainstay of bipolar pharmacologic treatment. It was first found to have antimanic properties in 1949 (Cade, 1999) but was not widely prescribed for bipolar disorder in the United States until the mid-1960s (Jefferson et al., 1987). Lithium demonstrates efficacy in the treatment of acute mania, depressive episodes, and prevention of recurrent episodes (Goodwin & Jamison, 1990). Side effects are reported in up to 75 percent of individuals that take lithium (Jefferson et al., 1987; Goodwin & Jamison, 1990). Lithium has demonstrated efficacy in suicide prevention, possibly from reducing "impulsive-aggressive" behavior (Benard et al., 2016). Side effects of lithium include excessive thirst, excessive urination, memory problems, tremors, weight gain, and drowsiness/tiredness (Lenox & Husseini, 1998). Rates of noncompliance range from 18 to 53 percent, and the side effect most often reported as the reason for discontinuing lithium is memory problems (Goodwin & Jamison, 1990). Toxic effects and overdose can occur and are more common with high serum levels. Monitoring of serum plasma levels is an important aspect of lithium treatment. Initially, close serum monitoring is required to find the optimal therapeutic dose and to avoid toxicity. It is recommended that renal and thyroid functions be tested regularly because lithium use may disrupt these processes (APA, 2002).

Other Mood Stabilizers

Valproate, an anticonvulsant, is another agent commonly used in the treatment of bipolar disorder. Valproate has demonstrated efficacy in the treatment of acute mania and some evidence of effectiveness in acute bipolar depression and maintenance (APA, 2002). Common side effects of valproate include sedation, gastrointestinal distress, tremors, increased appetite, and weight gain. There may be life-threatening adverse reactions, but such events are rare. Dosing is established through blood serum monitoring. Toxicity and overdose are not common with routine dosing. It is recommended that liver function and hematologic measures be assessed on a regular basis (APA, 2002). Other commonly prescribed mood stabilizers include carbamazepine and lamotrigine.

Antipsychotics

Beginning with olanzapine in 1999, all of the atypical antipsychotics have FDA approval for the treatment of bipolar disorder with the exception of paliperidone and iloperidone. This includes asenapine, lurasidone, aripiprazole, ziprasidone, risperidone, and quetiapine. The conventional antipsychotic chlorpromazine is indicated for the treatment of bipolar disorder. Traditionally, antipsychotics have been used to treat acute mania and psychotic symptoms. However, there is evidence that they can also treat depressive symptoms and prevent future episodes (Gutman & Nemeroff, 2007; Suppes et al., 2016). Unlike lithium and valproate, atypical antipsychotics do not require serum monitoring. Common side effects associated with the use of atypicals include drowsiness, sedation, dry mouth, constipation, dizziness, orthostatic hypotension, nausea, and possibly extrapyramidal symptoms (but reduced in comparison with conventional antipsychotics). Atypical antipsychotics can have negative metabolic effects such as an increased risk of weight gain, hyperglycemia, diabetes mellitus, and dyslipidemia. It is recommended that clinicians monitor weight, waist circumference, blood pressure, glucose, and lipids regularly in patients taking these medications (Hirschfeld, 2005).

Adjunctive Medications

Other medications that are used to treat bipolar disorder include benzodiazepines/tranquilizers, antidepressants, and other anticonvulsants. Benzodiazepines or tranquilizers are also used to treat acute mania because of their sedative effects. Antidepressants are used for bipolar depression; however, caution and close monitoring are required because these agents may induce mania (APA, 2002). There have been investigations into the use of other anticonvulsants such as topiramate and gabapentin in treating bipolar disorder (Wang et al., 2002; Vasudev et al., 2006). More research is needed to better quantify the beneficial effects of adjunctive medications.

Psychotherapeutic Interventions

The APA *Practice Guidelines for the Treatment of Bipolar Disorder* (2002) recommend the use of psychoeducation and psychotherapeutic interventions. The primary goals of these treatments are to decrease distress, improve functioning, and reduce the risk and severity of future episodes. While psychotherapeutic interventions alone are typically not effective in the treatment of acute mania, they do demonstrate efficacy with bipolar depression (Zaretsky et al., 1999; Vallarino et al., 2015). Treating bipolar depression without antidepressants can be especially beneficial to individuals who have antidepressant side effects, antidepressant-induced mania, or rapid cycling. In addition to individual therapy, individuals with bipolar disorder may also benefit from family therapy, group therapy, and support groups.

Vocational Impact of Bipolar Disorder

Bipolar disorder can result in significant difficulties in the workplace. Marwaha et al. (2013) report that 40 to 60 percent of people with bipolar disorder are employed. During a manic phase, symptoms such as grandiosity, distractibility, poor judgment, and excessive or inappropriate motivation can result in severe consequences on the job. A person experiencing manic symptoms has reduced interpersonal functioning, poor time management, difficulty maintaining attention, and may be distracting to coworkers. The individual may be unpredictable, unreliable, and irrational. At the most extreme, the individual experiencing mania can be dangerous to himself/herself and to others in the workplace. An individual experiencing a depressive episode may have lack of motivation, lack of energy, social withdrawal, and decreased ability to attend and focus (Fischler & Booth, 1999).

Reasonable Accommodations

Functional limitations and reasonable accommodations will vary according to the individual based on differences in episode, symptom severity, and effective coping strategies. Accommodations could include job sharing or job restructuring, putting all workplace communications in writing, and allowing time off for appointments and hospitalization, if needed. Increasing the structure of the workday and developing hourly goals can also be helpful. It is important to provide regular feedback on both job performance and interactions with others. Providing a quiet workstation with minimal distractions can improve attention and focus. Educating a supervisor or coworker about the early signs of mania could also be helpful in providing appropriate interventions early in the episode, thereby reducing functional impairment.

Costs of Bipolar Disorder

Bipolar disorder is a costly illness, in terms of both economics and impact on quality of life. Kleinman et al. (2003) report that lifetime costs of bipolar illness are estimated at $24 billion dollars. People with bipolar disorder utilize nearly three to four times more healthcare resources than those without bipolar disorder (Bryant-Comstock et al., 2002). The most costly intervention for bipolar disorder is hospitalization. It is estimated that 64 percent of individuals with bipolar disorder are noncompliant, meaning they do not take their medications as prescribed (Li et al., 2002). Direct health care costs rise in individuals who delay or do not take mood stabilizers during their first year of treatment (Li et al., 2002). Medication noncompliance can lead to relapse and rehospitalization—a costly cycle. While newer medications may be more expensive, there is some evidence that shows that they help to reduce overall costs, due to improved efficacy (Bergeson et al., 2012).

Obsessive-Compulsive Disorder (OCD)

Worry, doubts, and superstitious behavior are often a part of everyday experiences. Many people spend some time worrying, especially when psychosocial stressors are high. When worries become excessive or irrational or when certain actions are perceived as necessary to counteract these thoughts, then OCD is suspected. Important clinical features of OCD are that the thoughts and actions must be time-consuming (greater than 1 hour per day), cause marked distress, and significantly impair everyday activities (APA, 2013).

Epidemiology and Course of Illness

OCD was once considered to be a rare disease by mental health professionals. In the United States, the 12-month prevalence rate is reported at 1.2 percent of the population (APA, 2013). People with OCD come from all ethnic backgrounds. There are slight gender differences, where men have higher rates during childhood and women have higher rates during adulthood. Generally, the onset of OCD is any age between preschool and adulthood. Most people develop OCD by the age of 40 years (March et al., 1997). Up to 50 percent of individuals with OCD report that their symptoms began during childhood (March et al., 1997). OCD often goes unrecognized even after an individual seeks treatment. It is estimated that the average person with OCD sees three to four different doctors and spends 9 years seeking treatment before the correct diagnosis is made (March et al., 1997). Like other mental illnesses, OCD has genetic and physiological components. The symptoms are most likely due to an imbalance in neurotransmitters, as well as dysfunction in certain areas of the brain (March et al., 1997; Denys, Zohar, & Westenberg, 2004; APA, 2013). OCD symptoms are often chronic, although there may be periods of time when the symptoms are less severe.

Symptoms

Most people with OCD have both obsessions and compulsions. Obsessions are thoughts, images, or impulses that are persistent and perceived by the individual as unwanted, intrusive, and beyond control (APA, 2013). The obsessive thoughts are perceived as disturbing and result in high levels of distress and anxiety. Individuals experiencing obsessions often cope by ignoring or suppressing the thoughts or attempting to neutralize them through another thought or behavior, which is a compulsion. Therefore, compulsions are repetitive actions or thoughts that an individual performs in order to make obsessions go away. Compulsive behaviors in OCD are not pleasurable, but are used to reduce or prevent anxious feelings or worries (APA, 2013). Common obsessions include the following (APA, 2013):

- Fear of contamination (e.g., by touching a doorknob or shaking hands)
- Repeated doubts (e.g., wondering if the stove was left on or if a check was signed)
- Symmetry (e.g., lining up shoes a certain way, positioning canned goods according to size, type)
- Forbidden or taboo thoughts (e.g., aggressive, sexual, and religious obsessions)
- Harm (e.g., fear of harm of oneself or others)

Common compulsions include the following (APA, 2013):

- Repetitive behaviors (e.g., hand washing, ordering, checking, touching)
- Repetitive mental acts (e.g., praying, counting, repeating words or phrases)

Treatment

Treatment of OCD includes both medications and psychotherapeutic interventions. Most people require the use of both modalities, as only 20 percent experience symptom remission with medications alone (March et al., 1997). Treatment is divided into two phases: acute and maintenance. The respective treatment goals during the acute and maintenance phases are to end the current OCD episode and prevent future episodes. Most treatment occurs on an outpatient basis, as hospitalization is rarely necessary for the treatment of OCD. However, inpatient treatment may be an effective strategy for people with severe, chronic, treatment-resistant OCD (Boshen et al., 2008).

Pharmacotherapy

Antidepressants

Serotonin reuptake inhibitors (SRIs) are the mainstay of pharmacologic treatment of OCD. SRIs include clomipramine (a tricyclic antidepressant) and SSRIs such as fluoxetine, fluvoxamine, paroxetine, and sertraline. Antidepressants that do not have serotonergic properties are typically not effective in the treatment of OCD (Pies, 1998). Treatment response takes time. Most people will not have substantial improvement until they have been taking an SRI for four to six weeks, and it may take as long as 10 to 12 weeks of treatment. If OCD symptoms do not diminish after an SRI is initiated, it is recommended to increase the medication to the maximum tolerated dose within the approved dosage range (APA, 2007).

Adjunctive Medications

If patients do not respond to conventional treatment, then another strategy is the use of adjunctive medications. Commonly used adjunctive medications include clomipramine, benzodiazepines (e.g., clonazepam, alprazolam, lorazepam), antipsychotics (e.g., haloperidol, olanzapine, risperidone), and buspirone (an antianxiety agent) (APA, 2007). Adjunctive medications are not used alone, but added on to the existing medication regime. It is important to monitor for increased medication side effects or interactions when using multiple agents. Sedation is a common side effect of these medications, so it may be necessary to take them at bedtime.

Psychotherapeutic Interventions

Cognitive-behavioral therapy (CBT) is recommended for all individuals with OCD (APA, 2007). CBT techniques utilized in the treatment of OCD include exposure and response or ritual prevention. Exposure consists of having the individual come into contact with a feared stimulus (e.g., dirty objects, shaking hands, etc.). The goal of this technique is to reduce anxiety with each exposure session. Response or ritual prevention is another key element to this process. This technique is defined as preventing the individual from any actions that are used to reduce anxiety when exposed to the feared stimulus (APA, 2007), for example, not permitting the individual to wash her hands after touching something perceived as contaminated. Other CBT techniques used in OCD include thought stopping, distraction, and contingency management.

Individuals with OCD may also benefit from psychoeducation about the illness and ways to manage symptoms. Also, support groups can be helpful because they provide an outlet for individuals to share experiences and receive peer support. OCD has a negative impact on an individual's interpersonal relationships, and significant others may become part of the destructive symptom cycle by enabling rituals. In these cases, it is especially important to include significant others in the treatment plan, including the use of marriage and family therapy.

Vocational Impact of OCD

OCD can have a devastating impact on vocational functioning. Commonly, individuals with OCD will work at a slow pace as a result of coping with obsessions and compulsions. An individual may feel compelled to check and recheck his/her work or a need to do certain rituals while working that make ordinary tasks take an extended period of time to complete. Individuals with OCD have a lower tolerance for stress. Everyday occurrences such as shaking someone's hand or counting money might induce obsessive thoughts and compulsive behaviors. Also, a stressful work environment can contribute to the severity and frequency of OCD symptoms. Distractibility can occur because the individual with OCD is often preoccupied with symptoms, detracting from the ability to concentrate and focus.

Reasonable Accommodations

An individual with OCD will work better in an environment that offers predictability and routine. This can help keep stress levels to a minimum and reduce the need to make decisions throughout the day, which may prove difficult, especially when symptoms are moderate to severe. It may be helpful to allow some flexibility in the setup of the workspace. Providing hourly goals may help establish pace of work. A workstation that is not in close proximity to coworkers may decrease anxiety and distractibility. Last, flexible scheduling should be offered to accommodate medication management and CBT appointments.

Costs of OCD

In 1990, the total costs of OCD were estimated to be $8.4 billion, which was 5.7 percent of the estimated costs of all mental illnesses combined for that year ($147.8 billion) (Dupont et al., 1995). Another study reports that the projected direct cost of OCD treatment is $5 billion per year (Hollander et al., 1997). Lost wages and underemployment are large contributors to the economic costs of OCD. More current research is needed about the economic impact of OCD. In regards to quality of life, individuals with OCD have dysfunction in all areas. Hollander et al. (1997) reported that more than half of people with OCD experience moderate to severe impairment in family and social relationships and ability to study or work.

Schizophrenia

In 1896, Emil Kraepelin provided the first descriptions of the disease known today as schizophrenia (Wyatt, 2001). After decades of studying the mentally ill, Kraepelin began to categorize individuals by their course of symptoms. He used the term *dementia praecox* to describe individuals whose psychotic symptoms began early in life and continued on a deteriorating course (Wyatt, 2001). In 1911, Eugen Bleuler coined the term *schizophrenia* for the illness that Kraepelin called dementia praecox, because he thought it was a more fitting description of the illness. The word schizophrenia means a splitting (schizo) of the mind (phrenia), and not a split personality, which is a common public misperception about the illness (Wyatt, 2001).

Early treatments for schizophrenia such as hypoglycemic coma, seizure therapy, and frontal lobotomies were typically unsuccessful and even harmful for the patient. Schizophrenia treatment was revolutionized in the early 1950s with the introduction of the first antipsychotic agent, chlorpromazine (Thorazine), allowing many patients to be treated in the communities instead of in hospitals (Siegfreid et al., 2001). In the early 1990s, pharmacotherapy entered another more promising phase with the introduction of the first atypical antipsychotic agent, clozapine. New antipsychotics continue to be developed, broadening the treatment options for schizophrenia.

Epidemiology and Course of Illness

The ECA study found the annual prevalence rate for schizophrenia to be about 1.3 percent of the population (Robins & Reiger, 1991), translating into about 2.2 million people in the United States. The incidence rate is similar across diverse geographical, cultural, and socioeconomic categories. The onset of schizophrenia can be gradual or sudden, but many individuals display signs that something is wrong (e.g., decreased sociality, withdrawal, anxiety, depression, unusual behavior, problems at school or work) before actual psychotic symptoms are apparent (Larson et al., 2010). The age of onset is typically adolescence to early adulthood, with men typically having an earlier onset than women. It is unusual to develop schizophrenia after the age of 40 (McEvoy et al., 1999). Earlier onset is associated with poorer outcomes, which may be attributed to the loss of age-appropriate milestones in the areas of education, interpersonal relationships, and employment (Lay et al., 2000). The course of schizophrenia is often chronic and disabling. Individuals may have periods of acute psychosis alternating with periods of symptom remission or a constant level of residual symptoms that can greatly impair functioning.

Schizophrenia is primarily a problem of brain functionality rather than brain structure. While the role of dopamine imbalance has been well documented, other neurotransmitters appear to be involved in schizophrenia as well, including serotonin, acetylcholine, norepinephrine, glutamate, and GABA. While the causes of schizophrenia are unknown, scientists believe it is a combination of genetic predisposition and environmental factors that most likely occur in utero during the development of the brain. Psychosocial stressors such as living in an urban area and dysfunctional family communication may also play a role (Tsuang, 2000).

Symptoms

The two main categories of symptoms in schizophrenia are positive symptoms and negative symptoms. The term *positive* refers to occurrences that are added to one's ordinary experience, while the term *negative* refers to aspects of life that are taken away from one's ordinary experience.

Positive Symptoms

Positive symptoms include hallucinations, delusions, disorganized speech, and disorganized or catatonic behavior. Hallucinations can occur in all sensory modalities, but the most common are auditory. Auditory hallucinations are usually in the form of voices. A voice may provide a running commentary on a person's actions or thoughts; there may be two or more voices talking to each other or a single voice that commands a person to do things such as pray out loud or hide in the basement.

Delusions are false beliefs and may take on a bizarre quality such as believing one is from another planet or that one has two heads. Common categories of delusions include the following:

- Paranoid (believing one is being tracked by the CIA, is the victim of a communist plot, etc.)
- Grandiose (believing one is the president, a rock star, a religious prophet, etc.)

- Referential (believing that a song on the radio or popular novel is about oneself, etc.)
- Thought broadcasting (believing that one's thoughts are broadcasting out loud so that others can hear them)
- Somatic (believing one's teeth are soft or loose, that one's body is shrinking, etc.)

Negative Symptoms

Negative symptoms include flat affect (facial expressions of emotion are absent), alogia or poverty of speech (fluency and amount of speech are markedly reduced), avolition or lack of motivation or drive (decreased ability to initiate and continue goal-directed behaviors, little interest in any activity), anhedonia (loss of ability to feel pleasure, emptiness), anergia (lack of energy), and asociality (social isolation and withdrawal).

Associated Symptoms or Features

Other symptoms often found in schizophrenia include cognitive dysfunction (e.g., impaired memory, executive functioning, concentration, abstract thinking, etc.), inappropriate affect, dysphoric or depressed mood, anxiety, odd psychomotor activities (e.g., rocking, pacing), odd mannerisms or behaviors, lack of interest in eating and/or food refusal, and sleep disturbances (APA, 2013). Common comorbid conditions include substance abuse, depression, panic disorder, OCD, and post-traumatic stress disorder (Buckley et al., 2009). It is important to note that treatment noncompliance is very common and further complicates the clinical picture of schizophrenia.

Treatment Phases of Schizophrenia

There is no cure for schizophrenia. Treatment involves a broad range of interventions, both pharmacotherapy and psychosocial, designed to reduce the frequency and severity of symptoms and to improve functioning. The American Psychiatric Association has established treatment guidelines for schizophrenia (APA, 2004) and has conceptualized the treatment of schizophrenia into three phases: (1) acute phase, (2) stabilization phase, and (3) stable phase.

The acute phase is characterized by florid psychosis, where an individual has severe delusions, hallucinations, negative symptoms, and disorganized thinking. Individuals in this stage are often unable to care for themselves and may be violent, homicidal, or suicidal. The goals of treatment during the acute phase are to reduce the acute symptoms and improve functioning. Clients should receive care in the least restricted environment that will preserve safety and allow for effective treatment. Treatment should include the implementation of antipsychotic medication, as well as nonpharmacological treatments aimed at reducing stress and overstimulation and establishing a therapeutic relationship between the client and treatment team. Psychoeducation about schizophrenia should be provided at this phase to both clients and their families.

The stabilization phase typically lasts 6 months or more after the onset of the acute episode. Although the severity of the psychotic symptoms is reduced, symptoms are still present and can fluctuate in intensity. Functioning is improved, but some impairment remains. Treatment goals during the stabilization phase include minimizing stress, minimizing the likelihood of relapse, improving community functioning, and continued reduction of symptoms. During this phase, it is important to provide clients with psychoeducation regarding the importance of medication in reducing relapse. Pharmacologic interventions include the continued use of antipsychotics and other agents to reduce symptoms and relapse. The APA expressly discourages the reduction in dose or discontinuation of effective medications for at least 6 months after the resolution of the acute phase (APA, 2004). Psychotherapeutic interventions include psychoeducation about the course of illness, medication self-management skills, symptom self-management skills, and relapse prevention (APA, 2004).

The stable phase is characterized by relatively stable symptoms that are less severe than those experienced during the acute phase. Residual symptoms may be more nonpsychotic in nature, such as circumstantial thoughts or speech, overvalued ideas rather than delusions, and mild to moderate negative symptoms. Treatment goals during the stable phase include optimizing functioning and quality of life, minimizing the risk of relapse, and monitoring for medication side effects. Continuing antipsychotic treatment can reduce the relapse rate to less than 30 percent per year (APA, 2004). Pharmacologic interventions include maintenance therapy of effective medications (antipsychotics and others) while minimizing medication side effects. Nonpharmacological interventions include family interventions, supported employment, assertive community treatment, social skills training, relapse prevention education, and CBT (APA, 2004).

Treatment Refractory Schizophrenia

Treatment refractory schizophrenia remains a challenge to treat in the field of psychiatry. Around 10 to 30 percent of people with schizophrenia have little to no response to antipsychotic treatment and up to 30 percent of people only have a partial response (APA, 2004). The criteria for treatment refractory schizophrenia are as follows: (1) persistent, moderately severe, positive symptoms; (2) at least a moderately severe illness overall; (3) poor social/occupational functioning during the last 5 years; and (4) drug refractory, that is, lack of improvement on at least two conventional antipsychotics (Kane et al., 1988). Treatment refractory individuals are often highly symptomatic, with higher rates of service use and rehospitalization. Strategies for treating refractory schizophrenia include a trial of clozapine, adjunctive medications, higher antipsychotic dosing, ECT, CBT, and cognitive remediation (APA, 2004; APA, 2009).

Pharmacotherapy

Antipsychotics

First generation or conventional antipsychotics include perphenazine, haloperidol, loxapine, and pimozide. Second generation or atypical antipsychotics include clozapine, olanzapine, risperidone, ziprasidone, quetiapine, aripiprazole, and lurasidone. Conventional antipsychotics are associated with troublesome and serious side effects such as tardive dyskinesia (abnormal, involuntary movements commonly of the mouth, face, or extremities) and extrapyramidal symptoms (restlessness, tremors, muscle contractions, and rigidity). Common side effects associated with the use of atypicals include drowsiness/sedation, dry mouth, constipation, dizziness, orthostatic hypotension, nausea, extrapyramidal symptoms (but reduced in comparison with conventional antipsychotics), weight gain, and metabolic effects. Since their introduction, atypical antipsychotics have been recommended over conventional antipsychotics due to their decreased risk of tardive dyskinesia and extrapyramidal symptoms. However, there has been some debate about this recommendation due to some evidence of comparable efficacy with conventional antipsychotics and the serious metabolic side effects that can occur with atypical antipsychotics (APA, 2009).

The good news is that research continues into the development of effective antipsychotic treatment with tolerable side effects.

Adjunctive Medications

Commonly prescribed adjunctive medications in schizophrenia include anticonvulsants or mood stabilizers, antidepressants, benzodiazepines, and anticholinergics. Polypharmacy is becoming increasingly common, where a second antipsychotic is added with the goal of a greater or more rapid therapeutic response. When polypharmacy is in use, it is increasingly important to regularly monitor clinical response, as well as side effects (Barnes & Paton, 2011).

Anticonvulsants/Mood Stabilizers

Commonly prescribed anticonvulsants/mood stabilizers include valproate, carbamazepine, and lithium. These agents have shown some evidence of augmenting antipsychotic response, improving mood, and reducing agitation, hostility, and irritability (Citrome et al., 2004; Sajatovic et al., 2008). Anticonvulsants are generally well-tolerated agents. Carbamazepine may interact with other drugs, including reducing the serum levels of antipsychotics and benzodiazepines. Common side effects of anticonvulsants include neurological symptoms (e.g., double vision, blurred vision, fatigue) and gastrointestinal distress (e.g., nausea, indigestion, vomiting, and diarrhea) (Keck & McElroy, 1998).

Antidepressants

Depressive symptoms are common in schizophrenia. Estimates of the prevalence of depression in this population range from 7 to 65 percent (Bartles & Drake, 1988; DeLisis, 1990). Antidepressants are indicated when the depressive symptoms are severe, causing significant distress, or are interfering with functioning (APA, 2004). SSRIs may increase the serum concentrations of certain antipsychotics. Common side effects of SSRIs include gastrointestinal distress, insomnia/agitation, sexual side effects, headaches, extrapyramidal side effects, effects on weight, falls, serotonin syndrome, and discontinuation syndrome (APA, 2010).

Benzodiazepines

Benzodiazepines (e.g., lorazepam, diazepam, clonazepam, etc.) are often implemented during acute psychosis and may be continued in the stabilization phase. Benzodiazepines are used to treat sleep disturbances, anxiety, agitation, and catatonia (APA, 2004). Additionally, patients with certain motor disturbances, such as akathisia, may show improvement with the use of benzodiazepines (Siegfreid et al., 2001). Generally, benzodiazepines have few drug interactions. Common side effects of benzodiazepines include sedation, drowsiness, and risk of dependence (APA, 2004).

Anticholinergics

Anticholinergic medications (e.g., benzotropine mesylate, trihexyphenidyl hydrochloride, amantadine, etc.) are used to prevent and treat extrapyramidal side effects. It is commonly necessary to use anticholinergics in individuals that are prescribed conventional agents. The use of these agents should be reconsidered whenever a change in the antipsychotic dosage is made, as lower dosages may have reduced side effects (APA, 2004). Anticholinergics generally do not interact with other drugs. Side effects of anticholinergics include dry mouth, dry eyes, urinary retention, constipation, and memory disturbances (APA, 2004).

Vocational Impact of Schizophrenia

Employment is a critical aspect of reintegration into the community. In recent years, the importance of employment among individuals with schizophrenia has received renewed interest, and more supported employment programs are available. However, most people with severe and persistent mental illness remained unemployed. The National Alliance on the Mentally Ill (NAMI) reports that the employment rates for people with mental illness dropped from 23 percent in 2003 to 17.8 percent in 2012 (NAMI, 2014). There are many factors that contribute to such low rates of employment, including residual positive and negative symptoms, interpersonal skills deficits, cognitive impairments, relapse, lack of appropriate vocational programs, and stigma. However, the benefits of paid employment are far reaching, including an association with total symptom improvement, improvement in cognitive and negative symptoms, lower rates of hospitalization, and decreased rates of emotional discomfort (Bell et al., 1996; Bio & Gattaz, 2011). A study investigating the effects of paid work in individuals with schizophrenia found improvements in quality of life including increased motivation, sense of purpose, and empathy and decreased anhedonia (Bryson, Lysaker, & Bell, 2002).

Functional Limitations and Reasonable Accommodations

Functional limitations will vary according to the individual based on differences in symptoms (both severity and domain) and effective coping strategies. Positive symptoms can make it difficult for clients to concentrate, handle stress, and interact with others. Negative symptoms can result in lack of motivation and energy, difficulty with initiating and completing a work task, and impaired social skills. Cognitive symptoms have a negative impact on concentration, attention, memory, and ability to problem solve or learn new information. Additionally, cognitive symptoms can cause difficulties in a client's ability to prioritize, filter out irrelevant information, and function socially.

Reasonable accommodations for clients with schizophrenia will vary according to individual needs and may change over time. Typically accommodations are not costly, as they are not usually structural. Common reasonable accommodations for people with psychiatric disabilities include the following (MacDonald-Wilson et al., 2002):

- Flexible scheduling
- Job modification or restructuring
- Facilitating communication on the job
- Modifying employee training
- Providing training to staff or supervisors
- Modifying supervision
- Making policy changes
- Modifying the physical environment or providing special equipment
- Changing work procedures

Vocational Programs

Vocational program models include clubhouse programs, transitional employment, agency-sponsored or consumer-operated businesses, and supported employment. Supported employment has the most evidence as an effective employment strategy (Bond et al., 1997; Cook et al., 2005, 2008). Cook et al. (2008) found that people with schizophrenia who were enrolled in supportive employment had even better outcomes than people with other diagnoses in the control condition group. This is noteworthy given that at baseline, the schizophrenia group had more symptoms, more hospitalizations, lower education, earlier onsets, poorer work histories, and lower work motivation than the non-schizophrenia group. The basic tenet of supported employment is that any client can hold a job in the competitive workforce if provided the proper supports. Important features of supported employment include integration with treatment; client choice; ongoing, time-unlimited supports on- or offsite; and integrated settings.

Costs of Schizophrenia

In 2002, the overall U.S. cost of schizophrenia was estimated at $62.7 billion, with $22.7 billion in direct health care costs (Wu et al., 2005). Improving medication adherence could reduce the economic burden of schizophrenia by decreasing the rates of symptom relapse, rehospitalization, and overall need for services. The Clinical Antipsychotic Trials of Intervention Effectiveness (CATIE) found that 74 percent of patients had discontinued their medication within 18 months due to efficacy, side effects, or other reasons (Lieberman et al., 2005).

A review of 22 studies found that in most cases, the atypical antipsychotics were at least cost-neutral and may be cost-effective when compared with conventional agents (Hudson et al., 2003). However, the CATIE trial found similar efficacy of a conventional antipsychotic (perphenazine) with several atypical antipsychotics (risperidone, ziprasidone, quetiapine) (Lieberman et al., 2005). In this study, one atypical antipsychotic (olanzapine) did have better outcomes in terms of efficacy than the conventional agent. Since these studies were published, several atypical antipsychotics are now available as generics, which significantly reduces their costs. A study investigating cost-effectiveness of one of the newer atypical antipsychotics (lurasidone) found lurasidone to be more cost-effective than generic risperidone due to less hospitalizations and minimal cardiometabolic effects (O'Day et al., 2013). Clearly, more investigation is needed to better quantify the cost-effectiveness, efficacy, and quality-of-life benefits of the atypical antipsychotics in comparison with each other and the older agents.

Case Study

John is a 23-year-old single man who was diagnosed with schizophrenia at the age of 18. He has been hospitalized twice and attempted suicide at the age of 20. His primary symptoms include auditory hallucinations and delusions. The voices he hears often instruct him to do things such as "Don't go outside!" or "Don't eat that food, it's poisoned!" His delusions are mostly of a paranoid nature. He believes that he is monitored by the CIA through a chip implanted in his ear. When he walks down the street, he feels like others are staring at him. Sometimes he thinks that people are speaking in code about him at the supermarket. John also has a lack of motivation and drive. On a bad day, he stays on the couch for hours, barely moving. He sometimes has difficulty keeping up his hygiene. John often has trouble with his concentration and memory. To overcome this, he carries a small notebook with him everywhere he goes to remind him of things he needs to do such as appointments, grocery shopping, and laundry.

John takes many medications on a daily basis and requires the use of a medication organization box to keep track of them. Despite this, sometimes he still forgets his medication. John occasionally has delusions about his medications, believing that they are poisoned or hurting his body in some way.

Table 15.1 Example Life Care Plan

Medication/Supply Needs			
Medication/ Supply	*Age/Year Initiated*	*Age/Year Discontinued*	*Cost per Month*
Antipsychotic	18/2011	Lifetime	Generic = $10–$150/ month Brand name = $600–$1,100/month
Anticonvulsant/ mood stabilizer	23/2016	May be lifetime	Generic = $10–$200/ month Lab costs = $100–$200/lab
Antidepressant	20/2013	Minimum 9 months, then reevaluate	Generic = $5–$75/ month Brand name = $200–$300/month
Benzodiazepine	18/2011 20/2013	19/2012 21/2014 May be needed again if symptom relapse or rehospitalization occurs	Generic = $5–$30/ month
Anticholinergic	In conjunction with conventional antipsychotic, possibly with atypical antipsychotic	Unknown, dependent on symptoms	Generic = $5–$30/ month
Medication organizer	Age of onset	Lifetime	Nominal (about $5–$10); replace as needed
Acute and Facility Care			
Facility Description	*Description/Purpose*	*Length of Treatment*	*Costs per Day*
Hospitalization	Inpatient treatment; indicated if individual is a threat to himself or others; initiate medications and provide stabilization	Expect 1–2 weeks for stabilization; additional hospitalizations may be indicated in future	$700+/day

(Continued)

Table 15.1 (Continued) Example Life Care Plan

Option 1 Residential treatment	Supervised housing + day treatment; indicated if individual is unable to complete Activities of Daily Living (including taking medications as prescribed) without high level of assistance	Expect 1–6 months+, depending on symptoms; additional residential treatment may be indicated in the future	$230+/day
Option 2 Partial hospitalization/ day treatment	Day treatment; does not include housing; indicated if individual needs increased daily structure	Expect 1–6 months+, depending on symptoms; additional partial hospitalization may be indicated in the future	$100+/day
Option 3 Independent Living with Case Management	Live independently but in treatment center housing; includes medication management and case management	Expect 1–6 months+, depending on symptoms; additional independent living may be indicated in the future	$160+/day
Option 4 Group home	Living quarters and meals; no treatment provided	Expect 1–6 months+, depending on level of stabilization, may transition to living with a roommate without additional support services	$45+/day

He sees his psychiatrist once a month for medication management. He also attends individual and group therapy once a week. John has received social skills training, psychoeducation, and vocational counseling in the past. He lives independently with a roommate. Previously, he lived in a group home.

Although he had his first break at 18, John did complete high school. He has not had any other formal education. His work history is sporadic, with long periods of unemployment. He has worked as a grocery bagger, stocker, fast-food worker, pizza deliverer, and landscaper. He has morning sedation from his medications and is often late if he has to be at work before 11:00 a.m. His chronic lateness resulted in several job terminations. John is currently unemployed but wants to work. He wants to try vocational counseling again because he is having a hard time finding a job on his own.

John receives Social Security Disability Insurance (SSDI) payments and has Medicare. His parents also contribute substantially to his living costs. John's parents want funds set up for when they are deceased, so that John will continue to receive appropriate treatment. They want to hire a life care planner to help them create these plans. Table 15.1 provides a sample life care plan for schizophrenia based on the format published in Deutsch & Sawyer (2004).

Table 15.2 Life Care Plan Checklist for Mental Illness

- *Psychotherapeutic Interventions*: What types of therapy will be needed? Are there family or marriage issues that need to be addressed? How complex is the treatment plan? Will a case manager be needed to coordinate care? Are support groups available? Is substance abuse present? If so, what treatments will be needed?
- *Diagnostic Testing*: Often other illnesses need to be ruled out before a diagnosis of mental illness is made, especially in cases where symptoms might overlap with brain abnormalities (e.g., tumors). What tests are needed to rule out other illnesses? Will a psychological battery be needed? What level of education has the individual completed? Is separate educational testing needed as well?
- *Medication/Supply Needs*: Medication regimens can consist of multiple medications at various dosages. Some require blood serum monitoring, which will add to the overall cost. What medications are indicated (including daily dosages and how supplied)? Are they available in generic?
- *Routine Medical Care*: How often will the individual need to see a psychiatrist? In what kind of treatment setting will medication management take place? Will there be regular monitoring by other staff such as nurses? comorbid conditions are common in people with mental illness. Will annual health checks be performed by medical personal, including laboratory assessments?
- *Acute and Facility Care*: Is the illness at an acute stage where inpatient treatment is required? What is the expected course of illness? Are multiple hospitalizations likely? What impact do symptoms have on functioning? Is family present in the individual's life? Is the individual capable of independent living? If not, what level of support is required?
- *Vocational/Education Plan*: What is the individual's work history? What vocational services are offered in his/her geographical area? Has vocational potential been assessed? What are the costs of supported employment?

Conclusion

It is important to understand the complexity of mental illness when creating a life care plan. Factors to consider include the expected course of illness, chronicity of symptoms, and response to treatment. The most costly treatment modality is hospitalization. Individuals with a chronic, disabling course of illness may require multiple hospitalizations or longer-term stays. Treatment nonadherence is a major issue to consider, given that it is a widespread phenomenon and is associated with poorer outcomes and higher costs.

Despite the differences among various mental illnesses in symptoms, treatment, and degree of disability, there are common areas to consider when creating a life care plan for this population. The checklist provided in Table 15.2 can help the life care planner cover the various areas required to create a plan for individuals with mental illness. Given the high costs of mental illness in both direct costs and quality-of-life issues, life care planning is definitely a needed but untapped resource.

References

American College of Occupational and Environmental Medicine. 2002. *ACOEM Evidence-Based Statement, A Screening Program for Depression. Retrieved May 12, 2003, from* www.acoem.org/guidelines/ article.asp?ID=54.

American Psychiatric Association. 2002. *Practice Guidelines for the Treatment of Patients with Bipolar Disorder.* Washington, DC: Author.

American Psychiatric Association. 2004. *Practice Guidelines for the Treatment of Schizophrenia* (2nd ed.). Washington, DC: Author.

American Psychiatric Association. 2007. *Practice Guideline for the Treatment of Patients with Obsessive-Compulsive Disorder.* Arlington, VA: Author.

American Psychiatric Association. 2009. *Guideline Watch (September 2009): Practice Guideline for the Treatment of Patients with Schizophrenia.* Washington, DC: Author.

American Psychiatric Association. 2010. *Practice Guidelines for the Treatment of Patients with Major Depressive Disorder.* Washington, DC: Author.

American Psychiatric Association. 2013. *Diagnostic and Statistical Manual of Mental Disorders* (5th ed.). Washington, DC: Author.

Barnes, T. R., & Paton, C. 2011. Antipsychotic polypharmacy in schizophrenia: Benefits and risks. *CNS Drugs, 25*(5), 383–399.

Bartles, S. J., & Drake, R. E. 1988. Depressive symptoms in schizophrenia: Comprehensive differential diagnosis. *Comprehensive Psychiatry, 29*, 467–483.

Bell, M. D., Lysaker, P. H., & Milstein, R. M. 1996. Clinical benefits of paid work activity in schizophrenia. *Schizophrenia Bulletin, 22*, 51–67.

Benard, V., Vaiva, G., Masson, M., & Geoffroy, P. A. 2016. Lithium and suicide prevention in bipolar disorder. *Encephale, Epub ahead of print.* Retrieved on May 4, 2016 at http://www.ncbi.nlm.nih.gov/pubmed/27000268.

Bergeson, J. G., Jing, Y., Forbes, R. A. et al. 2012. Medical care costs and hospitalization in patients with bipolar disorder treated with atypical antipsychotics. *American Health Drug Benefits, 5*(6), 379–386.

Bio, D. S., & Gattaz, W. F. 2011. Vocational rehabilitation improves cognition and negative symptoms in schizophrenia. *Schizophrenia Research, 126*(1–3), 265–269.

Bond, G. R., Drake, R. E., Mueser, K. T., & Becker, D. R. 1997. An update on supported employment for people with severe mental illness. *Psychiatric Services, 48*, 335–346.

Boshen, M. J., Drummond, L. M., & Pillay, A. 2008. Treatment of severe, treatment-refractory obsessive-compulsive disorder. *CNS Spectrums, 13*(12), 1056–1065.

Bowden, C. L. 1996. Rapid cycling among bipolar patients. *Primary Psychiatry, 3*, 40.

Bryant-Comstock, L., Stender, M., & Devercelli, G. 2002. Health care utilization and costs among privately insured patients with bipolar I disorder. *Bipolar Disorder, 4*, 398–405.

Bryson, G., Lysaker, P., & Bell, M. 2002. Quality of life benefits of paid work activity in schizophrenia. *Schizophrenia Bulletin, 28*, 249–257.

Buckley, P. F., Miller, B. J., Lehrer, D. S., & Castle, D. J. 2009. Psychiatric comorbidities and schizophrenia. *Schizophrenia Bulletin, 35*(2), 383–402.

Burcusa, S. L., & Iacono, W. G. 2007. Risk for recurrence in depression. *Clinical Psychology Review, 27*(8), 959–985.

Cade, J. F. 1999. Lithium salts in the treatment of psychotic excitement. *Australian and New England Journal of Psychiatry, 33*, 615–618.

Center for Behavioral Health Statistics and Quality. 2015. *Behavioral health trends in the United States: Results from the 2014 National Survey on Drug Use and Health (HHS Publication No. SMA 15-4927, NSDUH Series H-20).* Retrieved on April 22, 2016 from http://www.samhsa.gov/data.

Citrome, L., Casey, D. E., Daniel, D. G. et al. 2004. Adjunctive divalproex and hostility among patients with schizophrenia receiving olanzapine or risperidone. *Psychiatric Services, 55*, 290–294.

Cook, J. A., Blyler, C. R., Burke-Miller, J. K. et al. 2008. Effectiveness of supported employment for individuals with schizophrenia: Results of a multi-site, randomized trial. *Clinical Schizophrenia & Related Psychosis, 2*, 37–46.

Cook, J. A., Leff, H. S., Blyler, C. R. et al. 2005. Results of a multisite randomized trial of supported employment interventions for individuals with severe mental illness. *Archives of General Psychiatry, 62*, 505–512.

DeLisis, L. E. 1990. *Depression in Schizophrenia.* Washington, DC: American Psychiatric Press.

Denys, D., Zohar, J., & Westenberg, H. G. 2004. The role of dopamine in obsessive-compulsive disorder: Preclinical and clinical evidence. *Journal of Clinical Psychiatry*, *65*, 11–17.

Deutsch, P., & Sawyer, H. 2004. *Guide to Rehabilitation*. New York, NY: Ahab Press.

DuPont, R. L., Rice, D. P., Shiraki, S., & Rowland, C. R. 1995. Economic costs of obsessive-compulsive disorder. *Medicine Interface*, *8*, 102–109.

Ferrari, A. J., Charlson, F. J., Norman, R. E. et al. 2013. Burden of depressive disorders by country, sex, age, and year: Findings from the global burden of disease study 2010. *PLOS Medicine*, *10*(11), e1001547. Retrieved April 22, 2016 at http://journals.plos.org/plosmedicine/article?id=10.1371/journal.pubmed.1001547.

Fischler, G., & Booth, N. 1999. *Vocational Impact of Psychiatric Disorders*. Gaithersburg, MD: Aspen Publishers.

Goodwin, F. K., & Jamison, K. R. 1990. *Manic-Depressive Illness*. New York, NY: Oxford University Press.

Greenberg, P. E., Fournier, A., Sisitsky, T., Pike, C. T., & Kessler, R. C. 2015. The economic burden of adults with major depressive disorder in the United States (2005 and 2010). *Journal of Clinical Psychiatry*, *76*(2), 155–162.

Gutman, D. A., & Nemeroff, C. 2007. Atypical antipsychotics in bipolar disorder. In Pharmacologic Management of Mania and Depression in Bipolar Disorder. Retrieved April 27, 2008, from www.medscape.com/viewprogram/6870_pnt.

Hasin, D. S., Goodwin, R. D., Stinson, F. S., & Grant, B. F. 2005. Epidemiology of major depressive disorder: Results from the national epidemiologic survey on alcoholism and related conditions. *Archives of General Psychiatry*, *62*, 1097–1106.

Hilligoss, N. 2003. Life care planning for people with severe and persistent mental illness: An overlooked practice setting? *Journal of Life Care Planning*, *2*, 56–72.

Hirschfeld, R. M. 2005. *Guideline Watch: Practice Guideline for the Treatment of Patients with Bipolar Disorder*. Arlington, VA: American Psychiatric Association. Retrieved on May 1, 2016 at http://www.psych.org/psych_pract/treatg/pg/pract_guide.cfm.

Hirschfeld, R. M., Lewis, L., & Vornik, L. A. 2003. Perceptions and impact of bipolar disorder: How far have we really come? Results of the National Depressive and Manic-Depressive Association 2000 survey of individuals with bipolar disorder. *Journal of Clinical Psychiatry*, *64*, 161–174.

Hollander, E., Stein, D. J., Kwon, J. H. et al. 1997. Psychosocial function and economic costs of obsessive-compulsive disorder. *CNS Spectrums*, *3*(S1), 48–58.

Hudson, T. J., Sullivan, G., Feng, W., Owen, R. R., & Thrush, C. R. 2003. Economic evaluations of novel antipsychotic medications: A literature review. *Schizophrenia Research*, *60*, 199–218.

Jefferson, J. W., Greist, J. H., Archerman, D. L., & Carroll, J. A. 1987. *Lithium Encyclopedia for Clinical Practice* (2nd ed.). Washington, DC: American Psychiatric Press.

Kane, J. M., Honigfeld, G., Singer, J., & Meltzer, H. 1988. Clozapine for the treatment-resistant schizophrenic. *Archives of General Psychiatry*, *45*, 789–796.

Keck, P. E., & McElroy, S. L. 1998. Antiepileptic drugs. In A. F. Schatzberg & C. B. Nemeroff (Eds.), *Textbook of Psychopharmacology* (2nd ed., Chap. 21). Washington, DC: American Psychiatric Press.

Kessler, R. C., Berglund, P., Demler, O. et al. 2005a. Lifetime prevalence and age-of-onset distributions of DSM-IV disorders in the national comorbidity survey replication. *Archives of General Psychiatry*, *62*(6), 5913–602.

Kessler, R. C., Chiu, W. T., Demler, O., & Walters, E. E. 2005b. Prevalence, severity, and comorbidity of 12-month DSM-IV disorders in the national comorbidity survey replication. *Archives of General Psychiatry*, *62*, 617–627.

Keller, M. B., Trivedi, M. H., Thase, M. E. et al. 2007. The prevention of recurrent episodes of depression with venlafaxine for two years (PREVENT) study: Outcomes from the 2-year and combined maintenance phases. *Journal of Clinical Psychiatry*, *8*, 1246–1256.

Kleinman, L., Lowin, A., Flood, E. et al. 2003. Costs of bipolar disorder. *Pharmacoeconomics*, *21*(9), 601–622.

Larson, M. K., Walker, E. F., & Compton, M. T. 2010. Early signs, diagnosis and therapeutics of the prodromal phase of schizophrenia and related psychotic disorders. *Expert Review of Neurotherapeutics*, *10*(8), 1347–1359.

Lay, B., Blanz, B., Hartmann, M., & Schmidt, M. H. 2000. The psychosocial outcome of adolescent-onset schizophrenia: A 12-year follow up. *Schizophrenia Bulletin*, *26*(4), 801–806.

Lenox, R. H., & Husseini, K. M. 1998. Lithium. In A. F. Schatzberg & C. B. Nemeroff (Eds.), *Textbook of Psychopharmacology* (2nd ed., Chap. 10). Washington, DC: American Psychiatric Press.

Li, J., McCombs, J. S., & Stimmel, G. L. 2002. Cost of treating bipolar disorder in the California Medicaid (Medi-Cal) program. *Journal of Affective Disorders*, *71*, 131–139.

Lieberman, J. A., Stroup, T. S., McEvoy, J. P. et al. 2005. Effectiveness of antipsychotic drugs in patients with chronic schizophrenia. *New England Journal of Medicine*, *353*, 1209–1223.

MacDonald-Wilson, K. L., Rogers, E. S., Massaro, J. M., Lyass, A., & Crean, T. 2002. An investigation of reasonable workplace accommodations for people with psychiatric disabilities: Quantitative findings from a multi-site study. *Community Mental Health Journal*, *38*(1), 35–50.

Manning, J. S., Haykal, R. F., Connor, P. D., & Akiskal, H. S. 1997. On the nature of depressive and anxious states in a family practice setting: The high prevalence of bipolar II and related disorders in a cohort followed longitudinally. *Comprehensive Psychiatry*, *38*, 102–108.

Marangell, L. B., Dennehy, E. B., Miyahara, S. et al. 2009. The functional impact of subsyndromal depressive symptoms in bipolar disorder: Data from STEP-BD. *Journal of Affective Disorders*, *114*(1–3), 58–67.

March, J. S., Frances, A., Carpenter, D., & Kahn, D. A. 1997. The expert consensus guidelines for the treatment of obsessive-compulsive disorder. *Journal of Clinical Psychiatry*, *58*, 2–72.

Marwaha, S., Durrani, A., & Singh, S. 2013. Employment outcomes for people with bipolar disorder: A systematic review. *Acta Psychiatrica Scandinavica*, *128*(3), 179–193.

McEvoy, J. P., Scheifler, P. L., & Frances, A. (Eds.). 1999. The expert consensus guideline series: Treatment of schizophrenia. *Journal of Clinical Psychiatry*, *60*, 3–80.

Mueller, T. I., Leon, A. C., Keller, K. B. et al. 1999. Recurrence after recovery from major depressive disorder during 15 years of observational follow-up. *American Journal of Psychiatry*, *156*, 1000–1006.

National Alliance on the Mentally Ill (NAMI). 2014. *Road to Recovery: Employment and Mental Illness*. Accessed on May 10, 2016 at https://www.nami.org/About-NAMI/Publications-Reports/Public-Policy-Reports/RoadtoRecovery.pdf.

O'Day, K., Rajagopalan, K., Meyer, K., Pikalov, A., & Loebel, A. 2013. Long-term effectiveness of atypical antipsychotics in the treatment of adults with schizophrenia in the U.S. *Clinicoeconomics Outcomes Research*, *5*, 459–470.

Pagnin, D., Querioz, V., Pini, S., & Cassano, G. B. 2004. Efficacy of ECT in depression: A meta-analytic review. *Journal of ECT*, *20*, 13–20.

Pan, Y., Knapp, M., & McCrone, P. 2012. Cost-effectiveness comparisons between antidepressant treatments in depression: Evidence from database analyses and prospective studies. *Journal of Affective Disorders*, *139*, 113–125.

Papakostas, G. I., Shelton, R. C., Smith, J. et al. 2007. Augmentation of antidepressants with atypical antipsychotic medications for treatment-resistant major depressive disorder: A meta-analysis. *Journal of Clinical Psychiatry*, *68*, 826–831.

Pies, R. W. 1998. *Handbook of Essential Psychopharmacology*. Washington, DC: American Psychiatric Press.

Price, L. H., Charney, D. S., & Heninger, G. R. 1986. Variability of response to lithium augmentation in refractory depression. *American Journal of Psychiatry*, *143*, 1387–1392.

Robins, L. N., & Reiger, D. A. 1991. *Psychiatric Disorders in America: The Epidemiologic Catchment Study*. New York, NY: Free Press.

Romera, I., Perez, V., Ciudad, A. et al. 2013. Residual symptoms and functioning in depression, does the type of residual symptoms matter? A post-hoc analysis. *BMC Psychiatry*, *13*, 51.

Rush, A. J. 2003. Toward an understanding of bipolar disorder and its origin. *Journal of Clinical Psychiatry*, *64*, 4–8.

Sajatovic, M., Coconcea, N., Ignacio, R.V. et al. 2008. Adjunct extended-release valproate semisodium in late life schizophrenia. *International Journal of Geriatric Psychiatry*, *23*(2), 142–147.

Sanchez-Moreno, J., Martinez-Aran, A., Taberes-Seisdedos, R. et al. 2009. Functioning and disability in bipolar disorder: An extensive review. *Psychotherapy and Psychosomatics*, *78*, 285–297.

Shelton, R. C., Tollefson, G. D., Stahl, S. et al. 2001. A novel augmentation strategy for treating resistant major depression. *American Journal of Psychiatry*, *158*, 131–134.

Siegfreid, S. L., Fleischhacker, W., & Lieberman, J. A. 2001. Pharmacological treatment of schizophrenia. In J. A. Lieberman & R. M. Murray (Eds.), *Comprehensive Care of Schizophrenia* (Chap. 4). London: Martin Duntz.

Steadman, K., & Taskila, T. 2015. *Symptoms of Depression and Their Effects on Employment*. The Work Foundation. Accessed on April 26, 2016 at www.theworkfoundation.com/Assets/Docs/Reports/Symptoms20(short20version)%20FINAL.pdf.

Suppes, T., Kroger, H., Pikalov, A., & Loebel, A. 2016. Lurasidone adjunctive with lithium or valproate for bipolar depression: A placebo-controlled trial utilizing prospective and retrospective enrollment cohorts. *Journal of Psychiatric Research, 10*, 86–93.

Trivedi, M.H., Fava, M., Wisniewski, S. R. et al. 2006. Medication augmentation after the failure of SSRIs for depression. *New England Journal of Medicine, 354*, 1243–1252.

Tsuang, M. 2000. Schizophrenia: Genes and environment. *Biological Psychiatry, 47*(3), 210–220.

U.S. Burden of Disease Collaborators. 2013. The State of U.S. Health, 1990-2010: Burden of Diseases, Injuries, and Risk Factors. *JAMA, 310*(6), 591–606.

Vallarino, M., Henry, C., Etain, B. et al. 2015. An evidence map of psychosocial interventions for the earliest stages of bipolar disorder. *Lancet Psychiatry, 2*(6), 548–563.

Vasudev, K., Macritchie, K., Geddes, J., Watson, S., & Young, A. 2006. Topiramate for acute affective episodes in bipolar disorder. *Cochrane Database System Review, 25*, CD003384.

Wang, P. W., Santosa, C., Schumacher, M. et al. 2002. Gabapentin augmentation therapy in bipolar depression. *Bipolar Disorder, 4*, 296–301.

Weed, R. (Ed.). 1999. *Life Care Planning and Case Management Handbook*. Boca Raton, FL: CRC Press.

Weed, R., & Field, T. 2001. *The Rehabilitation Consultant's Handbook* (3rd ed.). Athens, GA: E&F Vocational Services.

Wu, E.Q., Bimbaum, H.G., Shi, L. et al. 2005. The economic burden of schizophrenia in 2002. *Journal of Clinical Psychiatry, 66*(9), 1122–1129.

Wyatt, R. J. 2001. Diagnosing schizophrenia. In J. A. Lieberman & R. M. Murray (Eds.), *Comprehensive Care of Schizophrenia* (Chap. 1). London: Martin Duntz.

Zaretsky, A. E., Segal, S. V., & Gemar, M. 1999. Cognitive therapy for bipolar depression: A pilot study. *Canadian Journal of Psychiatry, 44*, 491–494.

Chapter 16

Life Care Planning for People with Chronic Pain*

Denise D. Lester

Contents

Introduction 469
Diagnostic Efforts in Workup 472
Approaches to Management of Pain 474
Life Care Planning and Chronic Pain 481
Psychological Considerations 482
Additional Considerations for Chronic Pain Management 482
Determining Patient's Functioning Level 485
Life Care Planning and Chronic Pain and Future Concerns 485
Case Study 486
Life Care Plan 486
Conclusion 493
References 494

Introduction

Significant pain can be experienced as a result of a multitude of medical problems. *Chronic pain syndrome* refers to pain that lasts more than 6 months, worsens with time, and is associated with major comorbidities, especially psychological (McMahon & Koltzenburg, 2006). Multidisciplinary therapy is often required. The Institute of Medicine (IOM) recently estimated that more than 110 million adults, over one third of the population of the United States, experience some form of chronic pain, with the symptom of pain being the most common reason for people to consult a primary care physician. It has an associated annual economic cost of $560 to $635 billion, and

* This chapter is adapted in part, and reprinted with permission, of Ward, T., & Weed, R. (2004). Life care planning issues for chronic pain. In R. Weed (Ed.) *Life Care Planning and Case Management Handbook* (2nd ed., pp. 455–481). Boca Raton, FL: CRC Press.

is a leading cause of disability worldwide (Institute of Medicine Committee on Advancing Pain Research Care and Education Board on Health Sciences Policy, 2011; Vos et al., 2012).

The most common pain complaint is low back pain. Eighty percent of adults experience low back pain at some point in their lifetime. It is the most common cause of job-related disability and a leading contributor to missed work days.

Objective definitions of pain have eluded researchers (Weed, 1987). No pain literature available to these writers has been able to satisfactorily define pain objectively. Pain appears to be a subjective experience measured by self-report (Skinner, 1938; Merskey, 1964, 1972; Sternbach, 1968, 1974; Engel et al., 1970; Melzack, 1973; Fordyce, 1976; Shealy, 1976; Bresler, 1979; IASP, 1979; Ramsey, 1979). Research indicates that the pain threshold is similar from person to person and culture to culture, but pain tolerance can vary dramatically (Shealy, 1976). Sternbach (1968) has simply stated that "pain is a hurt we feel" (p. l). It is defined by the International Association for the Study of Pain (IASP) as "an unpleasant sensory and emotional experience associated with actual or potential tissue damage or described in terms of such damage."

The biopsychosocial approach model to the pain experience encourages the realization that pain is a complex perceptual experience modulated by a wide range of biopsychosocial factors, including emotions, social and environmental contexts, and cultural background, as well as beliefs, attitudes, and expectations. As painful experiences transition into a chronic phenomenon, these biopsychosocial abnormalities become permanent (Apfelbaum et al., 2012). In this model, chronic pain affects all facets of a person's environment, at great expense to the individual and society. This multimodal etiology of pain requires a multimodal therapeutic strategy by the life care planner to allow optimal cost-effective treatment outcomes.

Monitoring the severity and duration of pain through thorough pain assessment improves patient care. The subjective nature of pain explains the difficulty with measurement. The same standards should not be used to measure pain in all circumstances. Quality pain care requires optimizing pain assessment (Green et al., 2003a). Disability, depression, and pain-intensity issues often complicate pain assessment and treatment. Most pain assessment tools rarely address the role of social determinants despite evidence that age, race, ethnicity, gender, and socioeconomic status influence communication and pain. The literature describes racial and ethnic differences in the ability to discuss pain complaints and negotiate pain treatment plans with physicians. Women and racial and ethnic minorities are at risk for receiving poorer quality pain care than are men. Physicians were more verbally dominant, engaged in less patient-centered communication, used less rapport building, rated conditions as less severe (even when there were no differences), and provided less information in encounters with racial and ethnic minorities than they did with whites (Green et al., 2002; Green et al., 2003b). Patient-physician communication that encourages patients to ask questions and express concerns, as well as racial concordance, has been shown to reduce disparities (Ghods et al., 2008).

Alanmanou (2006) described an algorithmic approach to pain assessment varying from the basic interventional formal structured inventories. Pain tools are either unidimensional or multidimensional. The latter take into consideration the motivation and affective dimensions of pain and are typically used when there is (1) persistent acute pain, (2) mixed acute and chronic pain elements, (3) significant psychosocial dysfunction, (4) initial chronic pain evaluations, and (5) disability evaluation addressing the role of sickness impact. The psychological and emotional impact of chronic pain varies among individuals and is more readily assessed using multidimensional pain tools. This impact may be severe, resulting in depression/sense of hopelessness and disruption of family and social roles.

A brief listing of unidimensional and multidimensional pain measurement tools would include (Ramamurthy et al., 2006):

Unidimensional: Verbal Descriptor Scale, Visual Analogue Scale, Numerical Rating Scale, and Pain Relief Scale

Multidimensional: McGill Pain Questionnaire, Brief Pain Inventory, Dartmouth Pain Questionnaire, the Minnesota Multiphasic Personality Inventory, West-Haven–Yale Multidimensional Pain Inventory, and the Quebec Back Pain Disability Scale

For purposes of this chapter, chronic pain can be described as daily pain that has lasted anywhere from 6 months to 1 year after the original pain incident. Although there is controversy regarding definitions, most physicians agree that *acute pain* is from the date of onset to 1 month, *subacute pain* is defined as daily pain lasting from 1 to 6 months, and *chronic pain* can thereafter be defined as lasting 6 months or longer (Cleveland Clinic, 2017). The American Society of Anesthesiologists Task Force on Chronic Pain Management and The American Society of Regional Anesthesia and Pain Medicine published "Practice Guidelines for Chronic Pain Management" in 2010. Their definition of chronic pain was "*pain of any etiology not directly related to neoplastic involvement, associated with a chronic medical condition or extending in duration beyond the expected temporal boundary of tissue injury and normal healing, and adversely affecting the function or well-being of the individual*" (Practice Guidelines for Chronic Pain Management, 2010).

Chronic pain and the subsequent costs to society, however, do not necessarily include all individuals who have had pain of some type or another for longer than a year. In general, the diagnosis of chronic pain becomes broader as it includes the psychological stress and disruption to the everyday quality of life of individuals who suffer from it. Each year millions of people seek relief at hospitals or pain clinics. The overall cost in lost workdays, medical treatment, and additional psychological counseling from back pain diagnoses alone has been estimated at $25 billion (Moreo, 2003). Counting back pain, migraine and headache pain, osteoarthritis, rheumatoid arthritis, fibromyalgia, failed surgical fusion lumbar or cervical spine, reflex sympathetic dystrophy, causalgia, diabetic neuropathy, and cancer pain, estimates exceed over $40 billion annually.

The history of pain management dates back to the first known practicing doctors. It has been said that 80 percent of patient problems prompting a visit to a physician are the direct result of some form of pain—acute, subacute, or chronic. However, most recently, with the advent of chronic pain management programs, more comprehensive multidisciplinary team management for chronic pain and the associated disability/psychological stress/depression and subsequent functional loss have developed. Pain management centers are present in nearly every major metropolitan area in the United States. Pain management is a subspecialty recognized by the American Medical Association, and numerous societies offer continuing medical education, seminars, legislative lobbying assistance, and national boards of directors to oversee the problems associated with the disease state now classified as chronic pain. Beginning in 1911, workers' compensation laws were enacted to require employers to assume the cost of occupational disability without regard to fault (Weed & Field, 2012). These laws have dramatically altered the recovery of the individual injured in the workforce since that time. However, additional aspects involving litigation have become more prevalent in the last 20 to 30 years. Because of litigation, an adversarial role between the workplace and the injured worker often develops.

Also of interest are the recent aggressive efforts to reduce health care costs. Injured workers suffering chronic pain ailments are often given little, if any, direct assistance, and anecdotally it appears that legal assistance through litigation has become necessary to allow the patient to pursue more comprehensive treatment of his or her chronic pain condition. It can be said that if a patient truly has significant chronic pain, it will disrupt every aspect of his or her life. This includes vocational as well as avocational pursuits, sleep, and routine daily activities such as dressing, bathing, hygiene, and self-care. Exercise, relationships, sexual relationships, and financial stresses will all ensue. In this way, a comprehensive approach to the treatment of the chronic pain patient embodies all the aforementioned areas, as it focuses attention on restoring the patient to a level of independence to the extent that it is possible. The long-range goal is to achieve a degree of independence of the patient from the health provider.

Diagnostic Efforts in Workup

In 2010 the American Society of Anesthesiology Task Force on Chronic Pain Management and the American Society of Regional Anesthesia published "Practice Guidelines for Chronic Pain Management" (2010). This was an update for the "Practice Guidelines for Chronic Pain Management" adopted by the American Society of Anesthesiologists (ASA) in 1996 and published in 1997. The goals of the guidelines were to utilize the highest level of published scientific literature to:

1. Optimize pain control, recognizing that a pain-free state may not be attainable
2. Enhance functional abilities and physical and psychologic well-being
3. Enhance the quality of life of patients
4. Minimize adverse outcomes

The guidelines have two categories:

1. Patient Evaluation
2. Multimodal/Multidisciplinary Interventions

Completion of the patient evaluation is the primary essential step for patient's suffering from pain of 6 months duration or longer. This includes review of diagnostic evaluations, medical and psychological consultations, and laboratory, radiological, and surgical intervention. It is important to ensure that indeed the patient's diagnosis is one of a chronic painful disease rather than an untreated acute pain. In the latter, it is prudent to determine if all acceptable treatment options have been offered or failed before considering the palliative symptomatic management of a chronic painful illness. This is important because the pain pathways and pathophysiology of chronic pain is very different from acute pain, thus the acute pain signal could be alerting the patient that a serious consequence of tissue injury is imminent. An example would be the dilemma of the acute pain syndrome known as recurrent acute angina with the propensity for a myocardial infarction requiring extensive cardiac evaluation with each episode of crushing chest pain, versus the chronic pain syndrome known as chronic intractable angina, which has similar symptoms but is typically treated palliatively. The scope of diagnostic evaluations of the patient with chronic pain is quite large. Typically, diagnostic strategies will depend on the painful area to be evaluated but usually include detailed medical history (including medical record review of all previous evaluations of chronic painful disease and detailed medication history), detailed psychiatric/psychological history, comprehensive physical examination (including signs of nerve injury), laboratory review, radiological review (including magnetic resonance imaging, or MRI, of the affected area [note: MRI is not appropriate in all patients, for example, those with pacemakers and/or ferromagnetic foreign bodies]; computed tomography, or CT, scanning; plain-film X-rays; and/or myelograms), electromyographic muscle examinations, and nerve conduction velocity. Radiologic imaging can be overused and costly. The following diagram is an adaptation from Ramamurthy & Alvarado (2006) that simply outlines the use of radiographs in a cost-effective algorithm.

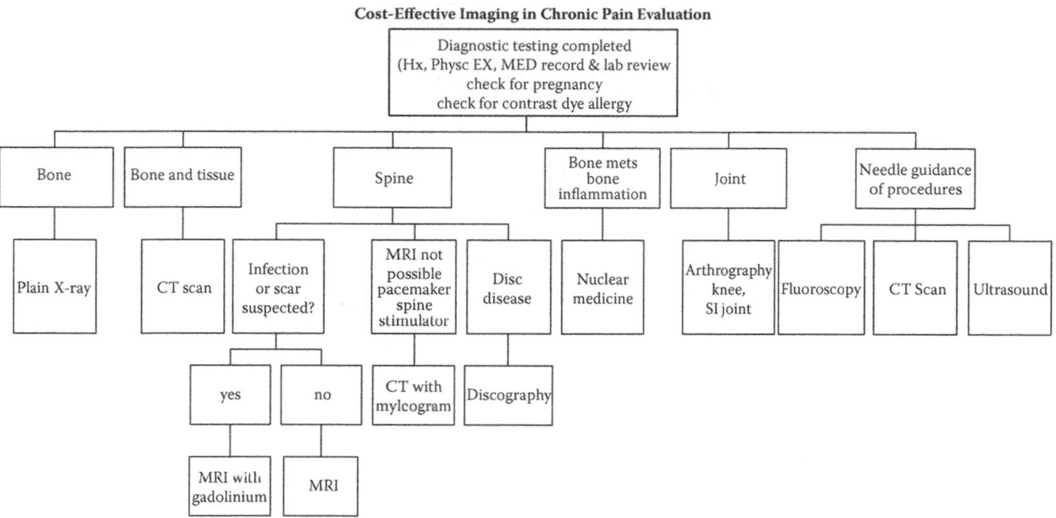

Often more invasive procedures will be necessary to support or refute a chronic painful diagnosis such as laparoscopic surgical evaluation or diagnostic spine injections (disc stimulation, facet joint nerve injections, nerve root injections) in the diagnosis of axial and radicular skeletal-related cervical, thoracic, or lumbar spine pain.

Occasionally multiple specialty consultations are required when differential diagnosis becomes elusive. An example of consulting during the diagnostic phase of care could include a psychologist for psychological testing (such as with the Minnesota Multiphasic Personality Inventory™ or other assistive testing), to determine a patient's psychological status as it pertains to his or her pain complaints. There are benefits of having several specialists evaluate the same patient. The overlap of clinical observations, including questionable symptom magnification with litigious patients with secondary gain in mind, will be noted from a variety of clinicians' vantage points. This would be helpful should questions arise regarding the authenticity of the patient's symptoms. It is sometimes difficult to show from the objective testing standpoint that pain has an organic cause that is immediately observable (Beecher, 1959). In these instances, chronic pain management specialists can add a further backdrop from which to define and further assess the patient's pain complaints. There are several sensory feedback loops to the central nervous system, including the sympathetic nervous system, bones, joints, ligaments, muscles, and, ultimately, the dermatomes of the peripheral nervous system. Despite the insurance company's desire to be shown where the pain is coming from, many times pain resulting from trauma does not reveal the presence of a herniated disk, fracture, or ruptured ligaments. In these instances, additional documentation or proof as to the nature of the patient's pain complaints will be required. There are many published algorithms available. For more information as well as a visual representation the reader is referred to the therapeutic algorithm for chronic spinal pain from Manchikanti et al. (2009) and "Evidenced Based Approach: An Algorithmic Approach for Clinical Management of Chronic Spinal Pain" (Von Korff et al., 2002). Using this algorithm, spinal pain is divided first into either somatic pain or radicular pain and then each of those categories receive diagnostic or therapeutic injections, minimally invasive spine procedures, and/or spinal implantable devices.

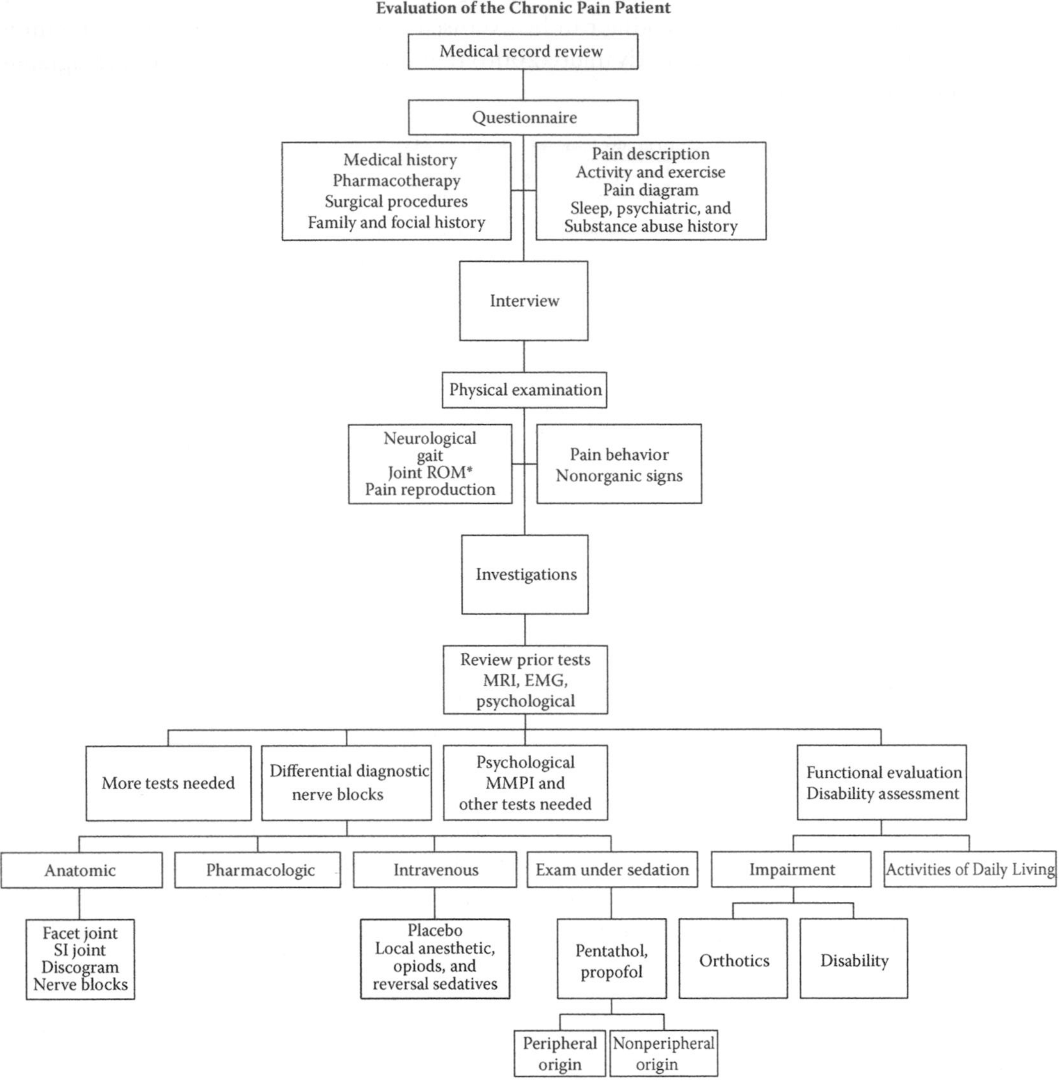

Approaches to Management of Pain

Once complete reviews of all diagnostic evaluations are performed, a list of differential pain diagnoses can be formulated. Although it would be more simple if the pain complaints were generated from a chronic painful illness of the same structure (e.g., a single herniated spine disc), it is more common that multiple pain generators contribute to a single chronic pain complaint. For example, axial back pain can exist on one side of the patient's low back and the patient may fixate on his or her knowledge that he or she indeed has a herniated disc at that level—but more likely the pain is the result of a combination such as facet joint spine arthritis, with myofascial disease and possibly sacroiliac joint disease. Additionally, the pain generators may be of different pathophysiology. Using the example of chronic foot pain patients, they indeed may have neuropathic pain from nerve injury resulting from chronic diabetic ischemic foot injury—but also may have coexisting nociceptive (tissue injury) pain from arthritis of the foot bones. Identifying the type of pain pathophysiology (nerve injury pain versus tissue injury pain) will direct the most appropriate types of pain management interventions for treatment. It is often difficult to differentiate which symptoms and signs are from which types of pain etiologies. Imaging alone cannot diagnose a specific pain generator because some imaging anatomic abnormalities are silent "red herrings." This has led to increased referrals to pain management clinics. An anesthesiologist, physiatrist, neurologist, psychiatrist, or other physician with special post-residency pain management training (pain algologist) typically manages these clinics. The pain management clinic is comprehensive in its evaluation and treatment of pain and often utilizes interdisciplinary specialists either by referral or directly within its clinic such as psychiatrists, psychologists, addictionologists, physical therapists, and social workers. Most of these clinics function in an outpatient setting or in the confines of a local hospital. The algologist has been trained to perform diagnostic injections of local anesthetic agents into different tissue regions, thereby blocking the local neuroanatomy and allowing for the cessation of the pain symptom complex. If performed properly (with minute volumes of local anesthetic and into the correct tissue planes), the patient will have a potential pain generator numbed—and if the pain is relieved, that will indirectly alert the provider that this anesthetized structure contributes to the patient's pain. There typically is a large placebo effect when performing injections of any type and therefore the provider often will perform two separate diagnostic injection trials with different local anesthetic duration of actions to be certain there is a true cause and effect relationship. Depending on the nature of the pain, its etiology, and its potential for catastrophic bodily injury (e.g., impending spinal cord injury), the patient may require surgical intervention bypassing more conservative treatment options. The surgeons most commonly involved in spine ailments are the neurosurgeons and the orthopedic surgeons. Specialists in these areas in most major metropolitan regions are familiar with causes and treatment of pain and will offer surgical remedies for their relief. In addition, in this setting in select patients, the pain management clinic algologist or the surgeon also offer minimally invasive spine interventions. Examples include the Minimally Invasive Lumbar Decompression (MILD) procedure where the algologist removes a small amount of ligamentous intraspinal tissue to decompress the spinal canal size. In the pain clinic setting, the comprehensive nature of the pain is addressed from several areas, including medications, sleep restoration, diet and exercise, orthotics, physical therapy, behavioral modifications (back school), electrical stimulation devices, and other neurological diagnostic workups. The decision as to which resource to employ is often selected by the patient.

Most patients in the authors' outpatient pain clinic have been injured for over a year and have already been evaluated by a surgeon. These patients typically have been referred by a primary care physician or surgeon because of extensive comorbidity (e.g., significant psychiatric disease, substance abuse, or end-of-life issues) or have been unmanageable despite standard of care conservative therapy. Many of them have already undergone surgical intervention, and the algologist will evaluate that and employ an interdisciplinary treatment plan. In general, chronic pain management should include the following, as noted by Von Korff and colleagues (Von Korff et al., 2002):

- Collaboration between physical therapist and the patient
- A personalized rehabilitation plan

- Tailored education of the patient on the nature of the problem
- Resolution of treatable barriers related to functional goal attainment
- Tailored instruction in independent management of pain
- Instruction in methods to prevent future problems
- Monitoring of outcome (achievement of patient goals)
- Monitoring of adherence to treatment
- Planned follow-up

It is important to note that *goal setting* is the important initial step in the development of the treatment plan. Goal setting is bidirectional, meaning that both health care provider for pain management and the patient–family unit participate in defining the goals of the interdisciplinary pain plan. These goals are very patient specific and can vary greatly from patient to patient. For example, a patient who was highly functional prior to an injury and has full brain function and mobility but cannot use his or her dominant upper extremity secondary to pain may establish goals of using that upper extremity in the future to return to work (e.g., typing, lifting, etc.) or perform Activities of Daily Living that utilize the dominant upper extremity (e.g., dressing, brushing teeth, writing). On the other hand, a patient who has had a significant cervical spinal cord injury with tetraplegia (also known as quadriplegia) and severe spasm and pain of the lower extremities may have just the goal of enough relief of pain and spasm to accept the appropriate lower extremity positioning for urinary bladder catheterizations several times per day. Simply stated, the first case represents a highly physically functioning patient's rehabilitation requests and goals versus the second case of little to no physical functioning rehabilitation goals. The issue of goal setting is not just for patient and provider satisfaction but also for cost-effectiveness. If the goals are not set or are unrealistic, excessive, unfounded treatments or unnecessary repeated diagnostics (e.g., MRI studies) may escalate costs and present potential harm to the patient. Goal setting is a dynamic process and must be reevaluated (and often readjusted) after the success or failure of each pain treatment.

The interdisciplinary treatment plan typically includes simultaneous introductions of medication management, interventional therapies, physical therapy, and psychosocial therapies. Figure 16.1 contains the Summary of Recommendations Regarding Multimodal and Multidisciplinary Interventions summarized from the "Practice Guidelines for Chronic Pain Management." Medication management must take into consideration that while many medications will relieve pain and suffering for a short period, many of these medications can have inappropriate side effects or consequences when delivered over a lifetime of chronic pain. Therefore, it is of utmost importance that not only the most effective pain reliever be considered but also the safest analgesic over the expected lifetime of the chronic disease. These authors often explain this issue to patients with the following analogy: "Inhaled anesthetic gasses can certainly relieve your pain for the short term—but would also require a ventilator and a breathing tube and therefore are not an option for your long-term pain strategies. In the same manner, high-dose injectable Ketorolac will certainly assist you with a pain exacerbation in the emergency room but would not be appropriate after more than a few days of your pain exacerbation because of bleeding risks." The decision to utilize specific types of oral analgesics often follows specific algorithms, such as the Analgesic Ladder in Figure 16.2, adapted from the World Health Organization Pain Relief Ladder (World Health Organization, 2009).

The interventional strategies include any treatments that are not considered an oral medication, but in the algologist setting they typically refer to minimally invasive injections of

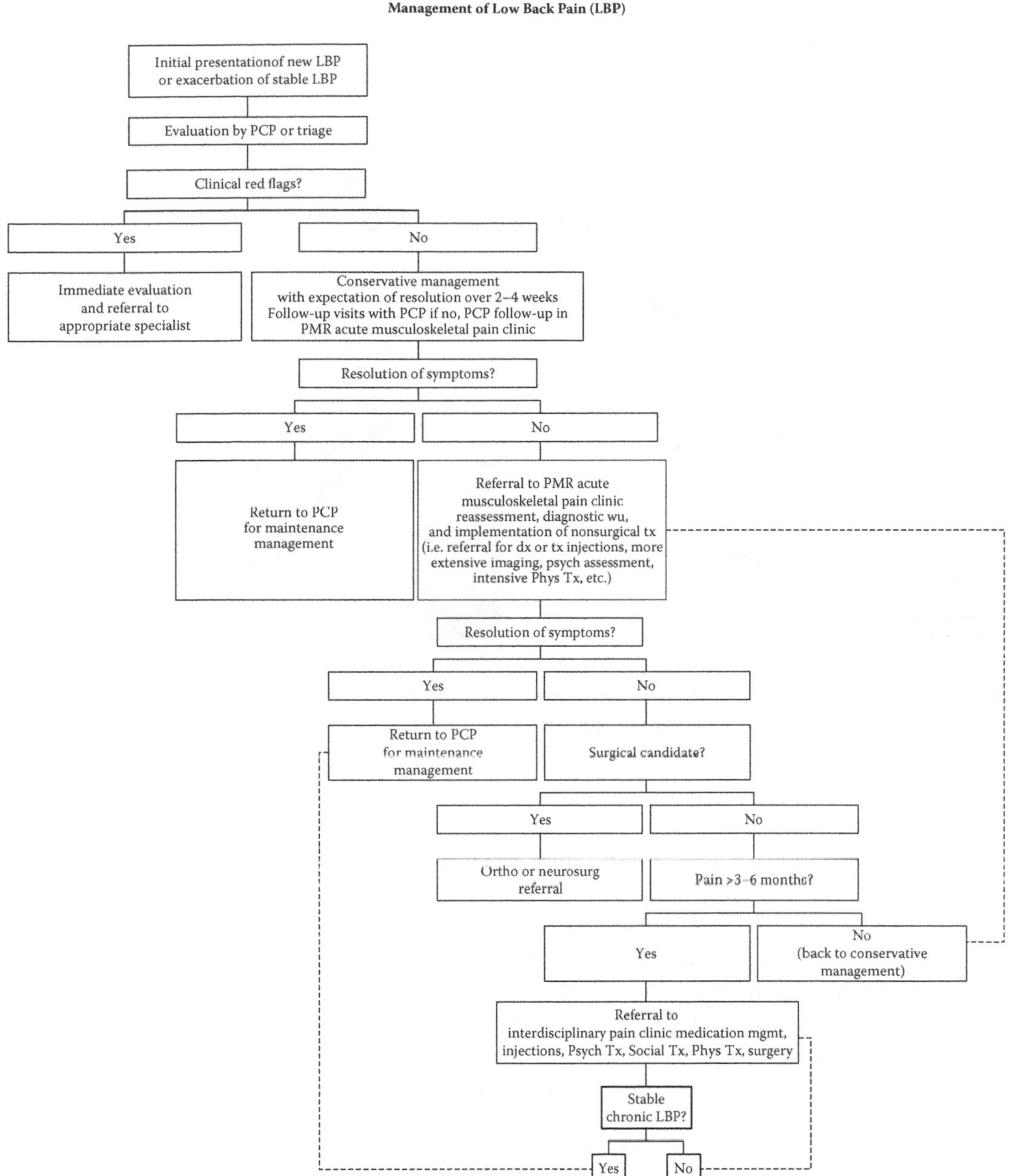

Figure 16.1 Multimodal and multidisciplinary interventions for pain.

nerve, muscles, or painful structures of the spine. Therapeutic injections are categorized into those that modulate painful tissues and those that neurolyse (kill tissue). Modulation of pain via therapeutic injections includes injecting local anesthetics and long-acting steroids into spine structures (e.g., epidural space, facet joints, sacroiliac joints, and spinal nerves), and injecting narcotics and other types of analgesics into various tissue planes (e.g., spinal fluid, brachial plexus,

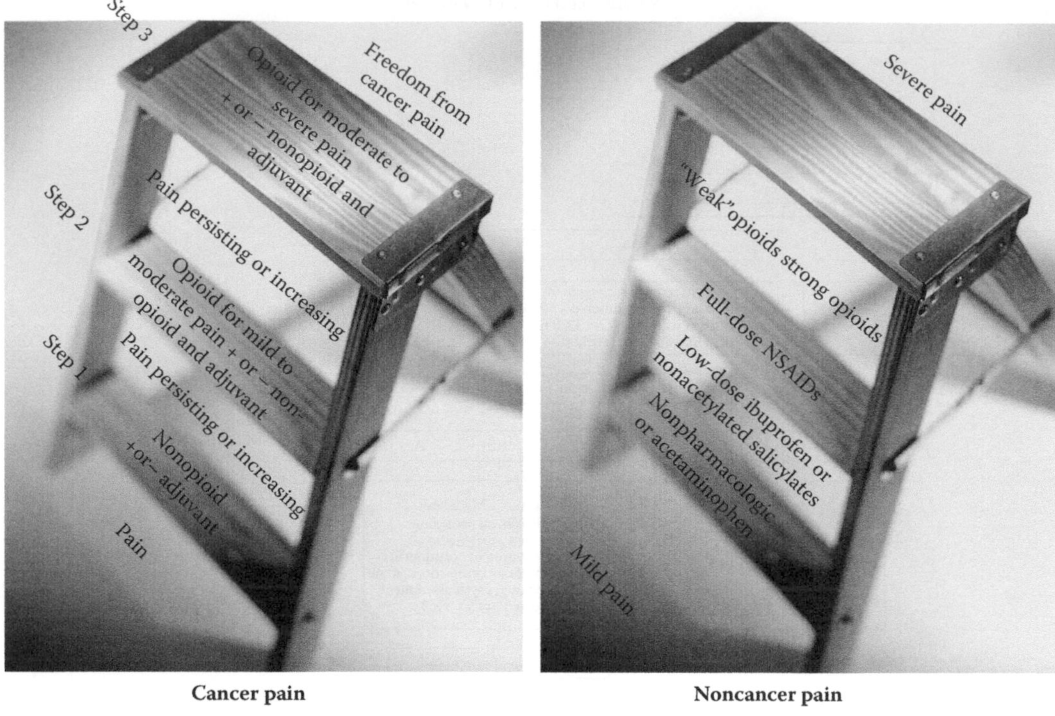

Figure 16.2 World Health Organization Analgesic Ladder.

epidural space). Additionally, modulating therapeutic types of injections include all types of electrical stimulation therapies for pain including implantable spinal cord stimulators, which are electrical wires implanted into the spine to control pain. Because neurolytic injections are often irreversible, they are provided after much consideration of the risk–benefit ratio. Examples of neurolytic injections include killing with heat (radiofrequency ablation of nerves or tissues), killing with cold (cryotherapy), or killing with chemicals (alcohol, phenol, glycerol, Sarapin tissue injections). A minimally invasive spine procedure provided by algologists and surgeons includes vertebral augmentation for bony spine fractures. In this technique algologists place cement or cement-like substances into the spine fracture via a needle, and this typically results in immediate resolution of pain. There are myriad additional interventional procedures that can assist with the therapy of chronic pain. One additional class of therapies is the implantable devices for pain. As introduced previously, these devices comprise two groups: implantable drug delivery systems (IDDS) and implantable electronic neuromodulation systems (IENS). The IDDS is a small catheter that is implanted into the spinal fluid and tunneled to the abdominal wall to a pump reservoir. This pump has a computerized motor that delivers minute amounts of opioids, local anesthetics, and other analgesics to the spinal fluid to control pain and limit side effects. It is typically considered in a very select group of patients who have failed all conservative therapies and have a life expectancy greater than 6 months. It is costly and additionally has the risk of infection of the spine, granuloma of the spine, or pump malfunction as well so it is placed only in a very select population of patients. It is totally implantable and requires a refill through a

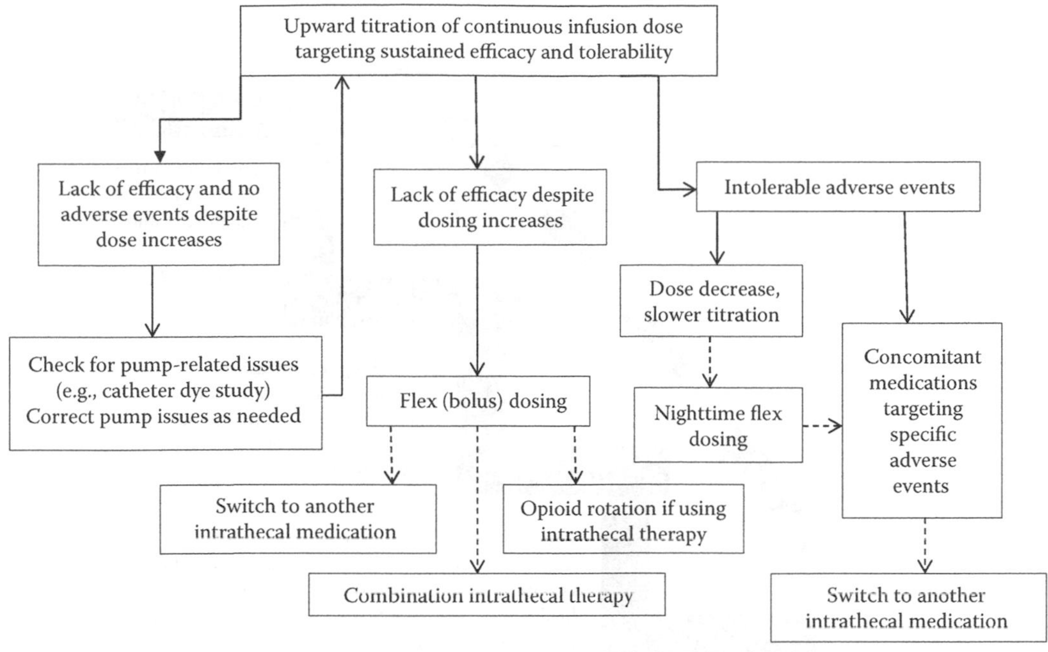

Figure 16.3 Long-term pain management using intrathecal therapy. Solid arrows: yes or desired outcome achieved. Dashed arrows: no or failure. (Adapted from Pope, J. Deer, T., Bruel, B., & Falowski, S. 2016. Clinical uses of intrathecal therapy and its placement in the pain care algorithm. *Pain Practice, 16*(8), 1092–1106.)

needle puncture through the skin about every 3 months. The IENS is also totally implantable, is a small wire that is placed into the epidural space, and is connected to a microcomputer that is indwelling in the abdominal wall or the scapula. The patient can manipulate the amount of electricity through a remote device through the skin. This therapy has its own associated risks and should only be considered after failing more conservative therapy and after several days of a trial period. Figure 16.3 demonstrates an algorithm for introducing implantable systems for pain (Pope et al., 2016).

Physical therapy interventions are often felt to be the strength of any good comprehensive pain management plan. In the authors' practice, the patients are expected to continue physical therapy (aquatic-based or land-based) as a lifestyle to remain an active patient in the pain clinic. While this is labor intensive to monitor for compliance, it has been demonstrated that those patients who remain compliant with physical therapy continue to maintain or restore physical function and have less additive pain syndromes related to the cycle of immobility-associated pain. Physical therapists may also employ other low-risk strategies such as transcutaneous electrical nerve stimulation (TENS units, which are devices that use electrical skin surface patches to remove pain), PROVANT (magnetic wave therapy units for home use) ultrasound therapy, cold, moist heat, traction, and paraffin wax therapy.

If an individual has already undergone several surgeries and a number of injections, then a physician may be reluctant to send him or her back for more invasive procedures. It is important that each patient undergo a thorough evaluation of his or her present condition to determine the

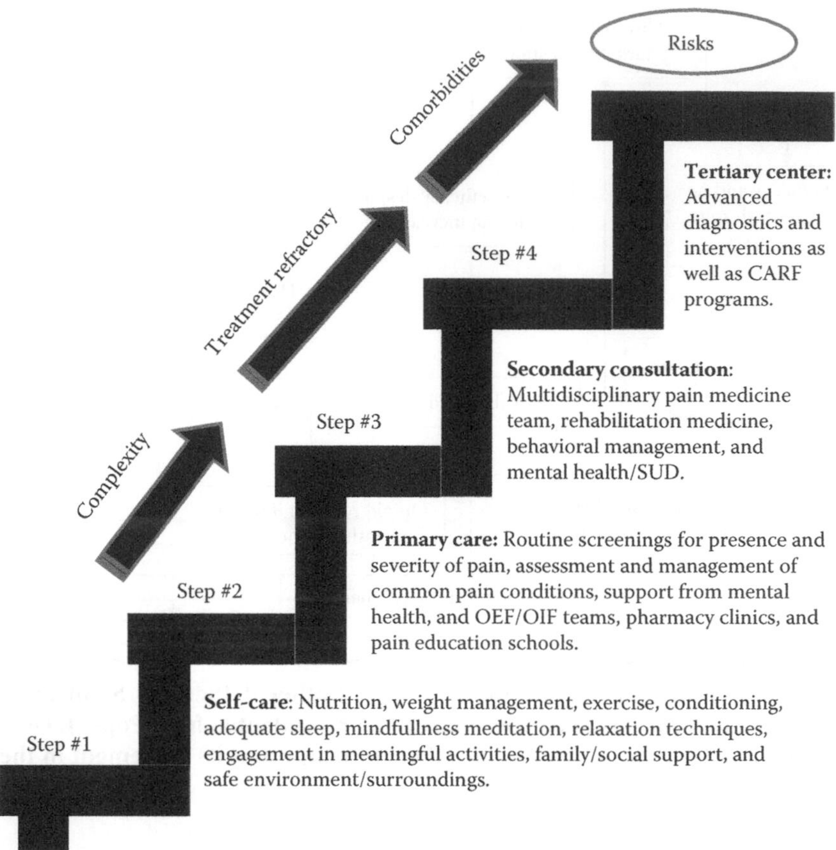

Figure 16.4 Illustration of the VA's stepped model for care of pain management. (Adapted from: Cosio D., & Swaroop, S. (2016). The use of mind-body medicine in chronic pain management: differential trends and session-by-session changes in anxiety. *Pain Management and Medicine.* 2 114. doi:10.4172/jpmme.1000114.)

etiology of the pain. If a patient's pain has not been evaluated for two or more years, despite a thorough documentation of the presence of a nonoperative lesion from the past, then it is quite possible that further evaluation and diagnostic X-ray information of perhaps a new pain problem may be necessary.

Multiple guidelines and algorithms have been published for specific painful disorders, including back pain, headache, and other chronic pain conditions commonly encountered in both specialty and primary care clinical practice (Bair et al., 2005; Weingarten et al., 2002). Many guidelines exist for opioid management, including the newest guidelines from the Centers for Disease Control (Agency Medical Directors Group, 2010, Chou et al., 2009; Department of Veterans Affairs and Department of Defense, 2010; CDC Guideline for Prescribing Opioids for Chronic Pain, March 18, 2016); however, there are limited published and widely accepted clinical practice guidelines for comprehensive measurement-based, stepped care for chronic pain beyond efforts by the Department of Veterans Affairs to streamline the treatment of pain within its health care setting. This gap persists despite published evidence that such a stepped care approach leads to better overall outcomes (Figure 16.4). Various studies in the published literature have evaluated the stepped care approach that hold promise for more standardized and widely accepted clinical practice.

Life Care Planning and Chronic Pain

Individual types of pain are especially variable and are almost beyond the scope of this short chapter. A listing of types of injuries that can result in chronic pain requiring lifetime medical care would include the following:

- Spinal cord injury: cervical, thoracic, lumbar with paraplegia, or tetraplegia (also known as quadriplegia)
- Cervical, thoracic, lumbar, or sacral spine bony traumatic injury (e.g., fractures, dislocations)
- Cervical, thoracic, lumbar, or sacral spine arthritis and degenerative disease states (e.g., degenerative disc disease, facet joint disease, spondylosis, disc herniations)
- Deafferentation pain syndromes (loss of sensation secondary to nerve injury with increased pain traffic: e.g., postherpetic neuralgia, phantom syndromes, post thoracotomy syndrome, diabetic neuropathies, HIV neuropathy, alcohol neuropathy, multiple sclerosis, central pain)
- Central nervous system and spinal cord infarctions (post stroke pain)
- Neuropathy (peripheral neuropathies, plexus neuropathies, cranial nerve neuropathies)
- Complex regional pain syndromes type 1 (reflex sympathetic dystrophy)
- Chronic regional pain syndrome type 2 (causalgia)
- Multiple orthopedic fractures and subsequent claudication injuries
- Cancer of any organ or any tissue type
- Traumatic brain injury
- Abdominal problems (e.g., inflammatory bowel disease, Crohn's disease, chronic pancreatitis)
- Genital/urinary problems (e.g., interstitial cystitis)
- Pulmonary problems
- Osteoarthritis
- Rheumatoid arthritis
- Systemic lupus erythematosus
- Fibromyalgia
- Trigeminal neuralgia
- Motor vehicle accidents
- Failed spinal surgeries
- Orthopedic joint replacement surgery, including hip and knee surgeries
- Vascular injuries, including angina
- Peripheral vascular injuries
- Peripheral vascular ischemia with crush injuries
- Headaches, including migraine, cluster, and tension headaches
- Pelvic inflammatory disease
- Environmental toxins and exposure

The medical needs and future care for these conditions run the gamut and require a coordinated effort of services that are individually determined. Some of the considerations are outlined in the following sections.

Psychological Considerations

In the comprehensive management of chronic pain, psychological testing and treatment for depression, anxiety, and stress are all components required for maximum improvement. All chronic pain patients should have psychological counseling and psychological testing in the course of their pain diagnosis or management. The family will also require assistance in coping with the patient's pain problems, as it is very disruptive to the normal activities of family life. Depending upon when the life care planner becomes involved in the case, an evaluation by a psychologist is commonly recommended, as well as subsequent further recommendations of biofeedback and stress management on a weekly basis for at least one year to improve the patient's ability to initiate and maintain a program that will benefit him or her for the lifetime of the complaint.

There are numerous additional resources for the chronic pain patient. Self-help groups and certain newsletters are available for individual diseases that the patient can access through the Internet. Local chapters, usually located by Internet searches, of the larger disease diagnoses that cause chronic pain may be available. These include rheumatoid arthritis foundation groups, fibromyalgia groups, spinal cord injury and recovery groups, brain injury recovery groups, multiple sclerosis groups, local diabetes foundations, and others.

It should be noted that self-treatment through alcohol or illicit drug use is a common feature of our society, which probably increases with the advent of chronic pain. Additional guidelines regarding patient self-medication have been released by the American Academy of Pain Medicine (www.painmed.org), the World Institute of Pain (www.-iapsar.org/WIP/WIP-base.htm), and the American Academy of Pain Management (www.aapainmanage.org). All entities now recognize the therapeutic use of chronic narcotic analgesia for chronic pain. However, medical societies in local as well as state medical boards are concerned about the use of chronic narcotic analgesia for chronic pain. This view seems to reflect our fears of addiction and the subsequent costs and problems that addiction has caused in our society. As this may be a national resource book for life care planning, it is likely that the reader may find in his or her locality a remaining bias toward the avoidance of use of chronic narcotic analgesia for the treatment of chronic pain. The CDC 2016 guidelines are excellent resources for decision making in opioid prescribing and monitoring.

Multidisciplinary pain programs that employ psychologists, social workers, anesthesiologists, orthopedic surgeons, neurosurgeons, neuropsychologists, physiatrists, and allied health professionals are often quite familiar with the local political flavor of the area and will be one of the better resources in determining what a patient's needs are in general, as well as giving him or her an understanding of what the trends throughout the nation are at that time.

Additional Considerations for Chronic Pain Management

As mentioned previously, a multidisciplinary team is the best resource for thorough and comprehensive management of chronic pain. Typically, the needs of the patient will require five or six comprehensive measures to maximize the outcome of the patient's ability to manage his or her own condition after a period of 6 months to a year. Most outpatient treatment of a chronic pain patient will result in a very brief 1- to 2-month period of intense evaluation and management followed by a middle period of 3 to 6 months of continued weekly monitoring or monthly monitoring and establishing of a management program that will fit the patient's needs. Biofeedback, stress management, counseling, psychological testing, and family counseling will be included. Additional areas for maximizing the patient's independence will include diet, weight loss, and exercise. Normally, most patients with chronic pain have a hard time functioning in the upright position and the normal gravity environment. For that reason, exercise programs, especially ones employing a pool, are very popular and quite prevalent and seem to best suit the needs of the chronic pain exercise program prescription.

A six-step comprehensive program in the treatment of chronic pain patients has been published in the prior edition of this text and is included below. Note that this program occurs in the rehabilitation setting, since the majority of the patients seen in this setting have already undergone pain clinic and surgical options. A comprehensive, conservative chronic pain management program would consist of the following areas:

- *Exercise*: A program including a pool for both strength conditioning and monitoring the effects of the central nervous system related to exercise with serotonin and norepinephrine release. Additional cardiovascular and pulmonary conditioning for weight-loss assistance is also a key element.
- *Diet*: A thorough review is usually achieved with a dietary journal kept by the patient for 2 weeks. After the journal is reviewed, recommendations are made with specific restrictions of foods that are clearly harmful to the patient's diet. For additional help with diet, reading materials and instructions are added for food selection, and a basic understanding of carbohydrates, fats, and protein is taught. Subsequently, the patient's weight is taken on a weekly basis for his next several visits and further assistance and encouragement are given.
- *Sleep Restoration*: Patients have difficulty managing daily stress of chronic pain without adequate sleep. Sleep achieves a degree of relaxation and resets the thermostat of the central nervous system. Deep sleep has also been shown to be the period in which growth hormone is released and significant tissue repair and restorative processes take place. Paradoxically, deep sleep is often shortened in the chronic pain patients, and very often the sleep additive medications paradoxically decrease deep sleep as well. The sleep-deprived patient will have more difficulty responding to minute-to-minute changes in his or her day and thereby will be much less adaptable to his or her chronic pain condition than those who are sleeping through the night. Pharmacological agents for this are often needed to restore the patient to a restful night's sleep. Of note, several studies suggest that psychological strategies (e.g., progressive relaxation) for managing the insomnia of the chronic pain patient are more effective than most prescribed sleep agents. Additional concerns would be for patients who have sleep apnea or other obstructive forms of sleep disturbance, which may require expensive equipment (BiPAP devices) to remedy the insomnia. Sleep centers are usually run and directed by a pulmonologist or neurologist and are available in most metropolitan areas. These physician authors have used these clinics as an assistive consultation in helping the patient return to a more restful night's sleep.
- *Pharmacological Agents*: The recitation of all medications that are prescribed and used in current pain management would be beyond the scope of this short chapter. There are five basic categories:
  - Antidepressants for pain relief (e.g., Duloxetine, Amitriptyline, Nortriptyline) and anxiolytics
  - Medications for the resolution of nerve pain, which consist of Pregabulin, Gabapentin, Tegretol, Dilantin, and Depakote
  - Muscle relaxants, consisting of Soma, Skelaxin, Robaxin, Flexeril, Baclofen

- Nonsteroidal anti-inflammatory drugs (NSAIDs) or other non-narcotic analgesics that also assist with the reduction in inflammatory joint changes. These would consist of ibuprofen (Advil, Motrin, and others), Releve, Relafen, Oravail, Tramadol, etc.
- Narcotic analgesia, which would depend on efforts of resolving the pain from all other measures and would follow the World Health Organization ladder to analgesics (previously cited in this chapter). Examples include Methadone, Oxycodone, Morphine, Fentanyl Patch, Levorphanol, etc.

- *Side Effects*: The medications listed commonly have side effects that affect patient compliance and comfort. For example, NSAIDs can cause gastrointestinal upset, ulcers, and liver and kidney damage. Opioids often result in physical dependence and cause dizziness, fatigue, concentration impairments, drowsiness, nausea, impaired vision, and constipation. Also, some of the newer medications can reach $100,000 per year in cost.
- *Physical Therapy and Outpatient Modalities*: Usually, patients who have chronic pain also have a sedentary lifestyle as a consequence of trying to avoid pain. A brief burst of physical therapy for 2 to 4 weeks following the intake of a new patient may prove useful. This is usually aimed at providing the modality that may have already been used in other efforts of physical therapy. The difference with the use of physical therapy at this time is to try other physical therapy prescriptions and also to allow patients the use of transcutaneous electric nerve stimulation (TENS) or percutaneous electrical stimulation (PES) units, or other locally available stimulation units to attempt to decrease their pain. Further sessions of physical therapy throughout the course of the patient's lifetime may also be necessary depending on brief or prolonged periods of inactivity, which will result in a loss of strength and function. In general, the nature of the comprehensive, conservative measures implemented for chronic pain management attempts to keep the patient from losing significant degrees of function for prolonged periods of time by instituting an exercise program. Nonetheless, a once-per-year physical therapy evaluation may be necessary to forestall more remedial forms of functional loss.
- For back pain and other selected central nervous system–generated pain, injections into the spinal canal area can provide relief, but often must be repeated regularly and can cause numerous side effects (e.g., nausea, vomiting, headache, transient weight gain, and infections).
- *Orthotics and Other Adaptive Equipment*: These products can usually be procured at the local orthotics or prosthetist or durable medical equipment supplier. There are a number of self-care adaptive aids, such as long-handled reachers, button hooks, and assistive devices for eating, grooming, and daily household tasks. In addition, under this heading would fall the grouping of spinal orthoses such as cervical pillows or orthopedic braces for sleeping and comfort in sitting, driving, walking, and moving about. From this standpoint, electric mobility devices, power chairs, assistive bathing devices, and personalized aids could all be considered for prescription. Throughout it should be mentioned that the patient's condition is not presumed to be static. Occasional retesting and obtaining X-rays and, in some cases, other surgical, neurosurgical, or orthopedic surgery interventions may be required.

In addition to the previously listed items, various surgical options may be available for structurally identifiable reasons and well-selected patients. Intrathecal morphine pumps, spinal cord stimulators, and repeat surgery are examples. Spinal fusions can total $18,000 to $25,000.

Implanted pumps can cost $15,000 to $32,000 for the surgery, an average of $300 per month for medication and other follow-up charges, and $10,000 to $21,000 for pump replacement. Spinal cord stimulation initially can be expected to reach $15,000 to $20,000 or more, and then another $2,500 per year for follow-up.

Determining Patient's Functioning Level

The patient's needs at the time of intake as a chronic pain patient and throughout life can be ascertained most effectively through an outside source of local physical therapy where functional capacity evaluations are performed. A functional capacity evaluation (FCE) (also referred to as a physical capacity assessment) is usually an 8-hour assessment that is typically performed over a 2-day period. During this assessment the patient's autonomic functions are evaluated, including heart rate, respiratory rate, and skin temperature. Other measurements, such as a visual analog scale of pain, may also be performed.

The majority of the testing includes performance of a variety of tasks that are observed and are also repeated in a number of different fashions to ascertain the patient's reliability from one task to the next. Typically, insurance companies and other health care providers will request these, as will the workplace at the time of a patient's disability. They are useful for disability determination, but are typically not adequate for disability rating. Disability ratings come under a different evaluation. Many times the consultants who have been working with the patient throughout the months are not capable or are not interested in performing disability evaluations. Determining individuals who are willing and capable to perform these assessments can be the source of difficulty in bringing the patient's legal problems to a close. The reader should be aware that the validity of FCE results has been challenged, particularly in litigation settings, and the value of the results may be only as good as the equipment used and the evaluator's expertise (King et al., 1998).

Life Care Planning and Chronic Pain and Future Concerns

In making preparations in the life care plan for the needs of a patient with chronic pain, it becomes necessary to take into consideration all of the measures listed previously. To this end, identifying someone who will follow the patient and participate in a comprehensive chronic pain management multidisciplinary team approach is preferred. If, however, that is not possible, then the needs from a chronic pain future life care plan would include all of the steps mentioned in the evaluation and treatment of a chronic pain patient at the initial intake. It should be noted that from a chronic pain standpoint, efforts are directed at making the individual with chronic pain self-reliant and avoiding constant medical intervention. Although this is the desired outcome, it is very time-consuming to achieve this goal, and as with any long-term disease problem, it becomes necessary for routine reevaluations and upgrades in the individual program. Cost estimates for chronic pain include medication and equipment repair and replacement, and 1- to 2-year reevaluations with X-rays, blood work, and consultations of the individual specialists will be necessary. It may also be necessary to include physical therapy and psychological counseling reevaluations. As the patient with chronic pain ages, additional evaluations and treatments with upgrades in equipment and possible surgical interventions may also be required. It once again becomes necessary to include in an exhaustive fashion a comprehensive listing of the patient's problems and some future prognosis as to the deterioration of these diagnostic considerations.

Case Study

The following example is a life care plan for a patient in the authors' clinic who traumatized her lower limbs after a massive saddle pulmonary embolus led to ischemic injury of both her lower limbs while she was on active military duty. This trauma eventually led to the development of complex regional pain syndrome type 1, and over time involved all four extremities. Initial attempts at conservative treatment and surgery were accomplished on several occasions with poor results over the years. Additionally, a multitude of pain specialists from a variety of disciplines (neurosurgery, anesthesiology, physiatry, neurology, and orthopedics) were consulted, and diagnostic and treatment strategies were implemented. Attempts at aggressive physical therapy failed because the patient was so hyperesthetic and dysesthetic to light touch in all four extremities. Her baseline pain management consisted of combinations of opioid medications, adjunctive antidepressant and anticonvulsant medications, physical therapy and psychotherapeutic strategies. She was referred to a specialist for a dorsal column stimulator, which failed to provide long-term relief. The patient had received mixed risk recommendations regarding spinal fluid pump placement because she required extensive anticoagulation. She later decided to defer that option of treatment for risk of spinal hematoma and worsening paralysis. At the time of the plan, she was completely a functional paraplegic requiring an electric wheelchair, and she remained essentially nonfunctional and did not drive, work, or clean her home. Her bed was relocated to the living room to avoid stairs or excessive movement. Her husband was supportive and actively assisted in her rehabilitation efforts.

Life Care Plan

Jane Doe

Table of Contents

Projected Therapeutic Modalities 487
Diagnostic Testing/Educational Assessment 488
Wheelchair Needs 488
Wheelchair Accessories and Maintenance 489
Aids for Independent Function 489
Orthotics/Prosthetics 489
Drug/Supply Needs 489
Home/Facility Care 490
Future Medical Care—Routine 490
Transportation 490
Health and Strength Maintenance 491
Architectural Renovations 492
Potential Complications 492
Vocational/Educational Plan 493
Future Medical Care/Surgical Intervention/Aggressive Treatment 493

		Life Care Plan			Client Name: Jane Doe Date of Birth: 1/1/62	
		Projected Therapeutic Modalities			Date of Injury: 7/7/2005 Date Prepared: 8/27/2007	
Therapy	*Age/Year at Which Initiated*	*Age/Year at Which Suspended*	*Treatment Frequency*	*Base Cost per Year*	*Growth Trends*	*Recommended by*
Pain support group; individual, couples, and crisis therapy; medication supervision	43/2005	Life expectancy	Group at $50/week for 48 therapeutic weeks. Individual at $125, 1 to 2 times/week for 2½ yrs., then 25 sessions/year (average) for life expectancy	$2,400 (group) $6,000–$12,000 (individual) $3,125 year to life expectancy	To be determined by economist	Dr. Lester and Dr. Litwack
Pain management program	43/2005	43/2005	3½ weeks	$7,000–$8,000	To be determined by economist	Dr. Lester and Dr. Litwack
Occupational therapy; included as part of inpatient pain program	43/2005	3–4 months	2 times per week, 1 hour per session as part of pain program	See pain program above	N/A	Dr. Lester and Dr. Litwack
Physical therapy	43/2005	3–4 months	2 times per week, 1 hour per session following pain program	$1,920–$3,200 at $80–$100/hour	To be determined by economist	Dr. Lester and Dr. Litwack

Source: Format adapted from Deutsch, P., & Sawyer, H. 2004. *Guide to Rehabilitation*. New York, NY: Ahab Press.

(Continued)

Diagnostic Testing/Educational Assessment						
Diagnostic Recommendation	*Age/Year at Which Initiated*	*Age/Year at Which Suspended*	*Per-Year Frequency*	*Base Cost per Year*	*Growth Trends*	*Recommended by*
Psychological testing, IQ and psychological status testing	43/2005	43/2005	Psychological evaluation	\$500–\$600	To be determined by economist	Dr. Lester and Dr. Litwack
Laboratory studies: (1) Opioid compliance (2) Assessment of therapeutic window for adjunctive analgesics	43/2005	Lifetime	4 times per year	\$600/year	To be determined by economist	Dr. Lester and Dr. Litwack
Radiologic studies: MRIs	43/2005	Lifetime	Range 1/year to 1 X every 4 years and as clinically appropriate	\$5,000 total	To be determined by economist	Dr. Lester and Dr. Litwack
Wheelchair Needs						
Wheelchair Type	*Age/Year at Which Purchased*	*Replacement Schedule*	*Purpose of Equipment*	*Base Cost*	*Growth Trends*	*Catalog or Supplier Reference*
Three-wheel power chair, rear-wheel drive (e.g., Pride)	43/2005	Every 5 years	Mobility, independence, and avoiding complications	\$3,000–\$3,500 Maintenance: \$150/year (avg.) after 1-year warranty	To be determined by economist	Adaptive Equipment Specialists

(*Continued*)

Wheelchair Accessories and Maintenance						
Wheelchair Accessory/ Maintenance	*Age/Year at Which Purchased*	*Replacement Schedule*	*Purpose*	*Base Cost*	*Growth Trends*	*Catalog or Supplier Reference*
Maintenance, carry bags, wheelchair batteries, and charger	43/2005	Yearly	Maintenance and supplies	$100/year average	To be determined by economist	Sammons-Preston
Aids for Independent Function						
Equipment	*Age/Year at Which Purchased*	*Replacement Schedule*	*Equipment Purpose*	*Base Cost*	*Growth Trends*	*Catalog or Supplier Reference*
Reachers or other aids	43/2005	Yearly	Aides for independent functioning	$50/year average	To be determined by economist	Sammons-Preston or other supplier
Orthotics/Prosthetics						
Equipment Description	*Age/Year at Which Purchased*	*Replacement Schedule*	*Equipment Purpose*	*Base Cost*	*Growth Trends*	*Supplier*
Right leg ankle/ foot orthosis Straps	43/2005 44/2006	Every 3 years Every 8–12 months	Support body weight, avoid falls, reduce complications. Attach ankle-foot orthosis (AFO) to leg	$406.64 $10	To be determined by economist	Butte Limb and Brace
Drug/Supply Needs						
Supply Description	*Drug (Prescription)*	*Purpose*	*Per-Unit Cost*	*Per-Year Cost*	*Growth Trends*	*Recommended by*
	Methadone, 10 mg, 3 times/day Ativan, 2 mg, 3 times/day	Pain control Antianxiety	$9.76/30 $12.62/90	$356 $153 Total = $509	To be determined by economist	Dr. Lester and Dr. Litwack
Note: Medications listed are representative of current and future needs. Specific prescriptions may change.						

(Continued)

Home/Facility Care						
Facility Recommendation	*Home Care/Service Recommendations*	*Age/Year at Which Initiated*	*Age/Year at Which Suspended*	*Hours/Shifts/Days of Attendance or Care*	*Base Cost per Year*	*Growth Trends*
	Companion, psychological support, aide, and house maintenance	2005	Life expectancy	Husband performs these functions; expect 2 days/week at $36/day if hired	$0 if continued marriage or $3,744/year if hired	To be determined by economist
Future Medical Care—Routine						
Routine Medical Care Description	*Frequency of Visits*	*Purpose*	*Cost per Visit*	*Cost per Year*	*Growth Trends*	*Recommended by*
Psychiatrist follow-up	As needed	Review of medications	See projected therapeutic modalities	N/A	N/A	Dr. Lester and Dr. Litwack
Neurological/orthopedic follow-up (not including X-ray, lab, or other diagnostic costs, e.g., MRI = $1,000–$1,200)	1 time/year to life expectancy	Prescribe braces, follow-up to back surgery, and prevent complications	$100 (average)	$100/year (average)	To be determined by economist	Dr. Lester and Dr. Litwack
Transportation						
Equipment Description	*Age/Year at Which Purchased*	*Replacement Schedule*	*Equipment Purpose*	*Base Cost*	*Growth Trends*	*Catalog or Supplier Reference*
Option 1 Handicap-accessible van with lift and hand controls	43/2005	Every 5–7 years (trade-in value to be determined by economist)	Mobility and independence	$42,000–$45,000	To be determined by economist (reduce by cost of average vehicle or by cost of client's vehicle trade-in)	Handicapped Services, Inc.

(*Continued*)

Option 2 Car with trunk lift and hand controls	43/2005	Every 5–7 years	Mobility and independence	$1,200–$1,750 ($400–$550 hand controls; $1,000–$1,200 trunk lift; car must be equipped with power steering and brakes)	To be determined by economist	Adaptive Equipment Specialists
Health and Strength Maintenance						
Equipment Description	*Special Camps or Programs*	*Age/Year of Purchase or Attendance*	*Replacement or Attendance Schedule*	*Base Cost*	*Growth Trends*	*Catalog or Supplier Reference*
Universal gym with physical conditioning components/ stationary bike/ weights		2005	1 time only	$500–$1,500	To be determined by economist	Sports Town

Architectural Renovations				
Accessibility Needs		*Accessibility Needs*		*Costs*
Ramping	X	Bathroom		Cost estimated at 10 percent over average home
Light/environmental controls	X	Sink	X	
Floor coverings (if wheelchair is used inside)	X	Cabinets	X	
Hallways	X	Roll-in shower	X	
Doorways	X	Temperature control guards		
Covered parking	X	Heater		
Kitchen		Fixtures		
Sinks/fixtures		Door handles		
Cabinets		Additional electrical outlets		
Appliances		Central air/heat		
Windows		Therapy/equipment storage	?	
Electric safety doors		Attendant bathroom		
Fire alarm	X	Single-story home; no steps	X	

Potential Complications		
Complications	*Estimated Costs*	*Growth Trend*
Rehospitalized for psychological/psychiatric care and crises management; electroconvulsive therapy costs approximately $1,000 each treatment	No duration or frequency available; costs not included in plan	
Failed back with additional surgery required		
Falls and reinjury		
Adverse reactions to medications		

(*Continued*)

		Vocational/Educational Plan				
Recommendation	*Age/Year at Which Initiated*	*Age/Year at Which Suspended*	*Purpose*	*Base Cost*	*Growth Trends*	*Recommended by*
Client appears unemployable; final determination deferred to vocational rehabilitation specialist based on progress in treatment						
		Future Medical Care, Surgical Intervention, or Aggressive Treatment Plan				
Recommendation (Description)	*Age/Year Initiated*	*Frequency of Procedure*	*Per-Procedure Cost*	*Per-Year Cost*	*Growth Trends*	*Recommended by*
Based on history, client likely to be rehospitalized for psychological reactions to disability.	Date unknown	Implanted pain drug delivery system 1 time.	$50,000	$150 for 5 times per year for refills?		Dr. Lester and Dr. Litwack

Source: Format reproduced with permission of Dr. Paul M. Deutsch. Adapted from Deutsch, P., & Sawyer, H. 2004. *Guide to Rehabilitation*. New York, NY: Ahab Press.

Conclusion

Chronic pain has the ability as a diagnostic entity to cause as much disruption in patient care as do the functional, psychological, and social losses involved in the original injury. It should be noted that as a specialty, chronic pain is developing and should be available in its broadest sense from the multidisciplinary approach nearly everywhere in the United States. A carefully arranged initial intake with subsequent development of the six categories outlined should place the life care planner in the position to expertly assess and recommend the appropriate level of care for patients with chronic pain. However, as with all diseases, individuals with chronic pain will suffer variable outcomes based upon their individual application of the programs outlined for them. The responsibility of the patient in chronic pain is not unlike that of a diabetic, who, although having undergone a comprehensive study and treatment program, nonetheless is left on a daily basis to provide the right type of treatment for his or her own condition. It is incumbent upon the patient to adopt new lifestyle measures, restrict activities, and habituate certain aspects such as biofeedback and relaxation, and not just do the easy thing, which is to take a pill or apply a TENS unit. Patient compliance in this regard is key, and assistance through psychological counseling and frequent monitoring is often the best hope for achieving some degree of success in modifying a patient's former lifestyle to include measures necessary for a chronic pain management program. The goal of chronic pain planning, therefore, is not to reduce the pain to the level it was before the injury, but to modify the pain such that the patient can enjoy an enhanced quality of life and maintain a reasonable degree of function. It is also pertinent to note that a comprehensive treatment plan that uses all six outlined areas will offer the best chance of success, rather than a patient selectively using two or three modalities. The goal is to reduce the patient's perceived level of pain to where certain activities that were prohibitive or restrictive are now possible. Clearly, this does not necessarily mean that the patient will be able to perform all activities. It is along these lines that the compromise between where the patient was and where the patient is now needs to be identified. In this context, the patient can be encouraged to achieve some degree of compromise with the condition of chronic pain and a future activity level that is beyond where he or she has been functioning. In light of these issues, the life care plan can be a valuable adjunct to assist the chronic pain patient.

References

Alanmanou, E. 2006. Pain measurement. In S. Ramamurthy, E. Alanmanou, & J. Rogers (Eds.), *Decision Making in Pain Management* (2nd ed., pp. 22–23). St. Louis, MO: Mosby Elsevier.

Agency Medical Directors Group. 2010. Interagency guideline on opioid dosing for chronic non-cancer pain: an educational aid to improve care and safety with opioid therapy. 2010 update. Cited March 7, 2012. Available at www.agencymeddirectors.wa.gov/Files/OpioidGdline.pdf.

Apfelbaum, J. L., Ashburn, M. A., & Connis, R. T. et al. 2012. Practice guidelines for acute pain management in the perioperative setting: an updated report by the American Society of Anesthesiologists Task Force on Acute Pain Management. *Anesthesiology. 116*, 248–273.

Bair, M., Richardson, K., & Dobscha, S. et al. 2005. Chronic pain management guidelines: a systematic review of content and strength of evidence. *Journal of General Internal Medicine. 20*(suppl 1), 62.

Beecher, H. 1959. *Measurement of Subjective Responses*. New York, NY: Oxford University Press.

Bresler, D. 1979. *Free Yourself from Pain*. New York, NY: Simon & Schuster.

Centers for Disease Control. 2016. Guideline for Prescribing Opioids for Chronic Pain.— United States, 2016. *Recommendations and Reports. 65*(1), 1–49.

Chou, R., Fanciulllo, G., & Fine, P. et al. 2009. Clinical guidelines for the use of chronic opioid therapy in chronic noncancer pain. *Journal of Pain. 10*, 113–130.

Cleveland Clinic. 2017. Acute vs Chronic Pain. Available at https://my.clevelandclinic.org/health/articles/12051-acute-vs-chronic-pain.

Cosio, D., & Swaroop, S. 2016. The use of mind-body medicine in chronic pain management: differential trends and session-by-session changes in anxiety. *Pain Management and Medicine. 2*, 114. doi:10.4172/jpmme.1000114.

Deutsch, P., & Sawyer, H. 2004. *Guide to Rehabilitation*. New York, NY: Ahab Press.

Department of Veterans Affairs and Department of Defense. 2010. VA/DoD Clinical Practice Guideline for Management of Opioid Therapy for Chronic Pain, Washington, DC. Available at https://www.healthquality.va.gov/guidelines/Pain/cot/VADoDOTCPG022717.pdf

Engel, G., MacBryde, C., & Blacklow, R. 1970. *Signs and Symptoms* (5th ed.). Philadelphia, PA: J. P. Lippincott.

Fordyce, W. E. 1976. *Behavioral Methods for Chronic Pain and Illness*. St. Louis, MO: C. V. Mosby.

Ghods, B. K., Roter, D. L., & Ford, D. E. et al. 2008. Patient-physician communication in the primary care visits of African Americans and whites with depression. *Journal of General Internal Medicine. 23*, 600–606.

Green, C. R., Anderson, K. O., & Baker, T. A. et al. 2003a. The unequal burden of pain: Confronting racial and ethnic disparities in pain. *Pain Medicine. 4*, 277–294.

Green, C. R., Wheeler, J. R., & LaPorte, F. 2003b. Clinical decision making in pain management: contributions of physicians and patient characteristics to variations in practice. *Journal of Pain. 4*, 29–39.

Green, C. R., Wheeler, J. R., & LaPorte, F. et al. 2002. How well is chronic pain managed? Who does it well? *Pain Medicine. 3*, 56–65.

IASP. 1979. International association for studies on pain, subcommittee on taxonomy. *Pain. 6*, 249–252.

Institute of Medicine Committee on Advancing Pain Research Care and Education Board on Health Sciences Policy. 2011. *Relieving Pain in America: A Blueprint for Transforming Prevention, Care, Education, and Research*. Washington, DC: The National Academies Press.

King, P., Tuckwell, N., & Barrett, T. 1998. A critical review of functional capacity evaluations. *Physical Therapy. 79*, 852–866.

Manchikanti, L., Helm, S., & Singh, V. et al. 2009. An Algorithmic Approach for Clinical Management of Chronic Spinal Pain. *Pain Physician. 12*, E231. Available www.painphysicianjournal.com

McMahon, S., & Koltzenburg, M. (Eds.). 2006. *Wall and Melzack's Textbook of Pain* (5th ed.). Philadelphia, PA: Elsevier.

Melzack, R. 1973. *The Puzzle of Pain*. New York, NY: Basic Books.

Merskey, H. 1964. An Investigation of Pain in Psychological Illness. *Unpublished doctoral dissertation*. Oxford, England: University of Oxford.

Merskey, H. 1972. Personality traits of psychiatric patients with pain. *Journal of Psychosomatic Research. 16*, 163–166.

Moreo, K. 2003. *Managing Low Back Pain*. Miramar, FL: Author.

Pope, J., Deer, T., Bruel, B., & Falowski, S. 2016. Clinical Uses of Intrathecal Therapy and Its Placement in the Pain Care Algorithm. *Pain Practice. 16*(8), 1092–1106.

Practice Guidelines for Chronic Pain Management. 2010. An Updated Report by the American Society of Anesthesiologists Task Force on Chronic Pain Management and the American Society of Regional Anesthesia and Pain Medicine 2010. *Anesthesiology. 112*, 1–24.

Ramamurthy, S., Alanmanou, E., & Rogers, J. 2006. *Decision Making in Pain Management* (2nd ed.). Philadelphia, PA: Mosby.

Ramamurthy, S., & Alvarado, E. 2006. Imaging studies. In S. Ramamurthy, E. Alanmanou, & J. Rogers (Eds.), *Decision Making in Pain Management* (2nd ed., pp. 24–25). St. Louis, MO: Mosby Elsevier.

Ramsey, R. 1979. The understanding and teaching of reaction to pain. *Bibliotheca Psychiatrica. 159*, 114–140.

Shealy, C. 1976. *The Pain Game*. Los Angeles, CA: Celestial Arts.

Skinner, B. F. 1938. *Behavior of Organisms*. New York, NY: Appleton-Century-Crofts.

Sternbach, R. A. 1968. *Pain: A Psychophysiological Analysis*. New York, NY: Academic Press.

Sternbach, R. A. 1974. *Pain Patients: Traits and Treatment*. New York, NY: Academic Press.

Von Korff, M., Glasgow, R. E., & Sharpe, M. 2002. Organising care for chronic illness. *BMJ. 325*, 92–94.

Vos, T., Flaxman, A. D., & Naghavi, M. et al. 2012. Years lived with disability (YLDs) for 1160 sequelae of 289 diseases and injuries 1990–2010: a systematic analysis for the Global Burden of Disease Study. *Lancet. 380*, 2163–2196.

Weingarten, S. R., Henning, J. M., & Badamgarav, E. et al. 2002. Interventions used in disease management programmes for patients with chronic illness: which ones work? Meta-analysis of published reports. *BMJ. 325*, 925.

Weed, R. 1987. Pain basics. *Journal of Private Sector Rehabilitation. 2*, 65–71.

Weed, R., & Field, T. 2012. *The Rehabilitation Consultant's Handbook* (4th ed.). Athens, GA: E&F Vocational Services.

World Health Organization. 2009. *WHO's Pain Relief Ladder*. Retrieved May 4, 2009, from http://www.who.int/cancer/palliative/painladder/en.

Chapter 17

Life Care Planning for Spinal Cord Injury

David J. Altman and Dan M. Bagwell

Contents

Introduction....498
Epidemiology....498
Anatomy.... 499
Spinal Cord Injury (SCI) Classification....501
Injury Classification.... 502
Preservation of Function by Neurologic Level of Injury.... 503
Common Complications of Spinal Cord Injury.... 504
Autonomic Dysfunction.... 504
Gastrointestinal Issues.... 505
Spasticity.... 506
Respiratory Complications.... 506
Pain.... 507
Genitourinary Dysfunction.... 508
Metabolic Changes....510
Integumentary Issues....511
Circulatory Disorders....511
Infections....512
Overuse Syndromes....513
Sexual Function and Reproduction....513
Psychological Issues....514
Home Modifications....514
Vehicular Modification....515
Powered Robotic Exoskeletons in SCI....516
Aging with Spinal Cord Injury and Personal Care Assistance Needs....517
Life Expectancy....518
Case Study....519
Acknowledgment....529
References....529

Introduction

Injuries to the spinal cord are among the most devastating of all neurological conditions, with profound, multidimensional consequences for both the individual and the family. An adult who has previously been independent is often devastated by his need for assistance with basic Activities of Daily Living, such as feeding, bathing, grooming, and carrying out bowel and bladder functions. Consequently, a team approach is needed for the care, treatment, and rehabilitation of individuals with spinal cord injury (SCI), with contributions from medical and surgical specialties, nursing, multiple therapeutic disciplines, medical case managers, and other health care professionals (Bagwell et al., 1996). The rehabilitation process extends for years after the injury. Furthermore, the aging process only compounds the effects of the spinal cord injury, necessitating proactive measures that include pharmacotherapy, physiotherapy, surgeries, counseling, environmental modifications, and an extensive array of adaptive devices, medical supplies, and durable medical equipment (Winkler et al., 2010).

Epidemiology

Data from the 2017 SCI Data Sheet, National Spinal Cord Injury Statistical Center (NSCISC), indicate that there are approximately 17,500 individuals each year who suffer a SCI, with an estimated 285,000 SCI survivors living in the United States (from 245,000 to 353,000 persons). Males still account for approximately 80% of new spinal cord injuries, but the average age is currently 42 years, an increase from 29 years during the 1970s. Motor vehicle accidents (including motorcycle accidents) remain the leading cause of injury, accounting for 38%, followed by falls (30.5%), violence, primarily gunshot wounds (13.5%), sports and recreation (9%), iatrogenic causes (5%), and other (4%).

While life expectancies of SCI survivors improved substantially during the 1970s and well into the 1980s relative to just two decades preceding the 1970s, further gains were beginning to plateau as we entered the 1990s, with little gain seen through the first decade of the 21st century. This leveling of the improvement trend caught the attention of many who are involved in the care of those with spinal cord injury, as well as the spinal cord injured population generally. Interesting observations were also being made about the prospects of a correlation with a greater influence of managed care initiatives to reduce the lengths of stay in the acute care and rehabilitation settings (DeVivo et al., 1999). Indeed, the average length of hospital stays in the acute care setting is currently less than half that of those who were injured in the 1970s, 11 days versus 24, and the average lengths of rehabilitation stay are currently just more than one third of those who received rehabilitation in the 1970s, 35 days versus 98 days (NSCISC SCI Data Sheet, 2017). This compression of acute inpatient hospitalization has correspondingly limited the amount of time for individuals with newly acquired spinal cord injuries to develop adaptation and coping skills that are necessary for successful transition to the community.

Death rates remain much higher during the first year post-injury when compared with subsequent years, particularly for those who sustain greater levels of neurologic impairment. Multiple studies have also identified a number of socioeconomic risk factors that are believed to be associated with increased mortality rates among those with SCI (Krause & Saunders, 2010). Despite a leveling of the gains in life expectancies for those with SCI, long-term survival has improved immensely since the 1940s, when survival was estimated at just 18 months. As a result of such gains, people with spinal cord injuries are living long enough to experience age-related health issues that are seen in the general population.

Data obtained from the 2016 NSCISC Annual Report indicate that diseases of the respiratory system remain the leading cause of death for those with SCI (21.9%), with the vast majority of these deaths due to pneumonia. The second leading cause of death was infective and parasitic disease (12.1%), of which 89.3% were the result of septicemia and usually associated with decubitus ulcers, urinary tract infections, or respiratory infections. Cancer (neoplasm) was the third leading cause of death in the SCI population (10.1%), followed closely by hypertensive and ischemic heart disease (10.0%), often due to unexplained heart attacks. Unintentional injuries were the sixth leading cause of death (6.7%), followed by disease of the digestive system (4.8%), cerebral vascular disease (3.6%), and suicide (3.1%). It should be noted that while diseases of the genitourinary system represent the leading cause of rehospitalization, they constitute only 3.0% of overall deaths (NSCISC Annual Report, 2016, Table 10).

During any given year, nearly one-third (30%) of spinal cord patients receiving care through the Spinal Cord Injury Model Systems of care are rehospitalized (NSCISC SCI Data Sheet, 2017). The average length of stay with rehospitalization is approximately 22 days. Far and away, the leading cause of rehospitalization within the first year continues to be diseases of the genitourinary system, at 46.3%. This is followed by diseases of the skin (18.7%) and diseases of the circulatory system (11.6%) for known or classified causes (NSCISC Annual Report, 2016, Table 96). The incidences of rehospitalization for diseases of the skin and respiratory system increase substantially over time, accounting for up to 28.9 and 16.9% of rehospitalizations respectively (NSCISC Annual Report, 2016, Table 96).

Spinal cord injuries usually occur during peak productivity years and survivors experience permanent disabilities that often impact employment opportunities. In fact, only 20.5% of SCI survivors are employed at 5 years post-injury and 27.1% at 10 years post-injury (NSCISC Annual Report, 2016, Table 43). Nearly half of these survivors (47.1%) have family household incomes that are less than $25,000 annually at post-injury year five, with only marginal changes from years 10 through 20 post-injury (NSCISC Annual Report, 2016, Table 50).

Anatomy

The spinal cord is the crucial conduit between the brain and the body, and its small surface area contains millions of neurons and axons which innervate motor, sensory, and autonomic functions. Injuries to the spinal cord cause temporary or permanent changes in motor, sensory, and/or autonomic function. The resulting damage to the cord impairs physiologic transmission of signals to and from the brain below the level of the injury. Even small injuries to the spinal cord can result in profound functional loss, and the higher the level of involvement, the greater the degree of disability.

The human spinal cord is divided into 31 segments, and each segment projects a pair of mixed sensory and motor nerves, which combine before passing through spaces (foramina) between the vertebrae. The spinal cord generally terminates at the level of the first lumbar vertebra (L1), below which nerve roots within the vertebral column are referred to as the cauda equina (so named because the elongated nerve roots have the appearance of a horse's tail). The terminal spinal cord is referred to as the conus medullaris.

The spinal cord is surrounded and protected by 33 weight bearing bones, referred to as vertebrae, which are in turn separated by gelatinous disks which act as shock absorbers and supported by ligaments (Figures 17.1 and 17.2). There are 7 cervical, 12 thoracic, 5 lumbar, 5 sacral, and 4 fused

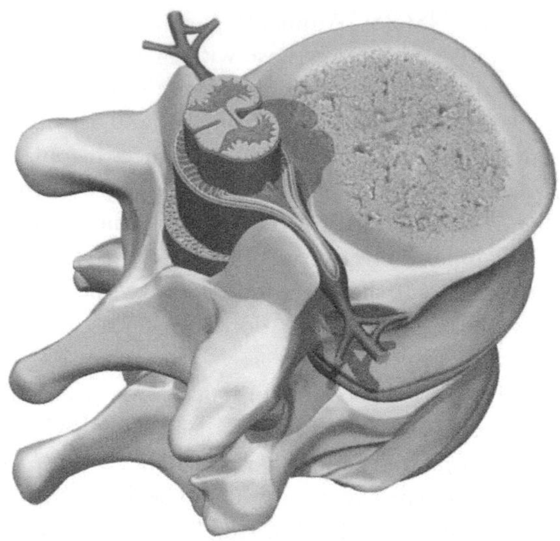

Figure 17.1 Vertebrae surrounding the spinal cord and other neural elements. (Dreamstime LLC. Reprinted with permission.)

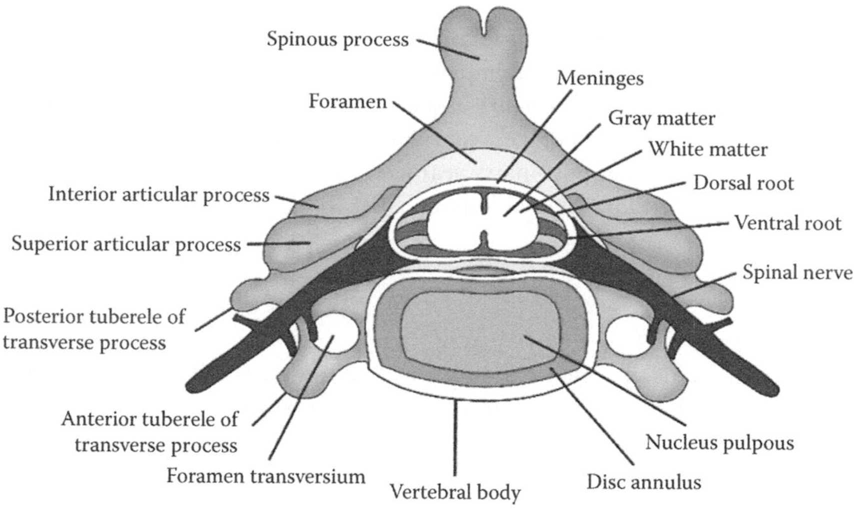

Figure 17.2 Cross section of vertebra surrounding the spinal cord and other neural elements. (Dreamstime LLC. Reprinted with permission.)

coccygeal vertebrae. The cervical and lumbar portions of the vertebral column have a great deal of flexibility relative to the rigid thoracic vertebrae.

Each segment of the spinal cord is associated with a pair of dorsal ganglia, which are situated just outside the spinal cord and which contain the cell bodies of sensory neurons (see Figure 17.3).

The spinal cord is organized somatotopically, such that the neurons that innervate muscles are located on its ventral portion, the fibers that carry proprioceptive and vibratory sensory modalities are positioned dorsally, and the nerve fibers that carry information for pain and temperature are

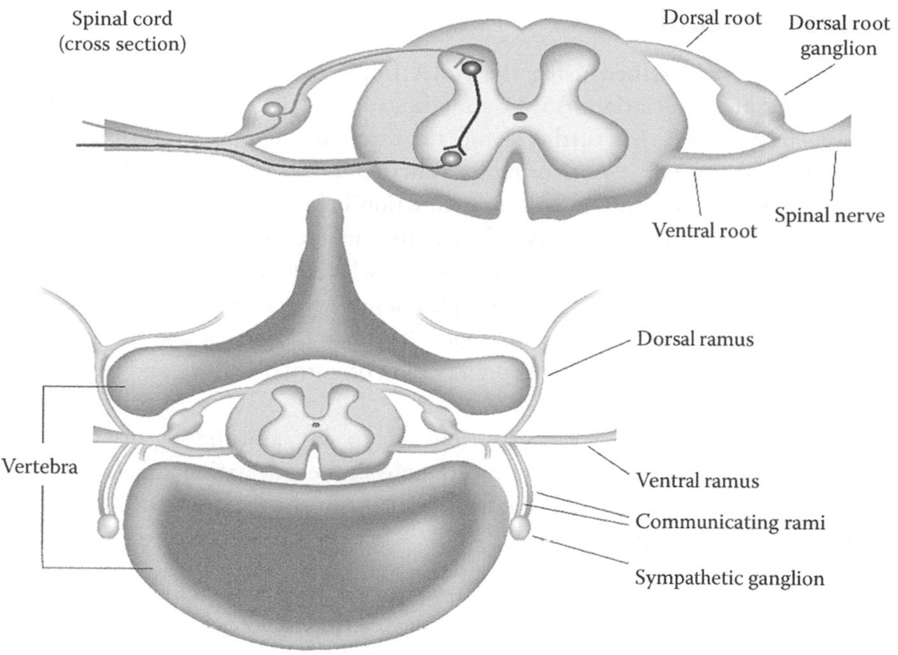

Figure 17.3 Cross section of the spinal cord. (Dreamstime LLC. Reprinted with permission.)

located laterally. Understanding the somatotopic organization of the spinal cord can often allow for localization of lesions based upon relative involvement or preservation of these modalities.

Anatomically, the spinal cord is protected by three layers of tissue, referred to as the meninges. The outermost layer (dura mater) forms a tough protective coating. Between the dura mater and the surrounding bone of the vertebrae is the epidural space, which contains adipose tissue and an intricate network of blood vessels. The middle layer of the meninges is the arachnoid (spider) mater, which is separated from the innermost delicate (pial) layer by the subarachnoid space, which contains cerebrospinal fluid. The pial layer is extremely delicate and intimately associated with the surface of the spinal cord. The spinal cord is stabilized by the denticulate ligaments, which extend from the pia mater laterally between the dorsal and ventral roots.

Spinal Cord Injury (SCI) Classification

The American Spinal Injury Association (ASIA) and the International Medical Society of Paraplegia have developed a worldwide nomenclature system which standardizes nomenclature and classification of spinal cord injuries, and which assists communication among clinicians, as well as clinical research and prognostic determinations. This system establishes a level of injury based upon the lowest neurological level that has intact sensory function and at least antigravity function. It is further classified through an A to E scale based upon the degree of preserved motor and sensory function below this level. These data are useful for the life care planner in projecting the type of medical and medically related goods and services that an individual with SCI will likely require, as well as providing a basis for projecting comorbidity and, where applicable, life expectancy.

Injury Classification

Spinal cord injuries are classified using the ASIA Impairment Scale (AIS) developed by the American Spinal Injury Association (ASIA), a modification of the Frankel Scale (see Figure 17.4). It has five levels from A to E that further define the extent of the injury (AIS). "A" is a complete lesion, based on the absence of sensory or motor function in the S4–S5 sacral segments. "B" is an incomplete lesion with sensation but no motor function below the neurological level. Sensation must be present in the S4 and S5 segments. "C" is an incomplete lesion with motor function present below the neurological level, and the majority of key muscles have a measured grade of strength less than 3 (5 is normal strength). "D" is an incomplete lesion with motor function present, and the majority of the key muscles below the neurological level has a muscle grade greater than or equal to 3. An AIS designation of "E" represents preservation of normal sensory and motor function on neurological examination (ASIA 2016).

Often, the sensory and motor levels vary from side to side, and the sensory and motor levels can be different on the same side of the body. The physical examination should record the most caudal sensory and motor level on each side which results in the recording of four levels (sensory and motor from both right and left).

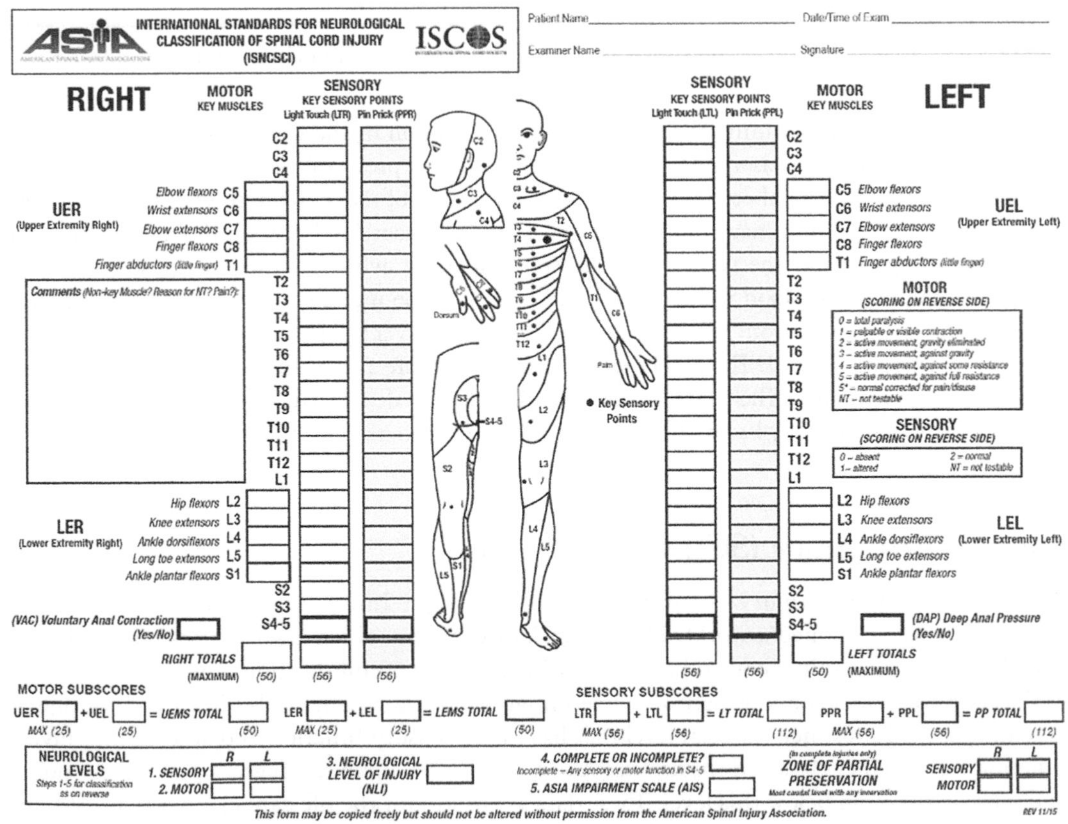

ASIA — INTERNATIONAL STANDARDS FOR NEUROLOGICAL CLASSIFICATION OF SPINAL CORD INJURY (ISNCSCI) — ISCoS

Patient Name ______ Date/Time of Exam ______

Examiner Name ______ Signature ______

RIGHT

MOTOR KEY MUSCLES | SENSORY KEY SENSORY POINTS: Light Touch (LTR), Pin Prick (PPR)

C2
C3
C4

UER (Upper Extremity Right)
Elbow flexors C5
Wrist extensors C6
Elbow extensors C7
Finger flexors C8
Finger abductors (little finger) T1

Comments (Non-key Muscle? Reason for NT? Pain?):

T2
T3
T4
T5
T6
T7
T8
T9
T10
T11
T12
L1

LER (Lower Extremity Right)
Hip flexors L2
Knee extensors L3
Ankle dorsiflexors L4
Long toe extensors L5
Ankle plantar flexors S1

S2
S3
S4-5

(VAC) Voluntary Anal Contraction (Yes/No)

RIGHT TOTALS (MAXIMUM) (50) (56) (56)

LEFT

SENSORY KEY SENSORY POINTS: Light Touch (LTL), Pin Prick (PPL) | MOTOR KEY MUSCLES

C2
C3
C4

UEL (Upper Extremity Left)
C5 Elbow flexors
C6 Wrist extensors
C7 Elbow extensors
C8 Finger flexors
T1 Finger abductors (little finger)

T2
T3
T4
T5
T6
T7
T8
T9
T10
T11
T12
L1

LEL (Lower Extremity Left)
L2 Hip flexors
L3 Knee extensors
L4 Ankle dorsiflexors
L5 Long toe extensors
S1 Ankle plantar flexors

S2
S3
S4-5

(DAP) Deep Anal Pressure (Yes/No)

LEFT TOTALS (MAXIMUM) (56) (56) (50)

MOTOR (SCORING ON REVERSE SIDE)
0 = total paralysis
1 = palpable or visible contraction
2 = active movement, gravity eliminated
3 = active movement, against gravity
4 = active movement, against some resistance
5 = active movement, against full resistance
5* = normal corrected for pain/disuse
NT = not testable

SENSORY (SCORING ON REVERSE SIDE)
0 = absent
1 = altered
2 = normal
NT = not testable

● Key Sensory Points

MOTOR SUBSCORES

UER ☐ + UEL ☐ = UEMS TOTAL ☐ MAX (25) (25) (50)

LER ☐ + LEL ☐ = LEMS TOTAL ☐ MAX (25) (25) (50)

SENSORY SUBSCORES

LTR ☐ + LTL ☐ = LT TOTAL ☐ MAX (56) (56) (112)

PPR ☐ + PPL ☐ = PP TOTAL ☐ MAX (56) (56) (112)

NEUROLOGICAL LEVELS (Steps 1-5 for classification as on reverse): R L — 1. SENSORY ☐ ☐ 2. MOTOR ☐ ☐

3. NEUROLOGICAL LEVEL OF INJURY (NLI) ☐

4. COMPLETE OR INCOMPLETE? ☐ Incomplete = Any sensory or motor function in S4-5

5. ASIA IMPAIRMENT SCALE (AIS) ☐

ZONE OF PARTIAL PRESERVATION (In complete injuries only) Most caudal level with any innervation: R L — SENSORY ☐ ☐ MOTOR ☐ ☐

This form may be copied freely but should not be altered without permission from the American Spinal Injury Association. REV 11/15

Figure 17.4 International Standards for Neurological Classification of Spinal Cord Injury. (© 2015, American Spinal Injury Association. Reprinted with permission.)

Muscle grades for testing motor power are:

- Grade 0—Complete paralysis
- Grade 1—Flicker of contraction present
- Grade 2—Active movement with gravity eliminated
- Grade 3—Active movement against gravity
- Grade 4—Active movement against gravity and some resistance described as poor, fair, moderate strength
- Grade 5—Normal power

Preservation of Function by Neurologic Level of Injury

With each progressive level of neurologic lesion identified below, the gain in additional preservation of function is identified:

- C1–3: Preservation of tongue movement and swallowing, as well as neck extension flexion, rotation, and side bending. There is paralysis of all muscles of the trunk, upper extremities, and lower extremities. There is also loss of diaphragmatic function necessary for respiration.
- C4: Shoulder elevation (shoulder shrug). Under most circumstances, there is sufficient diaphragmatic function to breathe without a ventilator. Upper cervical paraspinals are also preserved.
- C5: Scapular adduction; shoulder abduction (partial), flexion, extension, and rotation; weak elbow flexion and forearm supination.
- C6: Full rotation and abduction of shoulder; scapular abduction and upward rotation; shoulder horizontal adduction; full elbow flexion; wrist extension and tenodesis grip (passive thumb adduction on the index finger during active wrist extension).
- C7: Shoulder internal rotation, adduction, and depression; elbow extension; forearm pronation; wrist flexion; finger and thumb extension; partial finger flexion.
- C8: Full wrist extension with abduction and adduction and wrist flexion; full finger flexion; thumb flexion, abduction, adduction, and opposition; flexion at the metacarpophalangeals with extension of the interphalangeals (incomplete lumbricals).
- T1–6: Complete innervation of lumbricals for flexion of the metacarpophalangeals and extension of the interphalangeals; finger abduction and adduction at the interphalangeals; extension of the thoracic spine; upper intercostals innervated.
- T7–12: Trunk flexion and rotation; some pelvic elevation.
- L1–2: Full pelvic elevation and hip flexion.
- L3–4: Lumbar extension; knee flexion and extension, hip adduction; ankle dorsiflexion (weak).

There are a number of incomplete spinal cord syndromes that are also important to recognize:

1. *Central cord syndrome*: Central spinal cord swelling or formation of a central syrinx (a fluid filled cavity) is often characterized by relative weakness in the upper extremities, a "floating" loss of temperature, and pin prick sensation 1–2 levels below the level of the injury secondary to damage to the crossing spinothalamic tract fibers, and urinary retention.
2. *Brown-Sequard syndrome*: Hemisection of the spinal cord results in ipsilateral weakness below the lesion (as a result of damage to the descending corticospinal tract) and contralateral

sensory loss starting 1–2 levels below the lesion level (resulting from damage to the ascending and crossing spinothalamic tract fibers).

3. *Conus medullaris syndrome*: Injury to the terminus of the spinal cord results in bowel and bladder dyscontrol, sexual dysfunction, and paraparesis.
4. *Cauda equina syndromes*: Although not truly a spinal cord injury, lesions of the cauda equina result in loss of function to the lumbar plexus below the conus medullaris of the spinal cord. As such, it is a lower motor neuron lesion. These syndromes are characterized by sensory impairment in a saddle distribution, back pain, motor weakness of the lower extremities, neurogenic bowel and bladder, and sexual dysfunction.

Common Complications of Spinal Cord Injury

Spinal cord injuries result in numerous physiological changes that involve virtually every system of the body, which in turn can cause many complications. The life care planner must be very familiar with these complications in order to project the need for medical interventions, equipment, supplies, and medications for anticipated treatment, symptom amelioration, or as possible, prevention.

Autonomic Dysfunction

The spinal cord is a critical component of the autonomic nervous system, and injury can often lead to changes in the quality of hair, skin, and nails, as well as the ability of the individual to response to temperature changes (i.e., thermoregulation, including sweating). One of the most serious complications is autonomic dysreflexia, a syndrome associated with spinal cord lesions at or above the T6 level (Consortium for Spinal Cord Medicine, 2001). Lesions above this level block the central nervous system's ability to regulate the outflow of the sympathetic ganglia that are located within the intermediolateral cell column. This condition is often provoked by noxious stimuli (i.e., urinary tract infections, urinary retention, constipation, ingrown toenails, labor and delivery, and decubitus ulcers), and is characterized by the following signs and symptoms:

1. Severe headache
2. Diaphoresis
3. Piloerection
4. Hypertension
5. Tachycardia (occasionally bradycardia)
6. General malaise
7. Flushing or redness of the skin above the level of the spinal cord lesion

If unrecognized and untreated, autonomic dysreflexia can result in hypertensive cerebral hemorrhages, leading to severe disability and even death.

An opposite scenario is that of orthostatic hypotension, in which the individual with a spinal cord injury will experience sudden drops in blood pressure in response to position changes. This condition is characterized clinically by light headedness, dizziness, or even syncope. Proposed causes for orthostatic hypotension in the context of spinal cord injury include alterations in baroreflex receptor function, altered salt and water homeostasis, and impaired venous return from the lower extremities.

Poikilothermia is a condition that is defined by impaired thermoregulatory control. As individuals with spinal cord injuries are often unable to shiver, sweat, or otherwise appropriately regulate peripheral blood vessels, they are at relatively high risk for becoming hypothermic or hyperthermic. As such, it is critical that they are able to closely monitor and regulate their environments with accurate and responsive thermostats. While outdoors, cooling vests offer some protection against hyperthermia in warmer climates.

Gastrointestinal Issues

Gastrointestinal problems occur in 27–62% of individuals with spinal cord injuries, and symptoms include constipation, abdominal pain, incontinence, nausea, and diarrhea (Ebert, 2012). Furthermore, the individual with SCI is at greater risk for gastritis as well as gastric ulcers, particularly if the level of injury is at or above the T6 level. Another common complication, occurring in 17–31% of individuals with SCI is cholelithiasis, the underlying cause of which remains uncertain (Ebert, 2012). Complicating the situation is the fact that the clinical presentation of an acute abdomen is often subtle in this patient population, necessitating a low index of suspicion.

Neurogenic bowel can result from both upper (i.e., above the level of the conus medullaris) and lower motor neuron lesions (i.e., involving the conus medullaris and/or cauda equina). Most individuals with SCI experience an upper motor neuron syndrome, which is characterized by both the impaired sensation of rectal fullness as well as the inability to voluntarily relax the external anal sphincter. However, reflex bowel movements can still be triggered by intact nerve connections between the spinal cord, the colon, and the mesenteric plexus (Consortium for Spinal Cord Medicine, 1998). In this scenario, fecal incontinence occurs suddenly and without warning as part of a mass reflex. Conversely, those with lower motor neuron lesions involving the distal conus medullaris and cauda equina have voluntary control of part or all of their abdominal muscles, but there is neither spinal cord-mediated peristalsis nor external anal sphincter control. This syndrome is generally characterized by constipation and requires that the rectum be kept empty by digital evacuation of stool.

For most individuals with neurogenic bowel, a complete bowel evacuation every other day is satisfactory. Less frequent bowel movements may result in fecal impaction. Some patients require daily evacuation to avoid incontinence between bowel programs. A bowel evacuation program may take up to 2 hours to complete and should be completed at a time that is convenient for both the patient and the caregiver. Stool softeners and bowel evacuants, along with digital stimulation are usually needed to obtain a reasonable degree of continence (absence of frequent accidents).

Gastrointestinal motility can be further reduced by certain pharmacologic agents, such as narcotic analgesics and even some tricyclic agents. Where possible, these medications should be avoided. Broad-spectrum antibiotics may inadvertently alter gut flora and result in diarrhea. As patients with spinal cord injury often require these antibiotics, the bowel routine can be disrupted frequently, with need for replacement of normal gut flora with probiotic agents or other forms of lactobacillus, such as yogurt. The diet should also contain adequate amounts of water and fiber.

Most individuals with spinal cord injury experience constipation and an occasional fecal impaction. Younger individuals with SCI usually have fewer problems with chronic constipation than do older patients or individuals who are several years out from their injuries. Bowel programs generally change over time with changes in medication and the procedure used for bowel evacuation. However, most bowel regimens involve emphasizing the importance of adequate hydration and fiber intake to maintain proper stool consistency, as well as bowel training so that evacuation can occur at regular intervals. Other treatment options include the use of bisacodyl or saline enemas and oral medications such as cisapride, which facilitate the release of acetylcholine at the myenteric plexus (Badali et al., 1991), sacral nerve stimulation (Gstaltner et al., 2008), non-invasive magnetic stimulation, and surgical placement of a colostomy or ileostomy (Branagan et al., 2003).

Spasticity

Spasticity is defined as a velocity dependent increase in muscle tone resulting from hyperexcitability of the stretch reflex and is one of the hallmarks of spinal cord injury below the level of the lesion. The incidence of spasticity is reported to exceed 80% in the SCI population (Elbasiouny et al., 2010). Clinical findings include hyperreflexia (often with clonus), muscle spasms, and clasp-knife responses. While mild spasticity in the lower extremities can assist with weight bearing and the reduction in venous stasis, markedly increased tone can interfere with or prevent the performance of functional activities, such as range of motion exercises. When more pronounced, it can result in painful spasms that can negatively impact an individual's quality of life.

It is important to treat spasticity in order to prevent the development of tendon shortening across a joint (i.e., contracture) and permanent loss of function. Stretching exercises, often performed by a therapist in the clinical setting and caregivers in the home setting, can help to reduce spasticity severity. Without periodic stretching and range of motion exercises, spastic extremities develop tendon shortening and permanent contractures.

Oral antispastic medications, such as baclofen and tizanidine, are commonly prescribed as first lines of therapy, along with benzodiazepine medications (i.e., diazepam, clonazepam), and occasionally dantrolene, which directly reduces the contractility of muscle tissue. For individuals with more severe spasticity, oral medications will often be insufficient for adequate management, or the dosing required of these agents may result in intolerable adverse effects, such as sedation, mental confusion, or elevated liver enzymes indicative of liver damage. Under these circumstances, neuromuscular blockade with botulinum toxin can be extremely effective, with effects lasting for approximately 3 months between injections. Neuromuscular blockade can also be used adjunctively with orally administered antispastic agents.

Individuals with severe spasticity involving both upper and lower extremities may also benefit from the implantation of an intrathecal baclofen pump, a microprocessor controlled and programmable device that can administer miniscule quantities of medication through a catheter and into the intrathecal space, where spasticity can be greatly ameliorated with negligible systemic effects.

Respiratory Complications

The C3 through C5 nerve roots innervate the diaphragm through the phrenic nerves. Spinal cord injuries at or above these levels (particularly above C4) are usually associated with ventilator dependency. Ventilator dependency has significant implications for long-term post-injury survival and life expectancy. Even individuals who have sustained thoracic spinal cord injuries above T-12 can experience impaired ventilation and cough, leading to a restrictive pattern of pulmonary disease because of intercostal muscle dysfunction.

Respiratory failure is caused by either failure to ventilate, which is characterized by increased levels of carbon dioxide in the blood, or failure to oxygenate, in which there is reduced oxygen content within the blood. Global alveolar hypoventilation (GAH) is an insidious condition characterized by the gradual loss of pulmonary function as a result of reduced compliance from chronic hypoventilation. Its effects can be accentuated by comorbid scoliosis, kyphosis, and obesity. Individuals with vital capacities below 5 to 10 mL/kg are considered to be at highest risk for respiratory failure and may require assisted ventilation to support life. Other factors that can contribute to impaired respiratory status include pregnancy, scoliosis, spasticity, and syringomyelia.

Diseases of the respiratory system represent the leading cause of death for those with SCI, while it is the third most common cause of rehospitalization for the SCI population overall. For persons with tetraplegia, there is a much higher incidence of morbidity and rehospitalization due to diseases of the respiratory system, pneumonia in particular. As such, those with SCI should be given high priority for available flu and pneumococcal vaccines. All individuals with cervical or thoracic spinal cord injuries should undergo periodic clinical pulmonary assessments and pulmonary function testing and should receive both influenza and pneumococcal vaccinations in the absence of any contraindications.

Chronic ventilation may become necessary to sustain life for those with global alveolar hypoventilation, particularly with vital capacities that are less than 5 to 10 mL/kg. There are a variety of devices that are employed to assist individuals with respiratory function. These include ventilation assist machines such as continuous positive airway pressure (CPAP) and biphasic positive airway pressure (BiPAP), which can improve oxygenation and prevent hypercarbia. Phrenic nerve pacing (diaphragm pacing) is another option that electrically stimulates the diaphragm to produce more physiologic respirations. Phrenic nerve pacing provides many ventilator-dependent tetraplegics with freedom from total dependence upon mechanical ventilation. Even though many individuals with phrenic nerve pacing will still require periods of ventilator assistance throughout the day and night, the risk of death is diminished in the event of mechanical failure of the ventilator and affords time for backup measures to be put into place.

In higher and complete cervical spine injuries, ventilator assistance at some level is usually required and is administered through a tracheostomy tube. These individuals require 24-hour skilled nursing care to protect the airway, provide suctioning of secretions, pulmonary toilet, management of the tracheostomy tube, as well as to ensure accurate ventilator functioning.

Pain

Over the past 60 years, the literature has identified chronic pain as a serious concern for individuals who suffer spinal cord injury. Numerous longitudinal studies have been undertaken concerning the prevalence and types of pain encountered by persons with SCI. Approximately 70 to 80% of individuals with SCI report persistent pain (Cardenas & Felix, 2009). Approximately one third of persons with SCI report chronic severe pain that interferes with Activities of Daily Living and affects quality of life. In one study, a survey of the spinal cord injured revealed that approximately one third of individuals suffering from chronic pain were willing to trade the possibility of recovery from SCI for pain relief (Nepomuceno et al., 1979). Approximately two thirds of patients with upper extremity pain state that it interferes with their ability to transfer to and from a wheelchair, and rotator cuff tears are reported in 65% of those with chronic impingement syndrome with subacromial bursitis (Bagwell et al., 2010).

Wrist pain is reported in 53 to 64% of persons with chronic SCI and this is attributed to compressive loading during transfers with the wrist in extension (Bagwell et al., 2010).

Individuals with spinal cord injury can experience nociceptive, visceral, and neuropathic type pain. Nociceptive pain is defined pathophysiologically by the transmission of pain impulses through the normal peripheral and central pathways. Examples of this type of pain would include the inflammatory pain from overuse of compensating joints or musculoskeletal tissue injury, such as rotator cuff syndrome. Visceral pain is located in the abdomen or thorax and is generally described as a dull, aching, or cramping pain. It is most commonly associated with urinary tract infection, ureterolithiasis, cholelithiasis, or obstipation of the bowel with impaction. One of the particular challenges in caring for individuals with spinal cord injury is the often inchoate nature of their pain, which can mask serious underlying conditions, such as an acute appendicitis or nephrolithiasis. Neuropathic pain is caused by injury to the spinal cord or nerve roots and is believed to be the result of aberrant transmission of electrical impulses by damaged nerve pathways or by chronic electrochemical changes in the brain itself resulting from a spinal cord injury (Cardenas & Felix, 2009). While some individuals often describe this pain as "electrical," "stabbing," "shooting," or "burning," others may have difficulty articulating the specific nature of the pain. Another curious feature of neuropathic pain is the phenomenon of allodynia, in which a normally benign external stimulus (such as lightly stroking the skin) can be perceived as painful. Neuropathic pain itself can be further subdivided into pain at the level of a spinal cord injury and pain below the level of the injury. It is important to recognize neuropathic pain and to treat it aggressively, since delayed treatment is believed to contribute to the chronicity and refractoriness of the pain.

In contrast to the use of nonsteroidal anti-inflammatory medications and prescriptive analgesics for the management of nociceptive pain, the treatment of neuropathic pain generally involves the use of anticonvulsant agents (i.e., gabapentin, pregabalin, lamotrigine), tricyclic antidepressants, and serotonin-norepinephrine reuptake inhibitors (i.e., duloxetine). For persons whose neuropathic pain responds suboptimally to oral agents, other treatment modalities include topical analgesics (i.e., lidocaine or compounded analgesics), electrical neurostimulation, and neuroablative techniques.

A majority of individuals with spinal cord injuries also suffer from secondary nociceptive pain caused by joint inflammation, tissue injury, and muscle spasms at some point in their lives. Joint pain can arise from either disuse or overuse of limbs, which can cause contractures in the former situation and tissue disruption in the latter. Rotator cuff tendinitis and tears as well as entrapment neuropathies of the ulnar and median nerves are common manifestations of overuse syndromes that occur in association with dependence upon the upper extremities to propel manual wheelchairs and perform frequent transfers.

Genitourinary Dysfunction

Genitourinary dysfunction represents one of the most profound changes that occurs in spinal cord injury. Injuries that occur above the level of the conus medullaris (T12-L1) are associated with upper motor neuron dysfunction characterized by a spastic, hyperactive bladder, often with incoordination between the bladder musculature and the external sphincter, referred to as detrusor-external sphincter dyssynergia. If left untreated, this condition can result in renal injury from elevated pressures within the urinary tract. The understanding of this phenomenon in medicine, that is the secondary consequences to the upper urinary tracts due to high sustained intravesical pressures, and our ability to maintain low pressure systems in the management of neurogenic (neuropathic) bladders, has been one of the greatest influences on improved survivals and life expectancies for those with SCI. In the 1960s, renal failure was a leading cause of death in the SCI population with reports ranging from 37% to as high as 76%, while, as previously noted above, deaths as a result of diseases of the genitourinary system today are only 3.1% (11th leading cause). Renal failure in the general population is the 9th leading cause of death at 1.8% (NVSR, 2016).

Spinal cord injuries below the level of T12-L1 (lower motor neuron bladder) are generally associated with a flaccid bladder that expands greatly, resulting in overflow incontinence as pressure from the distended bladder overwhelms the sphincter. Intermittent catheterization represents the primary choice for urinary drainage in patients with neurogenic bladders. In most cases, this method reduces the incidence of recurrent urinary infection, urinary and ureteral reflux, and stone formation. Chronic indwelling catheterization is not generally recommended due to the increased risk for infection, bladder stones, urethral damage, increased risk of bladder cancer, and other complications, although this approach may be required when intermittent catheterization is not feasible. The surgical placement of a suprapubic catheter is another method of neurogenic bladder management; however, this procedure also contributes to increased risks for bacteremia and renal stone formation.

Proper urological management minimizes the risk of renal complications by reducing risk factors such as cystitis, pyelonephritis, vesicoureteral reflux, and trauma from the use of long-term indwelling catheters. The goals of treatment include establishment of a plan that maintains low detrusor pressures and allows complete bladder emptying. Continued urological follow-up is recommended to monitor for and reduce the risk of these renal, ureteral, and bladder complications.

Established protocols for follow-up and monitoring of the neurogenic bladder are listed in the following sections.

Baseline urological evaluation:

- History and physical examination
- Urinalysis
- Urine culture and sensitivity
- Renal scan and/or renal ultrasound
- 24-hour creatinine clearance or radionuclide scan
- Urodynamics
- CT urography or intravenous pyelogram (baseline assessment)

Subsequent routine follow-up:

- History and physical examination
- Urinalysis
- Urine culture and sensitivity
- KUB
- Renal scan or renal ultrasound annually. (Note: Some centers recommend renal scans annually as a preferred study to renal ultrasounds, which are performed when the renal scan suggests concern for obstructive disease, such as renal/ureteral calculi. Other centers recommend ultrasound annually with intermittent renal scans otherwise.)
- 24-hour creatinine clearance or radionuclide scan
- Urodynamic evaluations performed at one year and as needed thereafter, usually every other year if the bladder appears to be stable
- Urography: CT urography or intravenous pyelogram/cystourethrogram at approximately 3- to 5-year intervals
- Cystoscopy: Opinions on frequency vary greatly, but indications for cystoscopy include hematuria, recurrent symptomatic UTI, recurrent asymptomatic bacteremia with stone forming organism, i.e., *Proteus mirabilis*, episode of GU sepsis, eggshell calculus present with irrigating catheter, and management with long-term indwelling catheter

Diagnostic follow-up and treatment of neurogenic bladder is best performed by a urologist who is experienced with spinal cord injury and associated neurogenic bladder disorders. Improvements in the urological diagnostic investigation have reduced the incidence of progressive disease and death associated with end-stage renal disease (ESRD) for the SCI population. While the risk of ESRD remains slightly higher due to inherent complications with urinary tract infection, obstruction, and reflux, the incidence rates continue to decline such that it is approaching those of the general population.

Metabolic Changes

There are a number of important metabolic changes that occur after a spinal cord injury, including reduced energy expenditure and alterations in hormone levels that have important implications for the management of these individuals. As a result of the reduced energy expenditure, most with SCI experience weight gain that can further affect functional capabilities. For people with paraparesis, weight gain results in greater stress on upper extremity joints during transfers, increasing the risk for accelerated degenerative changes or overuse syndromes, such as rotator cuff injuries. Weight gain also has negative implications with regard to cardiovascular health. Furthermore, additional weight places more pressure on tissue during recumbence, substantially increasing the risk for decubiti (Consortium for Spinal Cord Medicine, PVA, 2008).

The most common hormonal changes that accompany spinal cord injury include insulin resistance and reduced levels of growth hormone and testosterone. The incidence of diabetes mellitus is approximately four times higher in SCI relative to the general population, with an incidence of nearly 25% (Winkler et al., 2010). Low levels of growth hormone and testosterone have been associated with accelerated loss of lean muscle mass, impaired cellular repair mechanisms, and prolonged healing.

Heterotopic ossification (HO) refers to the formation of new bone in the peri-articular soft tissue and occurs in approximately 20% of individuals who have sustained spinal cord injuries. The hips are commonly involved and those affected often present with impaired joint range of motion, associated with edema and warmth of the affected extremity. The diagnosis is typically made through the physical examination and X-rays, which clearly demonstrate the heterotopic bone formation.

SCI results in profound bone demineralization caused by the lack of weight bearing. Approximately 16 months after a spinal cord injury, bone homeostasis occurs at 50 to 70% of normal mineralization, which approaches the fracture threshold. Osteopenia is thereafter facilitated by osteoclastic activity associated with the aging process (Bagwell et al., 2010). This leads to hypercalcemia and hypercalciuria, which likely contributes to the development of not only heterotopic ossification but also nephrolithiasis (kidney stones). Another consequence of demineralization is osteoporosis, with the attendant susceptibility to fractures, which in turn can worsen overall disability. In fact, studies have reported that fractures occur in 21% of the SCI population and that the prevalence increases over time post-injury. The most common sites of fracture are the distal femur and proximal tibia (Bagwell et al., 2010). Common complications of these fractures include delayed union or non-union, pressure sores, and osteomyelitis. Individuals with SCI should undergo periodic monitoring (via DEXA scan) for the development of osteoporosis and should be maintained on vitamin D and calcium supplementation for prophylaxis. While some clinicians proactively prescribe bisphosphonates, recognizing the very high propensity toward long bone fractures, some studies have identified an association between the long-term use of this medication class with the development of osteonecrosis of the jaw (ONJ). Other options for prophylaxis include calcitonin and estrogen modulators (i.e., raloxifene).

Integumentary Issues

Spinal cord injury reduces or eliminates skin sensation in dermatomes below the injury site. Because the individual has either complete loss of sensation or impaired sensation, he or she may sit or lie for long periods of time on certain parts of his or her body. Due to associated muscle atrophy, the normal tissue padding that serves to cushion the skin is reduced. Normally, skin responds to pressure, mechanical stimulation, or inflammation with increased blood flow, but this reflex is blunted in SCI. Loss of this response not only adds to the vulnerability of the skin to pressure sores but reduces the ability of the skin to repair decubitus ulcers once formed.

Diseases of the skin constitute almost 20% of first year post-SCI admissions and approximately 30% of admissions at 15 years (NSCISC Annual Report). At any given time, approximately one third of persons with SCI in the community have a decubitus ulcer and 15% have a stage 3 or 4 ulcer. Once a pressure sore is encountered, the scarred tissue upon healing is more fragile; therefore, the risk of recurrence is heightened. Approximately 35% of those who have sustained a spinal cord injury will experience three or more admissions for this condition over their lifetime (Bagwell et al., 2010). About 75% will admit in follow-up studies to having at least three ulcers at stage 3 or worse (Bagwell et al., 2010).

Decubitus ulcers are potentially life threatening, but progression of these wounds to advanced stages is largely preventable. Great care must be taken to prevent injury to the integument from pressure by shifting sitting positions and frequent turning. If sensory feedback is poor or non-existent, many individuals use electronic devices such as watch alarms to provide timely cueing for lifting and repositioning. Special cushions for sitting and mattresses for extended recumbence have been developed to lessen the pressure upon bony prominences. Special seats that distribute the pressure are used in wheelchairs to prevent sacral decubiti. Vulnerable areas such as the heels must be padded. Sheep skin and other materials are often used for heel and foot protection, as well as orthotic devices to fully offload pressure on the heels, a common site for decubiti. If a decubitus develops, all pressure must be removed, or the decubitus can progress to loss of skin and tissues to the point of exposing bone. The sores must be kept clean or they can become infected. Extensive counseling and prevention education should be started early and continued in the years following the injury. Routine inspection by the patient, caregivers, and through periodic skilled nursing visits should usually identify the onset of these wounds in the earlier stages. Treatment of decubitus ulcers, once developed, requires extensive care and may lead to costly hospitalizations with or without the need for plastic surgery intervention.

Circulatory Disorders

SCI patients are at substantially elevated risk for cardiovascular disease as they age with the sequelae of their injuries (Lavela et al., 2012). In fact, cardiovascular diseases currently account for approximately 46% of all deaths in SCI persons who are greater than 30 years post-injury (Szlachcic et al., 2007). There are a variety of factors that are responsible, including reduced HDL cholesterol levels, higher incidences of obesity, and less exercise relative to the general population. Non-ambulatory individuals are also at risk for the development of phlebitis, deep venous thromboses, and pulmonary emboli, resulting from reduced sympathetic tone and diminished venous return. Therefore, it is critical that preventative measures be taken that include the frequent use of anti-embolic hose as well as frequent lower extremity exercises to reduce venous stasis. Individuals who are at particular risk for the development of deep venous thromboses may require chronic anticoagulation or even placement of devices within the inferior vena cava that can prevent clots from entering the pulmonary vasculature. Furthermore, the clinician should have a low threshold for ordering screening tests, such as Doppler ultrasonography to evaluate for the presence of clots that would necessitate more aggressive management.

One consequence of the reduced mortality from respiratory and renal complications is a relative increase in SCI deaths related to cardiovascular disease. The incidence of cardiovascular disease among those with SCI is greater than 200% of expected in age and gender matched controls (Kocina, 1997). Therefore, routine cardiac surveillance (i.e., periodic EKGs, echocardiography, Persantine stress test) should be instituted even in the younger SCI population, along with proactive recommendations that include aerobic exercise, weight control, and avoidance of tobacco products as well as other risk factors. Furthermore, those with spinal cord injury should anticipate the need for cholesterol lowering agents much earlier than the general population.

Individuals who are non-ambulatory are at substantially elevated risk for the development of various peripheral vascular complications, presumably secondary to the ineffective distribution of oxygenated blood and impaired venous return in the dependent regions of the body, especially the legs. One of the more common and serious conditions is the development of deep vein thrombosis (DVT). Studies on the incidence of DVT in this population are varied, ranging from as low as 7% to as high as 100% (Myers et al., 2007). Although the risk appears to be greatest during the first 6 months post-injury, DVT and thrombophlebitis remain lifelong concerns, particularly as the person ages. Risk factors include impaired mobility and reduced sympathetic tone, which contribute to venous pooling in the lower extremities. Once developed, DVT may continue to be problematic and require periods of prophylaxis and monitoring. With chronic changes in the peripheral venous system, the risk of venous pooling and thrombus formation again becomes a concern with aging.

Preventative measures include the use of anti-embolic hose to preserve the integrity of the peripheral venous system. Screening procedures include Doppler ultrasound, impedance plethysmography, and leg measurements. The definitive procedure for the diagnosis of DVT is venography, although this test is not without risk.

The most concerning risk of deep venous thrombosis is the development of a pulmonary embolism, which constitutes a significant cause of morbidity and mortality in the SCI population, with an incidence of approximately 5% in the first 3 months post-injury and 1 to 2% thereafter (Alabed et al., 2015). Pulmonary embolism may require diagnosis with the use of ventilation-perfusion (V/Q) scanning, although CT angiography of the pulmonary vasculature is today the most common diagnostic tool.

Infections

Infections of the respiratory and genitourinary tracts as well as the integument constitute the leading causes for hospital admissions for every post-injury year, and pneumonia is the leading cause of death from respiratory complications at 65.3% (NSCISC Annual Report, 2016, p. 9). The incidence rate of urinary tract infections alone is estimated at 1.5 to 2.2 per person, per year (Bagwell et al., 2010) and is even higher in those who have chronic indwelling catheters. Therefore, infections should be considered anticipated, not just potential complications. Individuals with higher level spinal cord injuries, particularly those with impaired respiratory function, are at substantially elevated risk for infections that can lead to sepsis. Other important risk factors for infection include the inability to weight bear and impaired mobility as well as the presence of bowel or bladder incontinence (Smith et al., 2007). Proactive measures, including pulmonary toilet, prevention of decubiti through frequent turning and skin surveillance, and the avoidance of chronic indwelling catheters can substantially reduce (but not eliminate) the incidence of infections. Other prophylactic measures include the administration of annual influenza vaccines and pneumococcal vaccination.

The life care planner should project the need for periodic courses of both oral and intravenous antibiotics and recognize that with many years post-injury, the organisms become more resistant to conventional pharmacotherapy, necessitating the use of newer generation (and more expensive) agents.

Overuse Syndromes

Overuse syndromes result from the repetitive, usually non-physiological upper extremity movements that attempt to compensate for deficits resulting from a spinal cord injury. These conditions are generally more prevalent in individuals who are living independently, without assistance. Examples include the propulsion of wheelchairs, the use of canes, walkers, as well as use of the arms for functional transfers. In one study (Curtis et al., 1999) 75% of subjects reported a history of shoulder pain since beginning wheelchair use. Such activities lead to accelerated degenerative changes, particularly in the shoulders but can also cause ulnar and median nerve entrapment syndromes at the elbow and wrist respectively, with wrist pain reported in up to 64% of persons with SCI (Cardenas & Felix, 2009). Diagnosis of shoulder injury (i.e., rotator cuff tear, bursitis, capsulitis) is usually made radiologically (i.e., MRI), while entrapment syndromes are definitively diagnosed by electrophysiological testing (i.e., EMG/NCV). Shoulder symptoms that prove refractory to conservative therapy or for which there is evidence of major structural pathology usually require arthroscopic surgery. Similarly, peripheral nerve entrapments that are not improved with orthotics and/or anti-inflammatory agents generally need decompression (i.e., ulnar nerve transposition, carpal tunnel release).

Sexual Function and Reproduction

Sexual function relies upon common neurologic pathways that innervate the bladder and bowel. Not surprisingly, spinal cord injuries that affect bowel and bladder function are likely to interfere with normal sexual function as well. Complete spinal cord injuries above the sacral segments produce a complete loss of psychogenic erectile function with relative preservation of reflex erectile functions. For males with erectile dysfunction caused by spinal cord injury, treatment modalities include the use of oral agents (i.e., Viagra, Levitra, Cialis), prostaglandin penile injections, MUSE (an intraurethral suppository), vacuum tumescence pumps, and penile implants. Testosterone levels should always be checked as well, as many men with spinal cord injuries experience deficiency of this hormone.

Females with spinal cord injury frequently experience disorders of genital sensation, arousal, and orgasm in addition to menstrual irregularities and even cessation of menstruation. Other comorbid conditions that impact sexual health include the presence of decubitus ulcers and bowel and bladder incontinence. The use of oral contraception for females with impaired mobility is relatively contraindicated secondary to the increased risk for deep venous thrombosis. Therefore, barrier contraception is generally recommended.

SCI also impairs both male and female fertility, and women who become pregnant have a higher incidence of premature and low birthweight babies. Nonetheless, for couples who desire biological children, assisted reproduction techniques are available. For men, vibratory ejaculation and electrical stimulation allow for retrieval of sperm in the vast majority of cases. More recently, testicular sperm extraction (TESE) is a technique that has a high success rate (Raviv et al., 2013). Other assistive techniques include intravaginal insemination, intrauterine insemination, and in vitro fertilization.

Most individuals with SCI who experience sexual dysfunction and/or infertility benefit from counseling, not only to address the emotional sequelae, but also to learn about the spectrum of treatment options.

The life care planner must be aware of how both sexuality and fertility are affected by spinal cord injury and incorporate this knowledge into the interview and evaluation process. As each life care plan is individualized, it is important to consider age, relationship status, and desire for children, understanding that these are fluid.

Psychological Issues

Perhaps one of the most profound consequences of a spinal cord injury is the emotional impact upon the individual and his family, particularly after discharge from the hospital or rehabilitation facility. People with chronic disabilities, including spinal cord injury, are at substantially greater risk for depression and anxiety as well as adjustment disorders. Not only can this result from the very significant physical limitations, but also from the debilitating effects of secondary complications, social isolation, and socioeconomic challenges that may limit access to adequate levels of health care.

While much of the literature references the greatest risk for depression occurring in the first months to one year following the onset of SCI, other longer-term follow-up studies have found ongoing problems with depression in SCI. For example, Anderson et al. (2007) reported depressive symptoms ranging from mild to severe in 27% of adults with childhood or adolescent onset of SCI, with 7% having suicidal thoughts in the prior 2 weeks, and 3% with symptoms consistent with probable major depressive disorder. It was concluded that depression is a significant problem among adults with pediatric-onset SCI and is associated with poorer outcomes and lower quality of life. Williams and Murray (2015) found the mean prevalence estimate of depression diagnosis after SCI was 22.2%, with a lower-bound estimate of 18.7% and an upper bound estimate of 26.3%. They concluded that the existing data on depression after SCI indicate that the prevalence of depression after SCI is substantially greater than that in the general medical population.

Family members are also subjected to social and psychological stress and may find themselves undergoing an adjustment process as they respond to changing roles and functions within the family unit. Depression and other psychological conditions are highly prevalent after SCI, and counseling should be offered to address issues such as the acceptance of impairment and the impact of the disability upon the family, as well as sexual and vocational roles. The psychologist or psychiatrist can assist other team members by clarifying the patient's behavior and recommending therapies that promote healthy adaptation. The judicious prescription of antidepressant medication is often appropriate in conjunction with adjustment counseling.

Home Modifications

Those with SCI require modifications of most residential settings for accessibility and function commensurate with the level of their handicapping conditions. The residence will need to consider safe and unobstructed access from the location of vehicular storage (garage or carport), as well as routine and emergency ingress and egress for a wheelchair dependent resident. Primary and emergency secondary egress ramping is recommended. Adequate storage space is required for supplies and the array of large and bulky durable medical equipment items, as well as sufficient space for living quarters and family circumstances for sleeping areas. Careful planning is required to construct a fully functional bathroom that is accessible by a roll-in shower chair and large enough to accommodate caregivers who may be required for assistance. The shower area will need to have sufficient interior space for transfers and turning in the shower chair, or gurney when applicable, and to enter and exit with the help of a caregiver when required. An area of the modified home will be required for home exercise programming, as well as a caregiver workstation. Standard doorways and hallways are usually too narrow to allow for ease of wheelchair access, or as may be required for maneuverability with other assistive devices. As such, personal injury, Sheetrock trauma, and damage to equipment can occur if this is not addressed during the planning phases. Proper architectural planning and construction consultation can alleviate many of these concerns and avoid unnecessary expense or potential injury to the wheelchair occupant or caregiver. Case management services can be most helpful to coordinate appropriate referrals for assistance with this process.

While the overall cost of medical care is generally higher for the tetraplegic than the paraplegic, it has been our experience that home modifications for the paraplegic individual are often more involved, and thus more costly than the requirements needed for most individuals with tetraplegia. This is because the paraplegic has full use of the upper extremities and has greater functional independence than the tetraplegic if the home environment is adequately modified. One example of this involves modifications of kitchens and laundry rooms. The tetraplegic, especially those above C6, will have greater dependence upon others for meal preparation and kitchen cleanup, thus potentially negating the need for some of the more extensive modifications of cabinets. Under most circumstances, the paraplegic can prepare meals and perform kitchen cleanup tasks if necessary items are located within reach at wheelchair level. This necessitates redesigning of cabinets, sinks, and counters, as well as acquisition and installation of ADA appliances that are accessible and functional at wheelchair level. Laundry rooms in most residential homes, more often than not, are smaller and not accessible for those in wheelchairs. There are, however, washers and dryers that are designed for ADA compliance by a host of manufacturers with wide front opening doors and eye-level controls. Again, sinks and counter tops in the laundry room need to be at appropriate heights for accessibility and the space will need to be adequate for maneuverability in a wheelchair. As such, those with greater functional potential at wheelchair level will have needs for home modifications beyond those who have greater dependence upon others without disability for basic Activities of Daily Living.

Another consideration in projecting the cost of home modifications is the location of the proposed project. Construction costs, particularly the costs for tradesmen and craftsmen, can vary widely from one region of the country to another. When making a decision to modify an existing residence, the age of the residence is an important consideration and applicable construction codes. An older residence may be required to undergo complete updates of electrical and plumbing throughout the entire house to bring the structure current with applicable codes, even if merely adding an addition to the home. This could be a "game changer" and should be investigated before incurring the cost of design, only to learn of this at the time of submitting plans for building permits.

Vehicular Modification

A wide range of vehicular modifications exists for individuals with spinal cord injury. The level of injury and preservation of motor and sensory function are key factors in the determination of appropriate modifications for independence with vehicular transportation. The young and otherwise healthy lower thoracic or lumbar paraplegics may choose to opt for hand controls only (see also Chapter 33 on vehicular modifications). This will offer them the greatest selection of vehicles and styles that may be important to their self-esteem, although this requires the physical ability to lift, hoist, and maneuver their wheelchairs into the interior of the vehicle while sitting in the driver's seat. Over time, the self-esteem derived from sports cars or trucks with lift kits usually gives way to the benefit of ease and efficiency of vehicular ingress and egress with comfort, convenience, and operational functionally, especially when inclement weather is a factor.

Independent vehicular operation is best accomplished with ramp vans. Well-known vehicular retrofitters, such as the Braun Corporation (BraunAbility—Rampvan, Companion Van, and Entervan) and Vantage Mobility International (VMI), provide safe and effective transportation. These vehicular adaptations provide for a ramp rather than an undercarriage power lift for entrance and egress. The vehicle can be raised or lowered hydraulically to reduce the angle of ascent or descent for ease of entrance and exit. Appropriate wheelchair securement is provided with multiple interior configurations available for driver and passenger location during transit. Modifications for vehicular operation may range from basic hand controls for the paraplegic to more sophisticated electronics with actuators, servo motors, touch screen controls, and joystick operation for the tetraplegic. The cost for modifications of ramp vans can range from $20,000 to $80,000 above and beyond the cost of the vehicle prior to modification. As one might expect, the sophisticated electronic control mechanisms needed for safe vehicular operation by tetraplegics above C6 are at the higher end of the cost spectrum; however, being able to enter, exit, and operate a vehicle without assistance offers those with SCI a tremendous sense of freedom and autonomy.

A newer concept meeting the needs for individuals requiring vehicular modification is provided by Mobility Ventures. While the more established companies modify vans produced by major automotive manufacturers, Mobility Ventures has taken a "ground-up" approach to manufacture the entire vehicle, called the MV-1. This process also results in less overall costs for the total package of the vehicle and modifications.

It should be noted that BraunAbility has recently partnered with Ford Motor Company to develop similar features available in popular minivans with a Ford Explorer. As such, individuals with disabilities now have an option for a sport utility vehicle. This is great news for many younger individuals who find it difficult to conceive the idea of driving a minivan.

The life care planner will need to consider that these modifications are required with each replacement vehicle purchased over time. In considering usual replacement cycles, it should be kept in mind that being stranded in a vehicle due to mechanical failure presents a very serious concern for individuals with paralysis relative to the able-bodied population.

Powered Robotic Exoskeletons in SCI

Achieving the ability to walk again is without a doubt among the top priorities for individuals with SCI. The added benefits of improving overall physical and mental health further support the desire to return to walking. Powered robotic exoskeletons represent major technological advances toward the goal of functional ambulation for many with thoracic level spinal cord injuries. These robotic exoskeletons are wearable orthoses that can be used as an assistive device to enable some individuals with SCI to walk or to augment rehabilitation.

On June 26, 2014, the FDA granted approval to Argo Medical Technologies (now marketed as ReWalk Robotics) for the sale of the ReWalk powered exoskeleton device for private use in the United States. With its initial release, the ReWalk was available in two versions, one for medical institutions for research and therapeutic applications under professional supervision, the ReWalk I, and another for personal use at home or in public, the ReWalk P. In early 2013, a newer version was released, the ReWalk Rehabilitation 2.0, featuring enhanced software for improved control and sizing options for taller individuals.

On March 10, 2016, the FDA granted Parker Hannifin permission to market and sell its Vanderbilt-designed Indego exoskeleton for clinical and personal use in the United States. It is marketed to be considerably lighter and less bulky than the other exoskeletons under development. The Indego is reported to incorporate functional electrical stimulation and adjust robotic assistance automatically for users who have some preserved muscle function, allowing use of their own muscles while walking.

On April 4, 2016, the Ekso GT Robotic Exoskeleton (Ekso Bionics Holdings, Inc.) was cleared by the FDA for use in the treatment of individuals with hemiplegia due to stroke, individuals with spinal cord injuries at levels T4 to L5, and individuals with spinal cord injuries at levels of T3 to C7 (ASIA D). The Ekso GT is the first exoskeleton cleared by the FDA for use with stroke patients.

Powered robotic exoskeletons can provide thoracic-level spinal cord injured individuals the ability to walk. They do require the use of a gait aid, such as forearm crutches, for support during walking. Individuals with lower thoracic lesions have greater preservation of truncal musculature, which helps with proficiency and speed of gait with less dependence upon their arms. Continued technological improvements will likely improve gait speed over time such that powered exoskeletal walking can be more efficiently used in the community and various terrains. The current cost of these power robotic exoskeletons ranges from $70,000 to $85,000 for the device alone. It should be noted that extensive training on the use of these devices is also required.

Aging with Spinal Cord Injury and Personal Care Assistance Needs

Every person who lives long enough will eventually experience a decline in function; however, for people who have sustained a spinal cord injury, this process is accelerated and compounded by comorbidities, such as overuse syndromes, accelerated osteoarthritis, chronic pain, decubiti, infections, and recurrent hospitalizations (Hitzig et al., 2008; Bauman & Waters, 2004). The individual with a spinal cord injury is typically younger at the time of his injury and experiences not only an immediate reduction in functional reserves but also in his financial resources. Since greater than 25% of all individuals with spinal cord injury are now more than 20 years post-event, health care professionals must be aware of these changes and be proactive in implementing services that can mitigate this functional decline. Similarly, life care planning must consider the need for and degree of personal care services based upon the age of the individual, the number of years since injury, the level of injury, the presence or absence of chronic pain, and other concomitant or comorbid medical conditions (Winkler, 2016). Among the more age-specific problems that are unique to or more pronounced in this population are the following:

1. Spasticity that contributes to pain and impaired function
2. Overuse syndromes (i.e., rotator cuff injuries, tendinitis, and peripheral entrapment neuropathies) related to wheelchair mobility and transfers
3. Recurrent decubiti from hypomobility
4. The need for frequent courses of both oral and intravenous antibiotics with the subsequent development of highly resistant strains of bacteria

The vast majority of individuals with tetraplegia and many of those with paraplegia require personal care assistance (skilled nursing care if they are ventilator dependent) regardless of age. For most individuals with tetraplegia, living alone is not a viable option. While the younger person with a lower thoracic paraplegia may initially require little personal care assistance and only modest homemaking and household services, as he or she ages, he or she will require increasing levels of personal care and homemaking assistance (Harrell & Krause 2002).

The Consortium for Spinal Cord Medicine develops and disseminates evidence-based clinical practice guidelines to professionals and consumers. Its membership consists of health care professional groups and payer and consumer organizations extensively involved with spinal cord injury. The Consortium publishes several clinical practice guidelines for health care professionals involved in the care and treatment of individuals with spinal cord injury. One such guideline is the Outcomes Following Traumatic Spinal Cord Injury published in July of 1999. This guideline is perhaps one of the most commonly used and cited guidelines for life care planners and case managers working with individuals with SCI. The guideline presents expectations of functional performance of SCI at one year post-injury and at each of eight levels of injury (C1–3, C4, C5, C6, C7–8, T1–9, T10-L1, and L2-S5). "The outcomes reflect a level of independence that can be expected of a person with motor complete SCI, given optimal circumstances. The categories presented reflect expected functional outcomes in the areas of mobility, Activities of Daily Living, Instrumental Activities of Daily Living, and communication skills. The guidelines were based on consensus of clinical experts, available literature on functional outcomes, and data compiled from Uniform Data Systems (UDS) and the National Spinal Cord Injury Statistical Center (NSCISC)."

The panel participants of the Consortium of Spinal Cord Medicine identified a series of essential daily functions and activities, expected levels of functioning, and the equipment and attendant care likely to be needed to support the predicted level of independence at one year post-injury. The panel also emphasized that the expected functional outcomes "must be individualized to the unique characteristics, circumstances, and capabilities of each person with SCI." Other qualifying information contained within the guidelines includes the following: "The hours of assistance recommended by the panel do not reflect changes in assistance required over time as reported by long-term survivors of SCI (Gerhart et al., 1993), nor do they take into account the wide range of individual variables mentioned throughout this document that may affect the number of hours of assistance required. The Functional Independence Measure (FIM) estimates are widely variable in several of the categories. One does not know whether the representative individuals with SCI in the individual categories attained the expected functional outcomes for their specific level of injury nor whether there were mitigating circumstances such as age, obesity, or concomitant injuries, that would account for variability in assistance reported. An individualized assessment of needs is required in all cases."

While the guidelines published by the Consortium for Spinal Cord Medicine provide valuable information to serve as a basis point for planning and estimating levels of assistance required by neurological level of injury, life care planners, case managers, and other health care professionals should always recognize that the unique needs of each and every individual must be considered carefully when projecting the level and intensity of personal care assistance, rather than a "one size fits all" approach.

Life Expectancy

The National Spinal Cord Injury Statistical Center (NSCISC) publishes data from the model system throughout the United States regarding life expectancies for the SCI population who are seen within these programs. Since there is a substantially higher mortality within the first year post-injury, these survival data are included in a separate table. For individuals who have survived greater than 1 year post-injury, the data are sub-divided by age, level of injury, completeness of the injury (e.g., AIS A-D), and the need for ventilator assistance. Not surprisingly, those who have sustained higher levels of injury or who have complete spinal cord lesions experience reduced life expectancies, as they are at much greater risk for the development of decubiti, respiratory complications, and recurrent hospitalizations and surgeries. However, just as the need for personal care and skilled nursing services is highly dependent upon individual factors, it is critical that when estimating life expectancies, the life care planner also considers more than merely the statistical data. For example, an important limitation of these data is the fact that they do not consider the level of medical care that SCI patients have received. Socioeconomic status can play an important role in access to care, and statistical data indicate that the average household income for those with SCI at 5 years post-injury is less than $25,000 per year. Since proactive measures and careful clinical surveillance can prevent many of the common complications that are associated with morbidity and mortality, the data likely underestimate life expectancies for those who are vigilant with medical follow-up and have adequate resources to procure appropriate levels of medical and skilled nursing care. Other important considerations include comorbid medical conditions, as well as the degree and severity of complications that the individual has experienced since sustaining his or her injury. For example, a person who has already experienced multiple hospitalizations for serious respiratory infections and decubiti has greater risks of recurrence that can impact long-term survival and life expectancy relative to another person who is the same age and with the same level of injury who has been relatively free of such complications.

Case Study

Joseph H. Name, a 30-year-old Caucasian male was involved in a motor vehicle injury on 01/02/13 when the vehicle in which he was driving was broadsided by a semi-truck. Mr. Name suffered multiple cervical vertebral fractures with 10 mm of anterolisthesis of C6 on C7 and associated injury to the spinal cord. He was transported to the acute care setting in Dallas, Texas where he underwent C5-T1 surgical stabilization with instrument fixation. Once medically stabilized, Mr. Name was transferred to a Spinal Cord Injury Model System program of care for acute SCI rehabilitation. His rehabilitation course was complicated by urethral trauma necessitating prolonged indwelling catheterization until adequate urethral healing could occur and allow for transition to intermittent catheterization. This likely contributed to problematic and recurrent urinary tract infections as well. Since transitioning to home, he also encountered recurrent episodes of autonomic dysreflexia with severe hypertension necessitating treatment in the emergency department. Ongoing problems requiring treatment and monitoring have also included chronic central neuropathic pain, a Stage I heel decubitus ulcer, and adjustment disorder.

At just over 13 months post-injury, Mr. Name's clinical presentation is consistent with C7 motor, T4 sensory AIS B tetraplegia. Further significant gains from additional physiologic recovery are not anticipated; therefore, his current clinical presentation represents permanent manifestations of his central neurologic injury. Consistent with his spinal cord injury, he has a neurogenic bowel and bladder, as well as erectile dysfunction and sexual dysfunction. Mr. Name is followed in the outpatient setting of the SCI Model System program where he continues to receive physical therapy three times weekly, occupational therapy twice weekly, and a gym-based quad exercise program with a personal trainer 2 days weekly. He is followed medically by his physiatrist, urologist, and primary care physician for SCI-related care. The status of his urethra is being followed closely by his urologist to determine if he will ultimately require urethroplasty. Despite catheterizations at five to six times daily, Mr. Name continues with high intravesical pressures and is undergoing intravesical botulinum toxin A injections via cystoscopy at 3- to 4-month intervals.

Mr. Name is married to his wife of 5 years and they have two children, ages 3 years and 19 months. Although Mr. Name has not been formally terminated from his pre-injury employment, he has not been able to return to work as a warehouse fork lift operator. He is not certain if his employer can offer him a position within his physical capability. He is a high school graduate. Mrs. Name has been a homemaker since their first child was born. She was pregnant with their second child when Mr. Name was injured. She is considering that she may have to return to work due to the pending significant loss of family income. She is also a high school graduate. Mr. Name has exhausted all leave benefits and they have drained their retirement savings.

LIFE CARE COST ANALYSIS
for
JOSEPH H. NAME

Date of Report: 02/12/14	Diagnoses:
Date of Birth: 10/01/83	S/P MVA 01/02/13;
Current Age: 30 Years	S/P C5-T1 Surgical Stabilization;
Gender: Male	C7 Motor, T4 Sensory AIS B tetraplegia;
Ethnicity: Caucasian	Neurogenic Bladder and Bowel;
Average Residual Life Expectancy: 47.7 Years	Autonomic Dysreflexia, Bladder Related;
Projected Residual Life Expectancy: 32.0 Years	Urethral Trauma; Recurrent UTIs;
	Erectile Dysfunction and 2° Sexual Dysfunction;
	Chronic Neuropathic Pain, Bilateral Hands;
	Stage I Decubitus Ulcer, Right Heel;
	Adjustment Disorder, Improved.

Service/Item	*Begin at Age*	*Duration Years*	*Frequency per Year*	*Average Unit Cost*	*Annual Cost*	*Lifetime Cost*
Outpatient Physician Services						
Physiatrist (PM&R)	30	2	4.5	$163.47	$735.60	$1,471.20
Physiatrist (PM&R)	32	30	2.5	$163.47	$408.67	$12,259.98

(*Continued*)

Service/Item	*Begin at Age*	*Duration Years*	*Frequency per Year*	*Average Unit Cost*	*Annual Cost*	*Lifetime Cost*
Internist/PCP (Additional)	30	32	2	$202.34	$404.67	$12,949.60
Urologist	30	2	3	$163.47	$490.40	$980.80
Urologist	32	30	2	$163.47	$326.93	$9,807.99
Podiatrist	30	32	3.5	$69.76	$244.16	$7,813.07
Other Physician Consultation	30	20	1/3	$317.35	$105.78	$2,115.69
Other Physician Consultation	50	12	1/2	$317.35	$158.68	$1,904.12
Therapeutic Services						
Disability Adjustment Counseling	30	2	30	$272.79	$8,183.73	$16,367.47
Intermittent Supportive Counseling	32	9	1/3	$5,322.55	$1,774.18	$15,967.65
Family Counseling	30	2	24	$182.21	$4,372.99	$8,745.98
Physical Therapy Evaluation	30	32	2	$173.88	$347.76	$11,128.21
Occupational Therapy Evaluation	30	32	2	$186.37	$372.75	$11,927.84
Physical Therapy, Treatment	30	1	54	$256.13	$13,831.13	$13,831.13
Occupational Therapy, Treatment	30	1	36	$269.52	$9,702.68	$9,702.68
Intermittent PT/OT	30	20	1/3	$5,279.71	$1,759.90	$35,198.09
Intermittent PT/OT	50	12	1/2	$5,279.71	$2,639.86	$31,678.28
Medical Case Management	30	2	9	$642.71	$5,784.38	$11,568.75
Medical Case Management	32	30	6	$428.47	$2,570.83	$77,125.00
SCI Driver Eval & Training	31	1	1	$1,300.00	$1,300.00	$1,300.00

(*Continued*)

Service/Item	*Begin at Age*	*Duration Years*	*Frequency per Year*	*Average Unit Cost*	*Annual Cost*	*Lifetime Cost*
			Home Care and Household Services			
CNA/HHA (8–12 hrs/day)	30	18	320	$200.00	$64,000.00	$1,152,000.00
CNA/HHA (Illness/ Convalescence 24 hrs/day)	30	18	45	$480.00	$21,600.00	$388,800.00
CNA/HHA (12–16 hrs/day)	48	14	300	$280.00	$84,000.00	$1,176,000.00
CNA/HHA (Illness/ Convalescence 24 hrs/day)	48	14	65	$480.00	$31,200.00	$436,800.00
Skilled Nursing Visits	30	18	24	$128.00	$3,072.00	$55,296.00
Skilled Nursing Visits	48	14	33	$128.00	$4,224.00	$59,136.00
Household Services	30	32	52	$112.50	$5,850.00	$187,200.00
			Medication			
Neuropathic Pain Agent	30	32	365	$8.80	$3,210.85	$102,747.21
Prescriptive NSAIDs	30	10	104	$3.84	$399.64	$3,996.36
Prescriptive NSAIDs	40	22	234	$3.84	$899.18	$19,781.96
Antidepressant, Intermittent	30	12	1/3	$1,597.27	$532.42	$6,389.09
ED Agent	30	20	130	$32.48	$4,221.88	$84,437.60
ED Agent	50	12	78	$32.48	$2,533.13	$30,397.54
Ditropan/ Equivalent	30	32	365	$6.12	$2,232.02	$71,424.76
Bowel Program						
Stool Softener	30	32	365	$0.27	$97.89	$3,132.58
Fiber Supplement/ MiraLAX	30	32	365	$0.57	$206.59	$6,610.88

(Continued)

Service/Item	*Begin at Age*	*Duration Years*	*Frequency per Year*	*Average Unit Cost*	*Annual Cost*	*Lifetime Cost*
Suppository	30	32	183	$1.85	$337.71	$10,806.66
Multivitamin/ Mineral	30	32	365	$0.08	$28.56	$913.96
Calcium with D	30	32	365	$0.14	$52.82	$1,690.10
Pneumovax	30	32	1/16	$124.63	$7.79	$249.27
Annual Flu Vax	30	32	1	$55.39	$55.39	$1,772.53
Topical Antibiotics/ Antifungals	30	32	4	$37.70	$150.78	$4,825.09
Oral Antibiotics	30	20	3.5	$141.05	$493.66	$9,873.20
Oral Antibiotics	50	12	4.5	$141.05	$634.71	$7,616.47
IV Antibiotics	30	20	1/4	$7,288.14	$1,822.04	$36,440.72
IV Antibiotics	50	12	1/2	$7,288.14	$3,644.07	$43,728.86
GI Protective	30	32	365	$5.94	$2,166.81	$69,337.93
Hyperlipidemia Agent	35	27	365	$5.97	$2,179.09	$58,835.34
Advair/Symbicort	50	12	12	$371.84	$4,462.08	$53,544.96
Combivent/ Equivalent	50	12	12	$259.57	$3,114.84	$37,378.08
Other PRN Medications	30	32	1	$312.50	$312.50	$10,000.00
			Diagnostics			
Urodynamics	30	2	1.5	$2,685.22	$4,027.83	$8,055.67
Urodynamics	32	30	2/3	$2,685.22	$1,790.15	$53,704.45
Renal Ultrasound	30	32	1	$523.72	$523.72	$16,758.95
Renal Scan (Nuclear Medicine)	30	32	1/3	$1,040.15	$346.72	$11,094.89
Urography (IVP)	30	32	1/4	$1,337.30	$334.32	$10,698.39
Abdominal Flatplate (KUB)	30	32	1	$138.48	$138.48	$4,431.29
X-ray (Limbs, Hips, or Spine)	30	32	1/3	$170.09	$56.70	$1,814.24

(Continued)

Service/Item	*Begin at Age*	*Duration Years*	*Frequency per Year*	*Average Unit Cost*	*Annual Cost*	*Lifetime Cost*
CT/MRI (Spine/Chest/Abd./Other Joint)	30	32	1/5	$1,893.23	$378.65	$12,116.65
Complete Blood Count	30	32	3.5	$42.69	$149.41	$4,781.13
Metabolic Panel (Comprehensive)	30	32	3.5	$71.84	$251.45	$8,046.30
Urinalysis	30	32	3.5	$24.99	$87.46	$2,798.71
Urine C&S	30	32	2.5	$163.47	$408.67	$13,077.32
Cultures (Other)	30	32	2	$112.71	$225.42	$7,213.35
Sedimentation Rate	30	32	1	$31.24	$31.24	$999.54
Creatinine Clearance	30	32	2	$81.21	$162.43	$5,197.61
Lipid Surveillance	30	32	2	$103.08	$206.16	$6,596.96
Chest X-ray	30	15	1/2	$162.43	$81.21	$1,218.19
Chest X-ray	45	17	2	$162.43	$324.85	$5,522.46
Pulmonary Function Studies	30	15	1	$447.71	$447.71	$6,715.66
Pulmonary Function Studies	45	17	2	$447.71	$895.42	$15,222.16
GI Review/Endoscopy	30	32	1/3	$2,205.04	$735.01	$23,520.46
EKG	30	32	1	$88.50	$88.50	$2,832.03
Cardiac Stress Test (Chemical)	40	22	1/3	$432.09	$144.03	$3,168.68
Duplex Venous Studies	30	32	1/5	$558.08	$111.62	$3,571.69
Bone Density Studies	30	32	1/3	$420.64	$140.21	$4,486.82
Supplies						
Sterile Catheter Kits (5–6/Day)	30	32	365	$21.34	$7,789.10	$249,251.20

(*Continued*)

Service/Item	*Begin at Age*	*Duration Years*	*Frequency per Year*	*Average Unit Cost*	*Annual Cost*	*Lifetime Cost*
Wet Ones/ Equivalent	30	32	365	$1.05	$384.18	$12,293.74
Skin Care Products	30	32	26	$44.50	$1,157.00	$37,024.00
Gloves Non-Latex (Clean)	30	32	19	$8.05	$152.95	$4,894.40
Lubricant Packets	30	32	2	$10.29	$20.58	$658.56
Heel Protectors	30	32	24	$10.93	$262.32	$8,394.24
Disposable Mattress Pads	30	32	365	$2.80	$1,021.15	$32,676.75
Wound Care Products	30	32	1	$237.50	$237.50	$7,600.00
Compression Stockings (3 Pair)	30	32	4	$156.00	$624.00	$19,968.00
Custom Hand Splints (Pair)	30	32	1/2	$462.50	$231.25	$7,400.00
Topical Pain Reliever	30	32	26	$8.42	$219.01	$7,008.21
Antibacterial Soap	30	32	32	$2.39	$76.48	$2,447.36
Disinfectant Spray	30	32	18	$5.28	$95.04	$3,041.28
Waterproof Mattress Pads	30	32	3	$57.50	$172.50	$5,520.00
Depends Guards for Men	30	32	365	$0.94	$344.08	$11,010.65
CPAP/BiPAP Supplies	50	12	4	$214.50	$858.00	$10,296.00
Equipment						
Electric Adjustable Bed	30	32	1/10	$3,198.00	$319.80	$10,233.60
Low Air Mattress Overlay	30	32	1/10	$9,354.38	$935.44	$29,934.00
Manual Wheelchair, Custom Seating	30	32	1/5	$4,325.00	$865.00	$27,680.00

(Continued)

Service/Item	*Begin at Age*	*Duration Years*	*Frequency per Year*	*Average Unit Cost*	*Annual Cost*	*Lifetime Cost*
Power Assist Rims (complete)	30	32	1/5	$8,715.00	$1,743.00	$55,776.00
Battery Packs for Rims	30	32	1/2	$1,099.00	$549.50	$17,584.00
Permobil C500 and Seating	30	32	1/5	$40,531.50	$8,106.30	$259,401.60
Backup Gel Cell Battery	30	32	1/2	$361.00	$180.50	$5,776.00
Battery Charger	30	32	1/5	$350.00	$70.00	$2,240.00
W/C Cushions, Jay/ROHO	30	32	2/3	$309.00	$206.00	$6,592.00
W/C Maintenance (Both Chairs)	30	32	1	$679.00	$679.00	$21,728.00
Stander	30	32	1/10	$5,350.00	$535.00	$17,120.00
Transfer Boards	30	32	3/5	$89.95	$53.97	$1,727.04
Clothing Adaptation	30	32	1	$780.00	$780.00	$24,960.00
Multi Podus Boots (Bilateral)	30	32	1/2	$301.00	$150.50	$4,816.00
Fleece Inserts, Multi Podus (Pair)	30	32	1	$145.00	$145.00	$4,640.00
Quad Trauma Shower Chair/ System	30	32	1/7	$5,211.72	$744.53	$23,825.02
Travel Bath Bench	30	32	1/5	$580.00	$116.00	$3,712.00
Exercise Table	30	32	1/5	$600.00	$120.00	$3,840.00
Exercise Mat	30	32	1/3	$159.50	$53.17	$1,701.33
Portable Ramp	30	32	1/7	$385.00	$55.00	$1,760.00
Ceiling Lift System/Equiv.	30	32	1/10	$8,170.00	$817.00	$26,144.00
Lift Slings	30	32	1/3	$295.90	$98.63	$3,156.27
Digital Scales for Lift Device	30	32	1/7	$1,529.95	$218.56	$6,994.06

(Continued)

Service/Item	*Begin at Age*	*Duration Years*	*Frequency per Year*	*Average Unit Cost*	*Annual Cost*	*Lifetime Cost*
Vital Signs Equipment	30	32	1/4	$156.50	$39.13	$1,252.00
CPAP/BiPAP	50	12	1/5	$1,599.00	$319.80	$3,837.60
ADL/Therapeutic Devices	30	32	1	$380.00	$380.00	$12,160.00
Other Equipment Maintenance	30	32	1	$262.50	$262.50	$8,400.00
Inpatient/Other Acute Care Services						
Botox via Cystoscopy for DSD	30	32	3.5	$1,650.36	$5,776.27	$184,840.74
Bacteriuria/ Problematic UTI	30	20	1/5	$38,607.48	$7,721.50	$154,429.93
Bacteriuria/ Problematic UTI	50	12	1/3	$38,607.48	$12,869.16	$154,429.93
Bacteremia, Urosepsis/Other	30	32	1/16	$108,397.90	$6,774.87	$216,795.79
Pneumonia/Other Respiratory	30	20	1/7	$89,095.62	$12,727.95	$254,558.90
Pneumonia/Other Respiratory	50	12	1/4	$89,095.62	$22,273.90	$267,286.85
Autonomic Dysreflexia (Outpt. ED)	30	20	1/3	$2,919.50	$973.17	$19,463.33
Excision, Ingrown Nails	30	32	7/32	$508.10	$111.15	$3,556.70
Wound Care, Outpatient	30	32	1/5	$10,110.00	$2,022.00	$64,704.00
Decubiti (non-operative)	30	32	1/10	$66,339.58	$6,633.96	$212,286.67
Decubiti (Operative)	30	32	1/16	$103,284.14	$6,455.26	$206,568.28
Overuse Syndromes	30	32	1/10	$31,518.98	$3,151.90	$100,860.73

(Continued)

Service/Item	*Begin at Age*	*Duration Years*	*Frequency per Year*	*Average Unit Cost*	*Annual Cost*	*Lifetime Cost*
Home and Vehicular Modifications						
Home Modifications	30	32	1/16	$70,125.00	$4,382.81	$140,250.00
Environmental Control/EADL	30	32	1/7	$11,775.00	$1,682.14	$53,828.57
ECU Software	30	32	1/4	$820.00	$205.00	$6,560.00
Vehicular Modifications (IMS Driver)	30	32	1/7	$33,912.50	$4,844.64	$155,028.57
Maintenance (Home Modifications)	30	32	1/2	$625.00	$312.50	$10,000.00
Maintenance (Vehicular Modifications)	30	32	1	$862.50	$862.50	$27,600.00
Potential Care Needs						
Fosamax/Boniva (Weekly/Monthly)	30	10	365	$4.71	$1,720.30	$17,203.00
Urethroplasty	30	2	1/2	$40,274.52	$20,137.26	$40,274.52
Penile Implant	30	1	1	$61,695.80	$61,695.80	$61,695.80
Penile Implant, Revision	30	32	1/10	$60,925.32	$6,092.53	$194,961.02
Deep Vein Thrombosis	30	32	1/16	$56,219.37	$3,513.71	$112,438.74
Bladder/Urinary Stones	30	32	1/16	$80,755.24	$5,047.20	$161,510.47
Syringomyelia	30	32	1/10	$75,153.24	$7,515.32	$240,490.37
Heterotopic Ossificans						
Diagnostic Follow-Up	32	5	1/5	$4,807.42	$961.48	$4,807.42
Medical Management	32	5	1/5	$3,653.45	$730.69	$3,653.45
Surgical Management	32	5	1/5	$52,759.41	$10,551.88	$52,759.41

COST ANALYSIS SUMMARY JOSEPH H. NAME		
Service/Item	*Lifetime Cost Totals*	*Percent of Total*
Outpatient Physician Services	$49,302.45	0.62%
Therapeutic Services	$244,541.08	3.10%
Home Care & Household Services	$3,455,232.00	43.75%
Medication	$675,931.12	8.56%
Diagnostics	$233,643.61	2.96%
Supplies	$419,484.39	5.31%
Equipment	$586,990.51	7.43%
Inpatient/Other Acute Care Services	$1,839,781.85	23.29%
Home & Vehicular Modifications	$393,267.14	4.98%
GRAND TOTAL	$7,898,174.15	100.00%
Potential Care Needs	$889,794.20	

Acknowledgment

This chapter is dedicated to the memory of Terry Winkler, MD, CLCP, for his contributions to the field of medicine, the practice of physical medicine and rehabilitation, and to his unsurpassed commitment to the advancement of knowledge and expertise in life care planning. Dr. Winkler served as the lead author of this chapter for all three prior editions. Very few have given so much and so unselfishly to the community of life care planners and to this specialty practice as Dr. Winkler. His presence and influence were realized throughout the evolution of life care planning for more than three decades, as it emerged from a concept to an internationally recognized area of specialization and certification. Dr. Winkler was a consummate educator with a unique ability to convey the necessary tools for critical thinking through the life care planning process. In addition to his extensive professional contributions, Dr. Winkler was a true gentleman and one of the finest human beings we have ever had the pleasure to know. We will continue to miss his encouraging attitude and his very special knowledge that has helped all of us in so many ways, but most importantly, we will continue to miss our friend. It is a tremendous honor and a humbling experience to take the baton from Dr. Winkler and to carry the chapter forward with the fourth edition.

References

Alabed, S. et al. Incidence of Pulmonary Embolism after the First 3 Months of Spinal Cord Injury. *Spinal Cord* 2015;*53*(11):1–3.

American Spinal Cord Injury Association. *International Standards for Neurological Classifications of Spinal Cord Injury (revised)*. Chicago, IL: American Spinal Injury Association, 2016.

Anderson, C. J., Vogel, L. C., Chlan, K. M., Betz, R. R., & McDonald, C. M. Depression in adults who sustained spinal cord injuries as children or adolescents. *J Spinal Cord Med* 2007; *30*(Suppl 1): S76–S82.

Badali, D. et al. A double-blind controlled trial on the effect of cisapride in the treatment of constipation in paraplegic patients. *Neurogastroenerol Motil* 1991; *3*:263–267.

Bagwell, D. et al. Team approach to life care planning: developing a blueprint of care for spinal cord injury. *Presented at the American Congress of Rehabilitation Medicine, 73rd Annual Meeting*; Chicago, IL, October 1996.

Bagwell, D., Winkler, T., & Reagles K. Long-term comorbidities in spinal cord injury: consideration for anticipated versus potential complications with life care planning. *Presented at the 2010 International Symposium on Life Care Planning*; Orlando, FL, September 13, 2010.

Bauman, W. A., & Waters, R. L. Aging with a spinal cord injury. In *Aging with a Disability: What the Clinician Needs to Know*. Baltimore, MD: Johns Hopkins University Press; 2004:153–174.

Branagan, G. et al. Effect of stoma formation on bowel care and quality of life in patients with spinal cord injury. *Spinal Cord* 2003; *41*:680–683.

Cardenas, D. D., & Felix E. R. Pain after spinal cord injury: A review of classification, treatment approaches, and treatment assessment. *PMR* 2009;*1*(12):1077–1090.

Consortium for Spinal Cord Medicine, Neurogenic Bowel Management in Adults with Spinal Cord Injury. Clinical Practice Guidelines, Paralyzed Veterans of America, March 1998.

Consortium for Spinal Cord Medicine. Outcomes following traumatic spinal cord injury: Clinical practice guidelines for health-care professionals. Paralyzed Veterans of America, July, 1999.

Consortium for Spinal Cord Medicine. 2001. Acute Management of Autonomic Dysreflexia. https://www.pva.org/CMSPages/GetFile.aspx?guid=2e9169c3-d2d9-4b4c-b3f1-c06f50aeba65.

Consortium for Spinal Cord Medicine, Paralyzed Veterans of America Preservation of Upper Limb Function Following Spinal Cord Injury. A Guide for People with Spinal Cord Injury. 2008.

Curtis, K. A., Drysdale, G. A., Lanza, R. D., Kolber, M., Vitolo, R. S., & West, R. Shoulder pain in wheelchair users with tetraplegia and paraplegia. *Arch Phys Med Rehabil* 1999;*80*(4):453–457.

DeVivo, M. J. et al. Recent trends in mortality and causes of death among persons with spinal cord injury. *Arch Phys Med Rehabil* 1999;*80*(11):1411–1419.

Ebert, E. Gastrointestinal Involvement in Spinal Cord Injury: A clinical perspective. *J Gastrointestin Liver Dis* 2012; *21*(1):75–82.

Elbasiouny, S. et al. Management of spasticity after spinal cord injury: Current techniques and future directions. *Neurorehabil Neural Repair* 2010;*24*(1):23–33.

Gerhart, K., Bergstrom, E., Charlifue S., Menter R., & Whiteneck G. Long-term spinal cord injury: Functional changes over time. *Arch Phys Med Rehabil* 1993;*74*:1030–1034.

Gstaltner, K. et al. Sacral nerve stimulation as an option for the treatment of faecal incontinence in patients suffering from cauda equine syndrome. *Spinal Cord* 2008;*46*:644–647.

Harrell, W. T., & Krause, J. S. Personal assistance services in patients with SCI: modeling an appropriate level of care in life care planning. *Topics in Spinal Cord Injury Rehabilitation: Life Care Planning* 2002; *7*:38–48.

Hitzig, S. L., Tonack M., & Campbell, K. A. et al. Secondary health complications in an aging Canadian spinal cord injury sample. *Am J Phys Med Rehabil* 2008;*87*(7):545–555.

Kocina, P. Body composition of spinal cord injured adults. *Sports Med* 1997;*23*(1):48–60.

Krause, J. S., & Saunders, L. L. Life expectancy estimates in the life care plan: Accounting for economic factors. *J Life Care Plan* 2010;*9*(2):15–28.

Lavela, S. L., Evans, C. T., Prohaska, T. R., Miskevics, S., Ganesh, S. P., & Weaver, F. M. Males aging with a spinal cord injury: prevalence of cardiovascular and metabolic conditions. *Arch Phys Med Rehabil* 2012; *93*(1):90–95.

Myers, J. et al. Cardiovascular disease in spinal cord injury. *Am J Phys Med Rehab* 2007;*86*(2):1–11.

National Spinal Cord Injury Statistical Center (NSCISC). 2016. *Annual Report for the Spinal Cord Injury Model Systems*; Birmingham, AL.

National Spinal Cord Injury Statistical Center (NSCISC). Spinal Cord Injury (SCI) Facts and Figures at a Glance. 2017 SCI Data Sheet.

National Vital Statistics Reports (NVSR). National Vital Statistics System, United States Department of Health and Human Services. Deaths: Final data for 2013. Feb 16, 2016. *64*:2.

Nepomuceno, C., Fine P. R., & Richards, J. S. Pain inpatients with spinal cord injury. *Arch Phys Med Rehabil* 1979;*60*:605–609.

Raviv, G, et al. Testicular sperm retrieval and intra cytoplasmic injection provide favorable outcome in spinal cord patients, failing conservative reproductive treatment. *Spinal Cord* 2013;*51*:642–644.

Smith, B. M. et al. Acute respiratory tract infection visits of veterans with spinal cord injuries and disorders: Rates, trends, and risk factors. *J Spinal Cord Med* 2007;*30*(4):355–361.

Szlachcic, Y., Carrothers, L., Adkins, R., & Waters, R. Clinical significance of abnormal electrocardiographic findings in individuals aging with spinal injury and abnormal lipid profiles. *J Spinal Cord Med* 2007; *30*(5):473–476.

Williams, R., & Murray, A. Prevalence of depression after spinal cord injury: a meta-analysis. *Arch Phys Med Rehabil* 2015;*96*(1):133–140.

Winkler, T., Weed, R. O., & Berens, D. E. Life care planning for spinal cord injury. In *Life Care Planning and Case Management Handbook*, 3rd ed. (Eds., R. O Weed, D. E Berens). Boca Raton, FL: CRC Press LLC; 2010:615–664.

Winkler, T. Spinal cord injury and aging. eMedicine. Updated April 21, 2016.

Chapter 18

Life Care Planning for Organ Transplantation

Dan M. Bagwell and Lisa Norris

Contents

Introduction ... 534
The Roots of Modern Transplantation ... 534
Life Care Planning in Transplantation ... 537
The Transplant Candidacy Process ... 537
Social Services and Psychiatric Consultation ... 540
Awaiting Transplantation ... 540
Kidney ... 541
Liver ... 541
Lung ... 542
Heart ... 542
Organ Procurement ... 543
Transplantation ... 544
Organ-Specific Postoperative Management ... 544
Immunosuppressive Therapy ... 546
Complications of Organ Transplantation ... 549
Infection ... 550
Other Complications ... 551
Long-Term Follow-Up ... 551
Graft and Patient Survival ... 552
Estimated Transplantation Costs ... 552
Retransplantation ... 553
Case Study ... 558
References ... 568

Introduction

Ancient writings reflect that over hundreds of years, attempts were made to transplant tissues from one human to another and from animals to humans in an effort to save lives or limbs. These efforts generally failed due to inadequate surgical techniques and tissue rejection. It was not until the twentieth century that medical science began to understand the role of the immune system and histocompatibility antigens responsible for rejection of genetically disparate tissues. With such enlightenment, along with advances in surgical techniques to connect blood vessels, the keys were discovered to unlock the secrets that had mystified medical scientists for centuries.

The Roots of Modern Transplantation

The following outline represents a timeline of significant events relating to transplantation:

- It is believed that as far back as 800 BC, skin grafting procedures were performed by physicians in India in an attempt to cover wounds.
- In the sixteenth century, the father of plastic surgery, Gasparo Tagliacozzi (Italy), improved on earlier skin grafting procedures from India using skin taken from the arms of patients to reconstruct their noses (rhinoplasty) that had been amputated during war. Tagliacozzi expanded this technique to reconstruct lips and ears. He is credited with early recognition of the immune response when donor skin obtained from a different host failed (rejection).
- In the beginning of the twentieth century, physicians in Europe performed kidney transplants with organs taken from animals in an attempt to save the lives of people dying from renal failure. None of these patients survived beyond a few days; however, in 1905, the first successful corneal transplant was performed by Eduard Zirm, an Austrian ophthalmologist, with restoration of sight in a patient who was blinded following an accident.
- In 1912, French-born surgeon Alexis Carrell was awarded the Nobel Prize in Physiology or Medicine for his work in vascular anastomosis, thus laying the groundwork to overcome a major hurdle in surgical technique for successful transplantation of an organ from a donor to a host. Carrell performed successful kidney transplants in dogs and developed methods for maintaining organ viability outside of the body.
- On April 03, 1933, Ukrainian-born Soviet surgeon Yurri Voronoy performed the first human allograft kidney transplant. Although the patient died after 2 days, much was learned from this experience about ABO incompatibility and the immunological characteristics of graft rejection.
- In 1954, American plastic surgeon Joseph Murray led a team of surgeons at Peter Bent Brigham Hospital in Boston, Massachusetts, performing the first successful kidney transplant in which a kidney was donated from an identical twin brother. The fact that the donor and recipient were identical twins provided support for the role of the immune response in rejection.
- In 1960, Brazilian-born British biologist Peter Medawar along with Australian Sir Frank Macfarlane Burnet received the Nobel Prize for their work in acquired immunological tolerance. Medawar is known for the discovery that graft recipients would form antibodies against the graft unless they had been exposed to similar foreign tissue early in life and that the body's rejection of foreign tissue was indeed an immune response. This led the way to tissue typing and the development of immune suppression drugs as a major breakthrough in successful cadaveric organ transplantation.
- Based on the work of Roy Calne with dogs, azathioprine was first used successfully in human transplantation 1962.

- In 1963, the first successful lung transplant was performed by American surgeon James Hardy at the University of Mississippi Medical Center in Jackson, Mississippi. On January 23, 1964, Dr. Hardy performed the first heart transplant, in which the heart of a chimpanzee was transplanted into the chest of a man as a last effort to try to save his life when no human heart was available. The patient died after 90 minutes and Dr. Hardy faced extensive criticism for performing the procedure; however he opened the door surgically for the prospects of human-to-human heart transplantation.
- The first successful simultaneous kidney–pancreas transplantation was performed in 1966 by surgeons William Kelly and Richard Lillehei at the University of Minnesota Medical Center.
- In 1967, American surgeon Thomas Starzl performed the first successful liver transplant at the University of Colorado.
- Also in 1967, the first successful human heart transplant was performed by South African surgeon Christiaan Barnard. While it was recognized that immunosuppressive drugs prevented rejection, the recipient of the first heart transplant died from complications associated with pneumonia after 18 days.
- In 1971, Jean-Francois Borel isolated a compound that would become known as cyclosporin. Borel found that cyclosporin, unlike other immunosuppressants known at the time, selectively suppressed helper T lymphocytes.
- By the late 1970s, Thomas Starzl began experiments with cyclosporine. The successes seen in graft and host survivals with the introduction of cyclosporine catapulted transplant surgery from an experimental process to a broadly recognized form of treatment for end-stage liver, kidney, lung, and heart disease. Starzl's successes and work in transplantation would earn him recognition as the "father of modern transplantation."

In the decades that followed, the first successful kidney transplant in 1954, organ transplantation emerged from an experimental process fraught with ethical dilemmas to an established medical science, with 33,606 transplants performed in the United States in 2016. This represented the fourth consecutive year of record high transplants performed in the United States, an 8.5 percent increase from 2015 and an increase of 19.8 percent since 2012 (UNOS, Jan 9, 2017). Despite the success rates of transplantation and continued improvements in graft and patient survivals, the number of individuals in need of a transplant continues to increase due to lower rates of organ donation relative to those in need of organs. Likewise, the waiting times and waiting list mortalities increase in tandem with survival rates after transplantation.

Until 1984, the allocation of organs for transplantation in the United States was largely unregulated and primarily coordinated by local organ banks scattered throughout the country. With the success of organ transplantation entering an era of wide recognition, congressional regulatory intervention was sought for the establishment of guidelines for a system of organ procurement and distribution. In 1984, Congress passed the National Organ Transplant Act, the first major legislative act concerning transplantation. From this Act, the Task Force on Organ Transplantation was formed resulting in the development of initial transplantation guidelines. Public Law (PL) 98-507 authorized the creation of qualified organ procurement organizations (OPOs), along with formation of the Organ Procurement and Transplantation Network (OPTN) and the Scientific Registry for Transplant Recipients (SRTR). The OPTN is comprised of a partnership between public and private sectors that serves as a system-wide link for all professionals involved in the system of donation and organ transplantation nationwide. The primary goal of the OPTN is to ensure the effectiveness, efficiency, and equity of organ sharing through a national system of organ allocation and to increase the supply of donated organs available for transplantation. The SRTR was established to ensure accurate and up to date transplant morbidity and mortality information. Through a contract with the Health Resources and Services Administration of the U.S. Department of Health and Human Services, the OPTN and SRTR were maintained by the United Network for Organ Sharing (UNOS). UNOS has maintained the OPTN contract since 1986 with successive contract renewals. UNOS performs many valuable functions, but it is best known as the "holder of the list": the nation's list of patients awaiting cadaveric organ transplantation.

All pre-transplant and post-transplant patients are registered with UNOS along with their health status. Laboratory results, rejection incidence, infections, and other data are reported to UNOS at periodic intervals throughout the life of the patient. The SRTR collates this information and maintains an elaborate informational database providing statistical information, such as waiting lists by organ type, graft and patient survival by individual transplant center, and volume and types of organs transplanted. The SRTR is provided data from the OPTN whose staff of scientists and statisticians is responsible for relevant evaluation of the scientific and clinical state of solid organ transplantation in the United States. The SRTR contract is maintained by Arbor Research Collaborative for Health with the University of Michigan. The body of statistical outcomes and analysis produced and published by the SRTR plays a critical role in OPTN policy development.

The entire organ transplant system benefits from transparency, consensus, and cooperation among all interested parties including the public, the SRTR, the OPTN, the Health Resources and Services Administration (HRSA), and the Advisory Committee on Organ Transplantation (ACOT). The current level of outcome transparency in the transplantation process is unparalleled in the national medical community. The data produced through these collaborative efforts is available to the public via the Internet in a manner that allows for national, regional, or transplant center specific review (www.ustransplant.org). The availability of this information allows members of the medical community, potential organ recipients, and payer sources the opportunity for transplant center specific research. Typical information frequently researched includes:

- Average length of time transplant candidates spend on the waiting list by blood group, race, transplant center, and/or region
- Number of organs accepted at a particular transplant center
- Number of organs declined at a particular transplant center and reasons declined
- Volume of transplants performed nationally and by transplant center
- One- and three-year survival rates; nationally, center-specific, by diagnosis, age of recipient, and length of time awaiting receipt of an organ

As of February 5, 2016, the number of UNOS-certified transplant centers in the United States was just under 250 (UNOS, 2016). UNOS certification is provided for transplantation programs that meet its strict standards for patient and graft survival rates, transplant volumes, surgeon and physician training, and nursing, laboratory, and hospital criteria. These standards are monitored through the OPTN to ensure that certified programs maintain compliance with certification criteria. Transplant centers are required to obtain and maintain certification for each transplant program it operates to include kidney, pancreas, pancreas islet cell, liver, intestine, multivisceral, heart, lung, and heart–lung transplantation (UNOS, 2016).

In 2007, the Centers for Medicare and Medicaid Services (CMS) published revised Conditions of Participation for transplant centers in the United States. While transplant programs can perform transplants as an abiding member of the OPTN, CMS approval is today viewed by most as a fundamental requirement for transplant programs. The CMS Conditions of Participation provide intense structure and requirements along with a reapplication process and on-site audit at 3-year intervals to maintain this highly regarded certification. While new Medicare approved transplant programs are added over time, some programs lose their approval status. The most current listing of Medicare approved transplant centers can be found at www.cms.gov/medicare/provider-enrollment-and-certification/certificationandcomplianc/downloads/approvedtransplantprograms.pdf.

As of June 17, 2016, the number of people awaiting organ transplantation in the United States was 120,311. However, in the prior calendar year, only 30,969 transplants (solid organ) were performed (UNOS, 2016). With less than 30 percent of those awaiting transplantation actually receiving an organ each calendar year, it is easy to understand the dilemma of a compounding effect of demand outpacing organ donation and why many people do not live to receive an organ. More than 80 percent of those on the waiting list are diagnosed with end-stage renal disease (ESRD) and are awaiting kidney transplantation. It is notable that the prevalence of end-stage renal disease in the U.S. population has risen from 1,321 per million in 2002 to 2,034 in 2013 (USRDS, 2015).

Primary etiologies of kidney failure are diabetes, hypertension, and glomerulonephritis. Hepatitis C and hepatocellular carcinoma account for most liver failures requiring liver transplantation. Chronic obstructive lung disease and pulmonary fibrosis represent the most common etiologies for the 1,423 individuals awaiting lung transplantation. Those awaiting heart transplantation are estimated at 4,091 with an equal distribution of primary disease caused by coronary artery disease and cardiomyopathy. The vast majority of people in the United States that comprise the national waiting list for all organs are adults, although the majority of intestinal transplants performed are pediatric transplant recipients.

Life Care Planning in Transplantation

Developing life care plans for individuals with end-stage organ disease requires a thorough understanding of organ specific disease processes. The client/patient's candidacy for organ transplantation must be determined, or at least projected within a reasonable degree of medical certainty, such that a logical projection can be made that transplantation will occur within the average waiting time for a suitable organ (cadaveric). While awaiting transplantation, the transplant candidate requires life-sustaining medical treatment and care. Depending on the specific organ involved and the extent of the disease, time can be an extremely important factor of patient survival. Those with end-stage renal disease can usually be kept alive for many years on renal dialysis; however, those with liver failure and advanced heart and lung disease do not have the same opportunity. As such, some of these individuals will die while awaiting transplantation.

To address the issue of deaths while awaiting transplantation, the OPTN seeks to allocate organs to those who need them the most. In the case of liver, heart, and lung failure, organs are allocated using a mortality risk score corresponding to the degree of medical urgency. Once candidacy is determined, comprehensive evaluations and ongoing follow-up are required until transplantation.

The Transplant Candidacy Process

Patients in need of transplantation are referred to transplantation centers in many different ways. Generally, referrals are made through physicians specializing in end-organ disease such as nephrologists, gastroenterologists, cardiologists, or pulmonologists. Patients may also be referred by claims representatives of health insurance companies who have developed contractual relationships with various "centers of excellence" or "transplant institutes." Individuals may also refer themselves to transplant programs by way of the Internet.

Prior to scheduling an initial evaluation, medical records are forwarded to the transplant center for review by a physician and a transplantation nursing coordinator. Patients are assigned to a pre-transplantation nurse coordinator at the time of referral to begin the process of determining candidacy through a program's transplantation evaluation protocols. The pre-transplantation nurse coordinator is an invaluable resource to the life care planner, as he or she can assist in the analysis of program-specific medical evaluations and diagnostic protocols in preparation for transplantation.

Indications for transplantation:

- End-stage organ failure not amenable to medical therapy
- Psychological stability and family support to sustain the patient through the transplant and complex post-operative regimen
- Age parameters: neonate to mid-70s (varies greatly from center to center)

Contraindications for transplantation:

- Morbid obesity (greater than 35 to 40 percent body mass index)
- Metastatic cancer
- Uncontrolled systemic infection
- Pregnancy
- Psychological instability that will make compliance difficult
- Ongoing elicit substance abuse (past substance abuse generally requires a period of at least 6 months abstinence and relapse prevention training or counseling)
- Positive for human immunodeficiency virus (HIV), except in some select centers
- Cardiac ejection fraction less than 20 percent (unless patient is a heart or combined heart-lung transplant candidate)

The underlying disease etiology is an important consideration, as certain disease processes may recur and threaten the transplanted organ. Membranoproliferative glomerulonephritis and focal segmental glomerulosclerosis have fairly high recurrence rates (25 to 50 percent) and represent a major challenge for transplant physicians (Crosson, 2007). For liver transplantation, the distribution of diagnoses at listing has been very stable since 2000. Non-cholestatic liver disease remains the largest single diagnostic category, representing about 72 percent of the waiting list. Hepatitis C is not cured by liver transplantation and recurs after transplantation, with 30 to 70 percent of patients exhibiting complications during the first post-operative year (Ohler & Cupples, 2008). Graft hepatitis may lead to fibrosis and cirrhosis in up to 30 percent of patients.

Following the initial interview and evaluation, transplant candidates will undergo rigorous medical testing to ensure the best possible outcomes during and following the transplant procedure. Typical diagnostics routinely performed during the pre-transplantation evaluation period for all transplant candidates include the following:

- *Routine Laboratory:* Blood type, white blood cell count (WBC), chemistry profile, serology studies (hepatitis A, B, and C; HIV; rapid plasmin reagin (RPR), histocompatibility leukocyte antigen (HLA) typing, 24-hour creatinine clearance (except for kidney transplant patients already on dialysis), and viral titers; cytomegalovirus (CMV), varicella, Epstein-Barr virus (EBV), HgBA1C
- *Other Basic Diagnostics:* Skin testing for tuberculosis, chest X-ray (posterior–anterior [PA] and lateral), electrocardiogram, and peripheral vascular studies such as duplex venous Doppler

- *Cardiac Evaluation* (based on symptomatology or per protocol): Echocardiogram, cardiac stress test, and possibly cardiac catheterization
- *Dental Consultation* (to rule out infectious agents)
- *Standard Cancer Screening:* Pap smear (women over age 18 or younger if sexually active), mammogram (women over age 40 or younger with positive family history), prostate-specific antigen (PSA) levels (men over age 40), and colonoscopy for men and women over age 50
- Social services consultation with possible psychiatric consultation
- Additional organ-specific diagnostics:
    - *Kidney:* Voiding cystourethrogram (optional) for diabetics or those with a history of urinary tract infections
    - *Pancreas:* C-peptide to ensure Type I diabetes
    - *Liver:* Abdominal computed tomography (CT) scan or magnetic resonance imaging (MRI) to rule out hepatocellular carcinoma, evaluate the portal vein, and measure the size of the liver
    - *Heart:* Cardiac catheterization for all patients to determine filling pressures and pulmonary resistance
    - *Lung:* Ventilation perfusion scan of each lung to determine the specific lung to be removed during transplantation; pulmonary function tests to establish pre-transplant baselines; CT scan of the chest to rule out lung cancer

Additional diagnostics may be required for further evaluation or interim treatment of a health problem prior to transplantation, if the typical diagnostics performed yield abnormal findings. Cardiac abnormalities found during echocardiography or cardiac stress testing may require cardiac catheterization for definitive results and treatment plans. Even in the absence of abnormal noninvasive cardiac testing, many transplant centers require cardiac catheterization to evaluate for small vessel disease and thus improve perioperative success. This is not an infrequent occurrence, as persons with end-stage organ failure often have multiple organ system problems.

Completion of the initial evaluation period may take a few days to months. Following the evaluation period, the patient's data are collected and presented to a committee, review board, or perhaps individual physician for review and determination of transplant candidacy. Once approved, the prospective transplant recipient is notified, and his data is forwarded for placement on the national waiting list for a cadaveric organ, or a living donation transplant is performed.

Living donation has expanded the donor pool for those waiting for liver and kidney transplant. Living donors can be spouses, friends, or "Good Samaritan" donors, also referred to as non-directed donors. Kidney paired donation (KPD) is also an option for candidates of a living donor who is medically able but cannot donate a kidney to their intended candidate because they are blood type or HLA incompatible. There are networks that now offer paired exchange, which allows an incompatible donor and recipient pair to be matched with another incompatible donor and recipient pair. Through this process, both recipients are able to receive living donor transplant. Unfortunately, living donation rates have dropped steadily in the past decade. For kidney, the rate of living donation has dropped from 4,340 in 2004 to 2,693 in 2014, and for liver, the rate of living donation has dropped from 323 in 2004 to 280 in 2014 (SRTR 2014). This decrease in living donation is probably multi-factorial; however, financial hardship and recent information regarding the long-term health outcomes of living donation has certainly played a part.

The options for living donation are presented to most kidney and liver pre-transplant patients and may also be offered to prospective lung, intestine, and pancreas transplant candidates at select programs. The primary mission for programs offering living donation is to first "do no harm" to the potential donor in an effort to help the recipient. This requires a thorough assessment of the living donor to ensure that he or she is in optimal health.

The donor evaluation will generally include the following studies:

- *Laboratory:* Blood type, WBC, chemistry profile, serology studies (hepatitis A, B, and C; HIV; and RPR), HLA typing with donor–recipient cross-match for kidney donation, and viral titers; CMV, varicella, EBV, urinalysis with urine culture, 24-hour creatinine clearance (two times), and, optimally, a glofil study to assess creatinine clearance for potential kidney donors.
- *Other Basic Diagnostics:* Skin testing for tuberculosis, chest X-ray (PA and lateral) and electrocardiogram, CT scan or arteriogram to evaluate renal arteries/veins, anatomy of kidneys, and CT or MRI scan of the liver for potential living liver donors; a liver biopsy is often requested by the transplant physician for prospective liver donors.
- *Cardiology Evaluation:* Based on the age of the donor, this may include echocardiogram and a cardiac stress test.

Social Services and Psychiatric Consultation

Throughout the donor evaluation process, transplant centers are required to provide an independent donor advocate or independent donor advocate team (IDAT) to ensure that the donors' rights are represented and they remain free from coercion. The members of the IDAT have a "legal responsibility" to remain independent of the transplant program. Following the donor evaluation, the results are often reviewed by a neutral physician that is not associated with the prospective transplant recipient. If the donor meets the requirements and is cleared for donation, then surgery is scheduled and performed.

Living donation remains a better choice for most patients, as shorter waiting times decrease morbidity and mortality. When the donor of a living related kidney and the recipient share histocompatibility antigens, significant improvements in long-term graft survival are seen.

Awaiting Transplantation

Median waiting times in the United States by organ type are presented in Table 18.1. The life care planner should consider that mean waiting times can be significantly impacted by blood type. For

Table 18.1 Median U.S. Waiting Times

Heart	4 months
Intestine	7.4 months
Kidney	5 years
Kidney/Pancreas	1.5 years
Liver	11 months
Lung	4 months
Pancreas	2 years

Source: Adapted from Gift of Life Organ Donor Program, 2016. *Average Median Wait Time to Transplant*. Philadelphia, PA. http://www.donors1.org.

example, the waiting time for a kidney in 2004 for blood type O was 1,881 days and 1,207 days for blood type A (OPTN, 2016). Waiting times may be extremely long for patients who are sensitized or patients with a significant degree of preformed antibodies for which the risk of immediate rejection is considerably high. Unfortunately, these antibodies are formed when an individual is exposed to other human antigens such as pregnancy, prior blood transfusions, and prior transplantation. Newer protocols have been established to enhance the opportunities for these sensitized patients through the use of gamma-globulin infusion and plasmapheresis, a process that helps to remove problematic antibodies from the blood. Some success has been seen with this process, but it has not been broadly adopted for general clinical utilization, as it remains constrained by the high cost of the therapy, which is not a covered service by Medicare and most managed care companies.

Kidney

Renal patients awaiting transplantation are followed at close intervals by their nephrologists through their respective dialysis units and nephrology offices. While awaiting transplantation, pre-kidney transplant patients will have blood specimens forwarded to the histocompatibility laboratories (HLA) at periodic intervals (at least quarterly) for cross-matching with prospective cadaveric kidney donors and for monitoring of antibodies associated with rejection. This represents an ongoing cost born by the recipient candidate until transplantation is accomplished. Likewise, the cost of donor evaluations and eventual organ procurement are assumed by the organ recipient. Patients on hemodialysis will continue to dialyze three times weekly for a period of 3 to 4 hours with each dialysis. Home hemodialysis has become more popular over time with nightly hemodialysis taking place in the patient's home.

In 2014, the OPTN announced a new kidney allocation system that gives higher priority to younger and healthier patients and minimizes racial and income disparities. It also promotes organ sharing across geographic areas and improves the chances of a transplant for those who have been previously sensitized. The prior system resulted in ever-increasing wait times without knowing the benefit to recipients.

Significant changes include:

- Counting wait time for a kidney from the date the patient started dialysis, rather than from the date the patient joined the kidney transplant list.
- Longevity matching, or matching kidneys expected to last the longest with patients expected to live the longest.
- Increasing priority and expanding transplant options for patients with rarer blood types. For example, blood type B patients can now receive kidneys from donors with blood type A2.
- Increasing priority on the wait-list for patients with higher amounts of Panel Reactive Antibodies, which can decrease their immune resistance and limit their transplant options.
- Elimination of "payback" requirements for hospitals receiving kidneys from organ procurement organizations outside their region (Putre, 2014).

Liver

Waiting periods for individuals with end-stage liver failure are variable and are determined on the basis of medical acuity of the prospective recipients. UNOS has assigned a methodology for rating liver transplant patients on the waiting list, the Model for End-stage Liver Disease, referred to as MELD. MELD is a "continuous disease severity scale that is highly predictive of the risk of dying from liver disease for patients waiting on the transplant list" (UNOS, 2006). This model incorporates the patient's bilirubin, international normalized ratio (INR), and creatinine in an equation that results in a patient score of up to 40 points. Liver organ candidates with higher scores are moved forward on the waiting list, thereby increasing their opportunity to receive an organ and hopefully reducing the number of deaths due to liver failure while awaiting transplantation. Exception points are available for certain conditions such as hepatocellular carcinoma (HCC). HCC is a growing indication for liver transplantation provided that the combined tumor size is below a specific threshold (generally 9 cm). In the setting of HCC, time is of increased significance, as the liver tumors may grow too large for transplantation to remain an option.

MELD laboratory values must be repeated at regular intervals and entered into the national waiting list for the patient to maintain his or her place on the list. When the patient has 25 points or greater, he must have laboratory studies drawn every 7 days, and the results must be entered into the UNOS database within 48 hours of laboratory draws. Liver organ recipient candidates with lower scores will have laboratory draws with frequencies ranging from every 30 days to as long as 12 months. In 2013, UNOS implemented Share 35, whereby regional candidates with MELD ≥ 35 receive higher priority than local candidates with MELD < 35. Under Share 35, the proportion of deceased-donor liver transplants allocated to recipients with MELD ≥ 35 increased from 23.1 percent to 30.1 percent. This has resulted in lower waitlist mortalities (Massie et al., 2015). Liver candidates may be followed medically by their own gastroenterologist in conjunction with a transplant center, or they may be followed solely by the transplant center.

Lung

Allocation of lungs is based on a model called the Lung Allocation Scoring (LAS) system. Candidates aged 12 and older are prioritized for donated lung offers by LAS (UNOS Bylaws, 2008) and are calculated using the following:

i. Wait-list urgency measure (expected number of days lived without a transplant during an additional year on the wait-list)
ii. Post-transplant survival measure (expected number of days lived during the first year post-transplant)
iii. Transplant benefit measure (post-transplant survival measure minus wait-list urgency measure)

Wait-list urgency measure and post-transplant survival measure (used in the calculation of transplant benefit measure) are developed using Cox proportional hazards models. Individuals suffering from end-stage lung disease are among the most acutely ill patients awaiting transplantation. Prior to transplantation, exacerbations of chronic obstructive lung disease may require frequent hospitalizations. Extended intubation and ventilation requirements are poor prognostic indicators for transplantation. A surgical approach is generally predetermined based on etiology, single lung transplant versus bilateral lung transplant, and projected outcomes.

Heart

Heart transplant candidates are ranked through a status criteria system with designations as 1A, 1B, 2, or 7 (UNOS bylaws 2008). To qualify as a status 1A, the recipient candidate must require mechanical circulatory support, mechanical circulatory support with objective medical evidence of significant device-related complications, mechanical ventilation, *or* continuous infusion of high-dose intravenous inotropic agents, *or* have an estimated life expectancy without a heart transplant of less than 7 days. To qualify for status 1B, heart transplant recipient candidates must have a left and/or right ventricular assist device in place and require intravenous inotropic medication. Those classified as status 2 do not meet the criteria for status 1A or 1B. Status 7 is applied to those patients deemed temporarily unsuitable for transplantation and are maintained in an on-hold status. As with patients awaiting lung transplantation, heart transplant candidates are also acutely ill and frequently require hospitalizations prior to transplant. It is not uncommon for these patients to require mechanical bridges to transplant, such as aortic balloon pump therapy or ventricular assist devices.

Individuals awaiting heart and lung transplants may have to relocate to live near their transplant centers, as the donor organs have a relatively short ischemic time and should be transplanted within 4 hours of organ procurement. If these organ recipient candidates reside at distances two or more hours from their transplant facility and do not have 24-hour coverage capability for emergency flight arrangements, then relocation to an area within the vicinity of the transplant center is necessary. At least one caretaker will need to be with the patient at all times to care for him/her, drive him/her to appointments, and be present at the time of transplant.

Finally, average waiting times for access to suitable organs vary from region to region, due to the length of the waiting lists and the volume of organs procured by each organ bank. The recipients' blood type is also a significant factor in the projected waiting times with regional variability. UNOS proposed two changes to the heart allocation system in 2016 in order to improve wait time: development of additional urgency stratifications based on relative waiting list mortality rates for all adult heart candidates and broadening of the geographic regional sharing to provide the most medically needy candidates access to donors.

The life care planner should research information available through the SRTR to review the transplant program where a specific client/patient is registered. Each organ procurement organization computes its data on average waiting times for each organ type.

Organ Procurement

Organs may be procured locally or regionally. The cost associated with cadaveric organ acquisition and procurement varies by the organ procurement organization with established standard acquisition costs (SAC). SAC fees are approved through the Medicare intermediaries of each state. These fees include charges from the donor hospital for testing of a donor after he or she has been declared brain dead. Typical charges include screening for infectious diseases, basic laboratory work, chest X-rays, hospital costs for use of the operating room and associated expenses for organ removal, surgical fees for organ removal, transportation of teams to outside hospitals by land (ambulance) or chartered air service, and the OPO's procurement coordinators and supplies. These SAC fees can be obtained by contacting the OPO in the region where the patient is listed for transplantation.

Transplantation continues to be a very successful treatment for end-stage liver disease. The number of liver transplants has increased steadily over the last decade, with 6,729 procedures performed in 2014. This growth may reflect a larger number of deceased donors, especially in the "expanded criteria donor" (ECD) and "donation after cardiac death" (DCD) categories. With the previous (3rd) Edition of this text, we reported that "Although the long-term outcomes for these recipients remain unclear, short-term benefits have been clearly identified. Patient and graft survivals for recipients of DCD grafts have continued to improve, with one-year survival rates for recipient grafts in 2004 virtually identical to those seen for recipients of standard criteria grafts"

(Bagwell & Milton, 2010). From 2005 to 2008, DCD liver transplantation was stable at 4 to 5 percent of all liver transplants. Unfortunately, more recent data since 2004 reflects an inferior outcome for DCD liver transplantation as compared to brain dead liver transplantation in terms of biliary complications, graft survival, and need for retransplantation (de Vera et al., 2009).

The DCD donor is not declared brain dead, but has generally suffered a massive traumatic brain injury. Either the patient appears to be lapsing into a persistent vegetative state and/or has lost all brain function except for some minimal brain stem activity, or the family does not wish to proceed with life support in the setting of such a devastating head injury. The family opts to withdraw life support, and the medical team pronounces death with the cessation of cardiorespiratory function. At the moment death is declared by the trauma or neurology team, the transplant team proceeds with organ recovery.

An ECD is defined as age 60 or older, or between the ages of 50 and 59 with at least two of the following conditions: history of hypertension, a serum creatinine level of greater than 1.5, and/or the cause of death was from a cerebrovascular accident. Long term outcomes are not as good with DCD and ECD. However, faced with certain death of individuals in the absence of a transplant, many transplant centers and patients accept the higher risk.

Transplantation

When a suitable donor becomes available, matching recipient candidates on the waiting list are notified and asked to come to the hospital. Upon arrival, consent forms are signed, blood work is drawn (CBC, chemistry profiles, HIV, hepatitis screens, CMV status, and HLA cross-matches for patients needing kidney transplants), a chest X-ray and EKG are performed, and a loading dose of immunosuppression is often given prior to transplantation. Frequently patients will be admitted and undergo the above described workups only to have the transplant cancelled, due to problems with the donor organ.

The diseased organ for transplanted patients involving the liver, lung, and heart will be removed (or in the case of single-lung transplantation, one diseased lung removed) and the new organ transplanted in its place. In the instance of kidney transplantation, the native kidneys remain in place unless they are removed for reasons of infection or intractable hypertension. The newly transplanted kidney is placed retroperitoneal in the lower abdomen adjacent to the bladder through an incision of the same location as an appendectomy. This position allows for fewer urological complications from ureter attachments and offers easier post transplantation biopsy. In children, kidneys are placed intra-abdominally. Hearts are sometimes being left in place when less optimal hearts are used for transplantation.

Immediately upon arrival to the ICU, extensive and specific postoperative monitoring is begun to include laboratory work, hemodynamic monitoring, fluid assessment, and administration of immunosuppressive medications, generally cyclosporine or Prograf. Daily drug levels will be drawn to monitor cyclosporine or Prograf levels in the blood. Patients receiving liver, lung, or heart transplants will remain on mechanical ventilation for at least a few hours. For many lung transplants, mechanical ventilation is required for as long as 3 days.

Organ-Specific Postoperative Management

Following kidney transplant, post-operative care focuses on monitoring urine output, replacing fluids, and maintaining normal electrolyte values. Foley catheters will be maintained for 3 to 5 days post-operatively. Transplanted kidneys may begin to function immediately, producing copious amounts of urine. Acute tubular necrosis may be seen, resulting from ischemia of the kidney tubules. Acute tubular necrosis necessitates an increased length of stay, along with dialysis for resolution and preservation of the patient's health.

Surgical complications from kidney transplantation are categorized into vascular, urologic, or lymphatic. Overall, surgical complications occur in less than 5 percent of kidney transplanted patients. Vascular complications include renal artery or vein thrombosis. The more common urologic complications seen postoperatively include ureteral obstruction, urinary leakage at the graft, and the occurrence of lymphoceles. These complications can involve a return to surgery for repair, although lymphoceles and obstructions caused by hematoma most often resolve with percutaneous drainage and sometimes without intervention (Ohler & Cupples, 2008). Renal artery thrombosis represents a very serious complication that may threaten graft survival. Ultrasonography of the new kidney is performed within the first 48 hours of transplantation to assess the status of the renal artery and vein and check for signs of ureteral obstruction.

Liver transplant patients begin their immediate postoperative period in much the same fashion as kidney transplants, although the focus of postoperative monitoring centers on the function of the new liver. Considerable blood loss and fluid shifts may have occurred in the operating room, often a result of the patient's pre-transplant medical condition. Signs and symptoms of hemorrhage will be carefully monitored, and coagulopathies may be corrected with fresh frozen plasma. In addition to the standard Foley, nasogastric tubes, and venous access lines seen with all transplanted patients, liver transplant patients will arrive with at least two Jackson–Pratt drains placed for drainage. Hemodynamically, the patients may have difficulty with hypertension and electrolyte imbalance. Typical vascular complications include hepatic artery and portal vein thrombosis and occur in approximately 10 percent of liver transplantation cases. These may require a return to surgery for repair.

Two to three days of mechanical ventilation can be expected following lung transplantation. When sufficient tidal volume is reached along with an adequate spontaneous ventilatory rate and an alert mental status, the lung transplant recipient can be extubated. Chest tubes placed during surgery are generally removed post-operatively between days six and eight. Complications following lung transplantation include the reimplantation response; a combination of ischemia, reperfusion, and injury; and lymphatic discontinuity that may contribute to pulmonary edema (Ginns et al., 1999). Ventilatory management is much the same as usual post-operative management, except for those who are transplanted for chronic obstructive pulmonary disease (COPD). These patients, who will continue with one hyperinflated lung in their chest, may be positioned with their native lung down to decrease mechanical pressure from the hyperinflated lung. Minimizing fluid intake is critical for these individuals, so as to reduce risk of pulmonary edema while maintaining hemodynamic stability.

Heart transplant recipients generally recover more quickly than patients undergoing open-heart surgeries. The hemodynamic monitoring and support of the transplant patient is similar to open-heart care. Bradycardia and junctional rhythms are not unusual in the transplant patient, and most patients will have pacing wires placed during the transplant procedure. Patients will also require small amounts of inotropic support for the first 2 to 3 days post-operatively. After a relatively short stay in the ICU for post-operative monitoring, the heart transplant patient can be moved to a general transplant ward for the remaining recovery period, typically 4 to 5 days. At the end of the first post-operative week, the patient will undergo an initial endomyocardial biopsy to monitor for rejection. The biopsy is performed in the cardiac catheter suite. The right internal jugular vein is catheterized, and bioptomes are advanced into the right ventricle for biopsy.

Throughout the entire hospitalization for patients receiving transplanted organs, transplant coordinators, social workers, and discharge coordinators are planning for and organizing a smooth transition to the home or alternative setting at the time of discharge. The average length of stay for transplant recipients has continued to shorten, as improvements in the entire transplantation process have been seen. Managed care influences have also contributed to shorter hospitalization stays. As a result, many transplant centers begin formal post-operative teaching classes prior to transplantation.

Immunosuppressive Therapy

Advances in organ transplantation have been largely due to improvements in and the general availability of immunosuppressants. Fifty years ago, total body irradiation was the only form of immunosuppression available following transplantation. High-dose irradiation was required to prevent rejection, and most patients died from secondary marrow aplasia or overwhelming infection. Azathioprine was introduced in the early 1960s, representing a major advance in kidney transplantation. With prolonged graft survival demonstrated, a dramatic increase in the number of kidney transplant units was seen throughout the world. Steroids were soon added in combination with azathioprine to treat rejection and subsequently for prevention of rejection. This regimen was typically followed during the 1960s and 1970s, until cyclosporin became readily available in the early 1980s. With the introduction of cyclosporin, another dramatic breakthrough in allograft survival was seen. Graft and host survival was improved not only in kidney transplantation, but in liver and heart transplants as well. Many new immunosuppressant agents are currently under investigation that are promising for yet further dramatic improvements in transplantation outcomes. The production of monoclonal antibodies that recognize different cell surface markers on lymphocytes expands the opportunity for increased specificity of immunosuppression.

Transplant recipients will require immunosuppressive therapy throughout their life or the life of the graft. Most will receive at least dual-agent therapy, although protocols vary to include triple and quadruple therapy, along with a variety of other medications. Immunosuppressants represent a significant proportion of the long-term outpatient expenses incurred by transplanted individuals beyond the first 12 months following transplantation. The cost of standard immunosuppression alone typically ranges from $10,000 to $14,000 per year (AOTA, 2016). Legislation expanded Medicare's coverage of immunosuppression through Part B and the advent of Medicare Part D coverage is having a tremendous impact on recipients' ability to afford transplant medication.

Managing immunosuppressant therapy can be a clinical challenge. Careful consideration is given to other necessary medications a patient may require for conditions other than end-stage organ disease. For example, there is increased metabolism of cyclosporine when administered with other medications such as phenytoin and Phenobarbital, thus decreasing its antirejection qualities. Conversely, drugs such as erythromycin and certain antifungal agents impair cyclosporin metabolism; therefore dosing must be adjusted accordingly. One of the major goals of the immunosuppressive regimen is to be nephron sparing.

Maintenance immunosuppressive agents commonly employed in today's transplant programs are listed in Table 18.2 and are identified by category, function, common side effects, and standard dosing.

Beyond maintenance immunosuppression, monoclonal or polyclonal antibodies add a new dimension to immunosuppression therapy and are utilized for induction therapy, as well as treatment of moderate to severe rejection (Table 18.3). These drugs are generally initiated in the hospital setting following transplantation, where patient response can be monitored. If well tolerated, they may be continued after discharge in the outpatient setting, although usually administered over a relatively short course (7 to 14 days). Should long-term monoclonal or polyclonal antibodies be required, a substantial increase in the cost of immunosuppression is seen with a single dose; average daily costs range from $595.86 to as much as $3,940.04.

Table 18.2 Maintenance Immunosuppression

Immunosuppressant	*Category*	*Function*	*Common Side Effects*	*Maintenance Dosage*
Prograf (Tacrolimus, FK 506)	Calcineurin inhibitor	Inhibits T cell function by impairing release of interleukin-2 (IL-2); binds to immunophilin FKBP (acute or cellular rejection prevention)	Hypertension Tremor Nephrotoxicity Diarrhea Hyperkalemia Insomnia Hyperglycemia	0.1– 0.3 mg/kg/day; generally given orally; may be given intravenously
Neoral (cyclosporine)	Calcineurin inhibitor	Inhibits T lymphocyte response by binding cyclophilin; also impairs IL-2 (acute or cellular rejection prevention)	Hypertension Tremor Nephrotoxicity Hirsutism Gingival hyperplasia Hypokalemia	5–15 mg/kg/day given in two divided doses
CellCept (Mycophenolate mofetil — MMF)	Selective antimetabolite	Blocks synthesis of guanosine, thus blocking T and B cell proliferation (acute and possibly humoral rejection prevention)	Diarrhea Nausea Abdominal discomfort Leukocytosis	1–3 g daily divided every 12 hours

(*Continued*)

Table 18.2 (Continued) Maintenance Immunosuppression

Immunosuppressant	*Category*	*Function*	*Common Side Effects*	*Maintenance Dosage*
Imuran (Azathioprine)	Antimetabolite	Inhibits T and B lymphocyte proliferation by inhibiting DNA and RNA synthesis	Leukopenia Thrombocytopenia Alopecia Anorexia Toxic hepatitis	1–3 mg/kg/day in a single daily dose
Rapamune (Sirolimus)	Macrolide antibiotic	Impairs capacity of cytokines to trigger T cells to enter cell division; inhibits B cell proliferation (possibly cellular and humoral rejection prevention)	Anemia Thrombocytopenia Leukopenia Hypertension Hypercholesterolemia	2–5 mg/day
Prednisone (Methylprednisolone, Solu-Medrol)	Corticosteroid	Inhibits lymphocyte proliferation; nonspecific anti-inflammatory agent	Increased appetite Cushingoid syndrome Hypertension Hyperglycemia Insomnia Mood swings GI upset Acne Osteoporosis Cataracts	5–10 mg/day for the treatment of acute rejection; may be given in doses up to 1–2 mg/kg IV

Table 18.3 Monoclonal and Polyclonal Antibodies (Immunosuppressive Induction and Rescue Agents)

Agent	*Category*	*Function*	*Common Side Effects*	*Dosage*
Simulect (Basiliximab)	Monoclonal antibody	Binds receptors of interleukin-2 (IL-2) complex; inhibits IL-2-mediated T lymphocytes	May predispose patients to infection or PTLD	Day of transplant: 20 mg IV Postoperative day 4: 20 mg IV
Campath-1H (Alemtuzumab)	Monoclonal antibody (off label)	Lymphocyte-depleting agent directed against CD52 antigen	Cytokine-release syndrome, neutropenia, anemia, thrombocytopenia, thyroid disease	20 mg × 2
Rituximab	Monoclonal antibody (off label)	Anti-CD20 agent for refractory PTLD and treatment of antibody-mediated and severe T-cell-mediated rejection		50 mg/m^2 to 375 mg/m^2
Thymoglobulin, ATG	Polyclonal immunoglobulin	Antibody may adhere to cell receptors, which reduces the amount of circulating T lymphocytes	Fever/chills Thrombocytopenia Leukopenia Myalgia Headaches	6.0–7.5 mg/kg

Complications of Organ Transplantation

Organ rejection and post-operative infection represent major complications following organ transplantation. Many other potential complications are also seen, and these are primarily the result of direct and indirect side effects of many of the necessary medications required for immunosuppression. Medical management of these individuals requires somewhat of a balancing act for transplant physicians, who strive to maintain viability of a transplanted organ through immunosuppressive therapy, while also attempting to reduce other potentially serious side effects these agents produce.

Rejection continues to represent one of the most common causes of graft failure. With an intact immune system, the body's natural response to a newly transplanted organ is rejection. Specific lymphocytes within the immune system recognize the genetic blueprint of anything that is not native to the recipient. As a result of advances in HLA typing and cross-matching, hyperacute rejection today is almost extinct, although chronic rejection remains a serious unsolved complication. Organs donated and received between identical twins are the only transplants that are widely accepted as not requiring comprehensive immunosuppression. Research continues on reaching immune tolerance through immunosuppressive withdrawal, as well as bone marrow transplantation at the time of solid organ transplant. A wide spectrum of improved immunosuppressive agents that have contributed significantly to a drastic reduction in the incidence of acute cellular rejection for most transplanted organs is now available.

The diagnosis and treatment of rejection varies by organ type. Table 18.4 identifies common signs and symptoms of rejection by organ transplant type and the most common diagnostics utilized to identify early rejection.

Infection

Infection is a major cause of morbidity and mortality for transplanted patients. It has been estimated that more than 60 percent of transplanted patients encounter some type of infection within the first post-transplant year (Rubin, 1999). Clearly, the risk of infection is exceptionally high with an immunocompromised host.

Within the first month following transplantation, bacterial infections are most common and are generally related to the surgery and invasive procedures such as intravenous lines, drain tubes, and indwelling catheters. Prophylactic antibiotic coverage begins pre-operatively at most transplant centers. Beyond the first post-operative month, the effects of sustained immunosuppression predispose the patient to viral infections, such as CMV, EBV, and hepatitis B and C. Post-operative CMV infection is common and represents a serious problem and concern in organ transplant patients. The host patient can be infected with this virus when CMV mismatched organs are transplanted such that a CMV-positive donor organ is transplanted into a CMV-negative recipient. CMV has been cited as a risk factor for acute rejection (McLaughlin et al., 2002) and chronic rejection (Weinberg et al., 2000). Most centers will preferentially treat with an intravenous antiviral agent for up to 30 days, then convert to an oral agent for long-term treatment or prophylaxis (Rubin, 2000).

Table 18.4 Signs and Symptoms of Rejection by Organ Type and Commonly Employed Diagnostics in the Detection of Rejection

Transplant Type	*Signs and Symptoms of Rejection*	*Common Diagnostics*
Kidney	Flank tenderness; diminished urine output; weight gain; edema; increased serum creatinine	Chemistry profile, specifically serum creatinine; immunosuppressive levels; kidney biopsy
Liver	Increased bilirubin and GGT; tenderness at operative site; usually asymptomatic of pain or discomfort	Bilirubin levels; GGT; immunosuppressant levels; liver biopsy
Lung	Increasing shortness of breath; infiltrates on chest X-ray; decreased FEV1; FEF 25–75 (PFTs)	Chest X-ray; exercise oximetry; pulmonary function tests; diagnostic bronchoscopy with bronchial lavage
Heart	Fatigue; peripheral edema; S3 gallop; pericardial friction rub; decreased ECG voltage	Rejection can only be monitored by endomyocardial biopsy

In combination with antivirals, CMV hyperimmune globulin may also be administered at periodic intervals. Opportunistic infections are also seen beyond 6 months post-operatively.

Prevention of bacterial, viral, and fungal infections is critical for graft and host survival. Therefore, prophylactic treatment, primarily for the first 3 months following transplantation, is standard practice. Thereafter, antibiotics and other antimicrobials are frequently prescribed with the onset of fever or other symptoms of potential infection.

Bactrim continues to be a mainstay in most transplant program protocols for prevention of pneumocystic pneumonia. For those sensitive to sulfa preparations, pentamidine inhalation treatments are administered in an outpatient setting on a monthly basis. CMV prophylaxis (ganciclovir/valganciclovir) is usually administered for the first 3 to 12 months following transplantation, as is acyclovir for herpes zoster prophylaxis. *Candida* prophylaxis (fluconazole, itraconazole) is also generally prescribed for the first 3 months after transplantation.

Other Complications

In approximately 75 percent of renal transplant recipients, hypertension is a problem following transplantation. Blood pressure monitoring is an integral part of follow-up. Patients are taught to monitor their own blood pressure and are sent home with blood pressure monitoring equipment. Commonly prescribed antihypertensives utilized by transplant centers include nifedipine, Norvasc, atenolol, clonidine, and hydrochlorothiazide.

Hyperlipidemia is commonly seen in many transplanted patients, with rates of occurrence ranging from 29 to 62 percent post-transplantation (Backman & Morales, 2000). Cardiovascular disease remains the leading cause of late mortality in renal transplant patients. A cholesterol-lowering agent, such as Pravachol, Lipitor, or Lopid, is usually included in the medication regime. There is also a high incidence of gastrointestinal ulcers, and many transplanted patients require long-term use of H2 receptor antagonists such as Pepcid, Zantac, Prilosec, Prevacid, Nexium, or Protonix.

Many patients require short-term insulin use following transplantation, although a small percentage will remain insulin dependent. The highest incidence of insulin dependency following transplantation is in the African American and Hispanic population groups. The reported incidence of new-onset diabetes after transplantation has varied between 2 and 53 percent, whereas the prevalence of diabetes in the general population is estimated at about 4 percent (Montori et al., 2002).

Transplanted patients also have a significantly heightened risk for malignancies. A 21-fold increased incidence of skin cancer has been reported in the transplanted population relative to the general population at large, along with a 28- to 49-fold increased incidence of lymphoproliferative disease (Penn, 2001). UNOS requires follow-up and mandatory tracking of all cancer and tumor incidents post-transplantation.

Long-Term Follow-Up

After discharge from the acute care setting, patients immediately begin their transplant clinic follow-up. With each clinic visit, laboratory studies are obtained to include CBC, chemistry profile, and immunosuppressant levels. Some transplant centers routinely biopsy transplanted kidneys annually or as indicated to monitor for rejection, while other centers biopsy within the first 12 months and only when there are demonstrable signs of rejection thereafter. Biopsies may be performed in an outpatient surgery setting under the guidance of ultrasound or through inpatient admission.

Heart transplant patients will undergo endomyocardial biopsy and follow-up chest X-rays. Heart biopsies begin at 7 to 10 days post-operatively. This is followed by weekly biopsies for 2 to 3 weeks, then monthly for 2 to 3 months, progressing to 60-day intervals, quarterly intervals, semiannual intervals, and, ultimately, biopsies on an annual basis.

Outpatient clinical follow-up with lung transplant patients will include laboratory monitoring, chest X-rays, and pulmonary function tests. Post-operative clinic visit intervals for these patients are generally scheduled weekly for 4 weeks, followed by 2-week intervals for approximately 8 weeks, monthly for 3 to 4 months, 60-day intervals for at least 4 months, and then quarterly. Patients are discharged with a handheld spirometer to encourage daily monitoring of pulmonary function.

Most transplant patients will average 20 to 35 outpatient transplant clinic visits during their first post-operative year. Assuming relative medical stability, clinic visits may be reduced and typically range from five to 15 per year thereafter. Hospital readmission is most common for infection or rejection, with the highest incidence of readmission for transplant complications following lung and kidney transplantation.

Graft and Patient Survival

Graft and patient (host) survival continues to improve in all transplant organ categories, despite the necessity of transplantation from donors with less than optimal HLA compatibilities due to a growing waiting list of individuals needing organs and a plateau in the number of donors. This has been particularly true for kidney transplantation, where the results of living donor kidney transplants continue to be superior to those achieved with cadaver donors. Longer-term graft and patient survival continues to be greatest for kidney transplants, while lung and combined liver and intestinal transplants have the shortest patient survival. Kidney transplanted patients also have the advantage of return to dialysis if the graft fails, and many have an opportunity for subsequent transplantation(s).

The U.S. Organ Procurement and Transplantation Network provides extensive and timely reports concerning graft and patient survival rates, as well as other valuable information concerning the transplantation and organ donation process in the United States. These reports are available to the general public on the Internet. Table 18.5 provides 1- and 5-year organ specific patient survival statistics following transplantation in the United States. OPTN data can also be researched extensively to extrapolate customized life expectancy projections by cohort to include the primary disease resulting in organ failure (Table 18.6).

Estimated Transplantation Costs

Hospitalization costs for organ transplantation can vary substantially, and this variation is usually complication dependent (post-operative), with varying lengths of stay. Standard deviations reported by reliable databases are generally in excess of $100,000. The sections above in this chapter have included pertinent information needed by the life care planner to develop a comprehensive life care plan for individuals suffering from the most common forms of end-stage organ diseases and awaiting organ transplantation.

As with other diagnostic groups, life care planning in transplantation must be individualized for each person, with consideration given to specific parameters applicable for the individual. Specific factors that should be considered in developing the life care plan include patient age, gender, blood type, transplant status, and transplant center, as these factors can affect recipient candidacy and specific waiting times

Table 18.5 Unadjusted 1- and 5-Year Patient Survival by Organ

Organ Transplanted	*1-Year Survival*	*5-Year Survival*
Kidney		
Deceased donor	98.4%	83.4%
Living donor	98.6%	92%
Pancreas alone	96.2%	91%
Pancreas after kidney	98%	88.6%
Kidney–pancreas	96.6%	88.7%
Liver		
Deceased donor	89.7%	74.3%
Living donor	91.3%	81.3%
Intestine	79.8%	60.3%
Heart	90.4%	76.8%
Lung	85.2%	55.2%
Heart–lung	76.1%	49.3%

Source: Adapted from Organ Procurement and Transplantation Network (OPTN) and Scientific Registry of Transplant Recipients (SRTR). *OPTN/SRTR 2011 Annual Data Report*. Rockville, MD: Department of Health and Human Services, Health Resources and Services Administration; Dec 2012.

for transplantation. Likewise, pre-operative and post-operative protocols can vary from one center to the next, although most OPTN-certified transplant centers are similar. Center- and organ-specific immunosuppressant protocols do tend to vary, which over time can have a significant impact on cost.

Table 18.7 provides an estimate of the number of transplants and the average billed charges per transplant in the United States for 2017.

Retransplantation

Graft loss is a possibility for all transplant recipients and for some, retransplantation is an option. In 2005, retransplants represented 12.4 percent of kidney, 9.0 percent of liver, 4.7 percent of heart, and 5.3 percent of lung transplants performed (Magee et al., 2007). The outcomes for those who have been retransplanted are poorer than those who have had a primary transplant with the exception of deceased donor kidney transplantation, for which the unadjusted 5-year allograft survival rate was the almost the same for first and second transplants (Rao & Ojo, 2008). Costs for retransplantation are much higher than for primary transplant.

Studies have shown that liver patients who were retransplanted encountered significantly longer hospital and intensive care unit stays than for those with primary transplants, along with associated increased costs (Azoulay et al., 2002). Retransplantation also raises an ethical concern in regard to the utilization of such scarce resources as transplantable organs.

Table 18.6 1-, 3-, and 5-Year Survival by Etiology of Organ Failure

Organ	*Cause of Organ Failure*		*Percent Survival*
Heart/Lung	Cardiomyopathy	1 Year	*
Heart/Lung	Congenital Heart Disease	1 Year	61.1
Heart/Lung	Coronary Artery Disease	1 Year	*
Heart/Lung	Cardiomyopathy	3 Year	*
Heart/Lung	Congenital Heart Disease	3 Year	50.1
Heart/Lung	Coronary Artery Disease	3 Year	*
Heart/Lung	Cardiomyopathy	5 Year	*
Heart/Lung	Congenital Heart Disease	5 Year	36.9
Heart	Cardiomyopathy	1 Year	89.4
Heart	Congenital Heart Disease	1 Year	82.2
Heart	Coronary Artery Disease	1 Year	87.1
Heart	Cardiomyopathy	3 Year	81.0
Heart	Congenital Heart Disease	3 Year	73.7
Heart	Coronary Artery Disease	3 Year	78.5
Heart	Cardiomyopathy	5 Year	74.2
Heart	Congenital Heart Disease	5 Year	68.2
Heart	Coronary Artery Disease	5 Year	71.8
Intestine	Functional Bowel Problems	1 Year	81.8
Intestine	Short Gut Syndrome	1 Year	77.3
Intestine	Functional Bowel Problems	3 Year	52.0
Intestine	Short Gut Syndrome	3 Year	59.5
Intestine	Functional Bowel Problems	5 Year	49.9
Intestine	Short Gut Syndrome	5 Year	45.6
Kidney	Retransplant/Graft Failure	1 Year	95.6
Kidney	Congenital, Rare, Familial	1 Year	98
Kidney	Diabetes	1 Year	93.6
Kidney	Glomerular Disease	1 Year	97.3
Kidney	Hypertensive Nephrosclerosis	1 Year	95.6
Kidney	Neoplasms	1 Year	98.1

(Continued)

Table 18.6 (Continued) 1-, 3-, and 5-Year Survival by Etiology of Organ Failure

Organ	*Cause of Organ Failure*		*Percent Survival*
Kidney	Polycystic Kidneys	1 Year	97.6
Kidney	Renovascular and Other Vascular	1 Year	95.7
Kidney	Tubular and Interstitial Disease	1 Year	96.2
Kidney	Other	1 Year	95.5
Kidney	Retransplant/Graft Failure	3 Year	89.9
Kidney	Congenital, Rare, Familial	3 Year	95.9
Kidney	Diabetes	3 Year	85.1
Kidney	Glomerular Disease	3 Year	94.0
Kidney	Hypertensive Nephrosclerosis	3 Year	89.0
Kidney	Neoplasms	3 Year	83.8
Kidney	Polycystic Kidneys	3 Year	94.0
Kidney	Renovascular and Other Vascular	3 Year	88.6
Kidney	Tubular and Interstitial Disease	3 Year	90.7
Kidney	Other	3 Year	90.0
Kidney	Retransplant/Graft Failure	5 Year	83.4
Kidney	Congenital, Rare, Familial	5 Year	93.1
Kidney	Diabetes	5 Year	73.9
Kidney	Glomerular Disease	5 Year	89.6
Kidney	Hypertensive Nephrosclerosis	5 Year	81.7
Kidney	Neoplasms	5 Year	79.8
Kidney	Polycystic Kidneys	5 Year	88.9
Kidney	Renovascular and Other Vascular	5 Year	79.3
Kidney	Tubular and Interstitial Disease	5 Year	85.8
Kidney	Other	5 Year	84.8
Liver	Acute Hepatic Necrosis	1 Year	81.6
Liver	Benign Neoplasms	1 Year	86
Liver	Biliary Atresia	1 Year	93.5
Liver	Cholestatic Liver Disease/Cirrhosis	1 Year	89.6

(Continued)

Table 18.6 (Continued) 1-, 3-, and 5-Year Survival by Etiology of Organ Failure

Organ	*Cause of Organ Failure*		*Percent Survival*
Liver	Malignant Neoplasms	1 Year	86.1
Liver	Metabolic Disease	1 Year	89.3
Liver	Non-Cholestatic Cirrhosis	1 Year	85.9
Liver	Other Liver Disease	1 Year	80.9
Liver	Other	1 Year	83.6
Liver	Acute Hepatic Necrosis	3 Year	72.6
Liver	Benign Neoplasms	3 Year	81.7
Liver	Biliary Atresia	3 Year	89.4
Liver	Cholestatic Liver Disease/Cirrhosis	3 Year	85.0
Liver	Malignant Neoplasms	3 Year	68.7
Liver	Metabolic Disease	3 Year	83.7
Liver	Non-Cholestatic Cirrhosis	3 Year	76.9
Liver	Other Liver Disease	3 Year	71.8
Liver	Other	3 Year	74.3
Liver	Acute Hepatic Necrosis	5 Year	69.6
Liver	Benign Neoplasms	5 Year	69.6
Liver	Biliary Atresia	5 Year	85.2
Liver	Cholestatic Liver Disease/Cirrhosis	5 Year	79.7
Liver	Malignant Neoplasms	5 Year	54.2
Liver	Metabolic Disease	5 Year	80.8
Liver	Non-Cholestatic Cirrhosis	5 Year	69.8
Liver	Other Liver Disease	5 Year	63.3
Liver	Other	5 Year	64.4
Lung	Alpha-1–Antitrypsin Deficiency	1 Year	85.5
Lung	Congenital Heart Disease	1 Year	76.2
Lung	Cystic Fibrosis	1 Year	86.1
Lung	Emphysema/COPD	1 Year	86.8
Lung	Idiopathic Pulmonary Fibrosis	1 Year	79.9

(*Continued*)

Table 18.6 (Continued) 1-, 3-, and 5-Year Survival by Etiology of Organ Failure

Organ	*Cause of Organ Failure*		*Percent Survival*
Lung	Other Lung Disease	1 Year	82.6
Lung	Primary Pulmonary Hypertension	1 Year	75.4
Lung	Retransplant/Graft Failure	1 Year	67.0
Lung	Other	1 Year	74.5
Lung	Alpha-1–Antitrypsin Deficiency	3 Year	61.1
Lung	Cardiomyopathy	3 Year	*
Lung	Congenital Heart Disease	3 Year	53.7
Lung	Cystic Fibrosis	3 Year	65.1
Lung	Emphysema/COPD	3 Year	65.9
Lung	Idiopathic Pulmonary Fibrosis	3 Year	56.4
Lung	Other Lung Disease	3 Year	61.1
Lung	Primary Pulmonary Hypertension	3 Year	60.2
Lung	Retransplant/Graft Failure	3 Year	40.7
Lung	Other	3 Year	69.8
Lung	Alpha-1–Antitrypsin Deficiency	5 Year	48.8
Lung	Cardiomyopathy	5 Year	*
Lung	Congenital Heart Disease	5 Year	40.9
Lung	Coronary Artery Disease	5 Year	*
Lung	Cystic Fibrosis	5 Year	50
Lung	Emphysema/COPD	5 Year	48
Lung	Idiopathic Pulmonary Fibrosis	5 Year	40.7
Lung	Other Lung Disease	5 Year	52.3
Lung	Primary Pulmonary Hypertension	5 Year	47.7
Lung	Retransplant/Graft Failure	5 Year	28.1
Lung	Other	5 Year	45.6
Pancreas	Retransplant/Graft Failure	1 Year	93.7
Pancreas	Diabetes	1 Year	95.9
Pancreas	Cancer	1 Year	*

(Continued)

Table 18.6 (Continued) 1-, 3-, and 5-Year Survival by Etiology of Organ Failure

Organ	*Cause of Organ Failure*		*Percent Survival*
Pancreas	Other	1 Year	78.8
Pancreas	Retransplant/Graft Failure	3 Year	91
Pancreas	Diabetes	3 Year	90.7
Pancreas	Cancer	3 Year	*
Pancreas	Other	3 Year	63.8
Pancreas	Retransplant/Graft Failure	5 Year	75.8
Pancreas	Diabetes	5 Year	82.2
Pancreas	Cancer	5 Year	*
Pancreas	Other	5 Year	41.7

Source: Adapted from 2014 OPTN National Data.

Note: The 2014 report was published in 2016. The 2016 Annual Report was not published until Jan 2018, long after this chapter work was finished.

Case Study

James H. Patient is a 39-year-old Caucasian male who was born on 03/15/1977. Neonatal screening performed shortly after birth revealed evidence of cystic fibrosis. James has been followed closely by pulmonary specialists, endocrinologists, gastroenterologists, and primary pediatrics throughout his life, and he received treatment available at the time for management of his disease and associated recurrent respiratory complications.

By the age of 38 years, James began to develop progressive pulmonary deterioration requiring frequent hospitalizations due to respiratory failure. He was ultimately diagnosed with end-stage lung disease and referred to a leading transplant center in Baltimore, Maryland, near his home. James continued to receive frequent medical interventions due to respiratory failure and was considered gravely ill. After 5 months on the transplant wait-list, a donor organ was identified for which he was determined to be a candidate. James was promptly scheduled and prepared to receive a double lung transplant.

In developing a life care plan for James, it is important to note that once he receives his new organ, the transplanted lungs will not have cystic fibrosis; however, after the transplant, James will still have cystic fibrosis and will contend with disease involvement of the sinuses, pancreas, intestines, sweat glands, and reproductive tract. The new lungs do not acquire cystic fibrosis, but immunosuppressive drugs may decrease the ability to fight bacterial infections, such as *Pseudomonas aeruginosa* and *Burkholderia cepacia* (*B. cepacia*), as well as the more serious viral and fungal infections for which all transplant recipients remain at risk due to the requirement for life long immunosuppressant therapy. The risk of infection for those with cystic fibrosis who are transplanted is greatest immediately after the transplant procedure when immunosuppressive agents are given at the highest doses to reduce the risk of acute rejection.

The literature consistently reports improved longevity and quality of life for those with cystic fibrosis who have approached end-stage lung disease when compared to those who do not receive a transplant. Complications post-transplant include rejection, obliterative bronchiolitis, medication side effects, and

Table 18.7 Estimated U.S. Average 2017 Billed Charges per Transplant

Transplant	*Estimated Number of Transplants*	*Estimated Billed Charges*[a]
Heart Only	2,725	$1,382,400
Single Lung Only	673	$861,700
Double Lung Only	1,397	$1,190,700
Heart–Lung	21	$2,564,000
Liver Only	6,158	$812,500
Kidney Only	16,804	$418,800
Pancreas Only	136	$347,000
Kidney–Pancreas	724	$618,100
Intestine Only	49	$1,547,200
Intestine With Other Organs	80	$1,844,700
Kidney–Heart	130	$1,840,300
Liver–Kidney	682	$1,229,700
Other Multi-Organ	35	$1,855,400
	Transplant (Other)	
Cornea	50,099	$30,200
Bone Marrow-Autologous	12,160	$409,600
Bone Marrow-Allogenic	9,284	$892,700

Source: Bentley, T.S., & Phillips, S.J. 2017 *U.S. Organ and Tissue Transplant Cost Estimates and Discussion*. Brookfiled, WI: Milliman, Inc. Online, available at www.milliman.com.

[a] Total charge estimates include medical costs incurred 30 days pre-transplant, organ procurement, facility and professional charges for hospital transplant admission and re-admission within 180 days post-transplant discharge, and all outpatient medications prescribed from discharge for the transplant admission to 180 days post-transplant discharge.

malignancy. The patient will also continue to need additional medications and nutritional support beyond those for transplant alone due to cystic fibrosis. In the best transplant centers, the 10-year survival post-lung transplant for patients with cystic fibrosis is up to 80 percent (De Boeck, 2016).

A recent study of patients with cystic fibrosis in Canada who underwent lung transplant between 1988 and 2012 found that the 5-year patient survival was 67 percent and that 50 percent of patients were alive more than 10 years post-transplant. The age at transplant, pancreatic sufficiency, and *B. cepacia* infection remained important determinants of survival post-lung transplant (Stephenson et al., 2015). The International Society for Heart and Lung Transplantation notes that of those who survived to 1 year after primary lung transplant performed between January of 1990 and June of 2013, the conditional median survival was higher for cystic fibrosis patients at 11.1 years. For lung transplants across all recipient groups in the same time range, the median survival for bilateral lung transplant patients was 9.7 years versus 7.9 years for unilateral lung transplant patients (Yusen et al., 2015).

LIFE CARE COST ANALYSIS
JAMES H. PATIENT

Date of Report: 04/06/16	Diagnoses:
Date of Birth: 03/15/77	End-Stage Lung Disease;
Current Age: 39 years	Cystic Fibrosis
Gender: Male	
Ethnicity: Caucasian	
Average Residual Life Expectancy: 39.7 Years	
Projected Residual Life Expectancy: 11 Years	

Service/Item	Begin at Age	Duration Years	Frequency per Year	Average Unit Cost	Annual Cost	Life Time Cost
TRANSPLANTATION AND FIRST POST-OPERATIVE YEAR						
Inpatient/Other Acute Care						
Double Lung Transplantation						
Hospitalization	39	1	1	$754,144.00	$754,144.00	$754,144.00
Surgeons (Recipient & Donor)	39	1	1	$41,756.61	$41,756.61	$41,756.61
Other Physicians (Includes Anesth.)	39	1	1	$49,856.09	$49,856.09	$49,856.09
Donor Organ (SAC Fee)	39	1	1	$38,550.00	$38,550.00	$38,550.00
Donor Organ (Transport Fee)	39	1	1	$12,575.75	$12,575.75	$12,575.75
Bronchoscopy w/ wo Biopsy	39	1	4	$5,997.17	$23,988.68	$23,988.68
Hospital Readmission						
Transplant Complications	39	1	1.5	$126,017.44	$189,026.16	$189,026.16
Diagnostics						
CBC	39	1	13	$42.89	$557.54	$557.54
Metabolic Profile w/ LFTs	39	1	13	$89.96	$1,169.47	$1,169.47

(*Continued*)

Urinalysis	39	1	13	$25.10	$326.36	$326.36
Coagulation Studies	39	1	4	$85.78	$343.10	$343.10
Lipid Panel	39	1	4	$104.60	$418.42	$418.42
Prograf Levels	39	1	15	$210.25	$3,153.81	$3,153.81
Therapeutic MMF (MPA) Levels	39	1	15	$203.98	$3,059.67	$3,059.67
Hgb A1c	39	1	4	$75.31	$301.26	$301.26
Vitamin D, 25 hydroxy	39	1	3	$243.00	$729.00	$729.00
Cultures, Other/ Fungal	39	1	4	$116.89	$467.58	$467.58
Cultures, Viral, General	39	1	4	$246.87	$987.46	$987.46
Chest X-ray	39	1	6	$157.95	$947.71	$947.71
EKG	39	1	2	$84.73	$169.46	$169.46
Echocardiogram	39	1	4	$1,245.83	$4,983.33	$4,983.33
High Resolution Chest CT	39	1	1	$1,800.23	$1,800.23	$1,800.23
Pulmonary Function Tests	39	1	2	$571.14	$1,142.28	$1,142.28
Cystic Fibrosis Specific Diagnostics						
Vit ADE Levels, Serum	39	1	1	$520.93	$520.93	$520.93
Oral Glucose Tolerance Test	39	1	1	$103.56	$103.56	$103.56
ABPA Screen	39	1	1	$262.56	$262.56	$262.56
Nontuberculous Mycobacteria Cx	39	1	1	$97.28	$97.28	$97.28
Sensitivities & Organism ID	39	1	2	$101.76	$203.53	$203.53
Flu Test	39	1	2	$52.30	$104.60	$104.60
Medication						
Prograf (Calcineurin Inhibitor)	39	1	365	$26.14	$9,540.55	$9,540.55

(Continued)

Mycophenolate Mofetil	39	1	365	$15.17	$5,535.69	$5,535.69
Steroid	39	1	365	$0.26	$95.65	$95.65
Fungal Prophylaxis	39	1	90	$154.95	$13,945.14	$13,945.14
Bactrim DS	39	1	156	$0.98	$152.41	$152.41
Mag Ox, Folic Acid, Vitamin	39	1	365	$0.62	$225.24	$225.24
Metoprolol	39	1	365	$1.05	$384.64	$384.64
Additional Cardiac Agent	39	1	365	$1.29	$470.52	$470.52
Antibiotics (Oral)	39	1	3.5	$232.13	$812.46	$812.46
Antibiotics (Intravenous)	39	1	1.5	$9,077.27	$13,615.90	$13,615.90
Nebulized Bronchodilators	39	1	2	$76.65	$153.30	$153.30
Valganciclovir/ CMV	39	1	210	$77.28	$16,228.55	$16,228.55
FluVax	39	1	1	$61.87	$61.87	$61.87
Triple Vaccination	39	1	1	$196.81	$196.81	$196.81
Insulin	39	1	12	$42.80	$513.60	$513.60
Statin Agent	39	1	365	$6.14	$2,242.26	$2,242.26
Creon/Equivalent	39	1	365	$77.84	$28,412.34	$28,412.34
Macrolides (azithromycin)	39	1	365	$0.93	$338.83	$338.83
Vitamin ADEK, Tabs	39	1	365	$1.20	$437.42	$437.42
GI Protective	39	1	365	$5.27	$1,924.13	$1,924.13
Bisphosphonate	39	1	365	$4.71	$1,720.30	$1,720.30
Calcium/Other Supplement	39	1	365	$0.14	$52.20	$52.20
Outpatient Physician and Therapeutic Services						
Transplant Surgical Follow-up	39	1	9	$223.85	$2,014.67	$2,014.67

(Continued)

Pulmonologist/ Transplant Physician	39	1	12	$226.29	$2,715.52	$2,715.52
Transplant Clinic Follow-up	39	1	12	$308.58	$3,702.98	$3,702.98
Nutritionist/ Dietitian	39	1	2	$313.81	$627.62	$627.62
Case Management	39	1	12	$733.93	$8,807.14	$8,807.14
Home Health Care and Household Services						
Nursing or Respiratory Therapy	39	1	46	$127.50	$5,865.00	$5,865.00
Household Services	39	1	52	$102.50	$5,330.00	$5,330.00
Equipment and Supplies						
Supplemental Nutrition	39	1	365	$2.02	$738.36	$738.36
Blood Glucose Monitor	39	1	1	$72.99	$72.99	$72.99
Glucose Testing Supplies	39	1	12	$71.16	$853.97	$853.97
Gloves, Nonsterile	39	1	36	$12.10	$435.60	$435.60
Disinfectants	39	1	12	$42.59	$511.08	$511.08
Nebulizer	39	1	1	$140.00	$140.00	$140.00
POST-TRANSPLANTATION AND SUBSEQUENT YEARS						
Inpatient/Other Acute Care						
Hospital Readmission						
Transplant Complications	40	9	1/3	$126,017.44	$42,005.81	$378,052.32
Transplant Complications	49	1	2	$126,017.44	$252,034.88	$252,034.88
Bronchoscopy w/ wo Biopsy	40	1	2	$5,997.17	$11,994.34	$11,994.34
Bronchoscopy w/ wo Biopsy	41	9	1.5	$5,997.17	$8,995.75	$80,961.78

(*Continued*)

Diagnostics						
CBC	40	10	7	$42.89	$300.21	$3,002.13
Metabolic Profile w/ LFTs	40	10	7	$89.96	$629.72	$6,297.16
Urinalysis	40	10	7	$25.10	$175.73	$1,757.35
Coagulation Studies	40	10	3.5	$85.78	$300.21	$3,002.13
Lipid Panel	40	10	3.5	$104.60	$366.11	$3,661.14
Prograf Levels	40	10	7	$210.25	$1,471.78	$14,717.78
Therapeutic MMF (MPA) Levels	40	10	7	$203.98	$1,427.84	$14,278.45
Hgb A1c	40	10	4	$75.31	$301.26	$3,012.60
Chest X-ray	40	10	6	$157.95	$947.71	$9,477.12
High Resolution Chest CT	40	10	1/2	$1,800.23	$900.12	$9,001.17
EKG	40	10	2	$84.73	$169.46	$1,694.58
Echocardiogram	40	10	1/2	$1,245.83	$622.92	$6,229.17
Cardiac Stress Test	40	10	1/2	$378.67	$189.33	$1,893.33
DEXA Scan	40	10	1/2	$420.51	$210.25	$2,102.54
Colonoscopy, Outpatient	40	10	1/3	$3,412.91	$1,137.64	$11,376.38
Skin Biopsies (Pathology)	40	10	1	$241.64	$241.64	$2,416.35
Pulmonary Function Tests	40	10	2	$571.14	$1,142.28	$11,422.76
Cultures, Other/ Fungal	40	10	4	$116.89	$467.58	$4,675.80
Cultures, Viral, General	40	10	4	$246.87	$987.46	$9,874.62
Cystic Fibrosis Specific Diagnostics						
Vit ADE Levels, Serum	40	10	1	$520.93	$520.93	$5,209.28
Oral Glucose Tolerance Test	40	10	1	$103.56	$103.56	$1,035.58

(Continued)

ABPA Screen	40	10	1	$262.56	$262.56	$2,625.56
Nontuberculous Mycobacteria Cx	40	10	1	$97.28	$97.28	$972.82
Sensitivities & Organism ID	40	10	2	$101.76	$203.53	$2,035.29
Flu Test	40	10	2	$52.30	$104.60	$1,046.04
			Medication			
Prograf (Calcineurin Inhibitor)	40	10	365	$26.14	$9,540.55	$95,405.53
Mycophenolate Mofetil	40	10	365	$15.17	$5,535.69	$55,356.91
Steroid	40	10	365	$0.26	$95.65	$956.48
Mag Ox, Folic Acid, Vitamin	40	10	365	$0.62	$225.24	$2,252.42
Metoprolol	40	10	365	$1.05	$384.64	$3,846.37
Additional Cardiac Agent	40	10	365	$1.29	$470.52	$4,705.22
Antibiotics (Predental/other)	40	10	2	$37.85	$75.69	$756.90
Antibiotics (Oral)	40	10	3	$232.13	$696.39	$6,963.90
Antibiotics (Intravenous)	40	10	1/2	$9,077.27	$4,538.63	$45,386.34
FluVax	40	10	1	$61.87	$61.87	$618.67
Flu Vaccine, Family/Other	40	10	1.5	$61.87	$92.80	$928.00
Triple Vaccination	40	10	1/5	$196.81	$39.36	$393.63
Insulin	40	10	12	$42.80	$513.60	$5,136.00
Statin Agent	40	10	365	$6.14	$2,242.26	$22,422.59
Creon/Equivalent	40	10	365	$77.84	$28,412.34	$284,123.42
Macrolides (azithromycin)	40	10	365	$0.93	$338.83	$3,388.30
Vitamin ADEK, Tabs	40	10	365	$1.20	$437.42	$4,374.16

(*Continued*)

GI Protective	40	10	365	$5.27	$1,924.13	$19,241.34
Bisphosphonate	40	10	365	$4.71	$1,720.30	$17,203.00
Calcium/Other Supplement	40	10	365	$0.14	$52.20	$521.95
Nebulized Bronchodilation/ Other	40	8	3.5	$76.65	$268.28	$2,146.26
Daily Nebulized Therapy	48	2	365	$6.80	$2,480.85	$4,961.70
Outpatient Physician and Therapeutic Services						
Transplant Surgical Follow-Up	40	10	2	$220.02	$440.03	$4,400.34
Pulmonologist/ Transplant Physician	40	10	4	$185.15	$740.60	$7,405.96
Transplant Clinic Follow-Up	40	10	7	$308.58	$2,160.07	$21,600.73
Cardiologist	40	10	2.5	$223.85	$559.63	$5,596.31
Dermatologist	40	10	1.5	$146.45	$219.67	$2,196.68
Endocrinologist	40	10	2	$185.15	$370.30	$3,702.98
Nutritionist/ Dietitian	40	10	2	$313.81	$627.62	$6,276.24
Individual Counseling	40	10	1/3	$5,570.16	$1,856.72	$18,567.21
Case Management	40	10	6	$733.93	$4,403.57	$44,035.71
Home Health Care and Household Services						
Nursing or Respiratory Therapy	40	10	30	$127.50	$3,825.00	$38,250.00
CNA (16–24 Hours/Day)	48	2	365	$470.00	$171,550.00	$343,100.00
Household Services	40	10	52	$102.50	$5,330.00	$53,300.00
Equipment and Supplies						
Supplemental Nutrition	40	10	365	$2.02	$738.36	$7,383.65

(Continued)

Blood Glucose Monitor	40	10	1/4	$72.99	$18.25	$182.48
Glucose Testing Supplies	40	10	12	$71.16	$853.97	$8,539.66
Gloves, Nonsterile	40	10	36	$12.10	$435.60	$4,356.00
Disinfectants	40	10	12	$42.59	$511.08	$5,110.80
Pulse Oximeter	40	10	1/5	$568.38	$113.68	$1,136.75
Oximeter Finger Probe	40	10	1/2	$184.50	$92.25	$922.50
Room Humidifier	40	10	1/3	$97.50	$32.50	$325.00
Nebulizer	40	10	1/3	$140.00	$46.67	$466.67
Nebulizer Circuits	40	8	2	$4.50	$9.00	$72.00
Nebulizer Circuits	48	2	24	$4.50	$108.00	$216.00
Stationary 5L Air Concentrator	48	1	1	$1,713.00	$1,713.00	$1,713.00
Portable Oxygen Concentrator	48	1	1	$3,973.37	$3,973.37	$3,973.37
Oxygen Tubing	48	2	4	$2.12	$8.48	$16.96
Electric Scooter	48	1	1	$3,817.50	$3,817.50	$3,817.50
Scooter Lift/ Hauler	48	1	1	$2,695.00	$2,695.00	$2,695.00
Manual Wheelchair	48	1	1	$2,585.64	$2,585.64	$2,585.64
Potential Care Needs						
Acute Humoral Allograft Rejection						
Addition of Monoclonal/Polyclonal						
Antibody Therapy (Acute Setting)	39	1	1	$77,008.80	$77,008.80	$77,008.80

COST ANALYSIS SUMMARY JAMES H. PATIENT		
Service/Item	*Life Time Cost Totals*	*Percent of Total*
Inpatient/Other Acute Care	$1,832,940.61	55.72%

(*Continued*)

Diagnostics	$154,666.29	4.70%
Medication	$678,148.88	20.62%
Outpatient Physician and Therapeutic Services	$131,650.12	4.00%
Home Health Care and Household Services	$445,845.00	13.55%
Equipment and Supplies	$46,264.98	1.41%
GRAND TOTAL	**$3,289,515.88**	**100.00%**
Potential Care Needs	*$77,008.80*	

References

AOTA. 2016 American Organ Transplant Association. Data. Online, available at www.aotaonline.org.

Azoulay D., Linhares, M. M., Huguet, E. et al. 2002 Decision for retransplantation of the liver: an experience- and cost-based analysis. *Ann Surg 236*(6), 713–21.

Backman, L., & Morales, J. M. 2000. Is nonnephrotoxic immunosuppression a possibility? *Transplantation 69*, 27–30.

Bagwell, D. M., & Milton, J. 2010. Life care planning for organ transplantation. In R. Weed, & D. Berens (eds.) *Life Care Planning and Case Management Handbook* (3rd ed.), Boca Raton, FL: CRC Press LLC. 665–699.

Bentley, T. S., & Phillips, S. J. 2017 *U.S. Organ and Tissue Transplant Cost Estimates and Discussion.* Brookfiled, WI: Milliman, Inc. Online, available at www.milliman.com.

Crosson, J. T. 2007. Focal Segmental Glomerulosclerosis and Renal Transplantation. *Transplant Proc 39*(3), 737–743.

De Boeck, K. 2016. Introduction: from the discovery of the CFTR gene in 1989 through to 2014. In A. Bush, D. Bilton, & M. Hodson (eds.) *Hodson and Geddes' Cystic Fibrosis*, (4th ed.), Boca Raton, FL: CRC Press. 12.

de Vera, M. E., Lopez-Solis, R., Dvorchik, I. et al. 2009. Liver transplantation using donation after cardiac death donors: long-term follow-up from a single center. *Am J Transplant 9*, 773–781.

Gift of Life Organ Donor Program, 2016. *Average Median Wait Time to Transplant.* Philadelphia, PA. http://www.donors1.org.

Ginns, L., Cosimi A. B., & Morris, P. 1999. *Transplantation.* Malden, MA: Blackwell Science.

Magee, J. C., Barr, M. L., Basadonna, D. P. et al. 2007 Repeat organ transplantation in the United States, 1996–2005. *Am J Transplant 7*(Part 2), 1424–1433.

Massie, A. B., Chow, E. K., Wickliffe, C. E. et al. 2015. Early changes in liver distribution following implementation of Share 35. *Am J Transplant 15*, 659–667.

McLaughlin, K., Wu, D., Fick, G. et al. 2002. Cytomegalovirus seromismatching increases the risk of acute renal allograft rejection. *Transplantation 74*, 813–816.

Montori, V. M., Velosa, J. A., Basu, A. et al. 2002. Posttransplantation diabetes: a systematic review of the literature. *Diabetes Care 25*, 583–592.

Ohler, L. & Cupples, S. 2008. *Core Curriculum for Transplant Nurses.* St. Louis: Mosby Elsevier.

Organ Procurement and Transplantation Network (OPTN) and Scientific Registry of Transplant Recipients (SRTR). *OPTN/SRTR 2011 Annual Data Report.* Rockville, MD: Department of Health and Human Services, Health Resources and Services Administration; Dec 2012.

Organ Procurement and Transplantation Network (OPTN) and Scientific Registry of Transplant Recipients (SRTR). *OPTN/SRTR 2014 Annual Data Report.* Rockville, MD: Department of Health and Human Services, Health Resources and Services Administration; January 2016.

Penn, I. 2001. Neoplasia following transplantation. In D. Norman, & L. Turka (eds.) *Primer on Transplantation.* Mt. Laurel, NJ: American Society of Transplantation, 268–275.

Putre, L. 2014. *Will a New Kidney Allocation System Even the Playing Field?* Medscape News, available at http://www.medscape.com/viewarticle/837112.

Rao, P. S., & Ojo, A. 2008. Organ retransplantation in the United States: Trends and implications. *Clin Transplant* 57–67. PMID: 19708446.

Rubin, R. 1999. Infection in the organ transplant recipient. In L.C. Ginns, A.B. Cosimi, & P.J. Morris (eds.) *Transplantation*. Malden, MA: Blackwell Science. 747–769.

Rubin, R. 2000. Prevention and treatment of cytomegalovirus in heart transplant patients. *J Heart Lung Transplant 19*, 731–735.

Stephenson, A. L., Sykes, J., Berthiaume, Y. et al. 2015. Clinical and demographic factors associated with post-lung transplantation survival in individuals with cystic fibrosis. *J Heart Lung Transplant 34*(9), 1139–1145.

UNOS. 2006. United Network for Organ Sharing, Data. Online, available at www.UNOS.org.

UNOS. 2016. United Network for Organ Sharing, Data. Online, available at www.UNOS.org.

UNOS. 2017. United Network for Organ Sharing, Newsroom. U.S. organ transplants, deceased donors set record in 2016. available at www.UNOS.org.

USRDS. 2015. United States Renal Data System. *Annual Data Report*. Available at www.usrds.org.

Weinberg, A., Zhang, L., & Hayward A. R. 2000. Alloreactive cytotoxic CD4+ responses elicited by cytomegalovirus-infected endothelial cells: role of MHC class I antigens. *Viral Immunol 13*, 37–47.

Yusen, R. D., Edwars, L. B., Kucheryavaya, A. Y. et al. 2015. The Registry of the International Society for Heart and Lung Transplantation: 32nd official adult lung and heart-lung transplantation report—2015; focus theme: Early graft failure. *J Heart Lung Transplant 34*(10), 1264–1277.

Chapter 19

Life Care Planning for the Visually Impaired*

Roger O. Weed and Rasheeda Wilkins

Contents

Introduction....571
Definitions....572
Epidemiology....572
Etiology....573
Functional Outcomes....574
Psychological Impact....574
Aids to Independent Function and/or Durable Medical Equipment for the Visually Impaired....575
Lighting....575
Personal Care and Homemaker Services....578
Formal Rehabilitation....578
Case Study....579
Conclusion....581
Appendix....582
References....590

Introduction

Visual impairment and blindness can have devastating effects on an individual, in all aspects of life, including emotionally, socially, and vocationally. Younger and Sardegna (1994) have pointed out that an individual's personality, past experiences with blindness, education, social and financial factors, mobility, occupation, cultural background, general physical condition, psychological readiness, and family support system will have an effect on how she or he is able

* Terry Winkler, MD, deceased, contributed to previous editions of this chapter. He was a wonderful person, practitioner, and educator. His contributions to the specialty practice of life care planning will be missed.

to deal with vision loss. The consequences of vision loss or impairment are all-encompassing, impacting *every* area of an individual's life. This demands that the rehabilitation professional develop a carefully thought-out life care plan that meets the needs of the individual over a lifetime through all of the various areas affected. In addition, vision impairment encompasses a continuum of problems from low vision to total blindness. The level of preserved vision will affect the recommendations of the life care plan. Technology is rapidly changing and continues to provide interventions that have a tremendously positive effect on a visually impaired person's life and vocation.

The goal of this chapter is to provide basic background information that the life care planner will need to initiate a lifelong plan for visually impaired individuals. In addition, and perhaps more importantly, the chapter provides references to assist in locating resources for the visually impaired. The life care planner must have a thorough working knowledge of visual impairment, its effect and impact, and expertise regarding the types of equipment and technological advances for the visually impaired.

Definitions

Visual impairment may be divided into two main categories: low vision and blindness. Low vision is much more common than total blindness. From an educational standpoint, the Social Security Act defines blindness as central acuity of 20/200 or less in the better eye. The Act also provides that we consider an eye that has a visual field limitation such that the widest diameter of the visual field subtends an angle no greater than 20 degrees as having a central visual acuity of 20/200 or less (Social Security Act [SSA], 2016). In education, low vision is defined as visual acuity better than 20/200 but worse than 20/70 with correction (PL101-476, Individuals with Disabilities Education Act). Additional important terminology distinctions are *severe visual impairment* and *legally blind*. *Severe visual impairment* is defined by Nelson and Dimitrova (1993) as the self- or proxy-reporting inability to read ordinary newspaper print even with the best correction of glasses or contact lenses. In other words, severe visual impairment is not based on test of visual acuity. Rather, it measures perceived visual problems. *Legally blind* is used to indicate entitlement to certain government and private agency services. Low vision is defined by the American Academy of Ophthalmology (2003) to exist if ordinary eyeglasses, contact lenses, or lens implants do not give clear vision. People with low vision still have useful vision; however, this vision can be improved with visual aid devices. In addition, vision impairment is defined as having 20/40 or worse vision in the better eye even with eyeglasses. In most states, 20/40 is the point at which people can no longer obtain unrestricted driver's licenses (Owsley & McGwin, 2010).

Epidemiology

A variety of estimates are available at various sources regarding the numbers of individuals with low vision or blindness. Definitions of blindness and low vision vary with different authors or sponsoring organizations. This results in some variability of the numbers that are reported. The Prevention of Blindness Database estimates that in 1990, 38 million people worldwide met the definition of blind (Tielsch et al., 1990) and more than one million in the United States with projections of increasing prevalence of blindness over time. About two-thirds are female (NIH, 2018). This was more than double the population reported in 1972 of 10 to 15 million. Thylefors et al. (1995) reported that 4.6 percent of the U.S. population met the definition for blindness and 14.4 percent met the definition of low vision. Nelson and Dimitrova (1993) reported a total number of U.S. citizens with blindness among civilian noninstitutionalized population of 4.3 million. They went on to say that they believed this number represented approximately half of all the individuals with visual impairments in the United States. Nelson and Dimitrova's (1993) discussion of severe visual impairment revealed that the five states with the highest number of individuals meeting the definition were California, New York, Texas, Pennsylvania, and Florida. Florida had the highest rate of severe visual impairment at 22.6 persons per 1000. It was estimated that approximately 1,000,000 to 1,250,000 were of working age between 18 and 64. For persons ages 40 or older, Iowa, South Dakota, and North Dakota had the highest prevalence (Owsley & McGwin, 2010). In the national picture in 1990, more than 17 of every 1000 persons in the civilian noninstitutionalized population of the United States were severely visually impaired. Slightly over half a million met the definition of blindness in both eyes, with approximately 100,000 children meeting the definition of severely visually impaired. The National Information Center for Children and Youth with Disabilities estimates that for individuals under the age of 18, 12.2 per 1000 have visual impairments and 0.06 per 1000 have severe visual impairments, that is, are either legally or totally blind (Teplin, 1995). Some studies indicate that visual problems are strongly linked to race. For example, Tielsch et al. (1990) and Owsley & McGwin (2010) reported that legal blindness is more common among black Americans than whites, and Hispanics have a higher prevalence of vision impairment than other races (Owsley & McGwin, 2010).

Etiology

A variety of conditions can lead to visual impairment. The most common causes of visual impairment vary with the age of the individual. Deutsch and Sawyer (2003) pointed out that the leading causes for children under the age of five include retrolental fibroplasia, neoplasm, infections, and injuries. The same is true for individuals ages 5 to 19. Over age 20, cataracts become the most common cause. During the 1970s, glaucoma was the second-leading cause of blindness. However, 1992 data indicate that the most common causes of blindness in the United States are cataracts, trauma (most common diagnosis for the life care planner), amblyopia, and macular degeneration, respectively. This likely reflects a greater awareness, early detection, and treatment of glaucoma.

Low vision may occur from a variety of causes, which include birth defects, inherited diseases, injuries, diabetes, dacryoma, and cataracts. The most common cause is macular degeneration, which is a disease of the retina and causes damage to the central vision. Peripheral vision, however, is not affected. There are different types of low vision according to the American Academy of Ophthalmology (2003). Reduced central or reading vision is the most common; however, decreased peripheral vision may occur, or a loss of color vision, or the ability to adjust to light, contrast, or glare. The different types of low vision may require different kinds of assistance.

Traumatic etiology of eye injuries occurs in a variety of ways. They may be the result of chemical or ultraviolet burns, direct penetrating wounds, abrasions, lacerations, or violent shaking-type injuries (e.g., brain injury), which can damage the retina. Burns to the eye, lacerations, and corneal abrasions can result in significant visual impairment. However, later scar tissue development can also be a complicating factor that leads to deteriorating vision. Detached retina can lead to blurred or altered vision, flashes of light, or total blindness in an eye.

Some medical conditions that are undiagnosed or not treated properly can lead to severe visual impairment. These include eye infections, glaucoma, cataracts, hydrocephalus, and vascular disease. The central causes of visual impairment would include stroke, traumatic brain injury, hydrocephalus, and tumors. A significant limitation to vision can occur from ocular motor injuries.

Functional Outcomes

The degree of visual loss may vary significantly with the more severe visual impairments leading to the most profound types of functional deficits. The age of onset and level of development before loss of sight occurs are critical factors in a person's ability to acquire skills and concepts. Vision may actually fluctuate or be temporarily influenced by factors such as fatigue, light glare, or inappropriate lighting. An understanding of the types of visual impairment is important, but generalizations about a person's visual functioning cannot be made solely on the basis of a diagnosis. Assessment of functional and vocational implications must be conducted on an individual basis, which in turn affects the nature of the final life care plan (LaPlante et al., 1992; Higdon, 2018).

The types of interventions that are required vary, depending on the nature of the visual impairment. For example, if peripheral vision is damaged, the person has tunnel vision and requires different interventions than an individual with macular degeneration, which would result in the loss of central vision with relative sparing of the peripheral vision. Or, an individual may have night blindness where he/she has very little vision in dimly lit areas such as in retinitis pigmentosa, or there is photosensitivity where vision is severely impaired in the bright sunlight.

Special issues occur in very young children with visual impairment (Dodson-Burk & Hill, 1989; Teplin, 1995; Matthews, 1996). In fact, the child's development depends upon the severity of the visual impairment, type of visual loss, and age at onset of the vision deficit. The National Information Center for Children and Youth with Disabilities reports that a young child with visual impairment has little reason to explore interesting objects in the environment and misses opportunities to have experiences to learn. This lack of exploring will continue until learning becomes motivating or until intervention begins. Children with visual impairment may be unable to imitate social behavior and understand nonverbal cues because they are unable to see peers or parents. This creates obstacles to a growing child's independence. It is imperative that children with visual impairment be assessed early and receive appropriate interventions. They will require ongoing assessment as they grow and develop. An interdisciplinary approach will be beneficial in teaching self-care and daily living skills, as well as approaching educational and vocational issues. Deutsch and Sawyer (2003) have pointed out that even relatively minor impairment can result in vocational handicaps that limit the range of job alternatives available to an individual and reduce earning capacity. An example is color blindness, which can reduce the range of job opportunities that would otherwise be available. The degree to which total blindness results in permanent impairment and loss of earning capacity varies with the individual and depends on many personal and vocational factors. An infant or young child who has sustained the loss of an eye will require multiple careful follow-up appointments with the placement and replacement of an ocular prosthesis and conformer to promote development of the orbit. Failure to do this will result in some deformity of the forehead and face and will not allow placement of a cosmetic prosthesis.

Psychological Impact

Few conditions are as feared as blindness. As stated in the introduction, an individual's reaction is affected by personality, past experience, education, social and financial factors, mobility, occupation, cultural background, general physical condition, psychological readiness, and family support. Common psychological reactions include anxiety, depression, anger, and, perhaps the most limiting of all, fear. The individual may experience the five emotional stages of loss as defined by Dr. Kübler-Ross (1975): denial, anger, bargaining, depression, and finally acceptance. While not all individuals will experience each of the stages, and the length of time per stage may vary a great deal, some part or all of these reactions may occur.

Deutsch and Sawyer (2003) described a variety of sensory distortions that can occur early on, including a loss of position sense such as a sensation of floating. This disorientation is often exacerbated by the psychological problems that accompany visual impairments. In addition, an individual who has a sudden onset of total visual impairment may have more acute or severe psychological reactions than an individual who has had a slow onset of blindness and has had time to adjust along the way. Varying degrees of independence will be lost, with some individuals experiencing a high degree of dependence on others. This cannot be viewed as a lack of motivation on an individual's part. It should be recognized, as previously stated, that there are multiple factors involved that dictate the ultimate functional outcome from visual impairment. Most will experience a great deal of social isolation, frequently having difficulty in establishing relationships. Some individuals have a substantial difficulty in communicating with sighted people after the onset of their visual impairments. If the visual impairment occurs at a very young age, certain concepts such as visual spatial arrangements can be extremely difficult to grasp.

Psychological counseling will be crucial for individuals with visual impairment to assist in dealing with the impact of the disability. In addition, a variety of specialized training and equipment can be utilized to help improve the person's independence, which will have a positive psychological effect.

Aids to Independent Function and/or Durable Medical Equipment for the Visually Impaired

This need can be divided into two broad general categories: high-technology and low-technology devices. Devices exist to help individuals with low vision and individuals with total blindness. Low vision aids are tools that aid those with vision to maximize their remaining vision. The American Academy of Ophthalmology (2003) cautions that no one device restores normal vision in all circumstances, so that different devices may be required for different purposes. Higdon (2018) reports that a rehabilitation professional should consider three types of aids for the visually impaired: tactile, auditory, and visual aids. Low-vision devices can be divided into optical and nonoptical devices. Low-vision optical devices use a lens or combination of lenses to produce magnification. Low-vision optical devices are task-specific. There are five categories: magnifying reading spectacles, hand magnifiers, stand magnifiers, telescopes, and video magnifiers (formerly called closed-circuit television). Nonoptical low-vision devices include locator bump dots, task lamps, reading stands, absorptive lenses, letter and envelope writing guides, talking watches and clocks, self-threading needles, bold black pens, bold line paper, large print keyboards, big button phones, large print address books, and so on.

Lighting

It is surprising to a lot of people that something as basic as adequate lighting can be so effective at helping those with vision loss to continue their everyday activities (www.Visionware.org, 2016). As one ages, the need for light to perform a task increases. On average, a 60-year-old person will need twice as much illumination as he or she needed at age 20. A person who is visually impaired may require complete renovation or modification of the entire lighting system in his or her home or office in order to best accommodate his or her disability. In some cases, having light sources that can be portable or moved close to the work area, such as high-intensity lights on adjustable arms, are beneficial. Hat brims or visors can be useful in blocking annoying overhead light, and absorptive lenses, which can help control glare, should be considered.

Gail Pickering, an assisted technology specialist, has published an excellent chapter regarding assisted technology for the visually impaired in the 1996 edition of *A Guide to Rehabilitation* by Deutsch and Sawyer. This chapter provides a comprehensive discussion of low-technology and high-technology devices and concludes with an exhaustive list of resources (Appendix 19.1) for obtaining the devices and information about their cost and use. In addition to Appendix 19.1 at the end of this chapter, see the related chapter on assistive devices in Weed and Field (2012). With the vast improvements in search techniques and logic via the Internet, the use of Google or other search engines to locate current assistive technology is easier than ever.

Examples of low-technology devices that should be included in a life care plan include check-writing guides, signature guides, watches that can indicate time by voice, tactile clues, or feeling, Braille, digital recorders, PenFriend (labler), timers, measuring cups, cooking devices, rulers, large-dial telephones, and so on. Hi-Mark Tactile Pen (commonly called "puff paint") is a 3-D writing tool that creates raised lines, dots, and shapes for labeling settings on appliances, canned goods, identifying clothing, and so on. Hi-Mark Tactile pen comes in a variety of colors and can be easily seen or felt by someone with normal hand sensation. Label makers can make labels that are large print, Braille, or talking labels that will allow a person to organize her closets and wardrobes, among other uses. Pill splitters, pill organizers, and liquid medication guides and measuring spoons are available. Individuals with diabetes and visual impairment will benefit from talking insulin-measuring devices such as Prodigy Voice or Sols V2, talking blood pressure monitor, talking weight scale, or perhaps a computerized insulin pump. Numerous kitchen devices are available, such as liquid-level indicators, elbow-length oven mitts to prevent burns, contrast cutting boards (black/white), double spatulas, and vegetable- and meat-slicing guides. There are self-threading needles, magnetic padlocks (that do not require a combination or a key to open but use a magnetic sensor), and letter-writing templates.

Higher-technology devices include portable Braille note takers, refreshable Braille displays that can integrate with TDD devices and some Braille displays with Bluetooth capability, and optical character recognition (OCR), which allows a blind or visually impaired person to scan printed text and that information is read back in synthesized speech. OpenBook is one example of OCR software. Descriptive video services are available that will allow a visually impaired person to receive key narrative descriptions of the visual portions of a television program or movie. In order to receive this service, the person must have DVD, or TV and a second audio program channel to receive the descriptive video service. These devices can be considered in every life care plan for a visually impaired person. Computers can be modified or adapted, such as utilizing a screen reader, a speech synthesizer to allow a visually impaired or blind person to access computer programs. Screen readers are available from Microsoft that will read the graphical portion of a computer program. Electromagnetic ovens can be used to heat food without flames or heating elements to reduce the risk of burns. Kurzweil readers, a computerized camera that scans print media and converts it to voice-synthesized output, are available.

Video Magnifiers (formerly called closed-circuit TV) will allow the person who is visually impaired to modify printed text to an enlarged image or to an image that has enhanced contrast so that it may be easier to read. Software programs are available that will scan books on disk for individual words or combinations of words.

Mobility devices are the most common aid, and the simplest is a white cane (or long cane). The proper length is important. An orientation and mobility specialist can assess an individual for the right size cane and provide the proper training needed to use the white cane effectively. White canes come in different styles, lengths, sizes, and weights. There are also various tips that can be attached the end of the cane.

The individual should flex the shoulder until the upper limb is parallel with the floor. The distance from the hand to the floor is the proper length for the cane. The cane should be lightweight, flexible, and easily collapsible, and the end of the cane is painted red to indicate to others that the individual has a visual impairment. High-technology mobility devices include a laser cane; examples are the Laser Cane, Sonic Mobility Device, and Handheld Mobility Device. These devices operate either by sonar or by light beams. Walkmate is an electronic mobility device that vibrates to indicate when an obstacle is in the path. Some individuals will benefit from the Night Vision Aid, which will provide improved vision by amplifying available light. Aids are available that will help to orient an individual or familiarize a person with the environment that he or she is in (Higdon, 2018). Examples would be three-dimensional maps or tactile aids, verbal recordings, and sight descriptions of travel routes. A contemporary high-technology device for mobility that continues to improve significantly in function since the previous edition is a Global Positioning System (GPS) device, which can literally help a person locate his position on the Earth accurate to within a few feet. These devices are available with verbal directions and are available in models that can be installed in cars or be handheld. If the individual has turned the wrong way, the device will alert him or her to this fact. Digitized compasses are available also. Some areas or cities have transmitters in public areas such as telephones, restrooms, street signs, ATM machines, elevators, and so on, which transmit information about the location.

Guide dog services are extremely beneficial for some individuals who are visually impaired. Most organizations provide a guide dog at no out-of-pocket cost to the person who qualifies. These organizations often have long waiting lists and fairly stringent criteria as to who may qualify to receive the animal. Although there may be no direct cost, there clearly are numerous expenses associated with a guide dog, including the cost of transportation to obtain the guide dog, training on how to use the animal, and lost wages if the individual is employed. The training varies from 2 to 4 weeks in length. Once the guide dog has been obtained, there are costs associated with maintaining the animal's health, tick and flea control, food, grooming, veterinarian care, and kennel stays. In addition, there may be some increased costs to maintaining the home. Appropriate modifications such as a fenced-in yard to allow the guide dog the opportunity to be out of the home during times when not working are essential. Periodic replacement of the guide dog's harness will also be required.

The individual with visual impairment typically will choose not to own a private vehicle and utilize public transportation or taxicab services for community mobility. Such costs must be included in the life care plan, though in personal injury litigation, a deduction for damages received for loss of earnings capacity associated with transportation will be appropriate. If a private vehicle is maintained or the person lives in a town that has limited public transportation, then the cost of hiring a driver should be determined.

There are times and situations where the individual with a visual impairment requiring community mobility is best assisted by using a sighted companion as a guide. Some individuals do not adapt well to canine guides or the use of assistive mobility devices. There may be emotional or cognitive factors (such as a brain injury) that demand a companion assist the visually impaired person with his or her community mobility. Indeed, in many cases, dependent on the activity level of the person, career choice, environment, and so on, all of the mobility aids mentioned will be required or used.

Personal Care and Homemaker Services

There are numerous activities that are required to maintain a home or to live with a measure of independence in the community. The life care planner must carefully evaluate the individual's unique situation and functional abilities and keep foremost in mind the safety of the person for whom the plan is being developed. In addition, it is important to recognize that marked changes in the person's functional status can occur with what would be otherwise relatively minor illnesses for sighted people. The life care plan should have adequate funding for personal care services and homemaker services to cover this eventuality. The individual who is visually impaired will benefit from some assistance in areas such as personal banking; identifying and marking bills for payments; labeling clothing; food shopping and storage; marking settings on the furnace, washing machine, microwave, and stove; some housecleaning; maintaining the home, lawn, and yard; and many other tasks.

When attending school, college, or seminars, note takers and readers may be required and should be considered in the life care plan (Hazekamp & Huebner, 1989; Panek, 2002). In most public school settings, these services may be provided by the school system with funding from the Individuals with Disabilities Education Act (IDEA). There are also funding sources available through state, federal, and non-profit resources if the person qualifies (Mendelson, 1987). Such funding can vary with jurisdiction and congressional funding.

Mobility training, available in many metropolitan areas, is essential for persons who are visually impaired and requires a time-intensive initial training period and then updates on an annual or as-needed basis. Mobility instructors will be required when there are any changes in the individual's life such as a new home or home modifications, a new job or change in one's present job, a move to a new city, or orientation to new stores and businesses that develop in the community. Changes in public transportation systems or bus routes may also require an additional training period. This is separate from orientation training that is required on an ongoing basis. For example, a visually impaired person will have times when strangers are required to be in the home, such as for home repairs, servicing for utilities, deliveries, and so on. Having a trusted sighted companion present in the home during these times may provide an extra measure of safety for the visually impaired person and his/her personal belongings. Depending on the visually impaired/blind person this may not be needed.

Formal Rehabilitation

For the newly blind or visually impaired, a formal rehabilitation program should be undertaken. Topics that should be addressed at a minimum include communication, accessing printed materials, personal adjustment counseling (blindness/low vision), Activities of Daily Living (money management, kitchen safety, cleaning, meal preparation, organization, shopping, etc.), Braille instruction, computer training, job readiness/job placement assistance if the individual is returning to work full-time or part-time, orientation, and mobility training (in the community or near the home). Mobility training should be refreshed at least on an annual or as-needed basis and is somewhat dependent on changes in the person's life. Additional areas to be addressed would include Braille instructions, typing lessons, vocational training, and psychological counseling or adjustment.

Case Study

The following excerpts of a life care plan are for a 49-year-old woman injured in a motor vehicle accident. She experienced a mild brain injury as well as blindness from a blood clot on her brain. The following is for illustration purposes only and does not constitute the complete life care plan. Outside of the information listed below the cost of formal rehabilitation training for a new blind/visually impaired person will likely cost $24,750 or more.

Recommendation	*Dates*	*Frequency*	*Expected Cost*
Aids for Independent Function			
BrailleNote NOTE: Depending on the client's needs, this device may be appropriate but is utilized more by students (high school and college)	2016–2040	Replace every 3 years	$2,000–$5,000
Braille Embosser	2016	Replace every 5 years	$2,500–$6,000
Duxbury Braille Translator for Windows	2016	Replace every 5 years	$595
KNFB Reader (iOS/Android device) print to speech app that takes a picture of printed material and converts it into text	2016	1 X only	$99.99 Update costs unknown
OpenBook—OCR (Optical Character Recognition) Software	2016	Replace every 5 years	$995
Personal computer, laptop	2016–2040	Update every 2 years	$500–$1,000
iPhone/iPad	2016–2040	Frequent upgrades	$399–$750
JAWS (Professional) Screen Reading Software JAWS software maintenance agreement (SMA)	2016–2040	1 X Yearly	$1,095 $200

Window-Eyes Screen Reader for Windows PCs version Office 2010 or later download Window-Eyes free of charge	2016	As needed	Free
Refreshable Braille display	2016–2033	1 X	$1,500–$2,800
Talking money identifier-Eye Note	2016	As needed	Free app iOS/ Android
Color ID (color identifier)	2016	As needed	Free
Maintenance for equipment	2010–2027	Yearly with deduction for warranty	$500 per year average
BARD Mobile (app for talking books, audio materials, etc., via the National Library Service)	2016	Must be a registered user with the National Library Service	Free
Guide Dog	2016	Every 7–8 years	$0 for dog $1,500 per year for food, grooming, veterinarian, and flea and tick treatments
Allowance for aids such as canes, talking clock and watch, kitchen timer, blood pressure cuff, talking weight scale, digital recorders, labeler	2016	Yearly	$250 per year
Home Care			
Housekeeper	2009–2033	Weekly	$2,080 per year
Handyman	2009–2033	Weekly	$2,080 per year
Lawn maintenance	2009–2033	Seasonally (32 weeks)	$700 per year
Personal assistance for shopping, etc.	2009–2033	10 hours per week	$6,240

Home security	2009–2033	1 time only	$1,500 + $25 per month maintenance and monitoring
Future Medical Care—Routine			
Physiatrist	2009–2033	3 times per year	$204 per year
Neurologist	2009–2033	1 time per year	$54 per year
Ophthalmologist	2009–2033	2 times per year	$224 per year
Lab tests, including UA, Tegretol, and blood	2009–2033	2 times per year	$156–$578 per year
Transportation			
Uber base fares in Atlanta ($2–$4 per mile) Lyft	2016	As needed	Unknown. Fares vary depending on type of car selected and time of day.
Cost of public transportation or paratransit service if client lives in a metro area Atlanta Cost: $8 roundtrip for paratransit service, if eligible for paratransit service, ride bus/rail for free Bus/Rail: $5 roundtrip	2016	As needed	Fares vary depending on the state

Conclusion

Visual impairments can be caused by disease, injury to the eye or brain, or the natural process of aging. Although total blindness is relatively rare, low vision or vision disturbance (such as neglect or field cuts) can adversely affect the person's ability to live independently or work. This chapter is designed to suggest life care planner topics and services that need to be considered when developing a comprehensive plan. Since the causes of visual impairment are varied, and specific functional limitations and medical care are individual, the life care planner should either have education or training in this specialized area or associate with someone who does. Fortunately, many resources and adaptive aids (see below) have been developed for enhancing the person's quality of life as well as productive functioning.

Appendix

Appendix 19.1 Selected Resources

General Information	
American Academy of Ophthalmology P.O. Box 7424 San Francisco, CA 94120-7424 (415) 561-8500, ext. 223 www.aao.org	Glaucoma Research Foundation 251 Post Street, Suite 600 San Francisco, CA 94108 (415) 986-3162 (800) 826-6693 question@glaucoma.org Fax: 415-986-3763 www.glaucoma.org
American Foundation for the Blind (Headquarters) 11 Penn Plaza, Suite 300 New York, NY 10001 (800) 232-5463 (hotline) (212) 502-7600 (212) 502-7662 (TDD) www.afb.org	Lighthouse Guild 15 West 65th Street New York, NY 10023 (888) 284-4422 www.lighthouseguild.org
Center for Assistive Technology and Environmental Access Georgia Institute of Technology 512 Means St., Suite 300 Atlanta, GA 30332-0156 (404) 894-4960 (V/TTY) Fax: 404-894-9320 http://www.catea.gatech.edu/	
Note: Formerly Lighthouse International; Jewish Guild Healthcare and Lighthouse International combined as one organization in 2013.	
Lighthouse International, Information and Resource Service (I&R) 111 East 59th St. New York, NY 10022-1202 (212) 821-9200 (800) 829-0500 (212) 821-9703 (TTY) Fax: 212-821-9707 www.lighthouse.org (also see info above for Lighthouse Guild)	National Association for Visually Handicapped 22 W. 21st St. New York, NY 10010 (212) 889-3141 Fax: 212-727-2931 http://www.navh.org

(*Continued*)

Appendix 19.1 (Continued) Selected Resources

National Eye Institute Information Office 31 Center Drive MSC 2510 Bethesda, MD 20892-2510 (301) 496-5248 Fax: 301-402-1065 www.nei.nih.gov	VISIONS/Services for the Blind and Visually Impaired Nancy T. Jones, VISIONS Board President 500 Greenwich Street, 3rd Floor New York, NY 10013-1354 Phone: (212) 625-1616 Toll Free: (888) 245-8333 Fax: (212) 219-4078 www.visionsvcb.org
Recorded Reading Materials	
American Printing House for the Blind 1839 Frankfort Ave. P.O. Box 6085 Louisville, KY 40206-0085 (800) 223-1839 (502) 895-2405 Fax: 502-899-2274 www.aph.org	Braille Circulating Library 2700 Stuart Ave. Richmond, VA 23220-3305 (804) 359-3743 Fax: 804-359-4777 http://bclministries.org
Associated Services for the Blind 919 Walnut St. Philadelphia, PA 19107 (215) 627-0600 Fax: 215-922-0692 www.libertynet.net/tildaasbinfo	Jewish Braille Institute of America, Inc. JBI INTERNATIONAL 110 East 30th Street New York, NY 10016 Telephone: (212) 889-2525 Fax: 212-689-3692 Toll Free: (800) 433-1531 www.jewishbraille.org
Braille Bibles International P.O. Box 378 Liberty, MO 64069-0378 Toll Free: (800) 522-4253 Fax: 877-822-4253 http://www.braillebibles.org info@BrailleBibles.org	Learning Ally National Headquarters Mailing Address: 20 Roszel Road Princeton, New Jersey 08540 (888) 221-4792 www.learningally.org/
Books On Tape, Inc. P.O. Box 7900 Newport Beach, CA 92658-7900 (800) 626-3333 www.booksontape.com	Library of Congress National Library Service for the Blind and Physically Handicapped 1291 Taylor St. NW Washington, DC 20542 (800) 424-8567 (202) 707-5100 (202) 707-0744 (TDD) Fax: 202-707-0712 https://www.loc.gov/nls/index.html

(*Continued*)

Appendix 19.1 (Continued) Selected Resources

Xavier Society for the Blind Two Penn Plaza, Suite 1102 New York, NY 10010-4595 (212) 473-7800/ (800) 637-9193 Fax: 212-473-7801 www.xaviersociety.com	
Large-Print Reading Materials	
American Bible Society 1865 Broadway New York, NY 10023 (212) 408-1200 www.americanbible.org	Doubleday Large Print Home Library Membership Services Center 6550 East 30th St. P.O. Box 6325 Indianapolis, IN 46206 (317) 541-8920 www.DoubledayLargePrint.com
American Printing House for the Blind 1839 Frankfort Ave. P.O. Box 6085 Louisville, KY 40206-0085 (800) 223-1839 (502) 895-2405 Fax: 502-899-2274 www.aph.org	John Milton Society for the Blind in Canada 40 St. Clair Avenue East Suite 202 Toronto, ON M4T 1M9 (416) 960-3953 (Local) (416) 960-3570 (Fax) bbrown@jmsblind.ca http://www.jmsblind.ca
Blindskills, Inc. P.O. Box 5181 Salem, OR 97304-0181 (503) 581-4224 (800) 860-4224 Fax: 503-581-0178 www.blindskills.com	
Note: John Milton Society for the Blind US closed in 2001.	
National Association for Visually Handicapped 22 West 21st St. New York, NY 10010 (212) 889-3141 Fax: 212-727-2931 www.navh.org	New York Times/Large Type Weekly 229 W. 43rd St. New York, NY 10036 (800) 631-2580 (large-type weekly subscriptions) (212) 556-1734 (office) Fax: 212-556-1748

(*Continued*)

Appendix 19.1 (Continued) Selected Resources

Ulverscroft Large Print (USA), Inc. P.O. Box 1230 West Seneca, NY 14224-1230 (800) 955-9659 (716) 674-4270 Fax: 716-674-4195 http://www.ulverscroft.com/contact.php	
Optical Reading and Illumination Devices	
Bossert Specialties 3620 East Thomas Rd., Suite D-124 Phoenix, AZ 85018 (602) 956-6637 (800) 776-5885 Fax: 602-956-1008 http://bossertspecialties.com	Enhanced Vision Headquarters: 5882 Machine Drive Huntington Beach, CA 92649 USA Phone: (714) 374-1829 Fax: 714-465-3401 (888) 811-3161 www.enhancedvision.com/low-vision-products.html
Eschenbach Optik of America, Inc. 904 Ethan Allen Highway Ridgefield, CT 06877 (203) 438-7471 (800) 396-3886 www.eschenbach.com	Humanware 1 UPS Way P.O. Box 800 Champlain, NY 12919 (800) 722-3393 Fax: 888-871-4828 E-mail: info@humanware.com www.humanware.com/en-usa/home
Membership Organizations	
American Council of the Blind 1155 15th St. NW, Suite 1004 Washington, DC 20005 (800) 424-8666 (800) 424-8666 (202) 467-5081 Fax: 202-467-5085 www.acb.org	National Federation of the Blind 200 East Wells Street (at Jernigan Place) Baltimore, MD 21230 Phone: (410) 659-9314 Fax: 410-685-5653 www.nfb.org
Blinded Veterans Association 125 N. West Street, 3rd Floor Alexandria, VA 22314 Phone: (800) 669-7079 Fax: 202-371-8258 www.bva.org	

(*Continued*)

Appendix 19.1 (Continued) Selected Resources

<table>
<tr><td colspan="2">Consumer Organizations</td></tr>
<tr><td>American Foundation for the Blind
National Technology Center
11 Penn Plaza, Suite 300
New York, NY 10001
(800) 232-5463
(212) 502-7773 (CTIB)
www.afb.org</td><td>Glaucoma Support Network
Glaucoma Research Foundation
200 Pine St., Suite 200
San Francisco, CA 94104
(800) 826-6693
(415) 986-3162
www.glaucoma.org</td></tr>
<tr><td>Association for Macular Diseases, Inc.
210 East 64th St.
New York, NY 10021
(212) 605-3719
www.macular.org</td><td>The Institute for Families of Blind Children
1300 N. Vermont Ave.
Suite #1004
Los Angeles, CA 90027
info@instituteforfamilies.org
(213) 669-4649
www.instituteforfamilies.org</td></tr>
<tr><td>The Foundation Fighting Blindness
7168 Columbia Gateway Drive, Suite 100
Columbia, MD 21046
E-mail: info@FightBlindness.org
Toll Free: (800) 683-5555
TDD: (800) 683-5551
Local: (410) 423-0600
Local TDD: (410) 363-7139
www.blindness.org</td><td>Lighthouse Guild
15 West 65th Street
New York, NY 10023
(888) 284-4422
www.lighthouseguild.org</td></tr>
<tr><td colspan="2">Note: Formerly Lighthouse International; Jewish Guild Healthcare and Lighthouse International combined as one organization in 2013.</td></tr>
<tr><td>Macular Degeneration Foundation, Inc.
P.O. Box 531313
Henderson, Nevada 89053
Tel: (888) 633-3937 (USA)
Tel: (702) 450-2908 (Intl)
www.eyesight.org</td><td>National Association for Visually Handicapped
22 West 21st St.
New York, NY 10010
(212) 889-3141
Fax: 212-727-2931
www.navh.org</td></tr>
<tr><td>National Association for Parents of Children with Visual Impairments, Inc.
Executive Director, Susan LaVenture
P.O. Box 317
Watertown, MA 02272-0317
T: (617) 972-7441
Fax: 617-972-7444
(800) 562-6265
napvi@lighthouseguild.org</td><td>National Organization for Albinism and Hypopigmentation (NOAH)
P.O. Box 959
East Hampstead, NH 03826-0959
(800) 473-2310
(603) 887-2310
Fax: 800-648-2310
www.albinism.org</td></tr>
</table>

(Continued)

Appendix 19.1 (Continued) Selected Resources

Adaptive Equipment Catalogs	
Independent Living Aids, LLC 137 Rano Street Buffalo, NY 14207 (800) 537-2118 www.independentliving.com	National Federation for the Blind Product Center 1800 Johnson Street Baltimore, MD 21230 (410) 659-9314 www.nfb.org
LSS Group P.O. Box 673 Northbrook, IL 60065 (800) 468-4789 www.LSSgroup.com	Perkins School for the Blind (Perkins Solutions) 175 North Beacon Street Watertown, MA 02472 (855) 206-8353 (Toll-free) (617) 972-7308 www.perkinsproducts.org/store/en/
Maxi-Aids P.O. Box 3209 Farmingdale, NY 11735 (800) 522-6294 www.maxiaids.com	
Dog Guide Resources	
Arizona Eye Dog Foundation for the Blind 8252 S. 15th Avenue Phoenix, AZ 85041-7806 (602) 276-0051 (Local) (800) 393-3641 (Toll-Free) eyedog@eyedogfoundation.org http://www.eyedogfoundation.org	**California** Guide Dogs of America 13445 Glenoaks Boulevard Sylmar, CA 91342 (818) 362-5834 (Local) 818-362-6870 (Fax) (800) 459-4843 (Toll-Free) mail@guidedogsofamerica.org http://www.guidedogsofamerica.org
California Guide Dogs for the Blind 350 Los Ranchitos Road San Rafael, CA 94903 (415) 499-4000 (Local) 415-499-4035 (Fax) (800) 295-4050 (Toll-Free) information@guidedogs.com http://www.guidedogs.com	**California** Guide Dogs of the Desert International 60740 Dillon Road Whitewater, CA 92282 (760) 329-6257 (Local) 760-329-2127 (Fax) Info@guidedogsofthedesert.org http://www.guidedogsofthedesert.org/

(*Continued*)

Appendix 19.1 (Continued) Selected Resources

Connecticut Fidelco Guide Dog Foundation 103 Old Iron Ore Road Bloomfield, CT 06002 (860) 243-5200 (Local) 860-769-0567 (Fax) admissions@fidelco.org http://www.fidelco.org	**Michigan** Leader Dogs for the Blind 1039 S Rochester Road Rochester Hills, MI 48307-3115 (248) 651-9011 (Local) 248-651-5812 (Fax) (888) 777-5332 (Toll-Free) (248) 651-3713 (TDD/TTY) leaderdog@leaderdog.org http://www.leaderdog.org
Florida Southeastern Guide Dogs, Inc. 4210 77th Street East Palmetto, FL 34221 (941) 729-5665 (Local) 941-729-6646 (Fax) (800) 944-3647 (Toll-Free) info@guidedogs.org http://www.guidedogs.org	**New Jersey** The Seeing Eye 10 Washington Valley Road P.O. Box 375 Morristown, NJ 07963 (973) 539-4425 (Local) 973-539-0922 (Fax) (800) 539-4425 (Toll-Free) info@seeingeye.org http://www.seeingeye.org
Hawaii Eye of the Pacific Guide Dogs and Mobility Services 747 Amana Street, #407 Honolulu, HI 96814 (808) 941-1088 (Local) 808-944-9368 (Fax) Info@EyeOfThePacific.Org http://www.eyeofthepacific.org/	**New York** Freedom Guide Dogs for the Blind 1210 Hardscrabble Road Cassville, NY 13318 (315) 822-5132 (Local) info@freedomguidedogs.org http://www.freedomguidedogs.org/
Kansas KSDS, Inc. 120 West Seventh Washington, KS 66968 (785) 325-2256 (Local) 785-325-2258 (Fax) ksds@ksds.org www.ksds.org	**New York** Guide Dog Foundation for the Blind 371 East Jericho Turnpike Smithtown, NY 11787-2976 (631) 930-9000 (Local) 631-930-9009 (Fax) (800) 548-4337 (Toll-Free) info@guidedog.org http://www.guidedog.org

(*Continued*)

Appendix 19.1 (Continued) Selected Resources

New York Guiding Eyes for the Blind 611 Granite Springs Road Yorktown Heights, NY 10598 (914) 245-4024 (Local) 914-243-2232 (Fax) (800) 942-0149 (Toll-Free) admissions@guidingeyes.org http://www.guidingeyes.org	**Quebec** Mira Foundation (Guide Dogs for the Blind) 1820 rang Nord-Ouest Sainte-Madeleine, PQ J0H 1S0 (450) 795-3725 (Local) 450-795-3789 (Fax) info@mira.ca http://www.mira.ca
Ohio Pilot Dogs 625 West Town Street Columbus, OH 43215-4496 (614) 221-6367 (Local) 614-221-1577 (Fax) http://www.pilotdogs.org	**Texas** Guide Dogs of Texas 1503 Allena Drive San Antonio, TX 78213 (210) 366-4081 (Local) 210-266-4080 (Fax) (800) 831-9231 (Toll-Free) http://www.guidedogsoftexas.org
Ontario Canadian Guide Dogs for the Blind 4120 Rideau Valley Drive North Manotick, ON K4M 1A3 (613) 692-7777 (Local) 613-692-0650 (Fax) cgdb@sympatico.ca http://www.guidedogs.ca	**Wisconsin** OccuPaws Guide Dog Association P.O. Box 45857 Madison, WI 53744 (608) 772-3787 (Local) 866-854-3291 (Fax) info@occupaws.org http://occupaws.org/
Ontario Lions Foundation of Canada: Canine Vision Canada 152 Wilson Street Oakville, ON L6K 3H2 (905) 842-2891 (Local) 905-842-3373 (Fax) (800) 768-3030 (Toll-Free) (905) 842-1585 (TDD/TTY) info@dogguides.com http://www.dogguides.com	**Wisconsin** Custom Canines Service Dog Academy 6610 Fieldwood Road Madison, Wisconsin 53718 Phone: (608) 444-9555 Fax: 608-834-1700 Email: info@customcanines.org Website: www.customcanines.org
Oregon Guide Dogs for the Blind 32901 SE Kelso Road Boring, OR 97009 (503) 668-2100 (Local) 503-668-2141 (Fax) (800) 295-4050 (Toll-Free) information@guidedogs.com http://www.guidedogs.com	

References

American Academy of Ophthalmology. 2003. *Low vision facts, questions and answers*. Retrieved May 16, 2009, from www.aao.org.

Deutsch, P. M., & Sawyer, H. W. 2003. *A Guide to Rehabilitation*. White Plains, NY: Ahab Press.

Dodson-Burk, B., & Hill, E. W. 1989. *An Orientation and Mobility Primer for Families and Young Children*. New York, NY: American Foundation of the Blind.

Hazekamp, J., & Huebner, K. M. 1989. *Program Planning and Evaluation for Blind and Visually Impaired Students: National Guidelines for Educational Excellence*. New York, NY: American Foundation for the Blind.

Higdon, C. 2018. The role of the SLP and assistive technology in life care planning. In R. Weed, & D. Berens (Eds.), *Life Care Planning and Case Management Handbook* (4th ed., 147–252). New York, NY: Routledge.

Kübler-Ross, E. 1975. *Death: The Final Stage of Growth*. Englewood Cliffs, NJ: Prentice Hall.

LaPlante, M. P., Hendershot, G. E., & Moss, A. J. 1992. Assisted technology devices and home accessibility features: Prevalence, payment, needs and trends. *Advanced Data from the Vital Health Statistics, 217*, 1–11. Hyattsville, MD: National Center for Health Statistics.

Matthews, D. J. 1996. Examination of the pediatric patient. In R. Braddom (Ed.), *Physical Medicine and Rehabilitation* (Chapter 2). Philadelphia, PA: W. B. Saunders.

Mendelson, S. 1987. *Financing Adaptive Technology: A Guide to Sources and Strategies for Blind and Visually Impaired Users*. New York, NY: Smiling Interface.

Nelson, K. A., & Dimitrova, E. 1993. Severe visual impairment in the United States and each state. *Journal of Visual Impairment and Blindness, 87*, 80–85.

NIH. 2018. *Vision Problems in the U.S.: Prevalence of Adult Vision Impairment and Age-Related Eye Disease in America*. Bethesda, MD: National Eye Institute, National Institutes of Health Available at https://nei.nih.gov/eyedata/blind.

Owsley, C., & McGwin, G. 2010. Vision and driving. *Vision Research, 50*, 2348–2361.

Panek, W. 2002. Visual disabilities. In M. Brodwin, F. Tellez, & S. Brodwin (Eds.), *Medical, Psychological and Vocational Aspects of Disability* (pp. 157–169). Athens, GA: Elliott & Fitzpatrick.

Social Security Act. 2016. Retrieved from https://www.ssa.gov/OP_Home/ssact/title16b/1614.htm.

Teplin, S. W. 1995. Visual impairment in infants and young children. *Infant Young Children, 8*, 18–51.

Thylefors, V., Negrel, A., Pararajasegaram, R., & Dedzieky, K. Y. 1995. Available data on blindness update, 1994. *Ophthalmic Epidemiology, 2*, 5–39.

Tielsch, J. M., Sommer, A., & Witt, K. 1990. Blindness and visual impairment in an American urban population. *Archives of Ophthalmology, 108*, 236–241.

Visionware.org. 2016. *It's surprising to a lot of people*. Retrieved from http://www.visionware.org/info/everyday-living/home-modification-/lighting-and-glare/123.

Weed, R., & Field, T. 2012. *The Rehabilitation Consultant's Handbook* (4th ed.). Athens, GA: Elliott & Fitzpatrick.

Younger, V., & Sardegna, J. 1994. *A Guide to Independence for the Visually Impaired and Their Families*. New York, NY: Demos Publications.

Chapter 20

Elder Care Management Life Care Planning Principles

Dorothy J. Zydowicz-Vierling*

Contents

Introduction 591
Benefits for Life Care Planning in Elder Care 595
Assessment 596
Plan Implementation and Monitoring 598
Maximizing Resources 599
Conclusion 599
Appendix 600
References 605

Introduction

There are 75 million baby boomers on the verge of retirement and for the next 20 years, an average of 10,000 people each day will reach age 65 and the "retirement" phase of life (Bernard, March 23, 2012). Aging is one of the most important of all demographic trends in the United States today (U.S. Administration on Aging, 2006). Between 1950 and 2010, the average American life expectancy went up 10 years and more than 40 million Americans are now 65 or older and the numbers continue to climb.

According to the U.S. Census Bureau (May, 2014), between 2010 and 2050 the United States is projected to experience a rapid growth in its aging population, largely due to aging baby boomers as they began crossing into this category in 2011 in addition to trends in immigration (U.S. Census Bureau, 2014). In fact, by 2050, the number of Americans aged 65 and older is projected to be 88.5 million, more than double its projected population in 2010 of 40.2 million. In addition, while the "oldest old" (ages 85 and older) currently constitute only about 15 percent of the population

* Portions of this chapter were adapted from the Third Edition co-authored by the current author, Dorothy Zydowicz-Vierling, and Patricia McCollom.

over 65, this number will likely constitute fully one-fifth of Americans over 65 by the year 2050 (Kellerman, 2014). The aging of our more racially and ethnically diverse population is having wide-ranging implications for the country and for health care professionals (Cohen & Van Norstrand, 1995; JAMA Network, 1990).

To meet the diverse needs of an aging population, United States President Lyndon Johnson signed into law the Older Americans Act (OAA) on July 14, 1965. The OAA set out specific objectives for maintaining the dignity and welfare of older individuals and created the primary vehicle for organizing, coordinating and providing community-based services, as well as opportunities for older Americans and their families. The Act requires reauthorization every 3 years.

On April 19, 2016 the President Barack Obama signed into law the Older American Reauthorization Act (OAARA as amended) unanimously approved by Congress (House Committee on Education and the workforce, 2016, National Council on Aging, 2016). The Reauthorization had not taken place since 2006 (Blancato, 2016). The OAARA reauthorizes services through 2019 and strengthens the law by:

- Providing better protection for vulnerable elders
- Streamlining and improving program administration
- Promoting evidence-based support
- Improving nutritional services
- Aligning senior employment services with the workforce development system

In most cases, it is well known that health care costs tend to rise as we age (JAMA Network, 1990). As human beings, our bodies experience a fairly predictable rate of decline as the incidence of illness, obstacles, malfunction related to wear and tear, and age related conditions begin to present themselves. When an injury, disease, or other abnormal condition is present the likelihood of complications, exacerbations, and obstacles begins to increase.

As this age shift occurs and retirement is frequently postponed, physiological aging is delayed, as compared to a century ago. With advances in medical treatment, persons are living longer and healthier into the sixth, seventh, and eighth decades, with greater periods of time in what is considered old age (U.S. Administration of Aging, 2008).

Aging is often compounded by the onset of chronic illnesses and disabling conditions, bringing with it the increased likelihood of functional loss and disability. Alzheimer's, a potential complication rising in prevalence as people live longer, can increase costs significantly (JAMA Network, 2003). The Family Caregiver Alliance (2015) reports the lifetime probability of becoming disabled in at least two Activities of Daily Living, or of being cognitively impaired is 68 percent for individuals age 65 and older. As a result, costs for care and services increase, sometimes dramatically. Examples of age-related changes on functional activities are summarized in Table 20.1.

Coupled with lifestyle, nutrition habits, physical environment, mental health, work history, and extended retirement, expected physiological change varies. For those with chronic conditions, prescribed medications add an additional variable that impacts long-term health needs. For example, individuals with elevated blood pressure may be prescribed medication that increases susceptibility to falls as a result of orthostatic hypotension.

Facing long-term health needs, elders requiring care management can benefit from the development of a life care plan. The life care plan becomes a distinct written resource for the individual and their support systems, listing community resources, payer sources, contacts, and eligibility variables. Using this tool in elder care management benefits the individual, the family, and the case/care manager, as services are provided over a continuum of care.

Table 20.1 Age-Related Changes on Functional Activities

Body System	*Expected Change*	*Disease/Illness*	*Functional Consequences*
		Senses	
Vision	Degenerative change to pupils, iris, sclera, retina; decreased elasticity, opacity, and flattening of lens	Macular degeneration; cataracts	Need for increased lighting; sensitivity to glare; diminished adaptation to light/dark; poor eye coordination; decreased peripheral vision; decreased visual acuity; decreased depth perception
Hearing	Thickening of ear drum; decreased sensory receptors; auditory nerve degeneration; extended exposure to sound/damage	Deafness; chronic vestibular effects	Diminished ability to participate in conversation; safety problems; social withdrawal
Smell/taste	Decreased sensitivity of neuroreceptors	Health impairments related to poor nutrition	Decreased appetite; safety problems
Touch	Decreased sensitivity of neuroreceptors	Impaired skin integrity related to pressure, pain, burns	Decreased response to tactile stimuli; safety problems
Musculoskeletal	Decreased muscle mass; loss of elasticity; decreased bone density; deterioration of articular cartilage; altered motor neuron conduction	Arthritis; muscle atrophy; bone fractures; chronic pain	Immobility; decreased strength and endurance; postural changes; impaired balance and coordination; decreased speed of movement and reaction time; body flexibility
Neurological	Decreased short-term memory; decreased processing of information; slowed reflexes; decreased response time; sleep pattern changes	Decreased cerebral blood flow; stroke; dementia; depression	Decrease in adapting to new information; decreased ability to problem solve and integrate new information; difficulty in remembering or memorization; need for rest periods; changes in ability to drive decreasing autonomy

(*Continued*)

Table 20.1 (Continued) Age-Related Changes on Functional Activities

Body System	*Expected Change*	*Disease/Illness*	*Functional Consequences*
Cardiopulmonary	Decreased pumping force of heart; blood pressure changes; weakening of respiratory muscles; decreased elasticity of cardiac valves; reduced chest wall function and vital capacity	Orthostatic hypotension; hypertension; cardiac failure; myocardial infarction; pulmonary infection	Reduced ability to exercise, work; need to pace energy; increase in fatigability; decreased endurance; shortness of breath
Integumentary	Decreased skin vascularity and thickness; diminished sweat glands; decreased thermo-regulatory control; nails thicken and become brittle; increased corns, callouses, nevi	Frequent bruising, skin tears; delayed healing time; infection of skin and nails; skin cancer	Poor body temperature control; susceptible to tissue damage
Gastrointestinal (GI)	Changes in teeth, gingivae; decreased saliva, gastric juices; decreased bowel motility; decreased blood flow to liver, pancreas, bowel	Nutrition deficits; dysphagia; constipation; elevated liver enzymes; weakening of wall of GI system; hiatal hernia; gastroesophageal reflux disease (GERD)	Decreased ability to maintain intake; swallowing problems; alternations in medication metabolism; change in protein metabolism
Endocrine	Reduced insulin secretion; decreased glucose tolerance; changes in hormone, enzyme production; impaired thyroid function	Diabetes; hypoglycemia	Decreased endurance; monitoring of blood sugar necessary; specific nutritional intake required; prescription medication necessary
Genitourinary	Decreased renal blood flow; decreased muscle tone; decreased glomerular filtration, resulting in changes in acid–base balance	Electrolyte imbalance; recurrent urinary tract infection; urinary retention	Frequency of urination; stress incontinence; severe systemic effects with nausea, vomiting, or diarrhea

In many cases, a life care plan is developed for litigation. In geriatric care, however, it is most likely compiled for long-term care planning, transitions, or family and support structure education. A life care plan in elder care management is distinguished from life care planning for litigation support in three ways:

1. The life care plan is an outcome of elder care/case management services.
2. The life care plan is developed in collaboration with the individual and support system without regard to personal injury legal parameters.
3. The life care plan identifies community resources and health care options from which the individual and family may choose.

Benefits for Life Care Planning in Elder Care

The life care plan created to support elder care is a living document (McCollom, 2000). It is intended to be useful to all parties involved in the individual's care, including family, friends, support services, community resources, and caregivers among the health care team. The plan defines, organizes, prioritizes, and mobilizes every aspect of the elder's care. It includes provisions for care coordination, family and support education, health care and financial decision-making, care advocacy, crisis intervention, support, and any other necessary services. The plan may, with the benefit of Life Care Planning Law Firms, include such services as estate planning, asset preservation, and public benefits qualification (Life Care Planning Law Firms Association, 2017).

Benefits for life care planning in elder care may be specified in five areas. First, a life care plan for elder care management *enhances individual and family education*. Information in the plan includes physician appointments, procedures, medications, needed diagnostic or monitoring tests, home health care services, and chosen options for ongoing services. The document clearly and concisely lists needed information that can be readily accessed.

Consider, for example, Robert R., age 81, who was diagnosed with lung cancer, with metastasis to the lumbar spine. His primary caretaker was an 85-year-old brother. His physician(s) prescribed over 17 medications to address Mr. R.'s health care needs. In the elder care management process, a life care plan was developed that included all medications, the reason for prescription dosage, time of administration, and potential side effects to note. The pharmacist's name, address, and telephone number were included for reference. Over the remaining 7 months of Mr. R.'s life, he and his brother used the life care plan medication list several times daily as a support tool, to answer questions and confirm accuracy of administration.

Second, a life care plan in elder care management *facilitates integration of public and private services*. A recent RAND Corporation study found improving the coordination of care for elderly patients with chronic diseases trims costs, reduces use of health services, and cuts complications (Hussey, March 17, 2014).

Coordination of care among specialties has been identified as a priority by the Institute of Medicine and the National Priorities Partnership. For example, findings published online by JAMA International Medicine, suggest that improving the coordination of patients with diabetes, congestive heart failure, or emphysema, could save Medicare alone as much as $1.5 billion per year (Agency for Healthcare Research and Quality, 2012; Hussey, March 17, 2014). Multiple options may exist for a given service to meet a specific need. When developing the plan in collaboration with the family and providers, options are identified and choices are made regarding available services (Eldercare Workforce Alliance, 2017). Services are therefore not duplicated and can be accomplished in the most cost effective manner.

In the life care plan of Mr. R., noted previously, coordination between specialists eliminated the potential for drug interactions. Supplemental nutrition services were needed, since he did not have the strength or endurance to prepare meals. Working with the family, a cooking and food-shopping plan was developed with neighbors, to assure food met his tastes and appetite. Use of a community program was declined, due to institutional-style meals, with little fresh fruit or vegetables included.

Third, use of a life care plan in elder care management results in *decreased stress* and peace of mind for the individual and family when the right choices are made to ensure loved ones are safe and getting necessary care. The plan not only delineates care and services, but also associates costs, identifying the payer source. Prepared in a concise, clear form, the structure of the plan allows the individual and family to locate specific information related to needs and to review the rationale for treatment and services.

In our example, Mr. R.'s extended family lived in a distant state. The life care plan's costs section assisted the family in supporting Mr. R.'s brother in decision making regarding home care assistance (Zydowicz-Vierling, 2008). Further, a plan was developed that included homemaker services and increasing services, as his condition worsened.

Fourth, the life care plan in elder care management *provides a continuing resource to the family* through delineation of needs, rationale and outcomes for programs and services, and measureable goals for evaluation of services.

With implementation of the life care plan for Mr. R., the recommendation was for homemaker services once weekly. Listed within the plan was the expected outcome of implementing this recommendation: laundry and household cleaning completed. Evaluation of this service by the care manager demonstrated lack of achievement of the outcome at 4 weeks. Services were increased to three times weekly, which demonstrated outcome achievement.

Finally, *access to community resources* is facilitated through life care planning in elder care management (Agency for Healthcare Research and Quality, 2012). The life care planner must locate and identify community resources consistent with the individual's needs and present the resources as options to consider.

When homemaker services were recommended to assist Mr. R. to remain in his home, such services were not covered by Medicare. Community options were identified and selection for services was made based upon comprehensive review of available options, rather than referral by hospital social service only.

The development of a life care plan in elder care management is based upon individual rights, choice, individual/family values, comprehensive assessment, appropriate resource use and planning, and implementing, monitoring, and evaluating recommended services. The plan is developed with the individual's informed consent or that of a guardian/conservator. Ideally, by addressing an individual's rights, values, and preferences, the life care plan is removed from a litigation model to a model recognizing individual autonomy. Individual preferences, community resources, and financial abilities determine the plan.

Assessment

A life care plan used in elder care management is driven by clinical data about the individual, which provides the rationale for resources used. A systematic assessment of the individual's functional skills, cognitive status, limitations, needs, strengths, abilities, and resources (personal and community) is required.

An assessment of functional skills is critical to life care plan development. During an assessment interview, consider questions about lifestyle, such as how does the individual spend the day and what activities take place outside the home (McCollom, 2000). Further questioning should define how the client shops and carries out financial and household management. It is often appropriate to consider and include formal functional evaluations performed by care providers.

Environmental assessment must be integrated with functional assessment, to provide safety-related recommendations in the life care plan. Americans with Disabilities Act Amendments Act (ADAAA) (ADA.gov, 2017) is a solid foundation for understanding environmental resources for the elderly with disabilities. For example, the 2012 Barrier Free Health Care Initiative focuses on access to health care information, technology, programs, service, and facilities. External risk factors may include social isolation, lack of a support system, degree of integration in the community, issues with transportation, or current geographic location. Internal risk factors for consideration in a life care plan include cognitive status, medications, depression, comorbidities, and mobility.

Life care planning in elder care often involves more than medical issues. The life care planner must be able to assess the individual's risk factors, potential problems, barriers, and options. Funding, community resources, geographic barriers, or family/cultural variables may make autonomy difficult.

Lifestyle, hobbies, and cultural implications must be considered. Life care planners must recognize when their values may come in conflict with the individual's or family's preferences and beliefs. They must strive to maintain objectivity to facilitate patient advocacy.

Ultimately, the outcomes of an individually driven life care plan include improvements in patient care, cost of services, patient and family satisfaction, education, and understanding of care options. Individual participation also increases involvement in care and service evaluation, which allows the individual some level of autonomy and control over a difficult circumstance. Furthermore, self-reliance and self-determination are promoted. For the patient and family to receive the best care possible, a well-directed multidisciplinary approach is essential (Zydowicz-Vierling, 2008).

Table 20.2 provides an assessment tool for use in life care planning in elder care management.

Table 20.2 Elder Care Management Life Care Plan Assessment Tool

1.	Records review — all specialties
2.	Contacts
3.	Guardian/conservator
4.	Health status • Past medical history • Review of all body systems • Medications • Pharmacist • Program medications • Nutritional status/eating habits • Cultural specifications • Illness impact • Protein needs • Height, weight

(Continued)

Table 20.2 (Continued) Elder Care Management Life Care Plan Assessment Tool

5.	Functional skills • Self-care • Cognition • Communication • Behavior • Mobility • Elimination • Safety • Household management • Community involvement • Evaluations completed
6.	Psychosocial status • Family/friends • Patient/family values • Community support • Mood, affect • Coping mechanisms • Level of education • Stressors • Substance use/abuse • Sleep patterns
7.	Environment • Architectural barriers • Health hazards • Sanitary conditions • Modification needs • Durable Medical Equipment • Transportation • Community resources used
8.	Financial status • Income • Assets • Monthly costs • Insurance • Power of attorney • Living will
9.	Risk factors • External • Internal

Plan Implementation and Monitoring

Implementation of the life care plan reflects action based upon information analysis and synthesis. The plan identifies formal and informal support mechanisms and encourages family and/or other support system involvement in the plan. Ongoing assignments are made to family, providers, or other resources for evaluation of ongoing needs and the efficacy of all services. Remember that the life care plan is a living document requiring constant assessment and reevaluation.

Maximizing Resources

Life care planning in elder care management typically involves budgeting from limited financial resources and the creative use of community or collateral resources. Care and service options may include community or service/church groups; volunteers; private, personal pay; federal or local programs; or alternative family resources.

Support services needed may include health screening through parish nurse programs or recreation programs. Respite care may be located through church or diagnosis-specific organizations.

Long-term care insurance policies may provide alternative services support, such as adult daycare, which may be incorporated into the life care plan.

Creativity in resource use and allocation must be incorporated in the plan and evaluated for continued usefulness.

Conclusion

Life care planning benefits at-risk geriatric populations (see Table 20.3). Those who are identified after assessment in medium- to high-risk categories are prime candidates for life care planning. As an outcome of care/case management, life care planning enhances individual/patient education, facilitates integration of services, decreases stress, and encourages use of and access to community resources. With an aging population, life care planning offers a valuable tool for those facing long-term health care needs resulting from catastrophic injury, chronic illness, or the effects of extended life expectancy.

Table 20.3 At-Risk Geriatric Population

Category	*High Risk*	*Medium Risk*	*Low Risk*
Characteristics	70 years or older, assisted living, 3 or more comorbidities, major functional limitations, 2 or more acute inpatient stays in past 12 months, multiple physician contacts, dialysis, day treatment, home health services, active progressive dementia/ Alzheimer's	Newly diagnosed chronic illness, 2 or 3 comorbidities, lifestyle changes, moderate functional limitations, early onset dementia/ Alzheimer's	Lifeline, support system in place, compromised financial status
Case management	Intensive	Active	Maintenance
Frequency	2 weeks or more	Monthly	6–8 weeks

Appendix

Appendix 20.1 Resources

AARP: Coping with Grief and Loss www.aarp.org/griefandloss
Accessible Home Modification Page www.homemods.org
ADA Amendments Act of 2008 https://www.eeoc.gov/laws/statutes/adaaa.cfm
Administration on Aging—Department of Health and Human Services www.aoa.gov
Agency for Health Care Research and Quality http://ahcpr.gov
Aging Network Services www.agingnets.com
Institute for Aging Research https://www.instituteforagingresearch.org/resources/news
AGS Foundation for Health in Aging http://www.healthinagingfoundation.org/
Allscripts Care Management Solutions www.extendedcare.com
Alzheimer's Association www.alz.org
Alzheimer's Disease Education and Referral Center at the National Institute of Aging https://www.nia.nih.gov/alzheimers
American Association for Geriatric Psychiatry www.aagpgpa.org
American Association for Homecare www.aahomecare.org
American Association of Homes and Services for the Aging www.aahsa.org
American Association of Retired Persons (AARP) www.aarp.org
American Bar Association Commission on the Legal Programs of the Elderly www.abanet.org
American Cancer Society www.cancer.org

(*Continued*)

Appendix 20.1 (Continued) Resources

American Geriatrics Society www.americangeriatrics.org
American Society on Aging www.asaging.org
ARCH National Resource Center for Respite Care and Crisis Care Services https://archrespite.org/
Arthritis Foundation www.arthritis.org
Assisted Living Federation of America www.alfa.org
Association for Gerontology in Higher Education www.aghe.org
Benefits Checkup www.benefitscheckup.com
Brookdale Center for Health and Longevity www.brookdale.org
Cancer Treatment Centers of America www.cancercenter.com
Cancer Net www.cancer.net
Caregiving Online www.caregiving.com
Caregiving Supplies—The Boulevard www.blvd.com www.coast-resources.com www.dynamic-living.com
Careguide@Home—Elder Care www.eldercare.com
CarePlanner—Clinical Tools www.careplanner.org
Case Management Resource Guide www.cmrg.com/index.htm
Centerwatch www.centerwatch.com
Clinical Trials www.clinicaltrials.com

(Continued)

Appendix 20.1 (Continued) Resources

Dorland Health http://dorlandhealth.com/
ElderCare Online www.ec-online.net
Eldercare Workforce Alliance https://eldercareworkforce.org/
Elder Support Network Association of Jewish Family & Children Agencies www.ajfca.org
Elderweb—Center for Eldercare www.elderweb.com
Estronaut—A Forum for Women's Health www.womenshealth.org
Family Caregiver Alliance—National Center on Caregiving www.caregiver.org
Fisher Center for Alzheimer's Research Foundation www.alzinfo.org
Gerontological Society of America www.geron.org
GriefNet www.griefnet.org
Guide to Retirement Living http://www.retirement-living.com/
Health and Age Also www.healthandage.com
Health Answers Education www.healthanswers.com
Health Care Financing Administration https://www.federalregister.gov/agencies/health-care-finance-administration
Healthfinder www.healthfinder.gov
Health Policy and Management www.hpm.umn.edu
Home modifications https://www.acl.gov/sites/default/files/news%202017-03/Home_Modification.pdf
Hospice Foundation of America www.hospicefoundation.org

(Continued)

Appendix 20.1 (Continued) Resources

Life Care Planning Law Firms Association https://www.lcplfa.org
Long Term Care Insurance Buyer's Advocate Alliance www.prepsmart.com
Mayo Clinic www.mayo.edu
Medicine Program http://themedicineprogram.com
MEDLINEplus www.nlm.nih.gov/medlineplus
Medscape from WebMD http://www.medscape.com/
National Academy of Elder Law Attorneys www.naela.org
National Academy of Social Insurance www.nasi.org
National Academy Press www.nap.edu
National Advisory Council for Long Term Care Insurance www.longtermcareinsurance.org
National Asian Pacific Center on Aging www.napca.com
National Association for Hispanic Elderly www.anppm.org
National Association of Area Agencies on Aging www.N4A.org
Aging Life Care Association http://www.aginglifecare.org/
National Association of State Units on Aging www.nasua.org
National Cancer Institute www.cancer.gov
National Caregivers Library www.caregiverslibrary.org
National Center on Elder Abuse https://ncea.acl.gov/
National Center on Addiction and Substance Abuse http://www.centeronaddiction.org/

(Continued)

Appendix 20.1 (Continued) Resources

National Committee to Preserve Social Security and Medicare www.ncpssm.org
National Council on the Aging www.ncoa.org
National Family Caregivers Association www.nfcacares.org
Office of Disease Prevention and Health Promotion www.health.gov/nhic
National Hospice and Palliative Care Organization http://www.nhpco.org/
National Hospice Foundation Also see www.nationalhospicefoundation.org
National Institutes of Health https://www.nih.gov/
National Institute on Aging https://www.nia.nih.gov/
National Policy Resource Center on Nutrition Physical Activity and Aging http://nutritionandaging.org/
National Rehabilitation Information Center www.naric.com
National Senior Citizen's Law Center www.nsclc.org
National Senior Games Association http://nsga.com/
Senior Link; Innovation in care collaboration www.seniorlink.com
SeniorNet www.seniornet.org
Senior Dating Websites www.seniorsites.com
Social Security Administration Online www.ssa.gov
The Eldercare Directory www.eldercaredirectory.org
Healthy Living for Women and Their Families www.thirdage.com
Caregiver Survival Resources www.caregiver911.com

(Continued)

Appendix 20.1 (Continued) Resources

Web of Care www.webofcare.com
A Place for Mom (Senior Care Referral Service) http://locate.aplaceformom.com
Senior Helpers http://www.seniorhelpers.com/
Administration on Aging https://aoa.acl.gov/

References

ADA.gov. 2017. *Barrier-Free Health Care Initiative.* Available at https://www.ada.gov/usao-agreements.htm.

Agency for Healthcare Research and Quality. 2012. *Coordinating Care for Adults With Complex Care Needs in the Patient Centered Medical* Home: Challenges and Solutions. Available at https://pcmh.ahrq.gov/page/coordinating-care-adults-complex-care-needs-patient-centered-medical-home-challenges-and

Bernard, D. March 22, 2012. *The Baby Boomer Number Game.* Available at http://money.usnews.com/money/blogs/on-retirement/2012/03/23/the-baby-boomer-number-game

Blancato, B. April 14, 2016. *The Older Americans Act Finally Clears Congress.* Available at http://www.forbes.com/sites/nextavenue/2016/04/14/the-older-americans-act-finally-clears-congress/#7b3f72e24afc

Cohen, R., & Van Nostrand, J. 1995. Trends in the health of older Americans: United States, 1994. *Vital Health Statistics* 3: 3–7.

Eldercare Workforce Alliance. 2017. *Care Coordination & Older Adults Issue Brief.* Available at https://eldercareworkforce.org/research/issue-briefs/research:care-coordination-brief/

Family Caregiver Alliance. January 31, 2015. *Selected Long-Term Care Statistics.* https://www.caregiver.org/selected-long-term-care-statistics

House Committee on Education and the Workforce. 2016. *The Older Americans Act Reauthorization Act of 2016 (as amended).* Available at http://edworkforce.house.gov/uploadedfiles/bill_summary_-_older_americans_act_reauthorization_act_of_2016.pdf

Hussey, P. March 17, 2014. *Improving Continuity of Care for Elderly Patients with Chronic Diseases Cuts Costs and Complications.* Available at http://www.rand.org/news/press/2014/03/17/index1.html

JAMA Network. 1990. *The Aging of America: Impact on Health Care Costs.* Available at http://jamanetwork.com/journals/jama/article-abstract/381638.

JAMA Network. 2003. *Alzheimer's Disease in the US Population: Prevalence Estimates Using the 2000 Census.* Available at jamanetwork.com/journals/jamaneurology/fullarticle/784558.

Kellerman, B. 2014. *Hard Times, Leadership in America.* Stanford University Press.

Life Care Planning Law Firms Association. 2017. *What is Life Care Planning: A New Approach To Elder Law.* Available at https://www.lcplfa.org/about-life-care-planning.

McCollom, P. 2000, January/February. Life care planning: A tool for elder care management. *Case Manager* 11(1): 37–40.

National Council on Aging. 2016. *House amendments to S. 192, Older Americans Act Reauthorization Act of 2016.* Available at https://www.ncoa.org/public-policy-action/older-americans-act/house/house-oaa-reauthorization-act-of-2016/

U.S. Administration of Aging. 2008. *A Statistical Profile of Older Americans Aged 65+.* Retrieved May 16, 2009, from www.aoa.gov.

U.S. Administration on Aging. 2006. *Modernizing Older Americans Act Programs.* Washington, DC: Author.

U.S. Census Bureau. 2014. *An Aging Nation: The Older Population in the United States.* Available at https://www.census.gov/prod/2014pubs/p25-1140.pdf.

Zydowicz-Vierling, D. 2008. Complimentary skills deliver exceptional results. *Prof Case Manag* 13(6): 344–346.

Appendix 20.1 (Continued) Resources

Web of Care [illegible]
A Place for Mom [illegible] [illegible]
Senior Helpers [illegible]
[illegible]

[illegible]

FORENSIC CONSIDERATIONS

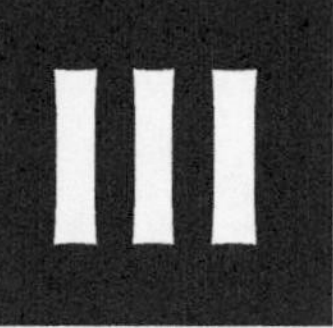

Chapter 21

Forensic Issues for Life Care Planners

Roger O. Weed

Contents

Introduction 609
Earnings Capacity Analysis 611
Hedonic Damages 612
Collateral Sources 612
The Life Care Plan (LCP) 612
Report Writing 613
    Rehabilitation Plan 614
    Access to Labor Market (Employability) 618
    Placeability 622
    Earnings Capacity 622
    Labor Force Participation 623
A Note to Nurses about Standards of Practice and Ethics 626
Conclusion 627
References 628

Introduction

This chapter will summarize some of the topics and issues that the life care planner must consider in order to practice in the area of forensic rehabilitation and may offer a somewhat different perspective than that offered in the chapters authored by attorneys. Although this chapter concentrates on forensic applications, clearly, the life care plan (LCP) is used for more than litigation (Weed, 1994; Riddick & Weed, 1996; Weed & Field, 2012; Deutsch & Sawyer, 2003; Weed, 2003, 2007). Historically, the care plan has been used in setting reserves for insurance companies, assisting workers' compensation companies with assessing future care costs associated with work-related disabilities, estimating the cost of future care for health care insurance companies, assisting Trusts with prioritizing and managing funds, and providing the client and family with an outline of future care (Weed & Field, 2012;

Deutsch & Sawyer, 2003). In the event that inadequate funding is available, the life care plan can become the road map for prioritizing care. In many instances, the future care plan may not be fully funded; therefore, the LCP can be used to prioritize treatment so that available funding is used most appropriately. In a simplistic way, the LCP is used to identify needs that can be translated into a budget so that the most important items are given the highest priority.

Since LCPs are used in a variety of jurisdictions, the appropriate "rules" must be considered. Probably the most comprehensive setting is in personal injury litigation (Weed & Berens, 2002). In the litigation arena, the LCP must consider the entire person and his or her situation. Only items that have economic value are included. For example, hedonic damages, such as the loss of pleasure of life or choice, are not included in this format. This chapter is not intended to provide a comprehensive analysis for items and issues that do not lend themselves to economic projections; the reader is referred to Brookshire and Smith (1990) for a more detailed discussion of this specialized area or the chapter in this edition by economist, Dr. Ev. Dillman. It must also be recognized that many states have different legal rules with regard to evidence and testimony. Indeed, federal rules are interpreted differently across the United States. This chapter is intended to address common issues and topics associated with civil litigation as applied to life care planning or forensic rehabilitation.

According to *Black's Law Dictionary* (Black, 1990), forensic rehabilitation refers to the practice of rehabilitation principles in legal settings. This short chapter will discuss the relationship between rehabilitation and the courts, expert witness roles, and selected terms that may be important to the rehabilitation consultant working within the legal system. An additional resource is the new contribution to this edition by Dr. Timothy Field, an exceptionally well regarded author and speaker, titled "Admissibility Considerations in Life Care Planning". His chapter summarizes historical information relating to qualifying as an expert in light of *Daubert*, *Kumho Tire*, and other rulings.

Rehabilitation experts are relatively new to the courtroom. Indeed, rehabilitation counselors historically were trained specifically to work in public agencies and were often shielded from acting as expert witnesses in personal injury litigation (Weed & Field, 2012). The first entry into the rehabilitation private sector, which involved nurses, was initiated on a larger scale in the late 1960s, when International Rehabilitation Associates, which later became Intracorp, was formed by an insurance company to help process and manage insurance claims. By the 1990s, private sector rehabilitation had extended into almost all areas of disability care, including workers' compensation, long-term disability, Social Security disability insurance, health insurance, railroad (Federal Employees Liability Act), longshore workers, Jones Act, and personal injury litigation (Weed & Field, 2012). Although there is considerable similarity across jurisdictions, there are a number of differences the rehabilitation expert should know before stepping into court, and even before beginning work on a case within a particular legal jurisdiction.

For example, the word *disability* is defined differently in various systems. In public rehabilitation, *disability* usually refers to the medical condition, which establishes eligibility for services, indicating that the client is able to perform work and benefit from vocational rehabilitation services (Weed & Field, 2012). When Social Security determines a person is disabled, the person is deemed unable to perform "substantial gainful activity" and may qualify for government support. In workers' compensation systems, some states have provision for disability that may be permanent or temporary, as well as partial or total. As with the word *disability*, terminology can make a significant difference, and it is important for the rehabilitation expert to understand the meaning of words used in the various disability systems and the courtroom.

Although this author recommends that the rehabilitation expert possess credentials related to life care planning consulting and testimony, it is not necessary for the rehabilitation professional to be certified or possess a certain level of education to be considered an expert. According to legal precedence (*Kim Manufacturing v. Superior Metal Treating*, 1976), an "expert witness is one who by reason of education or specialized experience possesses superior knowledge respecting a subject about which persons having no particular training are incapable of forming an accurate opinion or deducing correct conclusion." Therefore, an attorney may retain someone for personal injury litigation who would not necessarily be considered an expert in some states for workers' compensation or as a vocational expert (VE) for the Social Security system, but who fits this definition of expert witness.

Earnings Capacity Analysis

Often one element of damages is the loss of earnings capacity (Dillman, 1987; Field & Weed, 1988; Weed & Field, 2012; Weed, 2002b). If the life care planner is not independently qualified to opine about this aspect of the case either by education, training, or credentials, he or she may wish to associate with a vocational expert. In order to provide an expert opinion regarding the loss of potential earnings, the expert must be prepared to provide an assessment of the person's earnings capacity. Although a separate chapter addresses the details for what must be evaluated to arrive at a vocational opinion, generally accepted methods for determining loss of earnings capacity include the following:

- The most common method assumes the client has a work history. The rehabilitation professional scrutinizes vocational and medical records, perhaps supplemented by testing, and provides a professional opinion regarding preincident and postincident earnings capacity. See Table 21.3 for a description of the RAPEL methodology useful in determining earnings capacity. Obviously, this is not useful for a client who is too young to be of working age or for a client with limited or no work history.
- The Labor Market Access method, developed by Field and Field (1992), uses federal data regarding worker traits and the *Dictionary of Occupational Titles* (*DOT*) (U.S. Department of Labor, 1991). Although the Labor Market Access program is no longer available, a computer program (such as OASYS at www.vertekinc.com, or SkillTRAN at www.skilltran.com) can accomplish the same goal and can be used to help sort through more than 70 worker traits for the more than 12,000 job titles preincident versus postincident. This process identifies the number of preincident versus postincident jobs, preincident and postincident average earnings, and other information that can be used as a basis for the expert opinion. It is important to be aware that the O*Net (http://online.onetcenter.org) developed by the federal government *has replaced the DOT* for most career counseling purposes. However, at the time of this publication, there are numerous problems associated with using the O*Net in Social Security and personal injury pre- versus post-injury opinions, and the aging *DOT* remains the resource of choice.
- To determine earnings capacity for children and others who may not have ample work history, an extensive review of the client's background is useful. This may include school records, scrutiny of the parents and extended family with regard to work and education, and educational or neuropsychological testing. An extension of the RAPEL methodology, called PEEDS-RAPEL, has been developed to address factors specific to generating earnings capacity opinions for children (Neulicht & Berens, 2005). In acquired brain injury pediatric cases, preincident versus postincident ability to be educated can also be applied (Weed, 2000b).

- Another method, known as L-P-E, identifies the client's probability of life (L), probability of labor force participation (P), and probability of employment (E). For more information on this method, the professional is directed to *Economic/Hedonic Damages: The Practice Book for Plaintiff and Defense Attorneys*, by Brookshire and Smith (1990).
- A more contemporary methodology developed by Michael Shahnasarian (2007, 2015), is the *Earnings Capacity Assessment Form*, which has identified 14 factors to consider when developing opinions. At the time of this edition, little independent peer reviewed research has been conducted to assess the reliability and validity of the method, but the concept seems reasonable.

A more detailed explanation of some of these topics can be found in *The Rehabilitation Consultant's Handbook* (Weed & Field, 2012), the *Encyclopedia of Disability and Rehabilitation* (Weed, 1995), and chapters in this book relating to the roles of vocational expert and economist.

Hedonic Damages

Another domain that some rehabilitation experts address is the loss of pleasures or choices in life, known as hedonic damages. Methods include describing to the jury the client's situation regarding pain, loss of access to the labor market, psychological effects, loss of consortium, and other factors to provide the jury with guidelines. However, since hedonic damages cannot be specifically or directly translated into a dollar amount, this item is rarely a part of the LCP report.

Collateral Sources

In personal injury litigation, collateral sources have generally been very restricted in damage assessments (Field & Weed, 2015). However, in recent times based on the widely mandated Affordable Care Act (ACA) national requirement to purchase health care, some defense attorneys, most notably in California at the time of this update, are asserting the reasonableness of offsetting tort action damages with federally mandated coverages. Although these arguments are seemingly discounted by the court, life care planners nonetheless have been instructed to develop alternative plans considering ACA offsets. Field & Weed (2015) summarize many of the relevant issues and include a checklist of life care planning considerations including products and services that are not available through the ACA.

The Life Care Plan (LCP)

Regardless of the topic, the expert must be able to quantify damages in a way that provides the economist, if one is used, or the jury with the necessary information to project costs over time (Dillman, 1987; Weed, 2007). These data are used to help determine the amount of award to the client, if the party against whom the suit is lodged is found at fault. To ascertain the needs and costs of future care, particularly for serious medical conditions and catastrophic injuries, the LCP was originally published by Deutsch and Raffa in *Damages in Tort Action* (1981). This method organizes topics according to various categories (see Chapter 1 for an overview and Tables 21.1 and 21.2) that outline expected treatment, start and stop dates, costs, and other information that will

Table 21.1 Elements for Future Care Damages

When does treatment start?
What is the frequency of sessions?
What is the cost per session (if relevant)?
When does treatment stop?
Additional costs such as evaluations, tests, laboratory, or medications?
Any other needs/costs?

Table 21.2 Example Entry for Future Care Damages

Psychological evaluation in June 2008 at $600
Expect counseling to begin in July 2008 at 1 time/week, 1-hour session, for 26 weeks at $100/hour, then expect group counseling for 2 years (48 sessions) at $40/session
Expect medication, Prozac, 1 tablet of 20 mg/day for life expectancy, at $53.86 per month
Expect psychiatrist follow-up for medication 4 times/year beginning January 2009 at $150 for the initial visit, then $75 for each visit thereafter to life

provide the jury with an understanding of the treatment plan. The format is designed to develop a comprehensive rehabilitation plan that includes the necessary information to project the expense, usually with the help of an economist, in order to arrive at a "bottom-line" figure.

With specific respect to life care planning cases, there are two recent California medical malpractice citations that may become more relevant as time passes: *Markow v. Rosner* (2016) 3 Cal. App. 5th 1027 and *Cuevas v. Contra Costa County* (April 2017) 1 Cal App. 1st A143440 & A144041. Although there are several interesting topics, perhaps the portending issue was a successful defense appeal (*Cuevas v. Contra Costa County*) because the plaintiff's life care planner failed to include offsetting collateral financial resources that would probably be available to the plaintiff, which would mitigate the damages awarded by the jury. Specifically mentioned was the Affordable Care Act (ACA) as well as IDEA related services. Arguments that the ACA could not be relied upon (in part using President Trump's promise to repeal and replace) were rejected. It should be noted that in California, in 1975, the legislature enacted the Medical Injury Compensation Reform Act (MICRA) to address a crisis relating to rising costs of medical malpractice insurance (as cited in *Cuevas v. Contra Costa County*, 2017). This author believes that, although the successful appeals are located in California and are specific to medical malpractice litigation, life care planners throughout the United States should remain vigilant to jurisdictional rules changes.

Report Writing

Some general report-writing issues are discussed in other chapters. One important item to note here is that a potential shift in terminology has recently emerged within the area of forensic evaluations such that "the person who is the subject of the objective and unbiased evaluation" (Barros-Bailey et al., 2008, p. 7) should be referred to as the evaluee rather than client. Of other special interest, in this author's view, is the 1993 ruling known as the *Daubert* decision (*Daubert v. Merrell Dow*, 1993). This decision implied that any testimony in federal court offered by a scientific expert must be founded on a methodology or underlying reasoning that is scientifically valid and can be properly applied to the facts of the issue (also see the chapter in this edition by Dr. Field referenced earlier). Considerations included whether the theory or technique has been subjected to peer review and publication. This theory was extended to expert opinions by the *Kumho Tire Co. v. Carmichael* (1999). (Some states have adopted this federal court ruling, so experts may face a *Daubert* challenge in state court cases.) Although this topic has been addressed in preceding chapters, it is important to emphasize that proper foundations must be provided to a plan. Since many life care planners unfortunately either have failed to undergo specific training or do not follow published guidelines, the importance of continuing education, developing standards and methodologies, and publishing guidelines specific to our specialty practice is underscored (Feldbaum, 1997; Choppa et al., 2005; Field et al., 2006; International Academy of Life Care Planners, 2006; Weed & Johnson, 2006).

One important aspect of the report is inclusion of appropriate details for the jury to determine the cost of future care and effects on vocational opportunities, including earnings capacity. Assuming that an expert has developed all necessary data and opinions relative to damages in a personal injury case, it is appropriate to offer a rationale to encompass the issues that should be addressed in a written report. The RAPEL methodology (Table 21.3) is designed to address the relevant topics for personal injury litigation in a rational and commonsense way, as well as provide a format for displaying the information to the jury. A narrative description of each letter represented in RAPEL is in Table 21.3. Table 21.4 describes PEEDS-RAPEL, an earnings capacity analysis specific to pediatric cases. See Neulicht and Berens (2005) for a full description of PEEDS-RAPEL.

To enhance the comprehension and education of the reader of the report, another suggestion practiced by this author for cases which are complex due to numerous items, supplies and equipment needs such as one might see with tetraplegics, multiple amputations, severe brain injuries, and so on, is to add photographs. Displaying durable medical equipment, exhibiting supplies, photographing architectural problems/solutions (entry, hallways, ramps, etc.), presenting transportation needs, and any other visually appropriate aids of the needs evaluee can be enlightening. This author typically adds the visual images to the report as an appendix using PowerPoint, so that items can be identified and tagged with text and arrows as needed for clarification. Other professionals also include a list of references as support for recommendations contained within the rehabilitation or life care plan.

Rehabilitation Plan

This section includes the LCP that comprehensively outlines the expected future medical and related care of the client (see previous chapters for topics or *Life Care Planning: A Step-by-Step Guide,* Weed, 2007). This section may also include, as applicable, additional future testing, counseling, training fees, rehabilitation technology, labor market survey costs, job analysis, job coaching, placement, and other needs for improving the client's potential for employment.

For expert testimony, the life care planner is expected to follow established procedures and ethics (see Appendix I for peer-reviewed *Standards of Practice* published by the International Academy of Life Care Planners in 2002 and revised in 2015). Experts who elect not to be specifically certified in life care planning (such as CLCP or CNLCP) may not be subject to complaints that can be reviewed or disciplined by the certification board (Weed, 2000a). For example, one expert completed an updated life care plan for a client with a brain injury. Although the client had measurably improved from the first plan to the second, the updated plan (authored by the same person) was approximately double the cost of the first. Upon deposition, one explanation offered

Table 21.3 The RAPEL Method: A Commonsense Approach to Life Care Planning and Earnings Capacity Analysis*

Rehabilitation plan Determine the rehabilitation plan based on the client's vocational and functional limitations, vocational strengths, emotional functioning, and cognitive capabilities. This may include testing, counseling, training fees, rehab technology, job analysis, job coaching, placement, and other needs for increasing employment potential. Also consider reasonable accommodation. A life care plan may be needed for clients with catastrophic injuries or complex health care needs.
Access to the labor market Determine the client's access to the labor market or employability for jobs that exist in the labor market without regard to current economic or other conditions. Methods include the transferability of skills (or worker traits) analysis, disability statistics, and experience. Some professionals use computer programs to help manage large amounts of data. Access loss may also represent the client's loss of choice and is particularly relevant if earnings potential is based on very few positions.
Placeability This represents the likelihood that the client could be successfully placed in a job whereas employability or access to the labor market does not consider currently available jobs. This is where the "rubber meets the road." Consider employment statistics for people with disabilities, employment data for the specific medical condition (if available), economic situation of the community (may include a labor market survey), and availability (not just existence) of jobs in chosen occupations. Note that the client's attitude, personality, and other factors will influence the ultimate outcome.
Earnings capacity Based on the previous points, what is the preincident capacity to earn compared to the postincident capacity to earn. Methods include analysis of the specific job titles or class of jobs that a person could have engaged in pre- versus postincident, the ability to be educated (sometimes useful for people with acquired brain injury), family history for pediatric injuries, and computer analysis based on the individual's worker traits.
Special consideration applies to children, women with limited or no work history, people who choose to work below their capacity (e.g., highly educated persons who are farmers), and military trained.
Labor force participation This represents the client's work life expectancy. Determine the amount of time that is lost, if any, from the labor force as a result of the disability or retraining time. Issues include longer time to find employment, part-time versus full-time employment, medical treatment or follow-up, earlier retirement, etc. Display data using specific dates or percentages. For example, an average capacity of working 4 hours a day due to a brain injury may represent a 50% loss.

Source: Weed, R., & Field, T. *The Rehabilitation Consultant's Handbook*, 3rd ed., Athens, GA: Elliott & Fitzpatrick Vocational Services, 2001. With permission.

* In litigation the word *evaluee* may be more appropriate than "client." For a discussion on this related topic, the authors suggest reading Barros-Bailey et al. (2008). *Who Is the Client in Forensics*? Boise, ID: Authors (Contact Dr. Barros-Bailey at barrosm2002@yahoo.com).

was that he, the life care planner, was simply acting in an administrative role by writing down what the medical professionals told him. The second plan included opinions from a new expert, and the LCP author did not ask questions, collaborate, or otherwise participate in the *development* of the LCP (in either the first or second plan). As a result, at least one plan (and maybe both) was not an accurate representation of needs. Essentially, the life care planner reported that the attorney

Table 21.4 PEEDS-RAPEL Is Adapted for Pediatric Issues

Parental/Rental/Family Occupations Obtain family work history (occupations and skill levels). Include information from parents, older siblings, aunts/uncles, grandparents, or those adults that are likely to provide a role model for the child. Also include military experience, volunteer/community service, and/or avocational activities. Consider vocational assessment of parents, as appropriate, to determine a pattern of aptitudes or trait profile.
Educational Attainment Establish family patterns of educational attainment including information from the immediate and extended family. Determine not only the academic level/degrees earned, but the skills obtained through education and training. Administer or coordinate a referral for achievement, and/or intellectual assessment of parents as needed.
Evaluation Results Determine the child's functional capacities through interviews and formal assessment of physical, cognitive, emotional, and vocational capacity. Consider academic skills, interests, aptitudes, personality, assessment of independence/ADLs, and family patterns of hobbies/leisure activities. When appropriate, compare to preinjury status and function.
Developmental Stage Consider the normal developmental tasks of a particular age (e.g., ADLs, career development). Determine the effects of a disability on function and ability to achieve developmental milestones. Provide recommendations for remediation and/or accommodations to facilitate the optimum level of function for the child.
Synthesis Integrate results of the interview, parental/family occupations, educational attainment, evaluation results, developmental stage, and opinions regarding functional capacities to determine the impact of the disability and the likely options that are, within reasonable probability, available to the child.
Rehabilitation Plan Determine the rehabilitation plan based on the client's vocational and functional limitations, vocational strengths, emotional functioning, and cognitive capabilities. This may include testing, counseling, training fees, rehabilitation technology, job analysis, job coaching, placement, and other needs for increasing employment potential. Also consider reasonable accommodation. A life care plan may be needed for catastrophic injuries.
Access to the Labor Market Determine the client's access to the labor market. Methods include use of computer programs for transferability of skills (or worker trait) analysis, disability statistics, and experience. This may also represent the client's loss of choice and is particularly relevant if earnings potential is based on very few positions.
Placeability This represents the likelihood that the client could be successfully placed in a job. This is where the "rubber meets the road." Consider the employment statistics for people with disabilities, employment data for the specific medical condition (if available), economic situation of the community, availability (not just existence) of jobs in chosen occupations. Note that, where appropriate, the client's or family's attitude, personality, and other factors will influence the ultimate outcome.
Earnings Capacity Based on the previous points, what is the preincident capacity to earn compared to the postincident capacity to earn? Consider categories and examples of occupations (e.g., unskilled, semiskilled, or skilled as a result of elementary/middle school, high school, technical school, or college educational attainment) that are representative of the type of occupations a child could reasonably have been expected to perform pre- and post-injury. Determine the ability to be educated (sometimes useful for people with acquired brain injury). Utilize relevant research data and computer analysis, as appropriate, based on family work patterns or client's worker traits.

(*Continued*)

Table 21.4 (Continued) PEEDS-RAPEL Is Adapted for Pediatric Issues

Labor Force Participation	This represents the client's work life expectancy. Determine the amount of time that is lost, if any, from the labor force as a result of the disability. Issues include additional time to find employment, part-time versus full-time employment, medical treatment or follow-up, earlier retirement, etc. Display data using specific dates or percentages. For example, an average of 4 hours a day may represent a 50% loss.

Source: Neulicht, A. T., & Berens, D. E. PEEDS-RAPEL©: A case conceptualization model for evaluating pediatric cases, *Journal of Life Care Planning*, 4(1), 27–36, 2005. With permission.

should depose the experts on whom he relied to try and ferret out the reasons for substantial changes from the first LCP to the second. This stance seems to be an abdication of one of the major roles the qualified life care planner is expected to play. The qualified life care planner is expected to know what questions to ask, have enough knowledge about the disability to have a sense of what is reasonable, and be an active participant in the process. Further, according to one peer-reviewed article on the reliability of LCPs, professionals who conduct their life care planning practice according to published procedures should not observe significant differences between original and updated LCPs (Sutton et al., 2002; also see chapter of reprint on this topic).

In a second example, the plaintiff's life care planner compiled a future care plan without consulting, collaborating with, or soliciting recommendations from treating professions to which she had access. As a result, when the physicians were deposed, their recommendations were very different from those in the written plan. When deposed, the expert proclaimed that she had been doing LCPs for many years and did not need to consult with others.

In summary, the *qualified* life care planner is neither a secretary nor a know-it-all. (See Weed, 2002a, "The Life Care Planner: Secretary, Know-It-All, or General Contractor? One Person's Perspective," reprinted as an appendix for Chapter 1 for a more comprehensive discussion on this topic.) The expert needs to understand life care planning procedures, have knowledge about specific disabilities, and adhere to the profession's standards and ethics to develop a comprehensive and reliable LCP. When conducted properly, the LCP is a valuable road map of care that can also be utilized to resolve disputes.

Although ethics is covered in another chapter, there are LCP-specific issues and topics that may be relevant in this section. Certainly, within a reasonable range, professionals in the practice of life care planning can have differing opinions and philosophies. Some, particularly people who choose not to pursue specific life care planning education and training, seem to be most likely to push the boundaries (Berens & Weed, 2001). Indeed, in the Life Care Planning Summit of 2000, sponsored by several organizations and many different life care planning professionals, there were many topics that achieved consensus by all 100-plus participants present and was endorsed by seven participating organizations (Weed & Berens, 2001). One item that has wide acceptance is the need for a medical foundation for relevant plan entries. First, it must be explicitly noted that every LCP entry is not medical. Certainly nursing, allied health, vocational, psychological, case management, and other opinions can be offered by professionals who have the credentials to do so. However, many LCP needs are within the realm of physicians to prescribe. The ways to obtain a medical foundation are many. The most obvious is to collaborate with a qualified physician (or several if differing specialties are required). Other options include soliciting recommendations via letter or fax (keeping careful documentation), requesting the attorney to ask the physician questions in deposition if one does not have access to the physician (such as consulting for the defense), relying upon published medical research or clinical practice guidelines specific to the disability for standards and guidelines, and searching the client's medical records for documented recommendations.

Another issue common to life care planning is the methodology of the research conducted related to identifying costs for the needs identified in the document. It is common for facts and data on which the author of the LCP relies to come from a variety of sources such as physicians, allied health care professionals, consultants, catalogs, suppliers, pharmacies (actual patient records, online and brick and mortar), and others. It is also common for the author of the LCP to employ or subcontract a qualified individual who completes the necessary research. One caution is that the LCP author should provide specific direction to the person and supervise the research methodology so the document is reliable and can be effectively communicated by the author of the LCP within a litigation context. If one retains an independent consultant (rather than employing someone to help with the research), one must assure that the consultant is competent and willing to testify since it infers that the author of the LCP has delegated the duties to another person without the necessary oversight to fit the "direction and supervision" criteria. For example, in some life care plans, the durable medical equipment list may be extensive and complicated. In this instance, it may be reasonable to retain an expert consultant who can competently testify to the specifications, replacement schedules, and costs. On the other hand, researching the costs of medications may be within the realm of the life care planner's expertise, who may direct and supervise an employee or independent contractor on sources to contact and what information to obtain. Checklists and forms are helpful in this regard, as well as having clear and thorough documentation of the research conducted, contacts made, date of contact, name of resource and contact person, phone number or e-mail/web address, and so on.

When consulting with attorneys about another individual's LCP, one recommended strategy to help organize data and reveal the foundation for recommendations is a matrix of data containing a minimum of three columns. The first column is for each life care plan recommendation by the other expert, the second is for supporting documentation (medical records, depositions, report contents, interview information, day-in-the-life videos, etc.), and the third is for comments made based on the available information (see Table 21.5 for a basic example). In some cases, it may be appropriate to add a column for research-related information. It may also be useful to add a column when the expert's plan being reviewed has been updated. This will allow the reader to see at a glance what the changes are for each category from the initial plan to the updated plan. Also to be included are general comments at the end.*

For occasions where comparison of two opposing LCPs is desirable, the two plans can be displayed side by side, with a column for foundation. See Table 21.6 for a limited example where the plaintiff's life care planner did not collaborate with, or utilize, existing medical records and testimony from the treating physician for the LCP.

A third potential review technique is to compare the other expert's procedures (to the extent possible) with the published procedures. See Table 21.7 for the general outline.

Access to Labor Market (Employability)

In many litigation cases, an individual may very well be able to return to a job that is custom-designed around his or her disability or, as in the case of traumatic brain injury, with an employer who is interested in helping an employee with mild to moderate cognitive deficits (Weed, 1988; Weed & Field, 2012). However, the client may not have access to the same level of vocational choices he or she did prior to the incident. In essence, the client or evaluee might appear to have no particular loss of earnings capacity, but at the same time be at high risk for losing a job

* Thanks to Dr. Debbie Berens for the layout design for Tables 21.5 through 21.7.

Table 21.5 Example Basic Matrix for Determining the Foundation for Life Care Plan Recommendations

Plan Entry	*Recommendation Based on Records Review*	*Comment*
Counseling 1 time/week for 2 years	No recommendation found in records.	Unknown psychological foundation; the nurse consultant is *not* certified or licensed in a counseling field.
Physiatrist 4 times/year to life	Dr. Doodue's deposition of May 10, 2003, p. 33, line 20, says 2 times/year to life.	Dr. Doodue is the treating physiatrist and reported that she was not contacted with regard to her recommendations.
Attendant care 4 hours/day to age 60, then 8 hours/day	Dr. Doodue's deposition of May 10, 2003, p. 49, lines 18–20, says the L2 spinal cord injury (SCI) client will require "some attendant care for household activities."	SCI research for anticipated attendant care for an L2 level is 0–1 hour/day; see Blackwell et al., 2001, p. 246 (copy included).

Note: Records reveal a recommendation for ankle-foot orthoses (AFOs) for both legs, which was not included in the life care plan.

Table 21.6 Example Comparison Matrix of Future Care Recommendations

Recommendation	*Penny Money, PhD (Plaintiff's LCP)*	*Roger Weed, PhD (Defense LCP)*	*Medical Records/ Deposition of Boat Dock, MD (Treating Physiatrist)*
Physiatrist	2 times/year	1–2 times/year average to life expectancy	1–2 times/year for medication management
Primary care physician	Internist: 1 time initially, then 2 times/year to life expectancy	4–5 times/year to life expectancy (deduct average yearly medical care for general population)	4–5 times/year for general medical care (which includes a preexisting condition)
Orthopedic evaluation	1 time initially (by surgeon), then 1–2 times/year to life expectancy	Optional for complications, if any; year initiated and frequency unknown	*May need* if develops degenerative spine/joint disease and/or scoliosis; no need at present
Medical testing	No reference	Yearly lab tests to life expectancy Renal function studies every 3 months to life expectancy	Routine diagnostic testing Renal function studies every 3 months

Table 21.7 Comparison Matrix of Published Step-by-Step Procedures for Life Care Planning and Expert's Procedures

Published Step-by-Step Procedures for Life Care Planning (Derived from Step-by-Step Procedure for Life Care Planning, Table 1.3 of this volume.)	*Comments Regarding Expert's Procedures* (Based on records, report, deposition transcript, etc.)
Case Intake: 1. When you talked with the referral source, did you record the basic referral information? 2. Time frames discussed? 3. Financial/billing agreement? 4. Retainer received (if appropriate)? 5. Arrange for information release?	
Medical Records: 1. Complete copy requested including lab reports and X-rays	
Supporting Documentation: 1. Are there depositions of client, family, or treatment team that may be useful? 2. Day-in-the-life videotapes 3. And if vocational issues to be included in report—school records (including test scores)? 4. Vocational and employment records? 5. Tax returns, if appropriate?	
Initial Interview Arrangements: 1. Is the interview to be held at the client's residence? 2. Have you arranged for all appropriate people to attend the initial interview (spouse, parents, siblings)? 3. Did you allow 3–5 hours for the initial interview?	
Initial Interview Materials: 1. Do you have the initial interview form for each topic to be covered? 2. Supplemental form for pediatric cases, CP, traumatic brain injury (TBI), and spinal cord injury (SCI) as needed? 3. Do you have a copy of the life care plan checklist? 4. Example plan to show the client? 5. Camera or video camcorder to record living situation, medications, supplies, equipment, and other documentation useful for developing a plan?	

(Continued)

Table 21.7 (Continued) Comparison Matrix of Published Step-by-Step Procedures for Life Care Planning and Expert's Procedures

Consulting with Therapeutic Team Members: 1. Have you consulted with and solicited treatment recommendations from appropriate therapeutic team members (if appropriate)?	
Preparing Preliminary Life Care Plan Opinions: 1. Do you have information that can be used to project future care costs? 2. Frequency of service or treatment? 3. Duration? 4. Base cost? 5. Source of information? 6. Vendors?	
Filling in the Holes: 1. Do you need additional medical or other evaluations to complete the plan? 2. Have you obtained the approval to retain services of additional sources from the referral source? 3. Have you composed a letter outlining the right questions to assure you are soliciting the needed information?	
Researching Costs and Sources: 1. Have you contacted local sources for costs of treatment, medications, supplies, and equipment? 2. Or do you have catalogs or flyers? 3. For children, are there services that might be covered, in part, through the school system under IDEA?	
Finalizing the Life Care Plan: 1. Did you confirm your projections with the client and/or family? 2. Treatment team members (if appropriate)? 3. Can the economist project the costs based on the plan? 4. Do you need to coordinate with a vocational expert?	
Last But Not Least: 1. Have you distributed the plan to all appropriate parties (client [if clinically appropriate], referral source, attorney, and economist, if there is one)?	

and then having a significant problem locating suitable employment. As noted earlier in this chapter, access to the labor market can be determined through a variety of means. OASYS and SkillTRAN are two computer programs used as tools to *assist* in determining, based on worker traits, the client's ability to choose in the labor market. For example, one client may have a 50 percent personal loss of access to the labor market and another individual may have a 95 percent personal loss of access to the labor market. Obviously, an individual who has personal access to 5 percent of the labor market should be employable or placeable; however, the difficulty factor for suitable or sustained employment has increased significantly. By placing a loss of access percentage to the labor market, one can sensitize the reader or jury to the potential difficulty for placement. Generally, this is described in a particular percentage loss of access to the client's *personal* labor market rather than to the national labor market. Few unimpaired people have access to 100 percent of the labor market, and this is a common error assumed by the uneducated observer (Woodrich & Patterson, 2003).

Placeability

Placeability opinion represents the likelihood that the client will be successfully placed in a job with or without rehabilitation support or rehabilitation consultant assistance. One may need to conduct a labor market survey, job analysis, or, in pediatric cases, rely upon statistical data to opine about ultimate placeability. The economic condition of the community may also be a factor. It is important that the rehabilitation consultant recognize that the client's personality, cognitive limitations, and other factors certainly influence the ultimate outcome. For adults, the rehabilitationist may find that it is useful to include an opinion about jobs that are available (actual openings) in addition to jobs that exist but are not currently available to the client (employability)—if it is likely that the client will have worker traits that match various job titles. Matching to a job title does not suggest that the person can indeed be placed in a particular occupation. Other factors, such as location, experience, education, and personality, can adversely impact placement. Also, many jobs that may be appropriate for the client are difficult to obtain. The vocational opportunity may be highly competitive or there may be very few positions available. On the other hand, jobs may exist that the client with a disability may be able to do, even though on paper (through review of worker traits based on government statistics) it would appear to the contrary.

Earnings Capacity

Based on the rehabilitation plan, access to the labor market, and placeability factors, the client may or may not be employable in the labor market. If placement in a job is likely, an estimate of the earnings potential is important. In general, the difference between wage loss and earnings capacity analysis for an individual is that which he or she can reasonably attain and hold (also see Weed & Field, 2012 for more discussion on this topic). For example, consider a 17-year-old who delivers papers for an income when he is catastrophically impaired and is never able to work again. Certainly, the earnings history from the paper delivery does not represent the individual's capacity. On the other hand, a 55-year-old union truck driver may exhibit an earnings history that is consistent with his capacity. Considerations include whether the individual is a child or an adult and, if an adult, the industry for which he or she is best suited. For example, a drywall hanger of marginal intelligence may very well reach his earnings potential by the time he reaches his late twenties or early thirties. On the other hand, an attorney may not reach his or her potential until late in his or her career.

Labor Force Participation

This category represents an opinion about the client's anticipated work life expectancy. Usually an individual who has a reduced life expectancy will also be expected to have a reduced work life expectancy. At the other end of the spectrum, the client's participation in the labor force may be unchanged. An individual may also be expected to work 6 hours per day after the injury rather than 8 hours per day, which represents a 25 percent loss of normal work life expectancy. Some clients have demonstrated consistent extra income by working overtime, and this situation can be considered in this arena as well. Generally speaking, the consultant will express the opinion of loss by percentage or perhaps a number of years. It is usually the economist who makes the actual economic projections. This particular area is quite complicated, and most vocational counselors are not prepared to address the subtleties and complexities of economic projections (Dillman, 1987). However, for additional general information, though an aging resource, the consultant can obtain information about worklife estimates in *Worklife Estimates: Effects of Race and Education* (Bulletin 2254, U.S. DOL, 1986). Other privately produced worklife tables exist but, in this author's experience, controversy surrounds their usage so caution is urged.

In order to assure that experts cover the relevant areas and have the background to offer opinions, two checklists have been developed (see Tables 21.8 and 21.9).

Table 21.8 Checklist for Review of Life Care Plans

✓	**Was a complete set of medical and other relevant records provided with referral?** Did narrative report accompany LCP? Deposition transcripts of client, family, and/or treatment team provided? Day-in-the-life or other videotapes of client? Photographs of client? Deposition of life care planning expert?
✓	**Does LCP follow published standards and procedures?** Refer to IALCP website (www.IALCP.com) for published standards for life care planners. Use of published or standard checklists, forms, charts, etc.? Collaborative effort? Potential complications referenced on appropriate page and not included in LCP?
✓	**Are entries in LCP appropriate for disability/injury?** Input obtained from treatment team or consulting physician(s), if appropriate? Medical, psychological, or neuropsychological foundation established? Standards of care for the specific disability referenced, if applicable? Life care planner's recommendations within his area of expertise? Medical/therapeutic recommendations within respective providers' area of expertise? Preventive and rehabilitative goals? All areas related to disability included? Costs related to disability only and not related to general or routine care or preexisting conditions? Costs based on geographic area or other appropriate database?
✓	**Overlaps?** Are same or similar services listed more than once under different categories? Can one provider accomplish two recommendations and be more cost-effective (e.g., qualified speech therapist or occupational therapist to also do assistive technology evaluation, primary care physician to also do urinalyses, etc.)? Time frames for services chronological or mutually exclusive?

(*Continued*)

Table 21.8 (Continued) Checklist for Review of Life Care Plans

✓	**In-home/facility care?** For in-home pediatric care, are adjustments made for time child is at school and for time parents normally are expected to be available to parent a child? Adjustments made as child gets older and normally would require less assistance? Level of care appropriate to client's needs? (In general, minimum LPN for G-tube management, bowel/bladder program, trach care, medication administration, and cut/clean toenails; CNA/PCA/HHA for Activities of Daily Living (ADL), meal preparation, laundry, housekeeping, driving, and safety/supervision at home. Also refer to each state's Nurse Practice Act for specific requirements.) Do agencies surveyed provide CNA II or have state authorized special rules that allow trained CNAs to provide some skilled care under supervision of RN/LPN? Consideration made to potential negotiated cost reduction with home health agency if long-term contract? Parents/family expected to provide some of the care? Lawn/yard care and exterior/interior home maintenance included as adult? For residential community living program/facility, is average yearly cost of individual room and board deducted from per diem rate (if loss of earnings capacity is also a part of damages)?
✓	**Appropriate cost deductions made or noted to economist with regard to general expenses incurred without disability?** For wheelchair-accessible van, cost of average vehicle or trade-in value of family vehicle deducted if loss of earnings capacity is also a part of damages? Accessible home, cost of average home in local area deducted? Dental/medical care, cost of routine care recommended for general population deducted? Adaptive clothing allowance, average yearly cost of clothing for general population deducted? Adaptive leisure equipment allowance, average yearly cost of recreation/leisure activities of general population deducted? Total enteral nutrition, average yearly cost of food consumption for general same-age population deducted? Alternatively, is a distinction made that the recommended services in the plan are over and above those that are recommended for the general population?
✓	**Are costs calculated correctly?** Is the math correct? Source of cost information known or documented? If economic calculations are included, is life care planner qualified to make such calculations? Are costs of as-needed services/items included in plan? Are costs of potential complications included?
✓	**Vocationally relevant items?** Are vocational issues addressed or deferred to qualified vocational specialist for vocational considerations?
✓	**Plan confirmation?** Plan or relevant entries reviewed/confirmed/endorsed by physician(s) and/or treatment team, if access is available? Client/family, if access available? Future updates expected?
✓	**Aesthetics?** Are plan entries easy to read, follow, and understand? Does plan overall look professional and make sense? Minimal to no typographical errors or date errors? Is the information presented clearly, logically, and with sufficient detail? Consistency between narrative report, records, and plan entries?

Source: Debra E. Berens and Roger O. Weed.

Table 21.9 Checklist for Review of Life Care Planner Qualifications and Practices (aka Checklist for Selecting a Life Care Planner)

✓	Professional's **qualifications**?
	Education, including degrees and continuing education? If doctorate, was the university accredited? (Some so-called experts have mail-order degrees or diplomas from universities that are not accredited.)
	Training specific to life care planning?
	Work experience?
	Life care planning experience?
	Research knowledge and experience?
	Certifications or licenses? Generally accepted rehabilitation certifications include CLCP (certified life care planner), CNLCP (certified nurse life care planner), CRC (certified rehabilitation counselor), CDMS (certified disability management specialist), CVE (certified vocational evaluator), CRRN (certified rehabilitation registered nurse), CCM (certified case manager), diplomat or fellow ABVE (American Board of Vocational Experts), and CLNC (certified legal nurse consultant).
	Forensic experience (if appropriate)? Familiar with the rules pertaining to experts? Have they testified? Do they have a list of cases for which they testified at deposition or trial for the previous 4 years? Plaintiff/defense ratio?
✓	Prospective consultant's **awareness** of life care planning?
	Are they **certified** in an area relevant to life care planning? Refer to Commission on Health Care Certification website (www.ichcc.org) or contact the American Association of Nurse Life Care Planners (www.aanlcp.org) for a list of life care planners who are certified through either organization.
	Have they achieved the **certificate** in life care planning offered through one of the past or existing training programs such as Rehabilitation Training Institute, Intelicus, University of Florida, Kaplan University, Capital Law paralegal program, etc.?
	Have they completed **courses** or **continuing education** offered by past or present noted programs on life care planning (e.g., Rehabilitation Training Institute, Intelicus, Medipro, University of Florida, IARP, IALCP, Care Planners network, et al.)?
	Can they cite life care planning **references**?
	Do they know some of the **professionals** associated with life care planning publications and training?
✓	**Commitment** to the profession?
	Do they belong to professional **organization(s)** with focus on life care planning such as International Academy of Life Care Planners (IALCP), www.IALCP.com? Do they belong to a disability-specific organization? (Are they legitimate or fringe organizations such as a for-profit owned by an individual or group with little recognition or substance?)
	Do they **participate** in professional development?

(Continued)

Table 21.9 (Continued) Checklist for Review of Life Care Planner Qualifications and Practices (aka Checklist for Selecting a Life Care Planner)

	Have they **contributed** their time and effort by volunteering services to clients in need, speaking, holding office with professional organizations, writing articles, chapters, or books?
	Have they received **awards, honors, or peer recognition**?
✓	**Industry** experience?
	Workers' compensation or federal Office of Workers' Compensation Programs?
	Personal injury?
	Social Security?
	State rehabilitation?
	Longshore workers? Jones Act? Federal Employees Liability Act (FELA)?
	Long-term and short-term disability?
	Specialize in a particular disability?
✓	**Medical foundation** for opinions established?
	Use established published **checklists and forms**?
	Routinely consult with a **physician** as part of the team or have medical literature/ clinical practice guidelines relevant to client?
	Include other **health professionals** as appropriate (e.g., OT, PT, SLT, RT, audiology, neuropsychology, etc.)?
✓	Other?
	What and how do they **bill** for their services? Do they charge different rates for interview, records review, deposition, trial time, or rush cases?
	Current curriculum **vitae**?
	History of **ethics complaints or arrests**?

Source: Original checklist developed by Roger O. Weed, revised by Debra E. Berens, 2002.

A Note to Nurses about Standards of Practice and Ethics

The reader is referred to the chapter on ethics for a more comprehensive discussion on the topic, but there is an additional consideration that is relevant to this forensic chapter specifically for nurses. Professional life care planners represent a board cross section of disciplines. The two well-known certifications, Certified Life Care Planner (CLCP), for most life care planning disciplines including nurses, and Certified Nurse Life Care Planner (CNLCP), for nurses only* require foundation

* Another relatively recent specialty group, the American Academy of Physician Life Planners, offers certification for qualified physicians (see http://aaplcp.org/Membership/Membership.aspx). Some also hold the CLCP. Nonphysicians may join as associate members but will not be certified by that organization.

credentials (such as RN) in order to qualify for certification. Nurses may seek both the CNLCP and CLCP credential. However, the standards of practice and ethics foundation have many differences. The methodology employed also differs somewhat. Belonging to and being certified by more than one organization offering the same service with differing standards, methodology, ethics, and so on, is outwardly fraught with potential conflict. Seemingly, an astute attorney could utilize their skills to capitalize on that potential weakness.

Conclusion

This chapter offers a life care planning practitioner's view, hints, and opinions for enhancing one's success of testifying. The following chapters offered by experienced plaintiff and defense attorneys will be an essential addition to that goal. Furthermore numerous cases of successful and unsuccessful court challenges have appeared. Extensive summaries of examples up to 2006 are available in *Life Care Planning in Light of Daubert and Kumho* (Weed & Johnson, 2006) punctuated with comments, conclusions, and helpful hints. The chapter in this edition by Dr. Field regarding the *Daubert* Trilogy also addresses these sensitive topics. Examples include experts who have substantial experience but have been excluded based not on their work experience and background, but what they are planning on testifying about. In some cases, there appeared to be little or no foundation for opinions. Commonly, the expert failed to include a medical basis for recommendations. In other cases, the recommendations offered by the plaintiff's expert were contrary to the treating or plaintiff's medical expert's opinions.

The booklet by Weed and Johnson (2006) also includes examples of professionals who were deemed qualified. In general, successful experts utilized published standards of practice, adhered to published and peer-reviewed methodology, had evidence of training or continuing education specific to life care planning, and were able to show clear foundation for opinions and recommendations.

Other recommended publications related to the chapter topics are:

- *Damages in Tort Action*, Vols. 8 & 9 (Deutsch & Raffa, 1981)
- *Daubert Challenge: From Case Referral to Trial* (Choppa et al., 2005)
- *Depositions: The Complete Guide for Expert Witnesses* (Babitsky & Mangraviti, 2007)
- *Feder's Succeeding as an Expert Witness* (4th ed.) (Feder & Houck, 2008)
- *Methods and Protocols: Meeting the Criteria of General Acceptance and Peer Review under Daubert and Kumho* (Field et al., 2006)
- *The Comprehensive Forensic Services Manual: The Essential Resources for All Experts* (Babitsky et al., 2000)

In summary, this chapter has outlined many of the topics and issues that the life care planner must consider when developing opinions for civil litigation cases. The expert is in an excellent position to assist in resolving litigation by soliciting information that addresses almost all of the damage aspects of the case. Knowing the health care industry and effectively analyzing the needs and researching the future care and costs associated with a complex injury are specialized services that offer a true enhancement to the profession. When completed objectively and professionally, the care plan will assist the jury with a clear understanding of the needs of the client, as well as provide the road map of care for the client/evaluee and family or a client trust.

References

Babitsky, S., & Mangraviti, J. 2007. *Depositions: The Complete Guide for Expert Witnesses*. Falmouth, MA: SEAK.

Babitsky, S., Mangraviti, J., & Todd, C. 2000. *The Comprehensive Forensic Services Manual: The Essential Resources for All Experts*. Falmouth, MA: SEAK.

Barros-Bailey, M., Carlisle, J., Graham, M., Neulicht, A., Taylor, R., & Wallace, A. 2008. *Who Is the Client in Forensics*. Boise, ID: Authors.

Berens, D., & Weed, R. 2001. Ethics update for rehabilitation counselors in the private sector. *Journal of Applied Rehabilitation Counseling*, 32, 27–32.

Black, H. 1990. *Black's Law Dictionary* (6th ed.). St. Paul, MN: West Publishing.

Blackwell, T., Krause, J., Winkler, T., & Stiens, S. 2001. *Spinal Cord Injury Desk Reference: Guidelines for Life Care Planning and Case Management*. New York, NY: Demos.

Brookshire, M., & Smith, S. 1990. *Economic/Hedonic Damages: The Practice Book for Plaintiff and Defense Attorneys*. Cincinnati, OH: Anderson Publishing.

Choppa, A., Field, T., & Johnson, C. 2005. *The Daubert Challenge: From Case Referral to Trial*. Athens, GA: Elliott & Fitzpatrick.

Cuevas v. Contra Costa County. 2017. Contra Costa County Super. Ct. No. MSC09-01786.

Daubert v. Merrell Dow. 1993. 125 L Ed 2d 469.

Deutsch, P., & Raffa, F. 1981. *Damages in Tort Action* (Vols. 8 & 9). New York, NY: Matthew Bender.

Deutsch, P., & Sawyer, H. 2003. *Guide to Rehabilitation*. White Plains, NY: Ahab Press.

Dillman, E. 1987. The necessary economic and vocational interface in personal injury cases. *Journal of Private Sector Rehabilitation*, 2, 121–142.

Feder, H., & Houck, M. 2008. *Feder's Succeeding as an Expert Witness* (4th ed.). Boca Raton, FL: CRC Press.

Feldbaum, C. 1997. The *Daubert* decision and its interaction with the federal rules. *Journal of Forensic Vocational Assessment*, 1, 49–73.

Field, T., & Field, J. 1992. *Labor Market Access Plus 1992*. Athens, GA: Elliott & Fitzpatrick (computer program).

Field, T., Johnson, C., Schmidt, R., & Van de Bittner, E. 2006. *Methods and Protocols: Meeting the Criteria of General Acceptance and Peer Review under Daubert and Kumho*. Athens, GA: Elliott & Fitzpatrick.

Field, T., & Weed, R. 1988. *Transferability of Work Skills*. Athens, GA: Georgia Southern.

Field, T., & Weed R. 2015. Will the Affordable Care Act and Tort Reform Render the Collateral Source Doctrine Obsolete in Resolving the Issue of Damages in Cases Involving Personal Injury and Life Care Planning? *RehabPro*, 23(3), 133–148.

International Academy of Life Care Planners. 2006. Standards of practice for life care planners. *Journal of Life Care Planning*, 5, 123–129.

Kim Manufacturing, Inc., v. Superior Metal Treating, Inc. 1976. 537 S W Reporter, 2d 424.

Kumho Tire Co. v. Carmichael. 1999. 526 U.S. 137.

Markow v. Rosner. 2016. 3 Cal. App. 5th 1027.

Neulicht, A. T., & Berens, D. E. 2005. PEEDS-RAPEL©: A case conceptualization model for evaluating pediatric cases. *Journal of Life Care Planning*, 4, 27–36.

Riddick, S., & Weed, R. 1996. The life care planning process for managing catastrophically impaired patients. In S. Blanchett (Ed.), *Case Studies in Nursing Case Management* (pp. 61–91). Sudbury, MA: Jones & Bartlett.

Shahnasarian, M. 2007. Use of the Earnings Capacity Assessment Form in forensic rehabilitation evaluations. *Directions in Rehabilitation Counseling*, 18, 19–26.

Shahnasarian, M. 2015. *Assessment of Earning Capacity* (4th ed.). Tucson, AZ: Lawyers & Judges Publishing Company, Inc.

Sutton, A., Deutsch, P., Weed, R., & Berens, D. 2002. Reliability of life care plans: A comparison of original and updated plans. *Journal of Life Care Planning*, 1, 187–194.

U.S. Department of Labor. 1991. *Dictionary of Occupational Titles* (4th ed.). Washington, DC: U.S. Government Printing.

Weed, R. 1988. Earnings vs. earnings capacity: The labor market access method. *Journal of Private Sector Rehabilitation*, 3, 57–64.

Weed, R. 1994. Life care plans: Expanding the horizons. *Journal of Private Sector Rehabilitation*, 9, 47–50.

Weed, R. 1995. Forensic rehabilitation. In A. E. Dell Orto and R. P. Marinelle (Eds.), *Encyclopedia of Disability and Rehabilitation* (pp. 326–330). New York, NY: Macmillan.

Weed, R. 2000a. Ethics in rehabilitation opinions and testimony. *Rehabilitation Counseling Bulletin*, 43, 215–218, 245.

Weed, R. 2000b. The worth of a child: Earnings capacity and rehabilitation planning for pediatric personal injury litigation cases. *The Rehabilitation Professional*, 8, 29–43.

Weed, R. 2002a. The life care planner: Secretary, know-it-all, or general contractor? One person's perspective. *Journal of Life Care Planning*, 1, 173–177.

Weed, R. 2002b. The assessment of transferable work skills in forensic settings. *Journal of Forensic Vocational Analysis*, 5, 1–4 (special issue editorial).

Weed, R. 2003. Life care planning for workers with injuries. *Rehab News, January*, 13–21 (Georgia State Board of Workers' Compensation newsletter).

Weed, R. 2007. *Life Care Planning: A Step-by-Step Guide*. Athens, GA: E & F Vocational Services.

Weed, R., & Berens, D. (Eds.). 2001. *Life Care Planning Summit 2000 Proceedings*. Athens, GA: Elliott & Fitzpatrick Vocational Services.

Weed, R., & Berens, D. 2002. Ethics in life care planning. In P. Deutsch (Ed.), *The Expert's Role as an Educator Continues: Meeting the Demands under Daubert* (pp. 59–67). White Plains, NY: Ahab Press.

Weed, R., & Field, T. 2001. *The Rehabilitation Consultant's Handbook* (3rd ed.). Athens, GA: Elliott & Fitzpatrick Vocational Services.

Weed, R., & Field, T. 2012. *The Rehabilitation Consultant's Handbook* (4th ed.). Athens, GA: Elliott & Fitzpatrick Vocational Services.

Weed, R., & Johnson, C. 2006. *Life Care Planning in Light of Daubert and Kumho*. Athens, GA: Elliott & Fitzpatrick Vocational Services.

Woodrich, F., & Patterson, J. B. 2003. Ethical objectivity in forensic rehabilitation. *The Rehabilitation Professional*, 11, 41–47.

Chapter 22

A Personal Perspective of Life Care Planning

Raymond L. Arrona, and Mamie Walters,
as told to Anna N. Herrington

Contents

Introduction....631
Ray Arrona: My Daughter's Story....632
Mamie Walters: My Journey with Anita....637
Editor's Note....639

Introduction

This chapter is a brief account of Anita Arrona's story. On September 7, 1987, Anita was returning home from visiting her boyfriend when a drunk driver hit her. Her injuries were profound and included open brain trauma, severe brain contusion of the left and right frontal lobes, supraorbital fractures of her left and right eyes, multiple blunt trauma to the chest, hydrocephalus, pleural effusion of the left lung, fractured right clavicle, and severe spasticity with minimal control of bodily functions. By October 5, 1987, infected frontal lobe brain tissue was removed and a shunt was inserted to drain off excess fluid. Her left eye was unsalvageable. After 3 months and multiple surgeries, it became evident that Anita would never achieve independence, and the family's attorney retained the services of a life care planner to develop an outline of future expected care. Over the years, although severely brain injured, hemiparetic, and blind in the left eye, her medical situation has stabilized and she has learned to speak a few words. She resides in a wheelchair, which requires an attendant's service to move her. She is totally dependent on others for her well-being.

Anita's journey since her injury in 1987 has involved many factors: family and friends, high moral standards and strong values, and a solid plan. First, Anita's father, Ray Arrona, has been and continues to be her warrior in the many battles that must be fought to obtain what she needs. Mamie Walters, a family friend who has turned professional caregiver, has been devoted to seeking out creative therapeutic methods to enhance Anita's abilities and is committed to her growth. Second, Anita and Ray have had strong coping resources based on deep-rooted beliefs in optimism, honesty, perseverance, stubbornness, hard work, and faith in God. Last on Anita's journey has been the pragmatic vehicle—the life care plan. Anita's life care plan has been the essential road map, though detours are sometimes taken, of her often arduous journey.

Ray Arrona: My Daughter's Story

Let me begin with one of the codes by which I live my life: *be responsive*. A story I heard at a recent conference illustrates this well. There was a first mate that came to his captain advising him that the ship was going to be under attack and inquiring as to what to do. The captain told the first mate to run and get his (the captain's) red shirt. So he got the red shirt, they engaged in battle, and they won. About a week or two passed and the first mate returned to the captain and warned him of a pending battle with pirates. Once again the first mate asked, "What do you advise?" Again the captain replied, "I want you to bring my red shirt." So, they engaged in battle and wiped out all the pirates. When putting everything away the first mate was curious and asked the captain, "Can you please tell me about this red shirt? Every time you put this red shirt on we seem to do well. I wonder if there is some point in this." The captain told him that it "was the leadership thing." The captain explained that if he happens to get stabbed while under attack or is hit by a volley, "I don't want the men to see me get hurt and bleed so I can continue to lead them through the battle." That's pretty wise. Another month passes and the first mate rushed to the captain shouting, "Captain, Captain, I have news of yet another battle. There are pirates on starboard, on the bow, and on the port side! What shall I do?" So the captain says, "Will you please get me my brown pants?"

I tell this story to express the importance of a quick and smart response. I have found that being ready for the battle has been of immense importance in my life. I was born and raised in Miami, Arizona, a copper mining community about 80 miles east of Phoenix. Being Hispanic, I grew up in a strict and disciplined home. At home I learned the importance of a good attitude. I learned about making good choices and taking responsibility for those choices. I learned to believe strongly in myself. Now, I am 50 years old and I know these early lessons have assisted me through my life. I worked while attending college at Arizona State University and had plans to pursue a pre-med curriculum. That was in 1964. However, my plans changed when I met Anita's mother in 1965. Soon we were married and a year later, in November 1966, Anita was born.

I continued to work with my college employer, Wear-Ever, Inc., the first subsidiary of Alcoa, and later transferred to another subsidiary, Cutco. I have been associated with these two companies for nearly 30 years, though many changes have occurred. Our second child was another daughter, Andrea, who was born just about 11 months after Anita. Little did we know how short a time we would have with Andrea. Andrea, at 11 months, drowned in the bathtub. It was terrible. This tragedy was our first to experience as a family. I am not sure whether it prepared us for the future, but it certainly tightened the family.

Then there was the aftermath and our struggles. We had a son, my namesake, who was born on Christmas Day. You may remember the Apollo moonshot; it was somewhere around that time in 1968. Ray Jr. was 18 at the time of Anita's injury. (Ray is now married and has two children. He is in the Navy and lives in Seattle, Washington.) For many different reasons, our marriage did not work and we were divorced in 1971.

I later met and married (October 1974) Sheri, the love of my life. We just recently celebrated 22 years of marriage. At the time of Anita's accident Sheri was 38 years of age. My employer offered me a promotion to a position that required transferring across the country to Atlanta, Georgia. We moved in 1976. Alyson was born to Sheri and me a year later in May 1977. Alyson, Anita's younger sister, was 10 years old and was in fifth grade at the time of the injury. Alyson probably has the most anger in the family about Anita's disaster, even to this day. Ryan, whom Anita used to take care of often, was born 4 years later in October 1981. At the time of the accident, he was 5 and not really aware of what was happening.

It was during this period of time (1979) that Anita moved in with my parents in Miami, Arizona, because of difficulties she was having with her mother. However, Anita did not realize how strict her grandparents would be, and we soon realized that it might be best for her to move to Atlanta to be with me. Anita moved in with us and enrolled as a junior at North Cobb High School in Kennesaw, Georgia. She graduated in May 1984. Anita is a very determined person—she has not lost this trait. She is a hard worker and has not lost that drive either. After school she worked several jobs with the goal of eventually attending court-reporting school. During this time, she saved enough money to buy her dream car: a new, red, 1986 Toyota GT. Anita would not let anyone else drive or even touch that car. She loved that car.

It was Labor Day 1987, and since I am a football fanatic, I was glued to the television. At the end of the evening the news detailed Labor Day highway accidents. According to the report, the number of accidents was less than predicted. I thought, *This is really great.* Then the phone rang. The phone call was very similar to the one I received when I was working in Tucson and heard the news from an official at a local hospital about Andrea's accident. Although they would not say what was going on, I knew that something was terribly wrong. Anita had been visiting with her boyfriend, Dan, that evening of Labor Day and was on her way home. I called Dan and asked him what was going on. He did not know. Dan lived about half a mile from the hospital, and I asked him if he would please join me there. Upon arrival at the hospital, I was escorted into a private conference room, and as I walked in, I saw Dan talking with two professional men dressed in white. Later, I learned those were the neurosurgeons who were preparing for a lengthy, all-night operation on Anita. They informed me that Anita had been involved in a terrible auto accident that had crushed her skull. They said she was critical and was given only about a 20 percent chance to survive.

I felt all numb inside, as if I was living through a bad dream. That night was spent making emergency phone calls trying to find out what was happening because there was no information. I had a lot of support from Dan and his family; we prayed the rosary all night long together. We prayed that God would take care of Anita. The next morning the doctors came in and told us Anita had made it through the evening, but it was still touch-and-go. I was shocked when I went into the room. Tubes were inside of her, IVs, multiple machines that I had no idea what they were for, lights, monitors. I could barely find Anita because her body was very swollen. I felt a feeling of helplessness, not knowing what to do. I was overcome with feelings of despair, feelings of sorrow. As fate would have it, my mother had passed away the year before and Anita was planning to take a trip on that Labor Day to see my father. But the trip was postponed because of an American Legion conference that my dad, a veteran and an avid American Legion member, wanted to attend. So, there was this anger about why things could not have been different. There was a lot of grief.

During the next few weeks, I was not really aware of what was taking place. There were many visitors and everyone was trying to understand what happened. I can recall staying up all night, sleeping on the floor, and waiting to be awakened for any news that we would have of Anita. There were many life-threatening decisions on Anita's behalf that needed to be made. She had edema, which at that time I had no idea what that was. There was pressure being caused by the cerebral spinal fluid because it was not draining properly; so we learned what edema was. It was to plague us throughout the next several months. There were several needed operations that required removing part of the brain to relieve building pressure. We learned what a shunt was—something that was where the fluid needs to drain back—and we learned what operation that was going to take. We learned what the left brain does and what the right brain does. Throughout several months we were just hoping that all parts of her body would work. We were hopeful that she would have movement on the right side of her body. We did see that, and it gave us a lot of hope that things were going to be all right and that Anita could return, by the grace of God, to the original Anita. However, many problems continued to appear. So, the hope for survival was in and out, in and out, and the prognosis changed day by day. She had good days and bad days.

Many people told us that quite often in a crisis, your emotions and intelligence do not work together. All I know is that we learned to measure gains in inches and seconds and minutes. Anita was in the hospital ICU for 9 months. Everyone was distraught; there was a lot of sadness, but the family pulled together. The many prayers and visits from my extended family were invaluable. I believe in prayer. It brought hope to our family. We had so much support: from our family, church, friends, and business associates sending cards, making visits and calls, and saying prayers. The hospital staff was supportive, especially the ICU nurses and the physicians. We had legal and financial support. We were truly blessed.

However, our family was under tremendous stress. Our family had changed. Most of the attention was on Anita. All talk was Anita. Being a husband had to go by the wayside. Though I did the best I could, being a father to all my children was sacrificed. I really did not have any idea how it would affect the other children. There was a different schedule that was imposed upon us. New schedules, new decisions, and emotions we had not experienced before. As parents, we were obligated to take care of Anita, even though she was an adult. We had a lot of bills to pay, unaware of where the money would come from. My business is commission-based and, therefore, dependent on my being in the field to produce. Because I had become an independent contractor, I no longer had health insurance with the company. Our private-pay insurance did not cover Anita since she was not a full-time student. There were going to be a lot of things that were unclear to me. There were increased workloads for everyone in the family; we were stressed to the limit. We had no idea of what was ahead of us.

So what caused the accident? I can recall the second night that I was in ICU and a police officer came and talked to me. I thought he was very considerate to find out how Anita was doing. However, that was not his intention at all. The purpose of his visit was to serve me with a ticket, intended for Anita, for running a red light. Fortunately, there was an eyewitness who revealed the truth: Anita was broadsided by a college-age drunk driver who had run a red light. He was also on drugs at the time, and unfortunately, this was his third DUI offense.

I had no idea what was going to take place as far as Anita's litigation. The physician who had done the operation asked me if I had someone in mind, and I said no. He recommended an attorney who is very good with personal injury cases. However, I did not know he was good, I had never heard of him. My mind went through many things. I was unsure who to select and what to do, so I did what I was accustomed to doing and sought out other attorneys to see what their prices would be. I was told it would not cost me anything; however, it would be one third of whatever was awarded on a contingency basis. That blew my mind. I thought, *Anita needs all of this money.* I certainly can have an appreciation in retrospect. I did look for another attorney. I described the situation and he was willing to do it for a fixed cost and a certain percentage that was lower. However, as I talked with him, he thought we could make the records look like Anita was going to school at the time and work out something with the insurance. There was a part of me that was tempted to listen to that because I was desperate to find a way to preserve as many funds as I could. Thank God, I did not hire that individual. I found a good attorney, and it has worked out well in our case.

I learned how our courts work. There was to be a criminal trial and a civil trial. The criminal trial came first, and I do not know what effect the criminal trial had on our civil trial, but it was an ordeal. I came to the conclusion that our court system was not a justice system but an injustice system. Eyewitnesses had to be sought out to put together the actual scene of the accident, and we soon discovered the drunken driver who hit Anita was out of town on a vacation. He was out on bail. He never even spent one night in jail.

It was really hard for our family to sit in a courtroom with the man who hit Anita. He showed no remorse and neither did his family. That made it hard. Not once did they come and say they were sorry or anything at all. There were so many coincidental things that happened that would literally blow me away. One of the things is that the attorney that represented the defendant was a close friend of Anita's boyfriend. He did not know that Anita was the girl who had been hit, so he took the case. He happened to be an excellent attorney and I could not believe how things could be done in a way to make the innocent look guilty. There was a young lady in the ICU who really gave a lot of care to our daughter. She worked in another hospital and was a close friend of Dan's family. She transferred to Kennestone. As fate would have it, her brother was working for the defendant. It was very emotional and distressing. After about a week of trial, the defendant decided to plead guilty. We never had a civil trial. That was settled out of court. The young man was sentenced to 5 years for a third offense, and we heard later that he was given 2 years to serve and after about 18 months was up for parole. We took an active role to ensure he served his full 2 years.

Based on the life care plan, a settlement was reached with the defendant and I was made Anita's legal guardian. I opted to select an irrevocable trust. The reason I did so is that if something happened to me, I could pretty much dictate who would be in charge of the financial affairs for Anita and also avoid temptations by either myself or anyone else to misuse those funds. I have used the trust, my attorney, and the professional rehabilitation consultant as my second conscience. The professional rehabilitation consultant/professional expert was very involved in the life care plan. It is amazing how many things he was right on target with and how important that was in supporting Anita's case.

Would Anita be better off now if she had not lived through the accident? What is her life going to be like? That almost seems unfair. There was a lot of anger in dealing with this situation and probably always will be. Will we ever totally recover from the catastrophic effects to our family, let alone Anita? Since the accident, my daughter Alyson has had to deal with much residual anger. A positive aspect is that time and being vocal has helped to dissolve much of that anger. My dad is from the old school and wanted to be a vigilante and come and shoot the drunk driver. Many times the emotions speak instead of the intelligence. Occasionally I pop in and out of that anger. Dealing with the resentment is hard, too. Why Anita? A beautiful person, a bright future, why us? My Alyson cries for the sister she lost and I grieve for my daughter.

It was becoming evident that Anita was coming to the end of her hospital stay. The people at the hospital were telling me to look for a long-term facility. That is when I started doing research and making trips. I have a whole bunch of files on everything. I went to Tennessee to Rebound and was impressed. I went to Florida to see a program they had there. I had heard about Peachtree Re-entry here in Atlanta, but I was told they would not take her. I visited Texas, but that was too far away. We settled on a facility near Birmingham, Alabama.

Because of Anita's condition at the time of transfer, she went into a Birmingham hospital and was later transferred to an Alabama facility. The quality of care went down. My gut feeling after a while was that she was not getting the care we wanted. The people seemed to be superficial. That was the feeling I got. I was advised to get a case manager. I would offer the same advice. If you are ever in a similar situation, I urge you to hire an independent person or case manager that is your advocate and not use the facility's advocate.

Our case manager expressed dissatisfaction with the treatment that Anita was receiving and suggested we visit a brain injury program in Louisiana. We asked our initial life care planer to go with us and give us his professional opinion. We liked what we saw, so we moved Anita to Louisiana. Anita made many gains at the treatment facility. In fact, the first thing she ate since her accident was a communion, which was a great sign. A minister who worked at the facility administered this holy food. That is when Anita started eating.

A new facility had opened in Atlanta and I began to investigate the possibility of Anita returning "home." With the assistance of the initial life care planner, I obtained another case manager to study this possibility. When Anita was in Louisiana, it seemed as though the accident did not happen because she was a long distance away. Although I made trips, they could only be occasional, and we had to rely on and trust the quality of care of the facility. The family visitations were strained and the family seemed to be embarrassed of being with Anita in public. The involvement was guarded, and still is, though it is gradually getting better. A lot of it has to do with each family member maturing in his or her process of acceptance, as well as everyone remembering how much fun it is to be around Anita.

I have been very pleased with the things that I have obtained in the institutional setting, but I wanted something better for our daughter. We decided Anita's quality of life would improve if she lived in her own home. We tried to work with the doctors to set up a facility. There were many conflicts of interest that came about here in Georgia with doctors recommending clients to their own facilities, and we were hopeful that there would be a home environment. In trying to check out all our options, our life care planner and I made some more investigative trips. As it happened (God does work in mysterious ways) I was aware of a friend from work who had recently been outsourced (due to corporate downsizing). In fact, I was sending her resumes out throughout Atlanta trying to help her find a position because I was so convinced of her capabilities. Lightning struck my brain: What if I could convince our friend, Mamie Walters, to come to Atlanta and help us start a new program? Have Anita come out of Meadowbrook and go into her own home? Could we do this? Could we afford paying her? I confirmed the financial feasibility. We approached Mamie with the concept and she was interested. She came to Atlanta, and it has made a phenomenal difference.

There is hope for the future. One of the things we do in our business is to make measurable gains in a reasonable amount of time. That is by charting things, charting sales. We look for behavior that is going to enhance that increase. It requires positive thinking. Mamie and Anita have positive attitudes and it is evident by the progress Anita has made. She is tipping her chart.

So what about the future? Our long-term plans include the establishment of a licensed home with a home environment. However, as one might expect, there are obstacles (or a more positive interpretation is challenges). We want a home with a family atmosphere, a high quality of life, and a healthy, natural nutritional diet for the occupants. We are trying new ideas and approaches. I always laugh when I see Mamie coming up with something new and natural and noninvasive. I am so often humbled when her alternative therapies produce great results. Certainly there are going to be changes that are going to take place as time goes on. There are also many challenges that remain.

In conclusion, I would like to emphasize how much we all have learned from Anita during this whole ordeal. She has brought deeper meaning to perseverance, faith, determination, and love. One of the things that I always have done in my life is target areas in which there is control and in which there is potential for progress. I can look and find possibilities anywhere. I also like to identify areas in which there is no control and learn how to make adjustments or accept this lack of control. This concept is captured so well in the prayer of serenity.

> God grant me the serenity to accept the things that I cannot change,
> The courage to change the things that I can, and
> The wisdom to know the difference.
>
> — *Saint Francis of Assisi*

It is this prayer that has guided me throughout this ordeal and continues to be a source of comfort to me on my journey as Anita's dad.

Mamie Walters: My Journey with Anita

I remember 1 day a contractor was building a ramp at my home for Anita, and he made the comment to me that if this accident had happened to him, he would just want to be dead. He could not see himself in this position, going through what Anita goes through and having people do for her what has to be done. My answer to him was "You don't get to be dead. You just deal with this every day. You just live with it. You have to adjust to it because you did survive." And that is what I have seen Anita do. What an inspiration she has been to me.

My children's father had passed away (1994), and it was our first holiday (Thanksgiving) without their Dad. Ray's family, being the dear family that they are, invited us to their home. We had a wonderful time. It was about 11:00 on Thanksgiving evening and just out of the blue Ray started discussing the possibility of me moving to Atlanta and working with Anita. Even though I had never worked with this type of client before, I had worked with Ray for many years and knew that we have had great success in the past in what we tried to achieve. I decided if he was willing, so was I. If it did not work out, we would both know we gave Anita our best effort and that was what really counted.

Once I made this decision, I returned to Orlando. One of the assignments Ray and I had given ourselves was to set our goals and objectives for the program and for Anita. At our next meeting, in January, we compared notes. As it turned out, our goals and objectives were almost identical, including the time frames. That was really exciting. Our original plan was to have Anita in her own home by the end of the year (1995). We actually had her home in 6 months.

I had experience in corporate forecasting for a number of years, and Ray is one of these math wizards. He also had been doing forecasting for about 30 years. We knew what we were doing. However, I believe the key to our progress was being of the same mind-set. Our singular vision allowed us to focus our energies and to be expedient in the pursuit of our goals.

One of the first things we did was to arrange for me to come to Meadowbrook and work with Anita. I did so for 6 weeks. I wanted to observe Anita's care and have some supervised hands-on experience. This observation and experience was vital in preparing for Anita's weekend visits with me. When I first began working with Anita, and the facility staff was in agreement, I noticed that Anita was very depressed. She had no initiative. Her arms were always folded and her head stayed down unless she was watching television. If she liked you, she smiled.

This was the Anita that I met. Her speech therapist said she just did not try to do any work. Her interpretation was that Anita felt like there was no reason to bother. There was not a lot of progress at Meadowbrook. We believed that there were many things that are possible in a home environment that are either not possible or practical or just not done in an institution. Ray and I were very excited about the possibilities.

In March 1995, I brought Anita home 2 days a week; in April, we increased to 3 days a week, and we continued this schedule through the end of June. I would bring her home from Friday night until Monday morning. In March, I was doing the care, the meals, everything. In April, I realized with the increase of 3 days that I might not be able to handle the care alone. My 17-year-old daughter, Ana, helped out and soon became very interested in assisting with Anita's care. Anita's total transition time from institutional care, including her hospital stay, was 7 years. She has been home for almost 2 years now (Fall 1996).

My first objective for Anita, once she was home, was to increase her self-esteem. Without high self-esteem, she had little confidence. Without confidence, she had no initiative, and so it goes. I began by giving her control. Anytime I could give her control, I did. I bought different colored sheets so she could choose what color she wanted on her bed. I gave her a TV remote and CDs to choose for music. With more choice and independence, she began to have some self-respect and self-dignity. I let her know she was loved. As we worked together she gained trust and knew the things we were doing were for her own good (even the range of motion exercises, which she hated).

One of the challenges that Anita had was to drink enough fluids. She did not drink fluids. As a result, problems occurred. We wanted to increase her fluids. She drank V-8 juice but refused water and all other drinks, except sometimes a little pineapple juice. Currently Anita is drinking approximately 30 ounces of fluid a day, and she has been doing that for quite some time, and most of this is water. She has really come a long way with positive reinforcement and increased control. We took shopping trips so she could pick out some special drinking glasses for her water. Her favorite color is green, so we went on a shopping trip for green glasses. So simple, yet so effective.

Since Anita had a brain injury, I really did not know what she was capable of doing. I knew what I had been told. I knew that there was, supposedly, no place for her to go in her rehabilitation and progress. Her dad had taught her the word *hi*, and that was all she could say for about a year. Anita had not learned how to tap into her real voice, so her voice sounded really breathy. I would take her to the computer and she enjoyed it. I experimented and knew she could read. We made it fun. She has learned to type some words strictly from memory. This was a major accomplishment for Anita.

I believe this learning became possible with self-control, self-confidence, and the initiative to work. Once she started working and saw she could actually do things, she became more confident and more enthused about continuing to work. At this time she is reading a large number of words. We have an organization skills activity where she will group flash cards using the words in categories. Her proficiency is about 85 to 90 percent, sometimes better. Anita presently has a vocabulary of about 20 different words and syllables that she speaks with her true voice. This is something I felt could happen. She has worked very hard.

Her grandfather was coming for a visit from Arizona, and Anita dearly loves her grandfather. She is crazy about him. I asked her if she would like to greet her grandfather when he arrives. She nodded that she would work with me. In working with Anita I have learned how much she loves Elvis. We would practice to Elvis music. I did not know what I was going to get. We were having fun and were working at it. She started getting the "pa pa pa pa." From this we put a short sentence together. This was a giant step for Anita because of her severe apraxia. She eventually could say "Hi, Papa" and "Bye, Papa." I wondered if she would remember this when she saw her grandfather. A few weeks went by and we kept practicing. Her grandfather arrived and she said, "Hi, Papa," and when he got ready to leave she said, "Bye, Papa." There are some things money cannot buy because they are priceless, and that moment was one of them.

One of her words she learned was *hi*. We were working on the *pie* sound and I told her if she learned the word *pie* I would take her out to get some pie. I let her order it from the waitress. Her most current word is *sly*. That is because she is in love with Sylvester Stallone. Sometimes motivation gets easier and easier. Elvis is her romantic guy and Sylvester is her macho, hero guy. I told her if she could learn *sly*, I would take her to the movies. She worked and she said it, and so we went. I think it is important that if you do offer a reward, that it is given quickly. In her case, it has kept her going.

We have a Christian home where Anita lives. I believe that the mind, spirit, and body are intricately joined to make up the human being. In working with Anita I felt like the ball had been dropped in her spirituality. This is something Ray and I wanted to address. Today she enjoys Mass. She truly gets very excited about going to Mass. She loves gospel music. We try to address the spiritual side of Anita as a holistic approach to her care. Anita is very strong in her spirit and she is a survivor. I do not require my staff to go around saying Hail Mary's all day. They do not walk around with rosaries. We only provide for spiritual requests if the client wishes. I do ask the staff to play a rosary audiotape at nighttime for Anita because this is what she likes to hear. She likes gospel music, so they put in the tapes so she can hear that. These are the ways we are addressing her spiritual life. It is the belief in the importance of balancing the mental, the physical, and the spiritual.

When Anita came back to a home environment, her family visits increased. She dearly loves her family. Her strongest bonds are with her dad, her grandfather, her aunt, and her former boyfriend, Dan, who still comes to see her. Anita is quite social now and loves their visits. She also enjoys our emphasis on games, recreational outings, and community involvement.

Our home promotes prevention. One of the strongest results of our prevention approach has been the vast improvement in Anita's health through our nutritional program. Anita was plagued with upper respiratory infections, urinary tract infections, chronic conjunctivitis, and such. Now Anita experiences very few infections. Basically, we use only real food. There are no canned goods, no processed foods; our kitchen is stocked with fresh fruits and vegetables. We have eliminated meats, dairy products, and sugars from Anita's diet. Anita does not have a problem with swelling, her circulation is good, and she has had no skin breakdown since her return home. Her attention span has increased, her energy level has increased, and her stamina has improved. This has really helped with her therapy sessions.

If I had to select one aspect of the program that is essential, it would have to be teamwork. Teamwork started with the life care plan. That was our road map for Anita. When I came on board, it was essential that I have the life care plan available because my expertise is not in the medical field. I am not a certified case manager, rehabilitation specialist, or nurse. The life care plan was and is a main reference for Anita's life care. Also, the life care plan has been key in our financial success. We provide excellent care for minimal funds. The type of care we are providing costs approximately $250 to $300 per day. This does not include doctor visits, supplies, or medications. It does include 24-hour nursing care, bed pads and briefs, personal care for the individual, housekeeping duties, recreational and occupational reinforcement, and scheduled outings. We provide better care than the larger institutions with less money for this type and level of client.

Another vital aspect of our program is staff education and staff appreciation. If I explain to the staff the importance of why things need to be done, I find the job performance is good and their attitude is positive. I believe in staff recognition. The attitude at the home and the attitude of the staff is one of respect. We respect each other, we respect the clients, and we respect the guests coming into the home. We show a lot of dignity. The staff takes pride in what they are doing because they can see the results. We try to encourage each other, we try to encourage the client and not criticize.

We find that this attitude permeates the home and affects Anita's spirit. Although she continues to receive therapies and improvements are observed, the bottom line is that Anita is home—where she belongs.

Editor's Note

Since this account was initially published, in the first edition of this book, the family has moved back to Arizona where they are closer to family. Anita continued to successfully live at "home" with high quality of life with 24-hour care for several years. Sadly, we report that she has since died. However, this story underscores the value of a dedicated and supportive family. The family, particularly the father, was thrown into a complex arena with little preparation. The event has irrevocably changed the family's and Anita's lives. Without the caring and unwavering problem-solving dedication, as well as diligent pursuit for improving Anita's life, it is unlikely that progress in her situation would have occurred.

Chapter 23

A Plaintiff's Attorney's Perspective on Life Care Planning

Katherine A. Brown-Henry

Contents

Introduction ... 641
Interactions between the Plaintiff's Attorney and the Life Care Planner ... 642
Brief Overview of a Negligence Claim ... 643
The Life Care Planner's Role in the Litigation Process ... 644
What to Expect During the Pre-Trial Proceedings ... 645
Subpoena/Subpoena Duces Tecum ... 645
Requests for Production of Documents ... 646
Depositions ... 647
What to Expect at Trial ... 648
Challenges to the Admissibility of a Life Care Planner's Testimony and Opinions ... 650
Life Care Planner's Qualifications ... 650
Challenges to the Life Care Planner's Opinions ... 651
Hearsay ... 651
Variations in Foundational Opinions ... 652
Insurance, Medicare, and Medicaid Payment Rates and Collateral Sources of Payment ... 652
Conclusion ... 653

Introduction

To an attorney, a life care plan is a litigation tool in the catastrophic injury case. For the plaintiff's attorney, a life care plan is used to identify and prove future damages related to the injuries caused by the wrongdoer. For the defendant, its value is in setting insurance reserves and evaluating the risk of a large damages award. For both sides, a life care plan is a valuable settlement tool allowing both sides to evaluate offers and make counter offers based on more than just the past medical bills and pure speculation about the future.

Catastrophic injury cases present unique challenges for the plaintiff's attorney. Since these injuries typically involve a lifetime of medical and psychological care, vocational limitations, and additional impacts on the Activities of Daily Living, the plaintiff's attorney must assemble a team of experts to address the past and future damages suffered by the injured individual. This team usually includes medical doctors and therapists, an economist, a life care planner, and (sometimes) a vocational rehabilitation consultant.

Some plaintiff attorneys are better than others at coordinating their team of damage experts. Plaintiff attorneys come in all levels of experience and specialization. Some are the "jack of all trades" attorneys that handle everything from divorces to criminal cases to car crashes. Others specialize in a particular area of the law, like medical malpractice. Likewise, plaintiff attorneys come with varying levels of knowledge when it comes to working with life care planners. Some understand better than others what goes into creating a credible life care plan that can withstand the attacks of a defense attorney. Keeping that in mind, the goal of this chapter is to provide the life care planner with an overview of his/her role on the plaintiff's team of damage experts throughout the litigation process.

Interactions between the Plaintiff's Attorney and the Life Care Planner

When the plaintiff's attorney determines that a life care plan would benefit a case, the attorney should be responsible for making sure that the life care planner has adequate information to create the life care plan. Typically, this includes providing the life care planner with the injured individual's past medical records and bills. The attorney may also provide the life care planner with the depositions of the injured individual and his/her parents, spouse or children, as well as the depositions and reports his/her health care providers or other damages experts.

After reviewing the information provided by the attorney, the life care planner should work with the plaintiff's attorney to set up any meetings or phone calls with the injured individual and his/her family members, caregivers, and health care providers. If the life care planner sends out questionnaires to the health care providers, copies of any responses should be provided to the retaining attorney. The retaining attorney may eventually need to disclose these communications to the other side, and the attorney will want to track those communications for that purpose.

If the medical records or bills are incomplete, the life care planner will want to make arrangements with the attorney on who will be responsible for obtaining those documents. If the life care planner obtains any medical records or bills, he/she should provide a complete copy of the records to the retaining attorney. The documents considered by the life care planner in forming the life care plan may need to be disclosed to the opposing side.

The retaining attorney may seek input from the life care planner to determine if he/she needs to engage any additional damages experts. This typically occurs when the life care planner cannot independently give opinions about future medical, psychological, and vocational items that need to be included in a life care plan.*

* Some life care planners, based on their education, experience, and training are capable of making opinions other life care planners cannot. For example, a life care planner with a degree in vocational rehabilitation may be qualified to give opinions on future vocational needs, while a life care planner with a medical background would be unqualified to make such opinions.

The life care planner is responsible for preparing his/her opinions. The retaining attorney is responsible for making sure the opinions are admitted at trial. The attorney cannot assume that the life care planner understands the formality of the legal system. Every jurisdiction has its own set of legal constraints that must be addressed by the plaintiff's attorney. The plaintiff's attorney must also make sure that the life care planner is both qualified to give an expert opinion and that there is an adequate evidentiary foundation for the life care plan. There have been cases where the entire plan was thrown out, and the award with it, because the life care planner included medical expert opinions that were not given by a qualified physician.* On the other hand, other courts have recognized the admissibility of a life care planner's testimony when it reflects his/her training and expertise in projecting the costs of future treatments and procedures based on the facts from the medical records and opinions received from the physicians.† Therefore, a life care planner is expected and should be able to explain the source of each and every opinion contained in the life care plan. The best life care plans extensively footnote the source of information contained therein.

Brief Overview of a Negligence Claim

A life care planner is typically retained in negligence claims.‡ Negligence claims are sometimes referred to as "torts,"§ and the negligent party is sometimes referred to as the "tortfeasor." There are several different types of negligence claims, including medical malpractice, products liability, worker's compensation, premises liability, and so on. Regardless of the type of negligence claim, every claim for negligence alleges the failure to use reasonable care, which results in damage or injury to another. A person, company, or entity may be negligent by acting or by failing to act. When an individual is injured due to the negligence of another, he/she may bring a claim for compensation against the wrongdoer who caused those injuries.

There are two areas that every attorney must address in a negligence claim: proof of liability and demonstration of damages. Liability refers to whether or not a defendant was negligent and therefore a responsible cause of a plaintiff's injuries, harms, and losses. Damages refer to the amount of money that will fairly compensate a plaintiff. A plaintiff has the burden of proving both liability and damages.

Part of the damages a plaintiff is entitled to recover is his/her reasonable and necessary medical expenses. But "estimates of future medical charges are not as reliable as medical bills already incurred because the amount of future medical charges is usually debatable as to both the probability of the need for the treatment and the method of estimating its future cost."¶ Expert testimony is needed

---

* *Diamond R. Fertilizer v. Davis*, 567 So. 2d 451, 455 (Fla. Dist. Ct. App. 1990)(A rehabilitation counselor/life care planner established a program for medical treatment which would give her the discretion to oversee and supervise claimant's medical and nursing care. The court found that responsibility for establishing a treatment plan rests with a claimant's authorized physicians.)

† *Dan Cristiani Excavating Co. v. Money*, 941 N.E.2d 1072 (Ind. Ct. App. 2011)(" [The life care planner's] expertise was in compiling the reports and opinions of physicians to convey estimates and future projections based on facts and opinions she received from [the plaintiff's] doctors and her research and experience with medical costs. [The life care planner's] expertise was in estimating the costs of the treatments and procedures that the doctors told her about, described in their reports, or disclosed in their depositions. She did not attempt to craft a medical opinion, and the trial record is clear in this regard.")

‡ Other claims in which an attorney may retain a life care planner typically involve a division of assets between parties, such as a divorce.

§ Torts also encompass claims of fraud, libel, slander, battery, and assault.

¶ *Cook v. Whitsell-Sherman*, 796 N.E.2d 271, 278 (Ind. 2003).

to address the future medical damages because a judge or jury may not award damages on the mere basis of conjecture or speculation. Thus, the need for a life care plan.

The Life Care Planner's Role in the Litigation Process

The parties have two different methods available to resolve a negligence claim, through settlement or a trial. Sometimes settlements occur without having to initiate litigation. During pre-litigation settlement proceedings, an insurance adjustor and/or an attorney may represent the wrongdoer. There are no expert disclosure rules or rules preventing an opposing party from contacting a life care planner in pre-litigation proceedings. Therefore, a life care planner who has been brought in during the pre-litigation stage should establish a clear understanding with the retaining attorney if your identity or opinions will be disclosed and what contact is acceptable.

Once a lawsuit is filed, formal litigation has commenced, but a settlement can still occur. Often, the court will require the parties to attend mediation, where a neutral third-party attorney or judge (called a "mediator") will work with the parties to facilitate settlement negotiations. At mediation, the attorneys, insurance adjusters with settlement authority, and the parties are all present at one location to discuss settlement. Sometimes, financial advisors and lienholders may also be present. In catastrophic injury cases, the life care plan is a big part of the mediation discussions. It is used as a way of evaluating the value of the case and how to best allocate the available money with regards to negotiating how to pay lienholders while still considering that money has to be set aside for future damages.

When the parties cannot reach a settlement agreement, a judge or jury ends up making the decision for the parties. Before the parties see the inside of a courtroom, the parties must adhere to the typical pre-trial procedures and deadlines. The parties engage in discovery, which includes the exchange of information, photos, videos, and documents. Discovery can also include depositions. At a deposition, an attorney will question the deponent (usually a person who is a party to the lawsuit, a witness, or expert for the opposite side) under oath and a court reporter will take down a transcript of the questions and answers. The court usually requires the parties to finish discovery by a certain date and may set other deadlines, including deadlines to disclose the identity and opinions of any expert witnesses. Life care planners may be asked to be deposed or produce documents and will have to adhere to any expert disclosure deadlines set by the court.

At trial, the plaintiff must present expert testimony of future damages that is both helpful to the judge or jury and admissible into evidence. The life care planner will be brought to trial to explain the life care plan methodology, his/her credentials as a life care planner, and the specific plan developed for the catastrophically injured plaintiff. The opposing party's attorney will get the opportunity to attack the life care planner's testimony and the substance of the life care plan through cross-examination. After the parties have presented their cases, the judge or jury will decide whether or not the plaintiff is entitled to damages and the total amount of those damages.

There is a lot of uncertainty that comes with a trial. The common fear of the plaintiff's attorney is that the money award in the verdict (if any) will not be enough to care for the catastrophically injured client for the rest of his/her life. When there is insufficient money to fully compensate the injured individual, the life care planner may also be involved in the post-settlement or post-litigation proceedings on how to best allocate the money recovered. For example, many catastrophically injured individuals end up on Medicare, either due to the disability or age. The *Medicare Secondary Payer Act* requires the injured individual to consider Medicare's interests when it comes to the allocation and distribution of funds obtained by settlement or a judgment in a negligence claim.* This includes considering Medicare's interests when it comes to the payment of anticipated future treatment. The aim of this requirement is to prevent an injured individual from shifting the responsibility for payment of medical expenses from a primary payer (e.g., defendant's insurance policy) to Medicare. The life care planner may be asked to identify which items fall within the purview of Medicare's interests.†

What to Expect During the Pre-Trial Proceedings

Frequently, there are case management orders or rules of trial procedure that govern the pre-trial proceedings of a case. While these orders and rules vary from court to court, a life care planner can generally expect expert disclosure deadlines and requirements. For example, our federal courts require all testifying experts to produce final reports (draft reports are protected from disclosure), certain expert-attorney communications, a list of all cases where the expert has testified at trial or by deposition during the previous 4 years, a list of qualifications, including a list of all publications authored in the past 10 years, and a statement of the compensation to be paid for the expert's services.‡

Life care planners are subject to court-authorized discovery. There are usually deadlines for the parties to complete discovery, commonly referred to as the discovery cut-off date. If discovery is attempted after the deadline has passed, the recipient may not have to respond to the discovery. There are generally two types of discovery that a life care planner is subject to: requests for production of documents and depositions. A life care planner is compelled to comply with requests for production of documents or to attend depositions through the use of the subpoena.

Subpoena/Subpoena Duces Tecum

During the pre-trial proceedings, the opposing party uses subpoenas to compel the life care planner to sit for a deposition or produce documents. A subpoena can also be used to compel a life care planner to testify at trial. A subpoena that compels a witness to appear and give testimony is a *subpoena ad testificandum*, but it is typically just called a subpoena. A subpoena that compels a witness to appear and to bring specified documents is a *subpoena duces tecum*.§ It is not unusual for a life care planner to simultaneously receive both subpoenas so that the life care planner can be questioned about the documents produced during the deposition.

Subpoenas and subpoenas duces tecum should not be ignored. The term "subpoena" is Latin for "under penalty," and a life care planner is subject to court-ordered penalties if there is a failure to comply with a subpoena. Questions about the validity of a subpoena should be addressed to the attorney who retained the life care planner's services.

A quick word about testifying versus non-testifying experts. Just because a life care planner has been retained by an attorney or produced a report, that does not mean that the life care planner is subject to discovery. It is only after the retaining attorney has disclosed to the opposing party that he/she intends to offer the life care planner as a testifying witness at trial that the opposing party has the right to discovery. There is a limited exception to this rule. An opposing party can

* 42 U.S.C. § 1395y(b)(2).
† 42 U.S.C. § 1395(a).
‡ Fed. Rules of Civil Procedure, Rule 26(a)(2)(B) and 26(b)(4).
§ "Subpoena," *Black's Law Dictionary* (10th ed. 2014).

discover the facts known or opinions held by a life care planner upon the showing of exceptional circumstances under which it is impracticable for the party to obtain the facts and opinions on the same subject by other means. A subpoena issued to a life care planner who has not been disclosed as a testifying expert should be immediately brought to the attention of the retaining attorney.

Requests for Production of Documents

Subpoenas duces tecum may list the documents requested in the subpoena or may be accompanied by a separate request for production of documents. These requests for production may specify a date, time, and location for the life care planner to appear with the requested documents so that the opposing party can inspect and copy those documents. Alternatively, the request for production may require that copies of the documents be provided by a certain date, typically 30 days after the requests were served on the life care planner.*

The federal courts and most state courts require the opposing party to give the plaintiff's attorney advanced notice (sometimes called a "warning shot") when it intends to serve requests for production of documents on a life care planner. This notice is typically given 15 days prior to sending the requests to the life care planner. This allows the plaintiff's attorney time to dispute the scope of the requests or seek court intervention to quash or modify the subpoena if necessary.

Many jurisdictions also provide that the life care planner is entitled the reasonable costs of production. If the subpoena requests copies of documents, the reasonable costs typically include a reasonable copying fee and a reasonable fee for the time it took the life care planner to respond to the requests for production. If the subpoena compels the attendance of the life care planner, then the life care planner is usually entitled to a reasonable fee for the time it took to gather the documents and attend the request for production. It may also include mileage or reasonable travel expenses. Note that the federal courts require that the location for the production of the documents cannot be more than 100 miles from where the life care planner resides, is employed, or regularly transacts business in person.†

Requests for production of documents are not unlimited. There may be court orders or rules of procedure that limit the scope of discovery. For example, the Federal Rules of Civil Procedure were amended in 2010 regarding the scope of expert witness discovery. Under the current federal rules, an opposing party cannot obtain copies of draft reports. The opposing party is only entitled to a copy of the final report. Also, an opposing party cannot obtain copies of any documents reflecting communications between the retaining attorney and the life care planner, except for communications (1) related to the amount of compensation to be paid to the expert, (2) that identify facts or data that the retaining attorney provided and that the expert considered in forming his/her opinions, and (3) that identify any assumptions that the retaining attorney provided and the expert relied on in forming his/her opinions.‡ On the other hand, many state courts still provide that all communications between the attorney and life care planner are discoverable.

Privileged documents may also be excluded from production. If documents are withheld due to a claim of privilege or other protection, then the claim must be expressly made in the response to the request for production of documents. The life care planner may also have to give a short description of the nature of the withheld documents or communications in a manner that

* The date of service is the date that the requests are sent, not the day they are received. Most courts permit an extension of 3 days if the service is done by mail.

† Fed. Rule of Civil Procedure 45(c)(2).

‡ Fed. Rule of Civil Procedure 26(b)(4).

will enable the parties to assess the claim but without revealing information that is privileged or protected.* Any questions regarding the limits on expert production should be addressed with the retaining attorney.

Depositions

A deposition is nothing more than a formal exchange of questions and answers between the deposing attorney and the life care planner. A court reporter is always present to take down a transcript of the questions, answers, and any objections. A videographer may also be present. Any attorneys for the parties are permitted to attend and ask questions as well. The plaintiff(s) or defendant(s) may also be present, but this is uncommon. Some of the parties may not be physically present in the room but may be appearing by video teleconference or by phone. Some courts place time limits on depositions. In federal court, a deposition is limited to 1 day of 7 hours, unless the court permits additional time.†

A word about depositions that are videotaped. During the deposition, it is common for the life care planner to want to be engaged with the questioner. This leads to videos of life care planners who appear to be looking off to the side the entire deposition. The problem with these videos is that the audience may view the life care planner as avoiding the camera for some insidious reason. If there is any chance that the deposition is being videoed for the purpose of being used at trial, make sure to speak to the camera the same way you would speak to a jury from the stand.

There are typically two kinds of depositions that a life care planner will encounter: a "discovery" deposition or an "evidentiary" deposition. The "discovery" deposition is called by the opposing side. During these depositions, the opposing party is questioning the life care planner about his/her educational background, experience, and training, as well as the methodology used and the opinions reached by the life care planner. The opposing attorney will seek to learn what documents were reviewed, if any independent research was conducted, what communications took place with the injured individual, his/her family, caregivers, and health care providers, and any communications or opinions from other experts that the life care planner relied upon in developing the life care plan.

Prior to the life care planner's deposition, the retaining attorney may want to speak with the life care planner about his/her anticipated testimony. The substance of those conversations may be discoverable by the opposing side. There will also likely be questions about how much money the life care planner is being paid for his/her work, how often the life care planner has worked for the retaining attorney, how often the life care planner works for plaintiffs versus defendants, how the retaining attorney found the life care planner, how many cases and states the life care planner has testified in. Don't be surprised if requested to name past cases and other attorneys who have worked with the life care planner. The life care planner's report, especially any options included in the tables, may be discussed in detail. Be prepared for questions about how much insurance, Medicare, or Medicaid may affect the cost totals and why the tables utilize private pay costs.

The retaining attorney may or may not ask questions during a discovery deposition. If there are objections, they are stated for the record, but a judge is not present to rule on them. The life care planner will still respond to the objected question unless the objection is based on a privilege and the life care planner is instructed not to answer the question.

"Evidentiary" depositions are taken when the life care planner will be unable to attend a scheduled trial. The questioning is done in the same manner as actual trial testimony. Again, any

* See, for example, Fed. Rule of Civil Procedure 45(e)(2).
† Fed. Rule of Civil Procedure 30(d)(1).

objections are stated for the record and the life care planner still provides an answer regardless of the objection, unless a privilege is asserted. If the judge later rules that the objection is valid, that portion of the deposition is not presented to the jury. If there are exhibits that will be admitted during the life care planner's testimony, the attorney will typically go through the formal requests to admit the evidence in front of the court reporter even though the judge will later rule on the admissibility.

After the deposition has ended, the life care planner will be given the option to read the deposition to make sure that the court reporter accurately transcribed the life care planner's testimony. If the life care planner elects to read the deposition, he/she will be given 30 days to do so. Although many experts routinely waive reading and signing, it is recommended that one read and sign their sworn testimony for at least two reasons. The first reason is that occasionally court reporting errors occur which can change the intended testimony. For example, if the deponent is asked whether he/she contacted defense medical experts in the development of the plan and the answer is, "I did not contact defense medical experts," but it is recorded with the word "not" missing, that is, "I did contact defense medical experts." Another reason is to make sure the expert has a copy of their deposition in order to re-read prior to courtroom testimony to refresh one's memory. It is not uncommon for opposing attorneys at trial to quote from the expert's deposition with a slight twist or change of context which could compromise his or her testimony. When the expert elects to read and sign, an errata sheet is provided, and the life care planner will list any corrections to the transcript on it, state the reason for the correction, and then sign the errata sheet. A life care planner cannot materially change his/her testimony or add to his/her prior answers through an errata sheet. If this occurs, the courts typically allow an additional deposition to address the changed answers.

What to Expect at Trial

First and foremost, be prepared for the trial schedule to change. The dates of the trial may be postponed, or the attorney's presentation of evidence schedule may change. Attorneys aren't always the best at keeping experts updated on the trial schedule and appreciate it when the life care planner checks in on approaching trial dates. Once it is decided that the trial will proceed as scheduled, the retaining attorney (or his/her staff) will work with the life care planner to arrange a date and time for the life care planner's testimony. Flexibility in this scheduling is appreciated. The order of witnesses may change due to the availability of the witnesses and depending on how quickly the trial is actually proceeding.

If there has been a significant amount of time that has elapsed since the life care planner prepared the plan and the trial date, the life care planner should discuss updating his/her opinions with the retaining attorney. This will need to be done in advance of trial so that the retaining attorney can timely disclose any changes to the life care plan to opposing counsel. Also, the retaining attorney will work with the life care planner before his/her testimony to go over his/her anticipated testimony, any anticipated defense questions or challenges to the admissibility of the life care planner's testimony, and any orders of the court which may limit the life care planner's testimony.*

Some attorneys or life care planners like to use visuals during the life care planner's testimony. Visuals are a great way to help the jurors visualize the needs of the injured plaintiff. It makes the

* The courts often enter orders in limine, which are orders that limit or prevent certain testimony or evidence from being presented during trial.

testimony more interesting and helps keep the jurors from tuning out. Showing pictures of the durable medical equipment or home modifications can give the jurors a good idea of the challenges the injured individual faces when it comes to mobility issues or dealing with previously simple Activities of Daily Living. Blowups of the life care planning tables may be used to help guide the life care planner's testimony. Many courts require that these visuals must be disclosed to the opposing side prior to trial. The retaining attorney should discuss any visuals necessary for the life care planner's testimony well in advance of that testimony, or the risk is that the jury will never see the visuals.

There may or may not be a separation of witnesses order in place for the trial. This type of order means that the witnesses cannot sit in the courtroom and hear the testimony of other witnesses. If a life care planner is unsure of whether this type of order has been entered, the best bet is to wait in the hallway outside of the courtroom until called to give testimony.

Once the life care planner's name has been called to give testimony, the life care planner will be directed to the witness box. The judge will swear the life care planner in and may ask the life care planner to state his/her name and spell it for the record. If a break is called while the life care planner is still giving testimony, some courts hold that the attorney cannot speak with the life care planner regarding the substance of the testimony during breaks. Some attorneys will not speak with the life care planner during breaks just to make sure there isn't the look of impropriety.

Direct examination is conducted by the retaining attorney. The attorney will have to go through the legal formalities in order for the judge to recognize the life care planner as an expert. Expect direct examination to go through the life care planner's education, experience, and training, followed by an explanation of the purpose of life care plans in general before going into the specific opinions and details of the life care plan crafted for the injured plaintiff.

If the opposing side challenges the admissibility of all or part of the life care planner's testimony at trial, then the plaintiff's attorney may have to conduct an "offer of proof." In this scenario, the jury is taken out of the courtroom. The plaintiff's attorney will elicit testimony from the life care planner he/she intends to offer the jury and provide the judge with an explanation why the attorney believes the testimony is admissible. If the judge rules that the evidence is admissible, then the jury will be permitted to hear the testimony. If not, then the life care planner will not be able to testify about the excluded opinions before the jury.

The opposing side may also make other objections during the life care planner's testimony. If the judge *sustains* the objection, then the life care planner cannot answer the objectionable question. If the judge *overrules* the objection, the life care planner can answer the question.

After direct examination concludes, the opposing party has the opportunity to cross-examine the life care planner. Cross-examination is used to create doubt about an expert's testimony. Cross-examination usually comes in the form of leading questions that only seek a "yes" or "no" answer. Carefully listen to these questions and think about them before responding. The opposing attorney may attempt to misconstrue the life care planner's testimony or inadvertently misstate the facts. If "yes" or "no" does not accurately answer the question, feel free to explain the response. It may be difficult, but it is best to be courteous to the opposing attorney, even though questions may be asked with an inflection meant to rouse a negative emotional response. This is likely just part of the show for the jury, and your reaction is how the jury will judge your credibility at the end of the day.

It is not unusual for a discovery deposition or testimony from another case to be used by the opposing attorney during trial to "impeach" or discredit the life care planner. This occurs when the opposing party wants to point out facts that reflect poorly on the life care planner's credibility, inconsistencies with the life care planner's testimony, and any other evidence that reflects negatively on the life care planner's truthfulness or knowledge. The opposing party attempts impeachment by pointing out inconsistencies between the life care planner's discovery deposition and his/her trial testimony. He/she may also attempt to point out inconsistencies with the life care planner's past testimony in an entirely different case, with the methodology used by the life care planner, or with the authoritative writings of other life care planning experts.

The opposing party may also attempt to impeach the life care planner by pointing out some perceived bias. When a life care planner repeatedly works for the same attorney, the bias is that the life care planner gives the attorney what he/she wants to hear so that the life care planner will get repeat business. There is also a perceived bias when the life care planner only does work for plaintiffs. There is also the "hired gun" perception when all the life care planner does for his/her income is offer expert opinions for litigation purposes. There are many techniques that a life care planner can learn on how to deal with these impeachment challenges, but the best ones are honesty, consistency with the methodology, remaining objective, and refusing to be an advocate for one side or another.

Challenges to the Admissibility of a Life Care Planner's Testimony and Opinions

In order for the life care planner's testimony to even be heard by a jury, a judge has to determine that it is admissible in evidence. As an expert witness, the life care planner must qualify as such under the evidence rules in order to give expert testimony and opinions. Under the Federal Rules of Evidence, this includes Federal Rules of Evidence 702-705. The state courts all have their own rules of evidence, but state court evidence rules on expert testimony are typically similar to or mirror the federal rules. The retaining attorney can discuss the evidence rules and admissibility standards for expert testimony in his/her particular jurisdiction.

Life Care Planner's Qualifications

When there is a challenge to the qualifications of an expert to state an opinion, the trial court judge acts as a "gatekeeper." The judge determines if the expert is qualified to give the opinions and if the expert testimony is relevant and reliable.* Federal Rule of Evidence 702 is the rule concerning the qualifications of an expert to give an opinion. An expert witness qualifies as such based on his/her knowledge, skill, experience, training, or education. The expert is permitted to testify if:

1. The expert's scientific, technical, or other specialized knowledge will help the trier of fact (e.g., jury) to understand the evidence or determine a fact in issue;
2. The testimony is based on sufficient facts or data;
3. The testimony is the product of reliable principles and methods; and
4. The expert has reliably applied the principles and methods to the facts of the case.†

Daubert v. Merrell Dow Pharmaceuticals, Inc., concerns the application of Federal Rule of Evidence 702. It lays out a non-exhaustive list of factors that may be relevant in assessing the reliability of *scientific evidence*, including whether the theory or technique can be and has been tested, whether the theory has been subjected to peer review and publication, whether there is a known or

* *Conroy v. Vilsack*, 707 F.3d 1163 (10th Cir. 2013).

† This is the federal standard. State standards may differ.

potential error rate, and whether the theory has been generally accepted within the relevant field of study.* *Kumho Tire Co. v. Carmichael* expanded the applicability of *Daubert* to all types of expert testimony under Federal Rule of Evidence 702, including the testimony of a life care planner.†

A challenge to a life care planner's qualifications will likely be based on the education and training. If the life care planner lacks sufficient education to give an opinion, then that opinion may be excluded. All or part of the opinions may be excluded. Likewise, if it is found that the life care planner does not have sufficient training and experience in life care planning, the opinion may be excluded. Certifications in life care planning help obviate these types of challenges.

A word of caution: just because a life care planner thinks he/she is qualified to give an opinion does not mean that a judge will agree. Problems occur when life care planners give opinions regarding future medical needs without a sufficient medical education/background to give those opinions or who give vocational opinions without an educational background in vocational rehabilitation or consulting.

Challenges to the Life Care Planner's Opinions

Even when properly qualified to give an expert opinion, a life care planner's opinions may be excluded on other evidentiary grounds. These evidentiary challenges focus on the foundation for the opinions. In other words, whether the records and opinions relied upon by the life care planner are adequate.

Hearsay

A common challenge to a life care planner's testimony is that the life care plan is an impermissible attempt to insert hearsay into the trial. "Hearsay" is an out-of-court statement made by another, which is offered as evidence in a trial to prove the truth of the matter asserted in the statement.‡ Think of the game of telephone. If A tells B the light was red, B's attempt to convince a jury the light was red because A said so is an attempt to use hearsay. Hearsay is inadmissible unless it meets an exception under the evidentiary rules.§

Federal Rule of Evidence 703¶ permits a testifying expert to base an opinion on otherwise inadmissible facts or data that the expert has been made aware of *if* experts in the same field would reasonably rely on those kinds of facts or data in forming an opinion on the subject. It does not matter if the facts or data constitute hearsay or inadmissible evidence in this scenario. However, the expert cannot disclose the inadmissible facts or data to the jury unless the probative value in

---

* *Daubert v. Merrell Dow Pharmaceuticals, Inc.*, 509 U.S. 579, 113 S.Ct. 2786, 125 L.Ed.2d 469 (1993); *Turner v. State*, 953 N.E.2d 1039, 1048 (Ind. 2011); *Ervin v. Johnson & Johnson, Inc.*, 492 F.3d 901, 904 (7th Cir. 2007).

† *Kumho Tire Co. v. Carmichael*, 526 U.S. 137, 119 S. Ct. 1167, 143 L. Ed. 2d 238 (1999); *North v. Ford Motor Co.*, 505 F. Supp. 2d 1113, 1120 (D. Utah 2007).

‡ Fed. Rule of Evidence 801.

§ Fed. Rules of Evidence 802-804.

¶ Federal Rule of Evidence 703 states: An expert may base an opinion on facts or data in the case that the expert has been made aware of or personally observed. If experts in the particular field would reasonably rely on those kinds of facts or data in forming an opinion on the subject, they need not be admissible for the opinion to be admitted. But if the facts or data would otherwise be inadmissible, the proponent of the opinion may disclose them to the jury only if their probative value in helping the jury evaluate the opinion substantially outweighs their prejudicial effect.

helping the jury to evaluate the opinion substantially outweighs the prejudicial effect of having the jury hear otherwise inadmissible evidence.

A life care planner cannot testify about hearsay conversations with the injured plaintiff, his/her family member, caregivers, and health care providers to prove the truth of the matter asserted by those individuals, but they can be referenced by the life care planner in explaining the foundation for the life care plan opinions. For example, a life care planner can explain an opinion for the inclusion of a standing wheelchair for a quadriplegic based on conversations with the injured plaintiff and the recommendation of his/her physicians. Likewise, the pricing guides or calls to durable medical equipment providers would typically constitute inadmissible hearsay but can be referenced to explain the foundation for the pricing of items in a life care plan. The key is to explain that all life care planners rely on this type of hearsay information in formulating their opinions because that is the accepted methodology.

Variations in Foundational Opinions

It is not unusual for a defendant in a catastrophic injury case to retain physicians or other types of experts to opine on the plaintiff's injuries. Those experts typically will be disclosed when their opinions differ from the plaintiff's expert opinions. The life care planner should be made aware of any divergent expert opinions by the retaining attorney and should be prepared to discuss how the divergent opinions would affect the opinions contained in the life care plan.

A typical foundational challenge to a life care plan is based on a reduced life expectancy when the life care planner relies on the U.S. Life Tables for life expectancy. There may also be challenges to the foundation of the opinions based on a pre-existing condition of the injured individual. The life care planner should be prepared to discuss these variations and what, if any, impact the variations have on the life care planner's opinions.

Insurance, Medicare, and Medicaid Payment Rates and Collateral Sources of Payment

Another common challenge is to the costs associated with each item included in the life care plan tables. Insurance companies negotiate the amounts they will pay for medical services with each health care provider. Medicare and Medicaid set rates for payment of health care services. The amount that an insurance company, Medicare, or Medicaid pays likely varies from the private pay rate actually charged to the patient. The difference between the amount charged and the amount paid is called a write-off or adjustment. When it comes to past medical bills, some states permit the jury to hear evidence of the discounted rates, while others do not. Three states permit evidence of both the amount charged and the amount accepted.*

Since the disparities in the amounts charged and amounts paid may equal thousands of dollars when applied to a life care plan, defendants commonly argue that the life care planner must take into account the availability of insurance or public assistance when calculating the costs listed in a life care plan. The defense argues that a life care plan that only uses private pay costs does not reflect the actual value of any future medical expense. Therefore, the life care plan lacks foundation and reliability.

The passage of the *Patient Protection and Affordable Care Act* ("the ACA") in 2010 has bolstered this argument. Beginning in 2012, economists and defense attorneys focused on the ACA as a new

* *Patchett v. Lee*, 60 N.E.3d 1025, 1032 (Ind. 2016).

defense to a plaintiff's damages. Their position was simple. Under the ACA, an injured individual cannot be denied health insurance based on preexisting conditions,* including the conditions underlying their claim for damages against a tortfeasor. Therefore, the plaintiff's damages should be limited to their out of pocket expenses in purchasing the mandatory insurance coverage required by the ACA.† Defendants support their position by claiming that plaintiffs fail to mitigate their damages‡ if a life care plan does not account for health insurance coverage. Plaintiffs argue that the collateral source rule§ precludes discussions of private insurance in damage calculations.

The problem with the ACA is the same problem life care planners have faced when considering whether to use insurance, Medicare, or Medicaid rates in their calculations. There is no easy way to predict what coverage will be available to the injured individual or if the ACA will still be in existence in the foreseeable future. Also, it's called the insurance mandate, but an individual can always just elect to take the tax penalty instead.¶ The speculative nature regarding the continued existence of the ACA led one judge to remark:

> It would be an extremely unfair and prejudicial hardship on the plaintiff should he prevail on his claim against the defendants, and recover damages reduced on account of potential future ACA benefits, only to find that later he does not receive all such benefits that the jury considered. It is simply too speculative to determine whether and how much benefits [the plaintiff] will receive from an ACA insurer to permit the defendant to introduce such evidence for the purpose of persuading the jury to reduce the damages.**

The states have split decisions on whether or not information regarding ACA coverage comes into evidence. At least six states have permitted a life care plan's costs to be challenged or reduced based on the availability of ACA coverage or Medicare coverage. The life care planner should discuss with the retaining attorney if this type of evidence is permissible in the court where the case is proceeding. If so, the life care planner may be expected to delineate what items fall under the ACA coverage.

Conclusion

Due to the complex nature of catastrophic injury cases, the plaintiff's attorney will have to determine whether or not a life care planner's expertise will benefit the case. Listing the plaintiff's future medical, psychological, and rehabilitation needs through the life care plan not only provides an overview of the anticipated needs of the injured individual, but also helps establish a powerful base for other damages claims, such as claims for pain and suffering, loss of enjoyment of life, and

* 42 U.S.C. § 300gg-3.

† Congdon-Homan, Joshua, et.al. "Potential Effects of the Affordable Care Act on the Award of Life Care Expenses." College of Holy Cross, Department of Economics Faculty Research Series, Paper. 12-01 (Sept. 2012).

‡ Mitigation of damages is a legal doctrine wherein a jury can reduce the plaintiff's final damages award based on the plaintiff's failure to use reasonable care to avoid incurring an additional injury or loss.

§ The "collateral source rule" is a legal doctrine which prohibited defendants from introducing evidence concerning compensation received by the plaintiff from sources other than the defendant, such as insurance or worker's compensation. Some states have statutes which lay out exceptions to the collateral source rule.

¶ 42 U.S.C. § 5000A.

** *Dohl v. Sunrise Mountainview Hosp., Inc.*, 2015 WL 1953074 (Nev.Dist.Ct.).

the spouse's claim for lost services, love, and affection. When used in conjunction with the medical experts, vocational experts, and economic experts, the life care planner's report becomes part of a comprehensive presentation of the damages evidence.

It takes a coordinated effort between the plaintiff's attorney and the life care planner to ensure that the life care plan is accurate, reliable, and admissible into evidence. A well-designed, individualized life care plan paints a powerful picture regarding the injured individual's future. When properly presented by the plaintiff's attorney, the life care plan becomes a powerful tool of persuasion, whether persuading the defense to settle the case or persuading a jury to award a fair amount of damages.

Chapter 24

A Defense Attorney's Perspective on Life Care Planning

Tracy Raffles Gunn*

Contents

Introduction....655
Attacking the Plaintiff's Life Care Plan Qualifications....656
Qualifications as a Life Care Planning Expert Generally....656
Qualification to Present the Particular Life Care Plan....657
Foundational Objections, the *Daubert* Standard, and Other Preclusions....659
Cross-Examination of the Plaintiff's Expert....660
Financial Bias....661
Purpose of Retention....662
The Basis of the Opinions....662
Base Costing and Duplication....663
Application of the Collateral Source Rule....663
Licensing Issues....664
The Decision to Retain a Defense Rehabilitation Consultant....665
The Testifying Defendant Rehabilitation Consultant....666
Practical Considerations: The Effect on the Jury....668
Conclusion....668

Introduction

This chapter will address the defense perspective on life care planning. The basic purpose of a life care plan in personal injury cases is to assist in proof of the future cost of plaintiff's care

* Much of the information for this chapter appeared in the Second Edition chapter co-authored by Tracy Gunn and Lee Gunn.

and treatment. The plan is an efficient method for presenting this evidence since it consolidates future costs into a singular report. The plan is presented and explained to the jury by the life care planner as expert testimony.* The explanation of each feature of the plan allows the life care planner an opportunity to reinforce the extent of injury and associated impact on the plaintiff's life. An economic expert is able to "price" a life care plan which provides competent evidence supporting a jury verdict. A defendant must prepare opposition to the plaintiff's plan by evaluating the credentials of the life care planner, the foundation for necessity and reasonableness of each plan element, and the scope of the plan for inclusion of only legally recoverable damages. Effective cross-examination may demonstrate overreaching and cast a shadow of greediness over the plaintiff's case. In some cases, presentation of a defense plan may also be appropriate.

Attacking the Plaintiff's Life Care Plan Qualifications

The first step in attacking the plaintiff's life care plan is to determine whether the plaintiff's life care planner is, in fact, qualified to present the plan. This is a critical issue because an unqualified witness will not be accepted as an expert and will not be permitted to testify at trial. Thus, a successful attack on the plaintiff's life care planner's qualifications may remove the plan and associated economic cost from the jury's consideration.

There are two levels of qualification that will be required of a life care expert presenting a life care plan. First, the expert must be qualified generally in the area of life care planning. Second, the expert must be qualified to substantiate each element of the plan to the degree required under the particular jurisdiction's substantive law.

Qualifications as a Life Care Planning Expert Generally

Under the Federal Rules of Evidence,† an expert witness is qualified by reason of "knowledge, skill, experience, training, or education."‡ The use of the disjunctive "or" in this list of the grounds for determining a proposed expert's qualification has been consistently held to permit qualification as an expert based on any one of these five factors. Thus, a properly qualified expert may have no practical experience in the particular area about which he or she testifies.§ Similarly, a witness may qualify as an expert in a field in which he or she has no formal training, education, degree, or

* The Federal Rules of Evidence apply only in federal courts, and different requirements may apply in certain state courts. However, the majority of states have patterned their rules of evidence after the federal rules and have adopted the case law interpreting the federal rules as persuasive in their respective jurisdictions. As such, discussion of the admissibility of life care plans will focus on federal evidentiary standards.

† Federal Rule of Evidence 702, which governs the admissibility of expert testimony, provides as follows: "If scientific, technical, or other specialized knowledge will assist the trier of fact to understand the evidence or to determine a fact in issue, a witness qualified as an expert by knowledge, skill, experience, training, or education may testify thereto in the form of an opinion or otherwise."

Rule 702 serves several distinct functions. It establishes the authority to use expert testimony in general, sets forth the standard for admissibility of expert testimony in a given case, and addresses the qualifications necessary to accord a witness status as an expert. See generally *Coleman v. Parkline Corp.*, 844 F.2d 863, 865 (D.C. Circuit 1988); and *Sterling v. Velsicol Chemical Corp.*, 855 F.2d 1188, 1208 (6th Circuit 1988).

‡ See *Gardner v. General Motors Corporation*, 507 F.2d 525, 528 (10th Circuit 1974); *United States v. Viglia*, 549 F.2d 335 (5th Circuit 1977), cert. denied, 434 U.S. 834, 98 S.Ct. 121, 54 L.Ed.2d 95 (1977); *Friendship Heights Association v. Vlastimil Koubek*, 785 F.2d 1154, 1160 (4th Circuit 1986); and *Exum v. General Electric Company*, 819 F.2d 1158 (D.C. Circuit 1987).

§ *Jenkins v. United States*, 307 F.2d 637, 644 (D.C. Circuit 1962).

certification. In fact, at least one court has held that a skilled witness on a medical subject need not be duly licensed to practice medicine.* The determination of whether an individual qualifies as an expert is a decision for the trial court pursuant to Federal Rule of Evidence 104(a). This determination is left to the sound discretion of the trial court and will not be reversed on appeal absent an abuse of that discretion.†

Today, life care planning is a generally recognized area specialty. There are several credible organizations which offer educational programs and certification within the field.‡

Qualification to Present the Particular Life Care Plan

Rule 702 was written as a general grant of authority for the use of expert testimony and is therefore permissive in nature.§ Therefore, in many applications of the expert witness rule, the threshold issue is whether the field of expertise is proper for expert testimony in court. Expert testimony is generally proper in any scientific field that has reached a level of general acceptance. Most courts have at least implicitly recognized that life care planning itself has reached such a degree of general acceptance as to be the proper subject of expert testimony. Thus, expert testimony is generally permitted in conjunction with a life care plan.¶

Conversely, however, the particular substantive law controlling a given case may *require* expert testimony regarding a certain issue. In these cases, expert testimony is not only permitted by Rule 702 but also, in fact, required by the relevant substantive law.** For example, in cases involving claims of personal injury, courts around the country generally hold that expert testimony is required on the issue of whether treatment claimed as damages is medically necessary. Under this rule, many elements of a life care plan will often require qualified medical expert testimony in order to be

* *Salem v. United States Lines Co.*, 370 U.S. 31, 35, 82 S.Ct. 1119, 1122, 8 L.Ed.2d 313 (1962); *Grindstaff v. Coleman*, 681 F.2d 740, 743 (11th Circuit 1982); *Dunn v. Sears, Roebuck and Company*, 639 F.2d 1171, 1174 (5th Circuit 1981), modified on other grounds, 645 F.2d 511 (5th Circuit 1981); and *Mannino v. International Mfg. Co.*, 650 F.2d 846 (6th Circuit 1981).

† See *Fairchild v. United States*, 769 F.Supp. 964, 968 (W.D. La. 1991).

‡ https://www.ichcc.org/certified-life-care-planner-clcp.html; http://cnlcp.org/; and, http://bsch.phhp.ufl.edu/distance-learning/life-care-planning/. Consequently, it should be expected that the plaintiff will retain a legally qualified testimonial life care planner. Conversely, the defendant should prepare with the understanding that the court is likely to recognize the life care planner as a competent expert to testify subject to specific objections to the plan elements.

§ Note, however, that this general acceptance requirement can also impact the admissibility of a particular life care plan if the scientific bases for any elements of the plan are not generally accepted. This specific issue is discussed in more detail infra at notes 20 to 23 and accompanying text.

¶ See generally *International Brotherhood of Teamsters v. United States*, 431 U.S. 324, 97 S.Ct. 1843, 1851, 52 L.Ed.2d 396, 407 (1977) (recognizing that expert testimony is required in medical malpractice cases); *Randolph v. Collectramatic, Inc.*, 590 F.2d 844, 848 (10th Circuit 1979); and *Huddell v. Levin*, 537 F.2d 726, 726 (3d Circuit 1976); *M.D.P. v. Middleton*, 925 F. Supp. 2d 1272, 1275-76 (M.D. Ala. 2013)(Paul Deutsch is qualified to render opinions despite a lack of a medical degree and may rely upon medical opinions of others to support his plan opinions).

** *Diamond R. Fertilizer v. Davis*, 567 So.2d 451, 455 (Fla. 1st DCA 1990). In *Diamond Fertilizer*, the court held that it was reversible error to adopt a life care plan that was established by a rehabilitation counselor and that gave the counselor the discretion to oversee and supervise the claimant's medical and nursing home care, where the plan was supported solely by the counselor's own testimony without the testimony of any treating physician. The court emphasized that each element of a life care plan must be medically necessary and that, in most cases, medical expert testimony is required to establish medical necessity (567 So.2d at 455).

properly presented to the jury as a claimed element of damages. In the vast majority of cases, this foundation requires testimony of a physician.*

In many cases, plaintiffs seek to present a life care plan to the jury supported only by the testimony of a rehabilitation consultant or certified life care planner. The defense should take the position, and several courts have held, that each element of the life care plan must also be independently supported by a separately qualified expert's testimony as to that element's reasonableness and necessity in the given case. As one court stated, "The responsibility *for establishing a treatment* plan rests with a claimant's authorized physicians."† Unless such requirements are enforced, the use of the life care planning expert will enable the plaintiff to circumvent the threshold for admissibility of each claimed element of damages in the plan. Thus, once the life care planner is properly qualified as an expert in the field of life care planning generally, the court will next consider whether the proposed expert is qualified as an expert in the relevant field for each element of the life care plan that is not supported by other evidence or another expert's testimony.

Failure by the plaintiff to properly limit the scope of the life care planner's proposed expertise may result in the entire plan and the planner's entire testimony being precluded or stricken.‡ A life care planner testifying for the plaintiff must therefore ensure not only that he or she is qualified to testify as a life care planner generally, but that he or she is qualified to testify concerning the necessity of any individual elements of the plan that are not independently supported by appropriate medical or other expert testimony. In many cases the plaintiff's life care planner can best serve the client by enlisting the services of the proper medical experts, rather than by attempting to support

---

* *Runge v. Stanley Fastening Sys., L.P.*, No. 4:09-CV-130-TWP-WGH, 2011 WL 4903782, at *2 (S.D. Ind. Oct. 14, 2011) (life care planner's opinions based upon physician's reports admissible); *Hogland v. Town & Country Grocer of Fredericktown Missouri, Inc.*, No. 3:14CV00273 JTR, 2015 WL 3843674, at *29-30 (E.D. Ark. June 22, 2015) (future medical care opinions unsupported by a physician cannot be presented by a non-medical life care planner).

† See *Fairchild v. United States*, 769 F.Supp.964, 968 (W.D. La. 1991) (recognizing that each treatment element recommended by the life care planner must have independent record support); *First National Bank v. Kansas City Southern Railway Company*, 865 S.W.2d 719, 738 (Mo. App. 1993) (holding that a life care planner's testimony regarding the need for and costs of future attendant care should have been excluded due to the lack of a medical doctor's testimony establishing the need for such care on a medical basis) (analyzing the issue in terms of impermissible speculation on the question of damages); and *Timmons v. Mass. Transp. Authority*, 591 N.E.2d 667, 67071 (Mass. 1992) (holding that admission of vocational rehabilitation expert's opinion of future loss of earnings was prejudicial error because the expert assumed that the injury was permanent and this assumption was not supported by evidence). See also *Hobbs v. Harken*, 969 S.W.2d 318 (Mo. App. 1998); *Hines v. Sweet*, 567 S.W.2d 435, 438 (Mo. App. 1978). But see *National Bank v. Estate of Bollmeyer*, 504 N.W.2d 59, 65 (Minn. App. 1993) (holding that a qualified life care planner who has reviewed the plaintiff's medical records can testify to the plaintiff's need for future personal care services, and rejecting the argument that a medical doctor must testify regarding such need; the court did not state whether the medical evidence relied on by the life care planner established the plaintiff's need from a medical standpoint in the first instance). It should be noted that an appellate court may permit a trial court less discretion in determining the scope of the life care planner's expertise than in permitting the expert to testify in the first instance. See, for example, *First National Bank v. Kansas City Southern Railway Company,* 865 S.W.2d 719 (Mo. App. 1993) (allowing the trial court broad discretion in qualifying the expert but holding that the trial court committed reversible error in permitting the qualified life care planner to testify to matters requiring medical expertise).

‡ See *Reddish v. Secretary of the Department of Health and Human Services*, 18 Cl. Ct. 366, 375 (U.S. Claims Court 1991) (noting that life care plan incorporated needs outlined by treating physicians); *Neher v. Secretary of the Department of Health and Human Services*, 23 Cl. Ct. 508 (U.S. Claims Court 1991) (damage award reversed because elements of life care plan were speculative and were duplicated by other award); and *Ainos' Custom Slip Covers v. DeLucia*, 533 So.2d 862 (Fla. 1st DCA 1988) (reversing an order awarding the medical and nursing home services outlined in a life care plan where the testimony of the rehabilitation consultant was the sole support for the award and the medical witnesses testified that the claimant's current care was sufficient).

the plan based on his or her testimony alone.* A defendant's life care planning consultant can be of great assistance in helping defense counsel to identify any weaknesses in the plaintiff's proposed expert's qualifications to testify regarding the need for any given treatment element in the plan.

In general, a rehabilitation or habilitation expert will attempt to translate the physical or mental impairment into a disability in order to assess the effect upon the injured party's ability to participate in Activities of Daily Living. It is the role of the physician to establish the existence of a physical or mental impairment, and it is inappropriate for a rehabilitation consultant to present opinion testimony as to the existence of a medical condition or its likely progression. Rather, the foundation for the impairment must be laid by a physician, including any expected complications or progression. This medical opinion can then be translated by the rehabilitation consultant into the disabling effects.

It should be noted that there may also be limitations on the authority of a life care planner to oversee and supervise the plaintiff's treatment. In one case, the court reversed an award that placed a rehabilitation counselor in charge of supervising the claimant's medical and nursing home care where there was insufficient independent medical evidence to support the award:

> The award is patently erroneous insofar as it purports to give a rehabilitation company authority to oversee and supervise claimant's medical and nursing care. Such responsibility rests with a claimant's treating physicians. Furthermore, although [the rehabilitation expert] was apparently competent to testify concerning his rehabilitation services, his testimony was not sufficiently substantial to provide the sole support for such a far-reaching award of rehabilitative oversight and authority.†

Foundational Objections, the Daubert Standard, and Other Preclusions

In addition to challenging the plaintiff's expert's general and specific qualifications, defense counsel should be aware of other potential grounds to exclude the testimony. For example, an untimely disclosure of the intent to use a life care plan can bar its introduction at trial.‡

Likewise, even where there is no question regarding the expert's qualifications, the expert's opinion must be supported by an adequate factual foundation.§ The expert's proper role is to provide opinion testimony based on facts that are of record in the case. The lack of an adequate

* *Ainos' Custom Slip Covers v. DeLucia*, 533 So.2d 862, 864 (Fla. 1st DCA 1988), review denied, 544 So.2d 199 (Fla. 1989). See also *Alpha Resins Corp. v. Townsend*, 606 So.2d 506 (Fla. 1st DCA 1992) (court retained jurisdiction to determine which elements of the life care were medically necessary).

† In *Department of Health and Rehabilitative Services v. J.B.*, 675 So.2d 241 (Fla. 4th DCA 1996), the plaintiff's attorney represented to the defendant and to the court that he would not introduce a life care plan at trial, and subsequently attempted to introduce such a plan at trial. The court precluded the plaintiff from using the plan.

‡ *Randolph v. Laeisz*, 896 F.2d 964, 968 (5th Circuit 1990).

§ *American Bearing Co., Inc., v. Litton Industries, Inc.*, 729 F.2d 943, 947 (3d Circuit 1984), cert. denied, 469 U.S. 854, 105 S.Ct. 178, 83 L.Ed.2d 112 (1984); *Twin City Plaza, Inc., v. Central Surety and Insurance Corporation*, 409 F.2d 1195, 1200 (8th Circuit 1969) ("When basic foundational conditions are themselves conjecturally premised, it behooves a court to remove the answer from one of admissible opinion to one of excludable speculation"); and *Polk v. Ford Motor Company*, 529 F.2d 259, 271 (8th Circuit 1976), cert. denied, 426 U.S. 907, 96 S.Ct. 2229, 48 L.Ed.2d 832 (1976) (an expert's opinion must be based on matters sufficient "to take such testimony out of the realm of guesswork and speculation"). In *Randolph v. Laeisz*, 896 F.2d 964, 968 (5th Circuit 1990), for example, the court held that a properly qualified economist's testimony was inadmissible where the testimony was based on insufficient foundation. The economist had testified that lost wages should be reduced by a certain percentage due to market conditions. The court held that because such market conditions did not appear in the record, there was insufficient foundation for the expert's testimony. The court found that the testimony was improperly admitted because the expert's testimony served as substantive evidence rather than opinion interpreting facts in evidence.

factual foundation requires that the expert's testimony be stricken as based on speculation.* Such an issue may arise if, for example, the life care planner intends to testify regarding the cost of certain treatment but no medical evidence has been proffered to indicate that such treatment is reasonable, necessary, or caused by the relevant accident. Such foundational objections should be considered in cases where similar objections to the life care planner's qualifications have been overruled.

The speculative nature of a life care plan can also preclude its admissibility if the plan involves new or experimental treatments or novel theories of causation. Each element of the plan is subject to preclusion if it does not meet the *Daubert* standard for admissibility.† The defense should evaluate the plan for inclusion of therapeutic modalities which are not generally accepted as "necessary" for the treatment. For example, the use of long-term hyperbaric oxygen therapy for brain injury is controversial. A *Daubert* hearing will force the plaintiff to establish this therapy and the associated cost is admissible for the jury's consideration.

Defense counsel is advised not only to keep these potential exclusionary arguments in mind in analyzing the plaintiff's proffered life care plan, but also to ensure that any defense life care plan complies with each of these requirements and will be admissible.‡

Cross-Examination of the Plaintiff's Expert

As courts increasingly relax the formal requirements for qualifications of expert testimony, and as scientific advances render more elements of a life care plan generally accepted, it may not be possible to completely exclude the expert from testifying.§ Where the threshold requirements for qualification are met, any deficiency in the witness's knowledge, education, training, or experience is relevant only to the weight to be given his or her testimony, and not the admissibility of that testimony. Courts will often hold that a proposed expert of marginal qualification should be permitted to testify and the opposing party required to elicit the defects in his or her qualifications on cross-examination, rather than barring the testimony completely. Thus, when a life care expert is permitted to testify over defense objection, the expert should expect any weaknesses in his or her qualifications to be explored in detail on cross-examination.

Defense counsel will determine whether the plaintiff's expert is state certified in rehabilitation, habilitation,¶ vocational rehabilitation, workers' compensation, or other form of counseling.

* 293 F. 1013 (D.C. Circuit 1923).

† See, *Davidson v. U.S. Dep't of Health & Human Servs.*, No. CIV.A. 7:06-129-DCR, 2007 WL 3251921, at *1-3 (E.D. Ky. Nov. 2, 2007) (plaintiff's failure to demonstrate *Daubert* factors resulted in exclusion of care plan and associated economic cost).

‡ See, for example, *First National Bank v. Kansas City Southern Railway Company*, 865 S.W.2d 719 (Mo. App. 1993).

§ In the instance of rehabilitation, an individual has a known ability that is lost due to the impairment, creating a disabling affect. In the art of habilitation, the counselor is seeking to develop skills unknown to the injured party prior to the impairment. Accordingly, the techniques required to rehabilitate persons differ from those to habilitate individuals. In this chapter the term *rehabilitation counselor* refers to both rehabilitative and habilitative counseling, unless noted to the contrary.

¶ It should be noted that even where the relevant substantive law would permit compensation to the plaintiff for the fees of persons whose services were enlisted to obtain the award, a life care planner's fees may not be compensable. See *Southern Industries v. Chumey*, 613 So.2d 74 (Fla. 1st DCA 1993) (holding in a workers' compensation context that the life care planning services of a rehabilitation counselor and psychologist were not reasonably necessary to the procurement of benefits and therefore were not compensable expenses); *Frederick Electronics v. Pettijohn*, 619 So.2d 14 (Fla. 1st DCA 1993) (rehabilitation counselor and psychologist who developed life care plan did not qualify as a health care provider, and his services were therefore not reimbursable expenses in workers' compensation case).

A defendant will also find it helpful to determine whether the plaintiff's expert is a medical case manager. Often, plaintiffs will retain vocational rehabilitation consultants who have expanded their forensic practice into life care planning. Many plaintiffs' experts have never actively served as a patient advocate or coordinator of health services on behalf of an injured party. Establishing that the plaintiff's expert has done nothing more than read books and look at other life care plans in order to present a particular life care plan can be crippling to the plaintiff's case, even if the court finds the expert qualified to testify. A life care expert hired by the defendant to assist in preparing the defense case can assist his or her client by being familiar with all available training or education in the field, and making defense counsel aware of any such training or education that does not appear on the plaintiff's life care expert's resume.

Financial Bias

After the plaintiff's life care planner has overcome any qualification issues, the planner must avoid additional potential pitfalls. Financial bias is a common ground for defense efforts to discredit the plaintiff's experts, including the life care planner. The obvious financial bias of any expert is that he or she is being paid to present opinion testimony on behalf of the plaintiff.* Beyond the bias that all retained experts have, defense counsel will likely inquire about the amount of money received by the expert for litigation support services generally. Many jurisdictions require that the expert give a best estimate of the amount of money or percent of income received from litigation services as a whole. Under the Federal Rules (commonly referred to as Rule 26), the expert must disclose publications for the last 10 years, compensation paid for the study and testimony, and a listing of cases for which testimony was given in the last 4 years. Prior retention by the plaintiff's law firm is often a fruitful source of showing an ongoing business relationship that the life care planner presumably would not want to jeopardize by presenting conservative plans.

Another source of financial bias impeachment is the appearance of impropriety created by recommended self-referral. Some life care planners are involved in owned and operated rehabilitation centers. Where the life care plan is centered on such a program, this creates the appearance of a financial incentive on the part of the life care planner. In some egregious cases, defense counsel can successfully establish that the life care planner has engaged in self-referral of prior plaintiffs who have received settlements or judgment awards and entered into the life care planner's own facility programs. It can be devastating to the plaintiff's case for the jury to learn that the life care planner may receive a substantial amount of the life care plan funding by payment to a medical facility in which he or she owns a substantial interest.

Defense counsel should also be aware that the elements offered in the plaintiff's life care plan can impact other evidence and discovery in the case. For example, at least one court has held that where the plaintiff's life care plan included professional help to manage her assets, the plaintiff had put her economic condition at issue and was required to produce her personal financial records, which ordinarily would have been unavailable to the defense.†

---

* See *Compton v. West Volusia Hosp. Auth.*, 727 So.2d 379, 381 (Fla. 5th DCA 1999).

† Such issues apparently do not create enough speculation to preclude admissibility of the plan itself. See *Ballance v. WalMart Stores, Inc.*, 178 F.3d 1282 (unpublished disposition), 1999 WL 231653 (4th Circuit 1999) (trial court properly admitted life care plan testimony, despite defendant's claim that the life care plans are speculative because they are contingent upon future events and choices, such as whether the plaintiff has surgery and whether it is successful).

Purpose of Retention

It is useful to establish why the rehabilitation consultant was retained by plaintiff's counsel. The obvious purpose is to support the plaintiff's litigation by providing a life care plan that can be used by an economist as a foundation to support a present value of economic loss.

Rather than sharing such candor, some rehabilitation consultants will attempt to present themselves as an advocate for the client, who is allegedly seeking advice regarding his or her future care needs and how they can be met. Defense counsel will establish carefully the extent to which the rehabilitation consultant has furthered advocacy of the client beyond obtaining the information necessary to prepare the plaintiff's life care plan. In the usual instance, nothing has been done to advocate on behalf of the client beyond the preparation of the life care plan report. For example, rarely will the plaintiff's expert have contacted an insurer or public assistance program in order to qualify the client for services. Such a line of inquiry can be most effective in instances where an insurer, the public school system, or other resource has provided a medical case manager who has not recommended the various therapies or other aspects of the plaintiff's life care plan.

Another area of recent aggressive attack is the failure of the life care planner to look at the injured party's circumstances in any real-world sense. Defense counsels are increasingly inquiring of the history of the life care planner's clients who actually follow through with the life care plan after a court recovery or large settlement.* Often, the catastrophic case takes several years to resolve. Life care planners need to be prepared to respond to defense counsel inquiry as to how the injured party is being presently cared for and the current economic cost for that level of care. Obviously, the life care planner must be prepared to explain why the proposed life care plan markedly differs from the current care plan and thereby justify the increased costs of the more intensive care.†

The Basis of the Opinions

The basis of an expert's opinions is another potential area for criticism and cross-examination. In the discovery deposition, defense will establish the entirety of the work performed by the rehabilitation consultant in order to prepare the report and should determine that the work on the case is complete. Inquiry will be made regarding any interviews conducted and any authoritative text relied upon. A well-prepared life care expert will be able to demonstrate that he or she is familiar with all the relevant facts of the case.

Counsel should also determine at the time of the deposition that the rehabilitation consultant is not attempting to interpret any of the medical, psychological, or therapeutic assessments made, unless the

---

* Furthermore, the life care planner needs to be conversant regarding the stress being placed upon the current caregivers, especially when they are a spouse or parents, or some other family member. While the economist may talk about the economic cost to that caregiver, the role of the life care planner is to provide insight into the propriety of the care being given. In many instances, the life care planner will find that the parent or spouse is perfectly capable of giving adequate care with additional training and respite. In those situations, the life care planner should make that concession and remain objective. It is the role of the economist to extrapolate the cost to the family member of this type of care. In most jurisdictions, the court will allow evidence of the value of these services being provided by the family member and the jury will thus be able to consider the dollar value of this care in making an award.

† However, a defendant may be precluded from introducing evidence of the cost of an annuity to fund future medical expenses. See *North Broward Hospital District v. Bates*, 595 So.2d 578 (Fla. 4th DCA), rev. denied, 605 So.2d 1265 (Fla. 1992) (although evidence of the cost of an annuity to compute present value may be admitted in cases involving loss of future earning capacity and loss of support in wrongful death actions, the jury could not utilize an annuity approach in determining future medical damages).

rehabilitation consultant is qualified to do so. If the inclusion of some therapy, medical examination, diagnostic testing, or other aspect of the plan requires the opinion of a physician, psychologist, or other expert, it must be determined whether such a person has been contacted to validate those aspects of the life care plan. The more experienced rehabilitation consultant who is not a physician will have the life care plan reviewed by a physician in order to verify the inclusion of the various prescribed modalities. On the other hand, a life care planner who is a physician may very well require the support of a case manager, vocational counselor, psychologist, or other specialist if he or she cannot show specialized training in the area of damage-related opinions. If this is not done, it can be a fertile source of cross-examination and perhaps for striking some elements of the plan for lack of proper predicate.

Base Costing and Duplication

In most instances, the plaintiff's life care planner will attempt to identify a current cost for each aspect of the plan. Defense counsel will review the plan carefully to determine the reasonableness of each of these base cost assumptions. The defense rehabilitation consultant should also review the plan and point out any areas of weakness. Fertile ground for attack usually involves the failure of the plaintiff's plan to recognize the availability of bulk purchasing and long-term contractual rates. Many plaintiffs' plans will set forth an hourly rate for home health aides, nursing services, and household services. Such hourly rates are then extrapolated by the plaintiff's economist, resulting in exorbitant annual costs. It is not unusual to be able to demonstrate that the annual cost of hourly services is more than double the cost of negotiated contract rates.*

Plaintiffs' life care plans also commonly provide for many duplications of services and supportive items. Duplication not only is a basis for attack of the life care plan in argument to the jury, but also may result in the court striking all or part of the plan.† All costs of the life care plan should therefore be carefully assessed and a determination made of whether the plaintiff is recognizing the fixed costs that would not be relatable to the injury event. For example, where a plaintiff's injury requires a special diet, the cost of the special diet should be offset by the normally expected food cost incurred by any individual. In instances of special transportation requirements, it is important to establish whether the plaintiff's plan has offset those transportation expenses that would have been normally incurred. Where group home residency is being recommended, the plaintiff's plan should set off for typical housing costs. The group home rate often includes laundry, food, and other expenses that may also be included in some other aspect of the plaintiff's economic analysis, such as lost earnings capacity.

Application of the Collateral Source Rule

Defense counsel should also explore with the plaintiff's expert any consideration given to the availability of public programs or collateral sources.‡ It should be noted that the collateral source

* *Neher v. Secretary of the Department of Health and Human Services*, 23 Cl. Ct. 508 (U.S. Claims Court 1991) (damage award reversed because elements of life care plan were speculative and were duplicated by other award).

† See generally *Cates v. Wilson*, 361 S.E.2d 734 (N.C. 1987) (noting that the plaintiff's life care planner testified both in the plaintiff's case in chief and on cross-examination by the defense regarding the availability of public facilities to meet the needs outlined in the life care plan).

‡ See generally *Cates v. Wilson*, 361 S.E.2d 734 (N.C. 1987). See, *Brewington v. United States*, No. CV1307672DMGCWX, 2015 WL 4511296, at *4-6 (C.D. Cal. July 24, 2015)(Affordable Care Act benefits to be considered in a determination of future medical costs). Cf. *Joerg v. State Farm Mut. Auto. Ins. Co.*, 176 So.3d 1247, 1256 (Fla. 2015)(Medicare, Medicaid and other social legislation, are not a future benefit to be considered when determining damages for future medical costs).

rules of the particular jurisdiction may impact the permissible scope of such evidence.* In most states, the collateral source rule has been modified to allow defendants to set off insurance benefits provided without lien rights and benefits provided or available under public assistance programs from the damages awarded. The defendant's rehabilitation consultant should assist defense counsel in pointing out those matters called for by the plaintiff's plan for which there may be a government agency or other funding source not considered in the plaintiff's economic analysis.

For example, states receiving federal funds may be required to provide comparable education opportunities to severely handicapped children up to age 22. The public school system also makes available those therapies that are required to further the educational opportunities of the student. Therefore, the public school program is an excellent resource for cases of catastrophic injury to infants and young children. Defense counsel should establish the plaintiff's rehabilitation consultant's position with respect to the consideration of these public programs and be prepared to rebut the plaintiff's expected contention that such programs are substandard and inappropriate for the particular client. The failure of a plaintiff's life care planner to recognize and take into account the availability and suitability of charitable and other publicly funded programs can cast doubt on an otherwise objectively prepared analysis.

Licensing Issues

To this author's knowledge, no state has any specific licensing requirements for persons who author life care plans. As the majority of life care planning probably involves the medicolegal context, the lack of any standardized requirements and licensure makes the area fertile ground for those persons who wish to claim expertise for sale on the open market. Unlike recognized specialties that provide the planned care and are subject to licensing requirements, the planning field is open to the unscrupulous expert who views the life care plan as a device to sell in the forensic marketplace. The long-term solution is the creation of a national standards organization that becomes recognized by the states and lobbies for enactment of statutory licensing. Under the current state of the art, defense counsels are urged to point out any failure of the plaintiff's expert to obtain certification. For example, did the expert comply with ethics and standards as published by the International Academy of Life Care Planners, which publishes *Standards of Practice* guidelines?

In the absence of separate licensure, life care planners must be mindful of the limitations that are imposed by related and existing state licensure laws. In most states, persons are required to hold one or more licenses before they may prescribe or perform various therapies. For example, a licensed vocational rehabilitation counselor is not qualified in the State of Florida to prescribe or perform physical therapy. Moreover, therapists licensed to perform physical therapy may only do so subject to intermittent physician reviews. Life care planners must therefore be mindful not to misrepresent to the client or the jury the ability to recommend the various treatment modalities that the life care planner is not independently qualified to opine as reasonable and necessary.

A myriad of qualifications are typically seen on the life care planner's resume. The life care planner's formal training may be as a vocational rehabilitation counselor, nurse, certified case manager, mental health counselor, psychologist, occupational therapist, physical therapist, physician, or some combination of these and other professions. Thus, the ability of the life care planner to give specific opinions for care will vary with the type of case presented. For example,

* Life care plans are subject to the same requirements for pretrial disclosure as are applied to other evidence in the particular jurisdiction, and the life care plan may be stricken for failure to comply with such pretrial discovery requirements. See *Department of Health and Rehabilitative Services v. Spivak*, 675 So.2d 241 (Fla. 4th DCA 1996).

a vocational rehabilitation counselor who has no training in case management or nursing is not qualified to render a life care plan assessing the medical needs of a child with catastrophic birth-related injuries. The same life care planner may, however, be perfectly qualified to render a life care plan in the case of a less catastrophically injured plaintiff who simply requires modality seeking to reasonably accommodate the client in the workforce throughout his or her remaining work life. Conversely, a certified case manager with nursing experience in the long-term care of persons with impaired mobility would be well suited to the evaluation of the life care needs of the catastrophically injured child, and ill-equipped to assess the needs of the less catastrophically injured worker. Thus, the life care planner seeking to provide services in a medicolegal context should assess his or her own limitations and accept cases accordingly.

Moreover, a certified case manager may be very well qualified to opine as to future durable goods requirements and perhaps the nursing care coverage required for the type of injury presented. This same case manager would, however, be required to defer to a qualified physician the issue of future surgeries and attendant complications, prescription medication, and prescribed therapies. Similarly, this life care planner should defer to an orthoptist for the type of orthopedic bracing required and the various therapists involved in the care for the form and frequency of therapy provided. As the clinical care of the catastrophically injured person involves a multidisciplinary approach, the life care planner should not be hesitant to interact with and gain insight from these disciplines when creating a plan. In fact, the greatest service the life care planner can provide to a retaining attorney is to express the limitations of the planner to give opinions and encourage the retaining party's use of other experts to ensure a credible and legally sufficient foundation for the admission of the life care plan.

Many life care planners are unwilling to accept their own limitations for fear that it will erode their role. Such persons are encouraged to look at the other fields that are called upon to participate in the legal system. For example, economists were called upon to render opinions concerning future economic loss in catastrophically injured cases long before the assistance provided by life care planners was available. In order to properly perform this assessment, the economist would frequently review the opinions of the health care providers, the costs provided therein, and the extrapolations required based upon this foundation of information.

The life care planner's role is to take this analysis to the next step and include a more holistic approach. The weakness of the economist's analysis historically was that it was incomplete in its scope. It is submitted that the life care planner is best able to assist the legal professional by using experience to dictate the probable needs that will be involved with a patient's future care. This ensures that the life care planner and attorney will research and consider all aspects of care in creating the life care plan. Just as most of the economist's report of future economic losses is predicated by facts gained from others, there is no weakness in a life care planner's relying upon information gained from other sources. Such reliance may make the difference between admissibility and inadmissibility of the life care planner's testimony.

The Decision to Retain a Defense Rehabilitation Consultant

Because cases that are appropriate for plaintiff's use of a life care plan typically involve catastrophic physical injury or significant brain damage, the defense counsel is well advised to retain a defense rehabilitation consultant early in the case. Often courts do not require disclosure of experts' opinions until the months immediately preceding the trial.* As such, much of the discovery will be completed before the defendant has an opportunity to receive the plaintiff's life care plan.

* See Federal Rule of Civil Procedure 26(b)(4)(B).

In order to be properly prepared to rebut the plaintiff's plan and to determine whether to present a defense plan, it is vital that much of the groundwork be laid in the early portions of the case discovery. A defense rehabilitation consultant can provide early assistance by suggesting the various records that should be requested and identifying persons to be deposed in order to make the determinations necessary to evaluate the injured party's life care needs. In most cases, the defense rehabilitation consultant will not need to spend a significant amount of time or money to provide this initial assistance. Moreover, the dividends returned on this initial investment are paid in the form of easing the inevitably compressed final preparation toward trial.

The actual selection of a particular rehabilitation consultant requires a basic understanding of the types of injuries involved in the case and an investigation of those experts available and qualified to support the defense. The qualifications of any proposed rehabilitation consultant should be reviewed carefully by defense counsel. Most defense counsels will want to review the potential rehabilitation consultant's current curriculum vitae and rate sheet. Defense counsel will likely request referrals from other attorneys who have hired the counselor, in order to confirm both the expert's qualifications and his or her abilities as a witness.

Ultimately, defense counsel must exercise judgment in determining the practical interplay of the retained rehabilitation expert with the overall theme of the defense and the other experts. For example, if the plaintiff has no in-state experts, then the defendant's theme may be to retain only local experts on all issues in order to point out the need for the plaintiff to go to other jurisdictions to get experts to support the case. As with the selection of any expert, the overall picture of the case must not be lost and the rehabilitation expert must make a good fit.

The Testifying Defendant Rehabilitation Consultant

The initial scope of retention is usually limited to service as a consulting expert to assist defense counsel in the rebuttal of the plaintiff's life care plan. In some cases, the defendant may want to take the next step and hire his or her own life care planning expert to testify at trial. The decision of whether to call a defense rehabilitation consultant at trial is troublesome and must be made on a case-by-case basis. Several factors affect this decision. First, a credible life care planner, even though testifying for the defense, will likely validate at least some of the plaintiff's plan. Defense counsel must weigh the price of validation of some or all of the plaintiff's plan with the benefit of attacking the credibility of those portions with which the defense rehabilitation consultant has substantial disagreement. Just as a defendant intends to elicit substantial concessions from the plaintiff's rehabilitation consultant on cross-examination, so too the plaintiff's counsel anticipates being able to reinforce much of the plaintiff's theory of the case through cross-examination of the defense expert.

A second and perhaps more important factor in deciding whether to call a defense rehabilitation consultant as a testifying expert is the impact of this decision on the discoverability of the expert's work and opinions. In most jurisdictions, the contributions of consulting experts who do not testify at trial are protected by the work-product privilege. For example, under the Federal Rules, a party can discover facts known or opinions held by another party's consulting experts only upon showing "exceptional circumstances under which it is impracticable for the party seeking discovery to obtain facts or opinions on the same subject by other means."* Absent such a showing of exceptional circumstances, which is extremely rare, the expert's work is protected from discovery.

* See Federal Rule of Civil Procedure 26(b)(4)(A).

However, such protection is usually not afforded to experts expected to testify at trial. Thus, in instances where the rehabilitation consultant may be called upon to testify, both defense counsel and the life care expert should be aware that matters that would have been protected as work product if prepared by a consulting expert may be stripped of that protection. Notes, memorandums, research, and other matters held by the consulting expert may, by the decision to have the expert testify at trial, be transformed into the discoverable file materials of a testifying expert.* These materials may outline a great deal of the defense theory of the case. The cost of disclosing these materials to the plaintiff prior to trial may outweigh the benefit of having a defense life care planner testify at trial.

Furthermore, under the Federal Rules, a party must automatically disclose the identity of all testifying experts, and each testifying expert must provide the opposing party with a report that contains the following:

> A complete statement of all opinions to be expressed and the basis and reasons therefore; the data or other information considered by the witness in forming the opinions; any exhibits to be used as a summary of or support for the opinions; the qualifications of the witness, including a list of all publications authored by the witness within the preceding ten years; the compensation to be paid for the study and the testimony; and a listing of any other cases in which the witness has testified as an expert at trial or by deposition within the preceding four years.†

This report must be provided 90 days prior to the trial date or at such other time as the court requires.‡ Additionally, the opposing party may depose any testifying expert, and the opposing party is entitled to take that deposition after the disclosure of the expert's report.§ Such disclosure requirements and discovery opportunities are a substantial consideration in determining whether to retain a testifying life care expert for the defense.

In instances where the defense rehabilitation consultant will testify, it is imperative that a physical examination of the injured party occur, or that the court be requested to allow such an examination. Otherwise, the plaintiff will make the often persuasive argument that the defense expert has not even seen his or her client. As the provision of care to severely injured persons continues to become more complex and specialized, it is essential to recognize a multidisciplinary approach and to allow the defense rehabilitation consultant access to the depositions and, if possible, the actual persons involved in the care and treatment of the injured party.

In catastrophic injury cases, it is advisable for defense counsel to work with the rehabilitation consultant to engage the services of the specialized physicians and therapists necessary for the overall assessment of the life care plan. However, many jurisdictions have patient–physician or other privileges that preclude defense-retained experts from meeting with the plaintiff's physicians and therapists.¶ Additionally, many treating physicians and therapists do not want to become

---

* See Federal Rule of Civil Procedure 26(a)(2)(A),(B).

† See Federal Rule of Civil Procedure 26(a)(2)(C).

‡ See Federal Rule of Civil Procedure 26(b)(4)(A).

§ See McCormick, EVIDENCE, 98 at 244 n. 5 (noting that more than 40 states recognize a physician–patient privilege).

¶ Life care planning testimony may be relevant and helpful in cases other than personal injury cases. See, for example, *Urbanek v. Urbanek*, 484 So.2d 597 (Fla. 4th DCA 1986) (using life care testimony in a marital dissolution case to analyze the wife's changed circumstances in setting alimony amounts). Life care plans are often used to establish reserves in workers' compensation claims.

involved in litigation and therefore refuse to be informally interviewed by a defense-retained rehabilitation consultant. In such situations, compiling a defense team is the only approach that will ensure a complete evidentiary foundation for a defense life care plan. Plaintiffs obviously have a distinct advantage in having access to treating physicians. The defense must minimize this advantage by putting together its own team of experts and, if permitted under the laws of the relevant jurisdiction, explaining to the jury why such assembly was necessary.

Practical Considerations: The Effect on the Jury

It must be remembered by both plaintiff and defendant that the life care plan will not be presented in a vacuum. Issues of liability and causation can be affected by the credibility of the plaintiff's life care plan. Both plaintiff and defendant must be certain that they retain a well-qualified, knowledgeable rehabilitation or habilitation expert who will present an objective life care plan. Although the economic incentive to prepare an overreaching life care plan can be tempting to the plaintiff, the presentation of such a plan to the jury will often have a spillover effect on the overall view of the case. It may offend the jury and thereby swing a close liability case in favor of the defense. Defense counsel must therefore be prepared to take full advantage of the overreaching life care planner.

Conversely, the requirements of care for the injured party that are set forth in the life care plan directly affect the economic costs of the injury and indirectly affect the noneconomic losses by the life care plan's efforts at improving the quality of life. Defense counsel must therefore be cognizant that an attack on any aspect of the plan may be viewed as insensitive to the efforts at improving the plaintiff's quality of life. Just as the overreaching plaintiff can alienate a jury, the insensitive attack on elements of a plan for the benefit of the injured party can offend juries.

Conclusion

Defense counsel involved in the catastrophic injury case in which the plaintiff relies upon a life care plan is advised to aggressively attack damages. This attack begins with early retention of defense experts, including a rehabilitation consultant. At a minimum, the defense rehabilitation consultant will be instrumental in the preparation of early discovery and effective cross-examination of the plaintiff's expert. In instances where the plaintiff's life care plan warrants, the presentation of an alternative defense life care plan, and the early involvement and careful presentation of the defense rehabilitation consultant as a testifying expert, can enhance the overall credibility of the defendant's case and provide the jury with a more reasonable economic alternative.

Chapter 25

Life Care Planning and the Elder Law Attorney*

Terry C. Cox and F. Auston Wortman, III

Contents

Introduction 669
History and Development of Elder Law 670
The Nature of Elder Law Practice 670
Elder Law as an Emerging Specialty 672
The Holistic Approach (Forensic Life Planning) 672
Ethical Considerations 674
Elder Law Attorneys and Professional Life Care Planners: The Perfect Match 674
Case Study 676
State Statutes 678
References 679

Introduction

The practice of life care planning is familiar to members of the International Academy of Life Care Planners and others who regularly read their publication, the *Journal of Life Care Planning;* however, the practice of elder law as related to life care planning may not be as familiar. This chapter provides a description of and historical overview of the elder law forensic life planning function (not to be confused with life care planning as provided by the professional life care planner). For purposes of this chapter, rehabilitation professionals who practice life care planning are referred to as professional life care planners. In comparison, the life planning function of attorneys who concentrate in the field of elder law is referred to as forensic life planning. Beneficial collaboration between elder law attorneys who practice life planning and professional life care planners is discussed. Ethical considerations are also addressed.

* This chapter is in large part a reprint of the authors' article of the same name which appeared in the 2008 *Journal of Life Care Planning*, 6(3–4), 105–112. Reprinted with permission.

History and Development of Elder Law

The practice of law can be traced to the arguments and rhetorical speeches echoing through the halls of the Greek courts. Cicero, the Greek intellectual and philosopher, vividly describes the scenes of this primitive form of law practice (Sutton & Rackham, 1942). Since the days of Cicero, the practice of law has evolved into numerous areas of specialized practice.

Relatively speaking, elder law, as an identified area of practice concentration, is in its infancy in comparison to bedrock subjects including the law of property, crimes, torts, and contracts. Elder law became formally recognized as a specialty practice in 1988 with the founding of the National Academy of Elder Law Attorneys, Inc. (National Academy of Elder Law Attorneys, n.d.a). The NAELA serves as the "professional association of attorneys dedicated to improving the quality of legal services to the elderly" (National Academy of Elder Law Attorneys, n.d.a.). In addition to facilitating the enhancement of elder law practice, the NAELA serves as an interdisciplinary link between practicing elder law attorneys and those in other professions that serve the elderly.

In furtherance of its organizational mission, the NAELA board of directors formed the National Elder Law Foundation (NELF) in 1993. The NELF exists to improve the professional competence of elder law attorneys and to seek recognition of the specialty area of elder law practice by judicial authorities and the bar in general. To that end, the NELF created a program to certify qualified practitioners as elder law specialists. The specialty practice of elder law was officially recognized by the American Bar Association's House of Delegates in February 1995 (National Elder Law Foundation, n.d.).

The Nature of Elder Law Practice

As defined by the NELF,

> Elder Law is the legal practice of counseling and representing older persons and their representatives about the legal aspects of health and long term care planning, public benefits, surrogate decision-making, older persons' legal capacity, the conservation, disposition and administration of older persons' estates and the implementation of their decisions concerning such matters, giving due consideration to the applicable tax consequences of the action, or the need for more sophisticated tax expertise. (NELF, Rules and Regulations, n.d.)

Further, it is fundamental that elder law attorneys be capable of identifying, coordinating, and triaging issues that arise, or may arise, while advising and representing older persons. Elder law attorneys must be proficient in matters of health and life insurance, contracts, long term care, employment, retirement, and housing. Elder law attorneys address, from the forensic perspective, issues that arise during an elder's life transitions. These life transitions arise when the elder ceases to be solely in charge of health care, housing, personal care, and business decision making in favor of a team approach to life management involving a combination of persons like the caregiver, the attorney, the professional life care planner, and the geriatric care manager.

According to the board of certification of the NELF, an elder law attorney's knowledge must be broad; the attorney must know an assortment of topics, including, but not limited to, the following:

- Health and long-term care planning
- Public benefits (includes Medicaid, Medicare, and Social Security)
- Surrogate decision making (includes powers of attorney and guardianship)

- Older persons' legal capacity
- The conservation, disposition, and administration of the older person's estate (includes wills, trust, and probate of an estate) (Needham, n.d.)

As part of the forensic life planning function, an elder law attorney offers counsel on various subjects that arise in the context of the aging process:

Health and personal care planning, including the preparation and use of custom-designed advance medical directives (medical powers of attorney, living wills, and health care declarations), and providing counsel to older persons, attorneys-in-fact, and families about medical and life-sustaining choices, and related personal life choices

Pre-mortem legal planning, including the drafting and execution of wills, trusts, general powers of attorney, financial powers of attorney, real estate ownership, gifting, and the financial and tax implications of related transactions

Fiduciary representation, including the provision of counsel to one serving as executor, personal representative, attorney-in-fact, trustee, guardian, conservator, representative payee, or other formal or informal fiduciary

Legal capacity counseling, including advising how capacity is determined and the level of capacity required for various legal activities, and representing those who are or may be the subject of guardianship/conservatorship proceedings or other protective arrangements

Public benefits advice, including planning for and assisting in obtaining Medicaid, Supplemental Security Income, and veterans benefits

Advice on insurance matters, including analyzing and explaining the types of insurance available, such as health, life, long-term care, home care, COBRA, Medigap, long-term disability, burial/funeral policies, and dread disease coverage, which under certain life policies allow for advance payment of a portion of the death benefit when the insured develops certain fatal conditions or which under certain annuity contracts allows for accelerated payment of a portion of the accumulated value of the contract under such circumstances

Resident rights advocacy, including advising patients and residents of hospitals, nursing facilities, continuing care retirement communities, assisted living facilities, adult care facilities, and those cared for in private homes of their rights and appropriate remedies in matters such as admission, transfer and discharge policies, quality of care, and related issues

Housing counseling, including reviewing the options available and the financing of those options such as mortgage alternative, renovation loan programs, life care contracts, and home equity conversion

Employment and retirement advice, including pensions, retiree health benefits, unemployment benefits, and other benefits

Income, estate, and gift tax advice, including consequences of plans made and advice offered

Public benefits advice, including planning for and assisting in obtaining Medicare, Social Security, and food stamps

Counseling with regard to age or disability discrimination in employment and housing

Litigation and administrative advocacy in connection with any of the previously listed matters, including will contests, contested capacity issues, elder abuse (including financial or consumer fraud), fiduciary administration, public benefits, nursing home torts, and discrimination

The future of elder law practice portends dynamic change in two aspects. First, the scope of issues that confront the elder continues to grow with the increasing variety and complexity of the health care delivery system, housing options, personal financial products, and asset protection strategies.

Second, the needs of the elder client group have come to be recognized as largely comparable to those of persons with disabilities. Accordingly, some elder law attorneys are beginning to identify themselves as special needs counsel, a phrase that serves as an umbrella descriptor for any attorney who serves persons affected by aging or disability.

Elder Law as an Emerging Specialty

Given trends in contemporary society and based on the authors' opinion, the next 50 years of elder law practice in the United States will be driven by two phenomena: the rapid increase in the elderly population and the corresponding increased concentration of wealth among that generation. In the first phenomena, data from the U.S. Bureau of the Census and the U.S. Administration on Aging foretell a startling rate of growth in the older population (Popluation, n.d.). In 2011, the baby boomer generation began to turn 65, and by 2030, it is projected that one in five people will be ages 65 or older. It is expected that by the year 2030, there will be approximately 70 million Americans ages 65 or older (U.S. Census Bureau, 2000). In the second phenomena, in 1995, the median net worth of persons ages 65 to 69 was $106,408, the highest median net worth of any age group. It has been estimated that during the first decade of the twenty-first century, $6 trillion in wealth will change hands from parents to their baby boomer children (Takacs, 2007).

Despite increased wealth and longevity, the reality of the aging population is that "increases in life span do not guarantee a commensurate improvement in quality of life" (Takacs, 1998, p. 2). It has been hypothesized that the most prominent health problems for the elderly will likely be chronic conditions, such as heart disease, neuropsychiatric illness, and cancer. According to a study by Dr. Aevarsson (1996) reported in the *Journal of the American Geriatrics Society*, almost 10 percent of persons ages 85 to 88 will develop dementia each year. Dr. Aevarsson stressed that the danger of the elderly developing dementia is substantial (Aevarsson, 1996). The need to evaluate, assess, plan, and care for persons with dementia is, therefore, imperative.

Based on available data, the nursing home will be the residence for three out of every four elderly persons at some point during their lives (Takacs, 1998). The duration of nursing home stay for half of the elderly persons in a nursing home will be 6 months or less. The other half will, on average, stay in a nursing home 5 years or more. At any given time, 4.41 percent of the 65 and older population in the United States is in a nursing home. Recently, in the State of Minnesota, that number reached 7.95 percent (Takacs, 1998).

The Holistic Approach (Forensic Life Planning)

Statistics confirm what common sense inherently tells us: the elderly have a higher risk of poor health, disability, loss of income, and incapacity than the population in general. In recent years, the federal government and state governments have enacted legislation on almost a continuous basis in an effort to protect the elderly and expand benefits available to them. The elderly have become more aware of the benefits available to them. In this regard, the elderly and their caregivers have sought attorneys to assist them in planning matters to seek the benefits that are available and to advocate for the rights of the elderly.

While the typical attorney–client relationship generally involves two parties, the elder–client relationship is usually a three-sided affair, involving the elder, the attorney, and the family or caregiver, who often serves as the catalyst for engaging the attorney. In many cases, elder law attorneys welcome, and depend upon, the family's or the caregiver's participation in planning for the elder person. While this configuration presents obvious ethical challenges, such as identifying the elder as the client and serving the client's best interest even when that duty departs from the preferences of the caregiver, it recognizes the reality that effective assistance to elders requires a team effort, a multidisciplinary treatment, and a holistic approach (Morgan & Sabatino, n.d.).

Attorneys who follow the holistic approach characterize their practice model as a collaborative effort among the elder, the attorney, the geriatric care manager, the family, and various health care facilities and professionals, with the elder always being the primary focus. "Elder Law attorneys use a holistic, multi-disciplinary approach to help seniors, people with disabilities, and their families in a caring, compassionate way that seeks to preserve dignity for such individuals" (National Academy of Elder Law Attorneys, n.d.a). These attorneys have become affiliated in the newly organized Life Care Planning Law Firms Association. Most elder law practitioners that employ the forensic life planning model customarily represent the client over the balance of the client's lifetime. The forensic life planning process generally followed by elder law practitioners typically involves an evaluation, assessment, and continued reassessment of the following areas during the representation of an elder client or a client with a disability:

Housing arrangements: An assessment is performed to determine the level of care a client needs. The spectrum of living arrangements for clients varies from residing in the home to receiving skilled care in a nursing home. Between these two living arrangements lay home health care, continuing care retirement communities, independent living facilities, and assisted living facilities.

Asset protection strategies: An assessment of a client's assets is usually performed to determine what, if any, public benefits can be made available to a client. Strategies seeking Medicaid and Veterans Administration benefits eligibility are developed and reviewed with the client and implemented according to the client's desires.

Health care delivery assessment: A geriatric care manager assesses the client's current health status and care needs. In this regard, the geriatric care manager monitors the delivery of health care and anticipates future health care needs.

Financial management strategies: The client's monthly income and expenses are analyzed to maximize beneficial use of income and to control costs.

Estate planning assessment: An assessment of the estate planning strategies is necessary in order to maintain continued eligibility for public benefits. It is imperative to avoid any seemingly benign transaction that may nonetheless impair the client's eligibility for public benefits.

Advocacy and general representation: Often, it is necessary for an attorney to engage in the traditional legal role of advocating for the client. Advocacy skills are most important when communicating with benefits providers and insurance companies in order for the client to obtain the best possible outcome.

It has been insightfully observed that elder law is the only area of law practice that is identified by the unique legal needs of a particular client group and not necessarily by a body of substantive law, hence the need for comprehensive, personalized planning. The critical distinctive common to elder law practitioners who provide forensic life planning services is that they directly engage care managers in the development and execution of their plan. Prototypically, the practitioner utilizes the services of a care manager to meet with clients in their residential settings, assess clients' health care and housing needs, and assist and implement care plan decisions that are made. A former president of NAELA considers that his elder law practice addresses the personal, emotional, and legal needs of the client. He describes the goal of his practice as assisting clients in maximizing the quality of their lives (Takacs, 2007).

Table 25.1 provides a matrix that describes a holistic approach to life care planning for elderly clients. This distinctive, holistic approach recognizes care managers as professionals who bring a quality-of-life component to the process of developing and implementing a client's life care plan. It has been said, "The elder law attorney who practices life planning defines a satisfactory professional relationship with clients not in terms of resolving legal issues but … in how effective(ly) he [or she] has enabled his [or her] clients to 'maximize the quality of their lives'" (as cited in Takacs, 2007, pp. 1–21).

Ethical Considerations

In addition to the many ethical obligations inherent in the discharge of the professional duties of the professional life care planner and the elder law attorney, a body of complex ethical issues may arise when the life care planning/forensic life planning dichotomy is examined. Specifically, these issues, in their various fact-specific permutations, can spring from the dilemma of the impact of funds availability on future care planning. Elder law attorneys typically approach the forensic life plan from the standpoint of first quantifying existing financial resource availability and then developing a plan within the parameters of those financial constraints. Accordingly, forensic life plans for three clients with identical personal needs would be markedly different in light of the resource availability for each client. Where continuing court oversight of a plan of care is contemplated, as in the case of an adult under conservatorship or a minor under guardianship, the judge in charge of the case will take a balance sheet approach to approval of a proposed plan and to review of action taken in the implementation of an existing plan.

In sharp contrast is the ethical obligation of the professional life care planner to develop a care plan that is needs based rather than funds based (Commission on Health Care Certification, 2007). In such circumstances, the challenge for the elder law attorney who collaborates with the professional life care planner is twofold: first, to educate the party having authority to approve and oversee the implementation of a life care plan as to the wisdom of the needs-based approach; and, second, to advocate for the incorporation of flexibility in the evaluation of care plans. The professional life care planner can become a critical partner to the party having approval authority in defining the success of the care plan and, in so doing, can maintain adherence to the attendant professional standards and ethics of professional life care planners.

Elder Law Attorneys and Professional Life Care Planners: The Perfect Match

In consideration of the foregoing, it would appear that professional life care planners and elder law attorneys are positioned to work collaboratively to effectively assess, plan, advocate for, and deliver services to enhance or maintain the best possible quality of life for elderly persons or persons with disabilities.

Throughout the United States, local laws require that certain transactions involving legal awards of money to or for the benefit of persons who are under disability due to age or mental or physical infirmity must be court approved. Professional life care planners provide an invaluable service to the courts and the parties in developing an appropriate plan for the long-term uses of the funds awarded. Anecdotal information provided by experienced professional life care planners suggests that, at times, life care plans, even though court approved, unfortunately are not always fully implemented. One of the stated reasons for this dilemma is that there sometimes is no one on the care planning team who can help structure the plan so that it is legally enforceable and so that there is continuing accountability for implementation. The involvement of an attorney in the

Table 25.1 Professional Life Care Planner's Matrix for Collaboration with Forensic Life Planner Observing the Holistic Practice Model

			Persons Involved					
Activity	*Attorney*	*Caregiver(s)*	*Client*	*Health Care Provider(s)*	*Skilled Care Representative*	*Social Worker*	*Geriatric Care Manager*	*Life Care Planner*
Initial Consulation	**X**	**X**	**X (if the client is mentally able to participate)**					**X**
Physical Baseline Examination			**X**				**X**	**X**
Financial Status Review	**X**	**X**	**X (if the client is mentally able to participate)**					**X**
Pre-Admission Evaluation			**X**		**X**	**X**	**X**	
Strategic Asset and Resource Placement	**X**	**X**	**X (if the client is mentally able to participate)**					**X**
Residential Placement		**X**	**X**		**X (depending upon the placement of the client)**		**X**	**X**
Continuing Health Care Interventions				**X**			**X**	**X**
Quarterly Residential Placement Review		**X**	**X**				**X**	**X**
Periodic Review of Asset and Resource Placement Strategy	**X**	**X**	**X (if the client is mentally able to participate)**					

creation of the plan can contribute to the development of a strategy that will ensure that the plan is carried out long term. Another potential reason is that life care plans are often not fully funded and a qualified professional life care planner can be invaluable with prioritizing needs as well as attempting to locate alternative funding sources in the implementation of the plan.

As observed previously, the typical contexts in which the elder law attorney provides forensic life planning services generally are those that arise from the occurrence of a traumatic or acquired brain injury or other dementia where family involvement is a dependent element in successful planning. Elder law attorneys are not generally presented with the opportunity to serve persons with other disabling conditions (i.e., spinal cord injury, amputations, etc.) for whom personal independence in all aspects of life is a central issue and for whom there may be little, if any, involvement of family caregivers. The elder law attorney can provide much needed forensic life planning services for this population, particularly in the area of advocacy under state and federal statutory provisions ensuring accommodation and access in workplace, employment, and public facility settings. Professional life care planners working with such clients can add a dimension to the services they render by incorporating the assistance of a legal advocate.

The professional life care planner often does not have a means of reaching many in the potential client population who have need for life care planning. Within the forensic arena, the professional life care planner is typically engaged as a consequence of a catastrophic injury and the engagement typically is initiated by a liability insurance carrier, an insurance defense attorney, or a plaintiff personal injury attorney. Of course, there are other uses of life care planning outside the forensic arena such as hospital or nursing home discharge planning, estate planning, workers' compensation issues, and others. However, within the forensic setting, the term of the engagement generally is for the amount of time necessary to assess the injured person's needs and to design and present the plan for care; thereafter, the engagement of the professional life care planner typically ceases. The elder law attorney, however, is in contact with a vast pool of persons coping with issues related to aging and disability who have voluntarily sought the attorney's services for a long-term planning and management function.

In conclusion, the prospect of collaboration between the elder law attorney and the professional life care planner provides each the opportunity to expand the scope of his or her practice and the concomitant challenge to each to address serious and complex questions within the framework of his or her respective professional discipline. The attorney who seeks to provide forensic life planning for elders or persons with disabilities serves his or her client well when he or she incorporates the expertise of a professional life care planner throughout the course of representation.

Case Study

Facts: Carl and Imogene have been married for 40 years. Carl was a Navy veteran in World War II. Upon discharge, Carl began civilian employment. Imogene has a history of mental health problems. Her mental issues have at times strained their marriage. Imogene has, on more than one occasion, threatened Carl with a knife. When Imogene threatens Carl, he leaves the home and lives with a relative, usually one of their daughters.

Their assets include a jointly owned residence worth approximately $235,000 and joint bank accounts of less than $200,000. Carl's income consists of a retirement pension and Social Security. Imogene only receives Social Security. Together their income totals approximately $2,700 per month. Their joint expenses total approximately $2,500 per month, including groceries, utilities, insurance, mortgage, and other miscellaneous expenses.

At this time, Imogene has experienced a health downturn due to a stroke. She requires 24-hour at-home care. A daughter has taken Imogene into her home, where a home health care agency provides needed care. This caregiving arrangement has worked due to a long-term care insurance policy that Imogene purchased many years ago.

Issues presented:

1. *Financing Imogene's nursing home care.* Imogene's health continues to decline. The caregivers, Carl and his daughters, based upon the recommendations of the geriatric care manager and the life care planner, have decided to place Imogene in a skilled nursing facility. The average cost of skilled care can range from $170 to $225 per day. Even though Imogene's long-term care insurance policy will cover a portion of her skilled nursing cost, there will still be a difference to be paid by someone. As we can see from Carl and Imogene's financial portfolio, their current income will not cover the cost of Imogene's skilled care in a residential setting. Also, it would appear that Carl and Imogene's assets would render Imogene financially ineligible to qualify for public benefits through the Medicaid program or through the Veterans Administration to defray the cost of such care. The threshold considerations relative to placement in a skilled nursing facility are as follows:

   In considering an appropriate skilled nursing facility placement, it is imperative to consider Imogene's past behavioral issues. Many facilities may decline to accept her as a resident due to her past behavioral issues.

   Carl does not drive very much and cannot travel very far from their home to visit Imogene in the skilled nursing facility.

   Carl and Imogene's assets must be repositioned in forms that will cause those assets not to be categorized as countable resources under Medicaid criteria. Because a Medicaid benefits applicant can only have $2,000 in countable resources, the remainder of the assets must be allocated, spent, or invested in ways that are Medicaid compliant and thus are not included as countable resources when a Medicaid benefits application is considered. In the case of Carl and Imogene, several methods of asset repositioning should occur. The following asset repositioning strategy could be adopted to establish Medicaid benefits eligibility; it must be noted, however, that because the Medicaid program is administered in each state under state-specific rules and regulations, the calculations herein are representative only.

Standard maintenance amount	$1,711
Mortgage payment	$1,200
Property taxes	$167.33
Homeowners' insurance	$97.67
Utilities amount	$160
Total shelter cost (steps 2 through 5)	$1,625
30% of standard maintenance amount ($1,711 × .3 =)	$513.30
Excess shelter amount ($1,625 – $513.30 =)	$1,111.70
Total need of community spouse ($1,111.70 + $1,711 =)	$2,822.70
Total of community spouse's noninvestment income	$900
Total of institutionalized spouse's noninvestment income	$1,800
Personal needs allowance	$40
$1,800 – $40 =	$1,760
$2,822.70 – ($900 + $1,760) =	$162.70
$162.70 × 12 =	$1,952.40
$1,952.40/.3 (interest rate) =	$6,508.00

i. A portion of the couple's assets may be allocated exclusively to Carl: The amount of Imogene's assets allocated to Carl is $6,508.00.

ii. Next, a portion of Imogene's income may be allocated to Carl to cover his living expenses. Carl can request a fair hearing before the state agency charged with responsibility for administering the Medicaid program during which he can present proof of his living expenses so that a portion of Imogene's income may be allocated to him. It is possible for a portion of Imogene's income to be allocated to Carl so that his imputed income for purposes of Medicaid eligibility is $1,711, that is, the current standard maintenance amount. Thus, Imogene's imputed monthly income would be $989 and Carl's would be $1,711. The $989 amount that is allocated to Imogene under this calculation is the amount that must be paid to the skilled nursing facility as her personal contribution to the cost of her residential care. Medicaid will pay the remainder of the monthly cost of her residential care. The remainder of Carl and Imogene's monthly income in excess of the $989 amount may be retained by Carl and spent on his personal monthly living expenses.

2. *Seeking supplemental income for Carl.* Based upon Carl's military service, he may be eligible for Veterans Administration benefits because of Imogene's medical needs. If her medical needs are sufficient and if their assets can be positioned to establish benefits eligibility, Carl could qualify to receive roughly $1,000 per month, which could be spent on his living expenses or on Imogene's care. If Carl qualified for the VA benefit and if Imogene qualified for the Medicaid benefit, the Medicaid benefit for Imogene would be reduced by the amount of the VA benefit. The criteria and the corresponding calculations under which eligibility for VA benefits is determined are different from those that apply to establish Medicaid eligibility. A methodology similar to that set forth in Step 1 would be employed using the benchmarks set forth under separate and distinct VA eligibility criteria.
3. *Accommodating Carl's rehabilitation from his anticipated surgery.* Carl is scheduled to undergo hip replacement in the near future. This will impact his ability to visit Imogene and will create a temporary need for skilled nursing care for Carl. Care should be given to determine whether the skilled nursing facility selected for Imogene has the capability to care for Carl during his rehabilitation so that he may stay in Imogene's room during that time. Such arrangements can sometimes be made, resulting in economy in cost of rehabilitative care and reduction of demands upon family caregivers during Carl's convalescence.

State Statutes

- California: CAL. PROB. CODE §2504.
- Colorado: Colorado Court Rules: Colorado Rules of Procedure for Small Claims Courts: Chapter 27 Colorado Rules of Probate Procedure: Rule 16 Court Approval of Settlement of Claims of Persons Under Disability.
- Delaware: DEL. CODE ANN. Tit.12 §3901(k).
- Florida: FLA. STAT. ch. 768.25.
- Georgia: GA. CODE ANN. §29-3-3(e).
- Nevada: NEV. REV. STAT. 42.030.
- New Mexico: N.M. STAT. ANN. §39-1A-4.
- New York: N.Y. GEN. OBLIG. LAW §5-1706.
- Tennessee: TENN. CODE ANN. §29-34-105.
- Virginia: VA. CODE ANN. §8.01-424.

- Takacs, T. 1998. *Elder Law Practice in Tennessee* (1st ed.). Charlottesville, VA: Michie/Lexus Law Publishing.
- Takacs, T. 2007. *Elder Law Practice in Tennessee* (2nd ed.). Charlottesville, VA: Michie/Lexus Law Publishing.
- What Is NAELA. (n.d.). Retrieved August 4, 2007, from www.naela.com/public/whatisneala.htm.

References

Aevarsson, O. 1996. A population-based study on the incidence of dementia disorders between 85 and 88 years of age. *Journal of the American Geriatrics Society, 44*, 1455–1460.

Cicero. 1942. *Cicero on the Orator Books I-II* (E. W. Sutton & H. Rackham, Trans.). Cambridge, MA: Harvard University Press. (n.d.). Retrieved August 5, 2007, from http://app.e2ma.net/campaign/c0b945d040e2fc1968b fed18512be37d.

Morgan, R. C., & Sabatino, C. (n.d.). *Ethical Issues in Elder Law.* Retrieved August 15, 2007, from www.aarp-foundation.org/Friday/Workshops/EthicalIssues/Handout1.pdf.

National Academy of Elder Law Attorneys (n.d.a) About. Available at https://www.naela.org/Web/About/ImportTemp/About_NAELA_New.aspx?hkey=feb0efd3-bd62-4508-9ca4-20de373d4784.

National Elder Law Foundation (n.d.). Program for the Certification of Elder Law Attorneys. Retrieved August 5, 2007, from www. nelf.org/pdf/NELFRulesand%20Regs.pdf.

Needham, H. C. (n.d.). *Elder law comes of age.* National Elder Law Foundation. Retrieved August 5, 2007, from www.nelf.org/elderlaw.htm.

Population. (n.d.). Retrieved August 5, 2007, from www.agingstats.gov/Agingstatsdotnet/Main_Site/Data/2000_Documents/Population.pdf.

Rules and Regulations. (n.d.). Retrieved August 5, 2007, from www.nelf.org/randregs.htm.

Sutton, E., & Rackham, H. 1942. *Cicero: On the Orator.* Harvard University Press: Cambridge, MA.

Chapter 26

Day-in-the-Life Video Production in Life Care Planning

J. Mat Hunt, Jr.

Contents

Introduction....681
Moving Visuals Move People ... Especially If One Can Also Hear What's Moving....681
The Height of Bad Things Happening to Good People....682
Admiration ... Not Pity....683

Introduction

Moving Visuals Move People ... Especially If One Can Also Hear What's Moving

In this author's opinion, the day-in-the-life video can be one of an attorney's most effective tools to substantiate a client's injury, demonstrate ongoing difficulty, and put a name and a face on a case number. It is a legitimate opportunity to show what must be shown in a way that protects a client's dignity. Furthermore, videos can assert admiration in place of pity or misunderstanding, and can educate the viewer about very real circumstances in ways verbal or print communication rarely can. Indeed, video productions portray the essence of the client ... within a reasonable amount of time, in order to convey the message.

But it is not a cookie-cutter task, is rarely completed in a day, and some of the creative and emotional elements most people may believe would be the dramatic content of such a video just will not fly. Some content might just get thrown out if over the prejudicial line, so it is best to know where not to go, and then to not even go there.

First, one needs to know where to go, by determining the priorities necessary to be in the content. The single, most important planning tool to help accomplish this goal is a good life care plan.

After a number of years as a news feature reporter/producer/editor at a "#1-in-the-market" network affiliate television station, and after a couple of subsequent private sector years in the video business, mostly producing for ad agencies and businesses, I received my first opportunity to do a day-in-the-life video in 1984. I did not know the attorney at the time, but for some reason he believed I was the guy to call, and ever since then, it has been an evolving, fine-tuning mainstay of our company that is taken very seriously … because it truly matters to somebody. Many other attorneys have increasingly called upon our company over the years to provide this service, and each product is usually an improvement over the last. These demonstrative exhibits are considerably better when a life care planner is involved at the outset, but at the time of my initial assignment, I did not even know what a life care planner was. It was totally new territory, and there was much to learn in order to be credible.

Sharing some of that first experience may be a useful introduction for this chapter, because it is unforgettable. And I may be the only person who watched all of it, as many cases settle before the visuals are even put together. However, if the visuals are there, reality can be preserved in the event it is needed, and it is good to be prepared ahead of time. *You may only get one take.*

This first client was almost 300 miles away, in the middle of nowhere, and our work involved documenting the end result of an elderly minister's having been robbed and shot through his neck as he and his wife stopped to spend the night in a motel, on their way for him to preach in a revival in yet another state. He was medically unable to travel for court appearances in the resulting civil and criminal actions in another state's jurisdiction, due to his spinal injury and the resulting complications.

The Height of Bad Things Happening to Good People

Yes, we had a location light kit … we had a fine broadcast camera … and there was enough feature work experience to know something about doing a "warm and fuzzy" video in somebody's home. But there was much more to consider, and many of the creative things learned in the TV and ad business needed to be cast aside, because everything was potentially discoverable. In that planning process, there was the need to learn about the myriad of health care necessities that should be included in this video, in order to help a jury understand the difficulty and resulting expense. It had to be videotaped and later assembled in a way that made sense for the viewer … eventually consistent with somebody's live testimony. Writing a voiceover and presenting a self-contained narrated video in court was not an option. These visuals needed to substantiate testimony we did not yet have.

In producing day-in-the-life videos, nothing is staged. It is not necessary to stage, because the content is real. We did the location work, we got different angles, and we observed the client eating, taking his meds, the architectural modifications, therapy, the whole nine yards. I thought we had completed the important part and was personally moved that nobody was angry, especially under the circumstances. The client and his family had already dealt with that, and all their energy was devoted to day-to-day survival.

Our being present made our client's day even more exhausting and difficult. Concentration fatigue was very real, as everyone was working together to find solutions in dealing with this tragedy, and to set up specific shots in a way that made sense to a viewer who could not be there. In producing this first day-in-the-life video, there really was not an established standard or known precedent for reference. We found ourselves helping to set that standard as we developed this realistic visual that required no embellishment.

The next day was a secondary reason to justify the trip from my perspective, as it was not part of the day-in-the-life production. It was a simple video deposition at bedside to get our client's sworn *de bene esse* testimony for the criminal case. Both the public defender and prosecutor were present with the securely transported accused gunman, in order for him to be identified face-to-face as the assailant. This was simple, yet uneasy. Three attorneys, a court reporter with equipment, a videographer with more equipment, a handcuffed defendant, and yes … the client, bedside in a double-wide, with an added-on wheelchair-accessible bathroom.

After identifying the party who fired the shot that permanently disabled the client … a procedural necessity … the client did the sort of thing that makes a lawyer cringe when a client does such things: he forgave the man who shot him, right there on the spot … and on video.

No, he did not condone the action … there was no let-him-go-free mentality … but in this gentleman's pain, suffering, and permanently life-altering consequences, he freed himself of a burden … and likely cleared the way to get on with it for everybody. He also injected a strong dose of humanity in this procedural exercise. This client was Number One. Unforgettable.

Now it is not really known what settled the case, but in this first day-in-the-life, with no real guide to follow in the process, although the video work was an important process, it was not as important as the reality of this client. And as this case settled (as most of ours do), the video was never assembled for use at trial.

Admiration … Not Pity

In preparing a day-in-the-life video, the client's best interests are the first priority. The client should never be made an emotional star in an exciting, flashy video. In my opinion, after doing this work for more than 30 years, flashy is not good, and totally unnecessary. The work should credibly show what is really there. And to be credible, staging is unnecessary. Give the viewer the opportunity to be smart … and FEEL what is really there, without manufacturing drama to attempt to create a picture. Good images with natural sound can tell a credible story.

But that does not mean we should go with the flow with no planning. It does not mean don't move some furniture. And it does not mean no tripod, no lighting, and a quick overview with an "attorney's son's consumer camera," because it seems so easy when first discussed elsewhere.

When asked to produce a day-in-the-life video, especially if the initiating attorney has never retained a professional to complete one (or, occasionally, has never actually even seen one), the first step is to get on the same terminology page. *Make sure what we think we're being asked to do is what the attorney really wants.* For example, one may be asked to do a day-in-the-life video in a wrongful death case … and obviously, the client is no longer among the living. One may be asked to do a day-in-the-life video as if it were for trial, when it is really needed very quickly for a mediation just scheduled. Or the *day-in-the-life* term may be used to indicate settlement documentary … meaning one can more flexibly use music, photographs, unsworn interviews, and other demonstrative media to make it more interesting and credibly self-contained. The end use is a matter of editing. The day-in-the-life location work with the client is essentially the same, and ideally the videographer will be capturing credible visuals that can be used in many ways. The original location video can be the source media for a brief mediation visual, a segment in a settlement documentary, and/or a trial exhibit. Finding out what the attorney *means* procedurally can be more important than what the videographer is first told. *And one must ask.* One must ask specific visual questions that address what can realistically be covered in a video, and that can vary between legal processes and different jurisdictions.

It's important to ask these specifics in writing and get the answers in writing, especially when communicating through an attorney's paralegal or secretary. Perception is reality, and much can be lost in verbal translation.

When I am asked to produce a day-in-the-life video, the first question out of my mouth is "Do you have a life care plan?" In my opinion, the life care plan is the single most important startup tool for day-in-the-life video work, for without it you run the risk of missing the most important aspects of the client's life. You might totally overlook the most important cognitive issues that may impact the value of the case, if you are not equipped to recognize and document them when they occur, often unexpectedly. It may be wise to actually delay location work until a life care planner becomes involved, even if there is not a finished plan in time to meet the video deadline. The videographer can at least have some significant recommendations, a draft, or an outline from the life care planner with which to organize priorities. In the event a life care plan has not yet been drafted, at a minimum a telephone conference call can be a useful alternative in order to assess the life care planner's impressions and recommendations. This, of course, presumes that the life care planner has already met with the client and conducted at least an initial evaluation and assessment. An exception, of course, is if there is a need to document present reality, in anticipation of deterioration of condition before a life care planner is able to become involved.

Regardless of the tips and recommendations provided in this chapter, a day-in-the-life video is not a cookie-cutter project, and at this point there is no known, accredited, specific higher education course or templates on the Internet to adequately tell the reader everything to consider when working on such a video. What we have at the time of this writing are some basic acceptable standards, jurisdiction rules, and precedents to make sure the work is likely to be admitted in court, so it does not become a useless, expensive exercise in frustration. There are numerous, sometimes conflicting, court rulings on admissibility, and these standards vary from state to state and court to court (e.g., medical malpractice versus personal injury or state court versus federal court). Therefore, I will not reference specific rulings for purposes of this chapter. Instead, this chapter will be painted with a broad brush by stating some parametric considerations, and, along the way, offering some practical thoughts as to how to make it happen in the real world based on our experiences.

Basically, key consideration goals are as follows:

- Authentication
- Relevance
- Nonprejudicial portrayal
- Accurate portrayal

Within those goals, it is helpful to establish a chronology, including:

- Baseline: Normal life prior to life-changing event
- Event: Visuals that can substantiate or transition to the present
- Reality: Present-day life care visuals
- Conclusion: The final thought that summarizes the effects of the event

The baseline may be the most overlooked opportunity to make a day-in-the-life video effective. In order to show what a client has lost, establishing what they had to lose is key to making it real. For example, if the client was a computer technician, excelled in his or her work, got along with everybody, and made their boss a lot of money, with the resulting personal earning capacity. … and then a head injury impaired his ability to do the computer work, and also took away the most important purpose and enjoyment of everyday life. … Some qualified expert can write that conclusion in a report or testify to damages, like a college professor.

But wouldn't it be more effective to the jury pool, or a mediator, if you had pictures of the client working on computers? Better yet, some home, training, or corporate video, where one could also hear how swiftly he moved a keyboard, and possibly articulated expertise. He may look the same and may even appear quite normal. But a cognitive decline can be communicated much better if there is a baseline for comparison. Credentials, certificates, accepting performance awards, along with economic information can also visually help establish not only where the client was, but project where he would likely be now without the difficulty, and where he could have been expected to progress in the future.

Smart phone video files and still photographs are more available than ever, and part of the baseline job is to ask employers, coworkers, and family members what they have.... Then transfer and convert those files to your system. Many an attorney has found our looking under somebody's iPhone "rocks" to be an effective visual goldmine nobody expected.

The event may need to be communicated through testimony or documents, but production of a day-in-the-life is an opportunity to make that event more real with TV news reports one can hope the attorney or client has obtained. This can be very effective in mediation and can possibly have some limited use in trial. If the event was an accident and had some media coverage, these may be some of the most useful visuals one has. But often they are not just a phone call away.

In order to have access to this footage, an attorney may need a subpoena to obtain the media, if indeed it was even archived. Most news operations will require a subpoena to protect themselves, plus reasonable fees for their time to run it down and produce it. However, it is unlikely that the attorney will be able to get anything that did not air or was not published. Original footage, even if saved, will be procedurally difficult to obtain, even with a subpoena. Pushing for unedited footage that did not air may not be worth the risk of delaying production of aired video, which can be reviewed and used. In any event, the source should be properly credited with a brief graphic when used, if there is not already a station ID superimposed on the material.

Reality started after the event, and the videographer or editor may have become involved months or years into the process. Although family members have been stressed out for a long time while dealing with their new reality, some may have had the presence of mind to videotape coming home from the hospital, or some of the earlier days of recovery. As mentioned earlier, this "looking under the rocks" is worth the effort to locate a few well-selected seconds that can be a big help in substantiating real difficulty in the passing of time. That is something that may need to be requested repeatedly, and it is a good idea to inquire about videos that may be in the possession of friends. Still photographs are better than nothing, but moving video also gives the viewer ambient audio, and audio is often the foundation for feeling what is seen.

Another source of visuals, in addition to family members, is rehabilitation. Many rehabilitation facilities routinely videotape progress for such functions as walking, and, with the help of the attorney, that can probably be obtained. These recorded incidents add to the chronology.

It is now timely to address some of the day-in-the-life production that the reader may have thought was all there was to this process. But hopefully, after absorbing this chapter up to this point it is apparent there is more to a successful video than perhaps was first thought. Here are some suggestions in checklist form:

- This may sound self-serving on the part of the writer, but it is not a good idea for an attorney to hire a cousin, child, or neighbor to do this work, unless they are experienced. Neither should it be assumed that somebody who shoots sports or weddings is a good choice without some help. A National Court Reporters Association (NCRA) Certified Legal Video Specialist (see www.ncraonline.org) experienced in legal work beyond depositions should be a minimum requirement. And, if he or she has a broadcast television news background, that is even better. That person will know what a deadline is and is less likely to accumulate more material than you can manage. *Long is not good.*

- There should be at least two people involved on site, regardless of how the responsibilities are divided. The videographer needs to be able to totally concentrate on what is being documented, and another party should be producing … by anticipating what is next, helping with equipment, and dealing with family or other caregivers. The target is always moving, and the content being documented may be discoverable. Plus, there are some medical or rehabilitation procedures that must be captured correctly in one take.
- There should be no home video, except the already mentioned archives from family. Day-in-the-life work should be produced with professional equipment by experienced professionals. Minimal camera requirements should be a 3-Chip Broadcast or Industrial Camera, with at least a 10:1, preferably a greater-ratio optical lens. While some cameras have digital zoom capabilities, they can create artifacts that can distract from the closer shots that require a zoom ratio in the first place. Also, digital zooms are difficult to accomplish smoothly on location.
- Professional lighting is a must in order to assure normal skin tones in mixed or low-light environments. It may not be needed for every element, but it should be available with the expertise to use it. If a potential videographer says he/she does not have lighting because the camera is so good it's not needed, call someone else who is willing to work harder to get it right.
- This is probably the most important video in the client's life. Simply bouncing a light off the ceiling does not change reality, yet it may help eliminate color temperature discrepancies that detract. Remember, day-in-the-life videos are competing for an attention span with million-dollar-an-hour television programming coming into everybody's home, every day. Keeping it clean and natural does make a difference, even if the viewer does not think about it. If the end result is natural, one does not have to make excuses for it or think about it.
- The production professionals may be told "no sound." That is not what it means. The intended meaning is likely no narration, or don't have the client or the caregiver stand there and explain what they are doing because it likely cannot be used in court that way. Do record natural sound at all times, and make sure the levels are not too hot (audio recording where microphone volume is set too high) or on auto. This is especially important with the newer digital cameras, for the equipment is less forgiving than analog when levels are too high. Distortion occurs more easily with digital than analog, and it cannot be "undistorted" later. To be safe, audio levels should peak no higher than 12 dB, and one needs a camera with visible Volume Unit Meters in order to monitor audio levels. Good audio gives visuals presence. The viewer should hear machinery, somebody brushing her teeth, or a crutch hitting the floor if the client accidentally drops it. The crew should advise everybody that natural sound is being recorded, so unnecessary commentary is not taped. Always be aware that original footage may have to be produced to the other side.
- Whoever does day-in-the-life work should also be an experienced editor, and the attorney should see examples of his or her work before assuming competence. Reading trade magazines and knowing the language of the business is not sufficient preparation for what is likely the most important video in someone's life. A good editor is more likely to be on the lookout for what matters in the field. Be aware that editing is not cutting things out as much as it is putting in material that tells a story in a way that makes sense to and captivates the viewer. Editing is everything when there may be hours of material and an under-20-minute attention span. The importance of a talented, competent editor throughout the entire process cannot

be understated. Budget-wise, everything that goes into editing should be projected at about 2 hours per finished minute.

- This is not a process to be rushed.
- The location video process will be very tiring for a client. Those involved should be advised up front that eating, bathing, and other forms of caregiving may take three times as long as the usual painstakingly long time.
- Since this process is tiring for the client, restful downtime should be built into the anticipated schedule. It always takes longer than anticipated.
- Find something fun. Even though the situation at hand may be very sad, videos are works within an entertainment medium. If all the content is horrific, it becomes a tune out. The production crew should find and plan something fun that the client can do for enjoyment of life and take advantage of any light moments to contrast and balance the negatives. This will humanize the end product, will allow the viewer to relate, and may be one of the more beneficial things anybody does for the client's feelings.
- After obtaining permission to speak directly with the client or caregiver, establishing a trusting relationship is important. While the client may have been through years of personal intrusion … and while one may be very familiar with a video process … coming into someone's home or facility with a camera, equipment, and unknown people is a very big, potentially stressful event. It is not unlike going to court for the first time. Making people comfortable, and helping them understand that they do not have to clean up for company, can go a long way to pave the way to success.
- That may be complicated by a requirement in some jurisdictions that the other side be notified and allowed to be present. Fortunately, most judges do not consider day-in-the-life videotaping to be an inspection, and the intrusion of opposing counsel can usually be avoided. The presence of too many people is especially difficult if the client is in a hospital or nursing home (see next point).
- Day-in-the-life location work in a facility means numerous hurdles to proactively overcome before the production crew arrives. Not only is the client likely to be confined to one room, possibly semiprivate, but also access to even the least cramped of facilities can be a challenge. One cannot assume that because some family member said some nurse said it was okay for you to come make a video that it is okay to appear with your equipment when it suits the family. Regardless of whether it is a public or a private facility, there is likely an administrator who must run it by risk management, and risk management may be halfway across the country, if not on vacation. If the professional waits until the last minute to cross that bridge, the easiest immediate answer from risk management is always no, so in the process of asking for access, it is sometimes helpful to assert at the outset that (ideally) the facility is not a defendant, and the production crew is part of the process to obtain funding for care. Before being told that other residents or patients cannot be included, the facility should be informed that residents or patients will not be recorded. In fact, some facilities may prohibit including the participation of caregivers employed by the facility.
- Visuals should not be limited to someone lying still in a bed, as feeding, bathing, therapy, and other forms of care need to be part of the story. If videotaping employees is not feasible, perhaps family members or independent caregivers or therapists can be available. In any event, releases should be executed for each person appearing on camera, including family members.
- If facility access is problematic, an additional persuasion one may offer (with consent of the client's attorney) is to provide the facility with a "time code super" copy of all the video shot in the facility for their review prior to editing. This may need to be produced for the other side anyway, so proactively making it available to the facility should not be a problem. It then

becomes a simple matter for those in charge of the facility to confirm for their records that the footage is within reason, and if there is anything in doubt, they can advise in writing, referencing the on-screen numbers. It is probable that the attorney will not want to use any potential problem segment(s) anyway, so this process should be a positive exercise to accomplish what is needed. The writer has found that suggesting this safeguard, with consent of counsel, is useful in totally lowering the facility's shield. Most administrators truly want to help their patients … they just need to make sure their facility is protected, and that the video crew is not *60 Minutes* doing a hidden camera story on their type of facility. And if one ever needs to go back to the same facility in another case, trust is already established, and the process is made a lot smoother.

- More than likely, a day-in-the-life video will require significant videography in the home. A site check with no camera is time well spent to prepare the needs of the environment. If the videographer has come a long distance, perhaps a visit on the day of arrival, with no equipment, will break the ice and lower the shield of anxiety. It is a good opportunity to bond with the family by listening to their story first, and then showing them a cleared example of some of the professional's other work product. Providing an example not only lowers anxiety and creates confidence, but also opens a dialogue for practical suggestions to plan your location work. Then the crew can hit the ground running the next day, after anxieties are cleared and, hopefully, everyone has had a good night's rest. That's right … tell them to go to bed early.
- The site check also is a good time to plan the order of visuals and solicit the caregiver's input as to unique circumstances that might be important to know. One might plan a purpose for dressing by also planning a place to go, such as a doctor's office, grocery store, bowling alley, church, or wherever the client may actually go or enjoy going. This gives purpose for getting dressed and going out the door, and the documented arrival somewhere else does not necessarily have to be the same day. Under those circumstances, it is wise to plan for continuity by suggesting that the same outfit be worn each day.
- If a doctor visit or therapy appointment can be or is scheduled during the location work, that is yet another opportunity for a practical visual. Like any health care facility, getting clearance up front is a must, and the attorney or paralegal may be able to cut through the procedural red tape before the shoot. Again, if the client says the doctor will say it is okay, that does not necessarily mean it is okay. If permission is obtained ahead of time, that doctor or therapy visit is a great opportunity to substantiate how much difficulty the client has in accomplishing more basics than most people even need to consider. On-camera releases are still a must.
- If the field trip opportunity the client was dressed for is the grocery store, one may also need to obtain permission for interior location work. Frankly, it may not even be necessary to go inside a store. Getting in and out of a vehicle in the parking lot may sufficiently make the point.
- Most of what has been addressed to this point is active and moving. But the videographer with a good eye will also obtain visuals of the client doing nothing, possibly resting, possibly bored, possibly helpless. That is part of their day as well, and when that moment comes, a good videographer will know it and will not need to stage it. Throughout the process, there should be cutaways. Close-ups of medications, health care supplies, wipes, tubes, and machinery may have their place as visuals later in the edit. If there is a special bed, it is an expensive piece of equipment to document and justify.
- While it is tempting to want to show a lot of emotion, tight shots of extreme facial grimacing, too many noises, and anything that may be interpreted as overly dramatic should be avoided. If it is there, it's there, and one will know it without having to create it. The expectation is admiration, not pity.

- "Exaggerated difficulty" and "playing to the camera" should always be avoided, as should unnecessarily graphic footage. Such elements that can be interpreted as beyond the norm can invite challenges on grounds of prejudice.
- The videographer with a good eye and a heart will be thinking about what a client *can* do, or perhaps can do with a bit of difficulty. For example, the client with carpal tunnel syndrome may have difficulty opening a jar, but should be given the opportunity to open one, possibly with some help. Hugging children or grandchildren, or the inability to hug children or grandchildren, are visuals worth the effort. Not staged. ... natural ... they know how to do it ... or try to do it as best they can.

But whatever you do, protect the client's dignity. Just like you can video somebody walking down the street, framing from the waist up (à la *60 Minutes*), and you *know* even though you can't see them, the person has legs.... You can frame a caregiver inserting a catheter or doing a bowel program without exposing the private area. This is when you don't have to show everything and allow the viewer to be smart enough to get it and feel it.

This subject could have endless pages of different stories and situations, along with specific visuals that make the point. But since this is not a cookie-cutter process, a good videographer or editor will know what works without a checklist. However, there is also a need to be mindful of the legal process and what is within the bounds of those first priorities.

- *Authentication*: Make sure the party who did the work, or participated in the work, is credible, is available, and has integrity. Make sure the visuals accurately depict reality. No conflicts of interest.
- *Relevance*: Stay on point with purpose. Connect the baseline with the present situation and relate it to the event.
- *Nonprejudicial portrayal*: Prejudicial visuals are invitations for exclusion.
- *Accurate portrayal*: One should not make up or stage anything. Keep it real. Real is good, and it captivates. "Just the facts" increases admissibility.

In other words, the professional retained to develop the day-in-the-life video should use good judgment, exercise appropriate restraint, and save the creative, misleading, morphing effects for political commercials.

A day-in-the-life video is about substantiating something very real to somebody and does not need all the tricks that videographers know that they can do. But some modern-day effects are appropriate in order to protect the client's dignity, such as fuzzing or blurring out private areas in the edit, if they must be in the shot to communicate necessary care. The client deserves integrity, the best quality, the professional's concentration, and respect for dignity.

This type of personal yet professional work ... documenting the difficult ... may not be the most lucrative work one may produce, but it may very well be the most memorable and rewarding. It may or may not even be used in court, as the case may be resolved sooner than expected. But win or lose, one has accomplished something that truly matters, and the videographer may have done more to validate and help somebody get through a tragedy than any other professional brought into the mix, other than a hands-on caregiver. The product will have shared and seriously documented important personal time in *a personal* space.

So, in short, how does one do a day-in-the-life video?

It should be done the way one would like someone else to do it for somebody dear to them.

Chapter 27

Ethical Issues for the Life Care Planner*

Debra E. Berens and Roger O. Weed

Contents

Introduction 691
General Professional Duties within Health Care 693
Example Ethical Brushes 695
Suggestions for Success: Global 696
Suggestions for Success: Malpractice Insurance Related 697
Conclusion 699
References 700

Introduction

According to *Black's Law Dictionary* (Black, 1990), *ethics* is defined as (1) a set of principles of right conduct, (2) a theory or a system of moral values, or (3) the rules or standards governing the conduct of a person or members of a profession. A variation of this definition is found in *Merriam-Webster's Dictionary* (2009a), which defines *ethics* as (1) the discipline dealing with what is good and bad and with moral duty and obligation, (2) a set of moral principles or values, (3) a theory or system of moral values, (4) the principles of conduct governing an individual or a group, or (5) a guiding philosophy.

According to at least one study (Swartz et al., 1996), ethical decision-making undergirds all aspects of rehabilitation. This statement certainly holds true for the practice of life care planning as well, and this chapter will focus on ethics issues specific to the life care planner with suggestions for minimizing potential problems. Also included in this text is the Standards of Practice for Life Care Planners (2015, 3rd rev.) from the International Academy of Life Care

* Portions of this chapter have been adapted from Weed, R., & Berens, D. (2002). Ethics in life care planning. In P. Deutsch (Ed.) *The Expert's Role as an Educator Continues: Meeting the Demands under* Daubert, 59–67. Ahab Press: White Plains, NY.

Planners (IALCP) (see Appendix I). According to *Merriam-Webster's Dictionary* (2009b), a *standard* is defined as (1) something established by authority, custom, or general consent as a model or example; (2) something set up and established by authority as a rule for the measure of quantity, weight, extent, value, or quality; and (3) something that applies to any definite rule, principle, or measure established by authority. As can be expected from a review of these technical definitions, the interplay of ethics and standards is somewhat difficult to separate. However, based on the definitions, ethics-related observations directly related to life care planning are as follows:

- *Right Conduct:* This premise is perhaps the most understandable. Most professionals know right behavior from wrong behavior, yet many influences are exerted on the life care planner when faced with insurance referrals, client/evaluee advocacy, biased information provided by an attorney and/or other referral source, and so on (Banja, 1994). The attorney, for instance, is hired as an advocate for one side of the case or the other (i.e., plaintiff versus defense); however, the life care planner is ethically bound to be an objective professional who develops a future care plan based on the client/evaluee's needs regardless of who is paying the bill. It is especially relevant to clarify one's role at the outset, which can be done in the form of providing a professional disclosure statement. Some professionals provide professional disclosure verbally and some by handing out printed information fact sheets or statements about the role and function of the life care planner and what the person with the disability can expect from an evaluation. For example, in personal injury litigation, the life care planner might be retained as a defense expert to conduct an independent evaluation, or as a plaintiff's expert to provide life care planning opinions without any expectation of implementation of the care plan. In either instance, disclosure of the life care planner's role at the beginning of a case will help to minimize potential problems due to a lack of the client/evaluee's understanding or expectations of services provided. The Standards of Practice for Life Care Planners (IALCP, 2015) state that "Life care planners are expected to … adequately advise evaluees of the role of the life care planner…" Further, the Standards state, "Each evaluee should be fully informed about the role of the life care planner" (IALCP, 2015). The Code of Professional Ethics developed by the International Commission on Health Care Certification (ICHCC), under its principles and associated rules section, states that life care planners "… are obligated to clarify the nature of their relationship to all involved parties when providing services at the request of a third party," and "…will clearly define through written or oral means, the limits of their relationship, particularly in the areas of informed consent and legally privileged communications to all involved individuals" (ICHCC, 2015, R2.3).
- *Moral Values:* The above-referenced dilemma regarding maintaining objectivity regardless of whether the plaintiff or defense side has retained the services of a life care planner can be further influenced by the life care planner's view of the world. For example, a life care planner retained by the plaintiff may privately hold the belief that insurance companies are thieves that deprive people of their rightful recovery and there is a need to get as much as one can for the client/evaluee. Conversely, a life care planner retained by the defense may believe that plaintiff's attorneys get rich off the unfortunate circumstances of people with injuries and too many frivolous lawsuits are filed. These biases must be held in check with extra vigilance to ensure the life care planner provides a proper and objective evaluation and conclusion.
- *Rules or Standards of the Specialty Practice:* In an attempt to rectify some personal biases, industries and professions have developed agreed-upon rules or standards to govern professionals' behavior. Within the preview of the life care planner, there are many ethics codes and licensure laws that include rules regarding personal conduct. An example is

the Practice Standards and Guidelines and Code of Professional Ethics presented by the ICHCC, that include rules of professional conduct that are "exacting standards which provide guidance in specific circumstances" (Practice Standards and Guidelines, ICHCC, 2015, available at https://www.ichcc.org/images/PDFs/ICHCC_StandardsandGuidelines.pdf). Another example mentioned earlier in this chapter is the Standards of Practice for Life Care Planners developed by the IALCP (2015).

General Professional Duties within Health Care

Many ethics guidelines overlap with each other, and others have significant differences in detail. However, there are several concepts that appear to apply across the board. According to Banja (1994, p. 86) and Blackwell (1999), the four commonalities are as follows:

- *Autonomy*: The client's right to information and voluntary decision-making.
- *Nonmaleficence*: The client's right not to be harmed.
- *Beneficence*: The client will receive appropriate care or services.
- *Justice*: The client's right to receive unbiased and nonprejudicial treatment.

In accordance with these constructs, Shaw and Sawyer (1999) further divide the concepts into counseling and forensic environments. Although written for the certified rehabilitation counselor (CRC), several precepts apply to the life care planner. With regard to ethical priorities, Shaw and Sawyer (1999) assert that professionals who practice in the counseling environment emphasize autonomy, nonmaleficence, and beneficence, whereas the forensic counselor emphasizes justice. They also observe that there are many other variations in roles that can constitute challenges. In general, confidentiality does not exist in the legal case, but failure to maintain confidentiality in a counseling relationship is a clear breach of ethics. Within the legal environment, the consultant must be accountable to the jurisdiction in which the case is pending; whereas in the counseling environment, one is responsible to the client. The counseling relationship is expected to be supportive, whereas in the forensic setting the consulting relationship is evaluative in nature (Barros-Bailey et al., 2008).*

Furthermore, based on the authors' experiences and review of the literature, several scenarios are regularly observed. The first is associated by the life care planner going *outside of the area of expertise*. This can take the form of offering medical opinions, life expectancy projections, or economic valuations (distinguishing between economic summaries from present value calculations) without adequate knowledge, education, or foundation. Life care planners unfamiliar with the forensic setting may be seduced into offering opinions outside their area of expertise that can damage their credibility and, in a roundabout way, damage the case. In the event of a plaintiff's expert, this action also can cause harm to the client/evaluee.

A second scenario is associated with the life care planner who develops a relationship with the attorney such that he or she becomes the *hired gun*. This relationship can be cultivated with either plaintiff or defense attorneys where potential future referrals may be forthcoming. Also, some attorneys may be adept at providing biased information to the expert or inviting the expert to company parties or dinners just to form a more friendly or social relationship rather than a professional, working relationship. This statement is not intended to suggest that a life care planner

* For a discussion on this related topic, the authors suggest reading Barros-Bailey, M., Carlisle, J., Graham, M., Neulicht, A., Taylor, R., & Wallace, A. (2008). *Who Is the Client in Forensics?* [White paper] Boise, ID: Authors.

must not have a working lunch with a referral source, but that the ethical consultant should be aware of influences that may shade his or her professional opinion or give the perception of something other than a professional, nonbiased working relationship. In one case, a neuropsychologist admitted in deposition that she had invited the attorney who retained her services to her home for a lunch and swim party and that they had attended several personal social events together. In another case, a rehabilitationist compiled a plan for an injured worker during the same time frame that she was also married to the client's attorney. A third example is the case of a rehabilitation counselor who publicly claimed he was going to "kick the defense counsel's butt" in an upcoming trial. Although the reports and opinions by these professionals may very well have been appropriate and accurate, these statements and scenarios cast a shadow over the objectivity of the consultant's work.

A third scenario is the potential for errors and miscommunication because of *unclear expectations*. This is particularly a problem for the inexperienced life care planner who may take instruction from the referral source rather than have clear boundaries about his or her role. In general, it is more effective for the life care planner to assertively outline for the referral source what he or she is or is not qualified to do. In these writers' experience, it is better for the life care planner to clearly outline what the expectations are without relying on an attorney to direct the planner's activity and potentially influence the life care planner's objectivity.

Life care planners need to exercise *due care* by diligently reviewing case materials, seeking appropriate research and information, and following a process consistent with standards of the specialty practice that results in credible opinions and conclusions. Many consultants do not know what the established standards are (mostly because they are not members of the IALCP, are not certified in an area relative to the specialty practice, and do not attend conferences that offer life care planning topics), and therefore fail to follow the standards. It is reasonable to observe that a growing professional practice area, such as life care planning, will attract entrepreneurs who will learn through trial and error; however, this method of learning can damage the specialty practice unless effective intervention can occur, including education about accepted standards and procedures. (A wise person once said, if one learns by trial and error, they are likely to go on trial for one of their errors.)

Life care planners who are new to the specialty practice need to learn the specialty area (a.k.a., *literacy*). Unfortunately, many beginning care planners are seriously deficient in this area. There is a specialized methodology, vocabulary, and knowledge base that must be learned and understood in order to be an effective life care planner. Also, different jurisdictions have different rules with regard to the life care plan. For example, in forensic and workers' compensation areas, differences exist between state laws and regulations, as well as between state and federal rules of evidence, and it behooves the life care planner to be cognizant of the differences within the various jurisdictions in which he or she provides services. A case that the authors reviewed involved a life care plan developed as a result of a breach of contract lawsuit. Upon review of the plan and consultation with the attorney, it became apparent that the life care planner was not aware of, or perhaps not familiar with, the rules specific to breach of contract law such that the plan included recommendations and costs that were not allowable under this particular jurisdiction. Such lack of knowledge raised the question of accuracy of the life care plan and credibility of the life care planner who prepared it.

Another issue for the life care planner, even for the most experienced professional, is the potential problem with *dual relationships* (also related to dual roles or multiple relationships or roles). The term *dual* implies that the professional not only serves in his or her primary role, but also establishes a second (or multiple) role with the client/evaluee that may be viewed as harmful (Cottone, 2005). Although the issue of dual relationships historically has been a common topic in the ethics literature and is specifically addressed in the Standards of Practice for Life Care Planners (IALCP, 2015, reprinted in Appendix I), more recently the term *multiple relationships* has gained favor and implies two or more relationships with clients/evaluees that could impair professional judgment or increase the risk of exploitation (AAMFT Code of Ethics, 2001, subprinciple 1.3, as cited in Cottone, 2005). In the practice of life care planning, it may be common for the expert to develop a future care plan while also providing some case management and coordination services. Indeed, the ethics section of the Standards of Practice for Life Care Planners states that "serving in dual or multiple professional roles, such as case manager or treater, is permitted as long as the simultaneous roles are not used for the purpose of providing benefit to the professional (e.g., recommending continued use of the professional without justification)." Furthermore, "Each evaluee should be fully informed about the role of the life care planner... life care planners who have dual role responsibilities should clarify that the life care planning role is separate and should clarify what the limits of their participation might be" (IALCP, 2015). In other situations, life care planners may use counseling skills to facilitate information-gathering and reduce the client/family's psychological pain/anxiety when the real purpose is to obtain information to develop an expert opinion. In one example, a rehabilitation counselor proclaimed she was going to offer her services free to help an acquaintance in her divorce action because the acquaintance's "s.o.b. husband" was (in her opinion) mistreating her friend.

Cimino-Ferguson (2005) urges that it is critical for the life care planner to clarify the relationship with the client/evaluee at the outset. In the literature and as previously stated in this chapter, such disclosure is referred to as professional disclosure. Berens and Weed (2001) assert that a written professional disclosure statement signed by the client/evaluee is preferred and one of the best ways to uphold the life care planner's ethical obligation to inform clients/evaluees of the process and ensure the client/evaluee understands and gives consent to participate. The authors point out that professional disclosure such as this obviously applies to cases in which the life care planner has access to the client/evaluee and his or her designee. In cases where the life care planner does not have client/evaluee access or is serving as a consultant where no client/evaluee interaction is allowed or expected, professional disclosure generally is not made or required. (See also discussion at the beginning of this chapter regarding professional disclosure as promoted by the IALCP Standards of Practice for Life Care Planners and ICHCC code of ethics.)

Example Ethical Brushes

Court rulings provide insight into ethical issues related to rehabilitation professionals providing expert testimony (Weed, 2000). For example, in *Fairchild v. United States*, 769 R. Supp. 964 (W.D. La., 1991), the court awarded a sum of $150,000 instead of the $1.74 million requested because the rehabilitation plan was prepared by someone not considered an expert. The so-called expert reportedly had attended two conferences on rehabilitation counseling and had prepared only 25 life care plans. No other training or education within the field of rehabilitation counseling or life care planning had been completed.

In *Elliott v. United States*, 877 F. Supp. 1569 (M.D. GA., 1992), the defense expert's opinion was disregarded because the expert had been a rehabilitation consultant for only a short time, had completed only five life care plans, and had never implemented a plan. Additionally, the care plan reportedly did not include a physician contact or a conservative view.

In *Norwest Bank, N.A. and Kenneth Frick v. K-Mart Corporation*, U.S. District Court, Northern District of Indiana, South Bend Division (1997), the rehabilitation expert's opinion with regard to future care was excluded in part due to a lack of medical foundation, as well as an inability to produce evidence that the methodologies used to forecast the cost of future care were based on anything other than personal experience.

In a workers' compensation case, *Maria Teresa Palmer*, guardian ad litem for *J. Carmen Fuentes v. W. Brent Jackson d/b/a Jackson's Farming Company* (I.C. No. 859146, North Carolina),

> the life care planner did not travel to Mexico to evaluate plaintiff's home circumstances and was not familiar with the medical facilities which may be in the vicinity of plaintiff's home. Therefore, specific findings could not be made with respect to renovations which may be necessary to plaintiff's dwelling or specific medical and durable supplies and equipment. Further, while plaintiff would benefit from placement in a brain injury facility, there is insufficient evidence in the record on which any specific finding may be made of whether an appropriate facility is available for plaintiff.

However, in light of the unique contribution of the published procedures of a life care plan, the workers' compensation commission in this case concluded that a complete, current, and comprehensive life care plan would be beneficial.

In addition to published cases, there are other examples based on deposition testimony that are not readily available to the general reader. At least two cases reveal life care planners who admit no previous education specific to life care planning, few or no publications related to life care planning in their libraries, and no membership in professional organizations specific to life care planning. When asked about certification, at least one of the individuals claimed she does not need to be certified as a life care planner since she has years of experience and is certified in a related field. However, further examination of her credentials revealed she achieved certification as a case manager (CCM) and rehabilitation counselor (CRC) at the time the respective certifications were initially offered. Therefore, it may be presumed the individual was actually grandfathered in (i.e., took the certification exam but did not have to pass it in order to become certified).

Other examples of deponents' testimony include those that express claims that life care planners are only serving an administrative function where they, similar to a secretary, simply record what someone tells them (see also Weed, 2002, and Weed & Johnson, 2006, for many more examples). At the other extreme is the professional (who is not a physician) who asserts that he or she can develop a complex life care plan without consultation with medical or treating professionals (if he or she has access to them). Or a physician that develops a life care plan, including case management, nursing, vocational, and psychological opinions, without adequate corroborating foundation.

As noted in the Weed (2002) article, the competent life care planner is neither an administrative recorder nor a know-it-all. A better analogy may be a general contractor or one who knows the big picture and which questions are relevant to ask of which professionals while building the care plan from a sound foundation to a completed comprehensive structure.

Suggestions for Success: Global

In order for the life care planning specialty practice to thrive and expand, it is incumbent upon each individual life care planner to assume control and responsibility over his or her actions and to practice within the ethical boundaries of the industry. Some suggestions to enhance the life care planner's ethical practice include the following:

- Join a professional organization specific to life care planning that includes ethics and standards of practice (e.g., IALCP). Belonging to organizations that primarily are nursing, rehabilitation counseling, or related professions are useful but may not be helpful for specific issues associated with providing an ethical foundation in life care planning. Professional organizations specific to life care planning also offer a process by which life care planners can be held accountable to ethics and standards within the industry.

- Consider certification as a life care planner or become certified in an area related to life care planning. (Another option is to become a fellow of the IALCP.) Although it is a voluntary process, certification affirms that the professional has completed the requisite education, experience, and training and has passed an exam that demonstrates he or she possesses a minimum competency to provide services. Also, certification offers a process for ethics complaints and ongoing continuing education requirements. Having such requirements will assist the life care planner in maintaining a continuing focus on life care planning training, professional ethics and standards of practice specific to the industry. See also the chapter on credentialing in this text.
- Follow established standards of practice and ethics (see the Appendices at the end of this book) published by the IALCP or other organizations specific to life care planning.
- Expand one's knowledge base by attending conferences, summits, and specialty training specific to life care planning. Not only will the life care planner be kept current on the industry and acceptable practices (this is especially true if the consultant is not certified and has no continuing education requirements), but also leaders in the field will become part of his or her professional network.
- Subscribe to the *Journal of Life Care Planning* (and/or other relevant life care planning journals) to stay current with contemporary issues in life care planning. (Available by contacting the International Association of Rehabilitation Professionals at 888-427-7722 or www.rehabpro.org/ialcp/journal.)
- Be active in the specialty practice. Join a committee for program planning, offer an article to the *Journal* or other relevant publications, or conduct or participate in research projects; for example, do something that will enhance life care planning and give back to the profession.
- Develop a protocol for disclosing to clients/evaluees the various role(s) one might assume during the life care planning process.

Suggestions for Success: Malpractice Insurance Related

The following suggestions were offered by National Professional Group, a malpractice insurance carrier, as cited in Weed et al. (2003, pp. 47–54). Although there are many overlapping topics, these are specific to avoiding ethical brushes with insurance claims:

- *Role with Account/Referral Source*: It is very important for hiring parties to clearly define the rehabilitation professional's role and the type of evaluation or services being requested. It is preferable that these assignments be in writing.
- *Role with Client/Evaluee*: In cases where the consultant is hired by the insured party's insurance carrier, professional disclosure must be made with the client/evaluee and documented. The client/evaluee must clearly understand the role of the consultant (e.g., to evaluate and assist the client/evaluee with return to work, to case manage, or to develop a life care plan).
- *Written Documentation*: Many times the individual retaining the consultant may send a cursory retention letter outlining services requested. If not, it is incumbent for the consultant to get the necessary information verbally and follow up with a written confirmation to the referring party, preferably signed by both the referring party and the life care planner.

- *Scope of Service*: Misunderstandings can develop over the scope of service. Thus, the more accurate the consultant's documentation, the easier it is for a review committee or court to determine that the consultant acted appropriately.
- *Objectivity*: The consultant must remain objective and unbiased in the delivery of services and shall not accept assignments if the individual who retains the consultant's services attempts to influence the objectivity or outcome of the evaluation.
- *Contingency Fees*: Consultants shall not provide services on a contingency basis to prevent the appearance that the consultant's objectivity has been compromised at the prospect of financial gain.
- *Professional Fees*: If the consultant provides trial and deposition testimony, he or she will be cross-examined about professional fees. Fees should be standard for the services provided; exorbitant fees will compromise the consultant's credibility.
- *Communication*: Proper communication at all levels is critical, and it is important for the consultant to provide a clear explanation of what should be expected and the possible outcomes. Other areas of communication include ongoing progress, internal communication, external communication, fees, and fee structure. The consultant shall not tell a client/evaluee that a coworker (for a worker's compensation injury) made an error that caused the client/evaluee's injury or that the client/evaluee's problem could be worse.
- *Terminology*: Professionals have their own set of technical or industry-specific terminology, and it is easy to forget that laypeople may not completely understand those terms. It is important for professionals to use common terminology with clients/evaluees and maintain a speaking manner that ensures the client/evaluee is treated respectfully and that he or she understands what is being communicated. Provide booklets and pamphlets to encourage greater understanding among clients/evaluees and to encourage clients/evaluees to ask questions to avoid any confusion. Remember, the better the client/evaluee is educated and understands the role of the consultant, the lower the chances for misunderstandings and potential lawsuits.
- *Colleague Collaboration*: Quality collaboration helps detect areas of weakness in one's practice. An outside quality assessment from another professional perspective may help the consultant to recognize procedures that could be changed to benefit service delivery and potentially protect him or herself from malpractice claims.
- *Continuing Education*: It is important to keep abreast of new advances in technology within a particular area of specialty. Therefore, continuing education, whether required by any board or certification, is crucial.
- *Common Sense*: Good common sense always is valuable in dealing with people referred for services and in maintaining good solid business practice.
- *Records:* Do not alter a client/evaluee's record under any circumstances. Be careful about documentation and include the rationale for services or why in some cases a decision is made not to do something. Make sure to follow one's own policies and procedures in every case.
- *Client Respect*: Always treat clients/evaluees properly and with respect. Never let the client/evaluee feel he or she is unimportant or insignificant.
- *Consent*: Always obtain written informed consent from the client/evaluee when able. (For example, in defense referred cases, it generally is not possible to obtain written informed consent from the client/evaluee.)
- *Confidentiality*: Be extraordinarily careful about confidential information. Oftentimes, rehabilitation professionals may be in an environment where unsuspecting family members or others may overhear the content of information that potentially could be damaging to the client. Be aware of and comply with HIPAA guidelines as they apply to the practice of life care planning.

Conclusion

In summary, the case examples described earlier in this chapter underscore the need to adhere to ethics and standards that are agreed upon and followed by competent life care planning professionals. Ethics statements represent judgments about morality, what is right or wrong, good or bad, and how to deal with everyday situations. All possible situations or scenarios cannot be anticipated, and the life care planner with a solid ethics foundation will be able to approach those situations in a more ethical or correct manner, which likely will preserve his or her reputation and credibility while also minimizing the potential for ethics breaches or malpractice claims. In all instances, an ethical decision-making model is desired when confronted with an ethical dilemma.

As time passes, ethics statements seem to become more important. The Code of Professional Ethics for Rehabilitation Counselors (CRCC, 2017) essentially doubled in length from the previous code in an apparent continued attempt to address more issues based on a combination of ethics complaints, the evolution and growth of the rehabilitation industry, and anticipated problems. Additionally, continuing education requirements to maintain CRC certification historically were based solely on rehabilitation-related topics requirements; however, effective July 1999, standards for recertification were made stronger in the area of ethics, and now 10 hours of ethics continuing education are required (out of a total of 100 hours) for CRC recertification every 5 years. Similarly, the ICHCC continuing education requirements for certified life care planners include 8 of the 80 required recertification hours to be within ethics or "of ethical practice subject matter" (ICHCC, 2015). On a related issue, professional nurses are bound to a code of professional practice, promulgated by the American Nurses Association (ANA). Likewise, certified case managers (CCM) are professionally bound to practice under the Code of Professional Conduct for Case Managers published by the Commission for Case Manager Certification (CCMC®, 2015).

Life care planning professionals undergoing *Daubert* challenges or malpractice claims often will be held accountable to existing standards of practice regardless of whether they are certified or belong to a professional organization relevant to life care planning. On the other hand, if a life care planner commits an ethical violation but is not certified in a professional area related to life care planning, the certification board has no jurisdiction even if a complaint is lodged. Certainly, life care planners will face ethical dilemmas, and having knowledge and awareness of the accepted and published codes of ethics, as well as an established ethical decision-making model and a network of knowledgeable colleagues to call upon to work through problems, will reduce the risk of serious error. Indeed, knowledge reduces risk and fear.

A visual image one might keep in mind with regard to ethics is if the news crew from *60 Minutes* showed up at your office for an interview, would you feel comfortable with your opinions? Or, is your life care plan written so that experts from within the life care planning specialty practice will conclude that your work is reasonable and proper? Did you conduct yourself in a way that you would expect others to act toward you? If you can answer yes to these questions, perhaps the life care planner will be better positioned to avoid ethical complaints.

In closing, ethics is a critical area for life care planners and one that has evolved concurrently with the evolution of life care planning itself. With the advent of electronic communications, new considerations regarding dual (or multiple) relationships, HIPAA regulations regarding client/evaluee health information and confidentiality, and other contemporary events in life care planning, it is imperative for life care planners to regularly review their respective codes of ethics and standards of practice to maintain an ethical focus and remain current on ethical service delivery.

References

Banja, J. 1994. Professional or hired gun: The ethics of advocacy in life care planning. *NARPPS Journal, 9*, 86–90.

Barros-Bailey, M., Carlisle, J., Graham, M., Neulicht, A., Taylor, R., & Wallace, A. 2008. *Who Is the Client in Forensics?* [White paper] Boise, ID: Authors.

Berens, D. E., & Weed, R. O. 2001. Ethics update for rehabilitation counselors in the private sector. *Journal of Applied Rehabilitation Counseling, 32*, 27–32.

Black, H. 1990. *Black's Law Dictionary* (6th ed.). St. Paul, MN: West Publishing.

Blackwell, T. 1999. Ethical issues in life care planning. In R. Weed (Ed.), *Life Care Planning and Case Management Handbook* (pp. 399–406). Boca Raton, FL: CRC Press.

Cimino-Ferguson, S. 2005. Multiple relationships in the field of life care planning. *Journal of Life Care Planning, 4*(1), 11-16.

Commission for Case Manager Certification (CCMC®) (rev. 2015). Code of Professional Conduct for Case Managers with Standards, Rules, Procedures, and Penalties. Mt. Laurel, NJ: Author.

Commission on Rehabilitation Counselor Certification. 2017. *Code of Professional Ethics for Rehabilitation Counselors*. Schaumburg, IL: Author.

Cottone, R. R. 2005. Detrimental therapist-client relationships—beyond thinking of "dual" or "multiple" roles: Reflections on the 2001 AAMFT code of ethics. *The American Journal of Family Therapy, 33*, 1–17.

Elliott v. United States, 877 F. Supp. 1569 (M.D. Ga. 1992).

Fairchild v. United States, 769 R. Supp. 964 (W.D. La. 1991).

International Academy of Life Care Planners. 2015 rev. *Standards of Practice for Life Care Planners*. Retrieved December 27, 2017, http://c.ymcdn.com/sites/rehabpro.org/resource/resmgr/files/RehabPro/Standards_of_Practice_for_Li.pdf.

International Commission on Health Care Certification. 2002, rev. 2007, rev. 2015. *Code of Professional Ethics*. Retrieved December 27, 2017, from www.ichcc.org.

Merriam-Webster. 2009a. Ethics. Retrieved January 4, 2009, from https://www.merriam-webster.com/dictionary/ethics.

Merriam-Webster. 2009b. Standards. Retrieved July 31, 2003, from https://www.merriam-webster.com/dictionary/standards.

Shaw, L., & Sawyer, H. 1999. Ethics and forensic rehabilitation. Unpublished paper, University of Florida, Gainesville, FL.

Swartz, J. L., Martin, W. E., & Blackwell, T. L. 1996. Maintaining an awareness of ethical standards in guiding professional behavior. *NARPPS Journal, 11*, 27–32.

Weed, R. 2000. Ethical issues in expert opinions and testimony. *Rehabilitation Counseling Bulletin, 43*, 215–218, 245.

Weed, R. 2002. The life care planner: Secretary, know-it-all, or general contractor? One person's perspective. *Journal of Life Care Planning, 1*, 173–177.

Weed, R. O., Berens, D. E., & Pataky, S. K. 2003. Malpractice and ethics issues in private sector rehabilitation practice: An update for the 21st century. *RehabPro, 11*, 47–54.

Weed, R., & Johnson, C. 2006. *Life Care Planning in Light of Daubert and Kumho*. Athens, GA: E & F Vocational Services.

GENERAL ISSUES

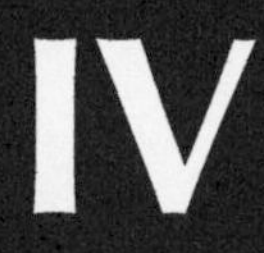

IV

Chapter 28

Reliability of Life Care Plans: A Comparison of Original and Updated Plans*

Amy M. Sutton, Paul M. Deutsch, Roger O. Weed, and Debra E. Berens

Contents

Reliability of Life Care Plans: A Comparison of Original and Updated Plans 703
Method Participants 705
Procedure 706
Results 706
Discussion 708
References 709

Reliability of Life Care Plans: A Comparison of Original and Updated Plans

To formulate an accurate depiction of an individual's current and future health care needs, a life care planner must integrate hundreds of pieces of information. This requires commitment to a consistent and unbiased process and reliance on fact, research, and expertise to formulate a plan that can predict future needs with accuracy and reliability. A life care plan (LCP) has been defined as "a dynamic document based upon published standards of practice, comprehensive assessment, data analysis and research, which provides an organized, concise plan for current and future needs with associated costs, for individuals who have experienced catastrophic injury or have chronic health care needs" (combined definition, 1998, as cited in Weed, 1999, p. iii).

---

* This peer-reviewed article originally appeared as Sutton, A., Deutsch, P., Weed, R., and Berens, D. (2002). Reliability of life care plans: A comparison of original and updated plans, in the *Journal of Life Care Planning*, 1(3), 187–194. Reprinted with permission.

According to Deutsch (1994), the development of life care plans came as a response to multiple professional concerns. First, persons with disabilities and their families need a concise summary to plan for future needs. Second, a communication tool is needed with which all parties involved in a catastrophic injury case will be informed of these needs. Third, a planning approach in the field is needed rather than the traditional reactionary approach. Fourth, through the life care planning process, disabilities could be broken down into basic components to more carefully identify complex concerns. Finally, concerns specific to the person with a disability and his or her family, such as geographic location, preferences, and personal goals, need to be incorporated into a plan of care to ensure a realistic implementation. In response to these concerns, life care plans have become important tools in a number of different settings, including complex disease management, establishing insurance reserves, worker's compensation case management, health insurance managed care, resolution of personal injury claims, and facilitating client and family understanding of the long-term costs and effects of injuries and illnesses (Weed, 1994). To meet the demands of preparing such a plan, certain skills provided by life care planning training and certification programs, in combination with expertise in numerous areas, are recommended. Brodwin and Mas (1999) outline 12 areas of expertise: medical aspects of disability, foundations of rehabilitation counseling, case management, psychosocial aspects of disability, behavioral interventions, preventative care, equipment and supplies, educational and vocational implications of disability, assessment and evaluation, community resources and services, rehabilitation facilities, and expert witness testimony. Similarly, the published life care planning model includes several subsections that should be addressed in a LCP in order to provide the most comprehensive plan possible. Subsections include (Weed, 1998):

- Projected evaluations
- Therapeutic modalities
- Diagnostic testing
- Wheelchair needs, accessories, and maintenance
- Aids for independent functioning
- Orthotics
- Home furnishings and accessories
- Medications and supplies
- Home/facility care
- Routine medical care
- Transportation
- Health and strength maintenance
- Architectural renovations
- Potential complications
- Aggressive treatment or surgical intervention
- Orthopedic equipment needs
- Vocational planning

It is from this knowledge foundation that life care planning professionals are able to make future projections and confer with multiple care providers to develop the most accurate care plan possible.

As the field of life care planning has become more defined through training programs, publication, and widespread use, a need for research that examines the reliability and validity of life care plans has emerged (Countiss & Deutsch, 2002). Although much research involving case management exists and numerous articles have been written on life care planning, little research has been conducted specifically to evaluate the reliability and validity of life care plans. Reliability is expected from a life care plan due to its influential role in the clients' future care management. Demonstrating reliability of life care plans also provides a foundation for establishing predictive validity. Due to the comprehensive and predictive nature of a LCP and the extreme variability of the population served (e.g., varying diagnoses, age differences, available support systems, treating professionals, etc.), it is a challenge to measure the reliability of a LCP (Deutsch, 2002). However, one study, by McCollom and Crane (2001), surveyed 10 clients with spinal cord injuries who had a life care plan developed for them several years prior to the study. The authors concluded that a clear consistency was found between projected and actual needs. In comparison, the study presented in this article measures LCP reliability by evaluating existing LCPs of clients who, for a variety of reasons, have had a second LCP written 1 to 5 years after the first plan was completed. These second LCPs were updated and revised versions of the original LCPs based on the status of the client and the interventions, services, and complications that arose following the original LCP. By comparing the two plans and determining what has been revised, a measurement of change can be generated that provides professionals with information regarding those areas of a LCP that likely are not subject to change and those areas that are sensitive to the passage of time. The two major areas analyzed in this study include Home/Facility Care and Routine Medical Care. These areas were targeted for two reasons: (1) they are common among virtually all LCPs and (2) they comprise the bulk of the needs that can be tied to measurable data and costs in nearly every LCP. Based on a review of the literature, the following two hypotheses were formulated:

- *Hypothesis 1*: There will be no significant difference between the Home/Facility Care costs of the original LCPs and the updated LCPs.
- *Hypothesis 2*: There will be no significant difference between the Routine Medical Care costs of the original LCPs and the updated LCPs.

Method Participants

A total of 130 life care plans from 65 anonymous cases were obtained and analyzed. Each case had an original LCP (LCP 1) and an updated LCP (LCP 2). The diagnoses for the participants included a wide range of traumatic as well as chronic medical conditions such as acquired brain injury, spinal cord injury, birth defect, and pain syndromes. There were 44 males and 21 females of various ethnic backgrounds. Ages of participants ranged from 2 to 75, with an average age of 28 years. The years between LCP 1 and updated LCP 2 were 1 to 5, with an average of 1.8 years. The LCPs were obtained from two experienced and certified life care planners in private practice, both of whom maintain a policy of strict adherence to published life care planning processes, procedures, and standards. Due to the limited number of cases available, all LCPs that fit the criteria were included in the study. To maintain anonymity to the researcher, all LCPs were purged of names and replaced with case numbers. The study methodology was submitted to the Institutional Review Board (IRB) of Georgia State University for approval of human subject's research. Approval was obtained before the study was initiated.

Procedure

Once all LCPs were reviewed, the projected needs outlined in the In-Home Care and Routine Medical Care subsections were extracted from each. A master list of all projected needs was generated and costs were assigned to the needs. The costs were obtained from a database of current health care costs from one specific region in the southeast United States during one specific time frame (2002). By using a consistent economic reference, all plans shared a common denominator with which they could be compared. As an example, the need for a home health aide was included in several LCPs, and an hourly rate for home health aide was determined from the database. Once all needs were assigned a cost, each LCP was again evaluated. If a LCP recommended a home health aide for 5 days a week for 3 hours a day, 15 hours was multiplied by the cost from the database and then multiplied by the number of weeks per year the client was to receive the service. Finally, a total cost per year for the home health aide recommendation was determined. This methodology was followed for each recommendation in the Home/Facility Care and Routine Medical Care subsections until a complete list of annual costs for the two subsections was obtained. The costs were then totaled to create an overall annual cost for the subsection comprising the variables Home/Facility Care Costs 1, Home/Facility Care Costs 2, Routine Medical Care Costs 1, and Routine Medical Care Costs 2.

While executing the aforementioned method, a number of challenges became apparent. First, many recommendations were presented as a range rather than a specific number. For example, follow-up visits with a neurologist were recommended four to six times per year. For the purposes of data analysis, recommendations were averaged in each case. The entry for neurologist visits from the above example was then recorded as five times per year. Second, some of the recommendations were reported as less frequent than annually. For example, if magnetic resonance imaging (MRI) was recommended once every 1 to 2 years, it was averaged on a yearly basis that equates to 0.66 MRIs per year. As each LCP is a unique plan that is tailored to the individual, other challenges materialized. Often, life care plans make recommendations for time periods such as "from age 20 to 30, age 31 to 55, and age 56 to life expectancy." For this study, one specific time frame was chosen so that data analysis was consistent across all plans. The time frame in the study was determined to be the first year immediately following the updated LCP regardless of when the original LCP was created, because some recommendations would have been concluded before the second plan was completed. As such, recommendations that were one time only (i.e., urology consult—one time only) were included in the annual calculations only if the recommendation was to occur in the first year following the second LCP. This eliminated the concern that certain recommendations in the first plan may have been completed before the second plan was developed, thereby creating an inaccurate discrepancy in the cost between plans. Finally, many LCPs offer multiple options within a subsection. For example, within the Home/Facility Care subsection, Option 1 commonly relates to the client being cared for at home and Option 2 for the client to be cared for in a long-term care facility. Statistical problems with averaging or totaling these different options, and the fact that some plans did not include both options, consequently led to the decision to consider only Option 1 in this analysis. With these procedural problems addressed, the data corresponding to the previously identified variables were analyzed using the Statistical Package for the Social Sciences (SPSS) and Excel. Three researchers, to ensure accuracy, performed the data extraction and data entry.

Results

Data points for the dependent variables did not fall into a normal distribution. Consequently, parametric tests such as analysis of variance, *t*-test, and repeated measures could not be used.

Figures 28.1 and 28.2 demonstrate this lack of normal distribution with the example of In-home Care and Routine Medical Care for the original life care plans (LCP 1). In particular, the distributions for each of the variables were skewed to the left, indicating that the majority of costs fell in lower-cost portions of the distribution, rather than the higher-cost ends. For this reason, the chi-square goodness-of-fit test is the most appropriate means of analyzing data that do not meet the

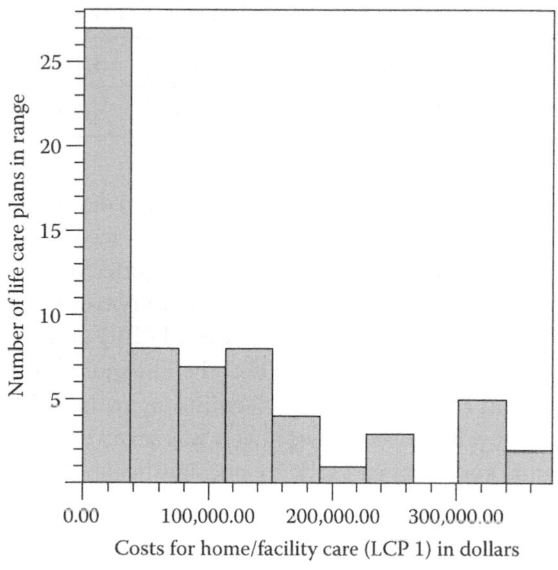

Figure 28.1 Distribution of actual costs for home/facility care in ranges for original life care plans (LCP 1).

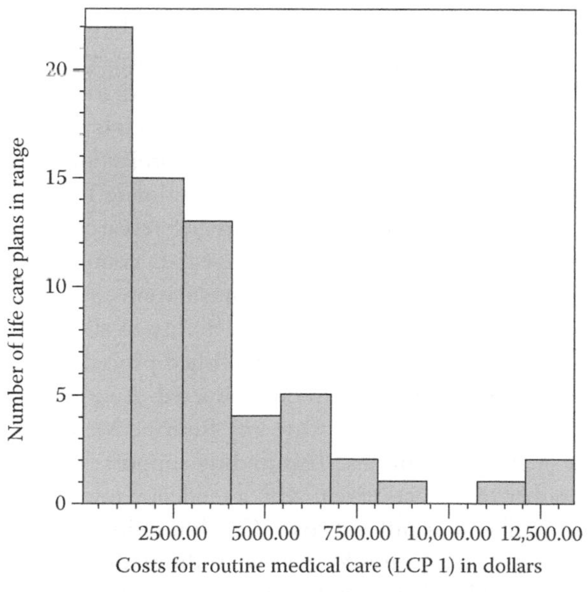

Figure 28.2 Distribution of actual costs for routine medical care in ranges for original life care plans (LCP 1).

Table 28.1 Means, Standard Deviations, and Minimum and Maximum Values of Routine Medical Care and Home/Facility Care Costs for Original and Updated Life Care Plans (in Dollars)

Variable	*Minimum*	*Maximum*	*Mean*	*Standard Deviation*
Home/Facility Care (LCP 1)	0.00	378,870.00	101,059.60	105,137.57
Home/Facility Care (LCP 2)	0.00	365,512.00	104,645.50	102,713.20
Routine Medical Care (LCP 1)	80.50	13,429.00	3,212.75	29,13.67
Routine Medical Care (LCP 2)	215.00	16,795.00	3,566.89	3,354.20

normal distribution criteria. This test compares distributions and determines significant differences between the distributions. Costs were categorized into 10 bins according to frequency, and these were then analyzed. It was necessary to use these 10 categories due to the large range of the variables, as well as the fact that absolute zeros were present in two of these ranges (see Table 28.1). The chi-square for Home/Facility Care variances between LCP 1 and LCP 2 was not significant at the .05 level (chi-square = .85, df = 9, $p > .05$). The chi-square for Routine Medical Care variances between LCP 1 and LCP 2 also was not significant at the .05 level (chi-square = 5.04, df = 9, $p > .05$). The critical value for both hypotheses was set at 16.919. These data indicate that differences between original and updated LCPs are not significant.

Discussion

Any number of complications or technological advances, which are relatively impossible to predict and plan for, may affect a client's prescribed needs and components of the LCP. Some degree of change, therefore, is entirely probable. However, an overall reliability is expected from a life care plan due to the large psychosocial, medical, and financial investments entrusted in the plan. The results of this study indicate that for the two subsections analyzed, life care plan needs are resistant to the effects of time and therefore reliably predictive. Although projections made by the life care planner cannot be specifically validated by this study, projections remained consistent even after 1 or more years had passed. In order to specifically validate LCP plan entries, the various recommendations relied upon would be subject to further research design and analysis across multiple life care planners. However, it is clear from these data comparisons of LCP 1 and LCP 2 that agreement on entries implies that over time recommendations were appropriate. It is also clear that the results of this study alone do not imply the reliability of all life care plans, especially for uncertified professionals or those who fail to use established procedures; however, the study can be a springboard from which more research can be conducted. Another interesting finding is that total costs for the subsections Home/Facility Care and Routine Medical Care tend to fall in the less expensive direction of the distributions. This finding supports the proposition that life care plans are needs-driven rather than cost-driven, with a tendency toward conservative estimates of expenditures as opposed to liberal or inflated costs. One limitation of the study is that there were only two life care planners providing cases for review. Additionally, both of the life care planners are considered experts in the field and may not be representative of all life care planners. Both assert that they remain consistent in their approach and committed to following published standards and methodology. Similar studies in the future will be more valuable if a larger sample of certified life care planners with varying levels of experience who also adhere to the published standards of practice participate. Future research should also include a large enough sample to evaluate plan reliability based on diagnoses, gender, and age, among other factors. Other studies may take a similar approach as this investigation but look at other subsections of the life care plan, particularly if enough samples can be identified for similar disabilities or gender, and to distinguish differences between children and adults.

Although a few of the updated life care plans in the study had marked variations from their original life care plans, these variations did not affect the overall results of the study. For future research, these cases could be investigated from a qualitative perspective to determine why these updated plans reflected greater change. Change may occur for any number of reasons, such as the development of another medical condition, complications due to unforeseen events, failure to comply with the life care plan, changed physician recommendations, and so on. Finally, a retrospective study to examine validity by determining what services were actually provided, what was needed, and what was projected would be valuable to determine recommendation validity.

This study underscores the effectiveness of future care forecasting where individual needs are identified and comprehensive treatment recommendations are documented when based on published models and procedures of life care planning. It appears that life care planners will benefit their clients by adopting a standardized approach to developing life care plans that is based on existing protocol designed for this specialized industry.

References

Brodwin, M., & Mas, L. 1999. The rehabilitation counselor as life care planner. *The Journal of Forensic Vocational Assessment*, 2, 16–21.

Countiss, R. N., & Deutsch, P. M. 2002. The life care planner, the judge and Mr. Daubert. *Journal of Life Care Planning*, 1, 35–43.

Deutsch, P. M. 1994. Life care planning into the future. *NARPPS Journal*, 9, 79–84.

Deutsch, P. M. 2002. Life Care Planning Validation Research. *Presentation at the Life Care Planning Summit 2002*, Chicago.

McCollom, P., & Crane, R. 2001. Life care plans: accuracy over time. *The Case Manager*, 12, 85–87.

Weed, R. O. 1994. Life care plans: expanding the horizons. *NARPPS Journal*, 9, 47–50.

Weed, R. O. 1998. Life care planning: an overview. *Directions in Rehabilitation*, 9, 135–147.

Weed, R. O., ed. 1999. *Life Care Planning and Case Management Handbook*. Boca Raton, FL: CRC Press.

Chapter 29

Americans with Disabilities Act (ADA): From Case Law to Case Management and Life Care Planning Practice

Lewis E. Vierling

Contents

Introduction....712
Bringing an ADA Perspective to the Practice of Case Management and Life Care Planning....713
National Council on Disability and ADA....714
ADA Definition of Disability and the Five Titles....715
ADA Restoration Act....716
The ADA Amendments Act of 2008....716
Major Life Activities and the Burden of Proof....718
Understanding the Development of Case Law....719
Precedent versus Persuasive Authority....719
The Effects of Supreme Court Decisions on Lower Courts....719
From Case Law to Practice: Integrating Court Decisions into the Practice of Case Management and Life Care Planning....720
The Role of Mitigating and Corrective Measures in Determining Disability....720
Single Job versus Class of Jobs....720
Toyota v. Williams Supreme Court Decision....720
Other Important Supreme Court Decisions....721
The Creation of a Nationwide Enforcement Campaign Under the ADAAA for Barrier-Free Health Care....722
Court Decisions and Their Impact on Rehabilitation and Life Care Planning Practice....723

Outcome of ADA Title I Cases 724
Comparison of the 1990 ADA and the ADA Amendments Act 724
Summary and Conclusions 725
Supreme Court Decisions 1998–2005 726
Important Websites 727
References and Additional Resources 727

Introduction

The Americans with Disabilities Act (ADA) of 1990 has undergone a major transition, as a result of the Americans with Disabilities Act Amendments Act of 2008. The purpose of this chapter is to provide the life care planner (especially one who opines about the vocational outlook) a framework for understanding the transition the ADA has experienced, especially in defining what it means to have a disability under the Act. The rehabilitation professional, whether case manager, life care planner, or vocational expert, is encouraged to have an understanding of these changes to best serve as an advocate for individuals with disabilities.

There has been a transition in the intent of ADA as well. Congress' original intent was that the Act should provide a clear, comprehensive mandate for the elimination of discrimination for individuals with disabilities. At the time of enactment, they suggested that the ADA should be a civil rights law that is inclusive and broadly interpreted. However, through its review by the Supreme Court, decisions have evolved to a very narrow interpretation. In fact, the Court stated in the *Toyota v. Williams* decision that the ADA should be "interpreted strictly to create a demanding standard for qualifying as disabled" (Vierling, 2002d).

The court's struggle with the definition of disability under the law is not necessarily a new issue. A search of the U.S. Code, which is the official compilation of federal statutes that are currently in force, identified 67 places where disability is defined. Of the 67 places, there were 26 references to definitions contained in other code sections. However, the definition of disability under the ADA has evolved from other disability legislation that had been consistently applied in the court system until the ADA was challenged in court. As a result of these court rulings, especially Supreme Court decisions, advocates introduced and passed legislation to restore the protection Congress originally intended (Vierling, 2000a, 2000b, 2000c, 2000d, 2001a). The ADA Amendments Act (ADAAA) signed by President Bush on September 25, 2008, was the result of those efforts and will be discussed in the context of the transition of the ADA in this chapter.

The unique nature of this transition is the more than 16 years of developing case law surrounding the 1990 ADA. The ADAAA was effective January 1, 2009. It was the purpose of Congress that the range of coverage and protection for individuals with disabilities expand significantly. A review of developing case law completed by the National Council on Disability (NCD, 2013) noted, "in the decisions rendered so far, the ADAAA has made a significant positive difference for plaintiffs." These findings were noted in a report to the President on July 23, 2013, by the NCD entitled "A Promising Start: Preliminary Analysis of Court Decisions Under the ADA Amendments Act."

In 2011, the Seventh Circuit Court of Appeals had issued two decisions interpreting the broader provisions of the ADAAA. In one case, a bridge worker's acrophobia was a disability under the law. The Court determined that a bridge worker's request that other employees substitute for him when called upon to work 25 feet in an extreme position was a reasonable accommodation. In another case, the Seventh Circuit upheld a jury award for almost $2 million that a teacher with seasonal affective disorder was a qualified individual with a disability. The teacher made numerous requests for a room with windows, but the school district failed to accommodate her request.

Other federal district courts have ruled that the following impairments rise to the level of a disability under the ADAAA:

1. Arthritis, hernia, rotator cuff issues
2. A high-risk pregnancy with complications that led to an emergency room admission
3. Asthma and high blood pressure
4. A knee injury which prevented squatting, kneeling, running, jumping, and climbing
5. An ankle injury making the employee unable to stand for more than an hour, but who could work with a special boot

Yet, in another case heard by the Tenth Circuit Court of Appeals, the decision was made that an employee with migraine headaches was not disabled under the ADAAA. In this decision, the Court made it clear that they were not opining that migraine headaches could not be considered a disability in other circumstances, only in this case.

Bringing an ADA Perspective to the Practice of Case Management and Life Care Planning

Catastrophic injury/illness did not necessarily equal disability under the 1990 Americans with Disabilities Act (ADA) as has been interpreted by the courts. After more than 16 years of enforcement and litigation, the courts struggled with the problem of proving whether an individual has a covered disability under ADA and therefore is protected against discrimination. In fact, in the words of a judge at the First Circuit Court of Appeals in a written decision, the word *disability* is considered to be a "term of art" (Heyburn, 2002). This clearly demonstrates the difficulty and subjectivity that has developed in the courts in defining disability under the 1990 ADA.

Even though four prominent pieces of legislation were influential in forming the basis of ADA, there has been no unified consensus concerning the meaning of a disability. For example, the Rehabilitation Act of 1973 (PL 93-112) provided for vocational rehabilitation services on a national scale to qualifying persons with disabilities. It also mandated employment of persons with disabilities in federal government jobs and most federally funded programs. Section 504 of the Rehabilitation Act, one of four sections, is considered to be "the underpinnings for the ADA" (Blanck, 1999). In summary, this section provides that people with disabilities have equal employment opportunities and prohibits the exclusion based on disability of otherwise qualified disabled persons from participation in any program or activity receiving federal financial assistance.

The Education for All Handicapped Children's Act, PL 94-142 (updated by PL 105-17 and termed the Individuals with Disabilities Education Act, or IDEA), had a strong influence in propelling the disabilities rights movement forward and was designed to educate and train children with severe disabilities who are likely to be placed into institutions (Blanck, 1999). Another important piece of legislation was the 1978 amendments to the Developmental Disabilities Assistance and Bill of Rights Act (PL 95-602). This legislation not only established a nationwide system of protection and advocacy but also created a program of comprehensive services for persons with developmental disabilities. The Fair Housing Amendments Act of 1988, 42 USC 3601-3631, made it illegal to discriminate on the basis of disability in housing, real estate transactions, zoning, and the operation and services of apartments and condominiums. Despite the fact that the road to ADA has a long legal history that includes over 27 pieces of legislation, there was still no social consensus regarding what it means to be disabled by 1999 (Diller, 1999).

Each year, the U.S. Supreme Court grants review to approximately 80 to 90 cases. The Supreme Court heard and provided decisions on 21 specific ADA cases since the law went into effect through the Court's 2007–2008 term. The Supreme Court reviewed numerous other ADA cases from lower courts and opined that the lower courts' decisions should stand, referred to as *stare decisis* (let the decision stand). Five of these 21 cases dealt with clarifying the definition of disability. As interpreted by the Supreme Court, however, it is absolutely clear that a medical diagnosis is not automatically considered to be a disability under the 1990 ADA. There has been an inherent paradox in how the courts have opined regarding the definition of disability. For example, individuals who are severely ill or disabled and unable to perform the essential functions of a job under Title I of ADA have not been protected. If an individual can do a particular job, he or she has not been considered disabled and therefore is not protected (Vierling, 2000a, 2000b, 2000c, 2000d, 2001a, 2001b, 2002a, 2002b, 2002c, 2002d).

National Council on Disability and ADA

In 1984, Congress established the National Council on Disability (NCD) to make recommendations to promote equal opportunity for persons with disabilities. In 1986, the NCD issued a report, "Toward Independence," recommending that a comprehensive law be passed. The NCD issued a follow-up report in 1988 entitled "On the Threshold of Independence," and the council published the draft bill of what was to become the ADA. A revised ADA bill was sponsored by Senator Tom Harkin and Representative Tony Coelho in 1989. President George H. W. Bush signed into law, on July 26, 1990, the ADA before an audience of more than 3,000 American leaders from disability rights movements gathered on the White House lawn (Editor's note: The author of this chapter was an invitee).

As previously indicated, the NCD reviewed court decisions following the passage of the ADAAA and submitted their findings in the report, "A Promising Start: Preliminary Analysis of Court Decisions Under the ADA Amendments Act." That report was provided to the President of the United States on July 23, 2013. In their findings, the NCD stated that "in the decisions rendered so far, the ADAAA has made a significant positive difference for plaintiffs in ADA lawsuits" (p. 8).

The NCD Report noted that in six of the seven Circuit Court decisions reviewed, the plaintiff "prevailed on the issue of establishing a disability." In the district court decisions reviewed, the "plaintiff prevailed on the showing of disability in more than three out of four decisions." Certainly, the first hurdle to overcome in presenting a disability discrimination case before the courts. It appears from the court decisions that the demanding individualized assessment as to whether or not an individual has a disability under the law is gradually diminishing. There is less emphasis in the courts on the individual proving a disability and more on whether or not an act of discrimination occurred in the case before the court.

Also in the NCD report, the agency offered 23 findings from their analysis of court decisions that provide not only a summary of the results of the court decisions, but also a detailed legal analysis of how the courts are reacting to the ADAAA in their decision process. Several of the findings are noted as follows:

- In most of cases, the plaintiff prevailed on the issue of having a disability under the new law.
- The courts appear to be reincorporating the principle that mitigating measures "shall not be considered in determining disability."
- A change in the focus of being "regarded" as having an impairment to whether or not the individual has been subjected to an action prohibited by the law. The new standard,

according to the findings, has been applied to allow plaintiffs to successfully make a case that they have been regarded as having a disability.

- The indication that the ADAAA has had a "dramatic impact in improving the success rate of plaintiffs in establishing disability in their court cases."
- The provision in the law that the determinations of whether or not the individual's impairment is a disability "should not demand extensive analysis," is witnessing a shift in this direction.
- The reduced need for individualized assessment because the law and revisions make it easier for some impairments to be recognized as disabilities.
- It should be noted that under the ADAAA, the determination of whether an impairment substantially limits does still require an individualized assessment.

ADA Definition of Disability and the Five Titles

Disability, as defined in the ADA, is a physical or mental impairment that substantially limits one or more major life activities; a record of such impairment; or being regarded as having an impairment (as cited in Vierling, 2002d). The Equal Employment Opportunity Commission (EEOC) issued guidelines for complying with the ADA law. Within the EEOC's regulations was an expansion of the definition that was within the original ADA legislation. However, the Supreme Court narrowed that definition considerably compelling Congress to rewrite the legislation.

The ADA took effect July 26, 1992, 2 years after the signing by President George H. W. Bush. Title I of the ADA prohibits private employers, state and local governments, employment agencies, and labor unions from discriminating against qualified individuals with disabilities in job application procedures, hiring, firing, advancement, compensation, job training, and other terms, conditions, and privileges of employment. The following is a review of each major emphasis under all five titles and is not meant to be a full description of Titles I through V (Vierling, 2002d):

Title I: Employment—affecting employers having 15 or more employees.

Title II: Public services—affecting all activities of state and local governments, with Subtitle B applicable to transportation provided by public entities.

Title III: Public accommodations and services operated by private entities—affecting privately operated public accommodations, commercial facilities, and private entities offering certain examinations and courses.

Title IV: Telecommunications—affecting telecommunications relaying services and closed captioning.

Title V: Miscellaneous provisions—including the relationship of ADA to other laws, the requirements for technical assistance, the role of the Architectural and Transportation Barriers Compliance Board, the coverage of Congress, and some additional definitions regarding coverage.

On October 11, 2016, the amended regulations for Title II and Title III of the ADAAA took effect (ADA.Gov, July 15, 2016). These regulations provide guidance from the Department of Justice and will help to clarify the interpretation and application of the ADAAA. The final rules under the regulations will coincide with Congress' mandate "that eliminating discrimination against people with disabilities requires an expansive definition of what disability means and who the law covers." It is the intent of the ADAAA to ensure that the definition of disability is interpreted consistently for these two Titles as has been done with Title I published by the EEOC. The ADA Accessibility

Guidelines for Buildings and Facilities (ADAAG) identify specific requirements regarding the removal of architectural barriers; new facilities have to meet the detailed requirement for fixed features of buildings and structures, i.e., entryways, doorways, stairs, elevators, floor surfaces, restrooms, parking areas, and curbs. While the ADA Standards for Accessible Design regulations were signed by the Attorney General on July 23, 2010, compliance with the Standards for Accessible Design was not required until March 15, 2012.

The problem of inaccessible medical equipment was attempted to be addressed through existing civil rights law, such as the ADA; however, significant barriers to the health and health care of people with disabilities still remain.

ADA Restoration Act

Because of the Supreme Court decisions limiting the scope of the ADA (Vierling, 2001a), there have been several attempts to restore the law's intended coverage by proposing numerous legislative changes through Congress. Twin versions of an ADA Restoration Act, S. 1881 and H.R. 3195, were introduced into Congress. The Restoration Act sought to address the problems with the ADA's definition of disability by eliminating the "substantial limitation" on a major life activity requirement and prohibiting courts from considering whether a person uses mitigating measures.

The NCD concluded in a series of comprehensive reports, *Righting the ADA* (2002–2004), that the Supreme Court's interpretation of the definition of *disability* altered the scope and coverage of the ADA. They concluded that "the majority of people with disabilities have no federal legal recourse in the event of discrimination, particularly in instances of employment discrimination" (as cited in Marat, Sept 12, 2013, p. 1). It was hoped that the Restoration Act would restore Congress' original intent when it enacted the ADA in June 1990 and that it should be a civil rights law that is inclusive and broadly interpreted.

The ADA Amendments Act of 2008

A compromise bill, the ADA Amendments Act of 2008, or ADAAA (S. 3406), was passed by both houses of Congress and on September 25, 2008, signed by President George W. Bush. The ADAAA significantly broadened the scope of protection intended by Congress to be available under the 1990 Act but had been severely limited by Supreme Court decisions over the last 10 years.

The purpose of the ADAAA was stated in the first line of the bill, "to restore the intent and protections of the Americans with Disabilities Act of 1990" (EEOC, 2008, p. 1). The ADAAA was effective on January 1, 2009. The Act retains the ADA's basic definition of *disability* as an impairment that substantially limits one or more major life activities, a record of such an impairment, or being regarded as having such an impairment. In terms of who is covered under the ADAAA, employers with 15 or more employees are required to comply with the new amendments.

The ADAAA focuses specifically on several main issues that have been narrowly interpreted by the courts. First, and most important, is the definition of disability. It retains the ADA's basic definition, but changes the way the statutory terms are interpreted (i.e., substantially limited and major life activities). It also addresses the controversial decisions regarding the use of mitigating measures. It clarifies that an impairment that is episodic or in remission is a disability if it would substantially limit a major life activity when active. The new law addresses "regarded as" cases and whether the medical conditions are transitory and minor and whether reasonable accommodations should be provided to those individuals determined to be regarded as disabled. Finally, Congress emphasized that the definition of *disability* should be interpreted broadly.

Congress found that the current, pre-ADAAA EEOC regulations defining the term "substantially limits" as "significantly restricted" are inconsistent with congressional intent by "expressing too high a standard." Therefore, EEOC was instructed to issue new regulations redefining "substantially limits" from its current definition ("significantly restricts") to comply with the ADAAA broader view. Various other agencies such as the U.S. Attorney General's Office and the Department of Transportation were instructed to issue revised regulations to serve as guidance in responding to the ADAAA.

Other changes include expanding the definition of *major life activities* (MLA) that have been delineated in the regulations by the EEOC and many activities that have not been recognized by the EEOC, for example, reading, bending, and communicating. The second list of major life activities in the new law includes those identified as major bodily function, for example, functions of the immune system, normal cell growth, and digestive, bowel, bladder, neurological, brain, respiratory, circulatory, endocrine, and reproductive functions.

The EEOC issued revised regulations that were published on March 25, 2011, implementing the new amendments (EEOC, 2011). Some of the more significant changes to the regulations from the statute are listed below:

To the major life activities identified in the ADAAA statute, the regulations added nine major bodily functions as noted above; immune system; normal cell growth; digestion; bowel and bladder functions; neurological and brain functions; respiratory functions; circulatory system; endocrine functions; and reproductive functions.

"Regarded as" coverage can be established whether or not the employer is motivated by fears, myths, or stereotypes. Evidence that the employer believed the individual was substantially limited in any major life activity is no longer required.

An employer cannot "regard a person" as disabled if the impairment the employer believes to affect the person is objectively both transitory and minor. The employer's subjective belief as to whether the impairment is transitory and minor is also no longer relevant.

The new regulations establish nine "rules of construction" to determine whether an impairment "substantially limits" an individual in a "major life activity."

The reader is encouraged to review the nine specific "rules of construction" for a better understanding of the process of determining whether an impairment substantially limits an individual in a major life activity.

The ADAAA took a major departure from the five Supreme Court decisions related to considering the use of mitigating measures in determining whether an individual is disabled under the law. The law now states that mitigating measures (medications, prosthesis, medical supplies, equipment, and other auxiliary aids or services) should not be considered in the determination of whether an individual has a disability. The exception is that prescription eyeglasses and contact lenses may still be considered in assessing whether an individual is "substantially limited." The ADAAA also states that an impairment that is episodic or in remission is a disability if it would substantially limit a major life activity when it is active.

Under the ADAAA, Congress declared that it provides a "clear and comprehensive national mandate for the elimination of discrimination" and "clear, strong, enforceable standards addressing discrimination" by reinstating a broad scope of protection (ADA.Gov, 2009, Section 12101). The law also defined the standard for being "regarded as disabled." That standard is defined as "establishing that the individual has been subjected to action prohibited under the ADAAA because of an actual or perceived physical or mental impairment whether or not the impairment limits or is perceived to limit a major life activity." In "regarded as" cases, employers do not need to provide reasonable accommodation to individuals who are considered to be regarded as or perceived to be disabled. The individual must now show that the employer perceived them as having a physical or mental impairment, not that the impairment substantially limits a major life activity. This is a major change from the case law surrounding "regarded as" cases.

The amendments also state that "regarded as" claims cannot be based on impairments that are transitory and minor. *Transitory* is defined as an actual or expected duration of 6 months or less.

It was hoped and has thus far been shown that the expanded definition of disability under the ADAAA will have an increasing effect on the number of individuals who will be considered "protected" by the new law. It is the intent that there will be less emphasis on the assessment of whether an individual is "qualified" under the law and more on whether an employer had unlawfully discriminated against that individual. The current advice given to employers because of the all-expansive list of what qualifies as MLAs: they will be better off to assume that an impairment qualifies as a disability.

Providing reasonable accommodations is becoming even more important for the employer. In doing so, the employer needs to consider not only the current effects of an impairment, "but also what the effects would be if the impairment were in an active state." The employer will find it even more advantageous to engage in the interactive process. Employers should now be prepared to engage either applicants or employees in conversations related to providing reasonable accommodations to qualified individuals to enable them to perform the essential functions of the job in question.

Major Life Activities and the Burden of Proof

The five specific cases that dealt with the definition of *disability* are *Bragdon v. Abbott* (1998); *Sutton v. United Airlines*; *Murphy v. UPS*; *Albertsons, Inc., v. Kirkingburg* (1999); and *Toyota v. Williams* (as cited in Vierling, 2002d). The precedent that had been established by the Supreme Court was that there needs to be clear evidence to assist the court with a three-part analysis to determine whether a plaintiff has shown that he or she is substantially limited in a major life activity. After hearing the plaintiff's evidence in his or her burden-of-proof phase, the court has applied the three-part analysis as follows (Vierling, 2002d):

1. The court must determine whether the plaintiff has an impairment under ADA.
2. It must identify the life activity on which the plaintiff relies in his or her case and determine if it constitutes a major life activity.
3. It must decide whether the impairment in question substantially limits the major life activity identified by the plaintiff.

It is important to note that the plaintiff must assert that he or she is substantially limited in a specific major life activity. Then it is apparent that the plaintiff must articulate with precision the impairment alleged and how that major life activity is affected by that impairment. This, however, appears to be less of a burden of proof under the ADAAA and the EEOC's regulations noted above. In addition, the courts have considered a number of other specific factors in their decision-making process. For example, when evaluating whether an impairment substantially limits a major life activity, the lower courts were guided by Supreme Court decisions to consider the nature and severity of the impairment; the duration or expected duration of the impairment; and the permanent or long-term impact or the expected permanent or long-term impact of, or resulting from, the impairment. Under the ADAAA, there is less emphasis on the assessment process and more on whether the employer met its legal obligations.

However, it should be noted that Supreme Court decisions can impact the regulations by the outcome of the case law directly related to their decisions. For example, under the ADA case law, the courts have required an individual assessment on a case-by-case basis. As a direct consequence of the *Sutton, Murphy,* and *Kirkingburg* decisions (as cited in Vierling, 2002d), the EEOC issued instructions for field offices regarding the analysis of ADA complaints and addressing the use of mitigating measures in considering whether a person is disabled (EEOC, 1999). These instructions changed the procedure for field office staff investigating individual complaints and appeared in the *Federal Register* in June 2000. The instructions to field offices summarized and explained how the Supreme Court cases impact the process of charges filed under ADA. The instructions emphasized "the individualized analysis that must be used in determining a charging party has a disability as defined by ADA and whether a person is qualified" (as cited in Vierling, 2002d). However with the new law, there will be less emphasis on the evaluation or assessment of a defined disability.

Another important aspect of the developing ADA case law has been that *individuals* are protected under ADA, not *specific disabilities.* Therefore, the Court has stated that each individual has to be evaluated on a case-by-case basis to determine if the individual has a disability and is therefore protected. But, as previously noted, under the ADAAA there will be less emphasis on this inquiry and more on whether acts of discrimination occurred.

Understanding the Development of Case Law

Precedent versus Persuasive Authority

A distinction needs to be made between precedent and persuasive authority. In a legal sense, a precedent is "an earlier decision relevant to a case to be decided" (Elias & Levinkind, 1999). Once a court decides how a law should be applied to a particular set of facts, this decision controls later decisions by that and other courts. It is only a precedent as to a particular set of facts and the precise legal issues decided in light of those facts. The more the facts of legal issues vary between two cases, the less the effect of the precedent. If the circumstances of a current case match an earlier one, the previous case is considered a precedent and binding on the court.

Persuasive authority, on the other hand, is not binding on other courts, but if a case contains an analysis of legal issues and provides guidance for any court referring to it, it has persuasive authority. Generally speaking, the higher the court level, the more persuasive a decision may be on other courts in similar types of cases.

In rendering an opinion, a court may apply the prevailing interpretation of similar cases to the case being heard in its court. These cases are said to establish a precedent. The principles that are derived from other court cases make up the body of case law applied in new cases. This is part of the legal tradition of common law.

As previously noted, applying the principles from an earlier decision is the doctrine of *stare decisis* (Vierling, 2002d). These principles are extracted from court decisions at a variety of levels. These decisions are pertinent to the field of rehabilitation. Case law further evolves as court cases are resolved.

The Effects of Supreme Court Decisions on Lower Courts

U.S. Supreme Court cases are precedent for all courts with respect to decisions involving the U.S. Constitution or any other aspect of federal law. Also, Appellate Court and Supreme Court cases are precedent with respect to future decisions by the same court. The cases of the U.S. Court of Appeals are precedent for U.S. District Courts within their 12 circuits, plus a Federal Circuit Court. Opinions of the U.S. District Courts are never precedent for other courts. However, the decisions may have persuasive authority on other district courts' decisions. As noted previously, the higher the court level, the more possibility for persuasive authority. State Supreme Court cases are precedent for courts only within that state.

From Case Law to Practice: Integrating Court Decisions into the Practice of Case Management and Life Care Planning

The Role of Mitigating and Corrective Measures in Determining Disability

In June 1999, the Supreme Court rendered opinions on a trilogy of ADA cases that had a major impact on determining who is disabled (Vierling, 2002d). These decisions provided a new legal standard that had been used for defining disability under the ADA. However, with the passage of the 2008 ADAAA new case law will preclude the standard. The most significant issue that the Supreme Court dealt with was affirming the use of mitigating measures such as medications, corrective lenses, prosthetic devices, and the body's ability to compensate for an impairment to determine disability. As noted, this inquiry will be of less concern because of the passage of the ADAAA. Now the inquiry is to be made without regard to the use of mitigating measures except for ordinary eyeglasses or contact lenses.

Single Job versus Class of Jobs

If a plaintiff is relying on demonstrating a substantial limitation in the major life activity of work, former EEOC regulations and case law stated that he or she will need to satisfy this definition: he or she must be significantly restricted in the ability to perform either a class of jobs or a broad range of jobs in various classes compared to the average person having comparable training, skills, and abilities. To satisfy this definition, the plaintiff and his or her representative who is preparing either a vocational evaluation or a life care plan has been required to present information on the number and types of available jobs from which he or she is disqualified that use similar training, knowledge, skills, or abilities and are within a reasonably accessible geographic area. This information has helped the trier of fact to decide whether the individual's impairment rises to the level of a disability and, therefore, falls within the protected class under ADA. Clearly, it has been crucial that the rehabilitation professional provide very specific information well beyond the medical diagnosis or medical information from a physician. The rehabilitation professional is encouraged to review upcoming governmental agencies' new regulations, specifically the EEOC as it relates to work as a major life activity with the passage of the ADAAA.

Toyota v. Williams Supreme Court Decision

In the *Toyota Motors v. Williams* case (2002), the question before the Supreme Court was: what is the proper standard for determining whether an individual is substantially limited in performing manual tasks? Performing manual tasks is a specific major life activity. As a part of her case, Ms. Williams claimed that she was covered under ADA because her cumulative trauma injury prevented her from doing tasks associated with certain types of manual jobs. However, the Supreme

Court said that the proper test for assessing whether an individual was substantially limited in performing manual tasks is whether the impairment prevents or restricts performing tasks that are of "central importance to most people's daily lives." In this decision, Justice Sandra Day O'Connor also made the distinction that routine or minor injuries not of a permanent or long-term nature are not protected under ADA.

Congress was very specific in the ADAAA in addressing the issues in the *Toyota v. Williams* decision. The Act stated that the decision in the *Williams* case "further narrowed the broad scope of protection intended to be afforded by the ADA." Congress' intent with the ADAAA was to restore a broader scope and expand the coverage that had been narrowed by this decision.

In the *Williams* case, work as a major life activity was again questioned by the Supreme Court. The court's response to work as a major life activity has diminished the value of claiming it as an issue in an ADA claim. In addition, the Supreme Court said that the plaintiff must prove a disability by offering evidence that the limitation is substantial in terms of her own experience, reinforcing the standard that such assessments must be on a case-by-case basis. This, of course, reemphasizes that a full evaluation, whether it is a case management report, vocational evaluation, or life care plan, must be made by the rehabilitation professional. This decision supports the legal standard relating to alleging a protected disability under ADA, if claiming a substantial limitation in the major life activity of performing manual tasks. Rehabilitation professionals will need to assess and review in their plan the individual's level of ability in performing manual tasks in his or her personal life. Manual tasks could include such things as ability to perform Activities of Daily Living (ADL), housekeeping chores, and the ability to care for oneself and other family members. These are the types of real-world activities that the courts have been looking to assess. It is unknown at this time what the impact of the ADAAA will be on the assessment of performing manual tasks.

In the *Williams* decision, published in January 2002, the Supreme Court stated that ADA should be "interpreted strictly to create a demanding standard for qualifying as disabled" (*Toyota Motors v. Williams*, 2002). As noted, this case law is refuted in the ADAAA but may indeed be challenged in future cases as the assessment process continues to be in transition because of the status of the ADA.

Other Important Supreme Court Decisions

There are two other decisions that have created case law with which rehabilitation professionals should be familiar. In June 1999, the Supreme Court published its opinion in the *Olmstead Commissioner, Georgia Department of Human Resources v. L.C.* case, which has particular relevance to life care planners. In this case, the question presented to the Supreme Court was whether the public service portion of ADA compels the state to provide treatment and habilitation services for persons with mental disabilities in community placement when appropriate treatment and habilitation can also be provided to them in state and mental institutions? The second issue was that if ADA does include providing treatment and habilitation in community placement, does that exceed the enforcement power granted to Congress?

In a vote of 6 to 3, the Supreme Court determined that states are required to place people with mental disabilities in community settings rather than in institutions when the state's treatment professionals have determined that community placement is appropriate. This would also be under the condition that transfer from institutional care to a community-based program would not be opposed by the individual and that the placement can be reasonably accommodated. The state must also take into consideration the resources available and the needs of other individuals within the state facility.

On June 18, 2001, President George W. Bush signed Executive Order 1.3217, titled "Community-Based Alternatives for Individuals with Disabilities." This order from the federal government helped states to implement the Supreme Court decision in Olmstead. The goal of these grants was to assist people with disabilities to do the following (Rubinger & Gardner, 2002):

1. Live in the most integrated community setting appropriate to their individual support requirements and preferences
2. Exercise meaningful choices about their living environments, the providers of services they receive, the types of support they use, and the manner by which services are provided
3. Obtain quality services in a manner as consistent as possible with their community preferences and priorities

As part of this initiative, President Bush proposed an increase in funding to help transition Americans with disabilities from institutions to community living. This is clearly another example of the integration of case law in providing valuable resources for rehabilitation professionals to assist their clientele.

The next decision to be discussed from the Supreme Court was *Cleveland v. Policy Management Systems Corporation* (1999). In this case, the question before the court was whether the application for, or receipt of, Social Security disability benefits precludes a person with a disability from bringing an ADA claim. The court recognized that there may be many situations in which the claim for Social Security disability benefits and an ADA claim may exist side by side. The court stated that because the qualification standards for Social Security benefits and ADA are not the same, an application for receiving Social Security benefits is not inconsistent with being a qualified individual with a disability under ADA. The court, however, did state that the plaintiff must provide an explanation that he or she can still perform the essential functions of the job with or without reasonable accommodations. The *Cleveland* case demonstrates to the rehabilitation professional the importance of providing reasonable accommodation under ADA. The rehabilitation professional should also be aware that there is the possibility that an individual receiving Social Security benefits would still be protected under ADA.

The Creation of a Nationwide Enforcement Campaign Under the ADAAA for Barrier-Free Health Care

In July 2012, the Department of Justice announced the Americans with Disabilities Act Barrier-Free Health Care Initiative by the U.S. Attorney's Office nationwide. It is a partnering of resources between the U.S. Attorney's Office and the Civil Rights Division of the Department of Justice. Health care providers are public accommodations under Title III of the ADA and, as such, are required to assure that individuals with disabilities have full access to all of the services and facilities including hospitals, HMOs and doctor's offices, diagnostic and treatment centers, physical therapy and rehabilitation centers, and E-Health providers. The initiative was originally focused on communications with deaf and hearing-impaired patients. However, specially included in the initiative was physical access to buildings, parking, examination rooms, and equipment for individuals with other disabilities. Another key target included websites, scheduling systems, and Internet-based services. The failure to make these facilities and services available has resulted in sometimes costly litigation.

This initiative has included investigations and settlements with a large number of health care providers, nursing facilities, dentists, doctors, hospitals, pharmacies, and mental health facilities.

In a report published by the NCD entitled The Current State of Health Care for People with Disabilities, the findings concluded that "people with disabilities experience significant health disparities and barriers to health care" (National Council on Disability Sept. 30, 2009, Executive Summary). The report also concluded that individuals with disabilities encounter a lack of coverage for necessary services, medications, equipment, and technologies. Even though the ADA requires equal access to health care, it does not require health care institutions or providers to have any specific type or types of equipment.

Court Decisions and Their Impact on Rehabilitation and Life Care Planning Practice

Whether rehabilitation professionals are serving in an advocacy role or as an objective evaluator, they have the responsibility to provide as accurate an assessment of the needs of the client as possible. Courts have provided specific guidelines in the form of case law to assist in making informed decisions in future cases. The life care planner needs to be knowledgeable about the case law to effectively provide appropriate data, particularly for vocational and expected future need opinions.

As already noted, court decisions affect EEOC's guidelines. The trilogy of ADA decisions in 1999 was the impetus for the publication of new instructions to the field offices regarding analyzing charges addressing disability and who is qualified under ADA. It was also the impetus for Congress to restore the protection afforded under the ADA that had been narrowed by the Supreme Court through the amendment legislation. Another example is the EEOC issuing new "Enforcement Guidelines on Reasonable Accommodation and Undue Hardship" under the Americans with Disabilities Act on October 17, 2002. These guidelines were a direct result of the Supreme Court decision in the 2001–2002 term on *U.S. Airways, Inc. v. Barnett* (2002). The updated enforcement guidelines revised the standard for reasonableness. The reasonableness of an accommodation is now evaluated by whether it is considered not only effective, but also feasible or plausible for the typical employer. In the *Barnett* decision, the Supreme Court suggested the possibility that special circumstances may exist for providing reasonable accommodations to an individual despite the seniority system. Without the existence of any special circumstances, the court determined that it would be unreasonable for an employer to reassign an employee to another job, which would violate the seniority system.

Under the standards from the *Barnett* decision, the plaintiff has the burden to prove that an accommodation is reasonable. Then the burden shifts to the employer to provide case-specific evidence proving the accommodation would cause an undue hardship. The guidelines also provide examples of what would be reasonable and unreasonable accommodations. The rehabilitation professional can be a valuable asset by understanding the ADA case law and new legal standards. Following are examples of case law pertaining to providing reasonable accommodations.

- Seniority systems prevail over reasonable accommodation. However, employees may identify special circumstances that lead to the employer providing reasonable accommodation.
- The concept of providing reasonable accommodation is to accommodate a person's disability rather than accommodate the person with the disability.
- The employer must make reasonable accommodations to the limitations of the disability rather than for those limitations.
- Reasonable accommodation applies to obstacles exclusively related to the workplace.
- Accommodations must be reasonable, feasible, and plausible.

- Employers have a mandatory obligation to engage in an interactive process with employees regarding making reasonable accommodation.
- The employer's obligation to be involved in the interactive process goes well beyond the first attempt and should continue when the employer is aware that the accommodation is not working.
- The duty to accommodate is a continuing duty that is not exhausted by one effort.

Outcome of ADA Title I Cases

Before the ADAAA, courts had decided in favor of employers in most ADA litigation cases. In a survey identifying court decisions from the year 2007, the *American Bar Association's Commission on Mental and Physical Disability Law Reporter* indicated that employees prevailed in less than 5 percent of the cases. It had also been noted that 80 percent of all employment cases are dismissed in motions for summary judgment. A motion for summary judgment is granted when the court believes no genuine issue of material fact exists. The party filing the motion is entitled to prevail as a matter of law. As a result, 80 percent of the ADA Title I cases never reach a jury. When they do, the vast majority of cases are won by employers. Since the period from 1992 to 2006, the average win for employers is 95.4 percent. However, with the passage of the ADAAA and the rewriting of Federal Regulations, results for employees have begun to improve in the court system.

Comparison of the 1990 ADA and the ADA Amendments Act

Following is a comparison between five specific issues addressed by Congress in its effort to restore the intent and protections afforded individuals with disabilities under the 1990 ADA:

Issue	*ADA (as Construed by the Courts)*	*ADAAA (as Amended)*
Mitigating measures	To be considered in the process of determining whether a person has an impairment that is substantially limiting.	Not to be considered in determining whether a person has an impairment that is substantially limiting except for ordinary eyeglasses or contact lenses.
"Substantially limits"	Impairment substantially limits an MLA if it prevents or severely restricts the individual from performing the activity.	EEOC and Supreme Court have incorrectly interpreted—have been rewritten to provide a broader scope of coverage.
The "major life activity" requirement	Must be an activity that is "of crucial importance" to most people's daily lives.	Expanded list of major life activities to also include the operation of major bodily functions.

(Continued)

Episodic conditions and multiple major life activities	Some courts have held that individuals must be limited in more than one major life activity. Other courts have held that episodic or intermittent impairments are not covered under the law.	An impairment that substantially limits one major life activity is sufficient. Impairments that are episodic or in remission are disabilities if limiting when the condition is considered active.
Regarded as having a disability	Covers individuals who are "regarded as" disabled. Courts have required individuals to show what employers were thinking.	Can establish coverage under the "regarded as" section by showing that they were subjected to an action prohibited by ADA based upon an actual or perceived impairment. No accommodations for those found to be "regarded as."

Summary and Conclusions

As of the 2007–2008 term, the Supreme Court heard and provided decisions in 21 specific ADA cases (Allbright, 2007). Five of the cases involved the definition of disability. These decisions have led to Congress passing the ADA Amendments Act of 2008 that seeks "to restore the intent and protections of the Americans with Disabilities Act of 1990." The ADA amendments focus specifically on several fundamental issues that have been narrowly interpreted by the courts. First and most important is the definition of disability. It retains the ADA's basic definition but changes the way the statutory terms are interpreted, for instance, substantially limited and major life activities. It also addresses the controversial decisions regarding the use of mitigating measures. It clarifies that an impairment that is episodic or in remission is a disability if it would substantially limit a major life activity when active. The new law addresses "regarded as" cases and whether they are transitory and minor and whether reasonable accommodations should be provided to those individuals determined to be regarded as disabled. Finally, Congress emphasized that the definition of disability should be interpreted broadly.

Of particular relevance is the *Olmstead* case, which may have implications for lifelong care of people with mental and developmental disabilities, since community-based programs may be legally required over institutional care. In addition, the vocational aspects of a life care plan may require a knowledgeable expert to ensure opinions are defensible.

These Supreme Court decisions have altered and, in many cases narrowed the definition of disability and, consequently, who is protected under ADA. Matthew Diller, Fordham University law professor, has stated, "The courts have seized upon the definition of disability as a way to stop cases, and in effect, shield an employer's conduct from scrutiny" (1999). The courts had taken the position that ADA should be strictly interpreted, creating a demanding standard for qualifying as disabled. The records indicate that was not the intent of the Congress. As demonstrated, only a very small number of cases dealing with the actual discrimination issues were heard by a judge or jury. The ADA Amendments Act was meant to correct this situation, and the recent research of court cases seems to support the change in the ability of individuals with disabilities to have their cases heard before a judge and/or jury.

Agencies given the authority to enforce the ADAAA have gradually published new regulations to restore the intent of the congress to broaden the coverage of the law and to provide a legal avenue for persons with disabilities to have their possible discrimination heard in front of a judge and/or jury.

Under the 1990 ADA, the plaintiff has had the burden to prove that he or she has a disability as a gateway step to presenting his or her case before a judge or jury. This has proven to be a difficult step. Congress' legislative goal with the ADAAA was to correct this and focus the emphasis on the possible act of discrimination rather than the assessment of whether the individual has a disability. The courts have provided very specific guidelines for presenting information within an evaluation to assist all parties concerned to understand the circumstances and needs of the plaintiff. In practice, a detailed assessment based on guidelines provided by ADA case law can be a valuable source of information for the judge or jury in adjudicating ADA cases. Some of this case law has been precluded by the ADA Amendments Act, adding yet another chapter to the intent of Congress to "provide a clear and comprehensive national mandate for the elimination of discrimination against individuals with disabilities and provide broad coverage." It has been demonstrated in this chapter that protection of people with disabilities under ADAAA has not been automatic, even if one is in a catastrophic impairment situation.

The unique nature of the ADA transition is the more than 16 years of developing case law surrounding its effective date of July 1992. The ADAAA was effective January 1, 2009. It is being identified that the range of coverage and protection for individuals with disabilities is expanding significantly. While it is essentially effective immediately, it is expected that areas of the ADAAA will be challenged, resulting in new case law. The case law regarding the ADAAA is continuing to develop positive outcomes in the court system, enabling the individual to have their case heard in the judicial system.

Supreme Court Decisions 1998–2005

- Available from www.law.cornell.edu/supct/search/index.html.
- *Albertson's, Inc., v. Kirkingburg,* No. 98-0591, June 22, 1999.
- *Barnes v. Gorman,* No. 01-682, June 17, 2002.
- *Board of Trustees of the University of Alabama v. Garrett,* No. 99-1240, February 21, 2001.
- *Bragdon v. Abbott,* No. 97-156, June 15, 1998.
- *Buchannon Board & Care Home, Inc., v. West Virginia Department of Health and Human Resources,* No. 99-1848, May 29, 2001.
- *Chevron v. Echazabal,* No. 00-1406, June 10, 2002.
- *Clackamas Gastroenterology Associates, P.C., v. C.V. Wells,* No. 01-1435 April 22, 2003.
- *Cleveland v. Policy Management Systems, Corp.,* No. 97-1008, May 24, 1999.
- *EEOC v. Waffle House, Inc.,* No. 99-1823, January 15, 2002.
- *National Railroad Passenger Corp. v. Morgan, Abner, Jr.,* No. 00-1614, January 9, 2002.
- *Olmstead Commissioner, Georgia Department of Human Resources v. L.C.,* No. 98-0536, June 1999.
- *Pennsylvania Department of Corrections v. Yeskey,* No. 97-634, June 15, 1998.
- *PGA Tour, Inc., v. Martin,* No. 00-0024, May 29, 2001.
- *Raytheon Company v. Joel Hernandez,* No. 07-749, December 2, 2003.
- *Spector v. Norwegian Cruise Line Ltd.,* No. 03-1388, June 6, 2005.
- *Sutton, Karen & Hinton, Kimberly, v. United Airlines, Inc.,* No. 97-1943, June 22, 1999.

- *Tennessee v. George Lane,* No. 02-1667, May 17, 2004.
- *Toyota Motors v. Williams,* No. 00-1089, January 8, 2002.
- *U.S. Airways v. Barnett,* No. 00-1250, April 29, 2002.
- *Vaughn L. Murphy v. United Parcel Service, Inc.,* No. 97-1992, June 22, 1999.
- *Wright v. Universal Maritime Service Corp.,* No. 97-0889, November 16, 1998.

Important Websites

- Department of Justice—ADA Home: www.usdoj.gov/crt/ada/adahom1.htm
- Equal Employment Opportunity Commission: www.eeoc.gov
- The Federal Judiciary: www.uscourts.gov
- Law News: www.law.com
- The National Council on Disability: www.ncd.gov/index.html
- U.S. Supreme Court Collection: www.supct.law.cornell.edu:8080/supct
- U.S. Supreme Court—Multimedia Media Database: http://oyez.nwu.edu
- U.S. Supreme Court of the United States: www.supremecourtus.gov
- *Washington Post* for Supreme Court News: www.washingtonpost.com

References and Additional Resources

ADA Amendments Act, S.3406. 2008, September 25. *One Hundred Tenth Congress of the United States of America, Public Law* 110–325.

ADA.Gov. 2009. *Americans with Disabilities Act Of 1990, As Amended.* Available at https://www.ada.gov/pubs/adastatute08.htm.

ADA.Gov. July 15, 2016. *Amendment of Americans with Disabilities Act Title II and Title III Regulations to Implement ADA Amendments Act of 2008.* Available at https://www.ada.gov/regs2016/final_rule_adaaa.html.

Albertson's, Inc., v. Kirkingburg, No. 98-0591, June 22, 1999.

Allbright, A. L. 2007. *Employment Decisions Under the ADA Title I: Survey Update, August, 2006.* Washington, DC: The Commission on Mental and Physical Disability Law Reporter.

Blanck, P. D. 1999. *Disability Law and Policy: A Collective Vision.* Washington, DC: ADA Commission on Mental and Physical Disability Law.

Bragdon v. Abbott. 1998, June 15. No. 97-156.

CESSI, *Federal Statutory Definitions of Disability, prepared for The Interagency Committee on Disability Research,* July 1, 2003.

Cleveland v. Policy Management Systems, Corp. 1999, May 24. No. 97-1008.

DBTAC: Southeast ADA Center, ADA Amendments Act of 2008 Summary and Resources, October 14, 2008.

Diller, M. 1999. *Judges Don't Understand the ADA.* www.raggededgemagazine.com.

EEOC. 1999, July 26. *Instructions for Field Offices: Analyzing ADA Charges After Supreme Court Decisions Addressing "Disability" and "Qualified,"* www.eeoc.gov.

EEOC. 2002, August 13. *Report: Study of Litigation Program Fiscal Year 1997–2001.* www.eeoc.gov.

EEOC. 2008, October. *Notice Concerning The Americans With Disabilities Act (ADA) Amendments Act of 2008.* www.eeoc.gov/ada/amendments_notice.html.

EEOC. 2011. *Fact Sheet on the EEOC's Final Regulations Implementing the ADAAA.* Available at https://www.eeoc.gov/laws/regulations/adaaa_fact_sheet.cfm.

Elias, S., & Levinkind, S. 1999, August. *Legal Researcher: How to Find and Understand the Law* (7th ed). Berkeley, CA: Bertelsmann Industry Services. www.nolo.com.

Federal Register, Vol. 65, No. 11. (2000, June 8). Rules and Regulations 36327: EEOC, 29 CFR Park 1630 Interpretive Guidance on Title I ADA.

Georgetown Law Federal Legislation and Administrative Clinic. 2008. *On behalf of the Epilepsy Foundation.*

Heyburn, J. G., Chief District Judge. *Cotter v. Ajilon Services, Inc.* 2002, April 25. *The Court of Appeals for the 6th Circuit*, No. 00-2041.

Lorber, L. 2008. *Get Ready to Relearn the ADA*. Retrieved December 27, 2008, from www.law.com.

Marat, J. P. Sept. 12, 2013. *Americans with Disabilities Act (ADA): From Case Law to Case Management and Life Care Planning Practice.* Available at http://tipsdiscover.com/health/americans-disabilities-act-ada-case-law-case-management-life-care-planning-practice.

Mental and Physical Disability Law Reporter 32.

National Council on Disability. 2009, September 30. *The Current State of Health Care for People with Disabilities.* Available at http://www.ncd.gov/publications/2009/Sept302009.

National Council on Disability. 2013. *A Promising Start: Preliminary Analysis of Court Decisions Under the ADA Amendments Act.* Available at https://www.ncd.gov/publications/2013/07232013.

Olmstead Commissioner, Georgia Department of Human Resources v. L.C. 1999, June. No. 98-0536.

Parry, J. 2008. *ADA Amendments Act of 2008: A Glass Half Empty or Half Full? Commission on Mental and Physical Disability Law*, American Bar Association, 2008.

Rubinger, H., & Gardner, R. 2002, May/June. Tearing down the walls: New freedom initiative. *Continuing Care*, 21, 24–31.

Sutton, Karen, & Hinton, *Kimberly, v. United Airlines, Inc.* 1999, June 22. No. 97-1943.

Toyota Motors v. Williams. 2002, January 8. No. 00-1089.

U.S. Airways v. Barnett. 2002, April 29. No. 00-1250.

U.S. DOJ (United States Department of Justice). 2003. ADA Definitions. Retrieved July 31, 2003, from www.usdoj.gov/crt/ada/.

Vierling, L. 2000a. The Americans with Disabilities Act: Implications of Supreme Court decisions for case managers part 1. *The Case Manager*, 11, 47–49.

Vierling, L. 2000b. The Americans with Disabilities Act: Implications of Supreme Court decisions for case managers part 2. *The Case Manager*, 11, 72–76.

Vierling, L. 2000c. The Americans with Disabilities Act: Implications of Supreme Court decisions for case managers part 3. *The Case Manager*, 11, 65–68.

Vierling, L. 2000d. The Americans with Disabilities Act: Implications of Supreme Court decisions for case managers part 4. *The Case Manager*, 11, 51–55.

Vierling, L. 2001a. The Americans with Disabilities Act: Implications of Supreme Court decisions for case managers part 5. *The Case Manager*, 12, 77–82.

Vierling, L. 2001b. Americans with Disabilities update. *The Case Manager*, 12, 20–21.

Vierling, L. 2002a. Americans with Disabilities update. *The Case Manager*, 13, 18–20.

Vierling, L. 2002b. Americans with Disabilities update. *The Case Manager*, 13, 21–23.

Vierling, L. 2002c. Americans with Disabilities update. *The Case Manager*, 13, 20–22.

Vierling, L. 2002d. *Court Decisions Involving the Americans with Disabilities Act: A Resource Guide for Rehabilitation Professionals.* Athens, GA: Elliott & Fitzpatrick.

Young, J. (Ed.). 1997, July 26. *Equality of Opportunity: The Making of the American with Disabilities Act. Appendix B: The Legal Road to the ADA.* Washington, DC: National Council on Disability.

Chapter 30

Life Care Planning Resources

Ann Maniha and Leslie L. Watson

Contents

Introduction 730
UCR and Recommended Pricing 731
H-385.923 Definition of "Usual, Customary, and Reasonable" (UCR) 731
Area Cost Analysis 732
The Art of Obtaining Information by Telephone and E-Mail 735
Locating Health Care Professionals 736
Useful Home Health Care Services Links 736
Other Useful Links 736
Vocational Rehabilitation Resources 737
Geographically Specific Wage Data 737
Schools/Educational Services 737
Health Club 737
Federal Information 737
Other Web-Based Resources 738
Life Care Plan Software 738
Selected Specific Resources 739
Paralyzed Veterans of America (PVA) 739
Veteran Benefits, CFR Title 38 739
Special Needs Trust 739
Northwest Regional Spinal Cord Injury System/NWRSCIS SCI Update Newsletter (University of Washington Department of Rehabilitation Medicine) 741
National Council on Disability (NCD) 741
HEATH National Clearinghouse on Postsecondary Education for Individuals with Disabilities 741
Viatical Resources 741
Through the Looking Glass: Resources for Parents with Disabilities 741

Telecommunications Accessibility....742
Summer Camps....742
U.S. Life Tables....742
Genworth Cost of Care Survey....742
General Information Sources....742
Topics in Spinal Cord Injury Rehabilitation....742
Exceptional Parent: The Special Needs Resource....742
Additional Resources (not all inclusive)....743
Journals....743
Books....743
Certification in Life Care Planning....743
Training Programs for Life Care Planning Certification....743
Utilizing Databases for Research....744
Medical Coding and Billing Software Subscriptions....744
EncoderPro.com....744
Find-A-Code....744
Super Coder....744
Medical Coding and Billing Resources....745
Coding Tips for Consideration....745
Important Crosswalks for the Life Care Planner....745
Reputable Databases....746
Facility....746
Physician/Other Health Care Professionals....746
DME....747
Anesthesia....747
Dental....747
American Hospital Directory....747
Context[4] Healthcare....748
FAIR Health....748
VA Reasonable Data Charges....748
H·CUPnet....748
Other Free of Charge Facility Databases....749
Zip Code (geo-zip)....749
Abeo Coder....749
Conclusion....749
Appendix 30.1: Area Cost Analysis Request Form....750
Appendix 30.2: Questionnaire....755
References....757

Introduction

One of the main objectives of the research phase of life care planning is to provide accurate and transparent costs and resources for the needs outlined in the life care plan (Sutton et al., 2002). The life care planner with the competitive edge is the one who has a multitude of data from a variety of reputable sources rather than just the basics involved in setting up the outline for the recommendations for the life care plan. Without proper resources that are easily accessible, understandable, and updateable, the task of completing a competent, thorough, and accurate life care plan can be formidable. It is important to remember that the money set aside is to care for this individual for the rest of their life and to provide and maintain their medical stability and quality of life.

The research and resources utilized in litigation related life care planning more often than not will be brought to question during deposition (Elliott, 2010; Raffles-Gunn, 2010). Using top-notch research and providing transparent costs will help the expert during deposition when asked to provide and explain the source, or during a telephone conference with a referral source, asking for specifics on services, products and other items referenced in the life care plan. Additionally, there are many topics not specifically covered in the life care plan itself that must also be readily available for conferencing, speaking, training, testifying, networking, and case managing.

This chapter will outline some of the resources that will enable life care planners to expand their horizons and base of information. This chapter is not designed to outline specific individual sources for a specific problem. Rather, this chapter will outline information that will provide the life care planner/case manager with the fact source(s) needed to be well-rounded and knowledgeable in all facets of the life care planning area of practice and that will provide a foundation upon which one can continually build a broad knowledge base.

The process of researching requires the life care planner to identify and define needed information and cultivate effective resources to locate the information. The life care planner needs to organize, store, and retrieve valuable information. In order to identify and define needed information, the life care planner must look at the client/evaluee specifics such as the injury, disability, and specific location of services. Client/evaluee needs based on the disability include medical services, nursing care and assistance, allied health services, therapies, residential needs, medications, supplies and equipment, educational and vocational needs, and miscellaneous services. Defining client needs goes hand-in-hand with identifying those areas for inclusion in the life care plan.

UCR and Recommended Pricing

When obtaining pricing for services and items, it is important that the costs be usual, customary, and reasonable (UCR) and not discounted. Usual and customary typically fall within the 75th or 80th percentile. Below is the AMA's (American Medical Association, 2013) definition of "Usual, Customary, and Reasonable" (not to be confused with insurance defined or other uses of UCR):

H-385.923 Definition of "Usual, Customary, and Reasonable" (UCR)

1. Our AMA adopts as policy the following definitions; (a) 'usual' fee means that fee usually charged, for a given service, by an individual physician to his [her] private patient (i.e., his [her] own usual fee); (b) a fee is 'customary' when it is within the range of usual fees currently charged by physicians of similar training and experience, for the same service within the same

specific and limited geographical area; and (c) a fee is 'reasonable' when it meets the above two criteria and is justifiable, considering the special circumstances of the particular case in question, without regard to payments that have been discounted under governmental or private plans.

2. Our AMA takes the position that there is no relationship between the Medicare fee schedule and Usual, Customary, and Reasonable Fees (AMA, 2013, p. 1).

It is important for the life care planner to make sure the appropriate amount of money is included in the plan to care for the individual for the rest of their life. One does not want to include the most expensive pricing found during their research but also not the least expensive; hence the importance of using UCR costs. Once the life care plan is developed, the case manager (or other person responsible for implementing the plan) is responsible to assist with cost savings that preserves the individual's funds. The care must provide for maintenance of medical stability and quality of life over the client/evaluee's lifetime.

In addition, the following consensus statement was promulgated by attendees of the 2015 Life Care Planning Summit (Johnson, 2015, p. 38):

98. Best practices for identifying costs in Life Care Plans include:

- Verifiable data from appropriately referenced sources
- Costs identified are geographically specific when appropriate and available
- Non-discounted/market rate prices
- More than one cost estimate, when appropriate

Medical necessity is a term associated with what is covered by the payor source (Medicare, insurance) and does not necessarily represent quality of life for a given client. Other terms such as out-of-pocket do not mean what the individual has actually paid but what the payor source feels they should have paid. If one paid $500 for a service and the payor source believes they should have only paid $50, then only $50 will be included as part of the out-of-pocket paid. Out-of-pocket also does not include premiums and, at times, does not include co-pays or deductibles. It is important to note that not all services that an individual requires for medical stability and quality of life are covered services. In addition, coverage does not, in and of itself, equate care.

The life care planner must be careful when utilizing the medical codes and databases to not use Medicare rules for the development of the pricing in the plan. Although Medicare may set the precedence for billing, this is not the same for all carriers.

Area Cost Analysis

When developing the life care plan, a helpful tool or blueprint to use is the Area Cost Analysis Request form (see Appendix 1). It is in using this form that the planner begins mentally constructing the plan as the requested cost information is outlined. By checking off the items that require costing research, the planner is also constructing the various recommendations contained within the plan.

The Area Cost Analysis Form provides information to include for the different sections/areas of the life care plan as described here:

The first section/area to be addressed will include the individual's name, age, gender, date of birth, disability, zip code for where they reside, zip code for where they will receive their services/care, area code, city, state, nearest metro area, today's date, and due date for the cost research to be completed.

Another section is medical care. This includes physicians, as applicable to the client, such as a general practitioner, internist, neuro-ophthalmologist, dentist, gastroenterologist, geriatric physician, neurologist, neuropsychologist, neurosurgeon, ophthalmologist, orthopedist, orthopedic surgeon, otolaryngologist, pain management specialist, pediatrician, physiatrist, plastic surgeon, podiatrist, psychiatrist, psychologist, pulmonologist, rheumatologist, and urologist, just to mention a few. One way to locate physicians includes searching for the website/professional organization of each specialty. These websites will usually provide a directory and searchable database for physician sources. An example for locating a physiatrist would be to access the American Academy of Physical Medicine and Rehabilitation website, www.aapmr.org, which provides a directory of physicians listed by location.

Home health care is another area commonly to be included in a life care plan. This section includes skilled nursing (LPN/LVN or RN), home health aide, homemaker services, and in-home physical, occupational, speech, or respiratory therapists. One will need to know if these services will be required hourly, as skilled visits or as live-in care. All of this will begin to come to light once the life care planner has gathered important information pertaining to the individual's medical, cognitive, and functional status. Examples of some of the questions to which life care planners commonly need answers are:

- Does the individual have a catheter and if they do, what type of catheter (Foley or suprapubic) or do they require intermittent catheterizations? If the latter is the case, do they perform self-catheterizations or require the assistance of a caretaker?
- Do they have a bowel program?
- Does this individual require infusion therapy, have a tracheostomy, have a G-tube requiring tube feeds, or are they on a ventilator?
- Require oxygen or suctioning?
- Are they totally dependent on others to perform their Activities of Daily Living?

These are just a few of the considerations the life care planner needs to be aware of because this will reflect the type of care and amount of care to be included in the life care plan. When obtaining costs, it is important to inquire about the laws of the state and each state's Nurse Practice Act that pertains to such information as what level of caregiver can administer medications (home health aides/CNAs or skilled nurses such as LPN/LVN/RN). Equally important is what level of caregiver can give G-tube feedings. One needs to know if the caregiver (skilled nurse or home health aide) is permitted to drive the client's vehicle to take them to appointments or what is the minimum and maximum time for a visit. As can be ascertained, it is important for the life care planner to be thorough and document effective notes when gathering data and resources for the life care plan.

Another section, allied health, includes specialties such as physical therapy, occupational therapy, speech therapy, aquatic therapy, hippotherapy, recreational therapy, nutritionist, massage therapy, adaptive driving evaluation and training, augmentative communication, respiratory therapy, assistive technology, and health and wellness. These allied health specialties can be found in hospital settings and outpatient or community settings.

Diagnostic testing may include any or all of the following tests in addition to others not listed: EEG, EKG, pulmonary function testing, renal scan, renal ultrasound, sleep study, swallow study, urodynamic studies, CT, MRI, X-ray, bronchoscopy, colonoscopy, cystoscopy, or another endoscopy. Diagnostic testing costs can be obtained through the hospital setting, at area radiology facilities, or by utilizing one of the databases such as American Hospital Directory. It is important to have the CPT codes when obtaining costs and to remember such details as a radiologist reading fee or technical fee associated with the test. The life care planner needs to determine all of the information associated with each diagnostic test when calling for charges. Lab testing may include such tests as a CBC, comprehensive metabolic panel (CMP), creatinine, culture, and sensitivity (i.e., blood or urine), liver function tests (LFT), lipid panel, urinalysis (UA), and chemical levels (i.e., magnesium or calcium). It is important to know what tests are included in the panels such as the CMP to avoid getting costs for duplicate tests. Cost for the lab tests can be obtained through the hospital setting or in the local community at such labs as Quest Diagnostics or Lab Corp. As with the diagnostic testing, it is helpful to have the CPT codes or lab test codes when calling for costs.

With regard to the next section, medications, the life care planner should obtain a list of medications the client currently takes and/or are prescribed by their treating physicians. There are several ways to obtain pricing for medications. Contact area pharmacies directly, www.goodrx.com and www.awpvaluerx.com. Be careful to include cost of medications without any discounts or coupon pricing as these discounts may not always be available for use into the future.

Household services include housecleaning, handyman services, yard services, and home modifications. Costs for these items can be obtained by directly contacting area businesses or utilizing area resources.

Educational programs include public school, private school, community college, vocational/technical school, college, tutor, summer program, and camps.

Vocational services include vocational evaluation, vocational/career counseling, job coaching, sheltered work, supported work, day/activity program, job placement activities, and, if applicable, tuition, fees, and so on, associated with college enrollment to enhance employability. Information for locating these programs can be obtained directly off the school websites and other websites for specific disabilities.

Facility care includes adult daycare day program for individuals with traumatic brain injury (TBI) or developmental/intellectual delay, assisted living facility, intermediate care facility (ICF) or group home, long-term care for individuals with TBI, skilled nursing facility, supported living, transitional living, neurobehavioral long-term care, chronic pain inpatient or outpatient care, spinal cord rehabilitation inpatient or outpatient care, spinal cord evaluation or reevaluation inpatient or outpatient. When speaking with the admissions department, the life care planner should consider the level of disability, age limits, hours of supervision, Activities of Daily Living, and client behavior. Additionally, is the client ambulatory, on a trach, vent dependent, continent, or verbal? Does the client need a day program or work program? All of these considerations will reflect the best resources for the client along with the estimated daily or monthly charge.

Surgeries and procedures include, but are not limited to, such items as epidural block, joint replacement, tendon release, hardware removal, contracture release, arthroscopy, scar revision, laminectomy, discectomy, scoliosis surgery, spinal fusion, spinal cord stimulator, morphine pump, baclofen pump, gastrostomy, PEG tube, trach revision, and shunt revision. This is not an exhaustive list but a list of some of the more commonly found procedures in life care planning. In addition to the more obvious surgeon charge for a surgery/procedure, facility fees can be obtained by contacting the area hospital or facility or utilizing one of the many databases that are discussed in this chapter. Another aspect of the charge for surgeries and procedures is the anesthesia charges. The life care planner should obtain anesthesiologist charges either through the anesthesiologist that the facility uses or anesthesia database.

Equipment/supplies may include environmental control unit (ECU), standers, wheelchair, cushions, ramp/lift, van conversion, assistive technology, augmentative communication device, pediatric equipment, orthotics and prosthetics, catheter supplies, gloves, lotion, diapers, supplemental formulas such as PediaSure, G-tube replacement, care and feeding supplies and visual aids, just to mention a few. The costs for equipment and supplies can be obtained by directly contacting local vendors or utilizing websites. The life care planner must make sure that a reputable vendor and/or Internet resource for costs is used, such as www.allegromedical.com, www.southwestmedical.com, www.spinlife.com, www.walgreens.com, and others, to name a few. Utilizing the Internet for cost resources can be a viable source, but remember not all information provided on the Internet is accurate. For that reason, it is important for the life care planner to determine the veracity or accuracy of the Internet costs by calling local sources for the same item to verify the costs are comparable.

The Art of Obtaining Information by Telephone and E-Mail

One of the most important parts of researching costs is to be prepared before making the contact with vendors and/or providers. Know the case, individual factors, and type of information needed. When contacting physician/provider offices, ask to speak with the billing department or office manager who oftentimes can more accurately provide charges for office visits and procedures. When surgeon fees are needed, ask for the billing department or surgery scheduling department. Remember the individuals to contact are typically busy performing their job and generally do not have time for multiple calls or to wait until the life care planner determines what information is needed. For example, the authors recommend that life care planners research the specific CPT code or codes used for the service that is being recommended before contacting the provider. And if contacting a treating provider, it is recommended to have the patient's date of birth readily available to provide if needed. An Authorization for Release of Personal Information, signed by the client/ patient, also is needed to be able to provide it to the treating provider.

When contacting hospitals to obtain costs, one good place to start is with the hospital's website. Many times, the website provides a list of departments and their telephone numbers which is helpful when trying to locate specific departments such as the therapy or radiology departments. Additional departments to research to obtain costs include financial counselor, admissions department, billing department, cost estimate line, or cashier's office.

Bear in mind that first impressions count when contacting others by telephone to obtain information for the life care plan. One's greeting and demeanor oftentimes will set the tone for the call and can impact the end result; that is, obtaining the necessary information. The authors suggest the following guidelines:

- Be positive and do not allow the person on the other end to dismiss the request by indicating that he or she does not know the answer. Be persuasive, but kind, and ask who can be contacted in order to obtain the information.
- Be complimentary and appreciative of the assistance you receive. It may be necessary to contact this source for more information and/or for another case in the future.
- Be persistent, patient, and persevere. One of the most important observations while researching costs is to think ahead and obtain as much information as possible during the contact. Obtain the contact person's name (first and last), department, and direct telephone number. This information is needed not only to document the research and contact made, but also is important for the life care plan resource list.

E-mail is another valuable tool especially when the life care planner is not able to speak directly with the intended contact. Instead of (or in addition to) leaving a voice mail, contact the front office and request an e-mail address for the person. Then compose a professional e-mail that outlines the requested information and includes the life care planner's return contact information. Keep in mind that professionalism, courtesy, and appreciation goes a long way for both telephonic and electronic/e-mail contact in order to get the requested information.

Locating Health Care Professionals

Below are useful tools that can assist the life care planner in finding specific specialists:

National Trade and Professional Associations Directory 2018. This text provides detailed information including over 8,000 associations, professional societies, and labor unions plus over 35,000 names and contact information for executives. The Directory is available online at www.AssociationExecs.com or www.associationtrends.com/store. The 2018 pricing for the Directory is $299.00; $269.10 for standing order; and $899.00 for online.

Columbia Books & Information Services (CBIS)
4340 East-West Highway, Suite 300
Bethesda, MD 20814
Phone: 1-888-265-0600
Email: info@columbiabooks.com

The Care Planner Network, http://careplanners.net/: Online community for life care planning and case management professionals, providing access to a directory of life care planners, valuable resources, professional forum, affiliates, and a bookstore.

IARP Internet Resources for Case Managers and Disability Manager, www.rehabpro.orgwww.rehabpro.org: Online list of Internet resources compiled by the International Association of Rehabilitation Professionals (IARP), including a list of links to disability management-related sites.

CMSA Care Management Industry Directory developed by MultiView for the Case Management Society of America (CMSA), www.caremanagementindustrydirectory.com: Online vendor search specifically designed for benefit of case managers.

Seniors Resource Guide, www.seniorsresourceguide.com: Comprehensive guide to national and geographic specific senior resources.

Useful Home Health Care Services Links

- Interim Healthcare: www.interimhealthcare.com
- ResCare: www.rescare.com
- Maxim Healthcare Services: www.maximhealthcare.com

Other Useful Links

- Brain Injury Facility Locator: www.biausa.org
- United Cerebral Palsy Services: www.ucp.org
- Spinal Cord Injury Information & Resources: www.spinalcord.uab.edu

- Commission on the Accreditation of Rehabilitation Facilities: www.carf.org
- Shepherd Spinal Cord Injury Program: www.shepherd.org
- Chronic Pain: https://theacpa.org
- United Spinal's Spinal Cord Injury Resource Center: www.spinalcord.org
- American Foundation for the Blind: www.afb.org
- University of Alabama at Birmingham Spinal Cord Injury Model System: https://www.uab.edu/medicine/sci/uab-scims-information

Vocational Rehabilitation Resources

- State Vocational Rehabilitation Programs: www.parac.org/svrp.html
- The Commission on Rehabilitation Counselor Certification (CRC) "Locate a Certified Professional": https://crcc.ebiz.uapps.net/PersonifyEbusiness/Default.aspx?TabID=168

Geographically Specific Wage Data

- Bureau of Labor Statistics: http://www.bls.gov/oes/current/oessrcma.htm (provides yearly metropolitan-area occupational employment and wage estimates):
- Occupational Outlook Handbook: www.bls.gov/oco/
- DME (Durable Medical Equipment) replacement frequencies: http://www.flcpr.org/Documents/Marini_Harper_JLCP_4_173-182.pdf

Schools/Educational Services

- Colleges and Universities: http://www.50states.com/college
- Preschools, public schools, private schools, and school boards: http://infospace.com/
- Tutors: http://www.sylvanlearning.com/ or https://www.wyzant.com/tutorsearch
- Special Needs Camp: http://www.acacamps.org

Health Club

- YMCA: http://www.ymca.net/

Federal Information

- Federal government: www.usa.gov
- Medicaid: https://www.medicaid.gov/
- Social Security Administration: https://www.ssa.gov/
- Federal Government Directory: https://www.usa.gov/federal-agencies/a

Other Web-Based Resources

- National Library of Medicine's Medline Database: https://www.ncbi.nlm.nih.gov/pubmed/
- National Center for Dissemination of Disability Research: www.ncddr.org
- Center on Knowledge Translation for Disability and Rehabilitation Research (KTDDR): www.ktdrr.org
- U.S. Department of Health and Human Resources: https://healthfinder.gov/

Life Care Plan Software

A life care plan database is an important aspect of what any successful life care planner/case manager will require, including using software that will allow storing, retrieving, presenting, and formatting information relevant to the life care plan. Following are several choices of products available:

LCP Stat, version 10, Pyxlglaze Digital Media, LLC (acquired from TecSolutions, Inc. in late 2009), www.lcpstat.com. Contact: Randall Nichols, 828-283-0109, randall@lcpstat.com.

LCP Stat 10 is designed for use on Windows and Macintosh operating systems and requires FileMaker Pro 12 (not included). The program is designed for life care planning and includes a resource database, contacts, and dashboard. One can access any resource without completely leaving the plan by clicking on the toolbar. The plan can be exported to pdf and stored within the program.

LCP Software, Legal Nurse Systems, LLC, http://www.legalnursesystems.com/life-care-planner.html. Contact: Sharon Martino, 440-285-7201, sharonmartino@legalnursesystems.com.

LCP Software has networking capabilities and a resource database. The software allows the life care plan to be customized to the individual client using templates, a plan profile, a plan log, electronic link to the CDC Life Tables, search features, math calculation capabilities, category selection, multiple cost reports, links to internal files, and the ability to create chapters, copy and paste a plan, and assemble the plan.

Life Care Planning for the PC. Contact: Ann Maniha, RN, CLCP, CMC, Certified Life Care Planner, Certified Medical Coder: ann.maniha@gmail.com.

Life Care Planning for the PC is authored and copyrighted by Ann Maniha, RN, CLCP, CMC, and is created in Word and WordPerfect file formats. The narrative and tables are all in one document. The software has the ability to be completely individualized to specific preferences. In addition, the software also has the ability to calculate within the tables. The format layout is easily understood and reasonably priced. The software comes with both a USB drive and an instruction manual. (*Editors' note*: For full disclosure, this program is the brainchild of one of the authors.)

Lifecarewriter.com: Online tools to assist planners in the preparation of life care plans. The tools require no software purchase or downloads and are accessed via a secure website. The finished plan is delivered in a Microsoft Word® document.

FormPro™ (currently—2018—in the process of changing name to InQuis Global, LLC and expanding services). Contact: sales@brightsuntech.com or info@brightsuntech.com.

FormPro was developed by Brightsun Technologies for life care planners, legal nurse consultants, paralegals, and plaintiffs or defense attorneys engaged in personal injury litigation. The software includes a customizable detailed Patient Care Needs Questionnaire, injury checklists, and relevant research, and it is available as an annual or monthly subscription.

Selected Specific Resources

Paralyzed Veterans of America (PVA) (www.pva.org)

The website includes access to the Consortium for Spinal Cord Medicine; Clinical Guidelines and Consumer Guides; Adaptive Sports Resources; Accessibility and Mobility; Accessible Housing Resources; Caregivers; Employment Resources for Veterans and All with Disabilities; General Medical Resources; Multiple Sclerosis; Spinal Cord Injury; Spina Bifida; Amyotrophic Lateral Sclerosis (ALS); Government Sites and Veterans Online Resources; and Directory of Chapters and NSO (National Service Officers) per state. Membership to the Paralyzed Veterans of America is free and open to qualified individuals.

Veteran Benefits, CFR Title 38 (www.ecfr.gov)

The Code of Federal Regulations (CFR) Title 38—Pensions, Bonuses, and Veterans Relief is composed of two volumes with the parts arranged in the following order:

- Volume 1, Chapter I—Department of Veterans Affairs, parts 0 to 17 and parts 18 to end
- Volume 2, Chapter II—Armed Forces Retirement Home, parts 200 to 299

Special Needs Trust

Special needs trusts (SNTs) have been in common usage since 1993 and have been used on behalf of individuals with disabilities in litigation since 1978. The trusts have received extensive attention lately and will continue to spark debate or changes over time.

Most trusts are established by court order for settlement or judgment proceeds received on behalf of a litigating party who is severely disabled but can also be established by a parent, guardian, or next friend. Dussault and Lauterbach (2002) recommend the trust be established by the court. One of the goals of the special needs trust is to preserve the individual's eligibility (when properly drafted and in the appropriate situation) for local, state, or federal benefit programs, including Supplemental Security Income, under Title XVI, and Medicaid under Title XIX, of the Social Security Act (42 USC).

Congress amended the Medicaid statute in the 1993 Omnibus Budget Reconciliation Act (OBRA), now codified at 42 USC 1396p(d)(4)(A), to expressly recognize the use of such trusts as a means of preserving Medicaid eligibility if certain conditions are met. The following is a description of the special needs trust per Dussault and Lauterbach (2002, p. 70):

> The special needs trust allows the disabled individual to preserve eligibility for Medicaid benefits while the assets in the trust go for other needs not provided by public programs. These include supplemental attendant care, home maintenance, transportation, schooling, job training and coaches, social interaction and recreation—all aspects of

> life taken for granted in the nondisabled world. In addition, trust funds may be used to enhance quality of life by paying for respite care for family caregivers, basic home furnishings, cable television, telephone service, computers, Internet access, and even some vacation opportunities. Finally, SNT assets may supplement Medicaid services with additional therapy, respite or custodial care, and may provide payment for cutting-edge medical advances or therapies not paid for by Medicaid. In many cases, only the coordination of public benefits and SNT assets allows individuals who experience a disability to live "normally."

It cannot not be stressed enough how important it is that the special needs trust be drafted by a qualified professional with complete knowledge of the disability delivery system and the requirements under federal law noted at 42 USC 1396p(d) (4) (A). There are several different kinds of special needs trusts. Although different, they all have the same goal.

Part of the intrigue of a trust is the Medicaid lien. The medical needs of a person with a disability are often funded in part by Medicaid after, say, an accident and before the resolution of the case. Medicaid may be the only source of payment while liability is being contested. All attorneys should know that the Medicaid lien must be satisfied and discharged as part of the settlement process. Usually this process was left to the end of a suit, with the hopes that Medicaid will offer a substantial discount (often 30 to 50 percent or more of the actual lien). However, this discount may no longer be available. One can no longer leave the treatment of the Medicaid lien to the conclusion of a case. Thus, to avoid the parties discovering at the end of a case that almost the entire recovery could go to the Medicaid lien, this lien must be examined at the front end of a case.

All of this is quite confusing. Each state is handled differently, so there is no blanket answer to questions often posed. It is suggested that the case manager/life care planner obtain additional information from William L. E. Dussault, Esq., Dussault Law Group, 2722 Eastlake Ave. E, Suite 200, Seattle, WA 98102; phone: 206-324-4300. Mr. Dussault was one of the first to publish data on the special needs trusts and has a network of professionals that specialize in this area. He received the 2012 Award of Merit, the Washington State Bar Association's highest honor, for his work on state and federal legislation to better the lives of individuals with disabilities.

Additionally, one can read more about special needs trusts in *Topics in Spinal Cord Injury Rehabilitation*, Vol. 6, Issue 4, Overlapping Legal & Medical Issues (Spring 2001), pp 27-51 (Thomas Land Publishers, Birmingham, Alabama) and *The Special Needs Settlement Trust: A Tool for the Catastrophically Injured*, by William L.E. Dussault.

Another helpful article can be found at:
http://www.mult-sclerosis.org/news/Feb2002/PlanningToolsForDisabled.html: This article is titled *Special needs trusts: Powerful planning tools for disabled individuals*, by Kate Dussault and Jeffrey R. Lauterbach.

A website that answers questions regarding special needs trusts can be found at:
http://specialneedsanswers.com/.

A presentation titled *The Future of Special Needs Trusts Under the ACA* can be found at this link:
http://www.pekdadvocacy.com/wp-content/uploads/2014/05/The-Future-of-Special-Needs-Trusts-Under-the-ACA.pptx.

Northwest Regional Spinal Cord Injury System/NWRSCIS SCI Update Newsletter (University of Washington Department of Rehabilitation Medicine), http://sci.washington.edu/info/newsletters/

The newsletter is published three times a year and includes articles regarding topics related to living with SCI, research news profiles, and medical journal abstracts. The NWRSCIS is centered within the Department of Rehabilitation Medicine at the University of Washington Medical Center and Harborview Medical Center; one of the model spinal cord injury centers in the country funded by the National Institute on Disability and Rehabilitation Research (NIDRR).

National Council on Disability (NCD) (http://ncd.gov)

The NCD is an independent federal agency charged with advising the president, Congress, and other federal agencies regarding policies, programs, practices and procedures that affect people with disabilities. The website provides a list of resources, at http://ncd.gov/resources, that includes information regarding Civil Rights, Education, Employment, Financial Assistance & Incentives, Health Care, Housing, Independent Living, International, Legal Assistance, Technology, Transportation and Youth Perspectives. The NCD publications section, http://ncd.gov/publications, lists publications and policy briefs by year and includes 2016 publications: *Implementing the Affordable Care Act (ACA): A Roadmap for People with Disabilities; The Impact of the Affordable Care Act on People with Disabilities: A 2015 Status Report;* and *Monitoring and Enforcing the Affordable Care Act for People with Disabilities.* Their quarterly newsletter can be found at http://ncd.gov/newsroom/newsletter.

HEATH National Clearinghouse on Postsecondary Education for Individuals with Disabilities (https://heath.gwu.edu/)

The HEATH Resource Center is managed by The George Washington University Graduate School of Education and Human Development and is an online clearing house on postsecondary education for individuals with disabilities, serving as an information exchange of educational resources, support services and opportunities. The site contains a link to a 192-page Guidance and Career Counselors' Toolkit titled *Advising High School Students with Disabilities on Postsecondary Options.* The resources section, https://heath.gwu.edu/resources, includes *Directory of Transition Websites*, Frequently Asked Questions, HEATH NYTC Newsletters, and other Links and Repository.

Viatical Resources (http://www.viatical-web.org/resources.htm)

A Viatical settlement is a unique financial resource that allows individuals facing a life-threatening illness to sell their life insurance policy for cash, which can then be utilized for treatment and resources required as a result of the disability.

Through the Looking Glass: Resources for Parents with Disabilities (https://www.lookingglass.org)

Founded in 1982 by Megan Kirshbaum, PhD, Through the Looking Glass (TLG) established as its goal to (1) bring a disability culture perspective to early preventive intervention with families with disability/medial issues in infant, child, or parent; and (2) bring awareness about families and parenthood to the independent living community.

Telecommunications Accessibility (https://www.fcc.gov/general/telecommunications-relay-services-trs)

With the advent of the Americans with Disabilities Act (ADA), each state is required to implement a telecommunications system that is accessible to people with disabilities to provide accessible telecommunications.

Summer Camps

Summer Camps, the online companion to *Guide to Summer Camps and Summer Schools* by Porter Sargent Publishers, http://www.collegexpress.com/articles-and-advice/summer-programs/.

Although the website shows the last edition as the 33rd edition published for 2012/2013, the site contains information pertaining to summer camps and summer schools for individuals with special needs.

U.S. Life Tables (http://www.cdc.gov/nchs/products/life_tables.htm)

Up-to-date U.S. Life Tables with information pertaining to life expectancy.

Genworth Cost of Care Survey (https://www.genworth.com/about-us/industry-expertise/cost-of-care.html)

The Cost of Care Survey is updated annually and provides nationwide and state specific information regarding cost of long-term care for: assisted living facilities, nursing homes, home health aides, homemaker, and adult daycare. There also is an app available for download.

General Information Sources

Topics in Spinal Cord Injury Rehabilitation (http://www.thomasland.com/about-spinalrehab.html)

This peer-reviewed journal is published quarterly and is devoted to multidisciplinary commentary on the management of persons with a disability because of an insult to the spinal cord. A special issue on life care planning, co-edited by Terry Winkler, MD, and James S. Krause, PhD, is found in Volume 7, Number 4, Spring 2002.

Exceptional Parent: The Special Needs Resource (http://www.eparent.com/)

Established in 1971, Exceptional Parent (EP) provides practical advice and up-to-date educational information for families of children and adults with disabilities and special health care needs, as well as information for physicians, allied health care professionals, and other educated professionals involved in their care and development.

Additional Resources (not all inclusive)

Journals

Journal of Life Care Planning (https://www.rehabpro.org)
The *Journal of Life Care Planning* is the official journal of the International Academy of Life Care Planning (IALCP), a Division of IARP, and is published quarterly by Elliot & Fitzpatrick (http://www.elliottfitzpatrick.com/). The journal is the premiere peer-reviewed journal for the specialty practice of life care planning.

Journal of Nurse Life Care Planning (http://www.aanlcp.org/)
The *Journal of Nurse Life Care Planning* is the official peer-reviewed publication of the American Association of Nurse Life Care Planners (AANLCP) and is published quarterly in spring, summer, winter, and fall.

Physical Medicine and Rehabilitation Clinics of North America, http://www.pmr.theclinics.com/, published quarterly by Elsevier. An issue of special importance is *Life Care Planning*, Volume 24, Number 3, August 2013, coedited by Michel Lacerte, MDCM, MSc, FRCPC, CCRC and Cloie B. Johnson, MEd, ABVE-D, CCM.

Books

Pediatric Life Care Planning and Case Management, Second Edition (2011), edited by Susan Riddick-Grisham and Laura M. Deming. Published by CRC Press, https://www.crcpress.com. This book is a comprehensive and unique reference including legal and financial aspects, life expectancy data, vocational and assistive technology with case samples of actual plans associated with specific conditions.

Certification in Life Care Planning

The Certified Life Care Planner (CLCP), International Commission on Health Care Certification, www.ichcc.org, is the first certifying body for life care planners and issued the first life care planner certification examination in March 1996. Later, the Certified Nurse Life Care Planner (CNLCP) certification was formed for nurses only and is available through the Certified Nurse Life Care Planner Certification Board, http://cnlcp.org/.

Training Programs for Life Care Planning Certification

- Institute of Rehabilitation and Education and Training (IRET): https://iretprograms.com/
- Capital University Law School: http://law.capital.edu/LifeCarePlannerProgram/
- Fig Services, Inc.: http://www.figservices.com/
- Kelynco: http://kelynco.com/

Utilizing Databases for Research

In addition to contacting a resource by telephone or e-mail, one may opt to utilize a reliable database available either in online subscriptions or published resources. When using databases, medical coding typically is required and it is important for the life care planner to have access to current information. An ideal situation is when the physician provides the necessary codes for the follow-up, treatment, and procedures he or she recommends; however, this is not always the case and it becomes the life care planner's responsibility to know what codes are associated with the treatment recommendations. In order to be effective, the life care planner needs to have an understanding of the medical coding system and how it works.

The process of looking up codes can be multi-layered, and many times life care planners will find that there are codes that are considered part of another code when utilized together. A resource that is helpful to identify such codes, specifically when it pertains to orthopedic surgery treatment and procedures, is the *Complete Global Service Data for Orthopaedic Surgery* published by the American Academy of Orthopaedic Surgeons.

When costing out implantable devices, most cost information provided by the manufacturers such as Medtronic, Zimmer, or Boston Scientific, to mention a few, include the Medicare allowable information. However, if one reads the fine print, there commonly is a disclaimer suggesting that interested persons contact the insurance carrier for information regarding coverage of such devices. It is important to note that "coverage" does not equate to "costs" when researching costs to include in a life care plan.

Medical Coding and Billing Software Subscriptions

EncoderPro.com (www.optum360coding.com)

EncoderPro is an online coding subscription available in several different versions including Standard, Professional, Expert, and Payer. In addition to the different versions, there are add-ons for an additional fee. The annual subscription range is from $299.95 to $1,495.95 depending on the version purchased. The crosswalk capabilities available with this software depend on the specific version; for example, the ASA Crosswalk is an additional cost (although partially included with the Payer version).

Find-A-Code (www.findacode.com)

Find-A-Code is another online coding and billing subscription that also is available in different versions with different features. This is another excellent resource with crosswalking abilities, depending on the version purchased and add-ons. The different versions include Essentials, Professional, and Facility with cost ranges from $4.95 to $89.95 per month. There is a $25 setup fee for the $4.95/month subscription. Add-ons cost an additional fee.

Super Coder (www.supercoder.com)

Super Coder is another online coding and billing subscription available in different versions with different features. Two of the versions are Physician Coder and Facility Coder, ranging in cost from $399.95 to $1,999.95 per year for the Facility Coder Power Pack. The versions/packages can be customized depending on the features included, and as with the other subscriptions, there are add-ons that can be purchased for an additional fee.

The difference between the above subscriptions depends mainly on the versions, features, and layout/format. All of the subscriptions have complimentary trial periods that allow the life care planner to explore and use the product prior to purchase. Discounts may be available through professional association membership, monthly versus annual billing subscriptions, or other affiliations, so it is important to always inquire about subscription fees. The subscriptions provide access to educational material associated with the medical coding and billing field, and the authors recommend that interested life care planners research and explore the program prior to purchase. Customization/packages are available depending on the features and add-ons, and some of the available add-ons include inpatient, outpatient, anesthesia, NCCI (National Correct Coding Initiatives), CPT Assistant, and dictionaries.

Medical Coding and Billing Resources

- *PMIC* (Practice Management Information Corporation): www.pmiconline.com, 800-633-7467.
- *Optum360:* www.optum360coding.com, 800-464-3649.

PMIC and Optum360 (previously known as Ingenix) have access to most publications associated with medical coding and billing (coding manuals) in addition to their own publications. As previously mentioned, do not forget to inquire about available discounts. Another word of caution is there are multiple companies that sell coding manuals and billing resources (www.medicalbooks.com and www.amazon.com), and the life care planner is advised to make sure the intended publication is being purchased.

Accessible information for costing research also is available for hospitals, physicians, dentists, other health care professionals/providers, health care services, and equipment. However, even though the information is available, one must know how to accurately and effectively utilize it.

Coding Tips for Consideration

All the code systems mentioned in this chapter are updated annually; it is therefore important for the life care planner to also update product manuals at this time. All the annual revisions are effective January 1 of the year except for the MS-DRGs and ICD 10 CM and ICD 10 PCS which become effective October 1 of the year prior; in other words the 2018 MS-DRGs revision became effective October 1, 2017.

When looking up codes to cost out for a life care plan, the process of "crosswalking" becomes important. Crosswalking is the process of taking a code and "crosswalking" it from one service, such as a physician service, to another service.

Important Crosswalks for the Life Care Planner

- *Anesthesia:* Procedure CPT to Anesthesia CPT
- *Outpatient:* CPT to APC (if you chose to use APCs)
- *Inpatient:* CPT to ICD 10 PCS, then ICD 10 PCS to MS-DRG
- ICD-10 CM to MS-DRG

Available free crosswalks include information from www.CMS.gov (Centers for Medicare and Medicaid); Addendum B of the OPPS (Outpatient Prospective Payment System) will crosswalk a CPT code to the appropriate APC; Addendum A of the OPPS will give the description of the APC. This data is updated throughout the year, and the life care planner will want the most recent and current version. However, it is important to note that the databases generally are approximately 2 years behind; therefore, the life care planner will want to identify what the current APC is and also identify the prior APC code, or the one utilized to find the facility cost, if the CPT is not available. Most of the databases described in this chapter utilize CPT codes for the search, but the American Hospital Directory includes an APC search and a CPT code search.

Reputable Databases

Reputable Databases all require at least an annual subscription, except for the VA Reasonable Data Charges and H·CUPnet. Below you will find some of the databases and the information they provide.

Facility

American Hospital Directory	www.ahd.com
Context[4] Healthcare	www.context4healthcare.com
FAIR Health	www.fairhealth.org
VA Reasonable Data Charges	https://www.va.gov/COMMUNITYCARE/revenue_ops/payer_rates.asp
H·CUPnet	http://hcupnet.ahrq.gov/

Physician/Other Health Care Professionals

Context[4] Healthcare	www.context4healthcare.com
FAIR Health	www.fairhealth.org
InGauge Physician's Fee and Coding Guide	http://www.coderscentral.com/
Medical Fees	http://pmiconline.stores.yahoo.net/
National Fee Analyzer	https://www.optum360coding.com
Physicians' Fee Reference	https://wasserman-medical.com/product-category/medical/
VA Reasonable Data Charges	https://www.va.gov/COMMUNITYCARE/revenue_ops/payer_rates.asp

DME

Context[4] Healthcare	www.context4healthcare.com
FAIR Health	www.fairhealth.org
VA Reasonable Data Charges	https://www.va.gov/COMMUNITYCARE/revenue_ops/payer_rates.asp

Anesthesia

Context[4] Healthcare	www.context4healthcare.com
FAIR Health	www.fairhealth.org
VA Reasonable Data Charges	https://www.va.gov/COMMUNITYCARE/revenue_ops/payer_rates.asp

Dental

Context[4] Healthcare	www.context4healthcare.com
FAIR Health	www.fairhealth.org
VA Reasonable Data Charges	https://www.va.gov/COMMUNITYCARE/revenue_ops/payer_rates.asp

With regard to published/hard copy resources, InGauge (previously known as Mag Mutual) *Physician's Fee and Coding Guide*, *Medical Fees*, *National Fee Analyzer*, and *Physicians' Fee Reference* are publications that can all be purchased from different sources. These publications are similar and all offer the ability to geographically adjust the fee. While *Medical Fees*, *National Fee Analyzer*, and *Physicians' Fee Reference* all present the fees per the 50th, 75th, and 90th percentile, *Physicians' Fee and Coding Guide* presents the fees in a range from low to high.

The descriptions of the databases listed below provide only a brief summary of the product. It is advisable to visit and explore each company's website to learn more about the products, including format, data sources, and pricing, prior to purchase.

American Hospital Directory

Phone:	800-894-8418
Website:	www.ahd.com

American Hospital Directory provides access to information regarding specific hospitals and their charges for inpatient and outpatient procedures. The information is only displayed if 11 or more of the procedures or MS-DRGs has occurred at the specific hospital during a specific time frame. Access to American Hospital Directory requires an annual subscription. Currently (2018) the cost for a subscription is $355 for life care planners annually. The data is updated throughout the year as it becomes available. American Hospital Directory also provides additional services and information.

Context[4] Healthcare

Phone:	800-783-3378
Website:	www.context4healthcare.com

Context[4] Healthcare has a Usual, Customary & Reasonable Benchmark Tool, DecisionPoint™ Health Payment System. This tool provides usual, customary, and reasonable (UCR) fee data for outpatient and inpatient facility, anesthesia, dental, HCPCS and medical (physicians and other health care professionals) for all geographic regions of the United States displayed in percentiles. Each category requires an annual subscription. The data are updated twice a year. Sources for the data and format can be found on the website.

FAIR Health

Account Manager:	Jeff Newbauer
Phone:	440-247-5720
Website:	www.fairhealth.org

FAIR Health has an online UCR benchmarking tool that provides UCR information for outpatient and inpatient facility, anesthesia, dental, HCPCS, and medical fee data. The information is presented in percentiles and is geographically specific. The International Association of Rehabilitation Professionals (IARP) has worked extensively with FAIR Health to make this information affordable for its members. The price depends on the number of searches purchased. A subscription provides access to all of the categories and lasts until the number of searches purchased is exhausted or for 2 years, whichever comes first. Some of the categories are updated twice a year and others are updated quarterly. Sources of the data and format can be found on the website.

VA Reasonable Data Charges (https://www.va.gov/COMMUNITYCARE/revenue_ops/payer_rates.asp)

According to the website: "Reasonable Charges are based on amounts that third parties pay for the same services furnished by private-sector health care providers in the same geographic area." The charges represent the 80th percentile and are for non-service related services provided to a veteran. The information included is very specific in nature and requires a formula to accurately calculate the charges according to the geo-zip (first three numbers of a zip code). The "Reasonable Data Charges Tables" include all the information to accurately calculate the charge for a specific service/item/hospitalization/outpatient procedure in a geographic area. There is no cost for this data. Instructions on how to appropriately calculate the VA charges are beyond the scope of this chapter.

H·CUPnet (http://hcupnet.ahrq.gov/)

According to the website, "H·CUPnet is a free, on-line query system based on data from the Healthcare Cost and Utilization Project (HCUP). It provides access to health statistics and information on hospital inpatient and emergency department utilization." The most recent update to the national inpatient information is for year 2014. This is another website where it is important to follow the prompts. The authors usually access the *State Inpatient Information* and the *National Inpatient Information* when the state information is not available. Not all states participate in the Healthcare Cost and Utilization Project and information for methodology, data sources, and definitions utilized are all found on the website.

Other Free of Charge Facility Databases

There are states that provide inpatient facility information per MS-DRG (Medicare Severity Diagnosis Related Group) and some APR-DRG (All Patient Refined Diagnosis Related Group, developed by 3M). One of the state databases is PricePoint. The states of Washington, Utah, Virginia, Wisconsin, Nevada, and Texas all utilize PricePoint. Other sources include the state's hospital association. Make sure when utilizing these databases that the information is presented as charges and not costs. A simple way to access the database is to perform a Google search for hospital charges for the state in which the cost research is being done and the information, if available for the particular state, may be available. For example, California provides data under the Office of Statewide Health Planning and Development (OSHPD), http://www.oshpd.ca.gov/chargemaster/Default.aspx. Be careful if using one of the hospital Chargemasters because a hospitalization will require more than just one item, usually multiple items. This applies to outpatient procedures as well.

The above list of available medical fee databases is not all inclusive. The life care planner is cautioned to be careful and make sure the information included in the database is reputable, provides data sources, and includes charges and not costs.

Zip Code (geo-zip) (http://www.zip-info.com/search/zipcode.htm)

To find the appropriate geographic area, the life care planner will need to know the appropriate zip code. The above noted website is invaluable to look up accurate zip codes for which database research can then be conducted.

Abeo Coder

Abeo Coder is an app for iPhone or Android operating systems. It requires a yearly subscription for full access. Abeo Coder crosswalks a CPT code to the appropriate anesthesia CPT code(s) in addition to providing the base units, time units and average time associated with the procedure.

Conclusion

This chapter on resources, including helpful databases, is designed to provide the life care planner with basic information to help with preparation of cost information for the life care plan. In the authors' opinion, the heart and soul of the life care planning process is the ability to quickly and efficiently locate reputable resources. Preparedness, thoroughness, and following the standard methodology of life care planning are the keys to a successful life care planning experience.

Appendix 30.1: Area Cost Analysis Request Form

This form is a sample that can be used as a blueprint for the life care plan.

Area Cost Analysis Request
Client: ___________________________________
Plaintiff: ___ Defense: ___ Age: ____ Sex: M F
Disability:___ Area Code: ___________
City: ___ Nearest Metro Area: _____________________
Today's Date:___ Date Due: ______________________
Medical Care
__ Dentist
__ Gastroenterologist
__ GP/internist
__ Neuro-ophthalmologist
__ Neurologist
__ Neuropsychologist
__ Neurosurgeon
__ Ophthalmologist
__ Orthopedist
__ Orthosurgeon
__ Otolaryngologist
__ Pain specialist
__ Pediatrician
__ Physiatrist
__ Plastic surgeon
__ Podiatrist
__ Psychiatrist
__ Psychologist
__ Pulmonologist
__ Rheumatologist
__ Urologist
__ *Other:* ___________________________

(*Continued*)

Home Health (See links to home health agencies)
Therapy: ____ PT, ____ OT, ____ ST, ____ Respiratory
Invasive procedures required? (Yes/No) Such as:
__ Catheter
__ Suction
__ IV therapy
__ Trach care
__ Tube feeding
__ Bowel program
Staffing
HHA ____ Hourly, ____Visit
LPN ____ Hourly, ____Visit
RN ____ Hourly, ____Visit
__ Live-in (available/definition/last time staffed this level?)
Allied Health Services
__ PT
__ OT
__ ST
__Respiratory therapy
__Aquatic therapy
__Therapeutic riding
__Recreational therapy
__Massage therapy
__Nutritionist
__Health and Wellness program (gym)
__Work hardening program
__Disabled driver
__Augmentative communication
__Assistive technology
__Other:

(*Continued*)

__Other:	
__Other:	
Household Services	
__Handyman service	
__Home modification	
__Housecleaning	
__Other	
Educational Programs	
__Public school	
__Summer program	
__Private school	
__College aid	
__Tutor	
__Camp__College: __AA __BA __Vocational/technical: ________________	
Vocational Services	
__Vocational evaluation	
__Vocational counseling	
__Job coaching	
__Sheltered work	
__Supported work	
__Day/activity program	
Wage data research required (if providing a loss of earnings report):	
Occupation:	
Programs/Facilities:	**Facility Care Level:**
__Adult daycare	Level of disability
__Day program __ABI __MR	# Hours of supervision
__Assisted living facility	ADLs:
__Other:___	Cues:
__ICF/MR or group home	Aggressive

(*Continued*)

__Long-term head injury	Ambulatory
__Skilled nursing facility	Continent
__Supported living	Verbal
__Transitional living __ SCI __ABI	PVS
__Neurobehavioral inpatient	Trach
__Chronic pain :__Inpatient __Outpatient	Vent dependent
__SCI rehab: __Inpatient __Outpatient	Tube fed
__SCI evaluation: __Inpatient __Outpatient	Bowel program
	Day program
__Other	Work program
Diagnostics	
__EEG	
__EKG	
__Pulmonary functions	
__Renal scan	
__Renal ultrasound	
__Sleep study	
__Swallow study	
__Urodynamic studies	
__CT	
__MRI	
__X-ray	
__Bronchoscopy	
__Colonoscopy	
__Cystoscopy	
__Endoscopy	
Labs	
__CBC (with diff.)	
__Comprehensive metabolic panel	
__Creatinine	

(*Continued*)

__C&S
__LFT
__Lipid panel
__UA
__Chemical levels (what medication): __________________
Medications
List of current medications:
Local pharmacy used:
Surgeries/Procedures:
__Epidural block
__SCI fertility program: M F
__Gastrostomy
__PEG tube
__Trach revision
__Shunt revision
__Hip subluxation
__Hip replacement
__Knee replacement
__Baclofen pump
__Morphine pump
__Spinal stimulator
__Scoliosis surgery
__Diskectomy (cervical/thoracic/lumbar)
__Laminectomy (cervical/thoracic/lumbar)
__Spinal fusion (cervical/thoracic/lumbar)
__Scar revision (length of scar: ___)
__Stump revision
__Arthroscopy
__Contracture release
__Tendon release
__Hardware removal

(*Continued*)

Equipment and Supplies
__ECU
__Standers
__Cushions
__Ramp/lift
__Van conversion
__Assistive technology
__Augmentative communication device
__Pediatric equipment
__Orthotics
__Prosthetics
__Visual aids
__Wheelchair
__Specialized equipment: ______________________

Appendix 30.2: Questionnaire

Appendix 30.2 is designed to be a questionnaire format used when contacting home health agencies on the services available and the related costs.

Nursing Research Format
Provider:
Telephone: ______________________ Fax:
Contact: ________________________ Title:
Areas of Service (Counties)
Is there a mileage charge in addition to hourly? ___Yes ___No If Yes: ___/Mile
Rates (Private-pay rate for all costs: ___Yes ___No)
HHA/hour: $_____ $_____ $_____
HHA/visit: $_____ $_____ $_____
LPN/hour: $_____ $_____ $_____
LPN/visit: $_____ $_____ $_____
RN/hour: $_____ $_____ $_____

(*Continued*)

RN/visit: $_____ $_____ $_____
Minimum # of hours per visit: _________
Live-in: ___Yes ___No Daily rate: $_____
Number of hands-on care hours per day with a live-in: _____
Number of uninterrupted sleep hours for a live-in per night: _____
Definition of live-in services as defined by this specific agency:
When was the last time this agency actually supplied a live-in?
Case Manager: $_____/hour
Therapies
PT ___ Yes ___No $_____/visit
OT ___ Yes ___No $_____/visit
ST ___ Yes ___No $_____/visit
Recreational therapy: ___Yes___No $_____/visit
Other
Transportation:
Can staff member transport patient? ___Yes ___No
Personal car? ___Yes ___No Patient's car? ___Yes ___No
Skill Responsibilities
Can Aide Level
Administer medications: ___ Yes ___ No
Perform bowel stimulation: ___ Yes ___ No
Administer G-tube feeds: ___ Yes ___ No
Insert catheter: ___ Yes ___ No
Trim finger/toe nails: ___ Yes ___ No
Can LPN Level
Perform trach care: ___ Yes ___ No
Perform vent care: ___ Yes ___ No

(Continued)

Trim finger/toe nails: ___ Yes ___ No
An agency may have a policy that aides, trained by RNs, can do certain invasive procedures such as bowel stimulation, catheter changes, etc. Under this arrangement, it is the specific RN training the aide who is ultimately liable and responsible for the activities of the aide. Therefore, in this agency, in practice, are the aides performing such services in their day-to-day activities?
Is RN Supervision (included with):
Live-in or aide care: one visit/_________ (week/month/quarter)
LPN care: one visit/_________ (week/month/quarter)
Is there an extra charge for the RN supervision visit? ___Yes ___ No
If Yes: $_____/visit
Comments
Research by: ______________________________ Date:

References

American Medical Association. 2013. *Definition of "Usual, Customary and Reasonable" (UCR) H-385.923.* Available at https://policysearch.ama-assn.org/policyfinder/detail/Policy%20H-385.923%20?uri=%2FAMADoc%2FHOD.xml-0-3242.xml.

Dussault, K., & Lauterbach, J. 2002. Special Needs Trusts: Powerful Planning Tools for Disabled Individuals. *Journal of Financial Planning, 15*(1), 70.

Elliott, T. 2010. A plaintiff's attorney's perspective on life care planning. In R. Weed & D. Berens (Eds.) *Life Care Planning and Case Management Handbook*, 3rd ed., 771–782. Boca Raton, FL: CRC Press.

Johnson, C. 2015. Consensus and Majority Statements Derived from Life Care Planning Summits Held in 2000, 2002, 2004, 2006, 2008, 2010, 2012 and 2015. *Journal of Life Care Planning, 13*(4), 35–38.

Raffles-Gunn, T. 2010. A defense attorney's perspective on life care planning. In R. Weed & D. Berens (Eds.) *Life Care Planning and Case Management Handbook*, 3rd ed., 783–797. Boca Raton, FL: CRC Press.

Sutton, A., Deutsch, P., Weed, R., & Berens, D. 2002. Reliability of Life Care Plans: A Comparison of Original and Updated Plans. *Journal of Life Care Planning, 1*(3), 187–194.

Chapter 31

Medical Equipment Choices and the Role of the Rehab Equipment Specialist in Life Care Planning

Paul Amsterdam

Contents

Introduction....760
Factors in Choosing Medical Equipment....761
Common Errors in Equipment Recommendations....761
Omissions....762
How Do You Avoid Omissions?....762
Problems in Wheelchair Choice....763
Wheelchair Choices....763
Questions to Consider....763
Accessories Required....765
Pressure Reduction....766
Custom Therapeutic Seating Systems....766
Mobility and Accessibility Features....766
Safety Features....767
Convenience and ADL Features....767
Exaggeration of Needs....767
Setting Standards of Protocol for Replacement Schedules of Medical Equipment in a Life Care Plan....768
Contributing Factors to Replacement Time for Wheelchairs....770
Age....770
Environment....771
Behavior....771

Body Type 771
Lifestyle 772
Replacement Allowance Worksheets 772
Estimated Replacement Schedule Assessment Form 772
Estimated Replacement Schedule Assessment Form 774
Use of References and Specialists 775
The Use of Rehabilitation Equipment Specialists as Consultants 775
Conclusion 776
Editors' Note 776
Appendix 31.1 776
The Medical Equipment Corner Paul Amsterdam, ATP 777
Making Correct Choices of Medical Equipment for a Life Care Plan 777
Factors in Choosing the Proper Wheelchair for Your Client 777
Standard Wheelchairs versus Complex Rehab 777
Why Is This an Important Consideration in Your Life Care Plan? 778
How Is the Correct Wheelchair Choice Made? 778
Appendix 31.2 779
The Medical Equipment Corner Paul Amsterdam, ATP 780
Proper Pricing Methodology for Your Life Care Plan 780
What about the Use of the Internet? 781
Use of Medicare Allowables in a Life Care Plan 781
Conclusion 782
Appendix 31.3 782
The Medical Equipment Corner Paul Amsterdam, ATP 782
Medicare's Current Status with Medical Equipment and Its Possible Effects on Life Care Planning 782
References 784

Introduction

The importance of medical equipment in the life care plan has always been a function of the physical impairment of the individual client. The greater one's physical impairments, the more dependent he or she will be on medical equipment and other assistive technology.

This chapter will address the need for accurate assessments of rehab medical equipment in a life care plan. It discusses the various factors that must be considered in choosing the correct models and types of equipment. Common errors of equipment planning are noted from the author's experience in reviewing life care plans, with some solutions toward achieving more accurate results. The role of the rehab equipment specialist (rehab technology supplier or assistive technology supplier [RTS or ATS]) is also discussed as a beneficial tool to the life care planner.

Medical equipment has parameters different from other factors of a life care plan. In almost all cases of permanent disability, if there is a need for certain medical equipment at the start of the plan that expense will continue throughout the client's life expectancy. Medical equipment choices are a very dynamic function of a life care plan as well. Allowances must be made for changes in the type of equipment that will be needed. Some of these changes in equipment will be due to the aging of a client, while others will be from expected physical deterioration of the client. A good example of the latter is the overuse syndrome that becomes common in spinal cord injury clients after years of propelling a manual wheelchair (O'Leary & Sarkarati, 2000).

Allowances must also be made for the repair and eventual replacement of each piece of equipment. Maintenance and replacement schedules vary for different types of equipment, and factors such as manufacturer's warranty, daily expected usage, and a client's environment will all play a part in assessing these variables (Graham-Field, 2002). Maintenance and replacement schedules will be addressed later in this chapter.

Medical equipment is only one area of assistive technology that should be considered for an individual client. According to the Technology-Related Assistance for Individuals with Disabilities Act of 1988 (Tech Act, 1988), an assistive technology device is "any item, piece of equipment, or product system, whether acquired commercially, off the shelf, modified, or customized, that is used to increase, maintain, or improve the functional capabilities of individuals with disabilities." Other areas of assistive technology, such as augmentative and assistive communication systems, environmental control units, computer interface technology, and visual impairment technology, may also be needed and considered for the client but are not primarily discussed in this chapter.

Factors in Choosing Medical Equipment

The predominant factor in choosing the correct medical equipment will be the client's *diagnosis* and overall medical assessment. A chronic lumbar sprain requires little in the area of assistive technology, whereas a spinal cord injury resulting in some level of paralysis may require considerable equipment depending on the extent of the injury. The need for equipment is somewhat commensurate with the level of the spinal cord injury. The higher the overall break in the neurological pathway, the more severe the client's physical involvement; consequently, there will be greater reliance on assistive technology to solve mobility, Activities of Daily Living (ADL), and other day-to-day independent functions.

Another factor in equipment needs is the *age* of the client. As previously noted, equipment will change as an individual ages, not only due to physical deterioration, but also as an individual's lifestyle changes. The 4-year-old born with cerebral palsy may start childhood using a therapeutic stroller for mobility, grow into a pediatric tilt-in-space manual wheelchair, and then, through increased function, graduate into a motorized wheelchair.

This also leads to another factor in determining correct equipment. What are the *mobility needs* for a particular client? Is the client able to manually propel a manual wheelchair, or is powered mobility going to be the primary option for independence? If an attendant must push the client, will a standard wheelchair frame meet his or her needs, or will he or she require something more specialized, such as a reclining or tilt-in-space wheelchair frame?

Often overlooked factors in determining the correct choice in equipment are the *environment* and *lifestyle* of an individual client. The equipment required for a T2 paraplegic who is living independently in a rural or urban environment and has a full-time vocation will be vastly different than that for a client with the same level of injury who resides in a skilled nursing facility with no occupation. Environment and lifestyle must also be considered when estimating correct replacement schedules for a client's wheelchair, which will be discussed later in this chapter.

Common Errors in Equipment Recommendations

The author has reviewed many life care plans for several years. The two most common errors found in the equipment recommendations are *omissions* and *exaggeration of need.*

Omissions

Omissions of equipment in a life care plan, especially in the plan created for the plaintiff, will hurt the client twofold. Primarily, by not including a needed type of equipment, the cost allowance for that equipment is not included in the client's immediate assistive technology needs. The omission is then multiplied as many as five times the current amount, by not being part of the economist's computations for replacements of the omitted item.

Omissions hurt the client in another way. A good life care plan is not just a list of medical costs but, as stated in the Life Care Planning Survey of 2002, is "a comprehensive plan for meeting the individualized and complex service needs resulting from the onset of a disability" (Neulicht et al., 2002). An omission of a certain type of assistive technology may lead a client away from a certain therapeutic road. For instance, the omission of any standing therapeutic aid from the plan for a quadriplegic may never guide the client toward a type of therapy that can be an important part of his or her daily life. As the benefits of standing have been shown to lessen the possibilities of skin breakdown, osteoporosis, and urinary tract infection, among other things (Stewart, 1992), the omission of the equipment needed for this therapy may very well alter the client's future physical health and need for additional medical services.

It should be noted that an omission in the plaintiff's plan does not necessarily mean the equipment should then be omitted in the defense plan. On the contrary, an objective plan should include all needed equipment necessary for proper functioning for the client, regardless of which side created the plan. In Glynn and Davis's (2001) article on physician-directed plans, they state there should be "no more variation from case to case" (whether plaintiff or defense requested).

How Do You Avoid Omissions?

A good first source to help objectively set some equipment choices for a life care plan is the expected functional outcomes tables assembled by the Consortium for Spinal Cord Medicine (1999). These tables delineate between different spinal cord levels of injury and what probable equipment would be needed for a variety of functional activities. These tables, however, are specifically limited to spinal cord diagnoses, and equipment choices are made in general terms, not specific ones.

Another way life care planners can avoid costly omissions in the type of equipment needed is to trace a day-in-the-life for their client. The idea here is to try and picture how the client must go through every aspect of his or her day.

When he or she wakes up in the morning, can he or she lift him-/herself out of bed? If so, how?

Does he or she require any sort of assistance, either a trapeze bar or safety rail, off the side of the bed?

Can transfers be done independently with the use of a transfer board, or is a caregiver required to use a hydraulic patient lift and sling?

Can he or she dress him-/herself, button his or her own shirts, and zip his or her own pants? How does he or she get to the closet or drawers to get the clothes in the first place?

Specific questions should be asked as the client goes into every room in his or her house. Functional mobility, independence in ADL, transportation, and bathroom safety must all be reviewed as the client goes through his or her daily routine. Vocational and quality of life interests must also be addressed to avoid costly omissions. Pressure relief issues, both in sitting and in the bed, must be reviewed; in addition, possible adjunct home exercise and therapies should be addressed. As each area of functional dependence is noted, there are a variety of equipment choices that can then be made.

Problems in Wheelchair Choice

The most common instances for omissions occur in the area of wheelchair choice. Because of the amount of complex variables when evaluating a client for a wheelchair, the lifetime choices of models and needed accessories must be examined carefully. There are many different types of manual wheelchairs: standard frames, lightweight, ultralight frames, and rigid ultralights. This does not include the more specialized frames such as recliners, super-low hemi-frames, and adult and pediatric tilt-in-space wheelchairs.

Motorized wheelchairs also are incredibly varied in model and overall function. As an example, in the year 2008, the three largest manufacturers of motorized wheelchairs in this country had more than 40 distinct models (Invacare Corporation, 2002; Pride Mobility Products Corporation, 2002; Sunrise Medical, 2002). The price of these chairs ranged from $3,000 to $30,000. If you are creating a plaintiff's plan, do all your clients with spinal cord injuries get a $30,000 chair? Likewise, can the defense hold that the least expensive $3,000 chair will meet all clients' power mobility needs?

The answer, of course, is that neither side should delegate choice of model by overall cost. Every client has a range of correct possible wheelchair models that must suit his or her physical and mobility needs. It is a function of the life care planner to determine either through his or her own research or the use of outside experts the correct types of wheelchairs needed and to be able to defend those choices.

Wheelchair Choices

For the purpose of funding durable medical equipment, the federal government's Medicare program created different allowances with numerical procedure codes and product groups to describe (and pay) for the different types of wheelchairs. These descriptive codes and group designations have now been almost universally used by most of the managed care organizations as a basis for their method of payment for wheelchairs. The codes (although we are not interested in the allowable prices associated with them) are a good method of breaking down wheelchairs into different descriptive categories for the life care planner to utilize as well. The planner should make an examination of his or her particular client's physical limitations, in regard to the choice of the correct wheelchair category. See also Tables 31.1 and 31.2 for manual and motorized wheelchair considerations.

Questions to Consider

- Can the client functionally propel a manual wheelchair?
- Will the use of a lighter-weight frame benefit overall mobility?
- Before advancing to a motorized chair, will the use of the manual wheelchair provide the client with the most probable means toward daily exercise, continued range of motion, and easier accessibility throughout the home and workplace, and via transportation?
- Will the client require customized programming or the use of specialized switches (e.g., sip and puff, or head arrays) that necessitate a motorized wheelchair with higher-end electronic capabilities?
- Would the need for power-actuated positioning systems such as power recline, power tilt-in-space, or a standing frame be substantiated, or would these functions be generally unused by the client and perhaps just make the chair overly heavy and cumbersome (not to mention far more expensive)?

Table 31.1 Manual Wheelchair Bases

Code Type	*Description*	*Utilization*	*Samples/Price Range*
K0001—Standard wheelchair	Weight = 36 pounds Width = 16 or 18 inches Depth = 16 inches Arms = fixed or detachable Footrests = fixed or swing-away	Clients who ambulate or are capable of standing pivot transfer; inexpensive choice for those who are not dependent on a wheelchair as their primary means of mobility, or must be pushed by caregiver	Standard frame from all manufacturers—Invacare Tracers, E&J Vista, and Traveler From $300–$700
K0002—Hemi (low-seat) wheelchair	Weight = 36 pounds Seat height = 17 or 18 inches Width = 16 or 18 inches Depth = 16 inches Arms = fixed or detachable Footrests = swing-away	Primary need for clients with hemiplegia; enables client to propel chair with one or both feet	Invacare Tracer EX From $500–750
K0004—High-strength lightweight frame	Weight = <34 pounds Width = variable Depth = 14 or 16 inches Lifetime warranty on side frame and cross-braces Back height = adjustable	For individuals who are unable to functionally propel a standard manual frame; excellent choice for older client or for nonpropellers with older caregivers who must lift chair	Invacare 9000 XT Quickie Breezy Series From $850+
K0005—Ultralight frame	Weight = <30 pounds Width = variable Depth = variable Lifetime warranty on side frame and cross-braces Adjustable rear-axle system	For highly active wheelchair user; spinal cord injuries, spina bifida, or any other client using a manual wheelchair as the primary means of mobility	Quickie 2 Quickie GPV and R2 Invacare MVP Invacare A4 and A6 All Tisport/Tilite Wheelchairs from $1,600+
K0009—Other manual wheelchair bases	May include tilt-in-space wheelchair frames or other custom-designed frames to meet individual needs	Clients with significant positioning issues, pressure issues, limitations in range of motion	Invacare Solara Quickie TS Freedom Design Libre From $3,000+ (does not include a seating system)

Table 31.2 Motorized Wheelchair Bases

Power Groups	*Description*	*Utilization*	*Samples/Price Range*
Group 1—Motorized wheelchairs	Frame = portable Electronics = little adjustablitiy or programmability	Client is not able to functionally ambulate or propel a manual wheelchair; client should have good upper-extremity control without cause for future progression	Invacare ATM
Group 2—Motorized wheelchair with programmable controls	Consumer Power chair group electronics must have limited programmability to adjust parameters for speed, tremor dampening, acceleration, and braking. This group does not allow for advanced switch options. Majority in this group have captain or van style seating.	Clients with orthopedic or respiratory conditions that present overall weakness. They are unable to self propel a manual wheelchair.	Invacare Pronto Series Wheelchairs Pride Jazzy models From $6,000+
Group 3—Motorized wheelchairs	Allow for advanced electronics; single or multiple power seating functions such as power tilt and recline.	Clients with neuro-muscular or progressive disorders that require more involved mobility functions and alternative drive controls. The client with poor trunk control or at a higher risk of skin breakdown is common.	Invacare TDX SP Quickie PULSE 6 or Rhythm models Permobil C300 Pride Quantum Series
Group 4—Motorized wheelchair bases	High-performance model motorized wheelchairs with advanced electronics and increased speed, designed for more outdoor use.	For the highly active clients utilizing their chairs as much or more outdoors than inside. (Note: These chairs are not approved for funding by Medicare.)	Invacare Arrow Quickie P-222 and S646 Permobil C500 Omega Trac Innovations in Motion 4 × 4

Accessories Required

By far the greatest omission seen in life care plans for wheelchair considerations is in the area of accessories. All of us have had the experience of wanting to buy a large item, such as an automobile. We may first be attracted to an ad claiming a very low sticker price. After going to the retailer, reviewing options and accessories, you could not drive out of the showroom without the automobile now costing you sometimes thousands of dollars more. There is little difference when having to purchase a new wheelchair, only in the case of the wheelchair, many of those options may truly be a medical necessity for the overall function of your client. These accessories fall into the following adjunct consideration categories.

Pressure Reduction

There are currently more than 200 different wheelchair cushions on the market. The prices of these may range from $20 to $2,000. In my experience, few will benefit from the quality of a $20 cushion, but just as few would ever require cushions in the $2,000 category. One excellent guide to proper cushion choice is the use of a skin assessment system, such as the Braden scale. When skin risk is determined, the range and type of possible cushion choices can be both narrowed down and substantiated.

When noting a cushion for the life care report, like the wheelchair itself, a replacement schedule must be set up. Inexpensive foam cushions will have a far shorter replacement life than some of the more expensive pressure equalization cushions, such as a Roho or Jay 2. It should be noted that many of the higher-priced cushions have far longer warranties as well. On many life care plans, I have often seen replacement of a Roho cushion after only 2 years, when the manufacturer fully warranties this product for the same 2 years. Additional cushion covers should also be taken into account. Providing an extra cover initially with a cushion will substantially extend the overall replacement needs for the cushion, as well as provide for needed cleanliness issues.

Custom Therapeutic Seating Systems

Many clients require the use of therapeutic seating in the wheelchair. Limits in range of motion, weaknesses or excessive muscle tone, trunk instability, or spinal deformities may all necessitate adding some range of customized seat and back systems. This may include other features, such as thoracic or pelvic supports, abductor wedges, chest harness, specialized head supports, or upper-extremity support trays.

How much therapeutic seating an individual client will need may be something the life care planner should research, with that client's former therapists or other rehab technology seating specialists, before noting it in the life care plan. (See also the section on utilizing references and outside experts at the end of this chapter.)

Prices for seating systems may be as low as $400 or more than $6,000. In many cases, it is equal to or more than the frame of the wheelchair. It should require references to modifications for growth, repairs, and replacements. Consequently, this is one aspect of the equipment report that cannot be omitted.

Mobility and Accessibility Features

Many of the features we commonly see on a wheelchair, such as the armrests and footrests, are not necessarily included in the base price of the wheelchair. Some chair models may include some of these as standard features, but there is a good chance the accessories needed by your client will not be the standard styles provided. A particular model of ultralight wheelchairs may have as many as six to eight different armrests or footrest configurations to choose from. This may add an additional $175 to $400 to the price of the chair.

The choice of wheels will vary from molded composite to lightweight spoke wheels. The choice of tires and front casters can make significant changes in both a wheelchair's performance and cost. Standard hand rims are made of either chrome or aluminum, but vinyl- or plastic-coated ones are also available. Projection hand rims in both vertical and offset styles may be a medical necessity for clients with limited fine-motor coordination. As noted on an ultralight wheelchair order form from TiSport Corporation (TiSport, 2002), there is currently a set of ultralight, highly durable wheel spokes under the brand name Spinergy that will add more than $600 to the base price of a wheelchair but may greatly enhance the suspension and mobility for some active clients.

Some mobility and accessibility features for motorized wheelchairs are not so obvious. One particular feature commonly recommended is a swing-away joystick mount. Without this device, most clients using a motorized wheelchair would be unable to bring the chair up to a dining table or desk. The device will in turn add an additional $300 to $400 to the base price of the power chair. Some clients may also benefit from a power seat actuator. At the push of a lever, this system will allow the seat of the power chair to raise about 8 to 11 inches from its standard height to enable the client to reach items that would normally be inaccessible.

Safety Features

Most accessories needed for wheelchair safety are usually not that expensive, but one would be negligent to omit them in the wheelchair order. Seatbelts and chest harnesses may be the first items that come to mind, but certainly most common is a pair of rear anti-tipping levers. As wheelchairs have gotten lighter and more adjustable, the anti-tippers have become more of a safety necessity. Clients who are amputees may also benefit from a chair that has been modified with amputee adapters to change the center of gravity on the rear wheels.

Convenience and ADL Features

There are many accessories that may not be considered medical necessities, yet they greatly enhance a person's ability to carry on with normal Activities of Daily Living. One must remember that a life care plan should reflect all necessary items and that services reflect their needs with consideration for the jurisdiction.

Some items that come to mind are backpacks and seat pouches for the client to easily carry items. Also available are fold-up luggage carriers and cup holders. For those who use a pair of crutches or cane for short-distance ambulation, a crutch or cane holder becomes a needed feature. One item overlooked in many life care plans for clients who actively propel wheelchairs is a good pair of wheelchair gloves. As the active user will wear out gloves quickly, at least two pairs per year should be allowed for in a plan.

Exaggeration of Needs

The second common error regarding equipment choices in a life care plan is exaggeration of needs. Gass and Gonzalez (2001) in their article discuss the overall effects of gross exaggeration to a life care plan. Where omissions may affect a plan by not allowing for certain needed equipment or specific features, gross exaggerations of equipment needs may affect the overall credibility of the entire life care plan.

A life care planner is not necessarily basing his or her equipment choices strictly on medical necessity but must be able to justify these choices in relationship to the functional needs and abilities of the client. For example, it would be difficult to justify a $12,000 alternating-pressure/low-air-loss mattress replacement system for a client with full skin sensation, ability to independently weight shift and transfer, and no previous history of skin breakdown. Likewise, an expensive high-performance ultralight titanium wheelchair is not the proper choice for a client who does not have the cognitive ability to self-propel a manual wheelchair.

As previously noted, the choices and price range of motorized wheelchairs are enormous. Unfortunately, this seems to encourage some in life care planning to pick only from the top end of this range, without regard to true individual need. This author has had to write an opinion on a plaintiff's life care plan that recommended a $30,000 motorized wheelchair with a power-actuated standing frame for a client who independently stands and ambulates with forearm crutches throughout his or her residence. It would only take a few examples of this type of gross exaggeration for a defense attorney to question the credibility of all the equipment choices and perhaps the credibility of the life care planner.

Setting Standards of Protocol for Replacement Schedules of Medical Equipment in a Life Care Plan

One controversial factor in life care plans has been the replacement schedule allowances for medical equipment (R. Weed, personal communication, April 20, 2002). As it is fundamental that all equipment have a usable life expectancy when listing medical equipment for a life care plan, it is likewise fundamental that each piece of equipment have a noted replacement schedule. This is especially true of the more major purchases such as beds, pressure support systems, and wheelchairs.

How crucial is the accuracy of the figures? As an example, consider the case of a 25-year-old tetraplegic who has a life care plan that lists a motorized wheelchair with a power-actuated tilt-in-space system and standing features, programmable controls, and other needed accessories. The manufacturer's list price is noted at $31,000. One life care planner projects replacement of the chair every 4 years, while the other life care planner says every 5 years. Based on a life expectancy of 69 years, the former planner allows for 10 replacement chairs; the latter only 8. The overall difference between the life care plans would be $62,000. This of course is not discounted to present value and does not take the economist's adjustments for inflation into account.

Even with less expensive equipment, such as a Jay pressure relief cushion with a list price of $425, the differences in replacement allowances can show some significant variances. In reviewing plans, the author has observed that replacement for these cushions ranges from 2 to 5 years. Continuing to use the previously noted client as an example, the 5-year allowance equates to eight replacement cushions at a total plan cost of $3,400. The 2-year allowance equates to 20 replacement cushions at a total price of $8,500 (not discounted to present value), for a difference of $5,100 between the two plans.

Even more problematic than the variance in costs between plans is the lack of any accurate standards to compute replacement allowances. This lack of any prescribed standards can easily allow an attorney to question not only the accuracy of the replacement costs of a particular plan, but also the accuracy of the methods of computation for all other medical equipment costs and allowances.

So what factors must be taken into account when figuring replacement schedules for equipment? The first factor to consider is the manufacturer's warranty of the particular piece of equipment being recommended. The implied expectation of any warranty is that the piece of equipment will last throughout the length of the warranty period. If the equipment is defective, the warranty allows for replacement or compensation with little to no cost to the user. In our homes most of us utilize equipment far beyond the expiration of the manufacturer's warranty. It is not uncommon to have the same refrigerator, stove, or washer for over 10 years, while the warranty on these items may expire after only 1 year.

In the author's experience, many life care plans include replacements of certain items that do not even meet or barely exceed the manufacturer's warranty of the product. The aforementioned

Jay cushion has a complete replacement warranty (other than the cover) for up to 2 years, and if properly maintained (occasional cleaning and kneading of the gel pad and replacements of covers), the cushion's life expectancy should at least double the warranty.

Most items referred to as durable medical equipment are well described. That is to say, they are quite durable. Most standard commodes, tub rails, tub benches, and folding walkers have a lifetime warranty; however, it should be noted that a lifetime warranty does not preclude a replacement allowance for these items. Over a period of time, any of these items will show excessive wear and tear. This is particularly true of any items with many moving parts that will become shaky with time, or items that have padding that can eventually tear or wear out. Some pieces of equipment such as a trapeze bar attached to a floor stand are so durable and their everyday usage sufficiently limited that their replacement can safely be expected to last 10 years or more.

In addition to the warranty and its relationship to replacement allowances, the life care planner must also take into account the need for repairs and maintenance to a piece of equipment. A pair of forearm crutches should last a client 3 years, but the crutch tips will have to be replaced perhaps twice a year. The Jay pressure relief cushion previously referenced has a longer life than many allow for, but the removable covers should be replaced yearly. (A better strategy is to allow for the purchase of two covers when first buying a cushion, in order to alternate their use while cleaning, and then allow for twice the replacement time, that is, 2 years for each cover.)

Repairs versus replacement becomes a far more complicated equation when one is considering more complex pieces of equipment with more parts, such as manual wheelchairs or power-actuated products, like electric hospital beds, air-powered support surfaces, and motorized wheelchairs.

When including a hospital bed in a life care plan, it is important to note that hospital beds have a lifetime warranty on all the welds of their frame (Invacare Corporation, 2002; Graham-Field, Inc., product warranty information, 2002). It is extremely rare for these frames to require repairs. Conversely, the mechanisms for adjustment, such as the shafts, motors, and hand controls, will require repair or replacement, and an allowance for maintenance should be made. Likewise, the mattress should be replaced every 4 to 5 years. There are certain factors that must be taken into account, such as the weight of the client, the daily usage of the bed (for less active clients), and the use of higher-end support surfaces or flotation mattresses that either put less stress on the mattress itself or entirely replace the standard hospital bed mattress. (The author has seen a number of life care plans allowing for replacement of hospital bed mattresses when the client is using none.)

Wheelchairs categorized as high-strength lightweight or ultralight must have a lifetime warranty on the side frame and cross-braces (Centers for Medicare and Medicaid Services, 1997). The other working parts of the chair are usually covered by a limited warranty of 1 year, excluding wear and tear or abuse. (The manufacturer many times upon return of a broken or defective part will determine if there was abuse of the product.) Likewise, there is a minimum of a 5-year-to-lifetime warranty for the frame of a motorized wheelchair, and the electrical components all have a life expectancy minimum of 1 to 2 years (Invacare Corporation, 2002; Pride Mobility Products Corporation, 2002; Product warranty information, 2002; Sunrise Medical, 2002). When recommending either a manual or motorized wheelchair, the life care planner should include maintenance and repair allowances, but after time must consider that the frequency of repairs and the overall wear on the frame will necessitate a replacement of the equipment.

Determining the replacement allowance for a wheelchair is a process that currently seems to lack any standardization or protocol. In Kendall and Deutsch's (2002) article on research methodology, the authors state that life care planning is a "standardized process" (p. 158). They further assert, "If Life Care Planning is a reliable tool in Case Management and the provision of patient care, then the results of a given LCP can be consistently replicated" (p. 157).

However, in reviewing life care plans, the author has observed that similar models of wheelchairs may be assigned a replacement with as little as 2 years or as great as every 10 years. Although there may be a valid reason for the 10-year replacement, such as a rarely used backup chair, the plan rarely includes any notation as to the justification for a replacement number given. As shown in the examples given earlier in the chapter, these variances, when multiplied by a young client's life expectancy, can add up to significant cost differences in opposing plans.

There are a variety of factors that will have an effect on the replacement allowance for a wheelchair. Some of these factors will reduce the life of a chair, while others will add to its life. It is necessary for the life care planner to consider which factors are inherent in an individual client's lifestyle and account for those factors in the life care plan. By using a standardized format, taking the factors noted in the following into a weighted scale for replacement allowance, both greater reliability for the individual life care plan and greater consistency, reliability, and validity for the life care planning process as a whole should be achieved.

Contributing Factors to Replacement Time for Wheelchairs

Age

The age of the client is the first contributing factor. Everyone's general activity level differs throughout different age ranges. The greater the activity level of an individual, the more wear and tear on the frame of a wheelchair.

Most children (4 to 16 years) are very active, and those children who are wheelchair dependent are no exception. They usually are attending school 5 days a week, and when not in classrooms, most are playing with other children. Athletic programs now include children in wheelchairs in a large variety of games and events. The Special Olympics and other athletic associations for children with disabilities are a part of many school and recreation programs nationwide.

Moreover, children grow. Growth is a factor that must be addressed in each child on an annual basis. This is not to say a child will require a replacement of the wheelchair each year, because the majority of pediatric wheelchair frames are built with adjustability for growth. A qualified RTS or ATS will always try to allow for a maximum amount of growth in relationship to the current measurements of a child. Sometimes, a child's measurements fall between two sizes of wheelchair frames, and less growth must be allowed for proper propulsion of a manual wheelchair. This is less of a concern in motorized wheelchairs, where the ability to reach a joystick is far more adjustable than the ability to properly reach two hand rims. In the author's experience, pediatric wheelchair frames generally will last the child from 4 to 5 years, with growth being modified and accounted for.

Growth also must be accounted for not just in the frame of a wheelchair, but also in any custom seating system for children. This too is easily accomplished through quality evaluations performed by rehabilitation professionals when first designing the seating system. All seating systems should have about 4 to 5 years of growth built into them. One exception to this rule is custom-molded seating systems, such as Contour U or the Otto Bock OBSS systems. As these systems are created utilizing an actual body mold of the child, there is far less available growth that can be built into them.

Young adults (ages 16 to 30) are also highly active, and from the teens through the early twenties, the average individual is still attending school. Many are propelling for longer distances, especially throughout college campuses. In general, this age group is far less sedentary, and the population who are wheelchair dependent are now spending far more of their time with able-bodied friends and out in the community than ever in the past. Most are in the same wheelchair for as much as 18 hours per day, 7 days per week. Some also have become involved in wheelchair sports on a far more aggressive level (although the more serious of these athletes will probably purchase or utilize a separate sports wheelchair for their particular game). Again, the greater the activity level, the more wear on the wheelchair overall.

Adults (ages 30 to 65) in general will tend to have a bit lower activity level. Many wheelchair-dependent individuals will be married, have families, and spend more time at home. Many who are working in offices are indoors in more confined spaces throughout the day, putting far less stress on the wheelchair frame. This is not to say that many individuals of this age range are not active in the community or their careers, but the stress on the wheelchair in this type of lifestyle is far less.

Senior citizens (over 65) as a rule have a lower activity level. Many who are using manual wheelchairs (even lightweight frames) may not have the endurance or strength as they age to manually propel the chair long distances or in more difficult outdoor environments. Many may not be able to self-propel at all and are pushed by an attendant. With such a lower activity level, the replacement schedule for the wheelchair should obviously decrease.

Environment

Where the wheelchair is being used will also affect its replacement allowance. A suburban and urban environment where there are mostly paved sidewalks, graded curb cuts between streets, and, thanks to the Americans with Disabilities Act, far more wheelchair-accessible buildings puts only limited fatigue on the wheelchair.

Clients who live in a more rural environment, with far less of the previously noted accommodations, will fatigue the frames of their chairs more quickly. Hills, rocks, and soft earth not only put more wear and tear on the frame, but also require more frequent repairs to the chair.

On the other hand, individuals who live in a skilled nursing facility will put far less stress on the wheelchair. The linoleum floors, fully accessible environment, and inferred lower activity level will increase the overall lifetime of the wheelchair.

Behavior

How an individual behaves in a wheelchair can greatly influence its replacement. This factor is more relevant for those in manual wheelchairs, as an individual with uncontrolled behavioral problems should probably not be driving a motorized wheelchair. The first instance to consider is whether your client can self-propel a manual wheelchair at all. If the client does not self-propel, due to either physical or cognitive deficits, his or her overall activity level in the wheelchair will usually be far less than that of those who functionally propel their chairs.

Some individuals may exhibit hyperactive, athetoid, or extreme self-stimulation behavior. All of these behaviors, which may result from developmental delays or clients with serious head injuries, will stress parts of a wheelchair frame. The author works with a large population of institutionalized clients who all incessantly perform some type of self-stimulation behavior in their wheelchairs. For example, they may slam their bodies back and forth in a rocking motion for hours while seated in a chair, and others, if not controlled, may beat the sides of the wheelchair with their fists, or, in transferring, will forcefully propel themselves into or out of the chairs. Any of these extreme behaviors will have an effect on the lifetime of the chair.

Body Type

Clients who are obese or are close to the weight limitations of a certain wheelchair frame will obviously put more overall wear on the chair. Most wheelchairs come with a 250-pound weight limitation; however, there are custom bariatric frames that are capable of supporting an individual weighing between 600 and 1,000 pounds. Obviously, the higher the weight limitation, the more it will compensate for this weight factor.

Lifestyle

How the client spends the majority of each week is another factor that should be considered. Does the client spend most of each day at home, or does he or she go into an office or a school 5 days a week? If so, how is the client transported? It should be noted that the very act of securing a wheelchair onto a van or school bus twice a day for a long ride will lead to some wear, as the vibrations on the frame will eventually cause the bolts to oval out the holes in the frame. Wheelchair manufacturers and research facilities routinely test their frames in a double-drum vibration sled to count how many cycles will lead to frame damage (Johnson, 1996; Vitek et al., 2001).

Lifestyle must also be reflected when choosing the appropriate model of wheelchair for the client. If the client is an active self-propeller, the chair prescribed should be a high-strength ultralight frame. Various studies have tested the durability and cost comparisons of different wheelchair frames, and it has been shown that ultralight rehabilitation wheelchairs are the most cost-effective over the life of the wheelchair, costing 3.4 times less (dollars per life cycle) than depot (standard frame) wheelchairs and 2.3 times less (dollars per life cycle) than the lightweight wheelchairs tested in the study (Cooper et al., 1997). Likewise, if the client is obese or exhibits self-stimulation behavior, a heavy-duty or even custom-reinforced frame is required. Similar appropriateness of correct model selection must be assured in calculating the replacement of a motorized wheelchair.

One note in considering a lifestyle should be when your client has both a motorized and manual wheelchair. In most cases, the manual wheelchair will be used as a backup, so consequently its overall use may be far more limited than the use of the motorized wheelchair throughout the week. This too must be taken into account when projecting replacement schedules.

Replacement Allowance Worksheets

The author first introduced the following worksheets to participants of the Life Care Planning Summit in Chicago, Illinois, on May 18, 2002. At that time, first drafts of the worksheets, based on available data, were sent to more than 20 life care planners throughout the country for their comments on both accuracy and ease of use. Initial changes were made, and the worksheets were then sent to another eight volunteers for additional comments. Responses from the life care planning community from both mailings were about 20 percent of all those sent.

It is hoped by the author that the worksheets will be considered a tool to improve the overall reliability of life care plans in the area of wheelchair replacement. By accounting for the factors described in this chapter, the assigning of a replacement value for a wheelchair can be better defended with a more objective basis. It is further hoped that this tool can be adjusted and improved with time by communication with the author as various life care planners utilize and perhaps supplement the worksheets based on the uniqueness of their individual cases.

Estimated Replacement Schedule Assessment Form

Manual Wheelchair

All medical equipment will eventually wear out and must be replaced. The frequency of replacement is dependent on the individual using the equipment and various factors in his or her life. Two assumptions must be made for this worksheet:

1. The wheelchair frame is appropriate for the lifestyle of the client (i.e., if he or she is an active self-propeller, this should be a high-strength ultralight frame). If the client is obese or exhibits self-stimulation behavior, a heavy-duty reinforced frame may be required.
2. Routine maintenance is done on an annual or as-needed basis.

The following worksheet will assist the rehabilitation consultant with evaluating the factors and how they affect the overall replacement schedule of each item. Each of the factors will either add to or subtract from the life of the equipment being used.

Identify factors that affect your client, and then apply them to the chart based on the *value* instructions. The adjusted replacement time in the lower-right-hand corner will be the estimated weighted replacement schedule for the particular piece of equipment.

Client Name: ____________________ Date of Birth: __________		
Average Replacement Time: 5 years		
Additional Determining Factors	*Value*	*Effect on Replacement Time*
Age: If client is …	Then +/–	From 5 years
4–16 years	–1 year	
16–30 years	–0.5 year	
30–65 years	No change	
>65 years	+1 year	
Environment: If client lives in …		
Suburban or urban	No change	
Rural environment	–0.5 year	
Skilled nursing facility	+1 year	
Behavior: If client …		
Can self-propel	No change	
Cannot self-propel	+1 year	
Has self-stimulation, athetoid, or other hyperactive behavior	+2 year	
Body Type: If client is …		
Over 250 pounds	–0.5 year	
Lifestyle: If client …		
Is highly active adult	–0.5 year	
Locks wheelchair into a van or school bus several times per week	–0.5 year	
Is using manual chair as a backup for a power chair	+2 years	
Adjusted Replacement Time	=	

Estimated Replacement Schedule Assessment Form

Motorized Wheelchair

All medical equipment will eventually wear out and must be replaced. The frequency of replacement is dependent on the individual using the equipment and various factors in his or her life. Two assumptions must be made for this worksheet:

1. The appropriate model of motorized wheelchair has been chosen to meet the lifestyle, environment, and weight capacity of the client.
2. Routine maintenance is done on an annual or as-needed basis.

The following worksheet will assist the rehabilitation consultant with evaluating the factors and how they affect the overall replacement schedule of each item. Each of the factors will either add to or subtract from the life of the equipment being used.

Identify factors that affect your client, and then apply them to the chart based on the *value* instructions. The adjusted replacement time in the lower-right-hand corner will be the estimated weighted replacement schedule for the particular piece of equipment.

Client Name: ____________________ Date of Birth: __________		
Average Replacement Time: 5 years		
Additional Determining Factors	*Value*	*Effect on Replacement Time*
Age: If client is …	Then +/–	From 5 years
4–14 years	–1 year	
14–30 years	–0.5 years	
30–65 years	No change	
>65 years	+1 year	
Environment: If client lives in …		
Suburban or urban	No change	
Rural environment	–0.5 year	
Skilled nursing facility	+1 years	
Body Type: If client is …		
Over 300 pounds	–0.5 years	
Very ataxic or has high muscle tone of upper extremities	–0.5 years	
Lifestyle: If client …		
Is highly active adult	–0.5 year	
Locks wheelchair into a van or school bus several times per week	–0.5 year	
Adjusted Replacement Time	=	

Use of References and Specialists

There are a variety of sources life care planners can use to create their list of the most optimal equipment and most accurate prices for their clients. One of the most common methods is to obtain the original list of equipment a client was provided when he or she left the rehab facility after the injury. Although this is an excellent first step, it may be far from a complete list of all the client's equipment needs. Some of the flaws with this method that must be recognized are as follows:

- *Time Factor:* If a great deal of time has passed since the original equipment was provided to your client, his or her physical condition may have changed (either better or worse).
- *Environment or Vocational Changes:* The client may have moved to a different home that requires other types of equipment, or the life care plan may be providing for a new, more accessible environment, which may change some of the equipment choices. Current or future vocational options must be considered as well.
- *Funding Issues:* When the original equipment was provided, the client's funding source may not have allowed for higher-quality models, or a large segment of equipment, such as independently controlled ceiling lifts, environmental controls, or computer interfaces built into the power wheelchair. The life care plan must address all equipment to provide the client with the highest possibility of independent function.

Prices for medical equipment are another area of possible contention in the report. As previously noted, by omission of various accessories, the price of a particular wheelchair may be vastly inaccurate. A more important point is what source a life care planner uses to acquire prices. The author has seen a variety of different sources used for price submission to the plan:

- Catalogs
- Internet sites
- Calls to medical equipment providers in the client's local area

There is a possible problem utilizing any of the previous sources to obtain prices. Many catalog and Internet sites are quoting extremely discounted prices for equipment. Some of these prices may be a result of overstocked merchandise or a particular price passed on by a manufacturer. When the client finally (possibly years later) receives a judgment on the case, and must now purchase his or her own equipment, he or she may not be able to receive an equivalent discount as to what was originally quoted. Likewise, when a life care planner calls a local vendor and requests a price, he or she may not be sure if the price has been discounted or possibly increased.

It has been the author's contention in past articles and lectures (Amsterdam, 2001, 2002) that the most objective price that should be used for a life care plan is the manufacturer's suggested list price (MSLP). As this price is provided by every manufacturer and is consistent throughout all 50 states, it provides the only true objective basis for accurate pricing. The MSLP is also always a price that the client should be able to obtain from any reputable equipment provider.

The Use of Rehabilitation Equipment Specialists as Consultants

If a client's physical disabilities are more involved, it may be beneficial to consult with a rehab equipment specialist. It is important to realize that the medical equipment industry, like all other branches of health care, has many areas of specialization. There are medical equipment companies that specialize in respiratory supplies, others strictly in the enteral or IV therapy business, and some whose primary income are as physician or hospital suppliers. Any of these companies can buy and distribute wheelchairs and other durable medical equipment, although they may have little, other than cursory, knowledge in proper evaluation of a rehab client.

Rehab technology suppliers (RTS) are individuals who specialize in the needs of clients with permanent disabilities. They are usually employed in a firm that is in the primary business of rehab medical equipment evaluation and distribution. An RTS can go through a national certification or credentialing process; the most recognized curriculum was developed through RESNA (the Rehabilitation Engineering and Assistive Technology Society of North America). Those passing this certification process attain the credentials of ATS (assistive technology supplier). A therapist who passes the same curriculum attains the credentials of ATP (assistive technology practitioner). If the individual is also a member in good standing with NRRTS (the National Registry of Rehabilitation Technology Suppliers; 2003), he or she may also be recognized through the trademarked credential of CRTS (certified rehab technology supplier). RESNA and NRRTS both provide a directory of certified specialists on their websites.

Certified ATS/CRTS specialists are working in rehabilitation hospitals, state developmental centers, and schools for children with disabilities, evaluating clients for equipment needs on a daily basis. Utilizing the expertise of a certified ATS will help you get the best idea of your client's current and future equipment needs. He or she can provide you with accurate pricing based on MSLP if requested, as well as help add greater defensibility to the equipment section of the overall plan.

Conclusion

For many with permanent disabilities, the lifetime use of rehabilitation medical equipment, such as a custom wheelchair, may be the one aspect that separates their lives from the rest of the able-bodied world. As technology improves, providing lighter materials and more functionality, new models of equipment will be continually introduced, and the job of the life care planner to include the correct type of equipment in a plan will only get more difficult. When equipment costs are a large segment of a particular life care plan, costly errors of omission and tendencies to exaggerate medical needs can be used by opposing attorneys as focal points of contention. Better systems of protocols must be used for replacement schedules, as well as the ascertaining of accurate prices. The use of rehab equipment experts is increasing in the life care planning industry, and life care planners who are working without such expertise may have a harder time defending their choices in a court of law.

Editors' Note

As the reader may know, sadly Paul Amsterdam succumbed to an extended illness and he was unable to update this valuable chapter. However, his wisdom will live on through his previous contributions to this text, as well as 2015 and 2016 *Journal of Life Care Planning* articles, three of which are reprinted here as appendices.

Appendix 31.1

Journal of Life Care Planning (2015), Vol. 13, No. 2, (29-30). Reprinted in accordance with member/subscriber guidelines. Publisher: International Association of Rehabilitation Professionals, 1000 Westgate Drive, #252, St. Paul, MN 55114, 888-IARPQaA (888-427-7722), webpage: http://www.rehabpro.org.

The Medical Equipment Corner Paul Amsterdam, ATP

Making Correct Choices of Medical Equipment for a Life Care Plan

This is the first of several planned articles focusing on issues associated with adding medical equipment to a life care plan. The need and choices for more complex equipment is usually directly proportional to the complexity of a client's disability and their associated loss of function. It should also be remembered that medical equipment must be viewed as a dynamic part of a life care plan, not only with the need for replacements formulated with some logical criteria (which we will discuss in upcoming articles), but the realization that equipment needs will change for clients as they age and/or suffer some physical deterioration. This initial article will focus more on how to differentiate the proper choices of more complex pieces of equipment when required versus more standard alternatives. It will also lead the planner on better possible roads in finding those correct choices. For those want to delve deeper than this article will allow, I would recommend my previous chapters in the Second Edition of the *Life Care Planning and Case Management Handbook*, edited by Roger O. Weed, and in the Third Edition, edited by Roger O. Weed and Debra E. Berens; as well as in the Second Edition of *Pediatric Life Care Planning and Case Management*, edited by Susan Riddick-Grisham and Laura M. Deming. Both of these textbooks offer a broader review of the entire subject with the ability to go into more specifics.

In a life care plan, medical equipment may be only a percentage of the possible assistive technology that a planner may want to include in a plan. Assistive technology may allow for a wide range of items such as augmentative communication systems, computer interface, and environmental control units. I have seen plans recommending service canines, as well as entire smart apartments. For the purpose of this article, we are focusing primarily on the more durable medical choices that need to be made. The most complex choice in this category can be wheelchairs, although beds and even bathroom equipment should be noted as well.

Factors in Choosing the Proper Wheelchair for Your Client

As noted above, when having to choose what medical equipment is required for a life care plan, the primary factor will be the diagnoses and associated loss of function of the client. If we are focusing on wheelchairs, then several other factors have to be taken into account:

- *Mobility*: Does the client have the ability to self-propel? If not, is a motorized wheelchair a first mobility solution? If self-propulsion is not a goal, then what other means of mobility will be needed to determine the proper choice?
- *Environment and lifestyle*: Does the client live in a rural or an urban neighborhood? Will the client be going to a job every day or a school or some other day program?
- *Positioning*: Is therapeutic positioning equally or more important than mobility (especially possible where self-propulsion is not an option)?
- *Pressure relief*: How will your choice of wheelchair help, if needed, solve pressure reduction needs?

Standard Wheelchairs versus Complex Rehab

I am using the above terms as this is how Medicare delineates wheelchairs. This is done for both manual and power chairs, primarily by use of HCPCS coding. They also have far more regulations pertaining to allowance of complex rehab equipment, requiring further justification, as well as the requirement of a credentialed ATP being part of the assessment process for these chairs. (For those who are unfamiliar with the term, an ATP is an internationally recognized specialist in assistive technology, credentialed through the Rehab Engineering Society of North America [RESNA].) In first assessing a client's need for a wheelchair, it is necessary to ask: When will a standard wheelchair do the job? Medicare classifies standard wheelchairs utilizing HCPCS procedure codes (K0001-K0004). These chairs may weigh from 32 to 45 pounds in comparison to ultralight-defined chairs (coded K0005); the standard models allow far fewer choices of sizes, seat heights, and overall options. They will also in some cases weigh considerably more than custom manual chairs. Most importantly, in terms of propulsion, the standard chair has no adjustment of the rear wheels, which is one of the defining features of an ultralight chair. What difference can this make to your client? A standard wheelchair, with no rear wheel adjustment, forces the client to literally pull themselves in a forward motion. If the wheelchair will be the client's only means of independent mobility, this can have significant consequences for the client: Far more difficult and repetitious pulls will be required to cover the same distance and far more probability of future overuse syndrome. Ultralight chairs all have the ability to move the rear wheels forward and, consequently, allow a true push on the hand rims which allows a true balance on the center of gravity of a person's weight and thereby significantly reduces strain and extraneous repetition of movement. Here, the rule of thumb should be that if your client is using a manual wheelchair as their primary means of independent mobility, then the need for an ultralight model is highly recommended.

Why Is This an Important Consideration in Your Life Care Plan?

When including costs in your plan, accuracy and reliability must be as certain as possible. Most importantly, the costs must hold up under scrutiny in court, especially given the life care plan presented by the opposing party in the case. If your choice of equipment shows glaring differences, this will become fodder for the opposing attorney to use against you. More important, if the equipment portion as a whole shows significant disregard for accuracy of choice and costs, this may place the reliability of your entire plan into question. How much difference in costs is involved? Take the above example of the need for either a standard wheelchair versus a custom-configured ultralight wheelchair:

- Invacare Tracer EX2 (STD K0001 wheelchair) $415 (MSRP-2015)
- Sunrise Medical Quickie 2 (K0005 Ultralight) base price only $2,050 (MSRP-2015)

It should be noted that this price reflects the base price only (Sunrise Medical, 2000); once the more common options, such as seating and accessories, are added to a custom-configured ultralight chair, the more likely price will be between $3,000 and $4,000. Given the probability of needed replacements, perhaps seven to 10 times in the life expectancy of a younger client, the difference in this initial choice becomes very significant (more than $26,000). This same choice becomes far more glaring when considering choices of motorized wheelchairs: The more simple of these chairs may have a list price of $3,800 when compared with a Group 4 power chair with full power-seating options (power tilt, recline, power center mount legs, and seat elevator) that will have an MSRP of well over $30,000. Doing the same comparison and adding in replacements, I have personally seen opposing plans with differences of more than $250,000.

How Is the Correct Wheelchair Choice Made?

Perhaps a better question is: Who should make these recommendations? If a client has simple needs, then an experienced life care planner may feel comfortable compiling a list of needed durable medical equipment. If the client is ambulatory and a wheelchair may just be for long-distance use and pushed by a caregiver, then the recommendation of a standard wheelchair may be more appropriate. If the life care planner decides that this same client should have a $20,000 motorized wheelchair with expensive seating options, I would suggest they have a specialist make this recommendation with a great deal of additional justification. Many planners will first use the recommendations of the physician who is consulting on their plan. It should be noted that even if you are using a physiatrist as your plan consultant, very few of these specialists have more than a rudimentary background of specific wheelchair and seating knowledge. Their preferred list may include general items, such as "manual or motorized wheelchair," but I have rarely seen them add more specifics, such as a particular model or appropriate options and therapeutic seating needs. Given the above choices noted in this article, more specifics are required with some justification of why that particular choice was made. Clients who need a more complex piece of medical equipment should have this optimally done during a mobility evaluation, also called a "wheelchair clinic." These clinics are usually found in better rehab hospitals. A therapist, usually with ATP credentials, should be part of this clinic. If there is not a clinic available, it is recommended that a certified ATP at least conduct a home evaluation with the client. To be certified now with Medicare, every complex rehab dealership must have a credentialed ATP on staff. You can also find a directory of ATPs under the RESNA directory at www.resna.org. This initial choice conundrum also must be made in other areas of durable medical equipment.

Noteworthy is the choice of bed for your client. If the consulting physician recommends a "hospital bed with pressure-relieving mattress," will this be manual or power? Is the client married or has [sic] a partner? Perhaps the need for a queen or king-size bed that still gives therapeutic positioning adjustments to the client's side of the bed would be a more appropriate choice to maintain their quality of life. Just as questionable may be the pressure-relieving surface. A simple alternating air mattress pad costs less than $200, whereas a full alternating low air-loss support surface may cost more than $6,000. How do you justify the choices between either of these options and so many possible solutions in between? This initial model selection is too often made carelessly. I have seen experienced life care planners (more often working on the plaintiff side) recommend equipment way beyond the needs and even the true wants of their client. In one case, this resulted in a judge virtually dismissing the entire report and forcing a settlement. On the other hand, clients who have some needs that will manifest more with aging are left with the barest of equipment recommendations and subsequent allowable funding, through a lack of forethought and knowledge of proper assistive technology solutions. As your life care clients' needs become more complex, recognize this first step of proper equipment selection. Make sure the proper level of chair is selected to meet the functional deficits of your client. Likewise, follow this procedure with all the other durable medical equipment in your plan. As the complexity arises, seek the proper specialists to insure your plan is both accurate and reliable. In future articles, other issues will be examined regarding proper costing issues, as well as replacement criteria, and a review of Medicare and its now questionable place in a life care plan.

Appendix 31.2

Journal of Life Care Planning (2015), Vol. 13, No. 3, (49-50). Reprinted in accordance with member/subscriber guidelines. Publisher: International Association of Rehabilitation Professionals, 1000 Westgate Drive, #252, St. Paul, MN 55114, 888-IARPQaA (888-427-7722), webpage: http://www.rehabpro.org.

The Medical Equipment Corner Paul Amsterdam, ATP

Proper Pricing Methodology for Your Life Care Plan

In the last issue of this journal, I wrote an initial article on how to first ascertain what level of medical equipment our client should have (either more standard versus the need for complex rehab) and various factors that go into that part of the choice. That article started to also note the disparity in pricing, especially over a life span of a client, if the wrong choice of equipment is chosen in the beginning. This article will start to focus on pricing methodology, where these incorrect choices can get more exaggerated, and worse, if done incorrectly, the accuracy of your life care plan can be questioned. I have been reviewing life care plans for well over 15 years, and in that time I have seen life care planners use the most ballpark methods for pricing of the equipment recommended. Before I start, you might want to consider for yourself, just how do you come up with the prices that you eventually publish in your individual plan? Do you use the following?

- Do you have your own reference material that you use as a basis for pricing?
- Are you calling a medical equipment dealer for all prices?
- Are you looking up individual prices over the Internet?
- Do you use a pre-packaged software for life care planners?
- Do you utilize Medicare or other public funding allowance coding as a price basis?

I have seen issues with each of these methods and will discuss the issue as well as other more accurate standards to consider instead. If you have your own reference materials, I would venture to guess much of them are outdated as you are reading this. I have an extensive set of both current catalogs and price lists direct from manufacturers, and the work required in keeping this up to date is daunting. As all major manufacturers display their products online, this job has been made easier, but I have found cases of life care planners offering equipment that is part of their past reference that is no longer available on the open market. One instance I reviewed several years ago was the recommendation of an IBOT power wheelchair. This amazing product was unique in being the first power wheelchair that could actually allow an individual to climb up and down steps! Unfortunately the plan recommendation came several months after the manufacturer of the product stopped production due to lack of sales. This lack of current information not only affected the choice of power chair for the plan but was the planner's basis for not looking at other mobility options to deal with the steps in the client's home. Calling a medical equipment supplier has been one of the time-honored ways of getting prices for the products you are recommending. It was through a phone call like this how I first found out about the life care planning industry. It was also how I understood that, in making these phone calls, life care planners many times were asking incorrect questions to sometimes the wrong people. Not all medical equipment suppliers specialize in the same area. If you are trying to get pricing on respiratory equipment from someone who never works with clients with ventilators, I will venture to guess your pricing may not be accurate. Likewise, many smaller dealers who have more of a retail surgical supply business never truly help evaluate or sell a complex power chair with alternative drive switches that allow the user to drive and recline their chair only through their head movements. They may be able to give you a somewhat roundabout figure—these chairs retail for more than $25,000. You must make sure the supplier you are requesting pricing from is familiar with the equipment you are recommending. Only a small percentage of suppliers sell and install stair glides or outdoor wheelchair lifts, so it is necessary to search out those more specialized dealers for more accurate figures. What price should you be asking for? In my previous chapters in both Roger Weed's and Susan Riddick-Grisham's textbooks, I recommended using the manufacturers' suggested list price (MSLP) as the most accurate basis for a life care plan. The reasoning for this has not changed since their original editions in 1999. A life care plan will ultimately set up a certain amount of money to be used, based on the recommendations in the plan. If your costs are based on discounted pricing, or on prices from a vendor far from your client's geographic area, or prices based on allowable of public funding such as Medicare, there is a very good chance your client will have to pay a significantly higher price from their local supplier.

What about the Use of the Internet?

The Internet can be an excellent source for some pricing, but certainly not everything. More importantly, use it with caution and reservation. If you are pricing some standard supplies, such as adult diapers or gauze pads, obtaining some average figures from notable Internet sites can be appropriate. I would recommend that you do not rely on just one in this case; take an average from perhaps three different sites. The reason here is, again, the large amount of discounts on the Internet. Discounts may be here today, but these same prices may not be available in the future. Understand that more major manufacturers are starting to clamp down on the pricing they are allowing Internet sites to publish. Many are insisting the sites follow an MAP (Minimum Advertised Price) for their items on a supplier's site. The company I work for, Sunrise Medical, recently terminated more than 20 Internet dealers from their account list for not respecting MAP pricing. If your life care plan used pricing for a wheelchair from one of these dealers, it would not be available for our client's use. More important is the type of equipment you are searching for on the Internet. I do not recommend using the Internet for pricing more complex equipment. Part of the reason, in terms of wheelchairs, will be discussed in future articles on building a complex wheelchair from the ground up. The other reason is that Internet sites, in my opinion, are truly not qualified to help evaluate, deliver, and then service more complex equipment. Most manufacturers of complex equipment only allow Internet sites to sell their more basic equipment, but there are motorized scooters and some power chairs available on sites today. Many people, after buying products online, find out their local dealer refuses to help adjust or service the equipment after they received it. This is not a situation you want to create in a life care plan. Prepackaged software for life care plans now has some equipment as part of the program. One should be careful that the prices quoted are both MSRP and currently up to date. Here again, the idea of complexity and the additional options, accessories, and need for possible custom seating may not be part of this prepackaged system.

Use of Medicare Allowables in a Life Care Plan

I have occasionally seen planners use Medicare as either a source of equipment pricing or as a means of moving all the equipment choices, based on the fact that the client will either immediately, or down the road, be covered primarily by Medicare. I cannot stress enough how wrong this method would be, not only for any accuracy of your plan, but to the total detriment of your client. Not only are the published allowables that Medicare provides to individual states highly discounted, but as of 2 years ago, the Medicare system for acquiring medical equipment is close to being completely broken. By July of 2013, Medicare put into effect a competitive bidding system throughout the entire country. Essentially, 95 percent of all the previous suppliers, and even small pharmacies that used to be able to rent and sell equipment through Medicare, are no longer able to do so. Imagine waking up tomorrow and finding that all the brand-named and other local coffee shops within a 20-mile radius were shut down except for one! That is where the nation now stands.

To get on the phone with a single supplier who is allowed to sell through Medicare may, in some urban areas, have a wait time of more than an hour; and because these suppliers are now being paid almost 50 percent less than the already discounted published prices, the quality and choice of equipment is extremely low. Although complex rehab equipment does not go through this competitive bidding process (at least for now), the amount of regulations and paperwork that Medicare requires for a complex power chair can realistically take 3 to 4 months to properly acquire from a specialized rehab dealer. As of next January (editor's note. When written the author was referring to January, 2016), if new legislation by Medicare proceeds, the options and accessories for these complex power chairs and complex manual wheelchairs will now be on the competitive bid price schedule; many dealers are already threatening to walk away from this funding if those prices go into effect. In a nutshell, Medicare should not be part of any pricing choice or methodology for a life care plan at this time.

Conclusion

Given all the issues above, what is a life care planner left with for proper price methodology? If you are calling a supplier, make sure it is someone who specializes and commonly sells the products you are trying to obtain pricing from. Always request an MSRP. Use the Internet sparingly and mostly for supplies rather than larger pieces of equipment that require more localized evaluation, setup, and future servicing. Medicare, or any other published insurance list of price allowables, should never be used as a source of pricing for a life care plan. Future articles will discuss adding all needed options and accessories to more complex pieces of equipment and how their omission reflects on total accuracy, so when you are creating a life care plan for an individual with more complex equipment needs, make sure there is a credentialed equipment expert you can turn to, if needed.

Appendix 31.3

Journal of Life Care Planning (2016), Vol. 14, No. 1, (87-88). Reprinted in accordance with member/subscriber guidelines. Publisher: International Association of Rehabilitation Professionals, 1000 Westgate Drive, #252, St. Paul, MN 55114, 888-IARPQaA (888-427-7722), webpage: http://www.rehabpro.org.

The Medical Equipment Corner Paul Amsterdam, ATP

Medicare's Current Status with Medical Equipment and Its Possible Effects on Life Care Planning

Through many years of consulting, I have observed instances of life care planners working Medicare pricing/costs into a life care plan. Some planners have curtailed services, especially for medical equipment as a client ages, noting that Medicare would at that point reimburse the cost of that medical equipment. This curtailment is inappropriate not only for several reasons, but mostly because when a client receives a legal settlement, that settlement becomes the evaluee's primary funding. The federal government then assumes a secondary role in funding medical services. As a matter of fact, if an evaluee used Medicare to pay for services previous to receiving a settlement, the evaluee is then required to reimburse Medicare for those previous payments upon case settlement.

What occurs more commonly, though, refers to the Medicare set-aside funds. These are funds, set aside in an interest-bearing account, to reimburse Medicare should the settlement in the future run short, and Medicare takes over as the secondary funding for the client. This is an appropriate deferment of some of the evaluee's settlement, although this presents a new problem: In terms of obtaining some standard and even more complex types of medical equipment, Medicare has broken its own system. More evaluees today, having Medicare as their primary funding, have lost accessibility to needed equipment, such as more complex wheelchairs, not to mention obtaining basic equipment, such as canes, walkers, and even hospital beds.

If you are not aware of this, it is because a series of new regulations, introduced 10 years ago by Centers for Medicare & Medicaid Services (CMS), has now come to a head in the last 3 years. In January 2016, these "new" regulations became effective; as a result, these regulations have exacerbated the durable medical equipment "problem" which has taken the program another step toward complete breakdown.

Ten years ago, CMS sent a memo to all medical equipment dealers, advising that it was considering employing a competitive bidding system in order to save the Medicare program money. This system would apply to all standard equipment that Medicare covers; e.g., standard wheelchairs, canes, walkers, oxygen, hospital beds, CPAP devices for sleep therapy, and so on. However, the competitive bidding system would not apply to custom wheelchairs, which is discussed later in this article. It should be noted that a couple of years before its initiation, Peter Cramton, a professor of economics at the University of Maryland, with a specialty in bids and auctions, explained in a letter to CMS and Congress, signed by 167 other auction experts, that this system had so many poor facets in its structure and certainly was not the correct way to set up a bid system and would ultimately fail.

Since the creation of this competitive bidding system 8 years ago, it went into full effect in July 2014 for more than 90 percent of the country. The day after its initiation, more than 93 percent of the medical equipment dealers in America were no longer able to bill Medicare for equipment. Think about the local pharmacy or small surgical supply dealer that sells canes or rents hospital beds; they no longer have that ability. Evaluees are forced to find on the Internet a list of the 10 to 20 closest Medicare-approved dealers now available to them. With any luck, one to three of those dealers on that list are located within 50 miles of the evaluee; the rest are located in other states or parts of the country.

You would then imagine that the few dealers who won bids are the luckiest in that they now have received a growth of over 400 percent in referrals. The only problem is, Medicare now pays these dealers 40 to 45 percent less than the already historically low allowable prices from the last 10 years for both rental and purchases of equipment. Even though the dealers' growth in sales is significantly higher, their actual profit is negligible. Also, along with this substantial growth was a need to hire more customer service representatives and billing personnel to intake the increased orders, as well as to obtain the even more regulatory paperwork that Medicare now demands before it pays an equipment claim.

So where has this led? Hundreds of small dealers who lost their bids have closed their businesses in the last 2 years; others are struggling to exist. Hospital discharge staff now routinely spends 30 to 50 minutes on hold just to take in orders with one of the few dealers left in the country. Equipment that used to be delivered on the same day now takes days for delivery; many times, the patient is asked to even pick up the equipment.

Another more telling example: One of the largest dealers in the Long Island area of New York (one of the most populous parts of the country) who won their bid found its growth in sales skyrocket so fast, they could not keep up with fulfilling orders. Within 1 year, the dealer closed because of total profit loss. This in turn has increased more pressure on the remaining dealers in the New York area to service its population.

For its part, Medicare has reported only positive outcomes from the competitive bidding system imposed, citing cost savings in the 100 million dollar range. It should be noted that the entire medical equipment industry accounts for less than 2 percent of the entire Medicare budget. Further, it has been surmised that had Medicare lessened by 2 percent, it would have saved the same amount or even more money without compromising evaluees' accessibility to services.

Ongoing, the Medicare program has continually written more regulations, demanding additional paperwork, necessitating inappropriate data and letters from doctors, who, in general, have little to no education or detailed knowledge about wheelchair mobility, as an example. Subsequently, this has led to delaying delivery of complex wheelchair orders 3 to 6 months before actual delivery of the product. Many times, through Medicare's audit process, the dealer neglected to dot an "I" or cross a "T," so Medicare simply subtracts what it pays for the chair (complex chairs can cost $15,000 to $25,000 with tilt and recline) and informs the dealer it can protest the rebate through an administrative proceeding. Currently, that administrative proceeding has a higher than 4-year backlog of more than 300,000 claims.

As of January 1, 2016, Medicare did what it was mandated not to do when it created the competitive bidding system: It utilized prices from bids for standard equipment instead of utilizing prices for complex manual and power chairs. Medical equipment dealers will now be paid on 119 parts and accessories prices that are now 25 to 40 percent lower than previous Medicare allowables. As of the printing of this article, there are many complex medical equipment dealers who do not know whether they will be able to either supply or repair an evaluee's power chair through the Medicare program.

How are these regulations affecting the life care planning industry? In terms of Medicare set-aside funds, planners are now partitioning some of an evaluee's settlement away, with the premise that Medicare may have to be reimbursed in the future for equipment purchases. This will be funds that the evaluee will be unable to use, yet there is a very strong likelihood (unless major changes are instituted) that the evaluee will never receive the appropriate equipment; or, even more problematic is the fact that the Medicare program only allows the evaluee a far lesser piece of equipment both in quality and medically needed features that the program no longer covers.

What can life care planners do to assure that the client will receive the appropriate, medically needed equipment? This article is merely a beginning to enlighten life care planners. It is vitally important that, when preparing life care plans, you approach your research process on including the appropriate equipment, the cost for that equipment, as well as including a strong rationale for the specific, appropriate equipment, thereby assuring that the Medicare set-aside funds are adequately funded. Another step that should be taken is by educating the industry as to what is occurring now as it pertains to the medically needed/appropriate equipment. By "industry," I am referring not only to life care planners, but also Medicare set-aside specialists, medical providers, insurers, attorneys, and mediators. Education comes in many formats, not only by this article, but also in future literature, at future conferences, by word of mouth, and to initiate petitions for change.

References

Amsterdam, P. 2001. Rehabilitation equipment needs in life care plans. *Academy Letter, International Academy of Life Care Planners*, *4*, 2–3.

Amsterdam, P. 2002. Setting standards of protocol for replacement schedules of medical equipment in a life care plan. *Journal of Life Care Planning, 1*, 275–283.

Centers for Medicare and Medicaid Services. 1997, June; reprinted July 2002. Manual wheelchair base definitions (Chap. 9). *DMERC Supplier Manual*. www.cms.hhs.gov.

Consortium for Spinal Cord Medicine. 1999. *Tables of Expected Functional Outcomes Clinical Practice Guidelines* (pp. 13–20). Washington, DC: Paralyzed Veterans of America.

Cooper, R., Gonzalez, J., Lawrence, B., Renschler, A., Boninger, M., & Van Sickle, D. 1997. Performance of selected lightweight wheelchairs on ANSI/RESNA tests. *Archives of Physical Medicine and Rehab, 78*, 1138–1144.

Gass, J., & Gonzalez, T. 2001. Using the life care plan to defend damage claims. In *General Cologne Re's Guide to Injury Management (Vol. 3), Life Care Planning* (pp. 27–29). www.gcr.com.

Glynn, G., & Davis, L. 2001. Physician directed life care planning: The concept, creation and challenge. In *General Cologne Re's Guide to Injury Management (Vol. 3), Life Care Planning* (p. 12). www.gcr.com.

Graham-Field. 2002. *Product Warranty Information*. Atlanta, GA. (800) 347-5678. https://www.medicalsupplydepot.com.

Invacare Corporation. 2002. *Product Order Form Information*. Elyria, OH. (800) 333-6900. www.invacare.com.

Johnson, D. 1996. Simplified strength tests for manual wheelchairs for developing countries. In *RESNA Proceedings* (p. 159). www.dinf.ne.jp/doc/english/Us_Eu/conf/resna96/page159.htm.

Kendall, S., & Deutsch, P. 2002. Research methodology for life care planners. *Journal of Life Care Planning, 1*, 157–168.

Neulicht, A., Riddick-Grisham, S., Hinton, L., Costantini, P., Thomas, R., & Goodrich, B. 2002. Life care planning survey 2001: Process, methods, protocols. *Journal of Life Care Planning, 1*, 97–148.

NRRTS. 2003. *CRTS Directory*. National Registry of Rehabilitation Technology Suppliers, www.nrrts.org.

O'Leary, J., & Sarkarati, M. 2000. Aging with SCI. *The Interdisciplinary Journal of Rehabilitation*. www.rehapub.com.

Pride Mobility Products Corporation. 2002. *Order Form Information*. Exeter, PA. (800) 800-8596. www.pridemobility.com.

Stewart, T. 1992. *Physiological Aspects of Immobilization and Beneficial Effects on Passive Standing*. www.lifestandusa.com.

Sunrise Medical. 2002. *Product Order Form Information*. Carlsbad, CA. (760) 930-1500. www.sunrisemedical.com.

Tech Act. 1988. Technology-Related Assistance for Individuals with Disabilities Act of 1988, PL 100-407, Section 3.

TiSport. 2002. *Product Information*. Kennewick, WA. (509) 586-6117. www.tisport.net.

Vitek, M., Cooper, R., Renschler, A., Algood, D., Ammer, W., & Wolf, E. 2001. *Static, Impact and Fatigue Testing of Five Different Types of Electric Powered Wheelchairs*. Department of Rehabilitation and Technology, University of Pittsburgh (RESNA slide presentation). www.wheelchairnet.org.

Chapter 32

Home Assessment in Life Care Planning*

Jim Karl and Roger O. Weed

Contents

Introduction 787
Home Assessment in Life Care Planning 788
Selection of Qualifying Professional or Company to Perform the Home Assessment 788
Home Assessment Process 789
General Assessment Overview 790
I. Entrance to Home, Covered Transfer Areas, and Fire Safety Exit 790
II. Access throughout the Home 792
III. Bedroom 793
IV. Bathroom 794
V. Kitchen 796
VI. Laundry Room 797
VII. Assistive Technology 797
Conclusion 797
References 798

Introduction

Of the originally published life care planning format, two pages or categories, Home Furnishings and Accessories, and Architectural Renovations, were dedicated to addressing requirements associated with living at home for clients with catastrophic injuries or complex chronic health care needs (Deutsch & Raffa, 1981; Deutsch & Sawyer, 1985). The category related to home furnishings is generally understood to incorporate equipment and supplies, typically of a "medical" nature, such as durable medical equipment and other required equipment. Examples include specialized beds

* Reprinted from Karl, J. & Weed, R. Home Assessment in Life Care Planning. *Journal of Life Care Planning*, 5, 159–171, 2007. With permission.

and skin care mattresses, patient lift systems, and portable ramps (Deutsch & Sawyer, 1985; Weed & Field, 2001; Weed & Berens, 2006). Similarly, the category related to architectural renovations provides for permanent alterations or modifications to a structure. Examples include accessible bathrooms, accessible entrances, wider doorways, modified kitchens, changed floor coverings, and so on. However, in many situations, an existing structure may require such extensive modifications that the task is impossible to achieve or the cost–benefit analysis results in a decision to design and build a new home that more appropriately fits the client's needs.

The life care planner must also recognize that some clients will not have the funding to fully achieve recommended modifications or housing design, and such home furnishings and architectural renovations recommendations should be prioritized based on the level of necessity to achieve maximum value. This chapter will offer an overview of a suggested life care planning process for home assessments, including the recommended qualifications of the professional on whom the life care planner may rely for appropriate home assessment recommendations.

Home Assessment in Life Care Planning

Qualified life care planners are trained to evaluate a client's needs for specialized housing and home modifications in addition to future medical care and other factors (Deutsch & Sawyer, 1985; Weed & Field, 2001; Grisham, 2004; Weed, 2004). Example conditions that may merit evaluation for specialized home equipment, renovations, or environmental requirements include spinal cord injury (Ford & Duckworth, 1987; Winkler & Deming, 2004; Winkler & Weed, 2004a), amputation (Meier, 2018; Meier & Weed, 2004), brain injury (Ripley & Weed, 2004; Savage et al., 2004; Weed & Berens, 2006), burns (Brown et al., 2004; Sheridan & Fox, 2004), cerebral palsy/neurodevelopmental disabilities (Neufeld et al., 2004), visual impairments (Winkler & Weed, 2004b), geriatrics/elder care (McCollom, 2004), and any other disability or condition that impairs daily living functioning. Requirements can range from relatively inexpensive equipment to a complete rebuild of the home.

Selection of Qualifying Professional or Company to Perform the Home Assessment

In the authors' opinion and based on their professional experiences, the assessment of home needs can be one of the most critical areas of the life care plan and can potentially be one of the most expensive. Proper design for function, safety, hygiene, independence, attendant care, transfer, and other activities need to be taken into full consideration. A general contractor, without appropriate knowledge, may look at the home and see the need for door widening, ramping, and possibly a roll-in shower, but likely will miss fire safety exits, adequate door header height for accessible van for covered transfer, interior flooring issues, accessible kitchen, office areas, client mobility and function, and so on.

In many cases, if not most, the entire home will need to be designed specifically to accommodate the client, giving consideration to their function, range of motion, and abilities. (Note: There may be occasions when a client will not require access to a second floor or a basement, so in some circumstances it may be justifiable to limit the assessment to the client's main living area.) Although the bathroom could be designed with a roll-in shower, the size of the shower will depend on the size of the individual, the type of shower chair, care attendant assistance requirements, and other factors. However, if the recommendation for the client is to include warm water therapy, then an

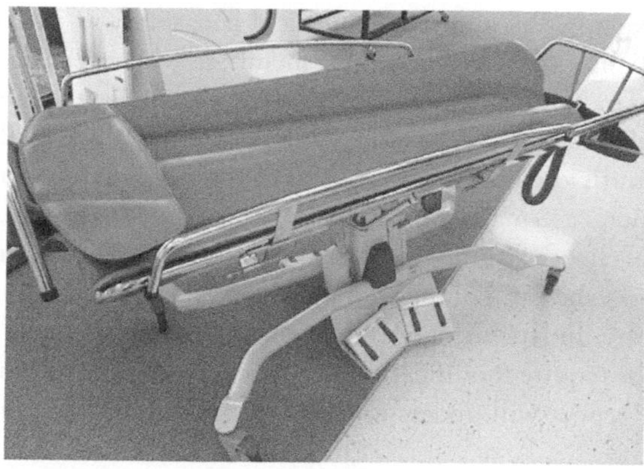

Figure 32.1 Shower Trolley. (Photo by Jim Karl.)

overhead transfer system and bathtub sized to accommodate the client would be the better option rather than a roll-in shower. Another option may be the Shower Trolley, the latest bath item for individuals who are tetraplegic who require full bathing assistance (see Figure 32.1). The Shower Trolley lays flat and will allow an attendant to turn the client on each side for full bathing and skin inspection. The trolley, which retails for $8,000 and up, requires a larger space than a roll-in shower plus a specific bathroom to accommodate care. An overhead transfer system is usually installed for transfer. The person performing the home assessment must be cognizant of such options.

As the reader may begin to understand, selecting a professional or company knowledgeable of all the options for home modifications and design is critical. Equally important is the professional's ability to have proper understanding of the client's situation in order to support their assessment report and defend it, particularly if the life care plan is utilized in personal injury litigation or workers' compensation cases. Suggested credentials for a home assessment professional include a Certified Environmental Access Consultant/CEAC (http://www.accesshomeamerica.com/ceac.asp), Accessible Home Improvement of America/AHIA (a division of VGM oversees its programs for certified providers and contractors; https://www.vgm.com/pages/who-we-are), or Certified Aging in Place Specialist/CAPS by the National Home Builders Association (www.nahb.org). There are also some architects and licensed general contractors (GC) who specialize in handicap accessible renovations or construction. Networking with peers who have had positive experiences with successful home assessments/modifications also may reveal good options.

Home Assessment Process

The home assessment should consist of a full overview of all the required modifications. To focus solely, as some less knowledgeable consultant might, on the bathroom and ingress or safety exits will leave one with a home that is not properly designed for the individual's function, safety, independence, and general mobility. One way to achieve a proper assessment is to consider that teamwork is a must. In these authors' opinion, it is important that the life care planner supply the home assessment consultant with as much information as possible, describing the client's physical functioning and range of motion, relevant mental or cognitive considerations, medical care recommendations, type of equipment used or recommended, level of home attendant care required, hobbies, and any other pertinent information. This information will assist the consultant in comprehensively surveying the home for function and safety. The home assessment should be discussed with the client and available family members whenever possible, to ensure that all relevant details regarding individual needs are considered and included. In the event that the client is temporarily residing elsewhere, such as a hospital or extended care facility, it is recommended that a meeting with the individual be arranged prior to the home assessment. A family member of the client, life care planner, case manager, occupational therapist, and, in some cases, an assistive technology expert and the client's attorney also may be included in the assessment process. Typically, the assessment will take on the form of questions and answers for each design area as to function, space, usable design, safety, independence, and attendant care assistance. In these authors' view, all home areas that do not require modification for the client should be so noted in the assessment so that the reader of the report will understand that the room or potential modification was not overlooked.

Based on the first author's experience, the usual time required for completion of a comprehensive on-site assessment generally will range from 2 to 4 hours. The typical assessment charged by the first author ranges from a flat rate of $1,800 to $2,800 and includes the time required for an on-site evaluation as well as researching design specifications and a written report. The difference in cost relates to the complexity and design sophistication requirements. When charging by the hour, the estimated range in the metropolitan Atlanta, Georgia, area is $150 to $180 per hour.

As the reader can imagine, trying to modify an existing home can be very challenging and, if the home is too small, adding on or designing a new home to properly allow maximum function, safety, and independence may be more cost-effective. However, with today's pricing, in the first author's experience, approximately 30 percent of the remodeling costs are for demolition and restructure to allow for the new modifications. In many cases, the funds directed toward demolition would be better spent on new construction since renovations and modification often have trade-offs and do not entirely meet the needs of the client. In addition, some homes, when modified, become much more expensive than other houses in the neighborhood, and this can complicate recapturing the home's value when resold. That is, the same modified home in a "better" neighborhood potentially would sell at a higher price.

General Assessment Overview

The following is a guide to a general *overview* of a home assessment and suggests possible modifications for each area. As noted earlier, client specifics will ultimately determine the actual home assessment report and the project cost range for each area. The authors note that the following list provides examples and is not inclusive of all options available to create the most accessible home.

I. Entrance to Home, Covered Transfer Areas, and Fire Safety Exit

A. Ramps

Areas with a rise of 30″ or less are appropriate for ramping. Several types of ramping can be developed and will be dependent on the style of home, location of ramp, and homeowners' association requirements, if applicable. Aluminum ramping with handrails is preferred to wooden ramping for longevity, ease of maintenance, and safety. Other types of ramping include concrete and other solid surface products. The general cost consideration for ramping is $150 per foot installed plus any additional site preparation work that may be required.

B. Porch Lifts

Areas over 30″ in height or with limited space, such as inside of a garage, can be modified by using a porch lift (see Figure 32.2). When using a porch lift, it is important to always have a permanent type of ramp that can be used as an emergency exit in the event the porch lift malfunctions or the power supply is cut. The cost of the porch lift is approximately $6,800 or more depending on height and site preparation. Basement access from a deck off the main floor is also possible using a porch lift. The unit can accommodate up to 12 feet. Basements are good options for storm protection.

C. Fire Safety Exits

Exits that require access through a kitchen, carport, or garage, or past a gas furnace that is sometimes located in a hall will not qualify as safety exits, as these areas are the most likely to be involved in a fire. A preferred location is directly out of the bedroom or within 25′ of the bedroom where the client sleeps. The cost to install a fire safety exit varies widely depending on exterior door installation requirements (moving electrical wire in walls, structural supports, brick or block exterior rather than wood or stucco, etc.), amount and style of ramping, and site preparation. At the low end, an uncomplicated exterior door installed would be about $2,400.

D. Covered Transfer Areas

The size of the client's van will determine the door header height of the garage. Keep in mind the size of the chair and age of the client as well. If the size of the chair or function of the

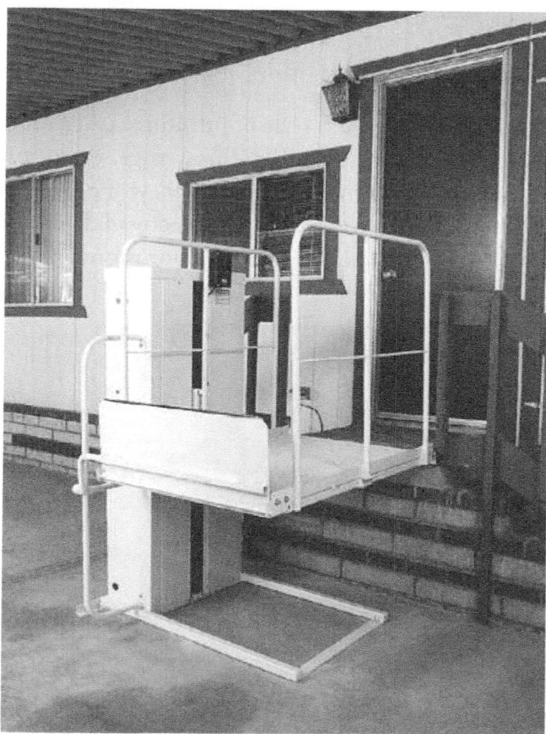

Figure 32.2 Mac's Porch Lift. (Photo from www.macslift.com.)

client will change or limit the movement of the head, the style of van and correspondingly the size of the covered structure (carport or garage) may change. In general, the garage door height should be designed for the taller van and would typically require at least a 9′ door header. Also, should the home be sold, the taller door header will open up the market to all clients with similar needs. Another consideration is that, due to the size of many handicap-accessible vans, additional concrete for backing up and parking likely will need to be installed to accommodate the reduced maneuverability of larger vehicles. Further, the van that has a side-landing platform will limit the space availability for another car in the garage, and the entry door location into the home will also determine the function of the van in the garage.

II. Access throughout the Home

A. Type of Mobility Equipment Used for Assistance

The type of floor covering, width of hall, width of door openings, and location of doors are considerations for using mobility equipment in the home. Not all areas of the home can be widened. Following is a description of possible options for in-home access.

B. Two-Story or Basement Access Required

Possible options for home access include stair lifts inside the home (see Figure 32.3), incline platform lifts, and elevators or porch lifts. As mentioned earlier, there should be a direct exit out of the client's living area without having to use the mechanical device for maximum safety.

C. General Maneuvering around the Home

The size of rooms will depend on the type and style of furniture, space for transfers, flooring, width and length of hallways and any turns, trip hazards, throw rugs, extension cords, and location of required controls (i.e., thermostats). Automatic door openers will provide major improvements for independence. Additionally, some clients will require voice-activated home automation systems (see, for example, assistive technology in the following sections for more on this topic).

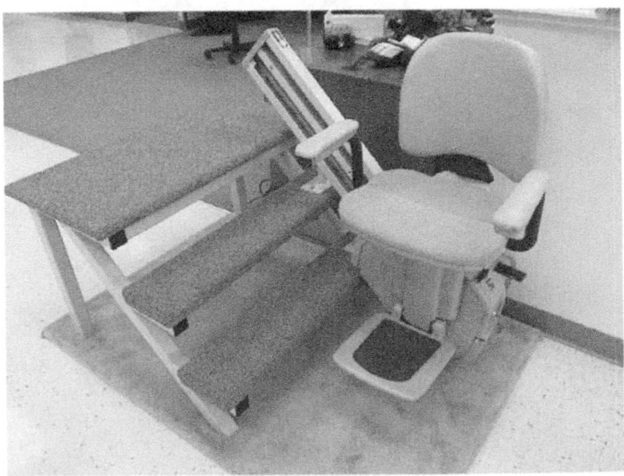

Figure 32.3 Stair Chair. (Photo by Jim Karl.)

III. Bedroom

The size and layout of the client's bedroom will be directly affected by the type of equipment required, size of the client's wheelchair, level of attendant care, and method of transfers. Following are some considerations to be addressed:

A. Adequate space by the bed is the first consideration because transfers can be assisted, unassisted, or involve specialty requirements that could increase the complexity of the room design. This would in turn necessitate special attention to room specifications.
B. Attention to possible specialty lighting requirements, additional heat sources, or additional electrical outlets for the client's equipment, and the location of each.
C. Some clients, such as one who is ventilator dependent, will require a backup generator for emergency power to operate equipment during a power outage.
D. Overhead transfer systems exist that can reduce the number of people needed to transfer a client to a chair, bathroom, or other locations in the home (see Figure 32.4). Certain designs allow for moving from room to room even with doorways between the rooms. Some lift systems have a hand control that a client with adequate function can use without assistance. Overhead lifts start at about $5,200 installed but will increase in cost based on the complexity of installation (such as ceiling supports and doorways), track, and run.

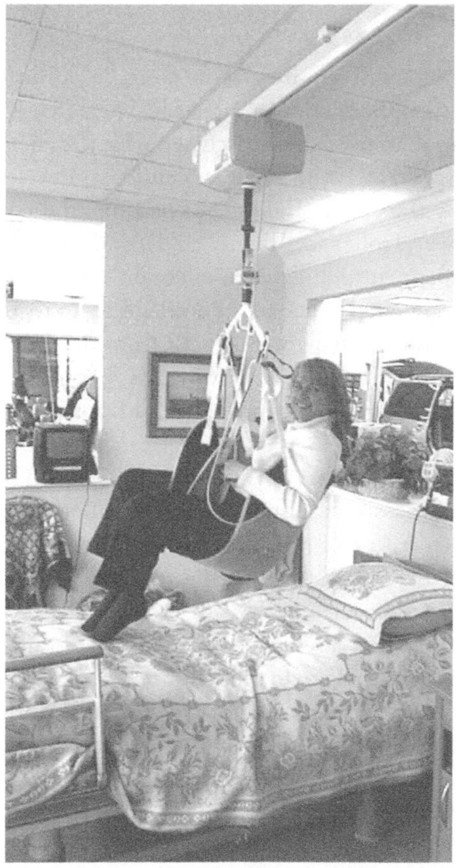

Figure 32.4 Ceiling-mounted powered lift with battery backup. (Photo by Jim Karl.)

E. For clients with adequate functional ability, clothing storage to include accessible closet and custom-designed dresser drawers will be needed. The dresser can be designed with easy pull-out drawers at wheelchair height and hanging rods that can be lowered or reinstalled in the closet at wheelchair height. The cost of the glides to be added to a drawer is about $50 per pair. Closets that incorporate motorized technology to reduce physical effort or enhance access can also be employed.

F. If extra space is required to accommodate therapy equipment that has been recommended by the OT and physician, a fold-down therapy table is an option that will reduce the amount of space needed. Cost of a fold-down therapy table depends primarily on size and can be expected to range from $850 to $1,800.

G. The home should have a fire safety exit that does not require going through the kitchen, through a garage, or past a furnace room. If a functional fire safety exit is not possible, a new home that provides a safe environment is strongly recommended. Many clients require substantially more time to exit a home (especially if in bed) or need an attendant to transfer. A plan for safe egress cannot be emphasized enough.

H. General room design to include a $14' \times 16'$ room size is a good reference point. Small rooms can limit wheelchair function beside the bed and access to storage in addition to increasing safety issues in patient transfers.

IV. Bathroom

The bathroom, like the bedroom, will require specific design modifications such as adequate room size, type of equipment, bathing options, and required assistance that is individualized to the client's specific needs. All of these variables need to be discussed with the client, health care providers, and probably family members (especially if the client is a child) to develop the bathroom design and safety of function required by the client. The type of bathing and equipment required, such as a tilt-back shower chair, a Shower Trolley (see Figure 32.1), and specialized care when bathing (i.e., clients who are ventilator dependent), all have an effect on the size and design of the bathroom. Due to convection cooling, a wet client who has reduced ability to regulate body temperature (such as a client with a spinal cord injury) likely will benefit from overhead infrared heat lamps if it is possible to install these. The cost of a tilt-back shower chair begins at about $2,100, and a Shower Trolley retails for $8,000 and up. Following are some additional considerations to be addressed in the bathroom:

A. Independence, or need for assistance and the level of functional ability, will affect the room dimension requirements. A rule of thumb is the more assistance that is required, the larger the room size. Additionally, the presence and location of specialized equipment for optimum use can dictate room dimensions.

B. Grab bars, if needed, will require careful assessment of their locations. Furthermore, most walls will require the installation of backing to properly anchor the bar. The standard grab bars range from about $50 to $60 and decorative models can cost up to $300, not including installation. Note that installation costs for most of the entries are not included because every situation is different. For example, a grab bar cannot be bolted to an older plastic tub or shower. Therefore, a rebuild of the tub or shower would need to be added to the cost of the grab bar.

C. Toileting options

   1. High-rise toilets can be stand-alone (expect about $285 plus installation) or specialized products that fit over existing toilets (cost ranges from $85 to $200). Also, electric toilet

lift seats that help a client rise to a standing position can be helpful to someone who has reduced function (e.g., elderly) and range in cost from $750 to $1,800.

2. The amount of space required for the client's wheelchair to be placed next to the toilet will be determined by method of client transfer. For example, a client with a spinal cord injury at, say, the T12 level, will likely be able to transfer him- or herself with the aid of grab bars by placing the wheelchair alongside the toilet. A client who needs some personal assistance such as "stand and pivot" to the toilet may need less room but will benefit from at least one grab bar. A client who utilizes a Hoyer or overhead lift will need enough room for two people (also see #3).
3. There are specific floor lifts that are designed for assisting caregivers with client toileting. The lift is designed to provide for seated to seated transfers with the function of the lift to raise the individual to a partial standing position. These specialty lifts greatly assist with the removal of garments in toileting and are known as standing aid lifts. The cost, at the low end, is about $3,800. The Barrier Free lift is another option and lists for about $6,800.
4. Open-bottom shower chairs have proven popular for double duty as a toileting aid, as well as shower assist. Cost begins at $980.
5. Overhead transfer systems may reduce attendant care requirements (previously mentioned since they can be useful in many areas of the home).

D. Bathing options
1. A walk-in bathtub with a high built-in seat adds increased safety for elderly persons or those with limited mobility/balance. However, the individual must have enough function to make a 3″ step into the unit. Cost is approximately $6,500 plus installation.
2. Roll-in showers are popular, but the dimensions will depend on the size of the client, required assistance in bathing, and type of shower chair. The minimum recommended size is 4′ × 5′. The shower unit by Best Bath is a modular unit that has several full roll-in model sizes available and has a ¾″ plywood reinforced wall structure to allow for installation of grab bars. Prices vary according to size and style but could be budgeted beginning at $4,400 plus installation costs.
3. If therapy bathtubs are recommended, the installation of an overhead transfer system is usually required for safe transfers. The system track design can be developed to allow for direct transfers from bed to therapy tub, thereby providing maximum ease, safety, and function.
4. As mentioned earlier, the newest item for bathing that facilitates client positioning and reduces attendant requirements is the Shower Trolley. This equipment allows care assistants to fully bathe and inspect all areas for skin breakdown and achieve maximum hygiene for individuals requiring this level of care. Due to the size and function of this unit, special attention is required during the bathroom design process to assure adequate room to maneuver the device with a client in a prone or supine position.

E. Additional storage area(s) for personal items, supplies, and equipment is a common need for individuals with a disability. An additional storage area should be designed for ease of independent usage, as appropriate, or according to the client's or caregiver's capabilities.

F. Roll-under sink and vanity area: The vanity area should have a cultured marble vanity top with a built-in sink to provide a smooth, flat surface to set and reach items, as well as a sink location. Cultured marble allows for a specific design and placement of the sink, which is an integral part of the product (no seams) and can be fabricated for clearance for roll-under access. The vanity should have full pull-out drawers for easy access, and the faucet can be located to the side of the sink if limited reach is an issue. Typically recommended is a single-lever faucet or an automatic turn-on faucet with a longer spout and angle to direct the water flow toward the center of the sink for easier water flow onto hands. The vanity mirror should be positioned to allow for seated viewing.

G. Flooring: Nonslip floor tile is the ideal surface as tile will generally withstand a wet environment without damage. Sheet vinyl floors typically will develop mold and mildew, as well as other problems, if not properly sealed and maintained. Allure is a solid vinyl that has no added backing and will not deteriorate like other vinyl flooring.
H. Minimum bathroom size is 10′ × 10′, although most bathrooms designed for clients are larger. The flooring should be moisture resilient and easily cleaned as hygiene issues and spills are likely to occur. Tile flooring is not recommended in areas outside bathroom as moving a wheelchair over grout lines causes jarring. Solid surface Allure Solid vinyl flooring is an excellent floor option.

V. Kitchen

The kitchen is an area that can be designed to provide for full function or a special function depending on the client's capabilities. The size of the kitchen will vary depending on the client's needs, as well as on the adjacent room. If the area is combined with, say, an eat-in kitchen and with open access, the kitchen may not require as much room as one that is in a room that is self-contained. In general, an open space of 5′ is needed for maneuverability and access. If the kitchen is self-contained, expect at least a size of 9′ × 14′. Areas of consideration for the kitchen are as follows:

A. Roll-under sink for clients who are wheelchair reliant but have enough functional abilities for independence.
B. Lowered food preparation surfaces so that clients can perform tasks from a seated position.
C. Roll-under electric cooktop is preferred. For safety reasons, a gas stove is not recommended for use by individuals with a disability or mobility impairment. The style of cooktop that is recommended by the first author is one by Fisher & Paykel, which will contain a spill of a half-gallon of liquid over the surface. This is an obvious major safety feature when cooking. Also, for clients who are able to cook, the controls must be located on the side so the person does not have to reach over the burners to operate the stove. The cost for a Fisher & Paykel cooktop is about $1,300. Look for one that has a small side trim around the top.
D. A raised dishwasher for easier function or the Fisher & Paykel dish drawer unit, which pulls out like a drawer, is recommended. The cost for a single-drawer model is about $1,100, and the two-drawer model is about $1,600.
E. A built-in oven with a side-opening door that is located at proper seated height (rather than a standard pull-down oven door) may be indicated depending on the client's abilities. Expect to pay $3,000 for a Bosch model.
F. Base cabinets with full pull-out extension drawers with taller than typical sides provide ease of access for clients. These are designed for dish and cooking utensil storage and pantry items and often have built-in guides for organizing utensils and dishes.
G. Switch controls for garbage disposal, lights, and so on, at the front of the cabinet for seated height, may be indicated.
H. Solid surface countertops for movement of items such as heated items and water may be required.
I. Adequate floor space and movement radius are critical and are dependent on client size, functional needs, and other factors.

VI. Laundry Room

This area can be designed for wheelchair function or for care attendant function or can be left as standard. Lowered roll-under folding surface to allow clients to sort and fold clothes from a seated position would be beneficial. Installing a wash sink is also recommended to assist with prep.

Types of possible modifications:

A. Raised front-loading washer and dryer units have become mainstream, and several models and features are available. Expect to pay about $2,000 or more for a pair, not including delivery. Pedestal style may be extra.
B. Lowered roll-under folding surface to allow client to sort and fold clothes from a seated position may be indicated.
C. Wheelchair-accessible hanging rack so client can reach and hang clothes to dry.
D. Accessible storage area for cleaning items.
E. Adequate floor space for ease of movement.

VII. Assistive Technology

The utilization of technology-based items can give independence back to individuals for specific functions that would otherwise not be possible (for more information on this topic, visit the Center for Assistive Technology and Environmental Access at www.catea.org). Environmental control units (ECUs), sometimes referred to as electronic aids for daily living (EADLs), are designed to allow individuals to perform daily routines and operate various household items in their home via technology-based products (Gilman, 2007). The technology, when incorporated with a computer system, can allow for complete home automation. Available computer system software packages can accommodate individual function including voice activation and automation, character recognition, control of household items, and much more. Some examples of independence through technology that can be achieved include turning on and off lights, dialing and answering the telephone, typing letters or other documents, sending a fax, taking care of personal finances, controlling the TV/DVD/CD player/stereo, opening outside doors, and adjusting the bed. By utilizing assistive technology, the client's level of independence not only reduces attendant care needs but also increases the client's self-worth and self-esteem as major benefits. Costs range from a few hundred dollars to more than $13,000 for full home automation.

Conclusion

The proper design of a client's living environment is critical for independence, function, safety, hygiene, and care attendance, as well as general enjoyment and quality of life. Sometimes an existing home will not accommodate the required modifications, or the expense for renovations will be unreasonable when considering demolition expenses or the house value after modification in relation to other homes in the neighborhood. On those occasions, the design of a new home will be more cost-effective and will provide for a much better level of safety and function. The new or modified home, depending on the client's specific factors and requirements, may be the home in which they reside to old age. The areas listed in this chapter may have the additional need to be designed to allow for the client's aging and deteriorating functional abilities and subsequent modifications.

In addition to aging considerations, the client's home, especially for one who has significant limitations, likely will be the environment in which most of his or her time will be spent. For this reason alone, safety, function, and comfort are of paramount concern. Adequate assessment not only provides the foundation to improve or modify the client's environment to meet essential needs, but can reduce the cost of care, decrease complications, provide safer surroundings, and improve one's quality of life and well-being, even as the client ages. This chapter was intended to familiarize the life care planner with the importance of utilizing an appropriately certified or qualified home assessment consultant who will consider and incorporate, as part of a comprehensive assessment, the topics and issues presented in this chapter.

References

Brown, M., Helm, P., & Weed, R. 2004. Life care planning for the burn patient. In R. Weed (Ed.), *Life Care Planning and Case Management Handbook* (2nd ed, pp. 351–380). Boca Raton, FL: CRC Press.

Deutsch, P., & Raffa, F. 1981. *Damages in Tort Action*. New York, NY: Matthew Bender.

Deutsch, P., & Sawyer, H. 1985, rev. 2005. *Guide to Rehabilitation*. New York, NY: Matthew Bender.

Ford, J., & Duckworth, B. 1987. *Physical Management for the Quadriplegic Patient*. Philadelphia, PA: F. A. Davis.

Gilman, D. 2007. *Electronic Aids to Daily Living*. Retrieved February 12, 2007, from www.abilityhub.com/ecu/index.htm.

Grisham, S. 2004. The role of the life care planner in pediatric life care planning. In S. Grisham (Ed.), *Pediatric Life Care Planning and Case Management* (pp. 47–91). Boca Raton, FL: CRC Press.

McCollom, P. 2004. Application of life care planning principles in elder care management. In R. Weed (Ed.), *Life Care Planning and Case Management Handbook* (2nd ed., pp. 591–611). Boca Raton, FL: CRC Press.

Meier, R. 2018. Life care planning for the amputee. In R. Weed & D. Berens (Eds.), Life Care Planning and Case Management Handbook (4th ed., pp. 335–365). New York: Routledge.

Meier, R., & Weed, R. 2004. Life care planning for the amputee. In R. Weed (Ed.), *Life Care Planning and Case Management Handbook* (2nd ed., pp. 281–312). Boca Raton, FL: CRC Press.

Neufeld, J., Monasterio, E., Livingston, L., Taylor, L., Grisham, S., & Taylor, R. 2004. Life care planning for children with neurodevelopmental disabilities. In S. Grisham (Ed.), *Pediatric Life Care Planning and Case Management* (pp. 421–486). Boca Raton, FL: CRC Press.

Ripley, D., & Weed, R. 2004. Life care planning for acquired brain injury. In R. Weed (Ed.), *Life Care Planning and Case Management Handbook* (2nd ed., pp. 313–350). Boca Raton, FL: CRC Press.

Savage, R., Klingbeil, F., & Fawber, H. 2004. Life care planning for the child with acquired brain injury. In S. Grisham (Ed.), *Pediatric Life Care Planning and Case Management* (pp. 529–552). Boca Raton, FL: CRC Press.

Sheridan, R., & Fox, L. 2004. Life care planning for children with burns. In S. Grisham (Ed.), *Pediatric Life Care Planning and Case Management* (pp. 637–657). Boca Raton, FL: CRC Press.

Weed, R. 2004. Life care planning: Past, present and future. In R. Weed (Ed.), *Life Care Planning and Case Management Handbook*, (2nd ed., pp. 1–13). Boca Raton, FL: CRC Press.

Weed, R., & Berens, D. 2006. Life care planning after TBI: Clinical and forensic issues. In N. Zasler, D. Katz, & R. Zafonte (Eds.), *Neurorehabilitation of Traumatic Brain Injury* (pp. 1223–1240). New York, NY: Demos Medical Publishing.

Weed, R., & Field, T. 2001. *The Rehabilitation Consultant's Handbook* (3rd ed.). Athens, GA: E & F Vocational Services.

Winkler, T., & Deming, L. 2004 Life care planning for the child with spinal cord injury. In S. Grisham (Ed.), *Pediatric Life Care Planning and Case Management* (pp. 375–420). Boca Raton, FL: CRC Press.

Winkler, T., & Weed, R. 2004a. Life care planning for spinal cord injury. In R. Weed (Ed.), *Life Care Planning and Case Management Handbook* (2nd ed., pp. 483–539). Boca Raton, FL: CRC Press.

Winkler, T., & Weed, R. 2004b. Life care planning for the visually impaired. In R. Weed (Ed.), *Life Care Planning and Case Management Handbook* (2nd ed., pp. 571–589). Boca Raton, FL: CRC Press.

Chapter 33

Vehicle Modifications: Useful Considerations for Life Care Planners*

C. Dan Allison, Jr.

Contents

Introduction 799
Safety Factors from a Historical Perspective 800
Structural Factors 801
Customization and Design Issues 803
Industry Safety Standards 803
Selected Cost Estimates 804
Case Study 805
Conclusion 807
Resources 809
References 811

Introduction

Most people with catastrophic injuries or complex health care needs that impact mobility will require specialized transportation adaptations. The needs range from minor modifications to very high tech and custom designed modified vehicles. This chapter, primarily based on a case study, will outline some of the basic issues associated with life care planning and transportation needs, with special emphasis on why some modified vehicles are very expensive to produce.

Transportation and vehicle modifications can be an essential part of the future care planning process to help a person with a disability return to as close to pre-injury status as possible, as well

* Partially adapted from Weed, R. & Engelhart, L. (2005). Vehicle modifications: Useful considerations for life care planners. *Journal of Life Care Planning, 4*(2&3), 115–125.

as provide appropriate transportation and access to the health care system. As noted by Deutsch in 1999, "Life care planning encompasses various topics that assure the effectiveness of the overall plan" (as cited in Weed, 2004, p. 5). An entry commonly included in a life care plan that contributes to the overall effectiveness of the plan is transportation, which often requires specialized evaluation and purchase of equipment (Pierce, 1999; McCaigue, 2004). McCaigue (2004) notes, "Great emphasis is placed on assessing a person's ability to drive," because independent transportation is a basic need for "access to gainful employment and community resources" (pp. 108–109). Additionally, adaptive mobility for people who are mobility-impaired and who will be either a passenger or driver can become a key and costly element in a life care plan. Needs can range from nothing special, to minimal modification (e.g., hand controls or spinner knobs), to vehicles with extensive structural modifications and sophisticated technology. This chapter will highlight factors for life care planners and case managers to consider both when evaluating what type of vehicle a client needs today and estimating his/her future needs and costs. An explanation of why some adaptive driving equipment options are considerably more expensive than others also will be given.

Safety Factors from a Historical Perspective

The history of the U.S. mobility equipment industry highlights safety as a prime factor in the cost of modified vehicles generally and structurally modified vehicles in particular. When adaptive equipment companies emerged as "garage shop" operations during the Vietnam war era, they primarily served veterans with disabilities, many of whom were willing to gain mobility by means that probably would be unimaginable today. For example, a person might have unsafely reclined his or her wheelchair to enter a vehicle and slouched to see through the windshield, or, moreover, did not have any mechanism for securing the wheelchair inside the vehicle. The Veterans Administration (VA) originally was the sole funding source for early vehicle modifications and they, along with some state vocational rehabilitation agencies, began to develop safety guidelines as early as 1972. However, regulation was inconsistent and slow to emerge. From the early 1970s to the mid-1980s, there were no significant changes in the way that a wheelchair driver accessed a vehicle. In the 1980s, the standard vehicle in the mobility industry was the full-size Ford Econoline van, modified either by adding a powered floor pan or by structurally lowering the floor. In 1992, Ford replaced the Econoline's dual front and rear fuel tanks with a single tank located in the center of the chassis to provide more crash protection. This precluded lowering the floor in 1992 and newer Ford E-Series vans. Reportedly, to avoid the appearance of ambivalence toward the disability community, Ford introduced an aft-of-axle fuel tank kit that allowed modifications, including lowered floors. Thus, for the first time in the history of the mobility industry, vehicle builders were able to use a crash-tested fuel system that complied with U.S. Federal Motor Vehicle Safety Standards (FMVSS). In addition, they were becoming increasingly aware of how essential these standards were to consumers' safety. Nevertheless, as the federal government improved accident data collection, it revealed the extent to which the mobility industry still was non-compliant with the FMVSS. The National Mobility Equipment Dealers Association (NMEDA) responded by developing a structural modifier certification, a "Quality Assurance Program," and by conducting crash tests of structurally modified vehicles. Since then, regulation has steadily increased, not only because of the availability of accident data and crash safety testing, but also due to the growing involvement of major automobile manufacturers and conversion vehicle specialists in the structural modification of vehicles. As a result, all types of modified vehicles are becoming safer, although their cost reflects the expense of compliance with rapidly evolving safety standards.

It is important to note that improving regulation and compliance have created a paradox, as reported in a recent *Wall Street Journal* article (Schatz, 2005) that cited "The Exemption from the 'Make Inoperative' Prohibition." This 2001 National Highway Traffic Safety Administration (NHTSA) rule created limited exceptions to the "Make Inoperative" statute, which prohibits the alteration or removal of motor vehicle safety equipment or features that are required pursuant to the FMVSS (National Highway Traffic Safety Administration, 2002). In other words, known safety devices cannot deliberately be altered or removed from a vehicle under ordinary circumstances. However, this exemption allows otherwise prohibited modifications, which, in essence, effectively allows people with disabilities to purchase adapted vehicles. The paradox is that while consumers can now enjoy the independence that mobility affords, their safety may be at stake. This is why it is essential for case managers and life care planners to identify the most technically knowledgeable and dependable modifiers, even though the cost of their products and services may be greater. In 2009, the National Mobility Equipment Dealers Association (NMEDA) established the Compliance Review Program (CRP) to verify that manufacturer's vehicles and/or components meet Federal/Canada Motor Vehicle Safety Standards (F/CMVSS). When a dealer uses vehicles and/or components that have passed the rigid Compliance Review Program process, they are assuring themselves and their customers the product being installed or delivered has been verified to comply with applicable safety standards (NMEDA, 2016).

Structural Factors

For purposes of the below discussion, the following definitions are provided as related to vehicle modifications:

- *Original Equipment Manufacturer (OEM)*: A vehicle manufacturer who performs all manufacturing operations on a motor vehicle up to the point that the vehicle is certified as complying with all applicable Federal Motor Vehicle Standards. (Most commonly referring to Ford, GM, Toyota, Chrysler, etc.)
- *Structural Modifier*: A company that completes alterations to the OEM structure of the vehicle, usually to facilitate access and/or increase headroom. Examples include: Braun, VMI, and ElDorado.
- *Mobility Equipment Dealer*: As used in this document, any individual or business that installs, sells, and services equipment or modifies vehicles for use by people with disabilities as a driver and/or passenger.
- *Non-Structural Modifications*: Include, but are not limited to wheelchair lifts, mechanical or electronic driving aids, wheelchair restraint systems, and interior modifications.
- *Driver Rehabilitation Specialist (DRS)*: An occupational therapist, other health care professional, driver educator, or other professional who is recognized as competent to perform clinical and on-road driver rehabilitation evaluations, as well as design and implement on-road training regimens.
- *Certified Driver Rehab Specialist (CDRS™)*: An individual who has obtained the necessary knowledge base and experience in the field of driver rehabilitation and who has successfully obtained and maintained certification requirements set forth by the Association for Driver Rehabilitation Specialists (ADED).

Most of the vehicles sold by today's mobility dealers are lowered-floor minivans, which dealers purchase from vehicle modifiers who typically use base vehicles manufactured by major automakers such as Ford, Toyota, Chrysler, Honda, and GM.

There are two different entry configurations for lowered-floor minivans: side entry and rear entry. Both have their advantages and disadvantages, which need to be considered for the specific needs of the client. It is important to note that only the side-entry vehicle can be independently driven by a person seated in a wheelchair. The amount that the floor is lowered (10 to 14 inches) effects the entry height which may vary from approximately 54 to 57 inches.

Side-entry minivans also have the advantage of delivering a person using a wheelchair onto various curb heights. Additionally, the person using the wheelchair can select varied locations in which to place the wheelchair inside the vehicle. Other benefits of side-entry vans include:

- *Seating for passengers*: Rear bench seat remains intact.
- *Remote access*: Most side-entry vehicles are accessed by one-touch remote systems.

Disadvantages of a side-entry minivan include:

- *Parking distance*: Most need 5 to 7 feet distance to enter vehicle from the side.
- *Price*: Typically more expensive than rear-entry vehicles.

Rear-entry minivans have the following advantages:

- *Price*: Typically less expensive than side-entry vans or other vehicle conversions.
- *Parking*: More flexibility in parking available as curb-side parking is not required.
- *Modifications*: Less process required for the conversion, lowering cost.

Disadvantages of rear-entry vans include:

- *Driver dependence*: Wheelchair users cannot get into the driver's position, thus are dependent on others to operate the vehicle.
- *Exiting*: The wheelchair user must exit from the rear of the vehicle, which may cause a safety factor in a busy parking lot situation.

Minivans are not the only option for the driver or passenger with a disability. For example, some people would just rather drive a truck. Fortunately, there are adaptations that can make that happen with a Turny or Lift-up Power Mobility Seat combined with a Power Lift mounted in the pickup bed. This solution handles the biggest power chairs (up to 350 lbs). There are even companies that modify pickup trucks and some SUV-type vehicles for occupied wheelchair users—even to be able to drive from while seated in their wheelchair. Even though the Ford Econoline full size vans are no longer in production, there are various new larger vans (Ford Transit, Dodge Ram ProMaster, and the Mercedes Sprinter) just making their way into the mobility industry. While at this time, these larger vans are not appropriate for wheelchair drivers, they are typically accessible without structural modification.

Remember, it is very important for any consumer to make sure and try *any* vehicle and consult with a NMEDA Mobility Equipment Dealer to find the solution suitable for their particular needs prior to purchasing a vehicle. The driver rehabilitation specialist can assist with vehicle selection based on a comprehensive evaluation process and the client's current and future needs.

Mobility equipment dealers sell these vehicles either "as is," or with additional non-structural modifications that are completed by the dealer to meet customers' unique needs as recommended with the help of a CDRS. Some dealers also continue to perform their own structural modifications, thereby "customizing" the vehicle for a particular person and their particular positioning needs.

Customization and Design Issues

The higher cost of a structurally modified van relates in part to the amount of time that engineers and mechanics spend on design requirements. A customer purchasing a vehicle that requires complex modifications will typically need 20 to 40 hours of driver training based on a comprehensive driver evaluation conducted by a driver rehabilitation specialist. Furthermore, once structural modifications are complete, the process of fitting the person to the vehicle is complex and time consuming, but critical to ensuring maximum safety and utility. A quarter of an inch in the location of mechanical or electronic driving aids can make a huge difference for a person with a disability. Therefore, driving aids must be positioned precisely to suit the physical capabilities of a person who may have limited strength or limited range of motion, or both, and even though a passenger vehicle may not present the complexities of a driver vehicle, the person still must be fitted to the vehicle. These driving aids are typically prescribed by a driver rehabilitation specialist based on a comprehensive evaluation and training program conducted with the client.

The delivery fitting is typically performed by the driver rehabilitation specialist, mobility dealer, and client. Fittings can take from a few hours to days and may include adjustments such as replacing the original equipment manufacturer's shoulder belt, or installing a new upper anchorage point for the shoulder belt if the door was raised, or if it required relocation due to the client's size or positioning of the wheelchair. For example, the vehicle had an automatic electric wheelchair lock-down device, and because the client used a powered wheelchair that had complex rehabilitation aids, the modifier spent 2 hours partially disassembling the wheelchair to install a bracket on the bottom. Additional time was required installing the device to the vehicle floor to allow precise placement of the client in his wheelchair.

In addition to ensuring proper vehicle fit, the person with a disability must learn how to get in and out of the vehicle and use equipment specially designed for him or her, and caregivers must be instructed about normal, as well as emergency, use of all equipment. This education process, typically included in the fitting appointment, includes reviewing owner's manuals and completing comprehensive delivery checklists, which ensures that the modifier has provided the purchaser with complete and accurate instructions.

Industry Safety Standards

In 2000, the American National Standards Institute (ANSI) and the Rehabilitation Engineering and Assistive Technology Society of North America (RESNA) jointly created "WC-19" (ANSI/RESNA, 2000). This is a voluntary industry standard for designing and manufacturing a wheelchair that will be used as a seat in a motor vehicle. The goal is to provide an equivalent level of passenger safety for those who ride seated in a wheelchair as is provided for those who sit in standard passenger seats and use standard safety belts.

A WC-19 wheelchair is strong enough to protect the wheelchair user in a wide range of crashes and vehicle maneuvers. To pass WC-19, a wheelchair must perform well in a crash test similar to the tests used to make sure vehicle seats and restraint systems are safe. In laboratory crash tests, a WC-19 wheelchair must not fracture, must provide a stable, supportive seat for the crash test dummy, and must remain well-secured to keep the wheelchair and rider in the vehicle.

WC-19 wheelchairs must also be equipped with four accessible points of securement. This securing method must be easily repeatable so it is relatively quick and easy to secure the wheelchair in the vehicle by the wheelchair user and/or their caregiver.

A WC-19 wheelchair has been checked for stability to improve safety during normal travel. Even if the vehicle is not involved in a crash, wheelchair riders can be hurt when a wheelchair tips over during vehicle turns or sudden stops. The WC-19 standard requires the manufacturer to measure and report the lateral stability of the loaded wheelchair when it is secured and tipped to 45 degrees.

A WC-19 wheelchair has been tested to determine compatibility with vehicle safety belts. Many current wheelchair designs do not allow for good lap/shoulder belt fit. For example, armrests and trunk supports can route vehicle-anchored lap belts away from the strong pelvis and over the soft abdomen, potentially causing injury. WC-19 requires belt fit quality to be measured and reported (using an ABCD scale) in the presale literature. This can help consumers and clinicians select wheelchairs that are safer for travel.

More information can be found at www.rercwts.org (Rehabilitation Engineering Research Center on Wheelchair Transportation Safety).

Considering the complexities of customization and modification, mobility equipment dealers cannot simply charge a fraction over a vehicle's cost. By definition, modifiers are low volume/high expertise businesses, and if they were to apply the standard automobile dealers' high volume/low margin distribution model, they could not deliver the customized service that today's mobility customers demand. In addition, carrying products' liability insurance is a significant consideration these days, even if a vehicle has not undergone extensive modification.

Selected Cost Estimates

According to *USA Today*, the cost of an average vehicle is approaching $34,000 (Healy, 2015). There is a wide variety of modifications that are available to a driver or passenger. Therefore, costs will vary depending on need. For example, a driver with limited arm use may only require a spinner knob for less than $100, while for a driver requiring hand controls the expected cost is between $1,500 and $1,800. Additional equipment or modifications made be required based on client need, for example a person driving with hand controls may also have spasticity, and a pedal block may need to be installed to prevent inadvertent acceleration or braking, or accidental entrapment of the person's foot under the brake pedal. This additional expense is about $475, plus installation. However, just as in all other fields, technology is advancing with hand controls. There are now floor-mounted options, electronic interfaced gas, and steering wheel-mounted accelerator controls. It is an ever-evolving field, and the driver rehabilitation specialists and mobility equipment dealer can provide information and recommendations that are best suited for the individual client's needs.

Modifications can be quite expensive, depending on client's conditions and needs. For example, a driver with C5–6 tetraplegia who can drive independently generally will require at least low-effort steering, a servo gas braking system, and a lowered floor in addition to the standard passenger devices, at a $30,000 to $50,000 higher cost. A driver with a C4–5 injury typically will require servo steering and servo gas brakes, at an estimated $50,000 to $80,000 more than the base cost. As can be seen, costs can easily exceed six figures to have a modified vehicle for an independent driver who uses the full spectrum of high-tech driving aids, such as a hand-operated joystick system and electronic touchpad.

In addition to the upfront costs of obtaining a modified or conversion vehicle, there are additional costs to consider. The annual maintenance costs for a high-tech passenger vehicle will only be slightly higher than for a more conventional vehicle. When the equipment is new and under warranty in years 1 to 3, there should be no cost unless the vehicle experiences extraordinarily hard service. In the author's experience, in year 4, an owner might pay $500 more for maintenance. Maintenance and repairs in year 5 could be an additional $800 should lift repairs be necessary; however, most problems are likely to be minor. Maintenance and repair costs in year 6 will depend on mileage and driving conditions, particularly if the lift and tie-down are exposed to dirt, and then costs could be considerably higher. Note: Some of the equipment, such as lifts and servo driving systems, have a service life expectancy and, due to liability issues, companies will not reinstall them into new vehicles even if they appear to be in good condition, nor repair them if they are beyond the service limits. Reportedly, new requirements for lift systems include cycle counters and a specific maintenance schedule.

Case Study

This case study is an example of how NOT to provide service to a client, but then rectifying it with an ideal outcome using the assistance of an entire team. Norm acquired a C5–6 spinal cord injury and associated inability to drive that resulted from a motor vehicle accident which functionally limits him equivalent to a high-level tetraplegic. He also has limited neck rotation to the left. If able to stand, Norm is approximately 6′2″ and uses a 4-year-old rear-wheel-drive power chair, in which his seated height is 56″.

At his initial driver's evaluation by a Certified Driver Rehabilitation Specialist (CDRS), the recommendations were:

1. Based on observations made during this assessment as discussed in the body of this report, formal driver training is recommended for Norm.

   - It is estimated that 12 hours of training will be appropriate (3 hours on equipment specification in training vehicle, and 9 hours after he gets his own vehicle).
   - Training should be provided by a CDRS or otherwise by an Occupational Therapist qualified in the field of Driver Rehabilitation.

2. At this point, Norm is advised not to drive outside of his formal training.
3. It is recommended that he be advised not to purchase a vehicle until successful completion of his driver training. After successful completion of training, adaptive equipment recommendations for his driving should be provided by the training facility.
4. It is recommended that he have a power wheelchair evaluation to acquire a WC-19 crash-tested wheelchair that is appropriate for his driving needs.

Four months later, before training was authorized, Norm was the recipient of a used wheelchair-accessible minivan from his employer, which was exactly what the previous evaluation recommended against. So, Norm was seen for a follow-up evaluation. While the van did have the appropriate dimensions to allow Norm clear access into the driver's station, it was more than 5 years old, which limited adaptive equipment choices for the servo controls. Had they waited to purchase the van until the training was completed, they could have made a more informed choice of vehicles that would have accommodated the needed adaptive equipment.

The recommendations at this time were:

1. Based on the results of this evaluation, it is recommended that Norm be considered a candidate to receive the adaptive equipment and vehicle modifications listed in the *Vehicle Modification Prescription* attached with this report.
   - The chosen vendor(s) may be contacted to obtain cost quotations and arrange installation and completion of the specified equipment and vehicle modifications.
   - The prescription should be provided in its entirety to the installing vendor.
   - Norm should be advised to have someone drive his vehicle from the vendor to his home after modifications are completed.
2. There should be a functional inspection of the vehicle once modifications are completed and before it is released to him.
   - The Certified Driver Rehabilitation Specialist (CDRS) and a member of the Vocational Rehabilitation (VR) Assistive Technology Division should be contacted by the vendor at least 2 weeks in advance to provide this service.
   - The inspection should include a behind-the-wheel session with Norm to confirm that the adaptive driving equipment is positioned properly for him.
   - The CDRS can be requested to attend any intermediate fitting meetings between Norm and the chosen vendor as needed.
3. Training: Based on observations made during this assessment as discussed in the body of this report, formal driver training is recommended for Norm.
   - It is estimated that 12 to 15 hours of training will be appropriate. This is to be completed in his van after modifications (to include a rental training brake on the right side).
   - Training should be provided by a Certified Driver Rehabilitation Specialist (CDRS) or otherwise by an Occupational Therapist qualified in the field of Driver Rehabilitation.

By the first functional fitting (8 months later), Norm had also received a new mid-wheel-drive wheelchair. While it was a crash-tested wheelchair, it was not suitable to drive from. Recommendations at that time were:

1. A convex mirror (like a FedEx truck) needs to be installed on the right front fender for Norm to be able to see to the left.
2. The air touch accelerator needs to be adjusted to be more sensitive; it has nearly an inch of travel before it is engaged.
3. Turn signals need to be adjusted on the gas/break (G/B) control or moved to the elbow switch.
4. The kneeling system is not working on his van.
5. The right ramp door will not automatically unlock, so Norm is not independent in getting into the van unless he leaves it unlocked.
6. Right armrest fabrication needs to be raised approximately 1.75″, and the elbow switch moved forward (will need to be trialed—but he is currently constantly hitting it).

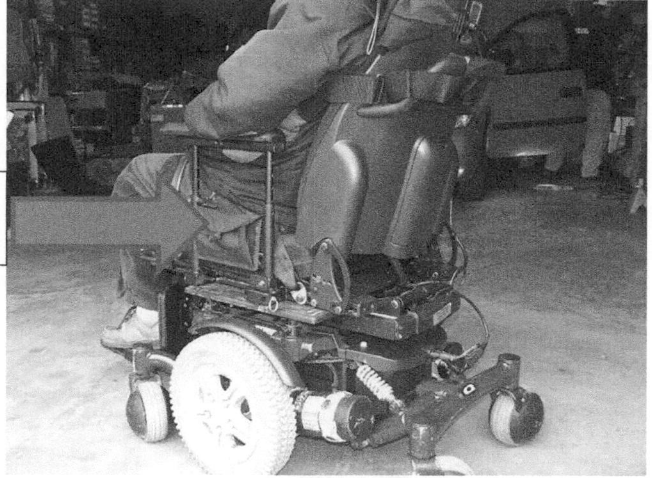
Twin post-style armrests
inhibit lap shoulder belt
path; not allowing seat belt

Figure 33.1 Armrest mount prevents appropriate seat belt path across pelvis.

7. Most importantly: His new power chair is still not safe for him to drive from: (a) the armrests do not allow the seat belt to be used when he drives, (b) now the joystick of the wheelchair hits the G/B control each time he enters—this will destroy either or both his joystick or the air touch; neither of which is a positive thing, and (c) the Ottobock-NuTec/TriQuality posture belt does not fit him correctly (too large) and does not correctly fit the wheelchair.

Three months later, the entire team was able to meet at the vehicle modifiers shop to do a final inspection. The team consisted of the client, the mobility equipment dealer and technician, the wheelchair supplier, the VR assistive technology specialist, and the CDRS.

At that time:

1. Norm's wheelchair armrests were replaced and adjusted so that they allowed for proper fit of his seat belt when in the driver's position.
2. Correct Smart view mirrors and front fender mirror were installed.
3. Vehicle armrest was replaced and adjusted appropriately.
4. Turn signal controls and G/B controls were adjusted correctly

This was an unusual case that lasted almost 2 years. While it is great to have the complete team present in person, this is not typical. It demonstrates the need to have the entire team involved from the initial evaluation. If the original recommendations had been followed, and the team had consulted, this case could have been completed at least a year earlier. This is where case managers can be so beneficial (Figures 33.1 through 33.4).

Conclusion

With the improvement in survival rates and life expectancy of individuals with catastrophic disabilities, as well as an increasing aging population, accessible vehicles are becoming more commonplace, and new products and services are abundant. There are many steps and factors

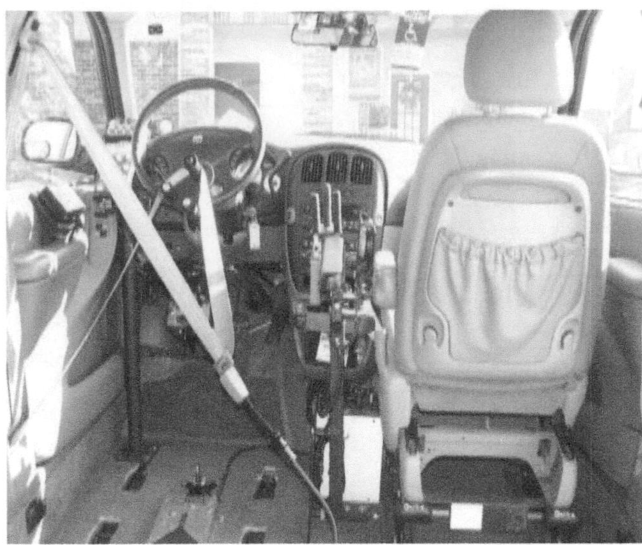

Figure 33.2 Final driver's station with seat belt positioned for Norm to be able to drive into (he is not able to buckle his seat belt independently).

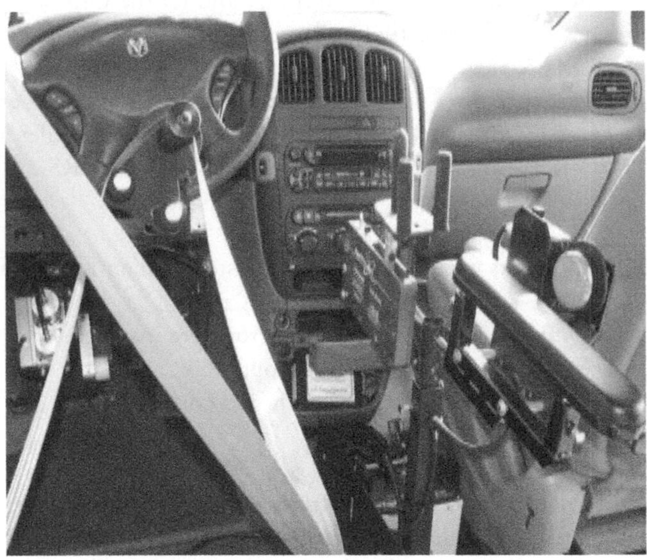

Figure 33.3 Right-side controls for G/B, with armrest, and switch for secondary controls.

involved in obtaining a mobility vehicle as every client brings a unique set of needs for consideration. It is important that the life care planner or case manager consult with all the members of the team when starting the process. Important team members include: physician, allied health providers, driver rehabilitation specialist, mobility equipment dealer, and funding source. Life care planners and case managers can play a key role in ensuring that team members are involved at the proper time in the process. Pediatric client needs, although not specifically included in this chapter, present additional deliberation since size of the child, seriousness of the effects of the disability on

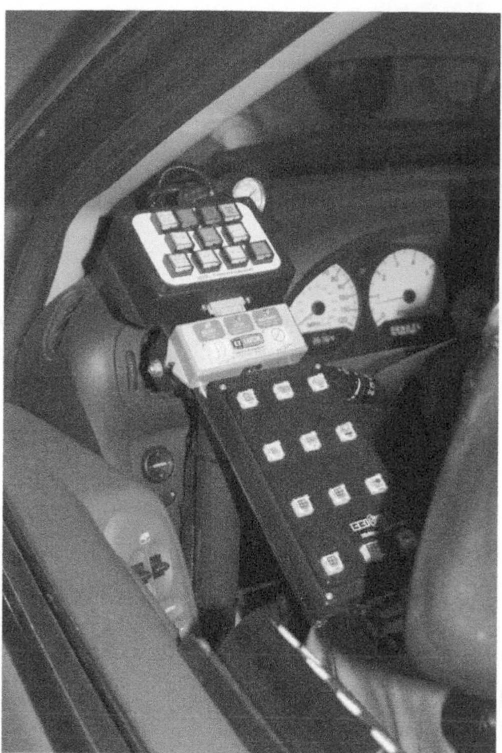

Figure 33.4 Left-side controls for shifter and other controls such as power windows, heat and A/C, and wheelchair docking release.

mobility, and growth factors will determine selection of a vehicle and appropriate modifications. For example, a child who relies on a wheelchair as a positioning seating system will likely require an accessible van earlier than one who can travel comfortably in a booster seat.

Professionalism dictates the importance of teamwork including consultation with a CDRS who can help to ensure that recommendations are appropriate and that competent vendors properly implement the specified modifications. As with any professional specialty area, the life care planner needs to assure competent recommendations with the client's and/or family's participation, when possible. Many life care planners may have the knowledge, experience, and expertise necessary to make transportation-related recommendations; however, regardless of the source of the recommendations, given the increasingly complex nature of this area, life care planners and case managers are encouraged to refer clients to accredited modifiers who comply with NMEDA standards, participate in the NMEDA quality assurance program (QAP) program, and are members of the Adaptive Driving Alliance.

Resources

Association for Driver Rehabilitation Specialists (ADED)—ADED was established in 1977 to support professionals working in the field of driver education, driver training, and transportation equipment modifications for persons with disabilities and persons experiencing the aging process. Through education, information dissemination, and a certification program for professionals,

ADED supports these professionals so that they may better serve these individuals. ADED stands ready to meet the professional needs of its members through educational conferences, professional development activities, and a professional certification program. The history of ADED reflects a unique blending of different professional fields into an organization dedicated to providing quality service in the field of driver rehabilitation, vehicle modifications for driving, transportation, and resources for alternative transportation.

www.aded.net
(866) 672-9466

National Mobility Equipment Dealers Association (NMEDA)—A non-profit trade association of mobility equipment dealers, driver rehabilitation specialists, and other professionals dedicated to broadening the opportunities for people with disabilities to drive or ride in vehicles modified with mobility equipment.

3327 Bearss Avenue
Tampa, FL 33618
(800) 833-0427

Adaptive Driving Alliance (ADA)—A nationwide group of vehicle-modification dealers providing van conversions, hand controls, wheelchair lifts, scooter lifts, tie downs, conversion van rentals, paratransit, and other adaptive equipment for drivers with disabilities and passengers.

111 Stow Avenue, Ste 103
Cuyahoga Falls, OH 44221
(330) 928-7401
http://www.adamobility.com

National Highway Traffic Safety Administration (NHTSA)—The federal government agency authorized to regulate the manufacture of automotive adaptive equipment and modified vehicles used by persons with disabilities.

National Highway Traffic Safety Administration
1200 New Jersey Avenue, SE
Washington, DC 20590
(888) 327-4236
(800) 424-9153 (TTY)
http://www.nhtsa.gov

Society of Automobile Engineers (SAE)—An international organization of engineers, business executives, educators, and students who share information and exchange ideas for advancing the engineering of mobility systems.

SAE World Headquarters
400 Commonwealth Drive
Warrendale, PA 15096-0001
(724) 776-4841
http://www.sae.org

Wheelchair Transportation Safety

http://wc-transportation-safety.umtri.umich.edu/ridesafe-brochure

References

ANSI/RESNA. 2000. *A New Transit Wheelchair Standard: ANSI/RESNA WC19*. Available at http://wc-transportation-safety.umtri.umich.edu/prescriber-resources/a-new-transit-wheelchair-standard-ansi-resna-wc19.

Deutsch, P. 1999. An overview of related care and services in catastrophic injuries. In P. Deutsch & H. Sawyer (Eds.), *Guide to Rehabilitation* (pp. 7.1–7.41). White Plains, NY: AHAB Press.

Healy, J. 2015. *Average new car price zips 2.6% to $33,560*. Available at https://www.usatoday.com/story/money/cars/2015/05/04/new-car-transaction-price-3-kbb-kelley-blue-book/26690191/.

McCaigue, I. S. 2004. The role of the occupational therapist in life care planning. In R.O. Weed (Ed.), *Life Care Planning and Case Management Handbook* (2nd ed., pp 89–144). Boca Raton, FL: CRC Press.

National Highway Traffic Safety Administration. 2002. *Exemption from the Make Inoperative Prohibition, 67 Fed. Reg. 38423*. Available at http://www.federalregister.com/Browse/Document/usa/na/fr/2002/6/4/02-13968.

National Mobility Equipment Dealers Association. 2016. Guidelines. Available at http://www.nmeda.com/wp-content/uploads/2016/01/QAP-103-2016-Guidelines.pdf.

Pierce, S. 1999. A comprehensive approach to transportation assessment. In P. Deutsch & H. Sawyer (Eds.), *Guide to Rehabilitation* (pp. 6C.1–6C.10). White Plains, NY: AHAB Press.

Schatz, A. 2005. *Joe's van: A tragic accident spotlights a hole in auto regulation*. Available at https://www.wsj.com/articles/SB110505136588019305.

Chapter 34

Credentialing and Other Issues in Life Care Planning

Debra E. Berens and Roger O. Weed

Contents

Introduction 813
Credentialing: General 814
Licensure 814
Certification 814
Registration 815
Accreditation 817
Conclusion 818
References 818

Introduction

Credentialing in support of one's professional work in health care-related fields has exploded with an increasing array of certifications, licenses, educational degrees, and registrations available. Many credentials are backed by research, accreditation, and role and function studies, while others seemingly appear overnight with no apparent foundation for establishing credibility. Included in the previous statement are the nonaccredited and, in some instances, bogus degrees (doctorates included). Nonetheless, life care planners seem to be attracted to enhancing their list of credentials and willingly pay the associated costs. Further complicating this issue is the apparent diversity of professional disciplines that is represented by the life care planners observed over the years (e.g., physicians, psychologists, certified rehabilitation counselors, nurses, occupational therapists, speech pathologists, social workers, and others). While this short chapter will not include a list of credible versus noncredible credentials, some hints or issues will be offered.

Credentialing: General

In the beginning, counselors, psychologists, and most other professions were unregulated. One could hang out a shingle advertising that he or she was, for an example, a barber and dentist. As time passed, more and more people formed organizations and set professional standards (T. Field, personal communication, November 7, 2007), or promoted protecting practice through implementation of laws or establishing certifications that would hopefully be required for employment in targeted settings. States began implementing laws intended to protect the welfare of their constituents. For example, all states require licensure to practice in the life care planning–relevant professions of physicians, nurses, and psychologists. Many states have licensure requirements for professional counselors, allied health therapists, prosthetists and orthotists, and others. However, there is no state that requires one to be licensed, registered, or certified to prepare life care plans, though some businesses may require specific credentials as part of their job requirements.

Licensure

Licenses, the most restrictive credential for rehabilitation professions, are issued by government entities and are expected to protect the health and welfare of citizens (Matkin, 1995). Licenses are typically thought of as being issued by states, but the federal government also grants licenses (such as the FCC). For purposes of life care planning, no state issues a license for life care planners, but an individual's credential *may* require licensure, such as physician, nurse, or psychologist. A few states require rehabilitation counselors to be licensed if they offer services within the scope of practice as defined by the state. Although most professionals reading this chapter will know whether they are covered by licensing laws and regulations, one will need to determine if there are different requirements with moves from one state to another state. The primary issue is that, unlike certification or registration, one who is required to be licensed to practice, but is not licensed, can be denied the opportunity to work within his or her profession. However, a person who completed medical school, for instance, but is not licensed as a physician could seemingly potentially be qualified to work as a life care planner as long as he or she does not practice medicine as defined by law. Note that some states have a title protection act and others have a practice protection act. In the state of Georgia, professional counseling has a practice protection law, which means that if one performs services as defined in the law as professional counseling, one must be licensed. In a title protection state, one may practice psychology, but may not call himself or herself a licensed psychologist unless licensed by that state.

Certification

Certification is described as a process by which an organization (governmental or nongovernmental) recognizes an individual for having met certain predetermined professional qualifications (Matkin, 1995). The organizational structure can run the gamut from being governed by a single individual or controlled by a group overseen by an outside organization. Some certifications can be related to meeting extensive qualifications and passing a written or oral examination or can be as simple as related to the work setting. For example, one of the authors was a "certified" educator by the National Council on Rehabilitation Education (NCRE), which means that he was employed 20 hours or more in an educational institution teaching rehabilitation counseling (no other credentials were required). While the membership structure of the NCRE was reportedly revised in 2008-09, NCRE considers itself the premier professional organization of educators dedicated to quality services for persons with disabilities through education and research. NCRE advocates up-to-date education and training and the maintenance of professional standards in the field of rehabilitation (NCRE, 2017).

Some organizations are structured such that the board or commissioners are selected from qualified applicants who possess the requisite credentials. For example, the Commission on Rehabilitation Counselor Certification (CRCC) is governed by a 12-person Board of Directors, each with the CRC credential (exception is the one public member director) who is charged primarily with the strategic, financial, and operational health of the organization (CRCC, 2017). Also, in terms of history, the CRC, established in the mid-1970s, is one of the oldest certifications in the rehabilitation consulting arena, predating the nationally certified counselor (NCC), among other well-established credentials. At the other extreme, some certifications are offered by organizations that are effectively controlled by one person, which may or may not have a board or a group of commissioners.

The point of this discussion is that most, if not all, life care planners possess at least one certification, and the person may acquire highly valued certifications with a substantial history, with an extensive research base (including role and functions studies), and which enjoy a credible reputation throughout the membership or by stakeholders. In the authors' opinion, one way to assure basic credibility is to determine if the certifying body or organization is accredited by the National Commission for Certifying Agencies (NCCA), the accreditation body of the Institute for Credentialing Excellence (ICE). Formerly known as the National Organization for Competency Assurance (NOCA), the name changed in 2009 to the Institute for Credentialing Excellence. Currently, ICE is an organization committed to advancing standards of excellence in the credentialing industry and advances credentialing through education, standards, research, and advocacy to ensure competence across professions and occupations. ICE's accrediting body, NCCA, evaluates certification organizations for compliance with the NCCA standards for the *Accreditation of Certification Programs* (NCCA, 2017). In these authors' opinion, it seems that if an organization is accredited by NCCA, then there is a mechanism by which the organization's standards, by-laws, policies and procedures, and overall credentialing process have been determined satisfactory (approved), and there is ongoing review and evaluation by NCCA for reaccreditation. There may be other accrediting bodies that support a certification, but one would be advised to make sure the statement "accredited by" has validity and is not simply another shell of an organization that is intended to give the impression of legitimacy. The authors recognize that other evidence of credibility can be located, and the expectation is that the reader will exercise due diligence before paying fees. One further note: certification does not stop one from practicing a profession but does prohibit what one can call himself or herself. For example, one may practice rehabilitation counseling, but may not call himself or herself a Certified Rehabilitation Counselor (CRC) unless the Commission on Rehabilitation Counselor Certification's requirements are met, and the individual has been granted certification status through the CRCC.

In general, the authors summarize the previous information within a checklist format in Table 34.1.

Registration

Registration is a term that can refer to someone who is either licensed or simply registered with an organization that represents a particular profession (e.g., Registered Nurse or Occupational Therapist/Registered). As Matkin (1995) observes, "Registration is closely related to certification and licensure, in that once these forms of credentials are issued, the professional becomes listed by name and other pertinent information among other similarly designated members of a specialty.

Table 34.1 Basic Questions before Seeking a Certification (with Authors' Comments)

✓ Is the organization not-for-profit or for-profit? (Comment: Not-for-profits on the surface enjoy an appearance of better credibility or face validity than for-profit organizations. However, that business structure by itself is not a determining factor.)
✓ Is the organization owned by an individual (profit or not-for-profit)? (Comment: An entity owned by an individual is less desirable.)
✓ Is the organization run by elected or appointed commissioners, or is it effectively run or controlled by an individual? Do the commissioners serve "at the pleasure of" the owner? (Comment: An independent board or group of commissioners is desirable.)
✓ Is the certification based on research and a reliable role and function study? (Comment: Preferably with approval and oversight by a university institutional review board.)
✓ Does one need to pass a legitimate examination to become certified? (Comment: Whether oral or written, there should be evidence that the exam, if one is required, is based on research. Attention should also be given to certificate holders who were "grandfathered in" at the time they were certified, which implies they did not have to pass an examination to obtain certification.)
✓ Do organizations that offer continuing education recognize the certification such that they offer credits for training? (Comment: If one attends several conferences and there are no available continuing education credits for a particular certification, it may mean that the credential is not valued.)
✓ Are policies and procedures accessible to review before seeking certification, and do they protect stakeholders by providing for due process? Or can the owner, board, or commissioners take action for purported transgressions without notice to, or participation of, the certified professional? (Comment: It seems reasonable to expect that a consistent due process policy is in force, and NCCA standards require due process. See next question.)
✓ Is the certification accredited by the National Commission for Certifying Agencies (NCCA) or another legitimate accreditation-related entity? (Comment: Although the authors do not believe that this provision is a necessity, the oversight is desirable for organizations that offer certifications.)

Thus, a registry is a document that assists the public to identify qualified practitioners or businesses to perform specific services" (pp. 396–397). For example, one of the authors is registered by the state in which she lives as a "registered rehabilitation supplier," indicating that she has met the requirements and is deemed eligible to provide rehabilitation services to injured workers who are receiving workers' compensation benefits under the state's workers' compensation laws. Although the state registration is voluntary and there is no examination specific to becoming registered, certain credentialing and educational requirements have to be met, including possession of one of the primary rehabilitation-related credentials (CRC, CCM, CDMS, CRRN, CLCP, etc.) which require sitting for and passing a national exam in order to become certified. Once registered, the state maintains a public listing of registered rehabilitation suppliers who are qualified to provide medical and vocational case management and related services to individuals injured on the job within that state. Similar to credentialing, registered providers must re-register annually by providing documentation of having continued certification in one of the accepted rehabilitation-related credentials (see above) and by paying an annual fee. Again, by requiring evidence of maintaining a primary credential (which requires evidence of ongoing continuing education credits), the state registration process is another resource to determine rehabilitation professionals in specific states who are qualified to work with individuals typically with a worker's compensation injury. Gianforte (1976, as cited in Matkin, 1995) noted that there can be state or national registries, with the advantage that national registration leads to reciprocity throughout the country whereas state registries may not extend beyond the borders of the respective state.

Accreditation

Accreditation can refer to educational institutions or other organizations. As noted previously, NCCA accredits organizations that meet certain standards. The operative word here is *organization* since the program or educational offerings are accredited whereas certification applies to individuals. Within educational institutions, accreditations can be numerous. For example, the university where both authors taught is accredited not only as a university, but the specific rehabilitation counseling program is also accredited by the Council for Accreditation of Counseling and Related Educational Programs (CACREP) (www.cacrep.org). Furthermore, some of the classes also meet the requirements for accreditation in school counseling, professional counseling, and school psychology. With regard to life care planning, the standards of rehabilitation counselor training identify knowledge content areas that include the mandate to teach life care planning elements as part of the rehabilitation counselor training program (CORE, 2008). As of October 2017, the Commission on Rehabilitation Counselor Certification (CRCC) has included life care planning under its Community Resources and Partnerships knowledge domain area such that individuals who sit for the national CRC exam are expected to know and be tested on concepts specific to life care planning (www.crccertification.com).

At the other extreme of programs accredited by well-established accreditation agencies are sham degrees offered by so-called universities that deliver, for a price, an impressive degree including, in some cases, transcripts (Bear & Bear, 2004). The degree may appear to be from an impressive university like Harvard, or a name very close to a recognized educational institution (in spelling or perhaps a slightly different name). Such degrees are obtained through highlighting one's experiences or attending a few classes that somehow meet the requirements for a doctorate. It is not uncommon for bogus degrees to claim they are accredited by equally bogus accreditation agencies. For anecdotal examples, the following is offered:

Several years ago, one rehabilitation-related organization began offering a doctorate but when state officials in which the business was located were notified, an investigation revealed that state requirements for an educational institution were not met and they were forced to close. In another case, a person who claimed that he possessed a degree from a university and had several years of testifying to such achievement was pressed to provide proof. As it turned out, he did not have the degree to which he testified, which unraveled several settled litigation cases. Last another testifying expert listed a PhD, which, when evaluated, was from an unaccredited program and the purported coursework additionally was not related to rehabilitation consulting or the area to which the PhD was claimed.

The authors hasten to add that despite some of the problems and issues listed previously, there are trustworthy and fully-accredited undergraduate, graduate, and doctoral programs, including emerging and established distant learning and online educational offerings. In summary, accreditation defines the requisite knowledge content areas to be offered by training and educational programs responsible for preparing individuals to enter an occupation (Matkin, 1985, as cited by May and Lubinskas, 2004).

Conclusion

For the specialty practice of life care planning, certifications abound and are not regulated by governmental agencies. Each has its own requirements—and costs—which in some cases simply constitute an economic enhancement to the person(s) who owns the business. Others are substantial, well-researched, long-standing certifications from organizations that are NCCA accredited or are well recognized within the rehabilitation profession. Furthermore, registries and educational institutions may or may not be legitimate. The authors recommend "caveat emptor," or let the buyer beware. Historically, in these authors' opinion, one could assert certain achievements and perhaps successfully work without being caught. However, with the vast improvements in searching the Internet and increasing abilities of rehabilitation professionals, attorneys, and others to discover these data, it seems increasingly difficult for life care planners to "fudge" their credentials. Before one commits to a certification, registration, or training program to support one's contention that they are qualified as a life care planner, it is suggested that some of the concerns, guidelines, observations, issues, and such items as previously listed be considered.

References

Bear, J., & Bear, M. 2004. *Degree Mills*. Retrieved January 3 2009, from www.quackwatch.org/04ConsumerEducation/dm0.html.

Council for Accreditation of Counseling & Related Education Programs. Retrieved December 27, 2017, http://www.cacrep.org/about-cacrep/

Council on Rehabilitation Education. 2008. *Standards for Rehabilitation Counselor Education Programs*. Schaumburg, IL: Author.

CRCC. 2017. *CRC Certification Guide*. Schaumburg, IL: Author.

CRCC. 2017. *CRCC Leadership*. Retrieved December 27, 2017, from Commission on Rehabilitation Counselor Certification, https://www.crccertification.com/leadership

Gianforte, G. 1976. Certification: A challenge and a choice. *Journal of Rehabilitation*, *42*, 15–17.

Matkin, R. E. 1985. *Insurance Rehabilitation*. Austin, TX: Pro-Ed.

Matkin, R. E. 1995. Private rehabilitation. In S. Rubin and R. Roessler (Eds.), *Foundations of the Vocational Rehabilitation Process* (4th ed., pp. 375–398), Austin, TX: Pro-Ed.

May, R., & Lubinskas, P. 2004. The Commission on Health Care Certification: Credentialing in life care planning service delivery. In R. Weed (Ed.), *Life Care Planning and Case Management Handbook* (2nd ed., pp. 761–809). Boca Raton, FL: CRC Press.

NCCA. 2017. *NCAA Accreditation*. Retrieved December 27, 2017, http://www.credentialingexcellence.org/p/cm/ld/fid = 65

NCRE. 2017. *The National Council on Rehabilitation Education Overview*. Retrieved December 27, 2017, https://ncre.org/ncre-overview/

Chapter 35

Admissibility Considerations in Life Care Planning

Timothy F. Field

Contents

Introduction 819
The *Daubert* Trilogy 820
Frye v. United States 820
Daubert v. Merrill Dow Pharmaceuticals 821
General Electric Company v. Joiner 823
Kumho Tire Company v. Carmichael 823
Case Discussion 825
    The *Daubert* Challenge and Credentials 825
Foundation and Methodology 827
Standards of Practice 828
Conclusion 830
References 831

Introduction

The admissibility of expert testimony in federal and state courts has evolved into a major issue related to civil cases of personal injury and life care planning (Elliott, 2010; Gunn, 2010). *In limine* motions to strike testimony are not uncommon and are usually directed toward the expert's credentials and/or methodologies relied upon in developing conclusions and opinions for presentation and trial (Elliott, 2010; Gunn, 2010; *Crouch v. John Jewel Aircraft*, 2016). This chapter discusses the history and development of rules and regulations which govern the testimony of an expert and clarifies some issues and confusion regarding the intent and meaning of recent court cases on this issue.

The *Daubert* Trilogy

Three U.S. Supreme Court cases are referred to as the *Daubert* trilogy (*Daubert v. Merrill Dow Pharmaceutical*, 92–102, US Sp Ct, 1993b; *General Electric Company v. Joiner*, 96-188, US Sp Ct, 1996, 1997; *Kumho Tire Company v. Carmichael*, 526 137, US Sp Ct, 1999). All three cases and the related U.S. District Court and U.S. Court of Appeals decisions leading up to the final rulings were meant to clarify and refine the guidelines for the admissibility of expert testimony in federal courts. The *Daubert* decision was a departure of the long-held decision of *Frye v. United States* (1923) and further emphasized the substantial importance of the *Federal Rule of Evidence 702* (FRE 702 was subsequently amended in 2000). The *Daubert* trilogy has had a significant impact on the parameters and meaning of such concepts as: What has changed from *Frye*? What are the criteria for admissibility that apply in any or all federal cases? And in particular, for the rehabilitation and life care planning community, what is acceptable methodology and testimony—especially in light of the *Daubert* criteria for admissibility? This chapter will review the various federal rulings, following which will be an examination of how the rules apply to life care planning experts. An analysis of several tort cases will be presented to illustrate how the courts have decided on issues of admissibility.

Frye v. United States

Frye involved the case of a defendant who was convicted of the crime of second degree murder. During the course of appeal, the defendant offered an expert who utilized a "deception test" based on the theory that "truth comes without conscious effort, while the utterance of a falsehood requires a conscious effort, which is reflected in the [systolic] blood pressure." The government objected to the presentation of the expert who conducted the test prior to trial, and the objection was sustained by the court. Given the fact that this "deception test" was relatively new to the scientific community, the court stated that

> the principle must be recognized, and while courts will go a long way in admitting expert testimony deduced from a well-recognized scientific principle or discovery, the thing from which the deduction is made must be sufficiently established to have gained general acceptance in the particular field in which it belongs.

Thus, the principle of "general acceptance" became the standard for admissibility of testimony from 1923 until *Daubert* was decided in 1993. However, as will become apparent, the *Daubert* ruling did not fully clarify the issue of admissibility since approximately one-half of the states still rely on *Frye* (as of this writing) as their standard for admissibility in their respective state courts. On another front, Feinman (2011) has raised the question of who decides the admissibility of a generally accepted principle or technique? And who decides who is the relevant scientific community? Feinman (p. 4) suggests that issues of science should be determined by adequately defined scientific research with controlled and randomized studies. The "opinions of respected authorities, based on clinical experience, descriptive studies, or reports of experts committees" should be the least likely path to establishing general acceptance. In the area of the soft sciences, such as life care planning, the same two questions apply: What is the agreed upon methodology, and is general acceptance by collegial experts sufficient for admissibility?

Daubert v. Merrill Dow Pharmaceuticals

Jason Daubert (and Eric Schuller) were born with deformities after their mothers ingested a drug named Bendectin during pregnancy. The issue before the court was whether Bendectin caused those deformities. The respondent, Merrill Dow Pharmaceuticals, was granted a summary judgment by the U.S. District Court (1989), and affirmed by the U.S. Court of Appeals, Ninth Circuit (1991). A summary of the District Court's ruling follows:

> The summary judgment based on a well-credentialed expert's affidavit concluding, upon reviewing the extensive published scientific literature on the subject, the material use of Bendectin has not been shown to be a risk factor for human birth defects. Although petitioners had responded with the testimony of eight other well-credentialed experts, who based their conclusion that Bendectin can cause birth defects on animal studies, chemical structural analyses, and the unpublished "reanalysis" of previously published human statistical studies, the court determined that the evidence did not meet the applicable "general acceptance" standard for the admission of testimony. The Court of Appeals agreed and affirmed, citing *Frye v. United States*, for the rule that expert opinion based on scientific technique is inadmissible unless the technique is "generally accepted" as reliable in the relevant scientific community. (*Daubert v. Merrill Dow Pharmaceuticals* Syllabus, 1993a, p. 1)

In *Daubert* (1993b), the U.S. Supreme Court summarized the expert testimony of both the petitioners and the defense. Steven Lamm, a physician and epidemiologist, testified that he had reviewed more than 30 published research studies involving more than 130,000 patients and had concluded that Bendectin "during the first trimester of pregnancy has not been shown to be a risk factor for human birth defects" (p. 1). The petitioners, on the other hand, presented eight experts who had "concluded that Bendectin can cause birth defects" (p. 1) based on animals studies that did find a link between Bendectin and malformations. The Court noted that the District Court (1989) had relied upon the *Frye* rule and found that the petitioners' evidence was not "sufficiently established to have general acceptance in the field to which it belongs." The U.S. Court of Appeals (1991) essentially reached the same conclusion that the petitioner's evidence did not reach the level of general acceptance. The Appeals Court affirmed the District Court's decision by rejecting the "petitioners' reanalysis as unpublished, not subjected to the normal peer review process, and generated solely for use in litigation" (p. 2).

The Supreme Court (1993) took the next step to address the issue by contending that the *Federal Rules of Evidence* (i.e., 401, 402, and 702) superseded the *Frye* test of 1923. FRE 402 established a baseline:

> All relevant evidence is admissible, except as otherwise provided by the Constitution of the United States, by Act of Congress, by these rules, or by other rules prescribed by the Supreme Court pursuant to statutory authority. Evidence which is not relevant is not admissible.

And FRE 401 defines the meaning of relevance:

> Relevant evidence is defined as that which has any tendency to make the existence of any fact that is of consequence to the determination of the action more probable or less probable than it would be without the evidence.

The Supreme Court further noted that the *Federal Rule of Evidence 702* governed expert testimony, and in doing so, that there was nothing in the rule that "established general acceptance as an absolute prerequisite to admissibility." In 1993, *FRE 702* defined the role of the expert as follows:

> If scientific, technical, or other specialized knowledge will assist the trier of fact to understand the evidence or to determine a fact in issue, a witness qualified as an expert by knowledge, skill, experience, training, or education, may testify thereto in the form of an opinion or otherwise.

The amended *FRE 702* (2000), in addition to the above, added the following narrative at the end of the above definition:

> if (1) the testimony is based upon sufficient facts or data, (2) the testimony is the product of reliable principles and methods, and (3) the witness has applied the principles and methods reliably to the facts of the case.

As a consequence, the Supreme Court noted that a rigid general acceptance requirement (i.e., *Frye*) would be at odds with the liberal thrust of the *Federal Rules of Evidence* and the [rules] general approach to relaxing the traditional barriers to opinion testimony. The standard of "general acceptance" for admitting testimony became incompatible with the *Federal Rules of Evidence*. The Court emphasized, however, that testimony or evidence must be both relevant and reliable. The court then took the next step to examine the issue of "knowledge" which is contained in *FRE 702*. Noting that knowledge can exist within three domains (scientific, technical, or other specialized), the Court argued that the "adjective scientific implies a grounding in the methods and procedure of science" (p. 4). As will become evident with the *Kumho* ruling is reviewed, technical and other specialized knowledge clearly differs from scientific knowledge, requiring a different approaching to evaluating a relevant and reliable methodology. The Court, in *Daubert*, a legal case involving an issue of science (i.e., scientific knowledge) suggested that

> Many factors will bear on the inquiry, and we do not presume to set out a definitive checklist or test. But some general observations are appropriate.

1. Scientific knowledge today is based on generating hypotheses and testing them to see if they can be falsified.
2. Another pertinent consideration is whether the theory or technique has been subjected to peer review.
3. In the case of a particular scientific technique, the court ordinarily should consider the known or potential rate of error.
4. Finally, "general acceptance" can yet have a bearing on the inquiry. The inquiry envisioned by FRE 702 is, we emphasize, a flexible one (p. 5).

In an endnote (#8) on the *Daubert* case (1993), the Court observed that "Rule 702 also applies to 'technical, or other specialized knowledge.' Our discussion is limited to the scientific context because that is the nature of the expertise offered here" (p. 9).

General Electric Company v. Joiner

Robert Joiner, working as a maintenance electrician on the city's Water and Light Department (Thomasville, Georgia), was exposed to a mineral-based dielectric fluid, a contaminate fluid with polychlorinated byphenyls (PCBs). Subsequently, Joiner was diagnosed with small cell lung cancer. The District Court granted a summary judgment to the petitioners (GE) for the following reasons:

> (1) there was no genuine issue as to whether Joiner had been exposed to furans and dioxins, and (2) the testimony of Joiner's experts had failed to show that there was a link between exposure to PCBs and small cell lung cancer. The court believed that the testimony of the respondent's experts to the contrary did not rise above "subjective belief or unsupported speculation." Their testimony was therefore inadmissible. (p. 2)

The Court of Appeals for the Eleventh Circuit held that the District Court "had erred in excluding the testimony of Joiner's expert witnesses" and reversed for two reasons: first, the jury should decide the correctness of an expert's testimony, and second, there was a genuine issue of the question of furans and dioxins. The U.S. Supreme Court (1997) disagreed and reversed, holding that the Appeals Court held a view of testimony that was too stringent and that under the *Federal Rules of Evidence* which now superceded *Frye*, the District Court is allowed to admit a much broader view of evidence. The gatekeeper role of the district judge has considerable discretion and latitude in admitting evidence at trial. The *GE–Joiner* decision is often referred to as the "discretion rule." The following paragraph best describes the essence of the *Joiner* decision:

> Most significant to experts was the Supreme Court's finding that the trial court properly excluded the plaintiff's expert's testimony because there was "simply too great an analytical gap between the data and the opinion proffered." In other words, the Court found the expert's opinion to be speculative because it could not be supported by the underlying methodology, even when the methodology itself was reliable. Furthermore, the Court noted that an expert cannot rely solely on his or her qualifications as validation that an expert opinion is reliable. (Pearson, 2014, p. 6)

Kumho Tire Company v. Carmichael

After a period of confusion by many as to what the Supreme Court actually meant and intended with regard to admissible testimony, the *Kumho Tire Company v. Carmichael* (1998, 1999) case was selected as a means to clarify and expand on this issue. Patrick Carmichael had purchased a used minivan with a significant amount of wear on the tires. While driving the van in 1993, a rear tire blew out causing a serious accident which resulted in one death and several injured. Carmichael sued Kumho Tire claiming that the tire was defective. Dennis Carlson, a tire construction expert, testified for the petitioner and concluded that a defective tire caused the accident when the tread separated from the carcass of the tire. The essence of his presentation to the court was a four-part criteria which he used in evaluating the tire that included "(a) tread wear on the tire's shoulder that is greater that the tread wear along the tire's center, (b) signs of a bead groove where the beads have been pushed too hard against the bead seat on the inside of the tire's rim, (c) sidewalls of the tire with physical signs of deterioration, such as discoloration, and (d) marks on the tire's rim flange" (p. 2). Note that the four-point *Daubert* criteria were not used in Carlson's analysis. With his own criteria, conclusions from two of which were observations, Carlson concluded that a defect must have caused the separation. The District Court (*Carmichael v. Samyang Tires Inc.*, 1996) found that Carlson's credentials were not at issue, but his methodology was when evaluated in light of the *Daubert* factors. The District Court "found that all those factors argued against the reliability of Carlson's methods, and it granted a [defendant's] motion to exclude the testimony. The plaintiffs argued that the court's application of the *Daubert* factors was too inflexible" (p. 3) and asked for a reconsideration. Observing the method used by Carlson used a visual inspection (observation) of the tire, the District Court again affirmed its earlier decision and found for the defendant in rejecting Carlson's methodology.

The U.S. Court of Appeals for the Eleventh Circuit (*Carmichael v. Samyang Tires, Inc.*, 1997) reversed the court's decision for applying *Daubert* factors as a means to establish reliability of a methodology. The Appeals Court was clear in their clarification of interpretation of the *Daubert* factors:

> The Supreme Court in *Daubert* explicitly limited its holding to cover only the scientific context, adding that "a *Daubert* analysis" applies only where the expert relies on "the application of scientific principles" rather than "on skill or experience-based observation." [The court] concluded that Carlson's testimony, which it viewed as relying on experience, falls outside the scope of *Daubert*, that the District Court erred as a matter of law by applying *Daubert* in this case, and that the case must be remanded for further (non-*Daubert*-type) consideration under FRE 702. (p. 3)

With the *Kumho* ruling, the Supreme Court took into consideration the following factors. First, *Daubert* does still apply, with an emphasis on reliable methods in evaluating scientific, technical, or other specialized knowledge. Next, a consideration must be made related to the proper manner in which a methodology is evaluated. There are several considerations to be made in this evaluation process. The FRE 702 "imposes a special consideration regarding both the relevance and reliability of evidence. In fact, FRE 702 is so central to the issue of admissibility that the U.S. Supreme Court basically predicated the decisions of the *Daubert* trilogy on this rule. The role of the expert begins with this rule and all else follows, i.e., credentials, the type of knowledge, emphasis on a reliable methodology. Next, a consideration must be made regarding the type of knowledge that is required in establishing a measure of evidentiary reliability. Not all knowledge is scientific (requiring an evaluation with the application of the four *Daubert* factors); some knowledge is technical or specialized (requiring relevant factors that fairly evaluate the nature of the knowledge and reliable methods relative to the facts of the case). The Court made it abundantly clear that the trial judge "may consider several more specific factors" (p. 5) other than the *Daubert* factors which, by way of emphasis, is within the domain of the gatekeeping role of the trial judge allowing (i.e., discretion). The Supreme Court concluded

> "that we can neither rule out, or rule in, for all cases and for all time the applicability of the factors mentioned in *Daubert*, nor can we now do so for subsets of cases categorized by category of expert or by kind of evidence" (p. 5); "whether *Daubert's* specific factors are, or are not, reasonable measures of reliability in a particular case is a matter that the law grants the trial judge broad latitude to determine" (p. 6), and "the relevant reliability inquiry should be 'a flexible one,' that its 'over-arching' subject should be validity and reliability, and that '*Daubert* was intended neither to be exhaustive nor to apply in every case.'" (p. 8)

Kumho, therefore, emphasized several factors that are the essence of admissibility, including FRE 702, the type of knowledge relative to the facts of the case, *Daubert's* requirement of relevance and reliability, gate-keeping discretion on the part of trial judge with considerable leeway in contemplating other factors (other than *Daubert*) in evaluating the reliability of a methodology. All of these considerations taken collectively provide ample opportunity for rehabilitation experts and life care planners to develop appropriate testimony without the threat of being disallowed in district courts. However, being able to sidestep the *Dauber*t criteria in no way alleviates the expert from due diligence in opinion development for depositions and trials. The *latitude* provided by *Kumho* offers much more flexibility for the gatekeeper role of the trial judge, and *may* involve different criteria in establishing reliability of a methodology use in evaluating the facts of the case. Note: The two words *latitude* and *may* were italicized for emphasis in the Supreme Court's summary of *Kumho*. This flexibility, however, can also serve as an unwanted pit-fall for those who fail to take the admissibility requirements seriously. In order to further clarify this issue for rehabilitation consultants offering technical or specialized testimony, a review of select cases follows to illustrate how some cases were adjudicated in this area.

Case Discussion

The Daubert Challenge and Credentials

The *Daubert* challenge is an *in limine motion to exclude* by either the plaintiff or defense usually directed toward an expert regarding the expert's credentials, attention to procedure, or methodology issues. The context of the importance of a *motion to exclude* is illustrated by the abstract from a case that was recently adjudicated (*M.D.P. v. Middleton*, 2013) which is very typical of nearly all challenges in federal courts. (A more detailed discussion of the importance of FRE 702 is presented by Field, 2011.)

The admissibility of expert testimony is governed by FRE 702 which provides:

> A witness who is qualified as an expert by knowledge, skill, experience, training, or education may testify in the form of an opinion or otherwise if: (a) the expert's scientific, technical, or other specialized knowledge will help the trier of fact to understand the evidence or to determine the fact at issue; (b) the testimony is based on sufficient facts or data; (c) the testimony is the product of reliable principles and methods; and (d) the expert has reliably applied the principles and methods to the facts of the case.
>
> As noted in *M.D.P. v. Middleton*, "in determining the admissibility of expert testimony under FRE 702, the trial court must conduct a rigorous three part inquiry considering whether: (1) the expert is qualified to testify competently regarding the matter he intends to address; (2) the methodology by which the expert reaches his conclusions is sufficiently reliable as determined by the sort of inquiry mandated in *Daubert*; and (3) the testimony assists the trier of fact, through the application of scientific, technical, or specialized expertise, to understand the evidence or to determine a fact at issue. (p. 2).

The following is a discussion of various motions to exclude a life care planning expert from testifying in trial for whatever reason. All of these cases reference FRE 702 as the basis for a decision on a challenge on expert admissibility, and a few specifically reference the *Daubert* decision in a secondary manner. In *Beavers v. Victorian* (2014) the defendant challenged both the qualifications of the life care planner (related to a specific opinion) and the reliability of a portion of the expert's life care plan. The defendants "challenge only [the life care planner's] expertise regarding the effects of plaintiff's traumatic brain injuries" and further argue that the [life care planner] "makes a 'speculative leap' between the [doctor's] findings and a need for assisted living services beginning at age 70 and through life expectancy" (p. 2). The Court rejected the challenge to the [expert's] credentials and determined that the expert relied on the medical opinions expressed making her opinions sufficiently reliable to be admissible. In *Worley & Worley v. State Farm Mutual Automobile Insurance Company*, (2013), a defendant's motion was presented to exclude or limit the testimony of a life care planner. The Court summarily determined that the expert was qualified to offer testimony. The defendant next challenged the expert's opinions as unreliable because the expert relied on a standard reference for costs of certain future medical costs. The Court required the expert to proffer "an adequate showing of reliability [of the reference] prior to testifying at trial." This decision by the Court is a good example of the latitude the judge has in determining the admissibility of evidence (i.e., *General Electric v. Joiner*, 1997). In *Mettias v. United States of America* (2015), the defendant's motion to exclude the testimony of a life care planner on the issues of qualifications and methodology was denied. The Court ruled that the expert was qualified and that "[expert's] testimony was highly relevant to the issue of [plaintiff's] future costs. Relying on FRE 702, the Court addressed the issue of reliability with regard to the expert's methodology in preparing a life care plan. The challenge centered on the argument that the [expert] had no expertise in the area of assessing the needs of a person disabled by gastric bypass surgery, that he conducted no independent research of the future needs of [plaintiff], and that he relied entirely on the opinions of [doctor]. In relying on the requirements inherent in FRE 702, the Court ruled "that [expert] does not have specific experience with assessing the needs of a person disabled with gastric bypass surgery, in particular, and does not make him unqualified as an expert" (p. 6). The expert stated that he "followed the accepted methodology and standards of practice in the field by looking to the medical providers to define the nature and extent of impairments and then translated those limitations and recommendations to the world of work, independent living, coordination of future medical and rehabilitation services, and the associated costs" (p. 6). The motion to exclude was denied. In *Ancar & Ancar v. Brown & TNE Trucking* (2014), as is sometimes the case, the expert's testimony is sometimes allowed under a challenge, in whole or in part. The expert in this case made recommendations regarding medication (allowed), physical therapy (allowed), weight-loss and home-exercise program (not allowed), and epidural steroid injections (allowed), but was subject to a vigorous cross examination as suggested by the *Daubert* ruling (509 US at 596) noting that "vigorous cross examination and other traditional safeguards are appropriate means of attacking shaky but admissible evidence."

Finally, in *Crouch v. John Jewell Aircraft* (2016), the Court, beginning with a reference to FRE 702, addressed the issues: failure by the expert to fully disclose information (*violations cited with reference to FRE 26 & 37*)—rules that outlined requirements for disclosure of a statement of opinions, facts and data considered by the experts in each case, exhibits, expert qualifications (including publications over the last ten years), a list of cases over the last 4 years, and whether or not the omissions were harmless to the current case. The defendant argued that the expert did not fully comply with the requirements of FRE 26, and when given the opportunity to supplement his testimony post-deposition, the expert failed to comply. There was also some confusion by the expert about which reports were used in forming his opinion. The Court found "that [expert's] reports were plagued with deficiencies" and the "most egregious is his failure to include the source(s) of the information used to formulate the costs utilized in the life care plan [for defendant]." Further, the expert "testified that he had a conversation with [physician], a rehabilitation medicine specialist, who suggested changes in Crouch's life care plan" which was not disclosed in the expert's report. The Court determined that [expert's] reports are stricken and [he/she] is prohibited from testifying at trial. This case illustrates the need for an expert to carefully prepare any testimony consistent with the rules related to admissibility. This being a federal court case, the *Federal Rules of Evidence* (Amended 2000) and the *Federal Rules of Civil Procedure* applied. In state courts, the appropriate state rules would apply.

Foundation and Methodology

Aside from the credentials an expert needs in order to qualify as a life care planner, the proper foundation that is utilized to develop a plan that will withstand a challenge and cross examination during trial is essential (see Weed, 2007; Weed & Johnson, 2006). Proper, relevant, and reliable methodologies are emphasized in *Kumho v. Carmichael* (1999) and the *Federal Rules of Evidence 702* (2000) (see also Field, 2011). In reviewing several legal cases (illustrated below), the second most common basis for a *motion to exclude* testimony is related directly to the experts methodology for forming an opinion (the first motion is usually related to the expert's credentials as previously discussed).

A frequent mistake made by an expert is the failure to rely on a proper foundation as the basis for a life care plan. In *Tucker v. Cascade General* (2014), the life care planning expert consulted with the plaintiff's physicians and medical providers who provided needed information regarding future medical care. "Based on these discussions, [expert] determined the need for future medical care and treatment, and its cost, in multiple disciplines for the remainder of his life. [The plan] included necessary medical services as well as other vocational and domestic assistance, and the costs of prescription medications." The primary treating physician "reviewed the [expert's] life care plan and agreed the services were necessary." This case is an excellent example of the proper approach a life care planner should take in developing a life care plan. Following a review of all the relevant reports and documents, the expert proceeded to develop a plan based on the medical evidence, and then ultimately had that plan reviewed by the primary physician. The methodology was sound and in keeping with the guidelines for plan development by the *Standards of Practice for Life Care Planners* (2015, pp. 5–10).

The defendant in *Sandretto v. Payson Healthcare Management, Inc.* (2014) argued, on appeal, that the life care planner's testimony for the plaintiff was allowed when it should have been denied, representing an error in discretion by the lower court (see *General Electric v. Joiner,* 1997 for a discussion on the abuse of discretion ruling). The specific complaint by the defendant was that the life care planning expert "did not provide proper foundation to testify about the cost of [plaintiff's] future medical care" (p. 6). Citing Arizona's *Rule of Evidence 703*, the court noted that "facts or data in the case that the expert has been made aware of or personally observed" (p. 6) serves as proper sources of information for expert opinions. Given the importance of relying upon a proper foundation for plan development, the following is a summary of the [expert's] own explanation to the court on her approach and cognizance of the foundation issue:

> [Expert] testified that she relied on her own observations and experience, as well as input from medical doctors, and readily-available pricing information for procedures, medications, and other line items. [Expert] also met with the plaintiff and the treating physician (on two occasions) and typically relied on physicians to provide medical justification for individual line items in the life care plan, and then she would determine the costs of the plan. [Expert]

> testified her expertise includes the calculation of the costs of the plan, but the doctors determined whether a particular line item was appropriate. (pp. 6–7)

The defendant continued to argue that the "[expert] was not candid in the preparation of her life care plan" (p. 7), but the Trial Court determined that this issue went to the weight of the evidence, not the issue of admissibility. On the issue of abuse of discretion by the Trial Court, the Appeals Court ruled that the "trial court did not err in admitting the [life care planner's] testimony and the life care plan" (p. 7); the motion for a new trial was denied.

The case of *Brown v. USA Truck, Inc. and Watkins* (2013) presents a situation involving differing medical opinions relied upon by the plaintiff's life care planner. As noted previously and as illustrated in the *Sandretto* case (2014), proper medical foundation is essential in developing life care plans (see also *Standards of Practice for Life Care Planners*, 2015). While no fault resides with the life care planner, the Court determined that the "preponderance of the evidence... is not sufficient to establish" (p. 3) the inability of the plaintiff to be employed in the future. Consequently, the Court ruled that the plaintiff was not "entitled to recover damages based on future lost income—a decision that negated the need for the plaintiff's life care plan."

In a case where the testimony of a life care planner was excluded, the issue of "foundation" for her testimony was the central focus. In *Taylor v. Speedway Motorsports, Inc.* (2003), the life care planner was excluded because the court found that

> "the witness wishes to express an opinion or numerous opinions without proper foundation ... the court finds that these opinions are entirely speculative" (p. 33). Relying on the federal rulings of both *Daubert* and *Kumho* that the "proffered testimony is unreliable and is not relevant ... and would not be helpful and will not assist the jury in understanding the evidence or determining the facts of the case, and the testimony (language adopted from FRE 403) is substantially outweighed by the danger of unfair prejudice, misleading the jury, and a waste of time." (p. 7)

The decision by the court in this case seems harsh and the decision clearly a firm rejection of the life care plan. However, this early case established a precedent that life care plans must be without speculation and developed with a proper foundation of relevant and reliable data and information. Preparation, or the lack thereof, was illustrated as well in a recent case (*CSC, Bryant and Cobbs v. USA*, 2013) where the life care plan for the defendant was found to be deficient. The Court determined that the life care planner never met the plaintiff or the child's parents, was not a certified life care planner, and relied only on the viability of the *Affordable Care Act* as too speculative as a funding source.

Standards of Practice

The *Daubert* trilogy ruling made it very clear that a relevant and reliable methodology was critical to the admissibility of opinion and testimony in federal courts (similar requirements also apply in state courts). The foundation for expert testimony is Federal Rule 702 which emphasized the three essential factors for the court to consider in determining admissibility:

> (1) the testimony is based upon sufficient facts or data, (2) the testimony is the product of reliable principles and methods, and (3) the witness has applied the principles and methods reliably to the facts of the case.

For the life care planner and testifying expert, in addition to the possession of proper credentials, methodology is central to the development of a life care plan. To further enhance and clarify the work of the life care planner is the important role professional associations play in providing guidance for the expert. The advantages of membership of such associations are the ongoing educational opportunities when attending regional and national conferences and the many opportunities for networking and/or collaborating with other professionals. However, one of the most valuable sources of information is the "standards of practice"—a document which has been developed over time by the very professionals who are also members of the professional associations. For example, the *Standards of Practice for Life Care Professionals* (2015) was most recently revised in 2015 by an advisory group and a revision committee (a total of 34 professionals), all of whom have been active life care planners for many years. These professionals have all earned graduate degrees in academic fields such as rehabilitation counseling, case management, and nursing; several have earned doctorates. In addition, all of the professionals have years of experience as life care planners, have been leaders and resource people at conferences, and possess a number of professional certifications in various practice areas related to rehabilitation and life care planning. Information on the *Standards* was first published by Weed & Berens (2001) and later expanded upon by Weed and Berens, (2010) and Preston (2002). The work of Neulicht, et al. (2002) resulted in an extensive survey on the life care planning process, methods and protocols which provided a much needed perspective from professionals who were developing life care plans. The *Standards* have been consistently reviewed and updated on alternate years ever since this initial effort by Preston (Johnson & Gamez, 2015; for a more complete discussion of standards for the life care planner, consult Weed & Berens, 2010).

The *Standards of Practice* provide a much needed guideline and resource for life care planners. The *Standards* serve as a basis for a consistent and comprehensive methodological approach which contributes significantly to reaching the needed levels of relevance and reliability for admissibility of testimony in state and federal courts. As a note of caution, however, in *Adams v. Laboratory Corporation of America* (2014), the Court addressed the issue on the extent to which a testifying expert could or should rely on a professional association's *Standards* in the preparation of a work product. The Court noted that *Standards* could be self-serving, are not objective findings, and that the District Court reliance on the *Standards* by permitting them as evidence for admissibility "was an abuse of discretion." The Court further noted that "neither *Daubert* nor *Kumho* permits a scientific or medical community to define a litigation standard that applied when its members are sued … but may consider the degree of acceptance of a scientific technique or theory in the relevant scientific community" (p. 2). It can be assumed that the same general admissibility standard would apply in cases involving "specialized or other technical knowledge" (i.e., FRE 702) such as would be present with life care plans. This ruling suggests that the *Standards of Practice for Life Care Planners* should serve as a guideline for both practice and the development of opinion and testimony in state and federal courts. The *Standards* should not be construed as the basis for admissibility, however. An excellent example of how this issue on *Standards* was considered for admissibility can be found in *Roach & Roach v. Hughes, Chicot, Chicot Sales, & Wheels* (2015) which included a *motion to exclude* the opinion of the life care planner in this case. The life care planning expert "followed the standards of the [professional association] in developing the life care plan and based her opinions on sufficient facts and data, including medical records, the opinions and recommendations of multiple medical providers, consulting with [plaintiff], and her own research. The Court finds that the principles and methodology utilized in the life care planning field are reasonable measures of reliability of [expert's] methodology and opinions" (p. 3). The motion was denied.

Conclusion

Professionals who are involved in the practice and development of life care plans should be familiar with and have a working knowledge of the following important areas of information:

1. The *Daubert, Kumho,* and *Joiner* federal rulings on admissibility
2. The *Federal Rules of Evidence* (i.e., 702, 401, 402, & 403) and the *Federal Rules of Civil Procedure* (i.e., 26)
3. *Standards of Practice*
4. Following current case law developments
5. Follow the suggestions in the Checklist shown in Table 35.1 as a guide in developing a life care plan

In addition, being active in one's respective professional association through such activities as attending conferences (for continuing education, certification credit, and networking), participating in leadership roles (committee memberships, presenting on topics, and representing the profession), and engaging in knowledge development (i.e., authoring for journals) will assist the professional with establishing a substantial foundation of knowledge on which to rely.

Table 35.1 Admissibility Related Topics Checklist

- Do you have appropriate life care planning–related specialized education, training, experience, and credentials?
- Do you have life care planning–relevant specialized training?
  - For example: Are you certified as a life care planner?
- Do you belong to and, even better, are you active in appropriate organizations that have life care planning education as part of their mission?
- Do you develop life care plans according to established and accepted standards of practice, ethics, and published methodologies?
- Do you make sure that life care plans include proper foundation (including medical)?
- Do you stay current with the parameters of the profession?
- Are you familiar with relevant life care planning literature?
- Are you intimately familiar with life care planning related *Standards of Practice*?
- Are you familiar with the rules of the jurisdictions in which you practice?
- Are you knowledgeable about applicable *Federal Rules of Evidence* when testifying in personal injury litigation?
- Is your report written to meet Rule 26 requirements? And do you have a list of all publications authored within the preceding 10 years and a listing of any other cases in which you have testified as an expert at trial or by deposition within the preceding 4 years?
- When you author a life care plan, are you an active participant/collaborator, rather than a "secretary" simply writing down whatever someone else recommends, or a "know-it-all" who believes he/she needs no participation from others? (*Editor's note*: See the reprint of a short article on this topic in Chapter 1, Life Care Planner: Secretary, Know-It-All, or General Contractor? One Person's Perspective.)
- Are you mindful about staying within one's area of expertise or scope of practice?
- Are you knowledgeable about the disability(ies) for which life care plans are developed?

Source: Adapted from *Lessons Learned*, Weed, R., & Johnson, C. 2006. Life Care Planning in Light of Daubert & Kumho. Athens, GA: Elliott & Fitzpatrick, p. 50.

References

Adams v. Laboratory Corporation of America, No. 13-10425, US Ci Ct of Appeals, 11th Cir (2014).

Ancar & Ancar v. Brown & TNE Trucking, No. 3:11-ev-595-DPJ-FKB, US Dist Ct for the So Dist of MA, No Div, (2014).

Beavers v. Victorian, No. CIV-11-1442-D, US Dist Ct for the W Dist of OK, (2014).

Brown v. USA Truck, Inc. and Watkins, No. CIV-11-856-D, US Dist Ct for the W Dust of OK, (2013).

Carmichael v. Samyang Tires, Inc., US Dist Ct, 923 F. Supp. 1514, 1521-1522 (SD Ala. 1996).

Carmichael v. Samyang Tires, Inc., US Eleventh Cir Ct, 131 F 3d 1433 (1997).

Crouch v. John Jewell Aircraft, Inc., No. 3:07-CV-638-DJH, US Dist Ct for the W Dist of KY, Louisville Div. (2016).

CSC, a minor, and Bryant and Cobbs v. United States of America, No. 10-910-DRH, US Dist Ct for the S Dist of IL, (2013).

Daubert v. Merrill Dow Pharmaceuticals, 727 F. Supp. 570, 572 SD Cal. (1989).

Daubert v. Merrill Dow Pharmaceuticals, 951 F. 2d 1128, US Ct of Appl, Ninth Cir. (1991).

Daubert v. Merrill Dow Pharmaceuticals Syllabus, 92-102, US Sp Ct. (1993a).

Daubert v. Merrill Dow Pharmaceuticals, 92-102, US Sp Ct. (1993b).

Elliott, T. (2010). A plaintiff's attorney's perspective on life care planning. In R. Weed & D. Berens (Eds), *Life care planning and case management handbook* (3rd ed., pp. 761–782). Boca Raton, FL: CRC Press, Taylor and Francis Group.

Federal Rules of Civil Procedure. Retrieved from www.law.cornell.edu/rules/frcp

Federal Rules of Evidence (Amended 2000). Retrieved from www.law.cornell.edu/rules/fre

Federal Rules of Evidence: Notes of Advisory Committee on Rules (2000). Retrieved from http://federalevidence.com/advisory-committee-notes

Feinman, R. (2011). *Evidence-based medicine: Who decides admissibility? The Frye standard.* Retrieved from http://rdfeinman.wordpress.com/2011/05/06/evidence-based-medicine.

Field, T. (2011). *Federal Rule 702 in Light of the Daubert, Kumho and Joiner Rulings on the admissibility of expert testimony.* Athens, GA: Elliott & Fitzpatrick.

Frye v. United States, 3968, 293 F 1013 DC Cir., (1923).

General Electric Company v. Joiner, 864 F. Supp. 1310, 1329 ND GA (1994).

General Electric Company v. Joiner, Ct of Appl for the Eleventh Cir, 78 F. 3d 524 (1996).

General Electric Company v. Joiner Syllabus, 96-188, US Sp Ct, (1997).

General Electric Company v. Joiner, 96 188, US Sp Ct, 1997.

Gunn, R. (2010). A defense attorney's perspective on life care planning. In R. Weed & D. Berens (Eds), *Life care planning and case management handbook* (3rd ed., pp. 783–797). Boca Raton, FL: CRC Press, Taylor and Francis Group.

International Academy of Life Care Planners, The Life Care Planning Section of the International Association of Rehabilitation Professionals. (2015). *Standards of practice for life care planners.* Glenview, IL: Author.

Johnson, C., & Gamez, J. (2015). What is the life care planning summit; and why should you attend the 2015 summit? *Journal of Life Care Planning, 13*(1), 19–22.

Kumho Tire Company v. Carmichael Syllabus, 97-1709, US Sp Ct, (1998).

Kumho Tire Company v. Carmichael, 97-1709, 526-137, US Sp Ct, (1999).

M.D.P. v. Middleton, No. 1:11cv461-WHA (wo), US Dist Ct for the Middle Dist of AL, So Div, (2013).

Mettias v. United States of America, Civ. No. 12-00527 ACK-KSC, US Dist Ct for the Dist of HI, (2015).

Neulicht, A., Riddick-Grisham, S, Hinton, L., Costantini, P., Thomas, R., & Goodrich, B., (2002). Life care planning survey 2001: Process, methods and protocols. *Journal of Life Care Planning, 1*(2), 97–148.

Pearson, W. (2014). What to expect when you're an expert: Admissibility of expert testimony. Retrieved from: www.ims-expertservces.com.

Preston, K. (2002). Standards of practice: What they can and cannot do. *Journal of Life Care Planning, 1*(2), 91–96.

Roach & Roach v. Hughes, Chicot, Chicot Sales, & Wheels, No. 4:13-CV-00136-JHM, US Dist Ct for the W Dist of KY, Owensboro Div, (2015).

Sandretto v. Payson Healthcare Management, Inc., No. 2 CA-CV 2013-0044, Court of Appeals of Arizona, Div Two, (2014).
Standards of Practice for Life Care Planners (3rd Ed.). (2015). Glenview, IL: International Association of Rehabilitation Professionals.
Taylor v. Speedway Motorsports, Inc, 01-CVS-12107, Mecklenburg Cty Sup Ct, NC, (2003).
Tucker v. Cascade General, 3:09-cv-1491-AC, US Dist Ct for the Dist of OR, Portland Div, (2014).
Weed, R. (2007). *Life care planning: A step-by-step guide.* Athens, GA: Elliott & Fitzpatrick.
Weed, R., & Berens, D. (Eds.). (2001). *Life Care Planning Summit 2000 Proceedings.* Athens, GA: Elliott & Fitzpatrick.
Weed, R., & Berens, D. (Eds.). (2010). *Life care planning and case management handbook* (3rd ed.). Boca Raton, FL: CRC Press, Taylor & Francis Group.
Weed, R., & Johnson, C. (2006). *Life care planning in light of Daubert & Kumho.* Athens, GA: Elliott & Fitzpatrick.
Worley & Worley v. State Farm Mutual Automobile Insurance Company, No. 3: 2012cv01041, 47 (M.D. FL, 2013).

Chapter 36

Cultural Considerations for Life Care Planning

Mary Barros-Bailey

Contents

Introduction 833
Foundations of Multicultural and Cross-Cultural Issues in Life Care Planning 834
Multicultural and Cross-Cultural Issues in Life Care Planning 836
  Individualistic and Collectivistic Cultures 836
  Acculturation and Enculturation 836
  Life Care Planner Cultural Competence 837
  Multicultural and Cross-Cultural Communication 837
  Methodological Framework for Cross-Cultural Life Care Planning 839
Conclusion 839
References 840

Introduction

Culture \'kəl-chər\ is a noun. *Merriam-Webster* (2018) defines it as, "the beliefs, customs, arts, etc. of a particular society, group, place, or time; a particular society that has its own beliefs, ways of life, art, etc.; a way of thinking, behaving, or working that exists in a place or organization" (Culture definition, 2018, para. 1). Sometimes, culture can be limited by ethnicity, country, or area of origin, and the definition goes no further to include other descriptive variables. In general terms, however, ethnicity or geography are only two of the potential delimiters of culture. Any unit of people in any society or region that share beliefs, lifestyles, ethnicity, or customs in common can be a cultural group.

Culture is the root term for two other important related definitions that carry the underlying structure of this chapter: multicultural and cross-cultural. Using *Merriam-Webster* (2018), the author defines multicultural as, "relating to or including many different cultures" (Multicultural definition, 2018, para. 1) within a society no matter regional or national boundaries, such as the culture of people with disabilities and the culture of allied health professionals in America or the culture of Aborigines and the culture of ex-patriots in Australia. The concept of multiculturalism is that the multitude of cultures is contained *within* a single society. The more cultures contained in such a society, the more heterogeneous it is in its beliefs, customs, arts, or other variables. Cross-culturalism, on the other hand, involves the interaction of people *between* more than one society instead of a single society or country. Using the *Merriam-Webster* source again, the author defines cross-culturalism as, "relating to and involving two or more different cultures or countries" (Cross-cultural definition, 2018, para. 1). Cross-cultural relationships may be when a person or group from one country interacts with an individual or group located in another country. As it involves life care planning, the terms used in this chapter are as follows:

- *Multicultural*: The life care planner provides services nationally in the country of residence and the evaluee/family comes from a different culture than the planner's (e.g., a life care planner in Canada develops a life care plan for a refugee residing in Canada).
- *Cross-cultural*: The life care planner provides services for the evaluee in another society than his/her own main country of residence (e.g., a life care planner in the United States [US] develops a life care plan for a South Korean national in the evaluee's country of residence).

Therefore, if the life care planner and the evaluee are within the same dominant culture, like a country, and the services are to be delivered within that dominant society, but the life care planner and the evaluee come from two different cultures, it is multicultural life care planning. However, if the life care planner is to develop and/or deliver services across societies, regardless of whether the life care planner and the evaluee come from the same or different culture, the fact that the life care planner will be interacting with individuals in other societies deems the relationship a cross-cultural one. Sometimes, in the latter example, this is also called international life care planning.

Foundations of Multicultural and Cross-Cultural Issues in Life Care Planning

The body of literature located in the life care planning specialty that directly addresses issues of culture in practice is nascent and emerging as this chapter is going to press (Barros-Bailey, 2017; Caragonne, 2016; Cosby, 2016; Phillips, 2016). The literature is explored along with the calls for consideration of cultural issues in practice.

There are some foundational documents and studies that allude to the knowledge of culture in life care planning practice. First, Pomeranz et al. (2010) performed a role and function study of life care planners to "help define a profession and provide an empirical basis for establishment of educational standards and certification requirements" (p. 57). As part of their study, they included the knowledge of multicultural issues within a composite question that also involved knowledge of family dynamics and geographical issues. This area was included in the needed knowledge required in Counseling and Services—or, the domain that of "items that represent the process of helping individual and/or family/caregivers adjust to the psychological and/or behavioral impact of disability" (p. 113).

Second, there are practice and ethical standards that include the consideration of cultural issues. One of the four Standards of Performance outlined in the *Standards of Practice for Life*

Care Planners (2015) is that the life care planner "considers cultural and linguistic factors that may influence assessment, development, and implementation of the plan" (p. 6–7). Specific to the broader professions from where life care planners may come, respective credentialing and professional bodies contain provisions for cultural considerations in practice. For nurse life care planners, for example, the standards of practice of the professional organization for all nurses, the American Nurses Association, address consideration of "cultural preferences, beliefs, and spiritual and health practices in plans of care" (p. 13, Cosby, 2016). In credentialing, the International Commission on Health Care Certification (ICHCC), for those in the United States and Canada, notes in its *Practice Standards and Guidelines* (2015) the adoption of a code of ethics that rests upon other codes, such as that of the Commission on Rehabilitation Counselor Certification (2016), that clearly outlines the consideration of cultural issues in clinical and forensic practice.

However, culture is missing from the collection of professional consensus statements in life care planning. The summits for life care planners from 2000 to 2015 (Preston & Johnson, 2012; Johnson, 2015) identified consensus on a variety of majority statements dealing with qualifications, professional and ethics standards, and methodological principles and procedures among members of the following organizations: American Association of Nurse Life Care Planners (AANLCP); American Association of Legal Nurse Consultants (AALNC); Care Planner Network; Commission on Disability Examiner Certification (CDEC); Commission on Health Care Certification (now, ICHCC); Case Management Society of America (CMSA); Foundation of Life Care Planning Research (FLCPR); Georgia State University; Intelicus; International Academy of Life Care Planners (IALCP); International Association of Rehabilitation Professionals (IARP); IARP-Canada; University of Florida; and Vocational Rehabilitation Association of Canada (VRA). None of these consensus statements directly address cultural issues in life care planning (C. Johnson, personal communication, November 16, 2016).

Regardless of the scant treatment of the topic of culture within the role and function study, in Standards of Practice, or in consensus statements, the fact that life care planners face multicultural and cross-cultural issues in life care planning is a fact. In their survey of life care planners and their processes and methods, Neulicht et al. (2010) asked respondents if they had provided services in the international arena in the preceding 5 years. A total of 25 (11.26 percent) respondents indicated providing life care planning in such a setting.

In 2016, Barros-Bailey performed exploratory research on multicultural and cross-cultural issues in life care planning by collecting data from life care planners who are members of AANLCP, IALCP, IARP, and the Care Planner Network. The results of the study suggested that in the multicultural area, the most significant issues encountered by life care planners were in communication; family; access/use of medical, mental health, or related care; housing; and advocacy. In cross-cultural life care planning, the most significant issues identified were in the access/use of medical, mental health, or related care; providers; legal; cost resources; communication; society; and referral source education. Therefore, it appears that generally from a multicultural framework, life care planners are more concerned with the relational and contextual factors whereas from a cross-cultural perspective, life care planners identified concerns more with resources for the life care plan development and, secondarily, with relational and contextual issues. Most recently, Barros-Bailey, Latham, and Mitchell (2017) and Barros-Bailey and Latham (2018a,b) studied multicultural ethical issues in life care planning and found dilemmas falling into some of the similar areas of practice identified in the Barros-Bailey 2016 study.

Multicultural and Cross-Cultural Issues in Life Care Planning

Individualistic and Collectivistic Cultures

The concept of life care planning, or what has been known in Canada as a Cost of Future Care Plan (Phillips, 2016), was developed in cultures that are considered individualistic, such as the United States. Conceptually, if the life care planner understands the difference between individualistic and collectivistic cultures, it could greatly assist in the approach, understanding, development, and services delivery across all types of groups across the life span. The definition of an individualistic society is one where "the culture focuses on the individual's needs and looks for happiness on an individual level before looking to the group" (Individualistic culture, para. 1, Reference*, 2018). On the other hand, collectivistic cultures are those that "emphasize family and work group above individual needs or desires" (Collectivist culture, para. 1, Reference*, 2018). Individualistic cultures are those such as Australia, Belgium, Canada, Ireland, Israel, New Zealand, Poland, Slovakia, South Africa, Sweden, the United States, and the United Kingdom. Collectivistic cultures are those such as Argentina, Brazil, Egypt, Ethiopia, Ghana, India, Japan, Korea, Mexico, Portugal, Russia, and Saudi Arabia.

How people cooperate (Boles et al., 2010; Nguyen et al., 2010; Marcus & Le, 2013), practice professionally (Shilo & Kelly, 1997), are treated over the lifespan (North & Fiske, 2015), how they behave ethically (Ralston et al., 2014), can be correlated with the type of society they come from. If life care planners can comprehend their socially constructed views and how those differ from those of the evaluee, it becomes the first step in bolstering potential areas of agreement or conflict in life care planning.

Acculturation and Enculturation

The United States has one of the most diverse societies on the planet, merging groups from individualistic and collectivistic cultures that have been studied and suggest that, long-term, there are no differences among immigrant groups to cultural assimilation (Vargas & Kemmelmeier, 2013). The immigrant adjustment process is dynamic and can happen in the short term, or over generations. The adjustment process is what is often referred to as acculturation.

Formally, acculturation is "the process of adopting the cultural traits and social patterns of another group" (dictionary.com, 2018, para. 1). This definition assumes that an individual started off in one culture, is being exposed to another culture, and is adopting some of the traits of the second culture. The distinction is different than when someone is born into a culture and undergoes the process of learning about his/her own culture; this is called enculturation. Various acculturation models exist, but generally involve how well someone is integrated or assimilated into the dominant culture, retains his/her own culture, and may also suggest whether the individual is segregated or marginalized by his/her own or dominant culture or society.

The level of someone's acculturation can affect how the individual communicates with those within the culture, or with other cultures. Members of a family can have different levels or rates of acculturation. Where people live, the kind of housing they choose, or the members within the household itself can be affected by the level of acculturation. Furthermore, how diverse members of a culture advocate for themselves or their loved ones can also be affected by acculturation. Important to life care planning is what health, mental health, other care or related services someone considers, administers, or participates in. These decisions can be substantially impacted by the evaluee's, caregiver's, or the family's level of acculturation.

Consequently, in multicultural matters, understanding the level of acculturation of the evaluee, as well as understanding one's own level of acculturation to the specific subculture, is a good second step to assessing the dynamic context in which the practitioner operates. Assessing someone's level of acculturation could be done informally first through the review of the records that might provide evidence as to these issues, and more directly as a part of the life care planning diagnostic interview and observation. If more formal assessment measures are needed to determine someone's level of acculturation, a variety of instruments exist. Celenk and Van de Vijver (2011) for example, summarize about 50 such tools that could be used with different populations.

Life Care Planner Cultural Competence

Beyond understanding the level of acculturation of the evaluee and his/her immediate support system, it is also important that the life care planning practitioner understand his/her own level of cultural competency. The competency standards for professional practice are outlined by a variety of organizations including those in counseling and psychology (Yoon et al., 2011), nursing (American Association of Colleges of Nursing, 2011; Beard et al., 2015), and social work (National Association of Social Workers, 2001), to name a few. Like tools to measure someone's level of acculturation, there are also a number of instruments that could be useful for a life care planner to test his/her level of cultural competency. One resource that may be helpful from the National Institutes of Health in the United States and its website on Tools for Assessing Cultural Competence (see https://www.ncbi.nlm.nih.gov/books/NBK248429/) includes direct access to such tools as the *Self-Assessment Checklist for Personnel Providing Services and Supports to Children and Youth With Special Health Needs and Their Families* and the *Multicultural Competent Service System Assessment Guide*. However, a Google™ search provides a multitude of different cultural competency checklists and guidelines specific to many cultural groups the life care planner may encounter in an individualized assessment.

Multicultural and Cross-Cultural Communication

Given that communication was the greatest concern for life care planners identified in the Barros-Bailey (2016) study, specific discussion of such communication—whether oral, bodily, or written—becomes important when addressing culture. In its simplest form, communication comes down to information that is expressed and received. How the information or thought is encoded by one individual and decoded by another person becomes increasingly complex when both people come from different cultures. This is due to how the context, words, or actions affect how the life care planner and evaluee/caregiver intend to communicate and how that intent is interpreted.

MindTools (2016) describes the 7 Cs of communication that may be helpful to the life care planner to ensuring expression and reception of information not only with evaluees and caregivers, but also with service providers, care team members, or others involved in the process. The 7 Cs are:

1. Clarity of message
2. Conciseness by sticking to the message and keeping it simple and brief
3. Concreteness of the message by giving a clear picture and presenting vivid facts
4. Correctness of the message and keeping it free of errors
5. Coherent messages that are logical and are connected together
6. Complete messages that include what the evaluee or caregiver needs to be informed about in order to make decisions
7. Courteousness of the message so that it is honest and friendly

Communication would be incomplete if the provision of translation and interpretation services within the life care planning process were not addressed. Both terms are used almost as synonyms, but they are different based on the medium used. In translation, it is text that is being transferred from one form of communication to another while interpretation is the oral transfer. Taking a medical record from one language to another is a translation. However, the individual in a medical appointment who takes the medical information from the physician and provides it in sign or other language to the patient is an interpreter. Typically, in life care planning, most practitioners will be using more interpreters than translators. Best practices in using an interpreter are (Refugee Health Technical Assistance Center, 2016):

- Introducing self to interpreter
- Acknowledge interpreter as the professional communicator
- Speak to the evaluee, not the interpreter
- Slow down the rate of speech so the interpreter can catch the totality and intent of what is being communicated
- Speech should be broken up in short segments and be at an even pace
- Assume everything being said is being interpreted
- Do not hold the interpreter responsible for what the evaluee says or does not say
- Understand that some concepts in one language have imprecise or nonexistent equivalents in another language; therefore, describing a concept in more than one way or asking for clarification from the evaluee to ascertain understanding may be necessary
- Give the interpreter time to relate information from both parties
- What may be personal or sensitive in one culture may not be so in another; therefore, be aware of the potential sensitive issues that might be important to explore through an interpreter in a variety of different modes of communication to obtain the information that is needed for the life care plan
- Avoid complex language or concepts; keep the communication clear and simple
- Encourage the evaluee, caregiver, or interpreter to ask questions
- Avoid patronizing or minimizing the evaluee
- Paraphrase, paraphrase, paraphrase to ensure you understand what the evaluee is expressing and that the evaluee interprets your communication correctly
- Allow extra time for the communication process, including a session with the interpreter beforehand that might provide insights about the communication

Professional interpreters are advised where there are linguistic differences. In situations where there may not be a professional interpreter and others may be used (e.g., friend, family member, community advocate), professional ethics should be contemplated and caution taken to verify the evaluee/caregiver understands the intent, purpose, or question and, in return, to confirm the life care planner's understanding of the information being collected or related.

With tools to effectively understand, measure, and interpret multicultural issues, the life care planner can best navigate the specific factors that may be present to the development of a plan. S/he may be better able to address social issues in the family and their relationship to the development and delivery of the life care plan, access and use of medical, mental health, or other care, advocacy or lack therefore, adequate housing or transportation, or any number of factors that may be present in the delivery of services.

Communication between cultures within a society may not be materially different than those in a cross-cultural setting. The difference may be that multiculturally, the life care planner and evaluee may be speaking the same language and the concepts being communicated may be the same or similar. The life care planner and evaluee may have been born in the same society, speak the same language, and have similar understandings of personal, geographical, societal, and other constructs, procedures, programs, or other factors although attitudes, beliefs, values, and customs may be different. In cross-cultural communication, the life care planner may be attempting to communicate in a society s/he has no or limited information about, even if the individual has lived in that society for a long time. Not just the language and ethnic or social culture may be different, but everything associated with the life care planner's culture that impact the development or management of the life care plan may be different. Therefore, the issues of communication cross-culturally may be more complex than multiculturally. The level of life care planner cultural competency, therefore, becomes more important in a cross-cultural setting. The 7 Cs of communication and the best practices identified previously are just as relevant in a cross-cultural environment; the life care planner just has to be more aware of the customs, attitudes, beliefs, and values of the society in which s/he is developing the life care plan.

Methodological Framework for Cross-Cultural Life Care Planning

No methodological frameworks were found in the literature specific to developing multicultural life care plans and only one in the cross-cultural context. In describing life care planning in such a setting, Caragonne (2016) states, "to be valid and truly useful post-litigation, a plan must exactly fit the cultural and health care infrastructure of the country where it will be used" (p. 18). Dr. Caragonne goes on to detail a useful 9-stage process for developing a cross-cultural life care plan including:

- Stage 1: Initial Request for Work: Determinations to Be Made
- Stage 2: Plan Translations
- Stage 3: Planner and Subject Safety
- Stage 4: Plan Research
- Stage 5: Skills and Familiarity in Equipment and Services for Disability
- Stage 6: Plan Documentation and Transparency
- Stage 7: Physician, Nursing, and Paraprofessional Validation
- Stage 8: Researching Quantitative Data Bases
- Stage 9: Representing Services Available through Federal Health Systems

Not only does Dr. Caragonne provide an important framework for the development of a life care plan cross-culturally, but also such multi-stage process could be modified to the development of a life care plan in a multicultural context. With its introduction into the literature, it throws open the door on the discussion of guidelines, procedures, and methods in the development and delivery of life care planning services multiculturally and cross-culturally.

Conclusion

Perhaps because the specialty of life care planning is relatively new, enjoying its fourth decade, and has been preoccupied with the activities relevant to the establishment of the specialty in practice across a host of different rehabilitation and allied health professionals, cultural factors in life care planning have not enjoyed attention, deliberation, and discussion in the professional literature until 2016. Yet, it is evident that such matters are facing life care planners on a regular basis. It is time to start the discussion and to delve deeply into those elements life care planners should be aware of in practice, whether these are within the multicultural or the cross-cultural context.

Much of the literature in the field focuses on the medical/mental/cognitive, functional, development, resource, or other immediate issues for the dominant culture. But, if someone is not a member of that culture, the life care planner is presented with a host of potential quandaries of how to develop or manage a life care plan. This chapter attempted to start at a very high level by introducing concepts into the life care planning literature that may help life care planners understand underlying dynamics that may be at play when two cultures meet—what kind of society one comes from or ascribes to (individualistic versus collectivistic), his/her level of acculturation or enculturation, modes of communication and the use of interpreters in that process, and a methodological framework for the development of a life care plan cross-culturally.

There are more topics that need to be explored. For example, from a very practical standpoint: What are some resources that could be used for the development of plans in these contexts? How are providers found? And, how does a life care planner effectively educate a referral source about the issues in a case, particularly if these vary from what is common in a life care plan where the same cultural questions do not exist? Those who provide life care plans in these contexts have anecdotal and practical experience that could benefit the entire profession. Comparisons of how life care plans are performed to those that have been developed in multicultural or cross-cultural contexts (e.g., Phillips, 2016) offer a starting point to focusing not only on philosophical or theoretical topics, but also on practical considerations in such life care planning practice settings. Let the discussion begin.

References

Acculturation definition. 2018. In *dictionary.com*. Retrieved April 19, 2018 from http://www.dictionary.com/browse/acculturation

American Association of Colleges of Nursing. 2011. *Tool kit for cultural competence in master's and doctoral nursing education*. Retrieved from http://www.aacn.nche.edu/education-resources/Cultural_Competency_Toolkit_Grad.pdf

Barros-Bailey, M. 2017. Cultural experience and international practices of life care planners: Results of an exploratory research study. *Journal of Life Care Planning. 15*(2), 7–12.

Barros-Bailey, M., Latham, S., & Mitchell, N. 2017. Multicultural ethics in life care planning: Research and practice. IARP Annual Conference, St. Louis, MO.

Barros-Bailey, M., & Latham, S. A. 2018a, March. *Multicultural ethics in life care planning.* Life is an Art: What are You Creating. American Association of Nurse Life Care Planners, St. Petersburg, FL.

Barros-Bailey, M., & Latham, S. A. 2018b, April. Ethics survey. The 2018 International Leisure and Learn Workshop: The Role of Evidence in Life Care Planning. Ajijic, Mexico.

Beard, K. V., Gwanmesia, E., & Miranda-Diaz, G. 2015. Culturally competent care: Using the ESFT model in nursing. *American Journal of Nursing, 115*(6), 58–62.

Boles, T. L., Le, H., & Nguyen, H. D. 2010. Person, organizations, and societies: The effects of collectivism and individualism on cooperation. In R. M. Kramer, A. E. Tenbrunsei, & M. H. Bazerman (Eds.), *Social Decision Making: Social Dilemmas, Social Values, and Ethical Judgments* (pp. 171–200). New York, NY: Psychology Press.

Caragonne, P. 2016. Life care planning in Mexico and Latin America. *Journal of Nurse Life Care Planning, 16*(3), 18–23.

Celenk, O., & Van de Vijver, F. 2011. Assessment of acculturation: Issues and overview of measures. *Online Readings in Psychology and Culture*, 8(1), 1–22. https://doi.org/10.9707/2307-0919.1105

Collectivist culture. 2018. In *Reference**. Retrieved April 19, 2018 from https://www.reference.com/world-view/examples-collectivist-cultures-ac597798cdac77fe

Commission on Rehabilitation Counselor Certification. 2016. *Code of professional ethics for rehabilitation counselors*. Retrieved from https://www.crccertification.com/code-of-ethics-4

Cosby, M. F. 2016. Cultural considerations for life care planners: Religious traditions and health benefits. *Journal of Nurse Life Care Planning, 16*(3), 13–17.

Cross-cultural definition. 2018. In *Merriam-Webster.com*. Retrieved April 19, 2018, from http://www.merriam-webster.com/dictionary/cross-cultural

Culture definition. 2018. In *Merriam-Webster.com*. Retrieved April 19, 2018, from http://www.merriam-webster.com/dictionary/culture

Individualistic culture. 2018. In *Reference**. Retrieved April 19, 2018 from https://www.reference.com/education/individualistic-culture-12e6b48e73cf5fd7

International Academy of Life Care Planners, International Association of Rehabilitation Professionals. 2015. *Standard of Practice for Life Care Planners* (3rd ed). Glenview, IL: Author.

International Commission on Health Care Certification. 2015. Practice standards and guidelines. Retrieved November 15, 2016 from https://www.ichcc.org/images/PDFs/ICHCC_StandardsandGuidelines.pdf

Johnson, C. B. 2015. Life care planning summit: Moving forward and looking ahead. *Journal of Life Care Planning, 11*(2), 27–33.

Marcus, J., & Le, A. H. 2013. Interactive effects of levels of individualism-collectivism on cooperation: A meta-analysis. *Journal of Organizational Behavior, 34*, 813–834.

Multicultural definition. 2016. In *Merriam-Webster.com*. Retrieved June 2, 2016, from http://www.merriam-webster.com/dictionary/multicultural

MindTools. 2016. *The 7 Cs of communication*. Retrieved November 16, 2016 from https://www.mindtools.com/pages/article/newCS_85.htm

National Association of Social Workers. 2001. *NASW standards for cultural competence in social work practice*. Washington, DC: Author.

Neulicht, A. T., Riddick-Grisham, S., & Goodrich, W. R. 2010. Life care plan survey 2009: Process, methods[,] and protocols. *Journal of Life Care Planning, 9*(4), 129–214.

North, M. S., & Fiske, S. T. 2015. Modern attitudes toward older adults in the aging world: A cross-cultural meta-analysis. *American Psychological Association, 141*(5), 993–1021.

Nguyen, H. D., Le, H., & Boles, T. 2010. Individualism-collectivism and co-operation: A cross-society and cross-level examination. *International Association of Conflict Management and Wiley Periodicals, Inc, 3*(3), 179–204.

Phillips, K. 2016. A comparison of Canadian and US life care planning. *Journal of Nurse Life Care Planning, 16*(3), 23–28.

Pomeranz, J. L., Yu, N. S., & Reid, C. 2010. Role and function study of life care planners. *Journal of Life Care Planning, 9*(3), 57–118.

Preston, K., & Johnson, C. 2012. Consensus and majority statements derived from life care planning summits held in 2000, 2002, 2004, 2006, 2008, 2010[,] and 2012). *Journal of Life Care Planning, 11*(2), 9–14.

Ralston, D. A., Egri, C. P., Furrer, O., Kuo, M. H., Li, J., Wangenhelm, F., Dabic, M., Naoumova, I., ... Weber, M. 2014. Societal-level versus individual-level predictions of ethical behavior: A 48-society study of collectivism and individualism. *Journal of Business Ethics, 122*, 283–306.

Refugee Health Technical Assistance Center. 2016. *Best practices for communicating through an interpreter*. Retrieved November 16, 2016 from http://refugeehealthta.org/access-to-care/language-access/best-practices-communicating-through-an-interpreter/

Shilo, A. M., & Kelly, E. W. 1997. Individualistic and collective approaches to counseling: Preference, personal orientation, gender, and age. *Counseling and Values, 41*(3), 253–264.

Vargas, J. H., & Kemmelmeier, M. 2013. Ethnicity and contemporary American culture: A meta-analytic investigation of horizontal-vertical individualism-collectivism. *Journal of Cross-Cultural Psychology, 44*(2), 195–222.

Yoon, E., Langrehr, K., & Ong, L. A. 2011. Content analysis of acculturation research in counseling and counseling psychology: A 22-year review. *American Psychological Association, 58*(1), 83–96. doi: 10.1037/a0021128.

Chapter 37

Life Care Planning in Canada

Dana M. Weldon

Contents

Background ... 844
What Is a Canadian Life Care Plan? ... 844
    Terminology ... 845
    Life Care Planning Process ... 845
    Who Prepares the Life Care Plan? ... 845
    Training for Life Care Planners ... 846
    How Do You Become a Canadian Certified Life Care Planner ... 847
    Life Care Planning Standards of Practice ... 848
    Types of Life Care Plans ... 848
        Catastrophic Life Care Plans ... 848
        Non-Catastrophic Life Care Plans ... 848
    Admissibility Rules in the United States and Canada ... 849
    Canadian Practice ... 850
    The Canadian Life Care Planner as Expert Witness ... 850
    Working with a Life Care Planner ... 851
    Canadian Supreme Court Judgments and the Life Care Planner ... 852
        Medically Justified ... 852
        Who Can Provide Evidence? ... 853
        Reasonableness ... 853
        Is It Likely the Item Will Be Used? ... 854
        Standard of Care ... 855
        Government Benefits ... 855
        Family Assistance ... 855
        PharmaCare Benefits ... 855
        Home or Institutional Care ... 856
        Double Compensation ... 856
        Failure to Mitigate ... 856
        Quantifying Care Provided by Family Members ... 856
        Attendant Care or Lifeline ... 857

Attendant Care—Will It Be Used? 857
Attendant Care—Overnight Security 857
Future Care Awards....858
The Role of the Treatment Team 859
Lack of Foundation....859
Institutional or Home Care....859
The Burden of Proof....859
Capacity.... 860
Orders for Examination by Nonmedical Practitioners 860
Double Recovery and Overlap 861
Government Funding and Future Care Costs....861
Conclusion.... 862
References 862
Case References.... 863

Background

As has been identified in print over the years in several rehabilitation publications, the earliest mention of life care planning points to the 1981 publication, *Damages in Tort Actions* by Paul Deutsch, and Fred Raffa (as cited in Riddick-Grisham & Deming, 2011).

An important figure in the history of life care planning is Paul M. Deutsch, PhD, who is widely credited for the creation of the professional credential of a life care planning practitioner (Physician Life Care Planning, 2017). His goal to establish and formalize the profession was accomplished through publications, the creation of curriculums, standards of practice, and involvement in a number of different organizations. (*Editors' note:* See Chapter 1 for a comprehensive summary of the history of life care planning.)

In the early 2000s there were merely a handful of certified life care planners in Canada, and at last count in the Spring of 2016 the number of Canadian life care planners is more than 130 from coast to coast.

What Is a Canadian Life Care Plan?

A life care plan is a dynamic document based on published standards of practice, comprehensive assessment, data analysis, and research that provides an organized, concise plan for current and future needs with associated costs, for individuals who have experienced catastrophic injury or who have chronic health care needs (Weed, 2010).

Canadian life care plans are based on the same principles and considered to be the benchmark when assessing future care costs for the injured individual. They have become useful to identify an individual's current needs, as well as to forecast the future care needs along with associated costs and the frequency in which services and goods will be needed.

The life care plan is customized to each individual and can cover a wide range of categories, which can include but is not limited to:

- Medical care
- Projected evaluations
- Projected therapeutic modalities

- Housekeeping and home maintenance
- Attendant care
- Home modification/Environmental adaptations
- Transportation
- Medication
- Mobility aids
- Assistive devices
- Leisure/recreational/fitness
- Vocational/educational plan
- Child care support
- Financial services

Terminology

"Future cost of care encompasses all post-trial expenses which the plaintiff will now incur, but which he or she would not have incurred" (Cooper-Stephenson, 1996).

In Canada, life care plans can be called Future Care Cost Assessments, Future Cost Analysis, Cost of Future Care Reports, or Future Needs Analysis, and so on. A life care plan by any other name is still a life care plan.

The individuals for whom the plan is prepared have a variety of labels such as evaluees, clients, claimants, or plaintiffs.

In its simplest form, a life care plan provides a road map to assist individuals and their families to obtain the necessary treatment, assessment, therapy, goods, and services in order to maximize their independence and function, as well as to prevent future complications.

Life Care Planning Process

Based on the procedures carried out in this author's practice, the following identifies creating the plan from start to finish:

1. Initial contact with referral source to discuss parameters of the referral
2. Obtain and review all available medical and other records
3. In person interview of evaluee and family
4. Contact treating health care practitioners
5. Consult with professionals outside of area of expertise if applicable
6. Retain correspondence with all providers in file
7. Outline recommendations
8. Identify costs
9. Identify relevant medical literature and statistical data
10. Prepare preliminary life care plan narrative and cost charts
11. Review findings with client (evaluee) and/or medical personnel
12. Complete final life care plan

Who Prepares the Life Care Plan?

Life care plans are most often prepared by rehabilitation professionals with specific training in life care planning who are identified as life care planners. In Canada, life care planners can come from a variety of health care specialties (case managers, rehabilitation professionals, occupational therapists, physiotherapists, nurses, social workers, etc.). The Certified Life Care Planner (CLCP) and Canadian Certified Life Care Planner (CCLCP) designations are the mark of competent, ethical, consultative professionals who go the extra mile, demonstrating their deep commitment to the field of life care planning. These designations are awarded by the International Commission on Health Care Certification (ICHCC) following successful completion of the certifying examination, but certification is not required to practice (Physician Life Care Planning, 2017).

To complete a life care plan, the life care planner must assess, as well as project an evaluee's current and future needs based on the sequelae of their disability. In order to do this, the life care planner must examine and analyze the medical documentation, as well as conduct interviews with the evaluee, family, treatment providers, and others involved in their care. Life care planning does not occur independently of others and is a collaborative practice that puts its weight in assessing, coordinating, evaluating, and projecting the services that are required for those with future needs as dictated by their level of disability.

The profession of the life care planner grew out of a need in the litigation arena, where there had not been any previous consolidated effort to summarize recommendations to use for future care in case settlements.

Through the integration of this new professional, there was definition in the form of a care plan that took into account the evaluee's situation. Essentially, the profession of life care planning was a response to an identified need in response to three central questions:

1. What is the medical status of the individual?
2. What is required based on their status?
3. How much will this cost over time?

Training for Life Care Planners

The life care planning training programs ensure life care planners will be qualified and knowledgeable of the methodologies, standards of care, ethical considerations, and best practices for the profession (Physician Life Care Planning, 2017).

Initially, a management company (Rehabilitation Training Institute) was contracted to set up training programs throughout the United States. Before the first flyers were fully distributed, the first of the organized tracks (scheduled for November 1993) was filled (Weed, 2010).

From the 1990s to the present the training program for life care planners underwent various changes in management including the University of Florida—Intelicus; the University of Florida—Medipro, and the University of Florida (UF) where it continued until 2016. The UF training program was acquired by the Institute of Rehabilitation Education and Training (IRET) in the spring of 2016 and continues under the IRET banner at this time, offering the onsite module in Canada once per year, in addition to the annual onsite module in the United States (Institute of Rehabilitation Education and Training, 2017).

For a few years in Canada, the Canadian Institute of Life Care Planning (CILCP) was formed and provided a training program from 2004 to 2008 through Carleton University in Ottawa, offering onsite training in Toronto, Vancouver, and Ottawa before it ceased operations.

Now, courses for life care planners are available at Capital University Law School and training specifically for nurses, such as FIG Services and Kelynco, to name a few.

The Institute of Rehabilitation Education Life Care Planning Pre-certification program is designed to prepare those who are seeking to become Certified Life Care Planners (CLCP) or

Canadian Certified Life Care Planners (CCLCP) with the knowledge necessary to successfully pass the certification exam offered by the International Commission on Health Care Certification (ICHCC).

How Do You Become a Canadian Certified Life Care Planner

Qualifying for the Certified Canadian Life Care Planner (CCLCP) credential is based on two factors: (1) meeting the definition of a "Qualified Health Care Professional," and (2) the applicant's education and training. Before reviewing the educational and training experience component, one must ensure that he or she meets the International Commission on Health Care Certification's definition of "Qualified Health Care Professional" (2017). The "Qualified Health Care Professional" definition and a listing of its criteria are detailed in the *ICHCC Standards and Guidelines Manual* available for download on the ICHCC website (www.ichcc.org). All certification candidates should have this manual in his or her library if certification is a true goal.

The ICHCC requires the following criteria to be met by all candidates in order to qualify to sit for the examination (International Commission on Health Care Certification, 2017):

- Each candidate must have a minimum of 120 hours of post-graduate or post-specialty degree training in life care planning or in areas that can be applied to the development of a life care plan or pertain to the service delivery applied to life care planning. There must be 16 hours of training specific to a basic orientation, methodology, and standards of practice in life care planning within the required 120 hours. The 120 hours may be obtained through online training/educational programs, as well as by attending onsite presentations and conferences. Additionally, the following educational components by a ICHCC approved CLCP program are required:
  - Life Care Planning Methodology (16 credit hours)
  - A course (module) in Catastrophic Case Management (of choice)
  - Vocational Rehabilitation Module
  - Legal component in life care planning with an onsite testimony/trial experience
  - Competency—preparation of a life care plan to be reviewed by an approved CLCP program or the ICHCC
- Applicants should have a minimum of 3 years work experience within their formal degree field and within the 5 years preceding application for certification. Final approval of any application with ambiguity regarding experience will be left to the discretion of the Commissioners following a thorough review of the respective applications. The opinion of the Commissioners is final.
- Training hours acquired over a time frame of 5 years from the date of application are counted as valid for consideration. Documentation of such coursework and participation verification is required in the form of attendance verification forms and/or curriculum documentation from the training agency. Each candidate must:
  - Meet the minimum academic requirements for their designated health care related profession
  - Be certified, licensed, or meet the legal mandates of the candidate's respective province that allow him or her to practice service delivery within the definition of his or her designated health care related profession
- Final approval of any applications with ambiguity regarding training and/or experience will be left to the discretion of the Commissioners following a thorough review of the respective applications. The opinion of the Commissioners is final.

- Each candidate must satisfy an experience component in one of the following options:
  - Submit one (1) life care plan with candidate's name displayed as author or co-author.
  - One (1) year of supervision with a Certified Life Care Planner. Supervision is to be registered for approval, and submission of quarterly supervision summaries are required detailing dates of meetings and a summary of discussions.
  - Graduation from an accredited training program which includes practicum or internship or which requires the development of an independent life care plan for review and critique by a faculty member who is a Certified Life Care Planner (CLCP).
- Each candidate must hold the entry level academic degree or certificate/diploma for their profession.

Life Care Planning Standards of Practice

There are several organizations that have provided substantial influence in the development of standards for the profession. These include the International Academy of Life Care Planners (IALCP), the International Association of Rehabilitation Professionals (IARP), the International Commission on Health Care Certification (ICHCC), and the Case Management Society of America, to name a few. In 2000, the first life care planning summit welcomed professionals from across the United States in a think tank format resulting in the release of the first publishing of the *Standards of Practice for Life Care Planners* (International Association of Rehabilitation Professionals, 2015). This proud tradition has continued over the years, and as of 2015 the *Standards of Practice for Life Care Planners*, Third Edition was released.

The Canadian Summit took place in Toronto in 2011, which allowed time for the Canadian life care planning profession to gather and discuss/debate issues in the field of relevance to Canadians (Lacerte & Johnson, 2013).

Types of Life Care Plans

In Canada, as in the United States, there are two main categories in which a life care plan would be requested.

Catastrophic Life Care Plans

Catastrophic life care plans are for individuals who have sustained permanent, lifelong physical and/or mental impairment, or those with chronic illness, who have lost significant capacity to perform some or all of the basic functions of daily living.

Non-Catastrophic Life Care Plans

Non-catastrophic life care plans are for individuals, who have sustained permanent, chronic, and/or structural physical impairment, or those with chronic illness, who have not lost significant capacity to perform some or all of the basic functions of daily living.

Whether the injury is catastrophic or non-catastrophic, the process for developing the plan remains the same as noted in the following list:

- Chronological record review
- Interview and assessment of the injured individual

- Summary of functional conclusions based on record review
- Contact with treating health care providers
- Future cost projections
- Detailed research
- Foundation sources

However, what is different in Canada is that referrals for the majority of cases requiring a life care plan do not come from the workers' compensation arena but rather mainly from the realm of personal injury litigation (Lacerte & Johnson, 2013).

Admissibility Rules in the United States and Canada

In order to evaluate expert witness testimony and to sort out junk science from relevant/reliable opinion, threshold standards have been set. (*Editors' note:* The reader is also referred to the chapter on admissibility by Tim Field in this textbook.)

In the case of *Frye v. United States,* 54 App. D.C. 46, 293 F. 1013 (1923), the U.S. Supreme Court ruled that the data and methodology of an expert witness must be "generally accepted" among others in the expert's field. Some states still rely on this ruling as their criteria.

That ruling was in place for 52 years until 1975, when Congress passed the *Federal Rule of Evidence 702* in order to let courts call on their own experts to sort out reliable from unreliable evidence.

In 1993, the Supreme Court created a new standard for the admission of scientific evidence into federal courts. In the case of *Daubert v. Merrill Dow Pharmaceuticals,* 509 U.S. 579 113 S. Ct. 2786, 125 L.Ed.2d 469 (1993), the Supreme Court made judges the "gatekeepers," charged with keeping junk science testimony away from the jury.

In the case of *Kumho Tire Company v. Patrick Carmichael,* 526, U.S. (1999), the Supreme Court ruled that reliability must be established in ALL types of expert testimony—both scientific and non-scientific/technical. The *Daubert* tests are to be applied to non-scientific testimony in a flexible manner that is appropriate to the situation. In their simplest form the *Daubert* criteria are:

- Can the theory or technique be tested?
- Has it been subjected to peer review and publication?
- Is there a known or potential rate of error?
- Is there a general acceptance in that particular discipline's community, similar to the former *Frye* test?
- Are there standards governing application?

Meanwhile in Canada in *R. v. Mohan* [2 S.C.R. 9] 1994-Ontario, admission of expert evidence was ruled to depend on the application of the following criteria:

- Relevance
- Necessity in assisting the trier of fact
- The absence of any exclusionary rule
- A properly qualified expert

In *R. v. J.L.J.* [Supreme Court of Canada] 2000, the Supreme Court expressly referenced *Daubert* as a relevant authority and referred to many of the same factors for analysis referenced by *Daubert* in the United States.

Canadian law has evolved in the area of expert evidence toward a much more stringent and analytic approach. *Daubert* has been referenced in Canada recently mainly in criminal cases but it has also been discussed with civil litigators, and recent changes in the rules of civil procedure in Canada definitely have reflected that recognizance.

Canadian Practice

Canada and the United States are similar in that the legal system is predominantly based on common law. Common law originated in England and is law that is derived from judicial precedent rather than statutes. There are a few places in Canada and the United States, such as Quebec or Louisiana, that operate on a civil code system, which can be traced to Napoleonic (French) law. In Canada, the word "lawyer" only refers to individuals who have been called to the bar or, in the province of Quebec, who are qualified as civil law notaries. Common law lawyers in Canada are formally known as "barristers and solicitors" and should not be referred to as "attorneys," since that term has a different meaning in Canadian usage (Hazard & Dondi, 2004).

Canada is comprised of 10 provinces and 3 territories that make use of federal and provincial systems of government that govern separate rights for the individual or entity. Due to the variety of their powers, depending on the subject matter, both federal and provincial level legislation must be considered. For example, when working with property, civil rights, and the administration of justice within its borders, the province is supreme. Even when provincial rules are in full force, differences between the provinces must also be considered because each province does not abide by the same set of rules.

The court system in Canada is broken up into three different levels but the most common for litigants is the Superior Court of each province. Within the Superior Court, there is division separating them into trial and appeal levels. Within certain courts, the trial level courts are still also referred to as the Court of Queen's Bench or the Supreme Court. The use of the word Supreme Court in Canada is not to be confused with the Supreme Court of the United States.

In Canada, there are rules known as the Rules of Civil Procedure (1990) that a life care planner should be familiar with in their scope of practice. In particular, those are the rules governing timelines and reporting requirements of expert's reports, which serve to ensure a high standard in the Canadian life care planning profession.

The Canadian Life Care Planner as Expert Witness

In Canada, going to trial as an expert witness in personal injury matters occurs on a more infrequent than frequent basis. However, the potential of a trial continues to be the premise around which all cases are structured. The expert's report and his or her subsequent evidence at trial will assist the Court in a better understanding of specific technical matters, which will ultimately assist in the rendering of a decision.

The judge is the fact finder and the gatekeeper. The expert is the educator. The role of the expert is to objectively inform the fact finder of the salient aspects of the case. The expert must be impartial, ethical, and credible. The expert must avoid being an advocate.

The role of an expert in Court has historically been determined by the case law ("common law") as opposed to by statute, regulation, or rules of Court. Experts are retained because they have special knowledge, which the trier of fact—judge or jury—requires to make an informed decision in a case (See *R. v. Mohan*, [1994] 2 S.C.R. 9.).

The life care planning expert must be cognizant of the legal climate and know the law of the land of each jurisdiction within which they practice. Within all of Canada, the cornerstone of quality life care plans is dependent on three pillars:

1. Preparation of a plan by those qualified/certified to do so
2. Adherence to the *Standards of Practice for Life Care Planning*
3. Foundation, foundation, foundation

The rules pertaining to expert reports are known as the Rules of Civil Procedure and govern the content of the expert's report (Rules of Civil Procedure, 1990). Dependent on the jurisdiction, specific forms and/or commentary need to be included with any expert report.

In Ontario, a general overview of Rule 4.1: Duty of Expert requires that an expert report must address the expert's qualifications, instructions, opinion, and the opinion's foundations. Furthermore, it must include an express acknowledgment of the expert's duty to the Court, as opposed to a party: to provide evidence that is fair, objective, and nonpartisan; to stay within the bounds of the witness' expertise; and to provide any additional assistance that the Court may require (Rules of Civil Procedure, 1990).

In addition, Rule 53.03, in effect January 1, 2010, set out certain basic requirements for an expert report. The former Rule 53.03 referred to expert reports merely including the author's name, address, and qualifications along with the substance of their testimony.

In British Columbia, the civil procedure Rule 40A (Rules of Civil Procedure, 1990. See also Supreme Court Rules, BC Reg 221/90, Rules 31–45) states:

1. A summary list of qualifications or a CV must accompany the report.
2. All reports and records relied on/or reviewed must be listed with dates and authors.
3. The report must clearly state who is responsible for drafting the opinion.
4. The facts and assumptions relied on by the expert must be clearly identified. An expert's report may be requested on behalf of either the plaintiff or defendant. Regardless of which side has retained the life care planner, it is imperative to provide an objective unbiased report based upon the facts ascertained in any particular case. Dependent on a combination of qualifications and experience, "weighting" is applied to testimony. Opposing counsel may challenge the life care planner's qualifications in order to affect the weight that testimony has given. A life care planning witness is considered an "expert" in their field if they have acquired the proper training, education, skill, or experience. The expert witness needs to be an educator and not an advocate while staying within their area of expertise when making their professional opinion known to the court.

Working with a Life Care Planner

When it becomes necessary to develop a life care plan, it is important to work with a skilled and knowledgeable life care planner who understands how to create a realistic framework of future needs. The plan should protect the evaluee's interests and their right to compensation for treatment, and it should be fair and objective so that the court is convinced that the described future costs will be reasonable and necessary.

A life care planner will need to do careful research to determine the anticipated needs of the evaluee for the rest of his or her life. The life care planner will take into account what the industry standard treatment is for the type(s) of injuries and will need to focus both on what the individual needs currently and what he/she may need in the future. The role of a life care planner can at times be difficult, but a knowledgeable expert will help create a life care plan to ensure all future care needs and costs are identified.

Canadian Supreme Court Judgments and the Life Care Planner

> "Future cost of care encompasses all post-trial expense which the plaintiff will now incur, but which he or she would not have incurred." (Cooper-Stephenson, 1996)
>
> "Assessing damages to meet the cost of future care is of paramount importance in personal injury cases." (Klar, 1995)

Provided below is a precis of the Canadian Supreme Court's judgments regarding life care planners and the evidence from their reports and testimony.

***Andrews v. Grand & Toy Alberta Ltd.*, 1978**

- Money alone cannot compensate.
- Plaintiff who has been gravely and permanently impaired would never have been put in the position if the tort had not been committed.

***Milina v. Bartsch*, 1985**

- Cost of future care award should not include amenities, which serve the sole function of making the plaintiff's life more bearable or enjoyable.
- Award should reflect what evidence establishes is reasonably necessary to preserve the plaintiff's health.

***Williams v. Low*, 2000**

- Not an exercise to save money.
- Analysis of how best to compensate the plaintiff for her grievous injuries and her loss of quality of life that occurred through no fault of her own but rather because of negligence of the defendant.
- This is not a discussion of retribution, but rather one of compensation.

Medically Justified

***Graham v. Rourke*, 1990**

- If real and substantial risk of incurring the expense, then plaintiff is entitled to compensation.
- Compensation for future loss is not all-or-nothing.
- The greater the risk of loss, the greater will be the compensation.

***Brennan v. Singh*, 1999**

- "Medically justified" is a less stringent test than "medically necessary."
- Many judgments can be found that highlight the importance of common sense.

***Penner v. ICBC*, 2011; *Harrington v. Sangha*, 2011**

- "A little common sense should inform claims under this head"

***Harrington v. Sangha,* 2011**

- Promote making an award at variance with recommendations of some of the expert witnesses, in favor of common sense.

Who Can Provide Evidence?

- Evidence from a medical doctor is not required.
- Evidence can come from some other qualified health care practitioner.

***Jacobsen v. Nike Canada Ltd.,* 1996**

- Rehabilitation expert accepted.

***Frers v. De Moulin,* 2002**

- Life care planner accepted.
- There must be evidence justifying the medical validity of items claimed in a cost of future care award (***Aberdeen v. Zanatta,* 2007**).
- Without an evidentiary foundation to show that recommendations are medically justified in the future, the court should reject the claim (***Job v. Van Blankers,* 2009**; ***Gregory v. ICBC,* 2011**).

Reasonableness

***Brito v. Wooley,* 2001**

- To meet the test of reasonableness, the proposed expenditure should be reasonable in the sense of what future care items were necessary in the context of the plaintiff's specific limitations.

***Forde v. Inland Health Authority,* 2010**

- In determining whether the inclusion of a future cost is reasonable, the Court must consider whether a reasonably-minded person of ample means would be ready to incur the expense.
- Consideration given of the level of care to be provided.
- Level of care must be moderate and fair to both parties.
- Moderation does not mean reducing a plaintiff to subsistence level.
- Court must determine what care is likely to be in the injured person's best interests.
- Plaintiff preferences as to the type and level of care should be considered.

***Bystedt v. Hay,* 2001**

- The expense should not be a squandering of money.
- Medical necessity is too stringent a test.
- What does the plaintiff reasonably need to expend for the purpose of making good the loss?

***Aberdeen v. Zanatta,* 2007**

- Life care planner drew a balance between providing care necessary for a quality lifestyle as opposed to complete pampering.

Is It Likely the Item Will Be Used?

***Izony v. Weidlich*, 2006**

- Considers the likeliness of incurring the expense.
- Not appropriate to make provision for items or services that the plaintiff has not used in the past.
- Not appropriate to make provision for items or services that the plaintiff is unlikely to use in the future.
- Other cases: *Coulter v. Ball*, 2005; *Predinchuk v. Spencer*, 2009

***Whetung v. West Fraser Holdings Ltd.*, 2007**

- Claim for sauna to alleviate pain rejected (amenity to be paid out of pecuniary damages).

***Gregory v. Insurance Corporation of British Columbia*, 2011**

- Some claims for cost of future care were rejected by the judge as there was no link between the physician assessment and the recommended treatment and care (as per OT report).

***Penner v. Insurance Corporation of British Columbia*, 2011**

- Plaintiff was awarded $120,325, on basis of an OT report which included sums for equipment such as cold packs, heating pads, bath mats, etc., until age 80.
- On appeal, award was reduced by $80,000 with the judge citing:

  "a little common sense should inform claims under this heading, however much they may be recommended by experts in the field."

***Travis v. Kwon*, 2009**

The judge's comments:

- "Damages for future care grew out of catastrophic injuries and were intended to ensure, so far as possible, that a catastrophically injured plaintiff could live as complete and independent a life as was reasonably attainable through an award of damages.
- "Passage of time has led to claims for items such as in this case, the present value of the future cost of a long-handled duster, long-handled scrubber, and replacement heads for the scrubber in cases where injuries are nowhere near catastrophic in nature or result."

***Jarmson v. Jacobsen*, 2012**

The judge criticized the life care plan citing that it was:

- "Not just a Cadillac; it is a gold-plated one, which goes far beyond reasonable."
- In this case, the judge did not accord the life care planner's recommendations very much weight in the assessment for the future care award.

***Tsalamandris v. McLeod*, 2012**

BC Court of Appeal upheld award for damages for the cost of future Pilates, and community center use:

- Pilates: Was found as medically necessary in assisting the plaintiff in managing chronic pain and chronic depression.
- Community center: Membership to access the pool was found as medically beneficial and reasonable as a future care treatment.

***Joinson v. Heran*, 2011**

Medical marijuana damages were awarded to help manage chronic pain. The judge's comments:

- Issue is controversial.
- More research required for the safe and effective use of marijuana.
- Medical evidence supports a finding that compensation for some medical use of marijuana is reasonably 8 ptnecessary in this case.

***MacEachern v. Rennie*, 2010**

- One of BC's largest awards—over $5.5 million dollars as a result of an MVA (plaintiff submission was for $10 million).
- 27-year-old woman with significant TBI resulting in need for care for the rest of her life.
- Total lifestyle approach used.
- Most costs allowed, except for hair services, home support (in group home), travel costs of care personnel to vacation with plaintiff—not considered medically justified.

Standard of Care

***Spehar v. Beazley*, 2002**

- Full compensation suggests a standard of care which allows the plaintiff, as far as possible, to enjoy a lifestyle like the one he or she would have enjoyed but for the injury.

Government Benefits

***Krangle v. Brsco*, 2002**

- If a government benefit scheme is available regardless of tort compensation, the scheme must be taken into consideration when determining an award.
- A government benefit scheme is therefore a factor in determining the plaintiff's available level of care.

Family Assistance

Does a future care award need to be reduced to take into account family who provides the care?

***O'Connell v. Yung*, 2010**

- Plaintiff is entitled to be compensated for the cost of care that is medically required.
- Law does not permit the defendants to pass off their responsibility to provide appropriate future care by suggesting that the plaintiff's husband should take care of her.

PharmaCare Benefits

***Harrington v. Sangha*, 2011**

- PharmaCare is not intended to be available to persons who have a tort claim for the cost of their medications.
- The plaintiff should be in a position, without relying upon the state, to pay the cost of the drugs she requires.

Home or Institutional Care

***Monych v. Beacon Community Services Society*, 2009**

- Plaintiff desire to stay in his own home should be acceded to.

***Dennis v. Gairdner*, 2002**

- Plaintiff expressed a wish to live on his own.
- Judge determined that plaintiff's desire to have his own dwelling ought to be acceded to as being reasonable in facilitating plaintiff's physical and mental needs.

Double Compensation

***Milina v. Barstsch*, 1985**

- Must be avoided.
- Potential overlap between cost of care and damages for loss of future income, specifically, with respect to the handling of expenses for basic necessities of life the plaintiff would have incurred regardless of the accident.
- Two approaches: total lifestyle approach or additional expense approach.

Failure to Mitigate

***Maltese v. Pratap*, 2014**

- Plaintiff chose not to undertake recommendations for treatment (active rehabilitation).
- In this case, the judge concluded an award for cost of future care would be inappropriate.

Quantifying Care Provided by Family Members

***Roberts v. Morana*, 1997**

- Brain-injured plaintiff was awarded future care costs including 12 hours/week of support at a cost of $65.00/hour for a rehabilitation support worker specializing in services for those with brain injuries.
- On the basis of what she had lost and not what she could "make do" with.

***Matthews Estate v. Hamilton Civic Hospitals*, 2008**

- Medical malpractice case.
- Although plaintiffs lost at trial, plaintiffs' contention was accepted that cost of care ought to be assessed at what it would have cost to purchase the services, and not on the fact that family members instead of health care professionals provided services because they could not afford to pay for professional care.
- "It is the nature and quality of the services provided and their value to the person injured rather than the professional qualifications of the provider that should govern the assessment."

***Parsons Estate v. Guymer*, 1998**

- Assessment of damages for the loss of services that the wife who was killed in an accident would have provided to her husband who had suffered a stroke unrelated to the accident.
- "In assessing the loss of Margaret's stroke-related care, the cost of replacing that care in the marketplace is an important measure…"

Attendant Care or Lifeline

***Morrison v. Greig,* 2007**

- Rejected Defense argument that a lifeline would be a more appropriate support than attendant care for Ryan Morrison who was catastrophically impaired by a spinal cord injury.
- Plaintiff Morrison awarded almost $12.5 million, with $8.8 million attributed to future care.
- "For example, if there were a fire and it was going to take a personal care worker half an hour to come to his residence the plaintiff might die in the meantime. This plaintiff is not one who only needs a nanny to pick up after him. He needs someone who can be there right away and someone who understands the limitations of a spinal cord injured person so that he can be assisted properly."

Attendant Care—Will It Be Used?

***Morrison v. Greig,* 2007**

- Rejected Defense argument that a much lower level of attendant care ought to be considered for Derek Gordon, who suffered a catastrophic brain injury, because Gordon was reluctant to accept assistance from caregivers and so unlikely to do so. Plaintiff Gordon awarded over $11 million, with $8.6 million attributed to future care.
- "There is no likelihood that Derek will recover and have no need for this form of care. Acquired brain injury is permanent. It affects his frontal lobe. To suggest that the recommended attendant care be reduced significantly or abandoned completely simply passes the task over to the family in the sense of dumping such responsibility on them."

Attendant Care—Overnight Security

***Desbiens v. Mordini,* 2004**

- Plaintiff's experts concluded that the paraplegic plaintiff required an overnight assistant to help with transfers from his bed to his wheelchair in the event of an emergency.
- Defendant's experts opined that there were other "common sense options" to address the overnight security issue.
- Court found plaintiff did require an attendant to provide overnight security but limited the cost for this service to minimum wage.
- "I agree that there probably are other "common sense practical options" to address the question of overnight security, however, the defendants failed to adduce any evidence of what they may be. It is true that the life care planner testified that the apartment building has a priority list as part of its fire safety plan. If Mr. Desbiens requested it, he could be placed on this list indicating the kind of assistance he requires. If the fire department attends the premises they look at this list to determine which tenants need special assistance. The defendants called no expert evidence to suggest that this adequately meets the overnight security needs of Mr. Desbiens. Furthermore, the defendants' own witness, Ms. Blaney, testified that if she had determined that Mr. Desbiens could not transfer in and out of bed independently, she would have made an allowance for overnight security in the same manner as the life care planner."

Future Care Awards

***Sandhu v. Wellington Place Apartments,* 2008**

- Largest personal injury damage award affirmed at the appellate level in Canada.
- Minor plaintiff fell from a fifth floor apartment building window and landed on the cement pavement below, resulting in catastrophic and permanent personal injuries and impairments including a severe brain injury.
- Plaintiff Sandhu awarded in excess of $17 million, including $10.9 million for future cost of care.
- Jury and trial judge awarded roughly $1.3 million more in future care than that put forth by plaintiff's counsel.
- Court of Appeal held that the plaintiff actually underestimated the hourly rates of caregivers and rehabilitation support workers, based on evidence from the defendants' expert economist about hourly rates charged by agencies employing these providers.

***Marcoccia v. Ford Credit Canada Limited,* 2009**

- Jury assessed the future cost of care award at $13.95 million, the highest cost of care award to date.
- Award upheld on appeal.
- "In our view, the jury's assessment of damages in this case was not "plainly unjust and unreasonable." Rather, it was based on expert evidence properly adduced at trial. No evidence was led at trial with respect to the alleged overlap in the calculations advanced by the respondent's expert. Although the parties' experts disagreed as to assumptions relating to the appropriate level and length of care required, it was open to the jury to prefer the respondent's expert on these points. Further, the jury did not simply adopt the figures advanced by the respondent's expert. Substantial reductions were effected to many of the claims, including a reduction in the claim for future care costs."

***Marcoccia v. Gill,* 2007**

- 20-year-old plaintiff sustained catastrophic and permanent personal injuries and impairments.
- Jury awarded more than 95 percent of the future care cost claims presented to it during the trial.
- "Further, for the purposes of assessing future claims, the family must be taken out of the picture. As such, it must be assumed that Robert may not continue to live with his parents. The jury award may allow Robert to live in an apartment with attendant care.... A family member may continue to act in a guardianship role but that will be very different than the multiple roles played to date by Mrs. Marcoccia as mother, housekeeper, cuing and prompting coach, behavior monitor, and attendant."

***MacNeil v. Bryan,* 2009**

- Largest award for future cost of care in Ontario's history.
- Plaintiff, a 15-year-old female passenger in a vehicle that resulted in catastrophic injuries including severe brain injuries, awarded $18,427,207.20.
- Largest portion of the judgment was $15,158,500.00 awarded for future care costs.

The Role of the Treatment Team

***Song v. Hong*, 2008**

- Defense counsel challenged testimony of three witnesses regarding future care needs (life care planner, housing expert, professor of health economics), in part because the witnesses' recommendations were informed by hearsay based on interviews with medical specialists.
- Judge allowed testimony with certain conditions: "If there is no evidence upon which the assumed fact may be determined by the jury, it may be that the opinion of the expert will not be heard. If, however, the Court is satisfied that there is some evidence before the Court now or that may come before the Court through the evidence of the remaining witnesses at this trial, the Court may allow the jury to hear the opinion of the expert."

Lack of Foundation

***Degennaro v. Oakville Trafalgar Memorial Hospital*, 2011**

- At trial, evidence of future care was entered by filing the life care planner's report as part of the plaintiff's document brief. No witnesses were called to give evidence.
- On appeal, the Court determined the report contained several unsubstantiated claims based on hearsay.
- "In several instances there was simply no evidence to support the claim set out. For example, the second life care plan report claims the need to recover an annual cost of $255.00 until age 75 for house painting. The assumption here is that, but for the injury, Ms. Degennaro would have painted 1,000 square feet of the house every five years until she reached the age of 75. There was no evidence by Ms. Degennaro that she had painted the house in the past or that there was a need for her to carry out this type of regular house painting until age 75."

Institutional or Home Care

***McErlean v. Sarel et al.*, 1987**

- Award reduced after a period of 20 years "by reason of several possibilities, such as the respondent's need for intermittent or permanent hospital care, staffing problems, and the lack of guardian supervision and provision of back-up care by his parents by reason of their incapacity or death."

The Burden of Proof

***Schrump et al. v. Koot et al.*, 1977**

- Court of Appeal undertook a comparison of the burden of proof required to establish whether or not the plaintiff would require future surgery.
- Plaintiff's expert predicted a 25 to 50 percent chance of occurrence and defendant's expert deemed the chance as remote.
- Plaintiff was awarded future care costs related to future surgery.
- "In assessing damages for personal injuries, the award may cover not only all injuries actually suffered and disabilities proved as of the date of trial, but also the "risk" or "likelihood" of future developments attributable to such injuries. It is not the law that a plaintiff must prove

on a balance of probabilities the probability of future damage; he may be compensated if he proves in accordance with the degree of proof required in civil matters that there is a possibility or a danger of some adverse future development."

***Graham v. Rourke*, 1990**

- Appeal allowed against the damages assessed at trial.
- "In arriving at a global figure which represents the non-pecuniary loss to the plaintiff, a trial judge will consider real and substantial future possibilities, both positive and negative, which could impact on the plaintiff's quality of life."

Capacity

***Lazaroff v. Lazaroff*, 2005**

- In certain circumstances, even if the person is capable of handling basic transactions and managing small amounts of money, a finding of incapacity may be made if that person is easily confused or taken advantage of by others.
- "Dr. Berry concluded that Caroline Lazaroff is not capable of managing her own property but is capable of managing her own person. The parties have accepted this assessment."

***Arnold v. Teno*, 1978**

- Supreme Court confirmed that in many cases plaintiffs will require the services of skilled financial advisors to assist them in the management of their capital sum.
- Therefore, it is appropriate to provide a sum for financial services or a management fee.

***Koch (Re)*, 1997**

- In all cases, the nature and degree of the alleged incapacity must be severe enough to warrant the Court's depriving the person of his/her right to live as he/she chooses.
- "On all of the evidence, I am satisfied that the patient would not be able to adequately appreciate the consequences of making expenditures on her limited income and is therefore incapable of managing her finances. It is also clear that the patient's insight into both of her disorders… is impaired."

Orders for Examination by Nonmedical Practitioners

***Ziebenhaus v. Bahlieda*, 2014**

- Plaintiff Alexander Ziebenhaus alleged he suffered a brain injury as a result of a skiing accident during an elementary school trip in 2001.
- Defendant sought an order requiring the plaintiff to undergo a vocational assessment by a certified vocational evaluator; so ordered by motion judge.
- Ground of appeal, that the motion judge lacked the jurisdiction to order the examination, rejected.
- "Accordingly, in my view, judges of the Superior Court of Ontario have the inherent jurisdiction to order that a party to an action undergo a physical or a mental examination by a person who is not a 'health practitioner'…"

***Jack v. Cripps and Reath*, 2014**

- Plaintiff Scott Jack alleged that as a result of a motor vehicle accident he sustained multiple serious injuries, including a "cerebral concussion."

- Defendants requested that plaintiff attend a functional abilities evaluation by a chiropractor; so ordered by motion judge.
- Ground of appeal, that the motion judge lacked the jurisdiction to order the examination, rejected.
- "Accordingly, in my view, judges of the Superior Court of Ontario have the inherent jurisdiction to order that a party to an action undergo a physical or a mental examination by a person who is not a "health practitioner"..."

Double Recovery and Overlap

***Ratych v. Bloomer*, 1987**

- Plaintiff should receive full and fair compensation.
- "The general principles underlying our system of damages suggest that a plaintiff should receive full and fair compensation, calculated to place him or her in the same position as he or she would have been had the tort not been committed, in so far as this can be achieved by a monetary award. This principle suggests that in calculating damages under pecuniary heads, the measure of the damages should be the plaintiff's actual loss. It is implicit in this that the plaintiff should not recover unless he can demonstrate a loss, and then only to the extent of that loss. Double recovery violates this principle."

***Watkins v. Olafson*, 1989**

- An issue that arises in traumatic brain injury cases is overlap between the cost of care and damages for loss of future income, specifically regarding basic necessities of life the Plaintiff would have incurred regardless of the accident.
- "In calculating loss of future earning capacity in cases where an award for future care is made, a deduction is made from the award for lost earning capacity for living expenses to avoid duplication between the two heads of damage."

Government Funding and Future Care Costs

***Boarelli v. Flannigan*, 1973**

- No difference in principle between social welfare programs and private insurance policies.
- Restricted to lost wages and not to cost of future care.
- "I do not think that there is any difference in principle between benefits received under our present social welfare legislation and those received by way of private or public benevolence. In such a case it may be said that the injured party has received a reward as a result of the injury. If that is so, in my view, it is no concern of the defendant and such matters should be dealt with by the appropriate legislative authority. In many statutes a right of subrogation for moneys received from an unsuccessful defendant is established. In this way the loss is borne by the tortfeasor, and the question of overlapping compensation is thereby avoided. However, in my opinion, it is for the appropriate legislative authority to determine whether the right of subrogation should be included in those statutes which are now silent in this respect."

***Stein v. Sandwich West (Township)*, 1995**

- First Ontario case that expressly dealt with the issue of awards of cost of future care for government-funded services.
- Refused to allow a deduction due to "the uncertain expectation of government help."

- "In the past some of the care and some of the equipment provided to John has been wholly or partly funded by government, that is the government of Ontario. It was, however, the evidence of the life care planner, whose evidence I accept, that these programs of government assistance really cannot be counted on to endure. It seems to me to be obvious that John Stein's award for future care should not be diminished based upon the uncertain expectation of government help."

***Lurtz v. Duchesne*, 2005**

- Awarded damages on the basis that the respondent would no longer have drugs paid for after the judgment.
- "The respondent should not be placed in the position of being uncertain whether those drugs will be paid for.... The trial judge was entitled to make the award on the theory that the tortfeasors, rather than the government, should be responsible for paying the cost of the medication. The trial judge was not required to reduce this part of the claim because of contingencies."

***Paxton v. Ramji*, 2006**

- Disallowed a deduction for publicly funded care.
- "A common disability that one can hardly imagine a government losing interest in assisting. Still, government policies change with the temper of the times, and Jaime has a long time ahead of her. I find she must have the benefit of the doubt, as government funding cannot be reliably predicted."

Conclusion

The practice of life care planning in Canada, although still in its infancy compared to our American cousins, continues to attract new rehabilitation professionals to this vital field. Life care planning in Canada is certainly at the forefront in the litigation arena. Life care planners are routinely utilized by plaintiffs and defendants alike to identify and project future care needs and associated costs for individuals with catastrophic and non-catastrophic injuries. As this practice continues to grow, it is essential for the practitioners in the field to abide by the standards of practice for the profession to ensure continued quality in providing this valuable service in the future.

References

Cooper-Stephenson, K. 1996. *Personal Injury Damages in Canada*, 2nd ed. Toronto, Ontario: Carswell.

Hazard, G., & Dondi, A. 2004. *Legal Ethics: A Comparative Study*. Stanford: Stanford University.

Institute of Rehabilitation Education and Training. 2017. *Welcome to the Institute of Rehabilitation Education and Training*. Available at https://iretprograms.com/.

International Association of Rehabilitation Professionals. 2015. *Standards of Practice for Life Care Planners—Third Edition*. Available at http://c.ymcdn.com/sites/rehabpro.org/resource/resmgr/files/RehabPro/Standards_of_Practice_for_Li.pdf.

International Commission on Health Care Certification. 2017. *Qualifications—Qualified Health Care Professional*. Available at https://www.ichcc.org/certified-life-care-planner-clcp.html.

Klar, L. N. 1995. *Remedies in Tort*. Toronto, Ontario: Carswell.

Lacerte, M., & Johnson, C. 2013. Life Care Planning. *Clinics Review Articles: Physical Medicine and Rehabilitation Clinics of North America*.

Physician Life Care Planning. 2017 *Life Care Planning A Natural Domain of Physiatry, Physician Life Care Planning.* Available at https://www.physicianlcp.com/LifeCarePLanningPhysiatry/.

Riddick-Grisham, S., & Deming, L. (Eds.) 2011. *Pediatric Life Care Planning and Case Management* (2nd Ed). Boca Raton, FL. CRC Press. (p. 845).

R.R.O. 1990, Reg. 194: Rules of Civil Procedure, under Courts of Justice Act, R.S.O. 1990, C.43.

Supreme Court Rules, BC Reg 221/90, Rules 31 to 45. Retrieved on *Aug 8*, 2016 from http://canlii.ca/t/kbpx.

Weed, R. 2010. Life care planning: Past, present and future. In R. Weed & D. Berens (Eds.), pp. 1–13. *Life Care Planning and Case Management Handbook* (3rd Ed). Boca Raton, FL: CRC Press.

Case References

- *Aberdeen v. Zanatta* (2007) BCSC 993; (2008) BCCA 420
- *Anand v. Belanger and State Farm* (Unreported) Oral Ruling: April 23, 2010, Court File
- *Andrews v. Grand & Toy Alberta Ltd* (1978), 2 S.C.R. 229
- *Arnold v. Teno* (1978) CanLII 2 (SCC)
- *Beasley et al. v. Barrand* (2010) ONSC 2095
- *Brennan v. Singh* (1999) B.C.J. No. 520
- *Boarelli v. Flannigan* (1973) CanLII 690 (ON CA)
- *Brito v. Wooley* (2001) BCSC 1178
- *Bystedt v. Hay* (2001) BCSC 1735
- *Coulter v. Ball* (2005) BCCA 199
- *Degennaro v. Oakville Trafalgar Memorial Hospital* (2011) ONCA 319 (CanLII)
- *Dennis v. Gairdner* (2002) BCSC 1289
- *Desbiens v. Mordini* (2004) CanLII 41166 (ON SC)
- *Frers v. De Moulin* (2002) BCSC 408
- *Graham v. Rourke* (1990) CanLII 2596 (ON CA)
- *Graham v. Rourke* (1990), 74 D.L.R. (4th)
- *Gregory v. Insurance Corporation of British Columbia* (2011) BCCA 144
- *Harrington v. Sangha* (2011) BCSC 1035
- *Izony v. Weidlich* (2006) BCSC 1315
- *Jacobsen v. Nike Canada Ltd.* (1996) B.C.J.
- *Jarmson v. Jacobsen* (2012) BCSC 64
- *Job v. Van Blankers* (2009) BCSC 230
- *Joinson v. Heran* (2011) BCC 727
- *Koch (Re)* (1997) CanLII 12138 (ON SC)
- *Krangle v. Brisco* (2002) SCC9
- *Lazaroff v. Lazaroff* (2005) CanLII 44834 (ON SC)
- *Lurtz v. Duchesne* (2005) CanLII 2555 (ON CA)
- *MacEachern v. Rennie* (2010) BCSC 625
- *MacNeil v. Bryan* (2009) CanLII 28648 (ON SC)
- *McErlean v. Sarel et al.* (1987) CanLII 4313 (ON CA)
- *Maltese v. Pratap* (2014) BCSC 18
- *Marcoccia v. Ford Credit Canada Limited* (2009) ONCA 317
- *Marcoccia v. Gill* (2007) CanLII 11322 (ON SC)
- *Matthews Estate v. Hamilton Civic Hospitals* (2008) CanLII 52312 (ON SC)
- *Milina v. Bartsch* (1985) 49 B.C.L.R. (2d) 33 (S.C)

- *Monych v. Beacon Community Services Society* (2009) BCSC 562
- *Morrison v. Greig* (2007) O.J. No. 225, 46 C.C.L.T. (3d) 212 (S.C.J.)
- *O'Connell v. Yung* (2010) BCSC 1764
- *Parsons Estate v. Guymer* (1998) CanLII 1378 (ON CA)
- *Paxton v. Ramji* (2006) CanLII 9312 (ON SC)
- *Penner v. Insurance Corporation of British Columbia* (2011) BCCA 135
- *Predinchuk v. Spencer* (2009) BCSC 1396
- *Ratych v. Bloomer* (1990) CanLII 97 (SCC)
- *Roberts v. Morana* (1997) CanLII 12201 (ON SC)
- *Sandhu v. Wellington Place Apartments* (2008) CanLII 46133 (ON SC)
- *Schrump et al. v. Koot et al.* (1977) CanLII 1332 (ON CA)
- *Slaght v. Phillips and Wicaartz* (2010) ONSC 6464
- *Song v. Hong* (2008) CanLII 10056 (ON SC)
- *Spehar v. Beazley* (2002) BCSC 1104
- *Stein v. Sandwich West (Township)* (1995) CanLII 1239 (ON CA)
- *Travis v. Kwon* (2009) BCSC 63
- *Tsalamandris v. McLeod* (2012) BCCA 239
- *Watkins v. Olafson* (1989) CanLII 36 (SCC)
- *Whetung v. West Fraser Holdings Ltd* (2007) BCSC 990
- *Williams v. Low* (2000) BCSC 345
- *Ziebenhaus v. Bahlieda* (2014) ONSC 138

Appendix I: Standards of Practice for Life Care Planners, 3rd Edition*

Standards of Practice Revision Committee 2013–2014

Kathie Allison, PT, MS, CLCP
Kansas City, Missouri, USA

Debra Berens, PhD, CRC, CCM, CLCP
Atlanta, Georgia, USA

Giovanna Boniface, BSc (Bio), BSc (OT), OT, OT(C), CCLCP
Boniface Consulting Occupational Therapy Services N. Vancouver, British Columbia, Canada

Patricia A. Costantini, RN, MEd, LPC, CRC, CCM, CLCP, LNCC, ABVE/D, CNLCP
Costantini Rehab, Inc. Pittsburgh, Pennsylvania, USA

Elizabeth Davis, MS, RN, CRRN, CLCP, CRC
Cedar Bluff, Virginia, USA

Sandra Impey, MHS, BScOT FACT
Services Grande Prairie, Alberta, Canada

Ann Neulicht, PhD, CLCP, CRC, CVE, CDMS, ABVE/D, LPC
Ann T. Neulicht PhD, PLLC Raleigh, North Carolina, USA

Karen Preston, PHN, MS, CRRN, FIALCP RNS
HealthCare Consultants, Inc. Sacramento, California, USA

* Source: *Journal of Life Care Planning* (2015), Vol. 13, No. 3 (pp. 31–36). Reprinted in accordance with member/subscriber permission guidelines from: International Academy of Life Care Planners, The Life Care Planning Section of The International Association of Rehabilitation Professionals. Publisher: International Association of Rehabilitation Professionals, 1000 Westgate Drive, #252, St. Paul, MN 55114, 888-IARPQaA (888–427–7722), webpage: http://www.rehabpro.org.

Christine (Chris) Reid, PhD, CRC, CLCP
Virginia Commonwealth University, Richmond, Virginia, USA

Sharon Reavis, RN, MS, CRC, CCM, FIALCP
Health Information Resources Richmond Virginia, USA

Susan Riddick-Grisham, RN, BA, CCM, CLCP
Life Care Manager, Richmond, Virginia, USA

Tracy Wingate, OTR/L, FIALCP, CCM, CDMS, MSCC
Life Care & Rehabilitation Consultants, Inc. Olathe, Kansas, USA

Steven A. Yuhas, MEd, CRC, CLCP, CCM, NCC, CBIS
The Directions Group, Inc., Mt. Pleasant, South Carolina, USA

Standards of Practice Advisory Group 2013–2014

Mary Barros-Bailey, PhD, CRC, CLCP, CDMS, NCC, ABVE/D
Intermountain Vocational Services, Inc., Boise, Idaho, USA

Hazel L. Bowles, BA, BHScOT, OT Reg. (Ont.), CCLCP
Occupational Therapist, Burlington, Ontario, Canada

Paul M. Deutsch, PhD, CRC, CCM, CLCP, FLCPR
Licensed Mental Health Counselor, Oviedo, Florida, USA

Reg Gibbs, MS, CRC, LCPC, CBIS, CLCP
Rocky Mountain Rehab, P.C., Billings, Montana, USA

Lois Hawkins, RN, CLCP
Hawkins Forensic Consulting, Mesa, Arizona, USA

Carolyn Wiles Higdon, PhD, CCC-SLP, F-ASHA
Wiles Higdon & Associates, LLC, Atlanta, Georgia, USA

Lori Hinton, DrPH, MPH, RN, CLCP
American Case Management, Houston, Texas, USA

Carol Hyland, MA MS CDMS CLCP
Lafayette, California, USA

Harvey E. Jacobs, PhD, CLCP
Harvey E. Jacobs, PhD LLC, Licensed Psychologist, Richmond, Virginia, USA

Vicky Jensen, BSN, RN, LNC, CLCP
Vocational Diagnostics, Inc., Phoenix, Arizona, USA

Cloie B. Johnson, MEd
OSC Vocational Systems, Inc., Bothell, Washington, USA

Joanne Latham, MA, CRC, MFT, CCM, ABVE/D, CLCP
Latham Vocational Services Inc., Encino, California, USA

Sarah Lustig, BSN, RN, CLCP, CNLCP
Lustig Consulting, LLC, Mount Pleasant, South Carolina, USA

Debbe Marcinko, RN, BSN, MA, CRRN, CCM, CRC, CLCP, CNLCP, MSCC, LPC
Pittsburgh, Pennsylvania, USA

Antony Ruddick, OT Reg (Ont.), CCLCP
Antony Ruddick Consulting, London, Ontario, Canada

Julie Sawyer-Little, MS, OT/L, CRC, CLCP, ABVE/F
Sawyer Consulting, LLC, Fuquay-Varina, North Carolina, USA

Maria Scaringi, MS, SLP (C), Reg CASLPO, RRP, CCCSLP, CCLCP
KIDSPEECH & Family Rehabilitation, Toronto, Ontario, Canada

Reema Shafi, BScOTReg (Ont), MA (Psych), CCLCP
Brampton, Ontario, Canada

Janet L. Smith, BScOT, MScOT, CCLCP, CCDP JL
Smith Occupational Therapy Services, Edmonton, Alberta, Canada

Roger O. Weed, PhD, CRC, LPC, CCM/R, CLCP/R, CDMS/R, FNRCA, FIALCP
Professor Emeritus, Counseling & Psychological Services, Georgia State University, Atlanta, Georgia, USA

Susan Wirt, MSN, RN, CRRN, CCM, CLCP, CNLCP
Wirt & Associates, LLC Catawba, Virginia, USA

Acknowledgment

Practitioners of life care planning are indebted to the pioneers who have worked tirelessly to promote professional life care planning practice and create a specialty that is recognized and respected. From the publishing of the first *Standards of Practice* in 2000 to today, life care planning has achieved many milestones of professional practice and is well positioned to continue this development into the future. This 3rd Edition of the *Standards of Practice for Life Care Planners* is dedicated to those who have given generously of their time and effort, and especially to the memory of Patricia McCollom, MS, RN, CRRN, CDMS, CCM, CLCP, FIALCP, who founded the International Academy of Life Care Planners in 1996. Her vision of ensuring a strong life care planning community for all practitioners led to IALCP becoming part of the International Association of Rehabilitation Professionals in 2006. This edition of the *Standards* exemplifies her legacy: alive, well, and thriving.

Standards of Practice for Life Care Planners

I. Introduction

A. Definition of Life Care Plan

"The life care plan is a dynamic document based upon published standards of practice, comprehensive assessment, data analysis, and research, which provides an organized, concise plan for current and future needs with associated costs for individuals who have experienced catastrophic injury or have chronic health care needs."

> (International Conference on Life Care Planning and the International Academy of Life Care Planners. (Adopted 1998, April). *Definition of Life Care Planning.* Presented at the Forensics Section meeting of the NARPPS [now known as the International Association of Rehabilitation Professionals] Annual Conference, Colorado Springs, Colorado.)

B. Historical Perspective

The development of an individualized plan of care has always been considered an integral part of the medical and rehabilitation process. This type of plan has historically been used by multiple disciplines. Rehabilitation professionals have created a rehabilitation plan. Nurses developed a nursing care plan. Physicians defined a medical treatment plan, and other professions developed plans specific to their practice. An integrated plan that includes all disciplines and specific costs of care has become an increasingly important aspect of the health care process due to rapid growth in medical technology and an increased emphasis on the cost of care. This process of developing an integrated plan and delineating costs has evolved over an extensive period of time and is now utilized by case managers, counselors, and other professionals in many sectors. These plans are also a valuable tool for rehabilitation planning, service implementation, management of health care resources, discharge planning, educational and vocational planning, and long-term managed care, among other areas.

C. Transdisciplinary Perspective

Life care planning is a transdisciplinary specialty practice. Each profession brings to the process of life care planning practice standards which must be adhered to by the individual professional, and these standards remain applicable while the practitioner engages in life care planning activities. Each professional works within specific standards of practice and regulatory requirements for his or her discipline to ensure accountability, provide direction, and mandate responsibility for the standards for which he or she is accountable. These standards include, but are not limited to, activities related to quality of care, qualifications, collaboration, law, ethics, advocacy, resource utilization, and research. In addition, each individual practitioner is responsible for following the *Standards of Practice for Life Care Planners.*

Furthermore, the individual practitioner must examine his or her qualifications, training, and experience as applied to each individual case. Therefore, knowledge of the medical diagnosis, disability, and future care considerations are necessary components of the practitioner's competency for each individual case.

II. Philosophical Overview/Goals of Life Care Planning

The life care plan is a document that provides accurate and timely information which can be followed by the evaluee and relevant parties. It is a detailed document that can serve as a lifelong guide to assist in the delivery of health care services. The life care plan is a collaborative effort among the various parties, when possible, and reflects goals that are preventive and rehabilitative in nature. As a dynamic document, the life care plan may require periodic updating to accommodate changes and should have quality outcomes as its goal.

Goals of Life Care Plans:

In life care planning, the evaluee is defined as the person who is the subject of the life care plan.

A. To assist the evaluee in achieving optimal outcomes by developing an appropriate plan of rehabilitation, prevention, and/or reduction of complications. This may include recommendations for evaluations or treatment that may contribute to the evaluee's level of wellness or provide information regarding treatment requirements.
B. To provide health education to the evaluee and relevant parties, when appropriate.
C. To specify services and the charges for those services needed by the evaluee.
D. To develop likely alternatives for care that take into consideration developmentally appropriate and least restrictive options for the evaluee.
E. To communicate the life care plan and objectives to the evaluee and relevant parties, when appropriate.

III. Standards of Performance

1. STANDARD: The life care planner has an educational background and professional preparation suitable for life care planning.
MEASUREMENT CRITERIA:
    a. Possesses the appropriate educational requirements in a rehabilitation or health care field as defined by his or her professional discipline.
    b. Maintains current professional licensure, provincial registration, or national board certification that is required to practice a professional rehabilitation or health care discipline.
    c. Demonstrates that the professional discipline provides sufficient education and training to assure that the life care planner has an understanding of human anatomy and physiology, pathophysiology, psychosocial and family dynamics, the health care delivery system, the role and function of various health care professionals, and clinical practice guidelines and standards of care. The education and training allows practitioners in the discipline to independently perform assessments, analyze and interpret data, make judgments and decisions on goals and interventions, and evaluate responses and outcomes.

d. Participates in specific continuing education as required to maintain the individual practitioner's licensure, registration, or certification within his or her profession.
e. Obtains continuing education and/or training to remain current in the knowledge and skills relevant to life care planning.

2. STANDARD: The life care planner shall practice in an ethical manner and follow the Code of Ethics of his or her respective professions, roles, certifications, and credentials.
MEASUREMENT CRITERIA:
a. Follows the Code of Ethics for his or her profession.
b. Follows the Code of Ethics for his or her professional roles, certifications, and credentials.

3. STANDARD: The life care planner uses the scientific principles of medicine and health care as a basis for life care planning.
MEASUREMENT CRITERIA:
a. Utilizes, and when possible, participates, in research relevant to life care planning practice.
b. Evaluates literature for application to life care planning.
c. Uses appropriate research findings in the development of life care plans.

4. STANDARD: The life care planner considers cultural and linguistic factors that may influence the assessment, development, and implementation of the plan.
MEASUREMENT CRITERIA:
a. Recommends care that is culturally sensitive.
b. Considers multiple evaluee-centered factors including ethnic, religious, sexual identity, and geographic.
c. Uses qualified interpreters.

IV. Standards of Practice

1. STANDARD: The life care planner practices within his or her professional scope of practice.
MEASUREMENT CRITERIA:
a. Remains within the scope of practice for his or her profession as determined by state, provincial, or national credentialing bodies. The functions associated with performing life care planning are within the scope of practice for rehabilitation and health care professionals.
b. Independently makes recommendations for care items/services that are within the scope of practice of his or her own professional discipline.

2. STANDARD: The life care planner must have skill and knowledge in understanding the health care needs addressed in a life care plan.
MEASURMENT CRITERIA:
a. Consults with others and obtains education when the life care planner must address health care needs that are new or unfamiliar.
b. Able to locate appropriate resources when necessary.
c. Provides a consistent, objective, and thorough methodology for constructing the life care plan, relying on appropriate medical and other health related information, resources, and professional expertise for developing the content of the life care plan.
d. Relies on state-of-the-art knowledge and resources to develop a life care plan.
e. Uses specialized skills including, but not limited to, the ability to research, critically analyze data, manage and interpret large volumes of information, attend to details, demonstrate clear and thorough written and verbal communication skills, develop positive relationships, create and use networks for gathering information, and work autonomously.

3. STANDARD: The life care planner performs comprehensive assessment through the process of data collection and analysis involving multiple elements and sources.
   MEASUREMENT CRITERIA:
   a. Collects data in a systematic, comprehensive, and accurate manner.
   b. Collects data about medical, health, biopsychosocial, financial, educational, and vocational status and needs.
   c. Obtains information from medical records, evaluee/family (when available or appropriate), relevant treating or consulting health care professionals and others. If access to any source of information is not possible (e.g., denied permission to interview the evaluee), this should be so noted in the report.
4. STANDARD: The life care planner uses a consistent, valid and reliable approach to research, data collection, analysis, and planning.
   MEASUREMENT CRITERIA:
   a. Identifies current standards of care, clinical practice guidelines, services and products from reliable sources, such as current literature or other published sources, collaboration with other professionals, education programs, and personal clinical practice.
   b. Researches appropriate options and charges for recommendations, using sources that are reasonably available to the evaluee.
   c. Considers appropriate criteria for care options such as admission criteria, treatment indications or contraindications, program goals and outcomes, whether recommended care is consistent with standards of care, duration of care, replacement frequency, ability of the evaluee to appropriately use services and products, and whether care is reasonably available.
   d. Uses a consistent method to determine available choices and charges.
   e. Uses classification systems (e.g., International Classification of Diseases, Common Procedural Terminology) to correlate care recommendations and charges when these systems are available or helpful in providing clarity.
   f. Uses and relies upon relevant research that should be readily available for review and reflected within the life care plan.
5. STANDARD: The life care planner analyzes data.
   MEASUREMENT CRITERIA:
   a. Analyzes data to determine evaluee needs and consistency of care recommendations with standards of care.
   b. Assesses need for further evaluations or expert opinions.
6. STANDARD: The life care planner uses a planning process.
   MEASUREMENT CRITERIA:
   a. Follows a consistent method for organizing data, creating a narrative life care plan report, and projecting costs.
   b. Develops and uses written documentation tools for reports and cost projections.
   c. Develops recommendations for content of the life care plan cost projections for each evaluee and a method for validating inclusion or exclusion of content.
   d. Makes recommendations that are within the life care planner's own professional scope of practice; seeks recommendations from other qualified professionals and/or relevant sources for inclusion of care items and services outside the life care planner's scope of practice.
   e. Considers recommendations that are age-appropriate, using knowledge of human growth and development, including the impact of aging on disability and function.

7. STANDARD: The life care planner seeks collaboration when possible.
   MEASUREMENT CRITERIA:
   a. Fosters positive relationships with all parties.
   b. Seeks expert opinions, as needed.
   c. Shares relevant information to aid in formulating recommendations and opinions.
8. STANDARD: The life care planner facilitates understanding of the life care planning process.
   MEASUREMENT CRITERIA:
   a. Maintains objectivity and assists others in resolving disagreements about appropriate content for the life care plan.
   b. Provides information about the life care planning process to involved parties to elicit cooperative participation.
9. STANDARD: The life care planner evaluates.
   MEASUREMENT CRITERIA:
   a. Reviews and revises the life care plan for internal consistency and completeness.
   b. Reviews the life care plan for consistency with standards of care and seeks resolution of inconsistencies.
   c. Provides follow-up consultation as appropriate and permitted to ensure that the life care plan is understood and properly interpreted.
10. STANDARD: The life care planner may engage in forensic applications.
   MEASUREMENT CRITERIA: If the life care planner engages in practice that includes participation in legal matters, the life care planner:
   a. Acts as a consultant to legal proceedings related to determining care needs and costs in the role of an impartial advisor to the court.
   b. May provide expert sworn testimony regarding development and content of the life care plan.
   c. Maintains records of research and supporting documentation for content of the life care plan for a period of time consistent with requirements of applicable authoritative jurisdictions.

Appendix

The Ethics section of the 2nd Edition of the *Standards of Practice* for life care planners is provided for reference and use until a separate Code of Ethics is available. This Appendix is to be removed at such time. Language in the Ethics section has not been changed from the 2nd Edition, except to use the term evaluee.

Ethical

Ethics refers to a set of principles of "right" conduct, a theory or a system of moral values, or the rules or standards governing the conduct of a person or members of a profession. The primary goal of ethics is to protect evaluees, provide guidelines to practicing professionals, and enhance the profession as a whole. Within the life care planning specialty, all practitioners are members of one or more professional disciplines and/or are licensed or certified. It is expected that life care planners follow appropriate, relevant, ethical guidelines within their areas of professional practice and expertise.

Life care planners are expected to maintain appropriate confidentiality, avoid ethically conflicting dual or multiple relationships, and adequately advise evaluees of the role of the life care planner, and maintain competency in the profession.

1. Confidentiality: Appropriate confidentiality is a sensitive and important concept. Some professionals will have communications protected by "privilege" which is statutorily based in each state or province. For example, although no "life care planners" are currently covered by privilege, many may be professional counselors, licensed psychologists or others who have the additional statutory protection. Litigation has the additional component of attorney work product that may have an effect on what information may be disclosed. The life care planner must be thoroughly informed on this topic.
2. Dual or multiple relationships: A personal relationship with an evaluee is not appropriate during the course of service. Developing life care plans for friends, coworkers, professional colleagues, or anyone where the objectivity and professionalism of the care plan is questioned should be avoided. Serving in dual or multiple professional roles, such as case manager or treater, is permitted as long as the simultaneous roles are not used for the purpose of providing benefit to the professional (e.g., recommending continued use of the professional without justification).
3. Evaluee advisement of role: Each evaluee should be fully informed about the role of the life care planner. For example, the evaluee should be fully informed about who is requesting the life care plan as well as the confidentiality of communications. Also, life care planners who have dual role responsibilities should clarify that the life care planning role is separate and should clarify what the limits of their participation might be.
4. Competency: The life care planner is expected to accurately represent any information received for a particular case. Recommendations are to have medical, rehabilitation, psychological, and case management foundations with appropriate medical specialist and treatment team collaboration when possible, with support from medical recommendations, clinical practice guidelines, research, and other current literature. Each case is unique and the life care plan must demonstrate professional judgment in bringing together data, supporting documentation, and the individual characteristics of the person addressed within the plan. The life care planner should possess knowledge of professional legal requirements including the legal principles of consent and confidentiality.
5. Life care planners are professionals, from varying educational backgrounds, who maintain professional conduct when addressing opposing life care plan consultants. Life care plan consultants should focus on methodology of plan development, supporting documentation for recommendations and plan content.

Appendix II: Consensus and Majority Statements Derived from Life Care Planning Summits Held in 2000, 2002, 2004, 2006, 2008, 2010, 2012, and 2015*

Cloie B. Johnson

The following statements were created by Life Care Planners at various Summits between 2000 and 2015, and are relevant and applicable to all life care planners:

1. Life Care Planners may come from a variety of disciplines, provided they have qualifications including 5 years' experience in a primary discipline, complete supervised time under a qualified life care planner, and belong to a life care planning professional association.
2. Life Care Planners shall seek out mentor relationships, educating students and unaffiliated professionals about life care planning training, education, experience, special knowledge, and required credentials.
3. Life Care Planners shall disseminate information regarding their area of practice through electronic collaboration, Websites, peer-reviewed journals, books, conferences and symposia, and professional associations.
4. Life Care Planning research shall be reviewed by peers through an objective and "blind" process that addresses methodology.
5. Life Care Planners shall understand the definition of reliability and consistently practice in such a manner.

* Source: *Journal of Life Care Planning*, (2015), Vol. 13, No. 4 (pp. 35–38). Reprinted in accordance with member/subscriber permission guidelines from: International Academy of Life Care Planners, The Life Care Planning Section of The International Association of Rehabilitation Professionals. Publisher: International Association of Rehabilitation Professionals, 1000 Westgate Drive, #252, St. Paul, MN 55114, 888-IARP (888–427–7722), webpage: http://www.rehabpro.org.

6. Life Care Planners shall explore markets for life care planning outside litigation.
7. Life Care Planners shall have knowledge of relevant laws and regulations, as well as local and national care standards.
8. Life Care Planners shall understand optimal outcomes achievable for particular injuries.
9. Life Care Planners shall promote and participate in a national organization for life care planners that serve as a single voice for the practice of life care planning and as a single repository for life care planning resources.
10. Life Care Planners shall complete 120 hours of training including courses that focus on disability issues and is specific to life care planning.
11. Life Care Planning programs shall be based on the latest knowledge and practices.
12. Life Care Planning programs shall cover certification-preparation, as well as advanced topics and complex issues.
13. Life Care Planning programs shall be promoted widely.
14. Life Care Planning programs shall be offered in accessible geographic locations and electronically.
15. Life Care Planning continuing education units shall be available at an increasing number of forums.
16. Life Care Planning continuing education units shall be available at forums that may not focus solely on life care planning.
17. Life Care Planners shall train themselves and recruit others to instruct educational programs.
18. Life Care Planner certification shall render its holder a qualified life care planner, provided that certification is maintained.
19. Life Care Planner certification shall be renewed every five years with the accumulation of 60 continuing education units.
20. Life Care Planners shall be licensed and/or certified in their professional discipline before being certified as a life care planner.
21. Life Care Planner certification standards shall be augmented.
22. The International Commission on Health Care Certification shall apply for National Commission for Certifying Agencies accreditation.
23. Life Care Planners shall hold a certification that has mechanism for complaints and resolution.
24. Life Care Planning certification shall flow from a practitioner-created core curriculum.
25. The Life Care Planning certifying body shall not be proprietary.
26. The Life Care Planning certifying body shall manage and disclose ethical complaints and violations.
27. Life Care Planning certification exams shall be developed and maintained by an advisory group.
28. Life Care Planning certification exams shall be administered by an autonomous entity independent of any organization that provides life care planning training and/or education.
29. Standards of Practice terminology shall be reviewed.
30. Standards of Practice terminology shall be defined.
31. Standards of Practice shall delineate educational requirements for entry into the practice of life care planning.
32. Standards of Practice shall assert the role and accountability of life care planners.
33. Standards of Practice shall be based on a study defining the role and accountability of life care planners.
34. Standards of Practice shall allow for individual judgment and expertise.
35. Standards of Practice shall be utilized in the development of the practice of life care planning.
36. Standards of Practice shall be applicable to current practices.

37. Life Care Planners shall accept referrals only in their area of expertise.
38. Life Care Planners shall draft life care plans under supervision for one year.
39. Life Care Planners shall maintain objectivity.
40. Life Care Planners shall maintain strict adherence to confidentiality practices.
41. Life Care Planners shall renounce inappropriate, distorted or untrue comments about peers.
42. Life Care Planners shall renounce inappropriate processes and training.
43. Life Care Planners shall disclose and differentiate between the roles in which they may be called upon to act.
44. Life Care Planners shall avoid dual relationships when objectivity may be challenged.
45. Life Care Planners shall better define dual relationships.
46. Life Care Planners shall establish themselves within their primary field of practice.
47. Life Care Planners shall objectively place their client's interests before any personal or professional consideration.
48. Life Care Planners shall adhere to relevant Codes of Ethics.
49. Life Care Planners shall have access to recourse/corrective action process for Ethical violations.
50. Life Care Plans shall be individualized.
51. Life Care Plans shall be objective and consistent.
52. Life Care Plans shall be lifelong and flexible.
53. Life Care Plans shall be clear, concise, and user-friendly document.
54. Life Care Plans shall be comprehensive and based on multidisciplinary data.
55. Life Care Plans shall utilize research for recommendations.
56. Life Care Planners shall consider the integrity of data.
57. Life Care Planning shall depend on data collection, analysis and synthesis.
58. Life Care Planners may request additional data, testing and evaluation if required.
59. Life Care Planners shall research condition, resources, services and costs.
60. Life Care Plans shall utilize established procedures.
61. Life Care Planning procedures shall be peer or organizationally reviewed.
62. Life Care Plans shall be developed in the client's best interest.
63. Life Care Plans shall include a basis for recommendations.
64. Life Care Planners shall utilize a reliable, consistent method for reaching conclusions.
65. Life Care Planners shall utilize adequate medical and other data for opinions.
66. Life Care Plans shall include an annotated list of requested and reviewed data/sources.
67. Life Care Planners shall utilize standardized procedures and tools for gathering and reporting information.
68. Life Care Plans shall feature standardized forms and formats.
69. Life Care Plans shall be consistent across similar cases.
70. Life Care Plans shall rely on medical/allied health professional opinions.
71. Life Care Plans shall be limited to the planner's expertise and scope of practice.
72. Life Care Planners shall methodically handle divergent opinions.
73. Life Care Planners shall properly inject personal expertise.
74. Life Care Planners shall utilize credible, evidence based guidelines.
75. Life Care Planners shall conduct an in-person interview whenever permitted.
76. Life Care Planners shall utilize protocols for cost research.
77. Life Care Planners shall gather geographically relevant and representative prices.
78. Life Care Planners shall utilize protocols for using local versus national resources.
79. Life Care Planners shall follow generally accepted methodology.
80. Differences in clinical judgment can result in different recommendations.

81. Life Care Planning databases, templates and software shall have appropriate foundation.
82. Life Care Planning products and processes shall be transparent and consistent.
83. Life Care Planners shall be involved in research.
84. Life Care Planners shall include research in life care plans.
85. Life Care Planners shall study the reliability, validity, and accuracy of life care plans.
86. Life Care Planners shall assess the reliability, validity, and accuracy of data and methods.
87. Life Care Planners shall conduct longitudinal studies.
88. Life Care Planners shall evaluate the cost effectiveness of life care plans.
89. Life Care Planners shall study the impact of life care plans upon quality-of-life.
90. Life Care Planners shall understand and explain research used in a life care plan.
91. Life Care Planners shall utilize research that is reasonable, relevant, and appropriate.
92. Life Care Planners may independently make recommendations for care items/services that are within their scope of practice.
93. Life Care Planners seek recommendations from other qualified professionals and/or relevant sources for inclusion of care items/services outside the individual life care planner's professional scope(s) of practice.
94. When the life care planner includes home care, both private-hire and agency-procured services are options to be considered.
95. The cost of private-hire home care includes caregiver compensation and associated expenses.
96. Life Care Planners shall consider the impact of aging.
97. Review of evidence-based research, review of clinical practice guidelines, medical records, medical and multidisciplinary consultation, and evaluation/assessment of evaluee/family are recognized as best practice sources that provide foundation in Life Care Plans.
98. Best practices for identifying costs in Life Care Plans include:
    - Verifiable data from appropriately referenced sources
    - Costs identified are geographically specific when appropriate and available
    - Non-discounted/market rate prices
    - More than one cost estimate, when appropriate
99. Life Care Planners will define terminology of our work product(s).
100. Life Care Planners have the option to use support staff under their direction and guidance in completing life care plans.
101. Life Care Planners shall identify conflicts of interest.
102. Life Care Planners shall identify the sources of their recommendations.

About the Author

Cloie B. Johnson, MEd, is a Rehabilitation Counselor and Case Manager providing life care planning service at OSC Vocational Systems, Inc. in Bothell, Washington. Cloie has chaired or co-chaired the Summits in 2010, 2011, 2012, and 2015. She is also a past Chair of the IALCP.

References

Johnson, C. (2015). Life care planning summit: Moving forward and looking ahead. *Journal of Life Care Planning, 13* (4), 27–33.

Preston, K., & Johnson, C. (2012). Consensus and majority statements derived from Life Care Planning Summits held in 2000, 2002, 2004, 2006, 2008, 2010 and 2012. *Journal of Life Care Planning, 11* (2), 9–14.

Appendix III: *Journal of Life Care Planning* Title Index*

Editor's Note: The Index is in reverse chronological order beginning with the most current publication year (2017) and ending with the inaugural issue of the *Journal* in 2002.

Journal of Life Care Planning, 15–4

- *Editor's Message*, Jamie Pomeranz and Nichole Stetten, 15(3), 1.
- *Introduction of the New Editorial Board*, Tanya Rutherford Owen, 15(3), 3–8.
- *The Role of the Occupational Therapist in Life Care Planning*, Nancy Mitchell, Courtney Mitchell, & Nichole E. Stetten, 15(3), 9–11.
- *Determining 24-Hour Supervision: A Scoping Review through a Canadian Legal Database*, Avelino (Jun) Maranan and Mathew Rose, 15(3), 13–17.
- *The Role of the Occupational Therapist in Valuing "Unpaid Work" and How It Impacts Wrongful Death Claims*, Carol Bierbrier and Hazel Bowles, 15(3), 19–23.
- *Memories of Paul Amsterdam, ATP – A Friend and Colleague*, Dianne Simmons Grab, 15(3), 25.
- *Ethics Interface*, Nancy Mitchell, 15(3), 27–31.

Journal of Life Care Planning, 15–3

- *Managing the Notion of UCR in a Life Care Plan*, Rebecca Mendoza Saltiel Busch, 15(3), 3–14.
- *Developing Life Care Plans for Cases Involving Multiple Plaintiffs*, Amber L. Allison & Aaron Wolfson, 15(3), 15–18.
- *2017 Life Care Planning Summit Proceedings*, Tracy Albee, Jamie N. Gamez, & Cloie B. Johnson, 15(3), 19–30.
- *Challenges and Practice Issues Faced by Canadian Life Care Planners*, Jodi Fischer & Melissa Jones Wilkins, 15(3), 31–36.

* Source: *Journal of Life Care Planning* Title Index from Inception through 2017. © Tanya Owen, PhD. Reprinted with permission. Tanya Rutherford Owen, PhD, CRC, CLCP, LPC, Owen Vocational Services, Inc. 1130 E Millsap, Fayetteville, AR 72703, (479) 695-1772. E-mail: owenvoc@gmail.com.

- *A Comparison of Life Care Planning Standards of Practice*, Jamie N. Gamez, Cloie B. Johnson, & Laura Stajduhar, 15(3), 37–44.
- *Ethics Interface,* Nancy Mitchell, 15(3), 45–54.

Journal of Life Care Planning, 15–2

- *2017 Life Care Planning Summit Proceedings at a Glance*, Jamie N. Gamez, 15(2), 3–4.
- *2017 IALCP Election Results,* 15(2), 5–6.
- *Cultural Experiences and International Practices of Life Care Planners: Results of an Exploratory Research Study,* Mary Barros-Bailey, 15(2), 7–12.
- *Eliciting Rehabilitation Recommendations during Forensic Life Care Plan Consultations*, Michael Shahnasarian, 15(2), 13–20.
- *The Opioid Epidemic and Its Effect on Life Care Planning*, Melissa Jones Wilkins, Amanda Connell, & Sandra Bullins, 15(2), 21–26.
- *The Inclusion of Cannabinoids and Medicinal Marijuana as a Treatment Option for Individuals with Disabilities in Life Care Plans,* Stephanie L. Lusk and Tanya Rutherford Owen, 15(2), 27–34.
- *Life Care Planning in a Country with For-Profit Medicine*, Rigel M. Pinon & Irmo Marini, 15(2), 35–38.
- *Trauma and Stress Related Disorders: Relevance to DSM-5 and Life Care Planning*, Melissa Jones Wilkins, Tanya Owen, & Brandy Kilpatrick, 15(2), 39–48.
- *Ethics Interface*, Nancy Mitchell, 15(2), 49–51.

Journal of Life Care Planning, 15–1

- *Complexities of Surgery Pricing and Implications for Life Care Planners,* Laura Woodard, Elizabeth Kattman, & Stella Spencer, 15(1), 3–8.
- *Assistive Technology in the Life Care Plan*, Chrissy Whiting Madison, Sandra Bullins, & Melissa Jones Wilkins, 15(1), 9–12.
- *Management of Hearing Loss in Adults: An Overview and Implications for Life Care Planning*, Rachel Glade & Amy Hunter, 15(1), 13–20.
- *2017 IARP/ISLCP Round-Table Summaries*, Carla Seyler, 15(1), 21–24.
- *Exploring Special Needs Adoptions and the Applicability of Life Care Plans*, Vicky Buckles & Jamie Pomeranz. 15(1), 25–34.
- *Ethics Interface*, Nancy Mitchell, 37–40.
- *Why Should You Attend the 2017 Life Care Planning Summit*, Jamie Gamez & Cloie Johnson, 15(1), 41–43.

Journal of Life Care Planning, 14–2

- *Differences among Life Care Planners and Physiatrists Regarding the Likelihood and Frequency of Secondary Complications for Persons with Spinal Cord Injury*, Noel A. Ysasi, Irmo Marini, Matthew Sprong, & Irasema Silva, 14(2), 3–37.
- *Revisiting Chronic Pain in the Life Care Plan*, David E. Stewart, Brian Jakubowicz, Kwadis Beard, George Cyphers, & Daniel V. Turner, 14(2), 39–45.
- *Ethics Interface*, Nancy Mitchell, 14(2), 47–48.

Journal of Life Care Planning, 14–1

- *A Comparison of Physiatrist Life Care Planners versus Non-Life Care Planner Physiatrists' Professional Opinions Regarding Secondary Complications of Spinal Cord Injuries,* Noel A. Ysasi, Irmo Marini, Danielle Leigh Antol, Kristin Maxwell, & Shelby Kerwin, 14(1), 3–24.
- *A Comprehensive Literature Review of Secondary Complications of Spinal Cord Injury,* Noel A. Ysasi, Shelby Kerwin, Irmo Marini, Bradley McDaniels, & Danielle Leigh Antol, 14(1), 25–58.
- *Physiatrists' Professional Opinions Regarding Secondary Complications After SCI,* Noel A. Ysasi, Irmo Marini, Bradley McDaniels, Roy K. Chen, Lisa Dunkley, & Shelby Kerwin, 14(1), 59–70.
- *Appendix: Life Care Planner Survey and Physiatrist Survey,* 14(1), 71–84.
- *LCP Practice Musings*, Robert H. Taylor, 14(1), 85–86.
- *The Medical Equipment Corner*, Paul Amsterdam, 14(1), 87–88.
- *The Canadian Circle and Beyond*, Dana M. Weldon, 14(1), 89–96.
- *Ethics Interface,* Nancy Mitchell, 97–101.

Journal of Life Care Planning, 13–4

- *Long-Term Outcomes of Pediatric-Onset Spinal Cord Injuries: Implications for Life Care Planning,* Lawrence Vogel & Kathy Zebracki, 13(4), 3–10.
- *Critical Elements of Home Health Service Provision for Life Care Planners*, Tanya Rutherford Owen, Melissa Jones Wilkins, & Brandy Kilpatrick, 13(4), 11–20.
- *Insights into the International Association of Life Care Planning Fellow Program: Question and Answers from Program Developers*, Michael Shahnasarian, 13(4), 21–26.
- *2015 Life Care Planning Summit: Moving Forward and Looking Ahead,* Cloic B. Johnson, 13(4), 27–34.
- *Consensus and Majority Statements Derived from Life Care Planning Summits Held in 2000, 2002, 2004, 2006, 2008, 2010, 2012, 2015*, Cloie B. Johnson, 13(4), 35–38.
- *2015 International Symposium of Life Care Planning (ISLCP),* Debra E. Berens, 13(4), 39–42.
- *Congratulations 2015 Life Care Planning Award Recipients,* 13(4), 43–46.
- *Prologue—The Collateral Source Rule and the ACA: Implications for Life Care Planning,* Cloie B. Johnson, Timothy F. Field, & Anthony J. Choppa, 13(4), 47–50.
- *LCP Practice Musings*, Robert H. Taylor, 13(4), 51–52.
- *The Canadian Circle and Beyond,* Dana M. Weldon, 13(4), 53–54.
- *Ethics Interface,* Nancy Mitchell, 13(4), 55–59.

Journal of Life Care Planning, 13–3

- *The Collateral Source Rule and the Affordable Care Act: Implications for Life Care Planning and Economic Damages*, Timothy Field, Cloie B. Johnson, Anthony J. Choppa, & John D. Fountaine, 13(3), 3–16.
- *An Attorney Perspective on Standards of Practice: A Weapon or a Shield?* Nathaniel Fick, Karen Preston, 13(3), 17–20.
- *Revision Process for the Standards of Practice for Life Care Planners*, Karen Preston & Christine Reid, 13(3), 21–30.
- *Standards of Practice for Life Care Planners, Third Edition,* 13(3), 31–36.
- *Life Care Planning for Burn Injuries*, Tanya Rutherford Owen, Melissa Jones Wilkins, Brandy Kilpatrick, & Teresia M. Paul, 13(3), 37–44.

- *Life Care Planning and Acquired Brain Injury: Determining Needs and Costs at the Dawn of the Patient Protection Affordable Care Act*, Harvey E. Jacobs, 13(3), 45–48.
- *The Medical Equipment Corner*, Paul Amsterdam, 13(3), 49–50.
- *The Canadian Circle and Beyond*, Dana M. Weldon, 13(3), 51–64.
- *Ethics Interface*, Nancy Mitchell, 13(3), 65–70.
- *Samples for Success: Life Care Plans from Practicing Life Care Planners, First Edition,* Victoria Powell, 13(3), 71.
- *2015 International Symposium on Life Care Planning Agenda,* 13(3), 72–73.

Journal of Life Care Planning, 13–2

- *Communication Sciences and Disorders: The Future of Speech-Language Pathology and Audiology*, Carolyn Wiles Higdon, 13(2), 5–6.
- *Neuroimaging Techniques to Help Patients with Neurological Complications*, Carolyn Wiles Higdon, 13(2), 6–8.
- *Transcranial Magnetic Stimulation/Transcranial Direct Current Stimulation*, Carolyn Wiles Higdon, 13(2), 9–10.
- *Laryngeal Imaging*, Carolyn Wiles Higdon, 13(2), 11–12.
- *Biofeedback for Acquired Apraxia of Speech*, Carolyn Wiles Higdon, 13(2), 13–14.
- *Audiology: The Future of Hearing*, Carolyn Wiles Higdon, 13(2), 15–20.
- *Technology: Smartphones and Apps for Hearing Impaired*, Carolyn Wiles Higdon, 13(2), 21–24.
- *Communication Sciences and Disorders: The Future of Speech-Language Pathology and Audiology*, Carolyn Wiles Higdon, 13(2), 25–26.
- *LCP Practice Musings*, Robert H. Taylor, 13(2), 27–28.
- *The Medical Equipment Corner*, Paul Amsterdam, 13(2), 29–30.
- *The Canadian Circle and Beyond*, Dana M. Weldon, 13(2), 31–32.
- *Ethics Interface*, Nancy Mitchell, 13(2), 33–38.
- *2015 International Symposium on Life Care Planning, September 19–20, 2015,* 13(2), 39–40.

Journal of Life Care Planning, 13–1

- *Introduction of the New Editorial Board, Costantini & Simmons Grab*, 13(1), 7–16.
- *2015 International Symposium on Life Care Planning: Change, Challenge, Opportunity,* Costantini & Simmons Grab, 13(1), 17–18.
- *What Is the Life Care Planning Summit; and Why Should You Attend the 2105 Summit?* Cloie Johnson & Jamie Gamez, 13(1), 19–22.
- *LCP Practice Musings*, Robert H. Taylor, 13(1), 23–24.
- *The Medical Equipment Corner*, Paul Amsterdam, 13(1), 25–26.
- *The Canadian Circle and Beyond*, Dana Weldon, 13(1), 27–28.
- *Therapeutic Swimming as a Community Based Program*, Corinne Slade & Dianne Simmons Grab, 13(1), 29–32.
- *Ethics Interface*, Nancy Mitchell, 13(1), 33–35.

Journal of Life Care Planning, 12–2

- *The Authors of Letter to the Editor Regarding "Life Expectancy Projections Supporting Life Care Planning,"* RP Bonfiglio & D Kasas in Volume 12, Number 1. Steven Day, Robert Reynolds, & Scott Kush, 12(2), 5–8.

- *Decubitus Ulcer Development in Individuals with Spinal Cord Injury,* Tanya Rutherford Owen & Melissa Jones Wilkins, 12(2), 9–24.
- *Urinary Tract Infections and Spinal Cord Injury,* Noel A. Ysasi, Irasema Silva, & Mariel Guerrero, 12(2), 25–31.
- *Neuropathic Pain: A Secondary Complication of Spinal Cord Injury,* Cynthia A. Serrata & Mary A. Rocha, 12(2), 32–44.
- *Cardiovascular Disease and Spinal Cord Injury,* Kim Nguyen-Finn, Jaime Lopez, & Matilde Barrera Alaniz, 12(2), 45–54.
- *Osteoporosis and Spinal Cord Injury,* Rachita Sharma, 12(2), 55–62.
- *Respiratory Dysfunction and Spinal Cord Injury,* Kim Nguyen-Finn & Danielle D. Fox, 12(2), 63–76.
- *Shoulder Injury and Pain among Person's with Spinal Cord Injury,* Noel A. Ysasi, Alicia Brown, & Irasema Silva, 12(2), 77–90.
- *Ethics Interface,* Nancy Mitchell, 12(2), 91–95.

Journal of Life Care Planning, 12–1

- *Estimating Life Expectancy: A Physiatric Perspective,* Bill Rosen, Reg Gibbs, & Ashley Crtalic, 12(1), 3–14.
- *Life Expectancy Projections Supporting Life Care Planning,* Richard Paul Bonfiglio & Dakota Kasa, 12(1), 15–20.
- *Life Expectancy and the Life Care Planner,* Robert Shavelle & David Strauss, 12(1), 21–30.
- *Life Expectancy for Life Care Planners,* Scott Kush, Steven Day, & Robert Reynolds, 12(1), 31–50.
- *Utilizing Research to Determine Life Expectancy: Applications for Life Care Planning,* James Krause & Lee Saunders, 12(1), 51–60.
- *Ethical Risks of Understanding Life Expectancy in Life Care Planning Practice,* Christine Reid, 12(1), 61–74.
- *Ethics Interface,* Nancy Mitchell, 12(1), 75–80.
- *Book Review,* Irmo Marini, 12(1), 81.

Journal of Life Care Planning, Volume, 11–4

- *18th Annual International Conference on Life Care Planning,* Heidi L. Fawber, 11 (4), 3–6.
- *Transcript of David Ball, Trial Consultant 2012 International Symposium on Life Care Planning: Persuasive Life Care Planner Testimony—Serving the Injured Client,* David Ball, 11(4), 7–18.
- *Recent Advances at Craig Hospital,* Kenny Hosack, Catherine Davis, & Candy Tefertiller. 11(4), 19–24.
- *Pediatric Traumatic Brain Injury, Before, During, and After: A Pediatric Physiatrist Point of View,* Richard Radecki, 11(4), 25–32.
- *Ethics,* Nancy Mitchell, 11(4), 33–38.

Journal of Life Care Planning, Volume, 11–3

- *Scrambler Therapy: An Innovative and Effective Treatment for Chronic Neuropathic Pain,* Frank Sparadeo, Cheryl Kaufman, & Stephen D'Amato, 11(3), 3–16.

- *Admissible Expert Testimony,* Tracy Albee & Douglas Gordon, 11 (3), 17–24.
- *Life Expectancy Determinations: Cerebral Palsy, Traumatic Brain Injury, and Spinal Cord Injury Analysis and Comparison,* Audrius V. Plioplys, 11(3), 25–38.
- *Organizational Viewpoints on Research in Life Care Planning,* Tanya Rutherford Owen, 11(3), 39–51.

Journal of Life Care Planning, Volume, 11–2

- *The 2012 Life Care Planning Summit: Third Time Is a Charm,* Cloie Johnson, 11(2), 3–6.
- *Consensus and Majority Statements Derived from LCP Summits Held in 2000, 2002, 2004, 2006, 2008, 2010, and 2012,* Karen Preston & Cloie Johnson, 11(2), 9–14.
- *Coding and Cost Research for the Life Care Plan,* Liz Holakiewicz & Marilyn Pacheco, 11(2), 15–26.
- *National Spinal Cord Statistical Center Cost Figures: A Comparison to the Life Care Planning Approach,* Tanya Rutherford Owen & Randall L. Thomas, 11(2), 27–34.
- *Life Care Planning in Wrongful Birth Cases,* Michele Nielsen, 11(2), 35–42.
- *Ethics,* Nancy Mitchell, 11(2), 43–44.
- *Book Review,* Tim Field, 11 (2), 45–46.

Journal of Life Care Planning, Volume, 11–1

- *Special Issue of the Journal of Life Care Planning on Summits,* Roger Weed, 11(1), 3–4.
- *Life Care Planning Summit 2000,* Debbie Berens, Roger Weed, 11(1), 5–31.
- *Life Care Planning Summit 2002,* Susan Riddick-Grisham, 11(1), 32–49.
- *Life Care Planning Summit 2004: The Progress Continues,* Debbie Berens, 11(1), 50–52.
- *Life Care Planning Summit 2006: Town Hall Meeting,* Debbie Berens, 11(1), 53–54.
- *Life Care Planning Summit 2006,* Susan Riddick-Grisham, 11(1), 55–66.
- *Life Care Planning Summit 2008,* Karen Preston, Jamie Pomeranz, & Carol Walker, 11(1), 67–75.
- *Life Care Planning Summit 2010,* Debbie Berens, Cloie Johnson, Jamie Pomeranz, & Karen Preston, 11(1), 76–86.
- *Canadian Life Care Planning Summit 2011 Proceedings,* Cloie Johnson & Michel Lacerte, 11(1), 87–109.
- *What Every Life Care Planner Should Know about the 2012 LCP Summit,* Roger Weed, Cloie Johnson, Susan Riddick Grisham, & Steve Yuhas, 11(1), 113–118.
- *Welcome to the 2012 Summit for Life Care Planners,* Cloie Johnson, 11(1), 119–125.

Journal of Life Care Planning, 10–4

- *Life Care Plan Implementation among Adults with Spinal Cord Injuries,* Tanya Rutherford-Owen & Irmo Marini, 10(4), 4–20.
- *Working and Care-Giving: The Impact on Caregiver Stress, Family-Work Conflict, and Burnout,* Karen R. McDaniel & David G. Allen, 10(4), 21–32.
- *Adult Care and Spinal Cord Injury: Usage Patterns and Perspectives for Those with Life Care Plans,* Tanya Rutherford-Owen & Irmo Marini, 10(4), 33–44.
- *Practical Matters Possibility versus Probability,* Irmo Marini, 10(4), 45–48.

- *Ethics Interface,* Nancy Mitchell, 10(4), 49–52.
- *Book Review,* Valerie J. Rodriguez, 10(4), 53–54.

Journal of Life Care Planning, 10–3

- *Editorial: A Decade of Thanksgiving,* Debbie Berens, 10(3), 1–2.
- *Canadian Life Care Planning Summit 2011 Proceedings,* Cloie Johnson Michel Lacerte, 10(3), 3–24.
- *Summary of Total Group Results for Canadian Life Care Planning Summit 2011,* Cloie Johnson, 10(3), 25–28.
- *Letters of Endorsement Professional Groups,* 10(3), 29–36.
- *How Life Care Planners Can Impact Legislation Through Legislative Tracking Technology,* Brandie Dawson & Carole Upman, 10(3), 37–44.
- *Synopsis of 17th Annual International Symposium on Life Care Planning (ISLCP),* Heidi L. Fawber, 10(3), 45–48.
- *Every Person Is Unique, Individual and Irreplaceable,* Anne Llewellyn, 10(3), 49–50.
- *Congratulations 2011 Life Care Planning Award Recipients,* Debbie Berens, 10(3), 51–52.
- *2011 International Symposium on Life Care Planning Gratefully Acknowledges their Vendors,* FLCPR, 10(3), 53–54.
- *2011 International Symposium on Life Care Planning Gratefully Acknowledges their Donors & Supporters,* FLCPR, 10(3), 55–56.
- *Ethics Interface,* Nancy Mitchell, 10(3), 57–60.

Journal of Life Care Planning, 10–2

- *Evaluation of Life Care Plans Developed by a Private Rehabilitation Consulting Agency for Victims of Abuse Utilizing the IALCP Standards of Practice as a Base,* Zarahi Nunez & Darlene M. Carruthers, 10(2), 3–14.
- *Book Review,* Carolyn Wiles Higdon, 10(2), 15–20.
- *Ethics Interface,* Nancy Mitchell & Mary Barros-Bailey, 10(2), 21–24.
- *BRONSON'S INC and TRAVELERS, Appellants, v. ROBERT MANN, Appellee.,* Debbie Berens, 10(2), 25–30.
- *SUMMARY: Bronson's, Inc. & Travelers v. Robert Mann, 2011,* Gerri Pennachio, 10(2), 31–32.
- *Comment on Bronson's Inc. & Travelers v. Robert Mann,* Timothy F. Field, 10(2), 33–34.
- *Life Care Planning Canadian Summit 2011,* Cloie Johnson, 10(2), 35–36.

Journal of Life Care Planning, 10–1

- *A Tribute to Cheryl "Sheri" Jasper,* Roger O. Weed, 10(1), 1–2.
- *Tributes to Sheri Jasper,* Sherry A. Latham, Terry Schramm, William R. Goodrich, Susan Riddick-Grisham, Julie A. Kitchen, & Karen Luckett, 10(1), 3–6.
- *Eulogy of Cheryl "Sheri" Jasper,* Paul M. Deutsch, 10(1), 7–10.
- *Eulogy of Sheri Jasper,* Terry Winkler, 10(1), 11–12.
- *A Dialogue with Sheri Jasper (reprinted),* Debbie Berens, 10(1), 13–16.
- *A Tribute to Tyron Elliott, Esq.,* Judy L. LaBuda, Ann T. Neulicht, & Roger O. Weed, 10(1), 17–18.

- *A Dialogue with Tyron Elliott, Esq. (reprinted),* Debbie Berens, 10(1), 19–22.
- *A Survey of Speech-language Pathologists: Long-term Speech Therapy Needs for Patients within Three Neurological Conditions,* Ayala, Marini, Luckett, & Blanco, 10(1), 23–46.
- *Ethics Interface,* Nancy Mitchell & Mary Barros-Bailey, 10(1), 47–50.

Journal of Life Care Planning, 9–4

- *Life Care Plan Survey 2009: Process, Methods and Protocols,* Ann T. Neulicht, Susan Riddick-Grisham, & William R. Goodrich, 9(4), 131–162.
- *Appendix to Life Care Plan Survey,* 9(4), 163–200.
- *Life Care Plan Survey at a Glance,* William R. Goodrich, Ann T. Neulicht, & Susan Riddick-Grisham, 9(4), 201–215.
- *Award Recipients Congratulations,* Debbie Berens & Jamie Pomeranz, 9(4), 216–217.

Journal of Life Care Planning, 9–3

- *Editorial: The Roles and Functions of a Life Care Planner,* Timothy F. Field & Roger O. Weed, 9(3), 55–56.
- *Role and Function Study of Life Care Planners,* Jamie Pomeranz, Nami Yu, & Christine Reid, 9(3), 57–106.
- *Ethics Interface,* Mary Barros-Bailey, 9(3), 119–122.
- *Book Review,* Karen Preston, 9(3), 123–124.

Journal of Life Care Planning, 9–2

- *Life Care Planning Summit 2010 Proceedings,* Debbie Berens, Cloie Johnson, Jamie Pomeranz, & Karen Preston. 9(2), 3–14.
- *Life Expectancy Estimates in the Life Care Plan: Accounting for Economic Factors,* James S. Krause & Lee L. Saunders, 9(2), 15–28.
- *Coping with Cancer, Quality of Life, and Return-to-Work,* Paul Bourgeois, 9(2), 29–36.
- *Reducing the Use of PRN Medication in In-Patient Psychiatric Hospitals,* George C. T. Mugoya & Charlene M. Kampfe, 9(2), 37–46.
- *Ethics Interface,* Nancy Mitchell, 9(2), 47–49.

Journal of Life Care Planning, 9–1

- *Rational Life Care Planning,* Wayne C. Kreuscher, 9(1), 7–13.
- *Reaction to Rational Life Care Planning,* Jeanne B. Patterson & Frank Woodrich, 9(1), 15–18.
- *An Irreverent Look at Life Care Planners,* Rodney M. Patterson, 9(1), 19–39.
- *Comments Regarding an Irreverent Look at Life Care Planners,* Roger O. Weed, 9(1), 41–44.
- *Life Care Plan of John Child, Jr.,* Charles A. Kincaid, 9(1), 45–51.
- *Ethics Interface,* Nancy Mitchell, 9(1), 53–54.

Journal of Life Care Planning, 8–4

- *Editorial: The Annual Student Paper Award*, Timothy F. Field, 8(4), 155.
- *Spinal Muscular Atrophy Type II, Implications for the Life Care Plan: A Case Study Involving Opposite-sex Siblings with Spinal Muscular Atrophy Type II*, Brandie Dawso.
- *Tools for Making Home Care Decisions: A Clinician's Worksheets*, Karen Preston.
- *Book Review - The CRCC Desk Reference on Professional Ethics: A Guide for Rehabilitation Counselors*, Roger O. Weed. 8(4), 157–193.
- *Tools for Making Home Care Decisions: A Clinician's Worksheets*, Karen Preston, 8(4), 195–198.
- *Book Review*, Roger O. Weed, 8(4), 201–202.
- *Book Review - Life Care Planning and Case Management Handbook*, Ann Neulicht, 8(4), 203–204.
- *Book Review - Medical, Psychosocial and Vocational Aspects of Disability, Third Edition*, Judith Parker, 8(4), 205–206.
- *Ethics Interface*, Nancy Mitchell, 8(4), 207–208.

Journal of Life Care Planning, 8–3

- *Editorial: Growing the Life Care Planning Literature Base*, Timothy F. Field, 8(3), 105.
- *A Survey of Physical Therapists: Long-Term Therapy Needs For Persons with Severe Disabilities*, Irmo Marini, Karen Luckett, Eva Miller, & E. Lisette Blanco, 8(3), 107–123.
- *Annual Student Paper Award — Brandie Dawson*, Debra Berens, 8(3), 124.
- *Life Care Planning in Bankruptcy Court: A Case Study*, Tracey Albee, 8(3), 125–134.
- *Ethics Interface*, Nancy Mitchell, 8(3), 135–138.
- *Congratulations, Terry Winkler — Recipient of the Life Care Planning Lifetime Achievement Award*, Debra Berens, 8(3), 139.
- *International Academy of Life Care Planning — Strategic Planning*, Cloie B. Johnson, 8(3), 145–148.

Journal of Life Care Planning, 8–2

- *Obesity and Disability: A Paradigm Shift in Workers' Compensation Rehabilitation*, Chad J. Betters, 8(2), 67–74.
- *Selvie Muse-Freeman, as duly appointed guardian of Linda Muse, Plaintiff v. Imran Bhatti, et al., Defendants,* Civil Action No: 75 07–3638 (AET), 8(2), 75–80.
- *Case: Selvie Muse-Freeman v. Bhatti, M.D.*, Trudy Koslow, 8(2), 81–82.
- *Replacement Cost Valuation of Production by Homemakers: Conceptual Questions and Measurement Problems*, Thomas R. Ireland & John O.Ward, 8(2), 83–92.

Journal of Life Care Planning, 8–1

- *New Developments in the Role of Neuropsychological and Psychological Assessments in Rehabilitation, Case Management and Life Care Planning,* Lisa Kohn, Elizabeth Hooper, Jessica Ballard, Alan Raphael, & Charles Golden, 8(1), 3–8.
- *Which Estimates of Household Production are Best?* John B. Douglass, Genevieve M. Kenney, & Ted R. Miller, 8(1), 9–30.

- *Market Valuation of Household Production*, Ronald A. Dulaney, John H. Fitzgerald, Matthew S. Swenson, & John H. Wicks, 8(1), 31–42.
- *Household Services: Toward a More Comprehensive Measure*, Frank D. Tinari, 43–56.

Journal of Life Care Planning, 7–4

- *Editorial: Expanding the Knowledge Base for the Life Care Planner*, 7(4), 161–162.
- *Bereavement and Mortality: A Methodology for Assessing Capacity and Functioning Following the Loss of a Spouse*, Timothy E. Field, Anthony J. Choppa, Cloie B. Johnson, Kent A. Jayne, John D. Fountaine, & Anna-Marie Smith, 7(4), 163–180.
- *Discounting the Cost of Future Care for Persons with Disabilities*, David Strauss, Robert Shavelle, Christopher Pflaum, & Christopher Bruce, 7(4), 181–190.
- *Life Expectancies for Person with Medical Risks*, Frank Slesnick & Robert Thornton, 7(4), 191–202.
- *Ethics Interface*, Nancy Mitchell, 7(4), 203–206.

Journal of Life Care Planning, 7–3

- *The Transgender Life Care Plan: A Case Report,* Mary Barros-Bailey & Jodi L. Saunders, 7(3), 97–104.
- *Recipient of the Life Care Planning Lifetime Achievement Award,* Julie A. Kitchen, 7(3), 105.
- *The Applicability of the Life Care Plan for Adopted Children with Disabilities: What Will Medicaid Pay?* Vicky P. Buckles, Jamie Pomeranz, & Mary Ellen Young, 7(3), 107–122.
- *Annual Student Paper Award,* Vicky P. Buckles, 7(3), 123.
- *Who Is the Client in Forensics?* Mary Barros-Bailey, Jeffrey Carlisle, Michael Graham, Ann T. Neulicht, Robert Taylor, & Ann Wallace, 7(3), 125–132.
- *Recipient of the Patricia McCollom Research Award,* Dr. James Krause 7(3), 133–134.
- *James McMillan, Claimant—against—The City of New York,* 7(3), 135–144.
- *Summary: McMillan v. City of New York*, Sharon Reavis, 7(3), 145–146.
- *A Comment: McMillan v. City of New York*, Susan U. Sheerin, 7(3), 147–148.

Journal of Life Care Planning, 7–2

- *Journal of Life Care Planning: A New Direction,* Timothy Field, 7(2), 45.
- *Life Care Planning Summit 2008 Proceedings*, Karen Preston, Jamie L. Pomeranz, & Carol Walker, 7(2), 49–60.
- *Research to Another Level: Medical Coding and the Life Care Planning Process: Part I*, Ann Maniha, 7(2), 61–72.
- *A Study of Quality of Life Issues for Individuals with Spinal Cord Injury Following Treatment and Financial Settlement*, Randy Salmons, 7(2), 72–83.
- *Ethics Interface*, Mary Barros-Bailey, 7(2), 85–87.

Journal of Life Care Planning, 7–1

- *Editorial: Life Care Planning…A Developing Process,* Debra E. Berens, 7(1), 1.
- *Identifying a New Area of Damages: Assessing Time Loss Associated with Bowel Management,* Nami S. Yu, Jamie L. Pomeranz, Michael D. Moorhouse, Linda R. Shaw, & Paul M. Deutsch, 7(1), 3–11.

- *A Dialogue with...Mary Barros-Bailey,* 7(1), 13–16.
- *Application of Life Care Planning to Psychiatric Cases (An Ontario Perspective),* Audrey R. Miller, 7(1), 17–26.
- *Ethics Interface,* Nancy Mitchell, 7(1), 26–29.
- *Innovations for Daily Living,* Klebine, P., 7(1), 31–34.
- *Book Review: Diplomate, American Board of Vocational Experts,* Weed, R. O. (2007). *Life Care Planning: A Step-by-Step Guide,* Ann T. Neulicht, 7(1), 35.
- *Book Review: Garland, W., & Anderson, L. (2008). Life Care Planning: A Method to Your Madness,* Roger O. Weed, 7(1), 37–39.

Journal of Life Care Planning, Vol 6–3&4

- *Editorial: A Legend in Life Care Planning,* Debra E. Berens, 6(3&4), 75.
- *In Memory of Patricia Lynne McCollom,* 6(3&4), 75–76.
- *Use of Scientific Research and Clinical Practice Guidelines: A Survey of Experienced Life Care Planners,* Pomeranz, Yu, Wemmer, & Watson. 6(3&4), 77–98.
- *A Dialogue with James S. Krause,* Debra E. Berens, 6(3&4), 99–103.
- *Life Care Planning and the Elder Law Attorney,* Cox & Wortman, 6(3&4), 105–112.
- *Report of the 2007 International Symposium on Life Care Planning: The Unity Conference,* 6(3&4)113–114.
- *Nami S. Yu, Annual Student Paper Award,* 6(3&4), 119–120.
- *Ethics Interface,* Mitchell, 6(3&4), 123–124.
- *Life Care Planning System Software Review,* DeFazio, 6(3&4), 127–129.

Journal of Life Care Planning, Vol 6–1&2

- *Editorial: "Sharpening the Saw..."* Debra E. Berens, 6(1&2), 1.
- *Determining Type and Quality of Household Services Required for persons with Disabilities: Using Time Use Survey Data,* Jodi Fischer, 6(1&2), 3–13.
- *International Classification of Functioning, Disability and Health: A Model for Life Care Planners,* Jamie L. Pomeranz & Linda R. Shaw, 6(1&2), 15–24.
- *Nursing Educational Requirements: Relevance to Life Care Planning Credentialing Policy,* Todd Van Wieren & Christine Reid, 6(1&2), 25–45.
- *Book Review,* Andrea Zotovas, 6(1&2), 49–52.
- *A Dialogue with Karen Preston,* Debra E. Berens, 6(1&2), 57–59.
- *Announcements and Educational Opportunities for Your Learning Pleasure,* Debra E. Berens, 6(1&2), 65–67.

Journal of Life Care Planning, Vol 5–4

- *Editorial: "Communication Is Key,"* Berens, 5(4) 141.
- *The Physical and Psychosocial Health Status of Clients with Spinal Cord Injury Awarded Damages in Litigation,* Irmo Marini & Eva Miller, 5(4) 145–158.
- *Home Assessment in Life Care Planning,* Karl & Weed, 5(4) 159–171.
- *Life Care Planning Tools, Websites and Resources: Summary of Relevant Presentations at the 2006 International Conference on Life Care Planning,* McDaniel, 5(4) 173–196.

- *A Dialogue with Sherie Kendall*, Berens, 5(4) 197–200.
- *Announcements: The 2007 International Symposium of Life Care Planning: A New Era for Life Care Planners*, Berens, 5(4) 201–202.
- *Ethics Interface*, Mitchell, 5(4) 203–204.
- *Announcements and Educational Opportunities for Your Learning Pleasure*, 5(4) 207–210.

Journal of Life Care Planning, Vol 5–3

- *Editorial: "Our Day Will Come,"* Berens, 5(3) 49–50.
- *To the Editor,* Deutsch, Weed, McCollom, & Grisham 5(3) 51–53.
- *Ethics Interface,* Mitchell, 5(3) 55–56.
- *2006 Life Care Planning Summit Proceedings*, Grisham, 5(3) 57–90.
- *The Life Care Planning RACE: Review, Analysis, Critique & Evaluation?* Neulicht, 5(3) 91–98.
- *Long-Term Neurobehavioral Characteristics after Brain Injury: Implications for Vocational Rehabilitation*, Witol, Sander, See, & Kreutzer, 5(3) 99–107.
- *Tools for Creating an Ethical Practice*, Preston, 5(3) 109–114.
- *Standards of Practice: The Weapon or the Shield?* Preston, 5(3) 115–120.
- *Foreword to the Revised Standards of Practice for Life Care Planners,* McCollom, 5(3) 121.
- *Standards of Practice for Life Care Planners*, 5(3) 123–129.
- *A Dialogue with Julie Kitchen*, Berens, 5(3) 133–136.
- *Announcements & Educational Opportunities for Your Learning Pleasure*, 5(3) 139–140.

Journal of Life Care Planning, Vol 5–1&2

- *Editorial: "Lead On…"* Berens, 5(1&2) 1–2.
- *Three Journal Life Care Planning Members Receive Prestigious Awards*, Berens, 5(1&2) 5–6.
- *Consensus among Life Care Planners Regarding Activities to Consider When Recommending Personal Attendant Care Services for Individuals with Spinal Cord Injury: A Delphi Study,* Pomeranz, Shaw, Sawyer, & Velozo 5(1&2) 7–24.
- *2006 Life Care Planning Summit/Town Hall Meeting: A Celebration of Life Care Planners… 10 Years Later*, Berens, 5(1&2) 25–26.
- *A Dialogue with Rick Bonfiglio, MD*, Berens, 5(1&2) 27–30.
- *Book Review,* Neulicht, 5(1&2) 31–32.
- *Book Review*, Isom, 5(1&2) 33–35.
- *Announcements & Educational Opportunities for Your Learning Pleasure*, 5(1&2) 37–40.

Journal of Life Care Planning, Vol 4–4

- *Editorial: Are You a Joiner?* Berens, 4(4) 157–158.
- *Technologies' Impact on Life Care Planners: A Pilot Study of Children with Cerebral Palsy,* Deutsch, Kendall, Raffa, Daninhirsch, & Cimino-Ferguson, 4(4) 161–172.
- *Empirical Validation of Medical Equipment Replacement Values in LCP*, Marini & Harper, 4(4) 173–182.
- *A Dialogue with Sharon Reavis*, 4(4) 183–184.

- *Life Care Planning Issues for Adult Swallowing Disorders,* Wiles Higdon, 4(4) 185–204.
- *Bilirubin Encephalopathy/Kernicterus & the Newborn Infant: Implications for Life Care Planner,* Deming, 4(4) 205–218.
- *The 2005 International Conference on Life Care Planning a Huge Success,* 4(4) 219–220.
- *Newly Elected Board Members for the IALCP Section of IARP,* 4(4) 221–222.

Journal of Life Care Planning, Vol 4–2&3

- *Editorial: Pockets of Knowledge,* Berens, 4(2–3) 65–66.
- *Field Review: Revised Standards of Practice for Life Care Planners,* McCollom, 4(2–3) 67–74.
- *A Quantitative Reappraisal of a Qualitative Survey to Assess Reliability & Validity of the Life Care Planning Process,* Kendall & Casuto, 4(2–3) 75–84.
- *Appendix A: Survey of Pediatric Life Care Planning Outcomes,* 4(2–3) 85–98.
- *Life Care Planning Issues for Pediatric Swallowing Disorders,* Wiles Higdon, 4(2–3) 99–114.
- *Vehicle Modifications: Useful Considerations for Life Care Planners,* Weed & Engelhart, 4(2–3) 115–126.
- *Americans with Disabilities Act: An Evolving Resource,* Vierling, 4(2–3) 127–138.
- *Accessibility—Are There Laws for Residences?* 4(2–3) 139–142.
- *A Dialogue with Fred Raffa,* 4(2–3) 143–146.
- *Book Review,* Isom, 4(2–3) 149–150.
- *Book Review,* Barros-Bailey, 4(2–3) 151–152.

Journal of Life Care Planning, Vol 4–1

- *Editorial: Season of Change.* Berens, 4(1), 1–2.
- *Perspective Medical Foundation Changing the Structure,* McCollom, 4(1) 3–8.
- *A Dialogue with Patricia McCollom,* 4(1) 9–10.
- *Multiple Relationships in the Field of Life Care Planning,* Cimino-Ferguson, 4(1) 11–16.
- *Lifelong Needs after Acquired Brain Injury: A Case of Study in Enhancing Community Awareness,* Guercio, Sanders, & Dixon, 4(1) 17–26.
- *PEEDS-RAPELL: A Case Conceptualization Model for Evaluating Pediatric Cases,* Neulicht & Berens, 4(1) 27–36.
- *What Life Care Planners Should Know,* Mitchell, 4(1) 37–50.
- *Book Review,* McCollom, 4(1) 51–52.

Journal of Life Care Planning, Vol. 3–4

- *Pain Hurts,* Weed, 3(4), 219–224.
- *Chronic Pain Assessment and Validation,* Lilly, Walker, 3(4), 225–244.
- *Life Care Planning for Pediatric Chronic Pain Patients,* Goldschneider-Ohme, 3(4), 245–258.
- *Spinal Cord Injury Related Pain: Diagnosis, Treatment, and Life Care Considerations,* Livingstone, 3(4), 259–270.
- *Life Care Planning for the Amputee with Chronic Pain,* Meier, 3(4), 271–290.
- *A Dialogue with Horace Sawyer,* Berens, 3(4), 292–296.
- *Book Review,* Deutsch, 3(4), 297–298.

- *Book Review,* Allison, 3(4), 299–300.
- *Thank You and Goodbye,* McCollom, 3(4), 301.
- *A Tribute to Patricia*, McCollom, Field, 3(4), 302.

Journal of Life Care Planning, Vol 3–3

- *Editorial: Life Care Planning: A Little Like Politics,* McCollom, 3(3), 129–130.
- *The Efficacy of Professional Clinical Judgment: Developing Expert Testimony in Cases Involving Vocational Rehabilitation and Care Planning Issues,* Choppa, Johnson, Fountaine, Shafer, Jayne, Grimes, & Field, 3(3), 131–150.
- *What a Forensic Economist Needs from a Life Care Planning Expert,* Ireland & Rizzardi-Pearson, 3(3), 151–162.
- *Aging with Early Onset Conditions: Post-Polio Syndrome, Spinal Bifida, Early Onset Neuromuscular Diseases, Down Syndrome, Brain Injury, and Juvenile Arthritis*, Mitchell, 3(3), 163–176.
- *Chronic Pain Medications: Current Trends for Life Care Planners*, Oakes, 3(3), 177–192.
- *Proceedings of the Life Care Planning Summit 2004 Atlanta, GA April 24–25, 2004,* Deutsch & Allison, 3(3), 193–202.
- *A Dialogue with Tyrone Elliott, Esq.*, Berens, 3(3), 203–206.
- *Book Review*, Winkler, 3(3), 207–210.
- *Book Review*, Casuto, 3(3), 211–212.

Journal of Life Care Planning, Vol 3–2

- *Editorial: Life Care Planning Summit III: Progress in Action,* McCollom 3(2), 65–66.
- *An Overview of the RAPEL Methodology for Life Care Planners in Tort Cases,* Weed, 3(2), 67–84.
- *Outcome Measurement in Life Care Planning: One Company's Approach,* Patterson, Murphy, & Masterson, 3(2), 85–92.
- *Aging with Cerebral Palsy, Spinal Cord Injury and Amputation: Implications for Life Care Planners,* Mitchell, 3(2), 93–104.
- *News Update…Nevada Amicus Brief and Impact on Life Care Planners,* Taylor, 3(2), 105–108.
- *Life Care Planning Summit 2004 the Progress Continues*, Berens, 3(2), 109–112.
- *A Dialogue with Linda Shaw*, Berens, 3(2), 113–118.
- *Certification for the CHCC CLCP Certification?* McKinley, 3(2), 119–122.

Journal of Life Care Planning, Vol 3–1

- *Editorial: A New Year of Growth,* McCollom, 3(1), 1.
- *Life Care Planning for the Client with Severe Spasticity: Intrathecal Baclofen Therapy,* Barker & Saulino, 3(1), 3–14.
- *Clinician's Perspective*, Winkler, 3(1), 15–16.
- *Augmentative and Alternative Communication (AAC) and Life Care Planning,* Hill, 3(1), 17–28.
- *Reliance on Objective Functional Testing to Identify an Individual's Needs for Home Support Services,* Fischer, 3(1), 29–34.

- *Fundamentals of Neuropsychological Evaluation for the Life Care Planner and Case Manager,* Bryant & McLean, 3(1), 35–44.
- *Neuropsychologist Questions,* Weed, Fraser, & Berens, 3(1), 45–46.
- *A Dialogue with Debbie Berens,* Weed, 3(1), 47–50.
- *An Update from the Commission on Health Care Certification,* McKinley, 3(1), 51–54.
- *Book Review,* Petgrave & Fountaine, 3(1), 55–56.

Journal of Life Care Planning, Vol 2–4

- *Editorial: In the Courts…The Beat Goes on!* McCollom, 2(4), 189–190.
- *Pathophysiology of Spasticity and Hypertonicity,* Winkler, 2(4), 191–194.
- *Augmentative and Alternative Communication (AAC),* Hill, 2(4), 195–204.
- *Supreme Court Decision: Cedar Rapids v. Garret, F. Impact on School Nursing and Life Care Planning,* Cosby, 2(4), 205–214.
- *Book Review: The Transitional Classification of Jobs,* Choppa, Jayne, & Petgrave, 2(4), 215–218.
- *A Dialogue with Timothy F. Field,* Berens, 2(4), 225–228.
- *Application of Life Care Planning Principles for Seniors Experiencing Catastrophic Injury,* Stolte-Upman, 2(4), 229–236.

Journal of Life Care Planning, Vol 2–3

- *Editorial: When Acting as an Expert…,* McCollom, 2(3), 141.
- *Tort Reform and Life Care Planning,* Powell, 2(3), 143–155.
- *A Dialogue with Bernie Kleinman,* Berens, 2(3), 157–158.
- *Obtaining Valid Informed Consent,* Hogue, 2(3), 159–162.
- *Strategies for Selecting or Being Selected as the Life Care Planner Expert – The Two-Way Street,* Fick, 2(3), 163–170.
- *Life Care Planning: Rehabilitation Education Curricula and Faculty Needs,* Isom, Marini, & Reid, 2(3), 171–174.
- *Report on the Amicus Curiae Brief,* Deutsch, 2(3), 175–176.

Journal of Life Care Planning, Vol 2–2

- *Editorial: What a Life Care Plan Can Do…,* McCollom, 2(2), 57.
- *Life Care Planning for People with Severe and Persistent Mental Illness: An Overlooked Practice Setting,* Hilligoss, 2(2), 59–72.
- *Life Care Planning Summit 2002,* Riddick-Grisham, 2(2), 73–102.
- *A Dialogue with Susan Riddick-Grisham,* Berens, 2(2), 103–106.
- *Book Review: An Introduction to the U.S. Health Care System,* Carter, 2(2), 107–108.
- *Case Study: Future Care Cost Analysis for a Post-splenectomy Patient,* Albee, 2(2), 119–124.
- *Brain Injury Rehabilitation for the Life Care Planner: A Look through the Family Kaleidoscope,* Jackson, 2(2), 125–134.
- *Caring for People with Disabilities: Prevention of Victimization*, Sandel, Isom, & Koch, 2(2), 109–118.

Journal of Life Care Planning, Vol 2–1

- *Editorial: The Open Road…,* McCollom, 2(1), 1.
- *Quality of Life Care Issues in Life Care Planning,* Brethauer & Brethauer, 2(1), 3–12.
- *A Retrospective Study of Pediatric Life Care Plan Outcomes: One Life Care Planner's Experience,* Casuto & Gumpel, 2(1), 13–24.
- *Workers' Compensation Settlements with Medicare Set-Aside Arrangements: Problem Solving the Issues,* Manley, 2(1), 25–32.
- *Historic Meeting Visioneering Case Management's Future,* Boling & Wolf, 2(1), 33–36.
- *Case Studies: Combining Life Care Planning and Case Management Services: One Practitioner's Thoughts,* Preston, 2(1), 37–42.
- *A Dialogue with Sherri Jasper,* Berens, 2(1), 43–46.
- *We've Come a Long Way – Perspective,* Knouse, 2(1), 47–50.
- *Life Care Planning in Ireland,* Brennan, 2(1), 51–52.

Journal of Life Care Planning, Vol 1–4

- *Editorial: Strategy for Quality,* McCollom, 1(4), 237.
- *An Educational Curriculum for Teaching Life Care Planning,* Isom & Marini, 1(4), 239–264.
- *Financial Diagnostic Tools and Comprehensive Life Care Planning,* Busch, 1(4), 265–274.
- *Setting Standards of Protocol for Replacement Schedules of Medical Equipment in a Life Care Plan,* Amsterdam, 1(4), 275–284.
- *Enhancing Credibility in the Courtroom,* Vierling, 1(4), 285–290.
- *A Dialogue with Terry Winkler,* Berens, 1(4), 291–292.

Journal of Life Care Planning, Vol 1–3

- *Editorial: Research: The Basis for a Life Care Plan*, McCollom, 1(3) 185–186.
- *Reliability of Life Care Plans: A Comparison of Original and Updated Plans*, Sutton, Deutsch, Weed, & Berens. 1(3), 187–194.
- *The Importance of Vocational Rehabilitation in Life Care Planning,* Field, 1(3), 195–202.
- *Case Study: Traumatic Brain Injury and Life Skills Training: A Cost Effective Treatment and Support Option*, McDonnell, 1(3), 203–208.
- *CHCC Grant Research at SIU: Exploring Life Care Planning Service Delivery,* May, 1(3), 209–212.
- *A Dialogue with Roger O. Weed,* Berens, 1(3), 213–214.
- *Hepatitis C: The New Epidemic,* McCollom, 1(3), 215–220.
- *Application of Life Care Planning Principles for the Individual with HCV,* McCollom, 1(3), 221–230.

Journal of Life Care Planning, Vol 1–2

- *Editorial: Standards of Practice: The Meaning, the Value,* McCollom, 1(2), 89–90.
- *Standards of Practice: What They Can and Cannot Do,* Preston, 1(2), 91–96.

- *Life Care Planning Survey 2001: Process, Methods and Protocols,* Neulicht, Riddick-Grisham, Hinton, Costantini, Thomas, & Goodrich, 1(2), 97–148.
- *A Dialogue with Ann Neulicht,* Berens, 1(2), 149–152.
- *Life Care Planning for Successful Outcomes: A Ten-Year Case Study,* Reavis, 1(2), 153–156.
- *Research Methodology for Life Care Planners,* Kendall & Deutsch, 1(2), 157–168.
- *Consistency of Hospital Pricing Data in Life Care Planning,* Rosenblatt, 1(2), 169–172.
- *Life Care Planner: Secretary, Know-It-All, or General Contractor? One Person's Perspective,* Weed, 1(2), 173–178.
- *Summary of the Life Care Planning Summit 2002,* Berens, 1(2), 179–182.
- *Developing the Education to Support the Growing Needs of Life Care Planners,* Jasper, 1(2), 183–184.

Journal of Life Care Planning, Vol 1–1

- *Editorial: A New Beginning,* McCollom, 1(1), 1.
- *Life Care Planning: Yesterday and Today,* McCollom & Weed, 1(1), 3–8.
- *Amicus Curiae Brief,* Countiss, 1(1), 9–34.
- *The Life Care Planner, the Judge and Mr. Daubert,* Countiss & Deutsch, 1(1), 35–44.
- *A Dialogue with Paul Deutsch, Berens,* 1(1), 45–48.
- *Standards of Practice,* Reavis, 1(1), 49–58.
- *Certification in Life Care Planning Is Alive and Well,* May, 1(1), 59–61.
- *Standards and Codes of Ethics,* 1(1), 62–72.
- *Bibliography of Life Care Planning and Related Publications,* Weed, Berens, & Deutsch, 1(1), 73–84.

Author Index

Note: Page numbers followed by "*fn*" indicate footnotes, and italics indicate figures and tables.

A

Adkins, R., 511
Aevarsson, O., 672
Agarwal, M., 66
Akiskal, H. S., 448
Alabed, S., 512
Alanmanou, E., 470, 471
Alexander, M. P., 377
Algood, D., 772
Allbright, A. L., 725
Almli, C. R., 376
Altmaier, E. M., 63
Alvarado, E., 473
Ammer, W., 772
Amsterdam, P., 775–776, 777, 780, 782
Anastasi, A., 46
Anderson, C. J., 514
Apfelbaum, J. L., 470
Archerman, D. L., 450
Arndt, S. V., 90, 377
Arnett, J. A., 381
Arrona, R. L., 631–636
Artiola i Fortuny, L., 87
Arvidson, H., 168
Ashburn, M. A., 470
Askay, S. W., 66
Atchinson, B. J., 106
Atkins, D. J., 347, 411
Azoulay D., 553

B

Babitsky, S., 627
Back, T., 380
Backman, L., 551
Badali, D., 506
Badamgarav, E., 480
Bagby, B. C., 273
Bagwell, D. M., 498, 507, 510, 511, 512, 544
Bair, M., 480
Baker, J. E., 382
Baldwin, N., 381
Ballachandra, B. B., 259
Bangen, K. J., 80
Banja, J., 692, 693
Barnes, M. P., 376
Barnes, T. R., 459
Barr, M. L., 553
Barr, W. B., 81, 87
Barrenas, M., 271
Barret, J. P., 407
Barrett, T., 485
Barros-Bailey, M., 613, *615*, 693, 834, 835
Barth, J. T., 368
Bartles, S. J., 459
Barza, M., 273
Basadonna, D. P., 553
Basford, J. S., 376
Basmajian, J. V., 71
Basu, A., 551
Bauby, J.-D., 159
Bauman, W. A., 517
Bay, C. R., 410
Bear, J., 817
Bear, M., 817
Beard, C. M., 384
Beard, K. V., 837
Beattie, B. L., 384
Beck, A. T., 71
Becker, D. R., 461
Beecher, H., 473
Beery, Q., 271
Belayev, L., 380
Bell, M. D., 460
Ben-Yishay, Y., 83
Benard, V., 450
Bendush, C. L., 273
Benitez, A., 80
Bennett, P., 368, 382
Berens, D. E., 7, 15, 33, 37, 55, 381, 411, 498, 510, 610, 611, 614, 617, *617*, 624, 626, 691*fn*, 695, 697, 703, 703*fn*, 731, 788
Bergeson, J. G., 452

Berglund, P., 445, 448
Bergstrom, E., 518
Berker, E., 374, 376
Bernard, D., 591
Berrol, S., 90
Berthiaume, Y., 559
Bess, F. H., 257, 258, 279
Betz, R. R., 514
Bhatnagar, S., 150, 151
Bienvenu, O. J., 66
Bigler, E. D., 80, 81, 376
Bilder, R. M., 81
Bimbaum, H. G., 461
Bio, D. S., 460
Bishop, D. V. M., 168
Black, H., 691
Black, K. L., 374
Black, M. A., 368, 376
Blacklow, R., 470
Blackstone, S., 174
Blackwell, T. L., 13, 24, 54, 55, 691, 693
Blakeney, P., 66, 403, 592
Blanck, P. D., 713
Blanz, B., 456
Bleiberg, J., 14
Bleuler, E., 455
Block, J., 163
Bloomfield, E. L., 376
Blount, M., 114
Blunt, B. A., 381
Blyler, C. R., 461
Boake, C., 374
Boles, T. L., 836
Bond, G. R., 461
Bonfiglio, R. P., 4, 22
Boninger, M., 772
Bonow, J. T., 71
Bontke, C. F., 374, 376, 377
Booth, N., 447, 452
Boshen, M. J., 454
Botterbusch, K. F., 44
Bowden, C. L., 448
Bowman, D. E., 87
Boyd, D., 221
Braddom, R. L., 21
Branagan, G., 506
Bresler, D., 470
Bresnick, M. G., 66
Brockway, J. A., 368, 377
Brodwin, M., 704
Brookshire, M., 610
Brown, A., 369
Brown, H. R., 370
Brown, M., 408, 788
Bruel, B., *479*
Brummett, R. E., 273
Brusselaers, N., 402
Bryant-Comstock, L., 452
Brych, S., 410, 411
Bryson, G., 460
Buckles, V., 14
Buckley, P. F., 457
Budnick, A. S., 273
Burcusa, S. L., 445
Burke-Miller, J. K., 461
Burton, L. A., 81, 87
Bush, G. H. W., 172, 714, 722
Butcher, J. N., 69
Butnik, S., 49, 51
Butters, Nelson, 81

C

Cade, J. F., 450
Cahill, L. M., 163, 165
Callahan, C. D., 87
Campbell, K. A., 517
Cantekin, E., 271
Caplan, B., 68
Caragonne, P., 834, 839
Cardenas, D. D., 507, 508, 513
Carlisle, J., 613, *615*, 693
Carpenter, D., 453, 454
Carroll, J. A., 450
Carrothers, L., 511
Casey, D. E., 459
Cassano, G. B., 446
Castle, D. J., 457
Celenk, O., 837
Chan G. M., 406
Chandra, V., 384
Chang-Quan, H., 275
Chang, E. W., 162
Charlifue, S., 518
Charlson, F. J., 445
Charney, D. S., 446
Chen, R., 881
Chesnut, R. M., 381
Chiu, W. T., 445
Chlan, K. M., 514
Cho, Y. S., 408
Choinière M., 406
Choi, S. C., 374
Choppa, A. J., 35, 331, 614, 627
Chou, R., 480
Chow, E. K., 542
Christensen, A. -L., 81
Chung, M. C., 65
Chwalisz, K., 382
Cicero, 670
Cifu, D. X., 368, 377, 382, 384
Cimino-Ferguson, S., 695

Ciorba, A., 275
Citrome, L., 459
Ciudad, A., 445
Claes, J., 273
Clifton, G. L., 374
Coconcea, N., 459
Cody, L., 13
Coelho, T., 714
Cohen, R., 592
Cohn, N., 67
Coleman, R. D., 67
Colpaert, K. E., 402
Congdon-Hohman, J., 331, 653
Connis, R. T., 470
Connor, P. D., 448
Conrad, D., 54, 55
Cook, J. A., 461
Cooper-Stephenson, K., 845, 852
Cooper, J. O., 24, 72
Cooper, R., 772
Cope, D. N., 376
Corrigan, J. D., 376, 381, 382
Corthell, D. W., 368
Cosby, M. F., 834, 835
Cosimi A. B., 545
Cosio D., *480*
Costantini, P., 762, 829
Cottone, R. R., 694–695
Countiss, R. N., 17, 34, 705
Crandell, C., 259
Crane, R., 705
Crean, T., 460
Cromes, G. H., Jr., 405, 408, 438
Crosson, J. T., 538
Culver, C. M., 24
Cupples, S., 538, 545
Curtis, K. A., 513
Cusick, C. P., 374, 378

D

Dabic, M., 836
Dahllof, A. G., 368, 378
Dakos, M., 43
Dalal, P. K., 66
Damasio, A. R., 80
Damasio, H., 80
Daniel, D. G., 459
Dannels-McClure A., 378
Darrow, S. M., 71
Daubert, V., 13
Davey, M., 66
Davis, B., 403
Davis, L., 762
Davis, R., 344
De Boeck, K., 559
De Broe, M. E., 273
Decoufle, P., 271
Dedzieky, K. Y., 572–573
Deer, T., *479*
DelGiorno, J., 409
DeLisa, J. A., 22
DeLisis, L. E., 459
Deming, L., 788, 844
Demler, O., 445, 448
Demling, R. H., 403, 404
Deneen, L., 45
Dennehy, E. B., 448
Denys, D., 453
DePompei, R., 382
Deutsch, P. M., 4, 13, 15, 17, 18, 33, 34, 42, 463, 487, 493, 573, 574, 575, 576, 609, 610, 617, 627, 703, 703*fn*, 704, 705, 731, 769, 787, 788, 800, 844
Devany, C. W., 374, 376
de Vera, M. E., 544
Devercelli, G., 452
DeVivo, M. J., 498
De Waele, J. J., 402
Diamond, P. T., 382
Diaz, A., 271
Dietrich, W. D., 380
Difede, J., 410
Dikmen, S. S., 368, 382
Diller, L., 83
Diller, M., 713, 725
Dillman, E., 55, 318, 325, 611, 612, 622
Dimitrova, E., 572, 573
Dirette, D. K., 106
Dobie, R. A., 273
Dobrkovsky, M., 407
Dobscha, S., 480
Dodson-Burk, B., 574
Dolske, M. C., 66
Dondi, A., 850
Dornan, J., 368, 382
Dougherty, A. M., 374
Downey, J. A., 22
Downs, M. P., 261, *269*
Doyle, W. J., 271
Drake, R. E., 459, 461
Dreisbach, L. E., 273
Drotar, D., 90
Drummond, L. M., 454
Drysdale, G. A., 513
Duckworth, B., 788
Duff, K., 66
Dunn, L., 167
DuPont, R. L., 455
Durrani, A., 452
Dussault, K., 739, 740
Dussault, W. L. E., 740

Dvorchik, I., 544
Dyster-Aas, J., 411

E

Eames P., 70
Ebert, E., 505
Edelman L. S., 406
Edwars, L. B., 559
Egri, C. P., 836
Ehde, D. M., 409
Eisenberg, H. M., 372, 374, 381
Elbasiouny, S., 506
Elias, S., 719
Elliott, T., 731, 819
Elovic, E., 369
Engel, G., 470
Engelhart, L., 799*fn*
Englander, J., 376, 377, 382, 384
Engrav, L. E., 410, 411
Ergh, T. C., 67
Esquenazi, A., 346, 347
Esselman, P., 410, 411
Etain, B., 451
Evans, C. T., 511
Evans, R. W., 49, 50, 376

F

Falowski, S., *479*
Fanciulllo, G., 480
Farmer, S., 408
Fauerbach, J. A., 66
Fausti, S. A., 273
Fawber, H., 788
Feder, H., 627
Feinman, R., 820
Feldbaum, C., 614
Felix, E. R., 507, 508, 513
Feng, W., 461
Ferrari, A. J., 445
Ferrucci, L., 274, 275
Fichtenbaum, J., 65
Fick, G., 550
Fick, N., 36
Field, J. E., 46, 611
Field, T. F., 4, 7, 9, 13, 14, 35, 42, 45, 46, 49, 53–55, 59, 331, 408, 444, 471, 576, 609, 610, 611, 612, 614, *615*, 618, 622, 627, 788, 814, 825, 827
Fine, P. R., 480, 507
Finger, S., 376
Fischler, G., 447, 452
Fisher, J. E., 71
Fisher, S. V., 404, 405
Fiske, S. T., 836
Fitzhugh-Bell, K. B., 80
Flanagan, S., 369
Fleischhacker, W., 456, 459
Fleminger, S., 90
Fletcher, C. F., 22
Flood, E., 452
Fogle, P., 268, 280
Follette, W. C., 71
Forbes, R. A., 452
Ford, D. E., 470
Ford, J., 788
Fordyce, W. E., 470
Forget R., 406
Foulkes, M. A., 374
Fountaine, J., 331
Fox, L., 788
Frances, A., 410, 453, 454, 456
Frank, R. A., 68, 273
Frank, T., 273
Fraser, R. T., 368, 382
Freemon, F. R., 80
French-St. George, J., 273
Frey, R. H., 273
Friedmann, L., 355
Fry, R., 382, 383
Fuller, D., 168
Furrer, O., 836

G

Gabel, S., 49, 51
Gabriel, V., 409
Gail, N. A., 344
Gallal, A. R. S., 408
Gamez, J., 829
Ganesh, S. P., 511
Ganio, M. S., 406
Gardner, R., 722
Garrel D. R., 406
Gass, J., 767
Gattaz, W. F., 460
Gavett, B. E., 81
Geckler C., 90
Geddes, J., 451
Gedye, A., 384
Gemar, M., 451
Geoffroy, P. A., 450
Gerber, D. J., 374
Gerhart, K., 518
Ghods, B. K., 470
Ghovanloo, M., 163
Gianforte, G., 817
Gibran, N. S., 410
Gibson, G., 58
Gibson, P., 408
Gillberg, C., 168
Gilman, D., 797
Ginns, L., 545
Ginsberg, M. D., 380

Giora, A., 90
Glasgow, R. E., 473, 475
Gleason, S., 170
Glynn, G., 762
Goebel, J., 273
Gonzalez, J., 772
Gonzalez, T., 767
Goodall, P., 368, 382
Goodglass, H., 81
Goodrich, B., 762, 829
Goodrich, W. R., 835
Goodwin, C., 404
Goodwin, F. K., 448, 450
Goodwin, R. D., 445
Goozee, J. V., 163, 164
Gopinath, B., 275
Govaerts, P. J., 273
Grafman, J., 370
Graham, M., 613, *615*, 693
Grant, B. F., 445
Greenberg, S. A., 85
Green, C. R., 470
Greist, J. H., 450
Grisham, S., 12, 788
Groswasser, Z., 379
Gstaltner, K., 506
Gudjonsson, G., 368, 378
Gulledge-Potts, M., 273
Gunn, R., 819
Gutman, D. A., 451
Gwanmesia, E., 837

H

Hadley, D., 372, 374
Haffey, W. J., 67
Haines, J. M., 66
Halbert J., 139
Hall, K. M., 368, 376
Halstead, W., 81
Hammond, F. M., 374
Hamm, R. J., 380
Hanks, R. A., 67
Harkin, T., 714
Harrell, W. T., 518
Harrison-Felix C., 378
Hartford, C. E., 403, 405, 409
Hartmann, M., 456
Hasin, D. S., 445
Hassenstab, J., 80
Hawkins, J., 271
Haykal, R. F., 448
Hayward A. R., 550
Hazard, G., 850
Hazekamp, J., 578
Healy, J., 804
Heckman, J. T., 340
Heilbronner, R. L., 66
Heilman, K. M., 80
Heimbach, D. M., 410
Helm, P. A., 404, 405, 408, 438, 788
Helm, S., 473
Hendershot, G. E., 574
Heninger, G. R., 446
Henning, J. M., 480
Henry, C., 451
Henry, J. A., 273
Herndon, D., 403
Heron, T. E., 72
Hessellund, T., 45
Hessol, N., 368, 376
Heward, W. L., 72
Heyburn, J. G., 713
Higdon, C., 574, 575, 577
Higgenbotham, J., 174
High, W. M., 368, 377, 384
Hill, E. W., 574
Hilligoss, N., 444
Hinojosa, J., 114
Hinton, L., 762, 829
Hirose, H., 162
Hirschfeld, R. M., 448, 451
Hirschhorn, N., 271
Hitzig, S. L., 517
Holavanahalli, R., 66
Holden-Pitt, L., 271
Hollander, E., 455
Holubkov, A. L., 368, 382
Honigfeld, G., 458
Horn, L. J., 368, 374
Horton, A., 384
Hoste, E. A., 402
Houck, M., 627
Howieson, D. B., 81, 82, 86, 88, 90
Hudson, T. J., 461
Huebner, K. M., 578
Huguet, E., 553
Humes, L. E., 257, 258
Husseini, K. M., 450
Hussey, P., 595

I

Iacono, W. G., 445
Ignacio, R. V., 459
Imagawa, H., 162
Ip, R. Y., 368, 382
Isom, R., 15
Iverson C., 139

J

Jacobs, H. E., 64
Jacobsberg, L., 410

Jamison, K. R., 448, 450
Jane, J. A., 372, 374
Jastreboff, P. J., 289
Jefferson, J. W., 450
Jenkins-Guarnieri, M. A., 70
Jeon, J. H., 408
Jerger, J., 271
Jerger, S., 271
Jette D., 139
Jiam, N., 274
Jing, Y., 452
Johnson, C. B., 4, 6, 13, 35, 55, 331, 614, 627, 696, 732, 827, 829, *830*, 835, 848, 849
Johnson, D., 772
Johnson, K., 70
Johnson, L., 271
Johnson, V. E., 88
Johnsrude, I., 275
Johnstone, B., 87
Jones, F. R., 268
Jorens, P. G., 273
Jorge, R. E., 377
Joshua, 653

K

Kahn, D. A., 453, 454
Kane, J. M., 458
Kapes, J., 46
Kapila, C. J., 87
Kaplan, E., 81
Kaskutas, V., 43
Katz, D. I., 377
Kaufman-Arenberg, I., 271
Kaufman, H. H., 368, 377
Kealy, G. P., 403, 405, 409
Keck, P. E., 459
Kellerman, B., 592
Keller, M. B., 446
Kelley, K. M., 66
Kelly, E. W., 836
Kelting, D. L., 374
Kemmelmeier, M., 836
Kendall, K. A., 162
Kendall, S., 769
Kennedy, P., 65
Kepler, K., 90
Kessler, R. C., 445, 448
Kewman, D. G., 65
Keyser-Marcus, L., 382
Khosh, M. M., 406
Kildal, M., 411
King, J., 598
King, P., 485
Kiritani, S., 162
Kirshbaum, M., 741
Kirshblum, S., 65
Kischer, C. W., 407
Kitchen, J., 4, 13
Klar, L. N., 852
Klauber, M. R., 372, 374, 381
Kleinman, L., 452
Klein, S., 90
Klingbeil, F., 788
Klock-Powell, K., 66
Knapp, M., 447
Knutsen, J. M., 273
Kobler, J. B., 162
Kocina, P., 512
Koehler, R., 83
Koele, S. L., 90
Kokmen, E., 384
Kolber, M., 513
Koltzenburg, M., 469
Kopelman, J., 273
Korsarek, E., 384
Kothari, S., 369
Kraepelin, E., 447, 455
Kramer, M. B., 273
Krause, J. S., 24, 498, 518, 742
Kraus, J. F., 368, 376
Kregel, J., 382, 383
Kreuter, M., 368, 378
Kreutzer, J. S., 90, 368, 374, 376, 377, 379, 382, 383, 384
Kroger, H., 451
Krugman, S., 408
Kübler-Ross, E., 67, 574
Kucheryavaya, A. Y., 559
Kuhn, C., 408
Kuiken, T. A., 352
Kuo, M. H., 836
Kuruvilla, M. S., 163, 164
Kwasnica, D., 369
Kwon, J. H., 455

L

Lacerda, C., 275
Lacerte, M., 848, 849
La Ferriere, K., 271
LaLonde, I. C., 404
Lance, K., 6
Lane, S. J., 72
Langrehr, K., 837
Lanza, R. D., 513
LaPlante, M. P., 574
LaPorte, F., 470
Larson, D. L., 407
Larson, E. B., 384
Larson, P. D., 65
Latham, S. A., 835

Lauermann, M., 273
Laukli, E., 273
Lauterbach, J., 739, 740
Lavela, S. L., 511
Lawrence, B., 772
Lawyer, H. L., 368, 382
Lay, B., 456
Le, A. H., 836
Le, H., 836
Lee, R. C., 66
Lees-Haley, P., 52
Leff, H. S., 461
Lehmkuhl, L. D., 376, 377
Lehrer, D. S., 457
Lenox, R. H., 450
Leonard, J. A., 346, 347, 349
Leskin, G., 14
Levin, H. S., 374
Levinkind, S., 719
Lew, H., 14
Lewis, L., 448
Lewis, P. R., 65
Ley, P., 368, 376
Lezak, M. D., 50, 81, 82, 86, 88, 90
Lezotte, D., 66, 410, 411
Li, G., 352
Li, J., 452, 836
Lieberman, J. A., 456, 459, 461
Liegeois, F., 159, 160, 164
Lien, E. J., 273
Lien, L. L., 273
Lin, F., 274, 275
Linares, H. A., 407
Lindgren, F., 271
Lindgren, S. D., 90
Linhares, M. M., 553
Lipsett, L. R., 273
Littlefield, L. M., 382
Livingston, L., 788
Lloyd, L., 168
Lock, B. A., 352
Loebel, A., 451, 461
Long, C. J., 43, 46, 49, 50
Lopez-Solis, R., 544
Lopez, E., 382
Loring, D. W., 81, 82, 86, 88, 90
Lovestone, S., 90
Lowin, A., 452
Lubinskas, P., 817
Lubkin, I. M., 65
Luria, A. R., 81
Luthe, M. A., 273
Luxton, D. D., 70
Lyass, A., 460
Lynch, J. K., 81
Lysaker, P. H., 460

M

MacBryde, C., 470
Macciocchi, S. N., 368, 382
MacDonald-Wilson, K. L., 460
MacDonald, M., 275
Machamer, J. E., 368, 382
Macritchie, K., 451
Magee, J. C., 553
Magyar-Russell, G., 66
Mair, L. W. S., 273
Malec, J. F., 376
Malone, J. M., 344
Manchikanti, L., 473
Mangraviti, J., 627
Maniha, A., 738
Mann, N. R., 368, 374, 376, 377
Manning, J. S., 448
Marangell, L. B., 448
March, J. S., 453, 454
Marcus, J., 836
Marini, I., 15
Marme, M., 42
Marquet, J., 273
Marshall, L. F., 372, 374, 381
Marshall, S. B., 372, 374
Martin, B., 71
Martin, K. O., 376
Martin, W. E., 691
Martinez-Aran, A., 448
Marwaha, S., 452
Marwitz, J., 90
Marwitz, J. H., 377, 384
Mas, L., 704
Mason, A., 404
Massaro, J. M., 460
Massie, A. B., 542
Masson, M., 450
Mastie, M., 46
Mateer C. A., 83
Matheson, L., 43
Matheson, V., 331
Matkin, R. E., 814, 815, 817
Matthews, D. J., 574
Max, J. E., 90
May, R., 817
May, V. R., 5
Maynard, F., 65
Mazmanian, P. E., 376
McAllister, T. W., 64
McCaffrey, R. J., 66, 81
McCaigue, I. S., 800
McCollom, P., 6, 16, 595, 597, 705, 788
McCombs, J. S., 452
McCracken, L. M., 71
McCrone, P., 447

McCroskey, B., 49, 58
McDonald, C. M., 514
McDonald, W. J., 273
McElroy, S. L., 459
McEvoy, J. P., 456, 461
McFarland, W. H., 268
McGwin, G., 572, 573
McKibben, J., 66
McLaughlin, K., 550
McMahon, B. T., 72, 383
McMahon, S., 469
McNaught T., 406
Meier, R., 788
Meier, R. H., 338, 340, 343, 346, 347, 349
Meltzer, H., 458
Melzack, R., 470
Mendelson, S., 578
Menter, R., 518
Merskey, H., 470
Meyer, G. J., 66
Meyer, K., 461
Miceli E., 139
Michaels, L., 129, 131, 132
Miller, B. J., 457
Miller, R., 271
Millis, S. R., 374
Milstein, R. M., 460
Milton, J., 544
Miranda-Diaz, G., 837
Miskevics, S., 511
Mitchell, N., 125, 126, 129, 835
Miyahara, S., 448
Monasterio, E., 788
Monstrey, S., 402
Montori, V. M., 551
Moore, W. S., 344
Morales, J. M., 551
Moreo, K., 471
Morey C., 378
Morgan, A., 159, 160, 164
Morgan, D., 408
Morgan, R. C., 673
Morris, P., 545
Morris S. E., 406
Morton, M. V., 368, 382
Moss, A. J., 574
Mueller, T. I., 445
Mueser, K. T., 461
Muir, C. A., 67
Mullaney, H. A., 87
Murdoch, B. E., 163, 164, 165
Murray, A., 514
Musngi, G., 410
Myers, J., 512
Mysiw, W. J., 376

N

Naoumova, I., 836
Needham, H. C., 671
Negrel, A., 572–573
Nelson, K. A., 572, 573
Nemeroff, C., 451
Nepomuceno, C., 507
Neufeld, J., 788
Neulicht, A. T., 55, 611, 613, 614, *615*, *617*, 693, 762, 829, 835
Nguyen, H. D., 836
Nguyen, S., 382, 383
Niemczura, J. G., 381
Norman, R. E., 445
North, M. S., 836
Northern, J. L., *261*, *269*
Novotney, A., 70

O

Oakes, M., 55
Occomore, L., 159, 160, 164
O'Day, K., 461
O'Donohue, W. T., 71
Ohler, L., 538, 545
Ojo, A., 553
O'Leary, J., 760
Oliver, D., 90
Olson, D. J., 273
Ong, L. A., 837
Oster, G., 49, 51
Ott, S., 408
Owen, R. R., 461
Owens, Jr., R. E., 168
Owens, T., 22, 26
Owsley, C., 572, 573

P

Pagnin, D., 446
Pait, T. G., 368, 377
Pan, Y., 447
Panek, W., 578
Papakostas, G. I., 446
Papandreou, K., 65
Papport, L. J., 67
Pararajasegaram, R., 572–573
Parente, R., 368, 382
Partridge, J., 410
Pasic, T. R., 273
Pataky, S. K., 697
Paton, C., 459
Patterson, D. R., 65, 66, 409, 410
Patterson, J. B., 622

Paul, G. L., 69
Pearson, W., 823
Peck, M., 408
Peers, C. J., 259
Penn, I., 551
Pepe, D., 271
Perez, V., 445
Perry, S., 410
Phillips, K., 834, 836, 840
Pickering, G., 576
Piek, J., 368, 374, 377
Pierce, S., 800
Pies, R. W., 454
Pikalov, A., 451, 461
Pike, B. R., 380
Pillay, A., 454
Pini, S., 446
Pliskin, N. H., 66
Pollard, C., 65
Pomeranz, J., 14
Pomeranz, J. L., 834
Pope, J., *479*
Pope, K. S., 69
Powell, S. H., 273
Powers, A. S., 69
Powers, L. E., 72
Preston, K., 36, 829, 835
Preveza, E., 65
Prevezas, N., 65
Price, L. H., 446
Pridgen, A., 370
Prohaska, T. R., 511
Pruitt, B., 404
Pruitt, L. D., 70
Ptacek, J., 410, 411
Ptacek, J. T., 410
Purdum, C., 381
Purisch, A. D., 81, 84
Putre, L., 541

Q

Queen, H., 14
Querioz, V., 446
Qu H. D., 405, 406

R

Rabe-Hesketh, S., 90
Rabin, L. A., 81, 87
Rackham, H., 670
Raffa, F., 4, 5, 42, 627, 787, 844
Raffles-Gunn, T., 731
Ragnarsson, K. T., 376, 377
Rainey, S. L., 409
Rajagopalan, K., 461
Ralston, D. A., 836
Ramamurthy, S., 471, 473
Ramsey, R., 470
Rao, P. S., 553
Rappaport, M., 374
Rasmussen, L., 65
Raviv, G., 514
Reagles, K., 507, 510, 511, 512
Reeves, D., 14
Reid-Arndt, S. A., 68
Reid, C., 15, 834
Reid, D. B., 368
Reiger, D. A., 445, 448, 456
Renschler, A., 772
Ricci, P. E., 374
Rice, D. P., 455
Richards, J. S., 65, 507
Richardson, E., 65
Richardson, K., 480
Riddick-Grisham, S., 33, 37, 762, 781, 829, 835, 844
Riddick, S., 4, 5, 7, 43, 609
Rimmer, R. B., 410
Ripley, D., 25, 64, 788
Ripley D. L., 378
Rivara, F., 410, 411
Roberts, M. A., 90
Robin, D. A., 90
Robins, L. N., 445, 448, 456
Robinson, R. G., 377
Roeser, R., 259
Rogers, E. S., 460
Rogers, J., 471
Rogers, L., 43
Rokaw, W., 368, 376
Romano, J. L., 24
Romera, I., 445
Rosenthal, M., 25, 90, 368, 376, 377, 381, 384, 384
Roter, D. L., 470
Rowland, C. R., 455
Rubinger, H., 722
Rubin, R., 550
Rudd, M., 84
Ruff, R. M., 376
Rumalla, K., 275
Rush, A. J., 448
Rusin, M. J., 68
Russell-Jones, D. L., 376
Russell, E. W., 81
Rybak, L. P., 273

S

Sabatino, C., 673
Saffle, J., 403

Saha, R., 66
Saito, H., 275
Sajatovic, M., 459
Salazar, A. M., 370
Sanchez-Moreno, J., 448
Sander, A. M., 379
Santosa, C., 451
Sardegna, J., 571
Sarkarati, M., 760
Sato, Y., 90
Saul, R. E., 81, 84
Saunders, L. L., 498
Savage, R., 788
Sawyer, H. W., 4, 463, 487, 493, 573, 574, 575, 576, 609, 610, 693, 787, 788
Sbordone, R. J., 81, 84, 88, 89
Schaffer, H. I., 273
Schanberg, S., 408
Schatz, A., 801
Scheifler, P. L., 456
Schellenberg, G. D., 384
Schentag, C., 368, 382
Schentag, J. J., 273
Schmidt, M. H., 456
Schmidt, N. D., 376
Schmidt, R., 55, 614, 627
Schneider J. C., 405, 406
Schoenberg, B. S., 384
Schumacher, M., 451
Schwab, K., 370
Sears, H. H., 346
Seelen, J., 69
Seel, R. T., 379
Segal, S. V., 451
Semlyen, J. K., 376
Sendroy-Terrill M., 378
Seok-Hyun, Y., 162
Serghiou, M. A., 408
Sessions, R. B., 273
Shahnasarian, M., 612
Shah P., 139
Sharpe, M., 473, 475
Shaw, L., 383, 693
Shealy, C., 470
Shelton, R. C., 446
Sheridan, R. L., 402, 788
Sherman, C. J., 344
Sherman, R. A., 344
Sherron, P., 382, 383
Shi, L., 461
Shilo, A. M., 836
Shiraki, S., 455
Shorvon, S. D., 376
Shoulson, I., 83
Shuman, D. W., 85
Siefker, J. M., 44, 46, 48, 49, 54
Siegfreid, S. L., 456, 459
Simmons, F. B., 268
Sinaki, M., 22
Singer, J., 458
Singh, S., 452
Singh, V., 473
Siosteen, A., 368, 378
Skinner, B. F., 470
Skord, K., 42
Slomine, B. S., 68
Sluis, A., 4, 13, 354
Sluis Powers, A., 13
Smith-Knapp, K., 381
Smith, B. M., 512
Smith, D. H., 88
Smith, J., 446
Smith, J. S., 409
Smith, K. R., 409
Smith, M. T., 66
Smith, S., 610
Smith, W. L., Jr., 90
Solberg, M. M., 83
Sommer, A., 572, 573
Sowers, J. A., 72
Spence, R. J., 66
Spivey, G. H., 271
St-Pierre D. M., 406
Stagliano, N., 380
Stahl, S., 446
Stancin, T., 90
Stapleton, M., 368, 382
Starkstein, S. E., 377
Steadman, K., 447
Stedman, T. L., 136
Stein, D. J., 455
Stender, M., 452
Stephenson, A. L., 559
Sternbach, R. A., 470
Stern, M. J., 379
Stevens, T., 72
Stewart, T., 762
Stewart, W., 88
Stiens, S., 24
Stimmel, G. L., 452
Stinson, F. S., 445
Stroup, T. S., 461
Studenski, S., 275
Sullivan, C., 368, 376
Sullivan, G., 461
Sullivan, M., 368, 378
Suman, O. E., 408
Summers, S. J., 376
Suppes, T., 451
Sutton, A., 15, 617, 703, 703*fn*, 730
Sutton, A. M., 33, 37
Sutton, E., 670
Swaroop, S., *480*
Swartz, J. L., 691

Sykes, J., 559
Szlachcic, Y., 511

T

Taberes-Seisdedos, R., 448
Takacs, T., 672, 673, 674
Taskila, T., 447
Tate, D. G., 65
Taylor, C., 55
Taylor, H. G., 90
Taylor, L., 788
Taylor, R., 613, *615*, 693, 788
Teasdale, E., 372, 374
Teasdale, G., 372, 374
Temkin, N. R., 368, 382
Teplin, S. W., 573, 574
Thase, M. E., 446
Theodoros, D. G., 163, 165
Thomas, R., 13, 762, 829
Thomas, R. L., 69
Thombs, B. D., 66
Thompson, J. D., 384
Thompson, W. L., 273
Thrush, C. R., 461
Thylefors, V., 572–573
Tielsch, J. M., 572, 573
Timberlake, G., 368, 377
Todd, C., 627
Tollefson, G. D., 446
Tonack, M., 517
Tonge, B. J., 168
Torres, M. M., 346
Trivedi, M. H., 446
Trudel, T., 381
Truthan, J., 49, 58
Tsuang, M., 456
Tuchel, T., 408
Tuckwell, N., 485
Tuokko, H., 384
Turk, D. C., 71

U

Uomoto, J. M., 68, 88, 368, 376

V

Vaiva, G., 450
Valenstein, E., 80
Valente, M. L., 273
Vallarino, M., 451
Van Bereijk, W., *269*
Van Berkum, C. M., 372, 374
Van de Bittner, E., 55, 614, 627
Van De Heyning, P. H., 273
Van de Vijver, F., 837
Vandewoude, K. H., 402
Van Loey, N. E., 65
Van Naarden, K., 271
Van Nostrand, J., 592
Van Sickle, D., 772
Van Son, M. J., 65
Vargas, J. H., 836
Vasudev, K., 451
Velosa, J. A., 551
Venkatagiri, H., 171
Ventry, I., 275
Vernon, S., 24
Vierling, L., 712, 714–716, 718–720
Viljanen, A., 274
Vitek, M., 772
Vitolo, R. S., 513
Voelker, J., 368, 377
Vogel, L. C., 514
Von Korff, M., 473, 475
Vornik, L. A., 448
Vowles, K. E., 71

W

Wade, S. L., 90
Wallace, A., 613, *615*, 693
Wall, J. R., 381
Walters, E. E., 445
Walters, M., 637–639
Wangenhelm, F., 836
Wang, P. W., 451
Ward, T., *469fn*
Warden, D., 370
Warden, G. D., 408, 411
Warner, P. M., 408, 411
Waters, R., 511
Waters, R. L., 517
Watson, S., 451
Wayne, R., 275
Weaver, F. M., 511
Weber, M., 836
Weed, R. O., 4, 7, 9, 11, 12, 13, 14, 15, 16, 22, 25, 26, 29, 30, 33, 37, 38, 42, 43, 45, 46, 49, 50, 51, 52, 53–55, *57*, 58, 59, 64, 354, 382, 383, 408, 411, 444, *469fn*, 470, 471, 498, 510, 576, 609, 610, 611, 612, 614, *615*, 617, 618, 622, 624, 626, 627, *691fn*, 695–696, 697, 703, *703fn*, 704, 731, 768, 781, 788, *799fn*, 827, *830*, 844, 846
Wehman, P., 368, 382, 383
Weichman, S. A., 409, 410
Weinberg, A., 550
Weingarten, S. R., 480
Weinstein, B., 275
Weintraub, A. H., 374
Westenberg, H. G., 453
West, R., 513

Wheeler, J. R., 470
Wheeler, S. D., 72
Whiteneck, G., 518
Whiteneck, G. G., 374
Wickliffe, C. E., 542
Wiechman, S. A., 65, 66
Wilhelm, E., 83
Wilkerson, J. M., 30
Willebrand, M., 411
Williams, A., 174
Williams, J., 382
Williams, N. R., 66
Williams, P., 403
Williams, R., 514
Wilson, L. G., 409
Winkler, T., 24, 498, 507, 510, 511, 512, 517, 571*fn*, 742, 788
Winn, H. R., 368, 382
Witt, K., 572, 573
Wolf, E., 772
Wolpe, J., 71
Wong, G. Y., 273
Wood, D. L., 374
Wood, R. L., 70, 368
Wood, W., 368, 382
Woodrich, F., 622
Wu, D., 550
Wu, E. Q., 461
Wyatt, R. J., 448, 455

Y

Yantz, C. L., 81
Yeates, K. O., 90
Yoon, E., 837
Young, A., 451
Young, M. E., 14
Younger, V., 571
Yousef, S. M., 408
Yu, N. S., 834
Yusen, R. D., 559

Z

Zafonte, R. D., 368, 374
Zaretsky, A. E., 451
Zasler, N. D., 368, 374, 376, 377, 382
Zeitels, S. M., 162
Zhang, L., 550
Zhao, W., 380
Zohar, J., 453
Zydowicz-Vierling, D., 596, 597

Subject Index

Note: Page numbers followed by "*fn*" indicate footnotes, and italics indicate figures and tables.

A

AAC, *see* Augmentative and alternative communication
AALNC, *see* American Association of Legal Nurse Consultants
AANLCP, *see* American Association of Nurse Life Care Planners
AAPdN, *see* American Academy of Pediatric Neuropsychology
AAPLCP, *see* American Academy of Physician Life Care Planners
ABA, *see* American Bar Association; American Burn Association
Abeo Coder, 749
Aberdeen v. Zanatta (2007), 853
ABI, *see* Acquired brain injury
AbilityHub.com, *224*
ABLEDATA, *224*
ABMCN, *see* American Board of Managed Care Nursing
ABOHN, *see* American Board for Occupational Health Nurses
Above-knee prosthesis, 358
ABR, *see* Auditory brain stem response
ABVE, *see* American Board of Vocational Experts
ACA, *see* Affordable Care Act
Acceptance, 67
Access, *197*
Access Board, *224*
Accessible Home Improvement of America (AHIA), 789
Access to labor market (employability), 54
Accommodations, reasonable
- under ADA, 718, 723
- for bipolar disorder, 452
- court decisions and, 723–724
- for major depressive disorder, 447
- for obsessive-compulsive disorder, 455
- required by Rehabilitation Act, 169
- for schizophrenia, 460
- undue hardship and, 723

Accountable health plans (AHPs), *197*
Accreditation, 15, 817; *see also* Certification/credentials
Acculturation, 836–837
ACLS-5, *see* Allen Cognitive Level Screen
ACOEM, *see* American College of Occupational and Environmental Medicine
ACOT, *see* Advisory Committee on Organ Transplantation
Acoustic immittance, 262–263
Acoustic impedance, *see* Acoustic immittance
Acoustic reflex measurements, 293
Acquired apraxia of speech, biofeedback for, 163–165
Acquired brain injury (ABI), 25, 85, 367–395
- age, 368, 369, 383–384
- anatomy of brain, 370–372, *373*
- case studies, 190, 384–395
- in children, 90–91
- classification, 372–374, *375*
- community reintegration, 381–382
- costs, 369–370
- definitions, 368–369
- epidemiology, 369
- etiology, 370
- Glasgow Coma Scale method, 374, *375*
- initial treatment, 374–376
- long-term impairments, 380–381
- medical complications, 376–379
- psychological issues, 67
- Rancho Los Amigos Scale of Cognitive Functioning, 379, *380*
- recovery from TBI, 379–380, *380*
- reevaluation, periodic, 90
- rehabilitation care, 376
- resources/websites, 738
- second impact syndrome, 382
- spasticity, 378, 380
- speech-language pathologist, 190–194
- vocational rehabilitation, 382–384
- *vs.* traumatic brain injury, 368

ACRM, *see* American Congress of Rehabilitation Medicine
Acronyms in communication, *232–234*

Activities of Daily Living (ADLs), 11, 21, 46, 108–114, 121
- under ADA, 721
- aides for, 121, 171
- checklist, 109–114
- effects of brain trauma, 50
- elderly and, 595
- electronic aids for daily living, 797
- features, 767
- Instrumental (IADL), 114–119
- occupational therapist evaluation, 108–114
- and rehabilitation, 26
- training, 382
- traumatic brain injury and, 64

Actual acquisition cost, *197*
Actual charge, *197*
Actual *vs.* average cost, 330
Acute care, *197*
Acute pain, 471
Acute pain syndrome, 472
Acute postoperative phase, 339
Acute tubular necrosis, 545
Acyclovir, 551
AD, *see* Alzheimer's disease
ADA, *see* Adaptive Driving Alliance; Americans with Disabilities Act
ADAAA, *see* Americans with Disabilities Act Amendments Act
ADA Accessibility Guidelines (ADAAG), 715–716
Adams v. Laboratory Corporation of America, 829
Adaptive Driving Alliance (ADA), 810
Adaptive sports excursion, 436
Adaptive work behaviors, 43
ADED, *see* Association for Driver Rehabilitation Specialists
Adjunctive medications, 446, 451, 454, 459
ADLs, *see* Activities of Daily Living
Administrative costs, *197*
Admissibility
- considerations, 819–829
- rules in United States and Canada, 849–850

Adolescents, SLP assessment, 167–168
Adult daycare, 599
Adult neuropsychological evaluations, 52
Advisory Committee on Organ Transplantation (ACOT), 536
AEPs, *see* Auditory Evoked Potentials
AER, *see* Auditory evoked response
Affordable Care Act (ACA), 331–332, 612, 613, 652–653, 741
Aged case, *197*
Agency-sponsored or consumer-operated businesses model, 460–461
Agency for Health Care Policy and Research (AHCPR), *197*
Aggressive treatment (future medical care), 359
Aging, 381, 591, 592; *see also* Elder care management; Elder law attorney
- with amputation, 351–352
- Certified Aging in Place Specialist, 789
- with disability, 124–126
- process, 434–435
- with spinal cord injury, 517–518

AHCPR, *see* Agency for Health Care Policy and Research
AHIA, *see* Accessible Home Improvement of America
AHPs, *see* Accountable health plans
Air conduction, 293
AIS, *see* ASIA Impairment Scale
Akathisia, 459
Albertsons, Inc., v. Kirkingburg (1999), 718
ALDs, *see* Assistive listening devices
Alerting devices, 280
All-payer system, *198*
Allen Cognitive Level Screen (ACLS-5), 108
Alliance for Technology Access, *224*
Allied health, 733
- professionals, *197*

Allodynia phenomenon, 508
All Patient Refined Diagnosis Related Group (APR-DRG), 749
Alpha testing, 177
ALR, *see* Auditory late (long latency) response
ALS, *see* Amyotrophic Lateral Sclerosis
Alzheimer's disease (AD), 384
AMA, *see* American Medical Association
AMA CPT, *see* American Medical Association Current Procedural Terminology
Ambulatory care, *198*
Ambulatory surgery, *198*
American Academy of Nurse Life Care Planners, 6
American Academy of Pediatric Neuropsychology (AAPdN), 84
American Academy of Physician Life Care Planners (AAPLCP), 6
American Association of Legal Nurse Consultants (AALNC), 37, 835
American Association of Nurse Life Care Planners (AANLCP), 6, 37, 743, 835
American Bar Association (ABA), 82
American Board for Occupational Health Nurses (ABOHN), 37
American Board of Clinical Neuropsychology, 84
American Board of Managed Care Nursing (ABMCN), 37
American Board of Vocational Experts (ABVE), *10*, 42
American Burn Association (ABA), 403, 404
American College of Occupational and Environmental Medicine (ACOEM), 447
American Congress of Rehabilitation Medicine (ACRM), 368
American Hospital Directory, 747
American Journal of Audiology, 287

American Medical Association (AMA), 731
American Medical Association Current Procedural Terminology (AMA CPT), 307
  Code Manual, 178
American National Standards Institute (ANSI), 803
American Occupational Therapy Association (AOTA), 106, 123
American Psychiatric Association, 446, 457
American Psychological Association (APA), 63, 82, 190
American Society of Anesthesiologists (ASA), 472
American Speech-Language-Hearing Association (ASHA), 153, 156, 257, 289–291
  SIGs, *154*
American Spinal Injury Association (ASIA), 501, 502
Americans with Disabilities Act (ADA), 59, 172, 712–727, 742
  ADA Amendments Act of 2008, 716–718
  ADA Restoration Act, 716
  case law development, 719
  from case law to practice, 720
  comparison of 1990 ADA and ADA Amendments Act, 724–725
  court decisions and impact on rehabilitation and life care planning practice, 723–724
  creation of nationwide enforcement campaign, 722–723
  of disability and five titles, 715
  life activities and burden of proof, 718–719
  mitigating role and corrective measures in determining disability, 720
  NCD and, 714–715
  outcome of ADA Title I cases, 724
  perspective to practice of case management and life care planning, 713–714
  precedent *vs.* persuasive authority, 719
  single job *vs.* class of jobs, 720
  Supreme Court decisions, 719–720, 721–722, 725–727
  Toyota v. Williams Supreme Court decision, 720–721
  websites, 727
Americans with Disabilities Act Amendments Act (ADAAA), 597, 712
  creation of nationwide enforcement campaign under, 722–723
Amitriptyline, 483
AMLR, *see* Auditory middle latency response
Amputation, 26
Amputees, 335–364; *see also* Prosthetic devices
  aggressive treatment, 359
  aging with amputation, 351–352
  aids for independent function, 357
  amputation surgery and reconstruction phase, 338–339
  architectural renovations, 359
  case example, 355
  diagnostic testing, 357
  drug/supply needs, 358
  future medical care, 358
  health and strength maintenance, 359
  home/facility care, 358
  home furnishings and accessories, 358
  LCP for, 356
  life care planning with physiatrist, 352–355
  limb amputation demographics, 343–344
  limb amputation levels, 344–345, *345*
  maximum medial improvement (MMI), 343
  newer surgeries for limb amputee, 352
  orthopedic equipment needs, 359–364
  orthotics/prosthetics, 358
  phantom and residual limb pain, 344
  phases of amputation rehabilitation, 337–343
  potential complications, 359
  projected evaluations, 357
  projected rehabilitation program, 356–357
  projected therapeutic modalities, 357
  prosthetic costs, 350
  prosthetic fabrication, 340
  prosthetic prescription, 345–351
  prosthetic replacement, 351
  prosthetic training, 340–341, *342*, *343*
  transportation, 353, 358
  vocational/educational plan, 359
  vocational rehabilitation, 342
  wheelchair accessories and maintenance, 357
  wheelchair needs, 357
Amyotrophic Lateral Sclerosis (ALS), 739
Analgesic Ladder, 476, *478*
Analog hearing aids, conventional, 282
Analog programmable hearing aids, 282–283
Anasognosia, *379*
Anatomy of brain, 370–372, *373*
Ancar & Ancar v. Brown & TNE Trucking, 826
Andrews v. Grand & Toy Alberta Ltd (1978), 852
Anesthesia, 745, 747
Anger, 67
Ankles and feet, 433
Anosognosia, 82
ANSI, *see* American National Standards Institute
Anticholinergics, 459–460
Anticonvulsants
  for bipolar disorder, 450, 451
  for schizophrenia, 459
Antidepressants, 459
  for bipolar disorder, 451
  for MDD, 446
  for OCD, 454
  for pain relief, 483
  for schizophrenia, 459–460
Antipsychotics
  for bipolar disorder, 451
  for MDD, 447
  for OCD, 454
  for schizophrenia, 458–459

Anxiety, 25, 30, 64, 65, 66, 87, *379*, 408–410
AOTA, *see* American Occupational Therapy Association
APA, *see* American Psychological Association
APDs, *see* Auditory processing disorders
Apple's Disability Solutions, *224*
APR-DRG, *see* All Patient Refined Diagnosis Related Group
Apticom, 48
Arachnoid mater, 370
Architectural renovations, 359
Area Cost Analysis, 732–735
Area cost analysis request form, 750–755
Arm amputee, 346
Armed Services Vocational Aptitude Battery (ASVAB), 48
ARN, *see* Association of Rehabilitation Nurses
Arnold v. Teno (1978), 860
Arrhythmias, 24
Arthritis, 447
ASA, *see* American Society of Anesthesiologists
ASD, *see* Autism/autism spectrum disorder
ASHA, *see* American Speech-Language-Hearing Association
ASHA CCC-SLP, 153
ASIA, *see* American Spinal Injury Association
ASIA Impairment Scale (AIS), 502
Asperger's syndrome, 168
Assertiveness training counseling, 300
Assessment; *see also specific conditions or tests*
  audiology, 292–293
  auditory processing disorders, 286–288
  balance (vestibular) system, 272–273
  chronic pain, 471–474
  elder care, 596–597, *597–598*
  home, 787–797
  pediatric and adolescent, 167–168
  return-to-work, 49–51
  speech-language pathology, 167
  vocational, 44–49
Assistive listening devices (ALDs), 278–281
  alerting devices, 280
  frequency-modulated systems, 278–280
  hearing aids, 278–280
  induction loop systems, 280
  infrared systems, 280
  one-to-one communicators, 280
  personal sound amplification products, 280
  resources/distributors, 305–307
Assistive technology (AT), 158, 170, 777; *see also* Augmentative and alternative communication (AAC); Medical equipment
  assessment by SLP, 160–161
  Center for Assistive Technology and Environmental Access, 797
  certifications, 776
  examples, 171
  federal mandates and policies, 168–171
  funding, *195*
  funding request (outline), 248–251
  for home, 797
  listening devices, 278–281
  manufacturers' roles, 177
  online resources and websites, 219–223
  periodicals/newsletters, 228
  Quick Reference Series, *224*
  resource directory, *239–248*
  services, 170
  speech-to-speech (STS) relay system, 175–177
  state programs, *235–238*
  vendor list, *204–205*
  for visually impaired, 575–577
Assistive Technology Funding and Systems Change Project (ATFSCP), *224*
Assistive technology practitioner (ATP), 776
Assistive technology supplier (ATS), 760, 776
Association for Driver Rehabilitation Specialists (ADED), 801, 809–810
Association of Rehabilitation Nurses (ARN), 31, 37
ASVAB, *see* Armed Services Vocational Aptitude Battery
AT, *see* Assistive technology
Ataxia, 372
ATFSCP, *see* Assistive Technology Funding and Systems Change Project
ATP, *see* Assistive technology practitioner
ATS, *see* Assistive technology supplier
Attorneys, 850; *see also* Forensic issues; Litigation
  defense, 655–668
  distribution of life care plan, 13
  elder law, 669–679
  life care planner's relationship with, 693–694
  plaintiff's, 641–653
Audiogram, 260–261
Audiologists, 256–313, 434; *see also* Hearing aids; Hearing loss
  acoustic immittance (tympanograms), 262–263
  assessment, audiological (aural) rehabilitation, 275–276
  assessment, pediatric, 264–267
  assistive listening devices, 278–281
  audiogram, 260–261, *261*
  audiological (aural) rehabilitation management, 276–277
  audiological (re)habilitation for children, 277–278
  audiological evaluation, 258–263
  auditory evoked response, 264–265
  auditory processing disorders, 286–288
  balance (vestibular) system assessment, 272–273
  case study, 301–303
  children behaviors at risk for auditory disorders, 297
  clinical process, 285–286
  cochlear implants, 284–285, *285*
  counseling, 299–300
  credentials, 291–293, *291*
  decibel ratings, 269

ear canal and cerumen, 259
funding issues, 299
hearing aids, 278–280
High Risk Registry, 265–266
implantable hearing devices, 284–286
licensure/certifications, 153, *153*, 291, 292, *292*, *304–305*
multicultural considerations, 270–273
neurophysiologic intraoperative monitoring, 271–272
nonbehavioral hearing assessment techniques, 264
otoacoustic emissions, 264
ototoxic drug therapy, 273–274
outcomes of services, 293–294
pressure-equalizing (PE) tubes, 269–270
pure tone audiometry, 259–261
referrals to, 292
resources, *305–307*
scope of practice, 289–291
specialties, 257–*258*
speech audiometry, 261–262
state requirements for audiologists, 304
superbill, *307–313*
test battery, 293
tinnitus management, 288–289
Audiology, 256, 257
Audiometry, conventional, 293
Auditory Evoked Potentials (AEPs), 293
Auditory brain stem response (ABR), 151, 265, 287
Auditory evoked response (AER), 264–265
Auditory late (long latency) response (ALR), 265
Auditory middle latency response (AMLR), 265
Auditory processing disorders (APDs), 293
assessment, 286–288
management, 288
Augmentative and alternative communication (AAC), 156, 158, 168, 171
CPT Codes, *179–181*
federal mandates and policies, 168–171
funding for, *195*
organizations, *251–252*
physical and communication impairments, *160*
speech-to-speech (STS) relay system, 175–177
websites, *205–213*
Autism/autism spectrum disorder (ASD), 168
Automobiles, *see* Vehicle modifications
Autonomic dysfunction, 504–505
Autonomic dysreflexia, 24, 504, 519
Autonomy, 693
Axial back pain, 474
Azathioprine, 534, 546
AZtech, Inc., *224*

B

Baccalaureate nursing curriculum, 17
Baclofen, 483, 506
Bacterial infections, 550
Bactrim, 551
Balance (vestibular) system assessment, 272–273
Bargaining, 67
Barnett decision, 723
Barona equation, 87
Baroreflex receptor function, 504
Barrier-free health care, ADAAA for, 722–723
Barrier Free Health Care Initiative (2012), 597
Barristers and solicitors, 850
Barthel Inventory of Self-Care Skills, 48
Basic Occupational Literacy Test (BOLT), 48
Bathroom, 788, *789*, 794–796
Shower Trolley, *789*, 789
Bayley Scales of Infant and Toddler Development, 108
Bayley Scales of Infant Development, 52
Beavers v. Victorian, 826
Bedroom, 793–794
Behavioral/behaviors, 49, 86
bio-social models, 69
contracting techniques, 72
observation, 48
psychologists, 63
testing, 264
Behavioral Observation Audiometry (BOA), 264, 292
Behind-the-ear (BTE), 282
Below-knee, 349
Beneficence (of care), 693
Benzodiazepines, 451, 459, 506
Beta testing, 177
Bias, financial, 661–662
BICROS, 282
Billing resources, 745
Bimodal distribution, 369
Bio-social models of behavior, 69
Biofeedback, 71, 163–165
Biopsies, 551
Biopsychosocial approach model, 470
Biphasic positive airway pressure (BiPAP), 483, 507
Bipolar disorder, 444, 445, 447–452; *see also* Mental disorders
costs, 452
depressive episode, 449
epidemiology and course of illness, 448
hypomania, 449
mixed episode, 449–450
pharmacotherapy, 450–451
psychotherapeutic interventions, 451–452
symptoms, 448
treatment, 450
vocational impact, 452
Black's Law Dictionary (Black), 610, 691
Blindness, *see* Visually impaired
Blood urea nitrogen (BUN), 24
BOA, *see* Behavioral Observation Audiometry
Board certification, 85
Boarelli v. Flannigan (1973), 861
BOLT, *see* Basic Occupational Literacy Test

Bone
  allograft, 352
  anchored hearing devices, 286
  conduction, 293
  homeostasis, 510
Boston Approach, 81
Botulinum toxin injections, 381
Bragdon v. Abbott (1998), 718
Braille note takers, 576
Brain
  anatomy, 370–372
  cerebellum, 372
  cerebral cortex, 370–372, *371*
  coverings, 370
  electrical activity mapping, 150
  imaging, 150
  midbrain, 372, *373*
  reading techniques, 161
  waves, 150
Brain-monitoring technology, 150
Brain injury, *see* Acquired brain injury (ABI)
Brain stem, 372
Brain stem auditory evoked response, 151
Brain stem implants, 286
Braun Corporation, 516
Breaking New Ground Resource Center, *224*
Brennan v. Singh (1999), 852
Brito v. Wooley (2001), 853
Broca's aphasia, 80
Broca's area, 80
Brown-Sequard syndrome, 503–504
Brown v. USA Truck, Inc. and Watkins, 828
BTE, *see* Behind-the-ear
BUN, *see* Blood urea nitrogen
Bupropion, 446
Burden of proof, 718–719
Burkholderia cepacia, 558
Burn care, 402–403
Burn depth, 404
Burn injuries, 65–66, 436
Burn patient, 401–438
  burn injury prevalence, 403–404
  classification of burns, 404–405
  complications, 411, *412–422*
  damage assessment checklist, 423–426
  follow-up, 409
  grafting, 406
  health and strength maintenance, 436–438
  life care plans, pediatric, 409
  major problems associated with, 405–409
  massage therapy, 408–409
  nutritional issues, 408
  outpatient services, 409
  pressure garments and splints, 407
  prosthetics, 407
  psychological issues, 409–410
  reconstruction, 407
  rehabilitation, 408
  role of skin, 405
  sample life care plan for John Doe, 426–436
  surgical procedures, 406
  total body surface area (TBSA) burned, 402–403
  vocational rehabilitation, 410–411
  World Burn Congress, 409
Bystedt v. Hay (2001), 853

C

CACREP, *see* Council for Accreditation of Counseling and Related Educational Programs
CAI, *see* Career Assessment Inventory
Calcineurin inhibitor, *547*, *561*
Calves, 433
Canadian Certified Life Care Planner (CCLCP), 846–848
Canadian Institute of Life Care Planning (CILCP), 846
Canadian life care plan, 844–860
  admissibility rules in United States and Canada, 849–850
  Canadian practice, 850
  Canadian Summit, 848
  Canadian Supreme Court Judgments, 852–862
  as expert witness, 850–851
  preparation, 845–846
  standards of practice, 848
  terminology, 845
  training for life care planners, 846–847
  types, 848–849
  working with life care planner, 851–852
Canadian Occupational Performance Measure (COPM), 107
Candida prophylaxis, 551
Cane, 577
CANS, *see* Central auditory nervous system
CAPDs, *see* Central auditory processing disorders
CAPS, *see* Certified Aging in Place Specialist
Carbamazepine, 451, 459
Cardiac abnormalities, 539
Cardiac evaluation, 539
Cardiology evaluation, 540
Cardiovascular complications, 377–378
Career Assessment Inventory (CAI), 48
Caregiver, 31
Care Manager, Certified (CMC), 37
Care plan development, 30–32
Carlson's testimony, 824
Carmichael v. Samyang Tires Inc., 824
CAs, *see* Communications assistants
Case law development (ADA), 719–720
Case management, 125, 437; *see also* Case manager
  ADA perspective to practice of, 713–714
  integrating court decisions into practice, 720–725
Case Management Resource Guide, 601
Case Management Society of America (CMSA), 736, 835

Case manager
 certifications, 37
 certified, 7, *10*, 37, 42, *625*, 696, 699
 nurse, 31
 organizations, 37
Cataracts, 573
Catastrophic cases
 disability in, 336
 life care plans in, 848
 special needs trusts in, 740
Catheterizations, 520
CATIE, *see* Clinical Antipsychotic Trials of Intervention Effectiveness
Cattelle Scales of Infant Development, 52
Cauda equina syndromes, 504
Cauda equine, 499
CBHSQ, *see* Center for Behavioral Health Statistics and Quality
CBIS, *see* Columbia Books & Information Services
CBT, *see* Cognitive-behavioral therapy
CCC, *see* Certificate of clinical competence
CCC-A, *see* Certificate of clinical competence in audiology
CCC-SLP, *see* Certificate of clinical competence in speech-language pathology
CCD, *see* Consortium for Citizens with Disabilities
CCLCP, *see* Canadian Certified Life Care Planner
CCM, *see* Certified Case Manager
CCMC, *see* Commission for Case Manager Certification
CDC, *see* Centers for Disease Control and Prevention
CDEC, *see* Commission on Disability Examiner Certification
CDMS, *see* Certified Disability Management Specialist
CDP, *see* Computerized dynamic posturography
CDRS, *see* Certified Driver Rehabilitation Specialist
CEAC, *see* Certified Environmental Access Consultant
Center for Behavioral Health Statistics and Quality (CBHSQ), 444
Center for Information Technology Accommodation (CITA), *225*
Center of Excellence (COE), 341
Centers for Disease Control and Prevention (CDC), 259, 266, 368, 370, 482, 403–404
Centers for Medicare and Medicaid Services (CMS), 299, 307, 536–537, 783
Central auditory behavioral tests, 287
Central auditory nervous system (CANS), 286
Central auditory processing disorders (CAPDs), 286
Central cord syndrome, 503
Central hearing loss, 292
Central nervous system (CNS), 287, 473
Central storming, 378
Cerebellum, 372
Cerebral cortex, 370–372, *371*
Cerebral palsy, 125
Cerebrospinal fluid, 151
Certificate of clinical competence (CCC), 292
Certificate of clinical competence in audiology (CCC-A), 292
Certificate of clinical competence in speech-language pathology (CCC-SLP), 153
Certification/credentials, 697, 816; *see also* Credentialing; Licensure
 assistive technology practitioner, 776
 assistive technology supplier, 776
 audiologists, 153, *153*, 291–292, *291*, *304–305*
 case manager, 7, 37, 42, 699
 certification, 814–815
 checklist of questions on, *816*
 Commission on Disability Examiner certification, 5
 definition of certification, 814
 International Commission on Health Care Certification (ICHCC), 5
 legal nurse, 37
 life care planning, 3, 4, 5, 15
 neuropsychologists, 83–87
 rehabilitation counselors, 699
 rehab technology supplier, 776
 speech-language pathologists, 153–165
 vocational rehabilitation counselors, 41
Certified Aging in Place Specialist (CAPS), 789
Certified ATS/CRTS specialists, 776
Certified Case Manager (CCM), 7, *10*, 37, 42, 696
Certified Disability Management Specialist (CDMS), *10*, 42
Certified Driver Rehabilitation Specialist (CDRS), 801, 805, 806
Certified Environmental Access Consultant (CEAC), 789
Certified Life Care Planner (CLCP), *10*, 16, 37, 626, 743, 846, 848
Certified Managed Care Nurse (CMCN), 37
Certified Nurse Life Care Planner (CNLCP), 37, 626, 743
Certified Occupational Health Nurse (COHN), 37
Certified occupational therapy assistants (COTAs), 119
Certified Physician Life Care Planner (CPLCP), 6, 37
Certified Rehabilitation Counselor (CRC), *10*, 42, 411, 693, 696, 815
Certified Rehabilitation Registered Nurse (CRRN), *10*, 31, 37
Certified rehab technology supplier (CRTS), 776
Certified Vocational Evaluator (CVE), *10*, 42
Cerumen management, 259
CFR Title 38, *see* Code of Federal Regulations Title 38
Checklist
 activities of daily living, 109–114
 burn damage assessment, *423–426*
 credentialing, questions on, *816*
 day-in-the-life video production, 685–689
 life care plan, *8*, *623–624*
 life care planner qualifications, *625–626*
 life care plan review, *623–624*
 speech-language pathologists LCP, *192–194*

Chi-square goodness-of-fit test, 707
Children
  audiological habilitation/rehabilitation, 277–278
  behaviors at risk for auditory disorders, 297
  developmental milestones for, *234–235*
  hearing loss risk factors, *267*
  individual education plans (IEPs), 169, 173
  individualized education program, 90, 120
  least restrictive environment, 169
  life care plans, 409
  No Child Left Behind Act, 173
  SLP assessment, 167
  visually impaired, 574
  wheelchair replacement, 770
Chiropractors, 318
Chlorpromazine (Thorazine), 456
Cholelithiasis, 505, 508
Cholesterol-lowering agent, 551
Chronic foot pain patients, 475
Chronic lumbar sprain, 761
Chronic obstructive pulmonary disease (COPD), 545
Chronic pain, 25, 469–493
  acute/subacute/chronic, definitions, 471
  Analgesic Ladder, 476, *478*
  case study, 486
  chronic pain syndrome, 469
  costs, 471
  determining patient's functioning level, 485
  diagnostic algorithms, 472
  diagnostic efforts/workup, 472–474
  and future concerns, 485
  life care planning, 481–493
  management algorithms, 482–485
  management approaches, 474–485
  psychological considerations, 482
  surgical interventions, 475, 485
  therapeutic injections, 477–478
CIC, *see* Completely-in-the-canal
CILCP, *see* Canadian Institute of Life Care Planning
Circulatory disorders, 511–512
Cisapride, 505–506
CITA, *see* Center for Information Technology Accommodation
Civil code system, 850
Claim, *198*
Claims Clearinghouse System, *198*
Clark v. Aqua Air Industries, 43
CLCP, *see* Certified Life Care Planner
Clearinghouse capability, *198*
Cleveland v. Policy Management Systems Corporation (1999), 722
Client advocate, 31
Client factors, 85
Clinical Antipsychotic Trials of Intervention Effectiveness (CATIE), 461
Clinical assessment techniques, 167
Clinical indicator, *198*
Clinical neuropsychology, 79–80, 83
Clinical Practice Guidelines, *198*
Clinic, pain management, 475
Clomipramine, 446, 454
Closed-circuit TV, 576
Closed-panel HMO, *198*
Closed captioning, 280
Closing the Gap, *225*
Clubhouse programs model, 460–461
CMC, *see* Care Manager, Certified
CMCN, *see* Certified Managed Care Nurse
CMP, *see* Competitive Medical Plan; Comprehensive metabolic panel
CMS, *see* Centers for Medicare and Medicaid Services
CMSA, *see* Case Management Society of America
CMV, *see* Cytomegalovirus
CNLCP, *see* Certified Nurse Life Care Planner
CNS, *see* Central nervous system
COBRA, *see* Consolidated Omnibus Reconciliation Act
Cochlear implants, 284–285, *285*
Cochleotoxicity, 273
Code of Federal Regulations Title 38 (CFR Title 38), 739
Code of Professional Ethics, 692–693
Code of Professional Ethics for Rehabilitation Counselors, 699
CODI, *see* Cornucopia of Disability Information
Coding, *see* Medical coding
COE, *see* Center of Excellence
Cognition, language *vs.*, *158*
Cognitive-behavioral psychologists, 63
Cognitive-behavioral therapy (CBT), 66, 71, 454, 446–447
Cognitive Abilities test, 52
Cognitive domains, 87
Cognitive factors, 65
Cognitive functioning, hearing loss impact on, 275
Cognitive rehabilitation techniques, 84
Cognitive remediation, 83
COHN, *see* Certified Occupational Health Nurse
Coinsurance, *198*
COJ, see Transitional Classification of Jobs
Collaborator, 31
Collateral source, 35, 612
  of payment, 652–653
Collectivistic cultures, 836
Columbia Books & Information Services (CBIS), 736
Coma, 369
Commission for Case Manager Certification (CCMC), 37
Commission on Disability Examiner Certification (CDEC), 5, 37, 692, 835, 846, 847, 848
Commission on Rehabilitation Counselor Certification (CRCC), 737, 815, 817
Communication, 150, 698
  with hearing-impaired people, 294–295
  impact of hearing loss, 274
  language *vs.* cognition, *158*
Communications assistants (CAs), 175

Communication sciences and disorders, 150
acronyms, *232–234*
biofeedback for acquired apraxia of speech, 163–165
checklist for life care planning, 192–194
laryngeal imaging, 161–163
research in, 161
SLP assessment process, 191
terminology in, 165–167
Community rating, *198*
Community reintegration, 341, 381–382
Comparable benefits funding, 174
Competency, 873
Competitive Medical Plan (CMP), *198*
Completely-in-the-canal (CIC), 282
Complex medical cases, 7
Complex mental functions, 80
Compliance Review Program (CRP), 801
Complications, 331
Comprehensive Major Medical Coverage, *199*
Comprehensive metabolic panel (CMP), 734
Computed tomography (CT), 81, 150, 374, 473, 539, 733
Computer access aids, 172
"Computerized" knee unit, 350
Computerized dynamic posturography (CDP), 272
Conditioned Play Audiometry (CPA), 264, 292
Conductive hearing loss, 292
Confidentiality, 873
Conjoint treatment, 70
Conroy v. Vilsack, 650*fn*
Consciousness, 372
Consensus and Majority Statements, 35
Consolidated Omnibus Reconciliation Act (COBRA), *199*
Consortium for Citizens with Disabilities (CCD), *225*
Consortium for Spinal Cord Medicine, 34
Consultant, 31–32
Consumer Price Index (CPI), 318
Context Healthcare, 748
Contingency management techniques, 72
Continuous positive airway pressure (CPAP), 507
Continuous Quality Improvement (CQI), *199*
Contract, *199*
Contractures, 379
Contralateral Routing of Signal (CROS), 282
Contributory, *199*
Conus medullaris syndrome, 499, 504
Conventional electroencephalography, 150
Cook v. Whitsell-Sherman, 643*fn*
Copayment, *199*
COPD, *see* Chronic obstructive pulmonary disease
COPM, *see* Canadian Occupational Performance Measure
Cornucopia of Disability Information (CODI), *225*
Cortical blindness, 372
Costs, 318
acquired brain injury, 369–370
actual *vs.* average annual, 330
annual increases, *329*
attendant/aide, 327
augmentative and alternative communication, 230–231
base costing and duplication, 663
bipolar disorder, 452
categories, 318–327
chronic pain, 471
consumer price index tables, 320–327
cost-per-case limits, *199*
earnings capacity analysis, 53–55, *53*
funding glossary, *196–204*
funding sources, *195*
of future care reports, 845
of hearing aids, 298–299
medical commodities, 319
medical services, 318–319
nonmedical commodities, 319, *320–321*, *322–323*, *324–325*, *326–327*, *328*, *329*
nonmedical services, 319
prosthetic, 350–351
retransplantation, 553
of schizophrenia, 461
sharing, *199*
shifting, *199*
speech-language pathology, 177–178
total lifetime values, 331
transplantation, 552–553, *559*
vehicle modifications, 804–805
vocational rehabilitation, 43
wheelchairs, 763, *764–765*
COTAs, *see* Certified occupational therapy assistants
Council for Accreditation of Counseling and Related Educational Programs (CACREP), 817
Counseling; *see also* Psychotherapy
audiology/hearing loss, 294, 299–*300*
theories and practices, 157–161
Counseling the Able Disabled (Deneen and Hessellund), 45
Couples therapy, 436
Court cases
Albertsons, Inc., v. Kirkingburg, 718
Bragdon v. Abbott (1998), 718
Crouch v. John Jewell Aircraft, 819, 826–827
Cuevas v. Contra Costa County, 613
Daubert v. Merrill Dow Pharmaceuticals, 821–822
Diamond R. Fertilizer v. Davis, 643*fn*
Drury v. Corvel, 55
Elliott v. United States, 695
Fairchild v. United States, 695
Frye v. United States, 820
Fuentes v. Jackson, 696
General Electric Company v. Joiner, 823
Kim Manufacturing v. Superior Metal Treating, 611
Kumho Tire Company v. Carmichael, 823–825
Murphy v. UPS, 718
Norwest Bank, N. A. and Kenneth Frick v. K-Mart Corporation, 695

Court cases (*Continued*)
Olmstead Commissioner, Georgia Department of Human Resources v. L. C., 721
Supreme Court decisions, 716, 719–722, 726–727
Sutton v. United Airlines, 718
Toyota v. Williams, 718
U.S. Airways, Inc. v. Barnett (2002), 723
Court of Queen's Bench or Supreme Court, 850
Covered transfer areas, 791–792
Cox proportional hazards models, 542
CPA, *see* Conditioned Play Audiometry
CPAP, *see* Continuous positive airway pressure
CPB/WGBH National Center for Accessible Media, *225*
CPI, *see* Consumer Price Index
CPLCP, *see* Certified Physician Life Care Planner
CPT codes, 733
CQI, *see* Continuous Quality Improvement
Cranial complications, 377
Crawford Small Parts Dexterity, 48
CRC, *see* Certified Rehabilitation Counselor
CRCC, *see* Commission on Rehabilitation Counselor Certification
Credentialing, 813–817; *see also* Certification/credentials
accreditation, 817
certification, 814–815, *816*
general, 814
licensure, 814
registration, 815–817
CROS, *see* Contralateral Routing of Signal
Cross-cultural communication, 837–839
Cross-culturalism, 834
Cross-cultural life care
planner, 834
planning, 839
Crosswalking, 745
for life care planner, important, 745–746
Crouch v. John Jewell Aircraft, 819, 826–827
CRP, *see* Compliance Review Program
CRRN, *see* Certified Rehabilitation Registered Nurse
CRTS, *see* Certified rehab technology supplier
CT, *see* Computed tomography
Cuevas v. Contra Costa County, 613
Cultural considerations, 833–839
acculturation and enculturation, 836–837
foundations of multicultural and cross-cultural issues, 834–835
individualistic and collectivistic cultures, 836
life care planner cultural competence, 837
methodological framework for cross-cultural life care planning, 839
multicultural and cross-cultural communication, 837–839
Culture, 833
Curbside consultation, 354
Current Procedural Terminology, 4th Edition (CPT), 178
Custom-molded seating systems, 770
Custom therapeutic seating systems, 766
CVE, *see* Certified Vocational Evaluator
Cyclosporin, 535, 546
Cytomegalovirus (CMV), 265, 538
organ rejection and, 550

D

DAI, *see* Diffuse axonal injury
Damages, 643
Damages in Tort Actions (Deutsch and Raffa), 4, 5, 612
Dan Cristiani Excavating Co. v. Money, 643*fn*
Dantrolene, 506
DAT, *see* Differential Aptitude Tests
Database, 35, 706, 733–734, 744
LCP Stat (version 10), 738
storing, retrieving, presenting, and formatting information, 738
Data collection, 15, 800, 871
Daubert analysis, 824
Daubert challenges, 34
and credentials, 825–827
Daubert decision, 613
Daubert rulings, 13, 820, 826
Rule 702, 822
Daubert trilogy, 820
Daubert v. Merrell Dow Pharmaceuticals, Inc., 613, 650, 821–822, 849
Day-in-the-life video
checklist, 685
impact, 681–683
key consideration goals, 684, 689
life care plan and, 684
production, 681–689
DCD, *see* Donation after cardiac death
Deafferentation pain syndromes, 481
Deaf people, communicating with, 295
Deception test, 820
Decibel ratings, *269–270*
Decubitus ulcers, 511
Deep full-thickness burns, 404
Deep partial-thickness burns, 404
Deep vein thromboses (DVTs), 377–378, 512
Deep venous thrombosis, 513
Defense attorney, 655–668
application of collateral source rule, 663–664
attacking plaintiff's life care plan qualifications, 656
base costing and duplication, 663
basis of opinions, 662–663
cross-examination of plaintiff's expert, 660–661
defense rehabilitation consultant, 665–668
effect on jury, 668
financial bias, 661–662
foundational objections, 659–660
licensing issues, 664–665
purpose of retention, 662
qualifications objections, 656–665

Degennaro v. Oakville Trafalgar Memorial Hospital (2011), 859
Degree of recovery, 90
Delivery period and amount, 327–330
Delivery system, alternative, *198*
Dementia development, 88
Dementia praecox, 447–448, 455
Denervation, 151
Denial, 67
Dennis v. Gairdner (2002), 856
Dental, 747
Denticulate ligaments, 501
Depakote, 483
Department of Health and Human Services (DHHS), 174, *200*
Depositions, 647–648
Depression, 67, 88, *379*, 409
Depressive disorder, 74
  bipolar disorder, 444, 447–452
  major depressive disorder, 444, 445–447
Depressive episode, 449
Depressive symptoms, 459
Depth-kymography, 162
Dermatologist, 434
Dermis, 405
Desbiens v. Mordini (2004), 857
Desensitization/exposure therapies, 71
Detached retina, 573
Detrusor-external sphincter dyssynergia, 508
Developmental Disabilities Assistance and Bill of Rights Act, 713
Developmental psychologists, 63
DHHS, *see* Department of Health and Human Services
Diabetes, 447
Diabetes mellitus, 510
Diagnostic efforts in workup, 472–474
Diagnostic spine injections, 473
Diagnostic testing, 733
Dialysis, renal, 537
Diamond R. Fertilizer v. Davis, 643*fn*
Diaphragm pacing, *see* Phrenic nerve pacing
Dichotic listening, 151
Dictionary of Occupational Titles (*DOT*), 41, 58, 611
Diet, 483
Dietary evaluation, 434
Differential Aptitude Tests (DAT), 48
Differential diagnosis, 167
Diffuse axonal injury (DAI), 374
Diffuse brain injuries, 374
Digital programmable hearing aids, 283
Dilantin, 483
Direct bone conduction, 286
Disability, 610, 713, 715, 716
  ADA Amendments Act of 2008, 716–718
  ADA Restoration Act, 716
  adjustment to, 67–68
  definition, 715–719
  major life activities and burden of proof, 718–719
  mitigating role and corrective measures in determining, 720
  National Council on Disability, 714–715
  parents with disabilities, 741
  physiatrist evaluation, 23
  postsecondary education for individuals with, 741
  reasonable accommodations, 169
  resources for parents with, 741
  as "term of art", 713
  transitory impairments and, 718
  vocational assessment tools, 47
Disability legislation, 712
DISABILITY Resources on Internet, *225*
Discharge planning, 7, 13–14, 868
"Discovery" deposition, 647
Discretion rule, 823
Distractibility, 455
District Court, 823, 824
DME, *see* Durable Medical Equipment
Do-It Internet Resources, *225*
Doctor of occupational therapy (DOT), 49, 119
Document production, requests for, 646–647
Doe, John, 426
  ankles and feet, 433
  burn injury, 427
  face and neck, 432
  forearms, elbows, and wrists, 432
  injury event, 428–430
  laser therapy, 433
  legs, 433
  massage therapy, 434–435
  personal interviews with John Doe and Jane Doe, 430–432
  pressure garments, 433–434
  psychiatric care, 435–436
  psycho/social issues, 435
  skin cancer, 433
  upper extremities and shoulders, 432
  web space releases, 432–433
Donation after cardiac death (DCD), 543–544
  donor, 544
Doppler ultrasonography, 512
Dorsal ganglia, 500
DOT, see Dictionary of Occupational Titles; Doctor of occupational therapy
Driver Rehabilitation Specialist (DRS), 801
DRS, *see* Driver Rehabilitation Specialist
Drug/supply needs, 358
Drury v. Corvel, 55
Dual relationships, 694–695, 873
Due care, 694
Duloxetine, 483, 508
Durable Medical Equipment (DME), 121, 737, 747, 769
Dura mater, 370
DVTs, *see* Deep vein thromboses
Dynamic optical coherence tomography, 162

Dynamic techniques, 150
Dysarthria, 164
Dysreflexia, 504
Dysthymia, *see* Persistent depressive disorder

E

Ear canal examination, 259
Ear infections, 269
Early Hearing Detection and Intervention (EHDI), 266
Early Hearing Detection and Intervention/Early and Periodic Screening, Diagnostic, and Treatment (EHDI/EPSDT), 155
Earnings capacity, 54, 622–623
Earnings capacity analysis, 53–55, 611–612
Earnings Capacity Assessment Form, 612
EASI, *see* Equal Access to Software and Information
Eastern Paralyzed Veterans Association Assistive Technology (EPVA Assistive Technology), *225*
Easter Seals, 34
EBV, *see* Epstein-Barr virus
EC, *see* Ethics Commission
ECA, *see* Epidemiologic Catchment Area
ECD, *see* Expanded criteria donor
ECochG, *see* Electrocochleography
E codes (speech-generating and non-speech generating devices), 178
Ecological validity, 88
Economic
  cost of burn injury, 403–404
  evaluation, 318
Economic/Hedonic Damages: The Practice Book for Plaintiff and Defense Attorneys (Brookshire and Smith), 612
Economist, 317–332
  actual or average annual, 330
  Affordable Care Act, 331–332
  attendant or aide costs, 327
  categories of costs, 318–329
  complications, 331
  consumer price index tables, *320–327*
  costs included in LCP, 319
  delivery period and amount, 327–330
  economy of effort, 330–331
  hospital services costs, *326–327*
  hourly earnings, historical, *328*
  increases for medical and care costs, annual, *329*
  marginal costs, 321, 325
  medical commodities costs, 319
  medical services costs, 318
  nonmedical commodities costs, 319
  nonmedical services costs, 319
  total lifetime values, 331
  value of items, 325, 327
Economy of effort, 330–331
ECT, *see* Electroconvulsive therapy
ECU, *see* Environmental control unit
ED, *see* Emergency department
Educational audiologist, 258
Educational programs, 734
Educational requirements, critical review of, 16–18
Education, child
  IDEA, 90, 173
  IEP, 90, 121
  NCLB Act, 173
Education for All Handicapped Children Act (EHA), 169–170, 713
Educator, 31
EEG, *see* Electroencephalogram
EEOC, *see* Equal Employment Opportunity Commission
EHA, *see* Education for All Handicapped Children Act
EHDI, *see* Early Hearing Detection and Intervention
EHDI/EPSDT, *see* Early Hearing Detection and Intervention/Early and Periodic Screening, Diagnostic, and Treatment
EITAAC, *see* Electronic and Information Technology Access Advisory Committee
Ekso GT robotic exoskeleton, 517
Elbows, 432
  disarticulation/above elbow, 348
Elder care, 591–605
  age-related changes on functional activities, *593–594*
  assessment, 596–597, *597–598*
  at-risk geriatric population, *599*
  benefits for life care planning in, 595–596
  life care planning principles, 591–605
  maximizing resources, 599
  plan implementation and monitoring, 598–599
  resources, 600–605
Elder law attorney, 669–679
  case study, 676–678
  elder law, defined, 670
  ethical considerations, 674
  functions of, 670–672
  holistic approach, 672–674
  increase in elder law specialty, 672
  NAELA, 670
  nature of elder law, 670–679
  and professional life care planners, 674, *675*, 676
  state statutes, 678–679
Electric prosthesis, 348
Electrocochleography (ECochG), 265
Electroconvulsive therapy (ECT), 446
Electroencephalogram (EEG), 150, 733
Electromagnetic ovens, 576
Electromyography (EMG), 151
Electronic aids for daily living (EADLs), *see* Environmental control units (ECUs)
Electronic and Information Technology Access Advisory Committee (EITAAC), *224*
Electronystagmography (ENG), 272
Electropalatography (EPG), 163, 165
Elementary and Secondary Education Act, 170

E-mail, obtaining information by, 735–736
EMDR, *see* Eye movement desensitization reprocessing
Emergency department (ED), 370
EMG, *see* Electromyography
Emotional difficulties, 88
Employability, 618–622
Employment, 460
EncoderPro, 744
Enculturation, 836–837
Encyclopedia of Disability and Rehabilitation, 612
End-organ disease, 537
End-stage renal disease (ESRD), 510
 kidney transplantation, 537
 life care planning, 537
Endocrine disorders, 377
Endocrinology, 377
Endocrinopathies, 377
ENG, *see* Electronystagmography
Enhanced Guide for Occupational Exploration, The (GOE), 58
Environmental controls, 172
Environmental control unit (ECU), 734, 797
EOB, *see* Explanation of benefits
EP, *see Exceptional Parent*
EPG, *see* Electropalatography
Epidemiologic Catchment Area (ECA), 445
Epidemiology, 572–573
Epidermis, 405
Epidural space, 501
Epstein-Barr virus (EBV), 538
EPVA Assistive Technology, *see* Eastern Paralyzed Veterans Association Assistive Technology
Equal Access to Software and Information (EASI), *225*
Equal Employment Opportunity Commission (EEOC), 715
Equipment
 adaptive, 46
 equipment/supplies, 734
 medical, 759–784
 medicine and rehabilitation, 21–22
Erectile dysfunction, 513
Ertl osteoplasty, 352
Erythromycin, 546
ESRD, *see* End-stage renal disease
Estate planning, 595
Ethical issues, 691–698
 example ethical brushes, 695–696
 general professional duties within health care, 693–695
 moral values, 692
 right conduct, 692
 rules or standards of specialty practice, 692
 suggestions for success: global, 696–697
 suggestions for success: malpractice insurance related, 697–698
Ethics, 154, 691, 872
Ethics Commission (EC), 123
Etiology, 573
Evaluation, initial, 684
Evaluee advisement of role, 873
"Evidentiary" deposition, 647–648
Evoked potentials, 151
Exaggeration of need, 761–762, 767–768
Exceptional Parent (EP), 742
Exclusivity clause, *199*
Exercise, 483
Expanded criteria donor (ECD), 543–544
Expenditures, *199*
Experience rating, *199*
Experiential therapy, 70
Expert witness, 18, 184, 258, 656, 850–851
Expert witness Canadian life care planner as, 850–851
Explanation of benefits (EOB), 174
Extended care, *199*
Eye injuries, traumatic etiology of, 573
Eye movement desensitization reprocessing (EMDR), 66

F

Facial movement, 372
Facility care, 734
Faciotomy, 406
FAIR Health, 748
Fair Housing Amendments Act (1988), 713
Family
 brain injury effects on, 90
 elder law attorney and, 672–673
 planning services, *199*
 systems, 157–161
Family therapy, 71, 436
FAPE, *see* Free Appropriate Public Education
FCC, *see* Federal Communications Commission
FCE, *see* Functional capacity evaluation
F/CMVSS, *see* Federal/Canada Motor Vehicle Safety Standards
FDA, *see* Food and Drug Administration
Federal/Canada Motor Vehicle Safety Standards (F/CMVSS), 801
Federal Communications Commission (FCC), *226*
Federally qualified HMOs, 200
Federal mandates and policies, 168–171
Federal Rule of Evidence 702 (FRE 702), 650, 822
Federal Rule of Evidence 703, 651
Federal Rules of Civil Procedure, 646
Fee-for-service, *200*
Feet, ankles and, 433
Fentanyl Patch, 484
FES, *see* Functional electrical stimulation
Fidelity, 124
Field cut, *see* Field of vision
Field of vision, 377
FIM, *see* Functional Improvement Measure
FIMS, *see* Functional Independence Measure Scores
Financing, *195*

Find-A-Code, 744
Fire safety exits, 791
First-dollar coverage, *200*
Fiscal agent, *200*
Fiscal intermediary, *200*
Fiscal year, *200*
Fixed battery approach, 86
Fixed fee, *200*
Flame, 404
FLCPR, *see* Foundation for Life Care Planning Research
Flexeril, 483
Florid psychosis, 457
Fluconazole, 551
FM systems, *see* Frequency-modulated systems
FMVSS, *see* U.S. Federal Motor Vehicle Safety Standards
Focal brain injuries, 374
Follow-up, 342–343, 409
Food and Drug Administration (FDA), 281
Forde v. Inland Health Authority (2010), 853
Forearms, elbows, and wrists, 432
Forensic audiologist, 258
Forensic issues, 609
  access to labor market (employability), 618–622
  basic matrix, *619*
  checklist for review of life care plans, *623–626*
  collateral sources, 612
  comparison matrix, *619–621*
  earnings capacity, 622–623
  earnings capacity analysis, 611–612
  elements for future care damages, *613*
  example entry for future care damages, *613*
  hedonic damages, 612
  labor force participation, 623
  placeability, 622
  rehabilitation plan, 614–618
  report writing, 613–623
Forensic life planning, 669
Forensic rehabilitation, 610
Forgetfulness, *379*
Formulary, *200*
Forward-looking life care plans, 22
Foundation for Life Care Planning Research (FLCPR), 6, 835
FRE 702, *see Federal Rule of Evidence 702*
"Free and appropriate education," 13
Free Appropriate Public Education (FAPE), 169
Freedom of Choice, *200*
Freestanding hospital, *200*
Frequency-modulated systems (FM systems), 278–279
Frequency-specific information, 293
Frers v. De Moulin (2002), 853
Frontal lobe, 370
Frontal lobotomies, 455–456
Frye rule, 821
Frye v. United States, 820, 849
Full-thickness burns, 404
Functional capacity assessment, *see* Functional capacity evaluation (FCE)
Functional capacity evaluation (FCE), 43, 107, 485
Functional electrical stimulation (FES), 517
Functional Improvement Measure (FIM), 107, 139, 518
Functional Independence Measure Scores (FIMS), 89
Functional mobility, 109
Funding, 155, *195*
  glossary, *196*
  source, 828
Funding sources, alternative, 177
Future Care Cost Assessments, 845
Future Cost Analysis, 845
Future Needs Analysis, 845

G

Gabapentin, 451, 483, 508
GAH, *see* Global alveolar hypoventilation
Gallstones, 24–25
Gamma-globulin infusion, 541
Ganciclovir, 551
"Garage shop" operations, 800
Gas/break control (G/B control), 806
Gastroesophageal reflux disease (GERD), 189
Gastrointestinal complications, 378
Gastrointestinal issues, 505–506
GATB, *see* General Aptitude Test Battery
Gatekeeper, *200*
G/B control, *see* Gas/break control
GC, *see* General contractors
GCS, *see* Glasgow Coma Scale
GE–Joiner decision, 823
General acceptance principle, 820
General Aptitude Test Battery (GATB), 48
General contractors (GC), 789
General Electric Company v. Joiner, 823
General Electric v. Joiner (1997), 826, 827
Generic substitution, *200*
Genetic abnormalities, 265
Genital/urinary problems, 481
Genitourinary complications, 378
Genitourinary dysfunction, 508–510
Genworth cost of care survey, 742
Geo-zip, 749
GERD, *see* Gastroesophageal reflux disease
Gil Crease v. J. A. Jones Construction Company, 42–43
Glasgow Coma Scale (GCS), 144
  method, 374, *375*
Glaucoma, 573
Gleason Act, 170–171
Global alveolar hypoventilation (GAH), 506–507
Global budget, *200*
Global Positioning System device (GPS device), 577
Glucose uptake, 408
Goal setting, 476

GOE, see Enhanced Guide for Occupational Exploration, The
Gonadal steroid production, 377
Government Services Administration (GSA), *224*
GPS device, *see* Global Positioning System device
Grab bars, 393, 794
Grafting, 406
Graham v. Rourke (1990), 852, 860
Gregory v. Insurance Corporation of British Columbia (2011), 853, 854
Group therapy, 70
GSA, *see* Government Services Administration
Guide to Physical Therapist Practice, 136, 137
Guide to Rehabilitation (Deutsch and Sawyer), 4, 576

H

H2 receptor antagonists, 551
Hallucinations, 456
Haloperidol, 458
Halstead–Reitan Neuropsychological Battery (HNRB), 81
Halstead–Reitan batteries, 51, 81, 86
Handicapped Infants and Toddlers Act (1986), 170
Harrington v. Sangha (2011), 852, 853, 855
HCC, *see* Hepatocellular carcinoma
HCFA, *see* Health Care Financing Administration
HCPCS, *see* Healthcare Common Procedure Code System
HCUP, *see* Healthcare Cost and Utilization Project
H-CUPnet, 746, 748–749
Health and strength maintenance, 359, 436
  case management, 437
  medication, 437
  personal attendant and home care, 437–438
  respite care, 437
  supplies, 437
Healthcare Common Procedure Code System (HCPCS), 307, 748
Healthcare Cost and Utilization Project (HCUP), 748
Health Care Financing Administration (HCFA), *200*
Health care professionals, 7
  locating, 736
Health club, 737
Health economy, 161
Health Insurance Portability and Accountability Act (HIPAA), 124, 174
  privacy rule, 174–175
  regulations, 699
Health maintenance organizations (HMOs), *198*
Health psychologists, 63
Hearing aids
  assistive listening devices, 278–281
  costs, 298–299
  first aid for, 295–297
  selection and fitting, 281–282
  special features for, 283–284
  styles of, 282
  types, 282–283
Hearing assessment, *see* Audiologists
Hearing level (HL), 260
Hearing loss
  audiogram, 260–261, *261*
  causes, 267–270
  communication suggestions, 294–295
  conditions with, 298
  decibel ratings, *269*, *270*
  degree of, *305*
  identification in newborn, 265
  impact, 274–275
  impact on communication, 274
  newborn/infant screening for, 266–267, *267*
  ototoxic, 273–274
  perinatal causes, 268
  postnatal causes, 268–269
  risk factors in infants and young children, *266*
  socioeconomic status, 271
  types, 292
Hearsay, 651–652
Heart transplantation, *see* Organ transplantation
HEATH National Clearinghouse on Postsecondary Education for Individuals with Disabilities, 741
Hedonic damages, 612
Hepatitis C, 538
Hepatocellular carcinoma (HCC), 542
Hester Evaluation System, 48
Heterotopic ossification (HO), 379, 405–406, 510
Hi-Mark Tactile Pen, 576
High-dose irradiation, 546
High-frequency speech sounds, 260
High-speed digital imaging (HSDI), 162, 163
High Risk Registry, 265–266
HIPAA, *see* Health Insurance Portability and Accountability Act
Hip disarticulation, 350
Hippocrates of Kos, 80
Histocompatibility leukocyte antigen (HLA), 538
HIV, *see* Human immunodeficiency virus
HL, *see* Hearing level
HLA, *see* Histocompatibility leukocyte antigen
HMOs, *see* Health maintenance organizations
HNRB, *see* Halstead–Reitan Neuropsychological Battery
HO, *see* Heterotopic ossification
"Holder of list," 536
Holistic approach, 638, 665, 672–674
Home assessment, 787–797
  access throughout home, 792
  assistive technology, 797
  bathroom, 794–796
  bedroom, 793–794
  conditions meriting home evaluation, 788
  entrance to home, covered transfer areas, and fire safety exit, 790–792
  kitchen, 796
  laundry room, 797
  in life care planning, 788

Home assessment (*Continued*)
overview, 790–797
process, 789–790
selection of qualifying professional/company, 788–789
Home care, personal attendant and, 437–438
Home/facility care, 358
Home furnishings and accessories, 358
Home health
care, 733
care services links, 736
Home modifications, 514–515
Hospitalization, 369, 409
Hospital services, 318
Household services, 734
HRSA, *see* U.S. Health Resources and Services Administration
HSDI, *see* High-speed digital imaging
Human immunodeficiency virus (HIV), 538
Human learning, 157–161
Hypercalcemia, 510
Hypercalciuria, 510
Hyperlipidemia, 551
Hypertension, 447
Hypertrophic scarring and contractures, 406
Hypoglycemic coma, 455–456
Hypomania, 448, 449

I

IADL, *see* Instrumental Activities of Daily Living
IALCP, *see* International Academy of Life Care Planners
IARP, *see* International Association of Rehabilitation Professionals
IASP, *see* International Association for the Study of Pain
ICD-10-CM, *see* International Classification of Diseases-10-Clinical Modification
ICE, *see* Institute for Credentialing Excellence
ICF, *see* Intermediate care facility
IDAT, *see* Independent donor advocate team
IDDS, *see* Implantable drug delivery systems
IDEA, *see* Individuals with Disabilities Education Act
IDIA, *see* Individuals with Disabilities Improvement Act
IENS, *see* Implantable electronic neuromodulation systems
IEP, *see* Individualized education program
IFSP, *see* Individualized family service plan
Immunosuppressive therapy, 546–549
Implantable drug delivery systems (IDDS), 478
Implantable electronic neuromodulation systems (IENS), 478–479
Implantable hearing devices, 284–286
"Impulsive-aggressive" behavior, 450
Independent donor advocate team (IDAT), 540
Independent function, 121
Individualistic cultures, 836
Individual Education Plan (IEP), 169
Individualized education program (IEP), 90, 120, 169, 173, 278
audiology services, 264, 294
OT evaluation, 121
Individualized family service plan (IFSP), 278, 294
Individualized written rehabilitation plan (IWRP), 174
Individual psychotherapy, 435–436
Individual's premorbid personality, 88
Individuals with Disabilities Education Act (IDEA), 13, 34, 90, 120, 278, 383, 572, 578, 713
assistive technology, 170, 172–173
audiology services for children, 170, 278
visually impaired definition, 572
Individuals with Disabilities Improvement Act (IDIA), 172
Individual therapy, 70
Individual Work Plan (IWP), *see* Individualized written rehabilitation plan (IWRP)
Induction loop systems, 280
Industrial audiologist, 258
Industry safety standards, 803–804
Infant development, assessment of, 52
Infant hearing screening, 253–255
Infant mortality rate, *201*
Infection, posttransplantation, 550–551
Infectious diseases, 265
Informational counseling, 300
Infrared systems, 280
Inhaled anesthetic gasses, 476
Inpatient hospital services, *201*
Inpatient rehabilitation facility (IRF), 376
Inpatient treatment, 70
INR, *see* International normalized ratio
Institute for Credentialing Excellence (ICE), 815
Institute of Medicine (IOM), 469
Institute of Rehabilitation Education and Training (IRET), 6, 743, 846
Institute of Rehabilitation Education Life Care Planning Pre-certification program, 846–847
Institutional Review Board (IRB), 705
Instrumental Activities of Daily Living (IADL), 114–119
Insurance, 652–653
malpractice, 697–698
plaintiff's attorney and, 652
viatical settlement, 741
Integumentary issues, 511
Intelligence assessment, 47, 52
Intensive care, *201*
Interdisciplinary treatment plan, 476
Interest assessment, 48
Intermediate care facility (ICF), 734
Intermediate care facility, *201*
Intermittent catheterization, 509
International Academy of Life Care Planners (IALCP), 5, 6, 15, 144, 692, 743, 835, 848
standards, 691–692, 695
International Association for the Study of Pain (IASP), 470

International Association of Rehabilitation Professionals (IARP), 6, 835, 848, 736, 748
International Center for Disability Resources, *226*
International Classification of Diseases-10-Clinical Modification (ICD-10-CM), 178
International Commission on Health Care Certification (ICHCC), *see* Commission on Disability Examiner Certification (CDEC)
International life care planning, 834
International normalized ratio (INR), 542
International Rehabilitation Associates, 610
Internet, 781
  cost resources, 735
  resources on, 219–223, 227
  search engines, 576
Interpersonal communication, 157–161
Interpersonal psychotherapy, 446–447
Interpretation (language), for tests, 87
Interprofessional Collaborative (IPC), 156
Interprofessional Education (IPE), 156–157
Interprofessional Practice (IPP), 156–157
In-the-canal (ITC), 282
In-the-ear (ITE), 282
In vivo desensitization, 71
In vivo therapy, *see* Experiential therapy
IOM, *see* Institute of Medicine
IPC, *see* Interprofessional Collaborative
IPE, *see* Interprofessional Education
IPP, *see* Interprofessional Practice
IRB, *see* Institutional Review Board
IRET, *see* Institute of Rehabilitation Education and Training
IRF, *see* Inpatient rehabilitation facility
ITC, *see* In-the-canal
ITE, *see* In-the-ear
Itraconazole, 551
IWRP, *see* Individualized written rehabilitation plan
Izony v. Weidlich (2006), 854

J

Jack v. Cripps and Reath (2014), 860–861
Jacobsen v. Nike Canada Ltd (1996), 853
JAN, *see* Job Accommodation Network
Jarmson v. Jacobsen (2012), 854
J. Carmen Fuentes v. W. Brent Jackson d/b/a Jackson's Farming Company, 696
JCIH, *see* Joint Committee on Infant Hearing
JEVS, *see* Jewish Employment and Vocational Service
Jewish Employment and Vocational Service (JEVS), 48
Job; *see also* Vocational rehabilitation
  Dictionary of Occupational Titles (*DOT*), 41–42, 46, 49, 58, 611
  market analysis, 55, *56*
Job Accommodation Network (JAN), 59, *226*
Job-lock, *201*
Job v. Van Blankers (2009), 853
Joinson v. Heran (2011), 855
Joint Committee on Infant Hearing (JCIH), 266
Journal of Life Care Planning, 6, 669, 697, 743, 776, 779, 782
Journal of Nurse Life Care Planning, 743
Justice, as ethical goal, 124, 693

K

K-ABC, *see* Kaufman Assessment Battery for Children
Kaplan University, 5, 6
Kaufman Assessment Battery for Children (K-ABC), 51–52
Ketorolac, 476
Kidney dialysis, 538, 539, 541
Kidney failure, etiologies, 667
Kidney paired donation (KPD), 539
Kidney transplantation, *see* Organ transplantation
Kim Manufacturing v. Superior Metal Treating (1976), 611
Kirkingburg decisions, 718, 719
Kitchen, 796
Knee disarticulation/above knee, 349–350
Knowledge Translation for Disability and Rehabilitation Research (KTDDR), 738
Koch (*Re*) (1997), 860
KPD, *see* Kidney paired donation
Krangle v. Brsco (2002), 855
KTDDR, *see* Knowledge Translation for Disability and Rehabilitation Research
Kuder Occupational Interest Inventory, 48
Kumho rulings, 13
Kumho Tire Company v. Patrick Carmichael, 614, 651, 823–825, 849

L

Laboratory and radiological services, *201*
Labor force participation, 54, 623
Labor market access, 618––622
  LMA method, 611
Labor market survey, 55, 56
Lamotrigine, 451, 508
Language *vs.* cognition, *158*
Lanternman Act, 34
Laparoscopic surgical evaluation, 473
Laryngeal imaging, 161–163
LAS, *see* Lung Allocation Scoring system
Laser-based technologies, 162
Laser therapy, 433
Last Minute Guide to Psychological and Neuropsychological Testing (Lees-Haley), 52
Laundry room, 797
Lawyers, 850; *see also* Attorney; Forensic issues
Lazaroff v. Lazaroff (2005), 860
L code, 351
LCP, *see* Life care plan
LCP Stat 10, 738
LEA, *see* Local education agency

Leadership Education in Neurodevelopmental and Related Disabilities (LEND), 156
Learning Disabilities OnLine, *226*
Least restrictive environment (LRE), 169
Legal issues, *see* Forensic issues
Legally blind, 572
Legal Nurse Certification, 37
Legal Nurse Consultant (LNC), 37
Legend drug, *201*
LEND, *see* Leadership Education in Neurodevelopmental and Related Disabilities
Levorphanol, 484
LFT, *see* Liver function tests
Liability, 643
Licensure, 814; *see also* Certification/credentials
  audiologists, *153*
  forensic issues, 664–665
Life care plan (LCP), 3, 4, 5, 15, 91, 317, 344, 356, 596, 609, 612–613, 641, 684, 703, 868, 869
  checklist, *8*
  checklist for mental illness, *464*
  checklist for selecting life care planner professional's qualifications, *10–11*
  defense attorney, 655–668
  entries, *185–188*
  future, 13–15
  historical perspective, 4–6
  implications for, 163, 165
  for John Doe, 426–435
  overview, 6–9
  pediatric, 409
  physical therapists contributions to, 142–144
  plaintiff's attorney, 641–653
  principles, 7
  software, 738
  step-by-step procedures, 9–13
Life care plan example
  for depressive disorders, *462–463*
  hearing loss/audiology, 301–303
  occupational therapist, 120–123
Life care planner
  audiology practices, 257
  burn care, 403
  competency, 873
  critical review of educational requirements, 16–18
  cultural competence, 837
  dual relationships, 694, 873
  due care, 694
  ethical issues, 691–698
  ethics-related observations, 692, 694
  OT to, 123, 127–132, 543
  relationship with attorney, 693–694
  selection of, 6, 7–8, 15, 617
  self-serving views, 16
  standards of performance, 869–870
  standards of practice, 865–873
  view, 18
Life Care Planner: Secretary, Know-It-All, or General Contractor? One Person's Perspective (Weed), 617
Life care planning; *see also* Certification/credentials; Training
  ADA perspective to practice of, 713–714
  admissibility considerations, 819–829
  case law to practice, 720–725
  chronic pain, 469–493
  consensus and majority statements, 875–878
  court decisions and impact on, 723–724
  cultural considerations for, 833–839
  cultural issues in, 834–835
  day-in-the-life video production, 681–689
  elder care management, 591–605
  historical perspective, 4–6
  holistic, 672–674
  home assessment, 787–797
  Journal of Life Care Planning title index, 879–895
  medical equipment, 760–784
  nurse, defi nition of, 37
  organ transplantation, 534–568
  overview, 136, 152, 443–464
  personal perspective, 631–639
  resources, 730–757
  role and functions of, 869
  SCI, 498–529
  scope of, 4–5
  in SLP, 152–153
  in transplantation, 537
  visually impaired, 571–589
Life Care Planning: A Step-by-Step Guide (Weed), 614
Life Care Planning for PC, 738
Life Care Planning Law Firms, 595
Life expectancy, 518–519
Limb amputation
  demographics, 343–344
  levels, 344–345, *345*
Limb amputee, newer surgeries for, 352
Lithium
  for bipolar disorder, 450
  for major depressive disorder, 446
  for schizophrenia, 459
Litigation; *see also* Attorneys; Forensic issues
  life care planner's role in, 644–650
  neurolitigation, 178–189
  plaintiff's attorney, 641–653
  speech-language pathologists, 178–189
Liver function tests (LFT), 734
Living donation, 539
LNC, *see* Legal Nurse Consultant
Local education agency (LEA), 170
Locked-in syndrome, 369
Long cane, *see* White cane
Long Term Acute Care Hospitals (LTACHs), 376
Long-term care, *201*
Long-term disability/short-term disability (LTD/STD), 43

Long-term impairments, 380–381
Long-term pain management, *479*
Louisiana, 850
Low back pain, 470
  costs, 471
  management algorithm, *477*
Lowered-floor minivans, 801, 802
Lower limb orthoses, 22
Low vision, 572–573
Loxapine, 458
L-P-E method, 612
LRE, *see* Least restrictive environment
LTACHs, *see* Long Term Acute Care Hospitals
LTD/STD, *see* Long-term disability/short-term disability
Lumbar puncture (spinal tap), 151
Lung Allocation Scoring (LAS) system, 542
Lung transplantation, *see* Organ transplantation
Luria–Nebraska batteries, 51
Lurtz v. Duchesne (2005), 862

M

MacEachern v. Rennie (2010), 855
MacNeil v. Bryan (2009), 858
Macular degeneration, 573
Magnetic resonance imaging (MRI), 150, *201*, 374, 472–473, 539, 706
Maintenance phases, 454
Major depressive disorder (MDD), 444, 445–447
  costs, 447
  epidemiology and course of illness, 445
  pharmacotherapy, 446
  psychotherapeutic interventions, 446–447
  symptoms, 445
  treatment, 446
  vocational impact, 447
Major life activities (MLA), 717, 718–719
Make Inoperative Prohibition, exemptions to, 801
Malpractice insurance, 613, 697
Maltese v. Pratap (2014), 856
Managed care, 14, *201*
Mania, 449
Manic-depressive insanity, 447–448
Manufacturer's suggested list price (MSLP), 775, 781
MAOIs, *see* Monoamine oxidase inhibitors
MAP, *see* Minimum Advertised Price
Marcoccia v. Ford Credit Canada Limited (2009), 858
Marcoccia v. Gill (2007), 858
Marginal costs, 321, 325
Markow v. Rosner, 613
Massage therapy, 408–409, 434–435
Matthews Estate v. Hamilton Civic Hospital (2008), 856
Maximum allowable cost, *201*
Maximum Medical Improvement (MMI), 343
MBTI, *see* Myers–Briggs Type Indicator
McCarron Dial System, 48
McCroskey Vocational Quotient System (MVQS), 58–59
McErlean v. Sarel et al., (1987), 859
MCT, *see* Motor Control Test
MDD, *see* Major depressive disorder
M.D.P. v. Middleton, 825
Mediator, 644
Medicaid, *201*, 299, 740
  buy-in, *201*
  payment rates, 652–653
Medicaid Management Information System, *201*
Medical audiologist, 257–258
Medical care, 358, 359, 733
Medical case managers, 403
Medical coding, 178, 745
  and billing software subscriptions, 744–745
Medical commodities costs, 319
Medical complications, 376–379
  cardiovascular complications, 377–378
  cognitive problems, 379
  cranial complications, 377
  endocrine disorders, 377
  gastrointestinal complications, 378
  genitourinary complications, 378
  musculoskeletal complications, 378–379
  neurological complications, 378
  pulmonary complications, 377
Medical equipment, 760–784; *see also* Assistive technology (AT); Wheelchairs
  accessories required, 765–766
  aids to independent function and/or durable, 575
  avoiding omissions, 762
  common errors in equipment recommendations, 761–768
  contributing factors to replacement time for wheelchairs, 770–772
  convenience and ADL features, 767
  custom therapeutic seating systems, 766
  exaggeration of needs, 767–768
  factors in choosing medical equipment, 761
  for general use, 319
  lighting, 575–577
  mobility and accessibility features, 766–767
  omissions error, 762–766
  pressure reduction, 766
  problems in wheelchair choice, 763
  replacement allowance worksheets, 772–775
  safety features, 767
  setting standards of protocol for replacement schedules, 768–775
  use of references and specialists, 775
  use of rehabilitation equipment specialists as consultants, 775–776
Medical Equipment Corner Paul Amsterdam, ATP, 777–784
  factors in choosing proper wheelchair for client, 777
  life care plan, 778
  making correct choices of medical equipment, 777

Medical Equipment Corner Paul Amsterdam, ATP (*Continued*)
  Medicare's current status with medical equipment and possible effects, 782
  proper pricing methodology, 780
  standard wheelchairs *vs.* complex rehab, 777–778
  use of Internet, 781
  use of Medicare allowables in life care plan, 781–782
  wheelchair choice, 778–779
Medical foundation for LCP, 617
Medical Injury Compensation Reform Act (MICRA), 613
Medical IRAs, *202*
Medical journals, 34
Medically needy cases, *202*
Medical records, copy of, 9
Medical Savings Accounts (MSAs), *202*
Medical services costs, 318
Medicare, 299, 652–653
  allowable reimbursement, 351
  allowables use in life care plan, 781–782
  current status with medical equipment and possible effects, 782
  pricing, 358
Medicare Severity Diagnosis Related Group (MS-DRG), 749
Medications, 86, 331, 437, 450
MEDLINE, 738
MELD, 541–542
Meninges, 501
Mental disabilities, community setting for, 721
Mental disorders, 443–464; *see also* Depressive disorders; Obsessive-compulsive disorder; Schizophrenia
  life care plan checklist, *464*
Mental functions, 80
Mental health, hearing loss impact on, 275
Mental illness
  impact, 444
  life care plan checklist for, *464*
Mentoring/life skills coaching, 72
Merriam-Webster's Dictionary, 691
Metabolic changes, from spinal cord injury, 510
Methadone, 484
Methicillin resistant staphylococcus aureus (MRSA), 355
Mettias v. United States of America, 826
MICRA, *see* Medical Injury Compensation Reform Act
Microprocessor foot/ankle technology, 349
Midbrain, 372, *373*
Middle latency evoked response (MLR), 287
MILD, *see* Minimally Invasive Lumbar Decompression
Milieu therapy, 70
Milina v. Bartsch (1985), 852, 856
Military personnel, injured, 14
Minimally Invasive Lumbar Decompression (MILD), 475
Minimally responsive, 369
Minimum Advertised Price (MAP), 781
Minivans, 802
Minnesota Multiphasic Personality Inventory (MMPI), 48, 473
Mirtazapine, 446
Mismatched negativity response (MMN response), 265, 287
Mixed episode, 449–450
MLA, *see* Major life activities
MLR, *see* Middle latency evoked response
MMI, *see* Maximum Medical Improvement
MMN response, *see* Mismatched negativity response
MMPI, *see* Minnesota Multiphasic Personality Inventory
Mobile mourning, 67
Mobility devices, 576
Mobility training, 578
Mobility ventures–1 (MV-1), 516
Modifiers, 804
Monoamine oxidase inhibitors (MAOIs), 446
Monoclonal/polyclonal antibodies, 546, *549*
Monych v. Beacon Community Services Society (2009), 856
Mood disorders, 445; *see also* Bipolar disorder; Major depressive disorder
Mood stabilizers, 451, 459
  for schizophrenia, 450, 459–460
Morphine, 484
Morrison v. Greig (2007), 857
Motor Control Test (MCT), 272
Motor neuron
  dysfunction, 508
  syndrome, 505
Motor vehicle accident (MVA), 144
Motrin, 484
MRI, *see* Magnetic resonance imaging
MRSA, *see* Methicillin resistant staphylococcus aureus
MS-DRG, *see* Medicare Severity Diagnosis Related Group
MSAs, *see* Medical Savings Accounts
MSLP, *see* Manufacturer's suggested list price
Multicultural communication, 837–839
Multicultural life care planner, 834
Multidimensional pain measurement tools, 471
Multidisciplinary pain programs, 482
Multiple relationships, 694–695, 873
Murphy v. UPS, 718
Muscle relaxants, 483
Musculoskeletal complications, 378–379
MV-1, *see* Mobility ventures–1
MVA, *see* Motor vehicle accident
MVQS, *see* McCroskey Vocational Quotient System
Myers–Briggs Type Indicator (MBTI), 48
Myoelectric control, 347–348
Myoneural, 151
Myopathy, 151
Myringotomy, 269

N

NACCM, *see* National Academy of Certified Care Managers
NAELA, *see* National Academy of Elder Law Attorneys

NAM, *see* National Academy of Medicine
NAMI, *see* National Alliance on the Mentally Ill
NAN, *see* National Academy of Neuropsychology
Narcotic analgesia, 484
NARIC, *see* National Rehabilitation Information Center
National Academy of Certified Care Managers (NACCM), 37
National Academy of Elder Law Attorneys (NAELA), 670
National Academy of Medicine (NAM), 156
National Academy of Neuropsychology (NAN), 87
National Alliance on the Mentally Ill (NAMI), 460
National Center for Health Statistics, 271
National certification, 155
National Clearing House of Rehabilitation Training Materials (NCHRTM), *226*
National Commission for Certifying Agencies (NCCA), 815, 816
National Council on Disability (NCD), 712, 714–715, 741
National Council on Rehabilitation Education (NCRE), 814
National Court Reporters Association (NCRA), 685–686
National Coverage Determination (NCD), 171
National Elder Law Foundation (NELF), 670
National Highway Traffic Safety Administration (NHTSA), 801, 810
National Institute of Deafness and Communication Disorders, 271
National Institute on Disability and Rehabilitation Research (NIDRR), *226*, 741
National Life Care Planning Summits, 6
Nationally certified counselor (NCC), 815
National Mobility Equipment Dealers Association (NMEDA), 800, 801, 810
National Organization for Competency Assurance (NOCA), 815
National Organ Transplant Act, 535–536
National Professional Group, suggestions from, 697
National Registry of Rehabilitation Technology Suppliers (NRRTS), 776
National Rehabilitation Information Center (NARIC), *226*
National Service Officers (NSO), 739
National Spinal Cord Injury Statistical Center (NSCISC), 498, 518–519
National Trade and Professional Associations Directory (2018), 736
Nationwide enforcement campaign, creation of, 722–723
NCC, *see* Nationally certified counselor
NCCA, *see* National Commission for Certifying Agencies
NCD, *see* National Council on Disability; National Coverage Determination
NCHRTM, *see* National Clearing House of Rehabilitation Training Materials
NCLB Act, *see* No Child Left Behind Act
NCRA, *see* National Court Reporters Association
NCRE, *see* National Council on Rehabilitation Education
Negligence claim, 643–644
NELF, *see* National Elder Law Foundation
Nerve blocks, 381
Nerve pain, 483
Neurogenic bladder, 22, 24
Neuroimaging, 80, 81
Neurolitigation, 178–189
Neurological complications, 378
Neurological control
  of bladder, 378
  center for body, 368
Neurological diseases, 190
Neurolytic injections, 478
Neuropathic pain, 508
Neuropathy, 151, 481
Neurophysiologic intraoperative monitoring, 271–272
Neuropsychological Assessment, 50, 64, 82–83
Neuropsychological evaluations, 49–52, 82, 382
Neuropsychological examination, 85–91
Neuropsychological testing, 50, 81, 82, 90
Neuropsychologists, 50, 63, 82, 382, *383*
  case study, 91–101
  clinical neuropsychology, 79–80
  neuroimaging, 80
  neuropsychological assessment, 82–83
  neuropsychological examination, 85–91
  neuropsychological testing, 81
  selecting, 83–85
Neuropsychology, 79, 81, 190
Neuroscience, 151
NHTSA, *see* National Highway Traffic Safety Administration
NIDRR, *see* National Institute on Disability and Rehabilitation Research
Night Vision Aid, 577
NMEDA, *see* National Mobility Equipment Dealers Association
NMEDA Mobility Equipment Dealer, 802
NOCA, *see* National Organization for Competency Assurance
No Child Left Behind Act (NCLB Act), 173
Nonbehavioral hearing assessment techniques, 264, 266
Non-catastrophic life care plans, 848–849
Non-directed donors, 539
Nonmaleficence (of care), 693
Nonmedical commodities costs, 319
  average annual increases for medical and care costs, *329*
  consumer price index for hospital services, *326–327*
  consumer price index for medical commodities, *322–323*
  consumer price index for medical components, *320–321*
  consumer price index for medical services, *324–325*
  historical hourly earnings for nonagricultural wage, *328*

Nonmedical services costs, 319
Nonphysician life care planners, 22
Nonsteroidal anti-inflammatory drugs (NSAIDs), 484
Northwest Regional Spinal Cord Injury System (NWRSCIS), 741
Nortriptyline, 483
Norwest Bank, N. A. and Kenneth Frick v. K-Mart Corporation, 695
NRRTS, *see* National Registry of Rehabilitation Technology Suppliers
NSAIDs, *see* Nonsteroidal anti-inflammatory drugs
NSCISC, *see* National Spinal Cord Injury Statistical Center
NSO, *see* National Service Officers
Nurse case managers, 29–38
  certifications, 37
  desirable traits, *33*
  organizations, 37
Nurse life care planning, defined, 37
"Nurse only" group, 6
Nurse Practice Act, 733
Nurses, 318
Nursing care plan, 30, 32
Nursing process, 30–32
Nursing programs, 17
Nutritional issues, 408
NWRSCIS, *see* Northwest Regional Spinal Cord Injury System
Nystagmus, 272

O

OAA, *see* Older Americans Act
OAARA, *see* Older American Reauthorization Act
OAEs, *see* Otoacoustic emissions
OASYS program, 611
Objective information, 85
OBRA, *see* Omnibus Budget Reconciliation Act
Obsessive-compulsive disorder (OCD), 444, 452–455
  costs, 455
  epidemiology and course of illness, 453
  pharmacotherapy, 454
  psychotherapeutic interventions, 454
  symptoms, 453
  treatment, 453
  vocational impact, 455
Occipital lobe, 372
Occupational Information Network (O*Net), 49, 58, 611
Occupational noise exposure ratings, *270*
Occupational Outlook Handbook (*OOH*), 58
Occupational therapist, 434
Occupational therapy (OT), 106–132, 144
  abbreviations in, 126
  activities of daily living, 108–114
  aging with disability, 124–126
  case study, 127–132
  educational requirements and specialization, 119–120
  ethical standards and considerations for occupational therapists, 123
  evaluation tools, 107–108
  instrumental activities of daily living, 114–119
  life care plan, 120–123
  life care planner, 106
  OT as consultant to life care planner, 123
Occupational Therapy Assessment Tools: An Annotated Index, 107
Occupational Therapy Practice Framework, 107
OCD, *see* Obsessive-compulsive disorder
O'Connell v. Yung (2010), 855
OCR, *see* Optical character recognition
"Odd lot" doctrine, 42
OEM, *see* Original Equipment Manufacturer
Office of Statewide Health Planning and Development (OSHPD), 749
Older American Reauthorization Act (OAARA), 592
Older Americans Act (OAA), 592
Omissions errors, 761–766
Omnibus Budget Reconciliation Act (OBRA), 739
One-Hand Typing, *226*
One-to-one communicators, 280
ONJ, *see* Osteonecrosis of jaw
Online assistive technology resources, *224–227*
OOH, see Occupational Outlook Handbook
Ophthalmologists, 318
Opioids, 484
OPOs, *see* Organ procurement organizations
Opportunity cost, 325
OPPS, *see* Outpatient Prospective Payment System
Optical character recognition (OCR), 576
Opticians, 318
OPTN, *see* Organ Procurement and Transplantation Network
Optometrists, 318
Oral antispastic medications, 506
Oravail, 484
Organ procurement, 543–544
Organ Procurement and Transplantation Network (OPTN), 535–536, 541
Organ procurement organizations (OPOs), 535–536
Organ transplantation, 534–568
  awaiting transplantation, 540–543
  case study, 558–568
  complications, 549–551
  estimated, 552–553
  graft and patient survival, 552
  immunosuppressive therapy, 546–549
  infection, 550–551
  life care planning in transplantation, 537
  long-term follow-up, 551–552
  1-, 3-, and 5-year survival by etiology of organ failure, *554–558*
  organ-specific postoperative management, 544–546
  organ procurement, 543–544
  roots of modern transplantation, 534–537

social services and psychiatric consultation, 540
transplantation, 544
transplant candidacy process, 537–544
unadjusted 1-and 5-year patient survival by organ, *553*
United Network for Organ Sharing (UNOS), 536, 543
Organ transplantation, 537, 543–545
Original Equipment Manufacturer (OEM), 801
Orthopedic equipment, 122, 359–364
Orthostatic hypotension, 451, 458, 504, 592
Orthotics, 122, 358, 484
OSHA Occupational noise exposure ratings, *270*
OSHPD, *see* Office of Statewide Health Planning and Development
"Osseous integration," 339, 352
Osteoarthritis, 354
Osteonecrosis of jaw (ONJ), 510
Osteopenia, 510
OT, *see* Occupational therapy
Otitis media, 271
Otoacoustic emissions (OAEs), 264, 293
Otolaryngology, 258; *see also* Audiologists
Ototoxic drug therapy, 273–274
OTR, *see* Registered occupational therapist
Outcomes/planning, 30
Outpatient modalities, 484
Outpatient Prospective Payment System (OPPS), 746
Outpatient services, 409
Overhead transfer systems, 793, *793*, 795
Overuse syndromes, 513
Oxycodone, 484

P

P300 response, 265
PA, *see* Posterior–anterior
Packed red blood cells (PRBC), 144
PAI, *see* Personality assessment inventory
Pain, 470, 507–508; *see also* Chronic pain
Analgesic Ladder, 476, *478*
assessment tools, 470
implantable devices, 478–480
management approaches, 474–481
management therapy, 71
multimodal and multidisciplinary interventions for, *477*
pathophysiology, 475
phantom and residual limb, 344
specialist, 434
threshold *vs.* tolerance, 470
Pancreas, 539
Panel Reactive Antibodies, 541
Paper-and-pencil tests, 50
Paralysis, 80
Paralyzed Veterans of America (PVA), 739
Paraplegia, 24
Parents with disabilities, 741
Parietal lobe, 370
Parsons Estate v. Guymer (1998), 856
Partial hand, 346
finger amputations, *348*
traumatic amputations of ring and little fingers, *348*
Partial/hindfoot, 349
Patellar tendon bearing (PTB), 349
Patient-centered collaborative practice, 156
Patient/client management model, 136
Patient evaluation, 472
Patient-physician communication, 470
Patient's functioning level, determining, 485
Patient-specific rehabilitation services, 408
Paxton v. Ramji (2006), 862
PCBs, *see* Polychlorinated byphenyls
PDD-NOS, *see* Pervasive developmental disorder
PDD, *see* Pervasive developmental disorder
Peabody Individual Achievement Test, 48
PEDI-CAT, *see* Pediatric Evaluation of Disability Inventory–Computer Adaptive Test
PEDI, *see* Pediatric Evaluation of Disability Inventory
Pediatric assessment, 264–267
Pediatric audiologist, 257
Pediatric Evaluation of Disability Inventory–Computer Adaptive Test (PEDI-CAT), 108
Pediatric Evaluation of Disability Inventory (PEDI), 108
Pediatric evaluations, 51–52
Pediatric issues
neuropsychological evaluations, 50
speech-language pathologist assessment, 168
Pediatric Life Care Planning and Case Management (2011), 743, 777
Pediatric life care plans, 409
PEEDS-RAPEL method, 55, 611, 614, *616–617*
Penner v. Insurance Corporation of British Columbia (2011), 852, 854
Percutaneous electrical stimulation (PES), 484
Perinatal causes of hearing loss, 268
Perphenazine, 458
Persistent depressive disorder, 445
Persistent vegetative state, 369
Personal attendant and home care, 437–438
Personal care assistance, 517–518
Personal FM systems, 278–279
Personal health information (PHI), 175
Personal injury litigation, 4
Personality assessment inventory (PAI), 48
Personal perspective of life care planning, 631–639
Personal sound amplification products (PSAPs), 280
Person-first language, 152
Persuasive authority, 719
Pervasive developmental disorder (PDD), 168
PES, *see* Percutaneous electrical stimulation
PET, *see* Positron emission tomography
PE tubes, *see* Pressure-Equalizing tubes
Phantom and residual limb pain, 344
Pharmacological agents, 483

Pharmacotherapy, 446, 450, 454, 458–460
adjunctive medications, 451, 459
anticholinergics, 459–460
anticonvulsants, 459
antidepressants, 459
antipsychotics, 451, 458–459
benzodiazepines, 459
lithium, 450
mood stabilizers, 451, 459
PHI, *see* Personal health information
Phrenic nerve pacing, 507
Phrenology, 80
Physiatrists, 43, 336, 434, 868
choosing right physiatrist, 23
evaluation process by physiatrist, 353
example case, 26
implications, 22–23
in life care planning, 21, 24
life care planning with, 352
medical scenarios, 24–26
physiatrist recommendation for life care plan, *27*
physician/other health care professionals, 746
potential complications, 354–355
prognosis, 26
services, 331
Physical capacity assessment, *see* Functional capacity evaluation
Physical capacity evaluation, *see* Functional capacity evaluation
*P*hysical condition, *u*pper limb, *l*ower limb, *s*ensory, *e*xcretory, *s*upport factors (PULSES), 48
Physical functioning, hearing loss impact on, 274–275
Physical medicine and rehabilitation (PM&R), 43, 376
Physical therapists (PTs), 136–146, 434; *see also* Speech-language pathologist (SLP)
case study, 144–146
life care plan, 142–144, 145–146
practice of, 137–138
in primary care, 138
in secondary care, tertiary care, health, and wellness, 138–139
standardized outcome measures in, 139–142
Physical therapy, 484
interventions, 479
Physicians, *see* Physiatrists
Pia mater, 370
Pimozide, 458
PL, *see* Public Law
PL 101-336, *see* Americans with Disabilities Act (ADA)
PL 89-10, *see* Elementary and Secondary Education Act
PL 94-142, *see* Individual Education Plan (IEP)
Placeability, 54, 622
Placebo effect, 475
Plaintiff's attorney, 641–653
challenges to admissibility of life care planner's testimony and opinions, 650–653
challenges to life care planner's opinions, 651–653
hearsay, 651–652
insurance, Medicare, and Medicaid payment rates and collateral sources of payment, 652–653
interactions and life care planner, 642–643
life care planner's qualifications, 650–651
life care planner's role in litigation process, 644–650
negligence claim, 643–644
pre-trial proceedings, 645–648
trial, 648–650
variations in foundational opinions, 652
Plasmapheresis, 541
Play therapy, 410
PM&R, *see* Physical medicine and rehabilitation
PMIC, *see* Practice Management Information Corporation
Pneumonia/pneumococcal vaccination, 512–513
Poikilothermia, 504–505
Polychlorinated byphenyls (PCBs), 823
Polypharmacy, 459
Porch lifts, 791
Positive emotional adaptive process, 341
Positron emission tomography (PET), 150
Post-acute care reconstructive surgery, 407
Post-transplant survival measure, 542
Post-traumatic amnesia, 374
Post-Traumatic Stress Disorder (PTSD), 344, 409, 435–436
Posterior–anterior (PA), 538–539
Postmorbid behaviors, 83
Postnatal causes of hearing loss, 268–269
Postural hypotension, 24
Powered mobility, 125
Powered robotic exoskeletons in SCI, 516–517
PPOs, *see* Preferred provider organizations
Practice Management Information Corporation (PMIC), 745
Practice Standards and Guidelines, 835
Practice variation, *202*
PRBC, *see* Packed red blood cells
Precedent authority, 719
Prednisone, *548*
Preferred provider organizations (PPOs), *198*, *202*
Pregabalin, 508
Prepaid Group Practice Plans, *202*
Preprosthetic phase, 340
Prescribed drugs, *202*
Prescription drugs and medical supplies, 319
Pressure-Equalizing tubes (PE tubes), 269
Pressure garments, 433–434
Pressure garments and splints, 407
Pressure reduction (wheelchair cushions), 766
Pre-transplantation nurse coordinator, 538
Pre-trial proceedings, 645–648
Preventative care programs, *202*
Primary care, *202*
Principle of Ethics II, Rule B, 154
Prior authorization, *202*
Private Health Plans, 299

Problem-solving therapy, 446–447
Productivity, 411
Professional disclosure, 695
Professional services, 318
Projected rehabilitation program, 356–357
Projected therapeutic modalities, 357
ProPAC, *see* Prospective Payment Assessment Commission
Prophylaxis, 510
Prospective financing, *202*
Prospective Payment Assessment Commission (ProPAC), *202*
Prostate-specific antigen (PSA), 539
Prosthetic devices, 345
  advantages and disadvantages of upper-limb prostheses, *347*
  elbow disarticulation/above elbow, 348
  hip disarticulation, 350
  below knee, 349
  knee disarticulation/above knee, 349–350
  partial hand, 346, *348*
  partial/hindfoot, 349
  prosthetic complications, 350
  prosthetic costs, 350–351
  shoulder disarticulation, 348
  wrist disarticulation/below elbow, 347–348, *349*
Prosthetics, 407
  complications, 350
  fabrication, 340
  in OT, 122
  replacement, 351
Prosthetic training, 340–341
  above-and below-elbow amputee, *343*
  above-knee amputee, *342*
Proteus mirabilis, 509
PROVANT, 479
Providers, *203*
PSA, *see* Prostate-specific antigen
PSAPs, *see* Personal sound amplification products
Pseudomonas aeruginosa, 558
Psychiatric care, 435
  adaptive sports excursion, 436
  couples therapy, 436
  family therapy, 436
  individual psychotherapy, 435–436
  psychiatry, 435
  transportation, 436
Psychiatric consultation, 540
Psychiatric illness programs, 444
Psychodynamic/psychoanalytic psychologists, 63
Psychodynamic therapy, 446–447
Psychological
  anxiety disorder, 435
  assessment, 64
  distress, 66
  flexibility, 71
  impact, 574–575
  interventions, 65
  issues, 65, 409–410
  testing, 473
Psychologists, 62–75, 318
  adjustment to disability, 67–68
  assessment and diagnosis, 68–69
  case example, 73–74
  choosing, 62
  client issues, 63–66
  credentialing and orientations, 62–63
  family issues, 66–67
  interface between life care planner and, 72–73
  items and services, 74–75
  methods of treatment delivery, 70
  therapeutic strategies, 69, 71
  treatment types, 69–72
Psychosocial counseling, 300
Psycho/social issues, 435
Psychosocial stressor, 445
Psychotherapeutic interventions, 446–447, 451–452, 454
Psychotherapy, 90
  for bipolar disorder, 452
  cognitive-behavioral therapy, 454
  for major depressive disorder, 447
  for obsessive-compulsive disorder, 455
  sessions, 91
Psychotic features, 448
PTB, *see* Patellar tendon bearing
PTs, *see* Physical therapists
PTSD, *see* Post-Traumatic Stress Disorder
Public Law (PL), 535–536
"Puff paint," *see* Hi-Mark Tactile Pen
Pulmonary complications, 377
  of acquired brain injury, 376
Pulmonary embolism, 512
Pulmonary embolus, 377–378
PULSES, *see Physical condition, upper limb, lower limb, sensory, excretory, support factors*
Purdue Pegboard, 48
Pure tone audiometry, 259–261
Pure tone hearing test, 259
PVA, *see* Paralyzed Veterans of America

Q

QAP, *see* Quality assurance program
Quadriplegia, *see* Tetraplegia
Qualified Health Care Professional, 847
Quality assurance program (QAP), 800, 809
Quality of life, hearing loss impact on, 275
Quebec, 850
Questions to ask life care planner, 9–12, *10–11*

R

Radiological diagnostic techniques, 151
Raloxifene, 510
Ramps, 790

Rancho Los Amigos Scale of Cognitive Functioning, 379, *380*
RAPEL method, 54, 611, 614, *615*
  PEEDS-RAPEL, 55, 611, 614, *616–617*
Rapid plasmin reagin (RPR), 538
RAs, *see* Remittance advices
Rate setting, *203*
Rational acceptance counseling, 300
Rational drug therapy, *203*
Ratych v. Bloomer (1987), 861
Raven Progressive Matrices, 47
Rear-entry minivans, 802
Reasonable accommodations, 169
Reasonable care, 643
Reasonable charge, *203*
Reasonable cost range, *201*
Reconstruction phase, 338–339
Reconstructive surgery, 405
Records
  copy of, 9–11
  review of, by SLP, 166–167
  subpoena of, 645–646
Regional Center and California Children's Services, 34
Registered occupational therapist (OTR), 119
Registration, 815–817
Registry, 816
Rehabilitation, 403, 408
  amputees, 337–343, *339*
  audiological (aural), 275–277
  burn patients, 403, 408
  care, 376
  for children, 277–278
  contributions, 32–34
  counselors, 18
  court decisions and impact on practice, 723–724
  desirable traits for, *33*
  equipment, 22
  equipment specialists, 775–776
  equipment suppliers, 776
  forensic issues, 609, 610, 614–618
  formal, 578
  functional capacity evaluation, 43–44
  life care planner qualifications and expertise, *37*
  model, 337
  neuropsychological assessment, 82–83
  nurse in life care planning, 29
  nursing process and care plan development, 30–32
  physicians, 23, 26
  plan, 54
  private sector, 610
  process, 253
  professional organizations and certifications, 5–6, 37
  psychologists, 63
  related certifications and organizations, 37
  research issues for, 34–35
  roles, 35, *36*
  team approach in, 22–23
  technology, 174
  technology supplier, 776
  vocational expert, *38*
Rehabilitation Act (1973), 169, 172, 174, 713
  amendment (1986), 172
  disability meaning under, 610
  reauthorization (1992, 1997), 174
Rehabilitation Consultant's Handbook (Weed & Field), 55, 612
Rehabilitation day programs, 376
Rehabilitation Engineering and Assistive Technology Society of North America (RESNA), 154, 776, 778, 803
Rehabilitation Measures Database, 139
Rehabilitation Training Institute, 4–5, 846
Rehabilitative care, 336
Rehabilitative/dispensing audiologist, 258
Rehab technology supplier (RTS), 760, 776
Relafen, 484
Relevant evidence, 821
Releve, 484
Reliability of LCP, 703–708
Remittance advices (RAs), 174
Renal artery thrombosis, 545
Renal dialysis, 537
Report writing, 613–623
Reputable databases, 746
  American Hospital Directory, 747
  anesthesia, 747
  Context[4] Healthcare, 748
  dental, 747
  Durable Medical Equipment (DME), 747
  facility, 746
  FAIR Health, 748
  H·CUPnet, 748–749
  physician/other health care professionals, 746
  VA Reasonable Data Charges, 748
Residual limb, 339
Residual limb pain, 344
RESNA, *see* Rehabilitation Engineering and Assistive Technology Society of North America
Resources for life care planning, 730–757
  Abeo Coder, 749
  additional resources, 743
  area cost analysis, 732–735, 750–755
  Certified Life Care Planner (CLCP), 743
  coding tips for consideration, 745
  crosswalks for life care planner, 745–746
  federal information, 737
  free of charge facility databases, 749
  geographically specific wage data, 737
  health club, 737
  home health care services links, 736
  information sources, 742–743
  links, 736–737
  LCP software, 738
  locating health care professionals, 736

medical coding and billing software subscriptions, 744–745
obtaining information by telephone and e-mail, 735–736
questionnaire, 755–757
recommended pricing, 731
reputable databases (list of), 746–749
schools/educational services, 737
specific resources, selected, 739–742
training programs for life care planning certification, 743
usual, customary, and reasonable (UCR), 731–732
utilizing databases for research, 744
vocational rehabilitation resources, 737
web-based resources, 738
zip code, 749
Respiratory complications, 506–507
Respite care, 437
Retransplantation, 553
Return-to-work assessment, 49–51
Revised Handbook for Analyzing Jobs, The (*RHAJ*), 55, 58
ReWalk, 22
RHAJ, see Revised Handbook for Analyzing Jobs, The
Robaxin, 483
Roberts v. Morana (1997), 856
Rorschach Inkblot Test, 48
Routine cardiac surveillance, 512
RPR, *see* Rapid plasmin reagin
RTS, *see* Rehab technology supplier
Rules of Civil Procedure, 850
R. v. J.L.J., 849
R. v. Mohan, 849

S

SAC, *see* Standard acquisition costs
SaddlePoint Software, 91
SAE, *see* Society of Automobile Engineers
Sandhu v. Wellington Place Apartments (2008), 858
Sandretto v. Payson Healthcare Management, Inc. (2014), 827
SAT, *see* Speech Awareness Threshold
Schizophrenia, 444, 455–464
associated symptoms or features, 457
case study, 461–462, *462–463*
costs, 461
epidemiology and course of illness, 456
negative symptoms, 457
pharmacotherapy, 458–460
phases, 457–460
positive symptoms, 456–457
symptoms, 456
treatment refractory, 458
vocational impact, 460–461
Schools/educational services, locating, 737
Schrump et al. v. Koot et al. (1977), 859–860
SCI, *see* Spinal cord injury
Scientific evidence, 650
Scientific Registry for Transplant Recipients (SRTR), 535–536
SCII, *see* Strong–Campbell Interest Inventory
SDS, *see* Self-Directed Search
Second impact syndrome, 382
Sedation, 454
Seizure therapy, 455–456
Selective serotonin reuptake inhibitors (SSRIs), 446, 447, 454, 459
Self-Directed Search (SDS), 48
Self-feeding, 109
Self-serving views, 16
Sensation, 372
Sensorineural hearing loss, 292
Sensory functions, 377
Sensory Organization Test (SOT), 272
Sensory Profile 2 (SP2), 108
Sensory stimulus, 151
Serotonin norepinephrine reuptake inhibitors (SNRIs), 446
Serotonin reuptake inhibitors (SRIs), 454
Serum plasma levels, 450
Service animals, 172
7 Cs of communication, 837
Sexual dysfunction, 378
Sexual function complications, 513–514
SGDs, *see* Speech Generating Devices
SHMOs, *see* Social health maintenance organizations
Shoulder disarticulation, 348
Shoulders, 432
Shower trolley, *789*
Shower Trolley, 789, *789*, 794
SIADH, *see* Syndrome of inappropriate diuretic hormone
SIC, *see* Standard Industrial Classification
Side-entry minivans, 802
SIGs, *see* Special interest groups
Silicone sleeve, 349
Single-photon emission computed tomography (SPECT), 150
Six-step comprehensive program, 483
16 Personality Factors (16 PF), 48
Skilled Nursing Facilities (SNFs), 376
SkillTRAN, 58
Skin
cancer, 433
role, 405
Skin/skin grafting, 406
Sleep
disturbances, 483
restoration, 483
study, 434
Slosson Intelligence Test, 47
SLP, *see* Speech-language pathologist
SNFs, *see* Skilled Nursing Facilities
SNRIs, *see* Serotonin norepinephrine reuptake inhibitors
SNTs, *see* Special needs trusts

Social adjustment, 88
Social health maintenance organizations (SHMOs), 299
Social Security, 610
Social Security Act (SSA), 572
Social Security Administration (SSA), 44–45
Social Security Disability Insurance (SSDI), 44, 45, 463
Social Security, retirement age, 44–45
Society of Automobile Engineers (SAE), 810
Song v. Hong (2008), 859
SOT, *see* Sensory Organization Test
Sound field, 293
Sound therapy, 289
SP2, *see* Sensory Profile 2
Spasticity, 378, 380–381, 506
Special interest groups (SIGs), 154
Specialist, *see* Physiatrist
Special needs trusts (SNTs), 739–740
SPECT, *see* Single-photon emission computed tomography
Speech and language, CPT codes, *179–181*
Speech audiometry, 261–262
Speech Awareness Threshold (SAT), 293
Speech banana, 260
Speech Generating Devices (SGDs), 170
Speech-language pathologist (SLP), 150–252; *see also* Assistive technology (AT); Augmentative and alternative communication (AAC); Physical Therapists (PTs)
  about, 150–152
  areas included, 150
  assessment process, 167, *191*
  case study, 190
  checklist for life care planning, *192–194*
  code of ethics, 154
  developmental milestones for children, *234–235*
  federal mandates and policies, 168–171
  functions/examinations performed by, 159
  funding and economic issues, 177–178
  funding and financing, *195*
  funding glossary, *196–204*
  funding request (outline), 248–251
  HIPAA rules, 174–175
  hot topics in SPL update, 189–190
  ICD-10-CM SLP Codes (2016), *181–184*
  imaging/diagnostic techniques, 150
  international sites, *227–228*
  internet resources, *219–223*
  life care planning, 152–153
  life care planning checklist, *192–195*
  medical coding, 178
  model superbill for, *228–232*
  neurolitigation, 178–189
  online assistive technology resources, *224–227*
  pediatric and adolescent assessments, 167–168
  periodicals/newsletters, *228*
  person-first language, 152
  privacy issues, 174–175
  qualifications and credentials of, 153–155
  research in communication sciences and disorders, 161–165
  review of records and intake, 166–167
  selected AAC websites, *205–213*
  SLP CPT Codes, *179–181*
  special interest divisions, 154, *154*
  speech-to-speech relay system, 175–177
  superbill, *228–232*
  terminology in communication sciences and disorders, 165–167
  toll-free phone numbers and hotlines, *213–219*
  training and preparation, 155–161
  vendor list, *204–205*
  voice disorders addressed by, *157*
Speech-language pathology, 150, 161, 190
Speech Reception Threshold (SRT), 293
Speech-to-speech (STS) relay system, 175–177
Spehar v. Beazley (2002), 855
Spinal cord injury (SCI), 12, 24–25, 64–65, 481, 498–529; *see also* Wheelchairs
  aging with, 517–518
  anatomy, 499–501
  autonomic dysfunction, 504–505
  case study, 519–529
  catheterization, 509
  circulatory disorders, 511–512
  classification, 501
  complications, potential, 504
  conus medullaris syndrome/injury, 504
  epidemiology, 498–499
  equipment, 575
  Frankel classification system, 502
  functional effects, 506
  functional electrical stimulation (FES), 517
  functional outcomes, 574, 762
  gastrointestinal issues, 505–506
  genitourinary dysfunction, 508–510
  home modifications, 514–515
  incomplete syndromes, 503–504
  infections, 512–513
  injury classification, 502–503
  integumentary issues, 511
  life care plans, 26, 125–126, 127–132
  life expectancy, 518–519
  metabolic changes, 510
  overuse syndromes, 513
  pain, 507–508
  powered robotic exoskeletons in, 516–517
  preservation of function by neurologic level of injury, 503–504
  psychological issues, 514
  respiratory complications, 506–507
  sexual function and reproduction, 513–514
  spasticity, 506
  vehicular modification, 515–516
SPSS, *see* Statistical Package for Social Sciences
SRIs, *see* Serotonin reuptake inhibitors

SRT, *see* Speech Reception Threshold
SRTR, *see* Scientific Registry for Transplant Recipients
SSA, *see* Social Security Act; Social Security Administration
SSDI, *see* Social Security Disability Insurance
SSI, *see* Supplemental Security Income
SSRIs, *see* Selective serotonin reuptake inhibitors
Stair chair, *792*
Standard acquisition costs (SAC), 543
Standard Industrial Classification (SIC), 56
Standards
  American National Standards Institute standards (ANSI), 259
  audiologists, 259
  cancer screening, 539
  ethical standards, 872–873
  goals/overview, 869
  historical perspective, 868
  IALCP guidelines, 691–692, 694
  life care planning, 3–20, 692, 868–872
  review of, 9
  scope of practice, 6–7, 869–870
  standards of performance, 872–873
  transdisciplinary perspective, 868–869
  wheelchairs *vs.* complex rehab, 777–778
Standards of Practice for Life Care Planners, 692, 695, 827, 834–835, 848
Stanford–Binet Scales, 47
Stare decisis, 714
State plan, *203*
Statistical Package for Social Sciences (SPSS), 706
Stein v. Sandwich West (Township) (1995), 861–862
Step-by-step procedures, 9–13
Steroids, 546
Stop loss, *203*
Strong–Campbell Interest Inventory (SCII), 48
Subacute pain, 471
Subarachnoid space, 501
Subjective information, 85
Subpoena ad testificandum, 645
Subpoena duces tecum, 645
Subpoena/subpoena duces tecum, 645–646
Substance abuse, assessment algorithm, 482
Suicidal ideation, 66, 68, 354, 449
Suitable employment, 45*fn*
Sulci, 370
Summer burn camp, 409
Summer camps/summer schools, 742
Super Coder, 744–745
Superficial burns, 404
Superficial partial-thickness burns, 404
Supplemental Security Income (SSI), 45, *203*
Supported employment model, 460–461
Support services
  legal, 175, *463*
  life care planning, *463*
Supreme Court decisions, 716, 719, 721–722, 726–727
  on ADA, 721, 722–723, 726
  effects on lower courts, 719–720
  impact on rehabilitation and LCP practice, 723–724
Surgical procedures, 406
Sutton v. United Airlines, *718*
Swallowing function, CPT codes, *179–181*
Symptom magnification, 473
Syndrome of inappropriate diuretic hormone (SIADH), 377
Systems theory, 157–161

T

Talk Radio, *226*
Tangible Reinforcement Operant Conditioning Audiometry (TROCA), 264
Tardive dyskinesia, 458
Targeted muscle reinnervation, 352
Taylor v. Speedway Motorsports, Inc., 828
TBI, *see* Traumatic brain injury
TBSA, *see* Total body surface area
TDD, *see* Telecommunication device
Team approach
  in life care planning, 22–23
  in rehabilitation, 62, 498
TeamRehab Report, *227*
Tech Act, *see* Technology-Related Assistance for Individuals with Disabilities Act
Technology-Related Assistance for Individuals with Disabilities Act (Tech Act), *169*, 172, *173*, 761
Tegretol, 483
Telecommunication device (TDD), 280, 576
Telecommunications accessibility, 742
Telecommunications Relay Service (TRS), 175
Telehealth services, 70
Telephone
  numbers and hotlines, *213–219*
  obtaining information by, 735–736
Telephone text (TTY), 280
Temporal lobes, 371
TENS, *see* Transcutaneous electrical nerve stimulation
Teratogens, 265
Testicular sperm extraction (TESE), 514
Testimony; *see also* Expert witness
  life care plan expert, 24, 644, 883
  of physiatrists, 24
Testing protocols, 69
Test of Visual-Motor Skills (TVMS-3), 108
Tests, 86
  neuropsychological, 88, 287
  psychological, 85
  vocational assessment, 47, 48
Tetraplegia, 24, 476, 481
Theory of brain–behavior relationships, 81
Therapeutic
  injections, 477
  substitution, *203*

Therapists, 318
Thighs and calves, 433
Third-party administrator, *203*
Third-party liability, *203*
Thoracic lumbar sacral orthotic (TLSO), 144
Threshold process, 259
Thrombus, 512
  deep vein thrombosis (DVT), 512
Through Looking Glass (TLG), 741
Thyroid dysfunction, 377
Ticket to Work, 174
Tinnitus management, 288–289
Tinnitus Retraining Therapy, 289
Tissue planes, 477
Title 38: Veterans' Benefits, 739
Tizanidine, 506
TLG, *see* Through Looking Glass
TLSO, *see* Thoracic lumbar sacral orthotic
Tongue movement, 372
Topics in Spinal Cord Injury Rehabilitation (journal), 742
Topiramate, 451
Tortfeasor, 643
"Torts," 643
Total body surface area (TBSA), 402–403
Total lifetime values, 331
Total Quality Management (TQM), *203*
Toyota v. Williams, 718
  Supreme Court decision, 720–721
TQM, *see* Total Quality Management
Trace Research & Development Center, *227*
Tramadol, 484
Tranquilizers, 451
Transcutaneous electrical nerve stimulation (TENS), 479, 484
Transfemoral, 349–350
Transferable skills analysis, 49
Transhumeral, 348
Transitional Classification of Jobs (*COJ*), 46, 49, 58
Transitional employment model, 460–461
Transitory, 718
Transplantation, *see* Organ transplantation
Transportation, 358, 436, 800
  in OT, 122–123
Transradial, 347–348
Transtibial, 349
Trauma, 381
  injuries, 430
Traumatic brain injury (TBI), 12, 64, 164, 368, 734
  model systems, 370
  recovery from, 379–380, *380*
Traumatic etiology of eye injuries, 573
Traumatic spinal cord injury, 518
Travis v. Kwon (2009), 854
Trial Court, 828
Tricyclic antidepressants, 508
TROCA, *see* Tangible Reinforcement Operant Conditioning Audiometry
TRS, *see* Telecommunications Relay Service
Truncal musculature, 517
Tsalamandris v. McLeod (2012), 854
TTY, *see* Telephone text
Tucker v. Cascade General, 827
Tumors, acquired brain injury from, 267
TVMS-3, *see* Test of Visual-Motor Skills
Tympanograms, 262–*263*
Tympanometry, 262, 293

U

UA, *see* Urinalysis
UAW, *see* United Automobile Workers
UCR, *see* Usual, customary, and reasonable
UDS, *see* Uniform Data Systems
UF, *see* University of Florida
Ulcers, decubitus, 511
Ultrasonography, 545
Unidimensional pain measurement tools, 471
Uniform Data Systems (UDS), 518
United Automobile Workers (UAW), 299
United Network for Organ Sharing (UNOS), 536, 543
Universal access, *203*
Universal coverage, *204*
University of Florida (UF), 846
  Distance Education program, 6
University of Washington Spinal Cord Injury Update, 741
UNOS, *see* United Network for Organ Sharing
Upper extremities and shoulders, 432
Urinalysis (UA), 734
Urologic complications, 545
U.S. Airways, Inc. v. Barnett (2002), 723
U.S. Centers for Disease Control and Prevention, 369
U.S. Federal Motor Vehicle Safety Standards (FMVSS), 800
U.S. Health Resources and Services Administration (HRSA), 266, 536
U.S. life tables, 742
U.S. Organ Procurement and Transplantation Network, 552
Usual, customary, and reasonable (UCR), 731–732, 748
Utilization review, *204*

V

VA, *see* Veterans Administration
Vaccinations, 507
Valid assessment of hearing, 264
VALPAR, 48
Valproate, 451, 459
Value of items, 325, 327
Vanity board, 84
Vantage Mobility International (VMI), 516
VA Reasonable Data Charges, 748
Vascular complications, 545

V codes, 178
VDARE, *see* Vocational Diagnosis and Assessment of Residual Employability Process
VE, *see* Vocational expert
Vegetative state, 369
Vehicle modifications, 515–516, 799–810
armrest mount, *807*
case study, 805–807
cost estimates, 804–805
customization and design issues, 803
final driver's station with seat belt, *808*
industry safety standards, 803–804
left-side controls, *809*
resources, 809–810
right side controls, *808*
safety factors, 800–801
structural factors, 801–803
VEMPS, *see* Vestibular-Evoked Myogenic Potentials
Vendor, *204*
list, *204–205*
payments, *204*
Ventilatory management, 545
Veracity, 124
Vertebrae, 499–500
Vertebral column, anatomy, 499–500
Vertek, Inc., 58
Vestibular-Evoked Myogenic Potentials (VEMPS), 272–273
Vestibular ocular reflex (VOR), 272
Vestibular system assessment, 272–273
Vestibulotoxicity, 273
Veterans, 739
Veterans Administration (VA), 800
VHIT, *see* Video Head Impulse Test
Viatical resources, 741
Video Head Impulse Test (VHIT), 273
Video Magnifiers, 576
Videonystagmography (VNG), 272
Videostroboscopy, 162
Video technology, 272
Vineland Adaptive Behavior Scales, 52
Vineland Social Maturity Scale, 48
VIPR, *see* Vocational interest and personality reinforcer
Vision, 574
Visually impaired, 571–589
aids/medical equipment for, 575–577
assistive technology for, 154
Braille, 576
case study, 579–581
epidemiology, 572–573
etiology, 573
functional outcomes, 574
Global Positioning Systems (GPS) device, 577
guide dog services, 577
legally blind, 572
mobility training, 578
personal care and homemaker services, 578
psychological impact, 574–575
recorded reading materials, 583
rehabilitation, formal, 578
resources, 582–589
Visual Reinforcement Audiometry (VRA), 264, 292
VMI, *see* Vantage Mobility International
VNG, *see* Videonystagmography
Vocational Diagnosis and Assessment of Residual Employability Process (VDARE), 56
Vocational/educational plan, 359
Vocational expert (VE), 611
Vocational interest and personality reinforcer (VIPR), 58–59
Vocational issues
access to labor market (employability), 618–622
assessment/evaluation, 44–49
assistive technology services, 154
of bipolar disorder, 452
earnings capacity, 622–623
labor force participation, 623
of MDD, 447
occupational therapist, 106
of OCD, 455
placeability, 622
resources, 58–59
return-to-work assessment, 49–51
of schizophrenia, 460–461
transferable skills analysis, 49
Vocational rehabilitation, 342, 382–384, 410–411
acquired brain injury, 368
amputees, 340, 341
burn patients, 403
legislation, 155
resources, 737
spinal cord injury, 676
wage data, geographically specific, 737
Vocational Rehabilitation Association of Canada (VRA), 835
Vocational rehabilitation counselors, 41, 42
adult evaluations, 52
assessment/evaluation, 44–49
collaborating with rehabilitation nurse, 57
job analysis, 55
labor market survey, 55, 56
life care planning questions regarding vocational needs, *57*
neuropsychological evaluations in return-to-work assessment, 49–51
neuropsychologist questions, *51*
pediatric evaluations, 51–52
resources, 58–59
as team member, 42–44
vocational resources, 58–59
wage loss and earnings capacity analysis, 53–55
Vocational services, 734
Voice disorders, 157; *see also* Speech-language pathologists

VOR, *see* Vestibular ocular reflex
VRA, *see* Visual Reinforcement Audiometry; Vocational Rehabilitation Association of Canada

W

W3C, *see* World Wide Web Consortium
Wage data, geographically specific, 737
Wage loss analysis, 53–55
Wait-list urgency measure, 542
Waiver, *204*
Walkmate, 577
Wall Street Journal, 801
Warning shot, 646
Watkins v. Olafson (1989), 861
WBC, *see* White blood cell count
WC-19 wheelchair, 803–804
Web-based resources, 738
Websites, *205–213*, 727
Web space releases, 432–433
Wechsler Intelligence Scales, 47
WeeFIM System II, 107
Wellness programs, *see* Preventative care programs
West Virginia Rehabilitation Research and Training Center (WVRRTC), *227*
Wheelchair cushions, *see* Pressure reduction
WheelchairNet, *227*
Wheelchairs, 357, 769–772
  accessories, 121, 357
  choice in, 778–779
  choice, problems in, 763
  clinic, 779
  convenience and ADL features, 767
  custom therapeutic seating systems, 766
  maintenance, 121, 357
  manual, *764*
  motorized, *765*
  motorized, replacement schedule, 768
  questions to consider in choosing, 777
  replacement issues, 770–772
  safety features, 767
  transportation safety, 810
  warranty, 768
Whetung v. West Fraser Holdings Ltd. (2007), 854
White blood cell count (WBC), 538
White cane, 576–577
WHO, *see* World Health Organization
Wide range achievement test (WRAT), 48
Williams v. Low (2000), 852
Witness, expert, *see* Expert witness
Woodcock–Johnson Psychoeducational Battery, 48
Woodcock–Johnson Tests, 52
Word Recognition Ability, 293
Workers' compensation laws, 471
Work Incentive Improvement Act (1999), 174
Worklife Estimates: Effects of Race and Education, 623
Work life expectancy, anticipated, 623
Work sample, 46, 48
WorkWell Systems FCE, version 2, 107
World Burn Congress, 409
World Federation of Occupational Therapists, 107
World Health Organization (WHO), 156
World Wide Web Consortium (W3C), *227*
Worley & Worley v. State Farm Mutual Automobile Insurance Company, 826
Wound care, 405
WRAT, *see* Wide range achievement test
Wrists, 432
  disarticulation/below elbow, 347–348
  "I-Hand" without coverage of cosmetic glove, *349*
Write-off or adjustment, 652
WVRRTC, *see* West Virginia Rehabilitation Research and Training Center

Z

Zero-reject principle, 170
Ziebenhaus v. Bahlieda (2014), 860
Zip code, 749

Printed and bound by CPI Group (UK) Ltd, Croydon, CR0 4YY
17/10/2024
01775694-0015